HANDBOOK OF NUTRITIONALLY ESSENTIAL MINERAL ELEMENTS

CLINICAL NUTRITION IN HEALTH AND DISEASE

Series Editor

LAWRENCE J. MACHLIN

Nutrition Research and Information, Inc.
Livingston, New Jersey

Additional Volumes in Preparation

HANDBOOK OF NUTRITIONALLY ESSENTIAL MINERAL ELEMENTS

edited by

Boyd L. O'Dell
Roger A. Sunde

University of Missouri
Columbia, Missouri

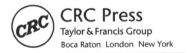

CRC Press
Taylor & Francis Group
Boca Raton London New York

CRC Press is an imprint of the
Taylor & Francis Group, an **informa** business

CRC Press
Taylor & Francis Group
6000 Broken Sound Parkway NW, Suite 300
Boca Raton, FL 33487-2742

First issued in paperback 2019

© 1997 by Taylor & Francis Group, LLC
CRC Press is an imprint of Taylor & Francis Group, an Informa business

No claim to original U.S. Government works

ISBN-13: 978-0-8247-9312-8 (hbk)
ISBN-13: 978-0-367-40106-1 (pbk)

Library of Congress Cataloging-in-Publication Data

Handbook of nutritionally essential minerals / edited by Boyd L.
O'Dell, Roger A. Sunde.
    p. cm. — (Clinical nutrition in health and disease ; 2)
    Includes bibliographical references and index.
    ISBN 0-8247-9312-9 (hc : alk.)
    1. Minerals in human nutrition. I. O'Dell, Boyd L. II. Sunde,
Roger Allan. II. Series.
QP533.H36   1997
612.3'92—dc21

97-55
CIP

**Visit the Taylor & Francis Web site at
http://www.taylorandfrancis.com**

**and the CRC Press Web site at
http://www.crcpress.com**

Preface

Essential mineral elements play a major role in the nutrition of humans and all animals. In fact, the number of essential mineral elements exceeds the number of vitamins or amino acids that are essential to the diet; however, their quantitative requirements are far less than those for protein, fat, and carbohydrate. Because life evolved in a milieu composed primarily of inorganic molecules, primitive organisms took advantage of the available inorganic elements to serve as catalysts, even as signaling agents, in the support of metabolism. Later, many of the elements were incorporated into protein constructs (typically metalloezymes) that improved their efficiency.

Modern approaches to the determination of mineral nutrient requirements began in the 1920s with the development and use of semipurified diets, but elucidation of the biochemical roles of these nutrients, particularly of the micro (trace) elements, did not emerge until the 1970s. This occurred with the unraveling of now well-established metabolic pathways and protein structures, detailed membrane and subcellular composition, and biochemical mechanisms by which genes are expressed. Over the past 20 years mineral elements have been shown to play key roles at nearly every step of the many life processes. These range from the role of calcium as a second messenger, to the role of zinc and "zinc fingers" in gene transcription, to the selenium-specific codons and insertion elements in mRNA translation. The integration of "mineral nutrition" and molecular biology creates the need for a handbook that encompasses molecular mineral nutrition—a book that provides a single source of advanced and integrated knowledge about all the essential mineral elements.

For historical reasons, the essential mineral elements are commonly divided into macro and micro categories. There is some excuse for this separation based on function, but in general such classification is unjustified; for example, calcium is a major component of bone but micro quantities serve as a second messenger. The number of micro elements recognized as nutritionally essential has increased dramatically since 1948, the end of the era of vitamin discovery. Because of the extraordinary interest in trace elements during the past four decades, numerous reviews and books related to this subject have appeared. In contrast to the coverage of micro elements, there are few books that cover the nutritional properties of the macro elements (calcium, phosphorus, potassium, sodium, chloride, and magnesium). In fact, this may be the first single volume that encompasses the roles of both macro and micro elements in nutrition, physiology, and biochemistry. Obviously such broad coverage demands exclusion of some information, but this book distills the essence of knowledge related to the physiological and biochemical functions of all essential mineral elements. To achieve this distillation, the expertise of internationally recognized scholars in their respective areas of mineral nutrition has been assembled.

While the handbook is designed primarily for students and professionals in nutrition (clinical, applied, and basic), it is a valuable source of information for students, teachers, and researchers in all areas of biology, including biochemistry, physiology, pharmacology, and medicine. In addition to the roles of mineral elements in animal nutrition, their analogous roles in plants and microorganisms are discussed where appropriate to provide coverage of the full range of biological functions. Recent work with prokaryotes and plants has provided valuable insights into mineral element function. Consequently, modern molecular nutrition is not restricted to higher animals.

The contributors have prepared and freely incorporated models and figures that can be used in the classroom to present basic concepts. Not only have the authors presented much detailed and specific information, but they have also provided comprehensive references for those who wish to pursue the subject. The editors wish to express their sincere appreciation to the authors for their cooperation and patience as well as their excellent contributions.

Boyd L. O'Dell
Roger A. Sunde

BIBLIOGRAPHY

Burk, R. F. (Ed.). *Selenium in Biology and Human Health*. Springer-Verlag, New York, 1994.
Ciba Foundation Symposium. *Biological Roles of Copper*. Excerpta Medica, New York, 1980.
Mertz, W. (Ed.). *Trace Elements in Human and Animal Nutrition, Fifth Edition*. Vols. 1 & 2. Academic Press, Inc. New York, 1986.
Mills, C. F. (Ed.). *Zinc in Human Biology*. Springer-Verlag, New York, 1989.
Nordin, B. E. C. (Ed.). *Calcium in Human Biology*. Springer-Verlag, New York, 1988.
Prasad, A. S., Oberleas, D. (Eds.). *Trace Elements in Human Health and Disease*. Vols. 1 & 2. Academic Press, New York, 1976.

Contents

Contributors

Manfred Anke Department of Nutrition and Environment, Friedrich Schiller University, Jena, Germany

W. Arnhold Friedrich Schiller University, Jena, Germany

John L. Beard Nutrition Department, Pennsylvania State University, University Park, Pennsylvania

Yitshal N. Berner Harzfeld Geriatric Hospital, Kaplan Medical Center, Gedera, Israel

Felix Bronner Department of BioStructure and Function, University of Connecticut Health Center, Farmington, Connecticut

Edith M. Carlisle[†] School of Public Health, University of California—Los Angeles, Los Angeles, California

Florian L. Cerklewski Department of Nutrition and Food Management, Oregon State University, Corvallis, Oregon

John K. Chesters Division of Biochemical Sciences, Rowett Research Institute, Bucksburn, Aberdeen, Scotland

Harry D. Dawson Nutrition Department, Pennsylvania State University, University Park, Pennsylvania

C. Drobner Friedrich Schiller University, Jena, Germany

K. Eder Institut für Ernährungphysiologie, Technische Universität München, Freising-Weihenstephan, Germany

M. Glei Friedrich Schiller University, Jena, Germany

Mary-Ellen Harper Department of Biochemistry, University of Ottawa, Ottawa, Ontario, Canada

[†]Deceased.

Edward D. Harris Department of Biochemistry and Biophysics, Texas A&M University, College Station, Texas

Basil S. Hetzel International Council for Control of Iodine Deficiency Disorders, Adelaide, Australia

H. Illing Friedrich Schiller University, Jena, Germany

M. Jaritz Friedrich Schiller University, Jena, Germany

Jean L. Johnson Department of Biochemistry, Duke University Medical Center, Durham, North Carolina

M. Kirchgessner Institut für Ernährungphysiologie, Technische Universität München, Freising-Weihenstephan, Germany

Roland M. Leach, Jr. Department of Poultry Science, Pennsylvania State University, University Park, Pennsylvania

M. Müller Friedrich Schiller University, Jena, Germany

Forrest H. Nielsen Grand Forks Human Nutrition Research Center, Agricultural Research Service, United States Department of Agriculture, Grand Forks, North Dakota

Boyd L. O'Dell Department of Biochemistry, University of Missouri, Columbia, Missouri

Esther G. Offenbacher St. Luke's–Roosevelt Hospital Center, New York, New York

John Patrick Department of Biochemistry, University of Ottawa, Ottawa, Ontario, Canada

Linda N. Peterson Departments of Physiology and Paediatrics, University of Ottawa, Ottawa, Ontario, Canada

F. Xavier Pi-Sunyer Division of Endocrinology, Diabetes, and Nutrition, St. Luke's–Roosevelt Hospital Center, New York, New York

A. M. Reichlmayer-Lais Institut für Ernährungphysiologie, Technische Universität München, Freising-Weihenstephan, Germany

U. Schäfer Friedrich Schiller University, Jena, Germany

M. Seifert Friedrich Schiller University, Jena, Germany

Maurice Edward Shils Department of Public Health Sciences, Bowman Gray School of Medicine, Wake Forest University, Winston-Salem, North Carolina

Richard M. Smith Division of Human Nutrition, CSIRO, Adelaide, Australia

Barbara J. Stoecker Department of Nutritional Sciences, Oklahoma State University, Stillwater, Oklahoma

Roger A. Sunde Department of Nutritional Sciences and Biochemistry, University of Missouri, Columbia, Missouri

Maurice L. Wellby Department of Clinical Chemistry, The Queen Elizabeth Hospital, Adelaide, Australia

John S. Willis Department of Cellular Biology, University of Georgia, Athens, Georgia

Kurt R. Zinn Department of Radiology, University of Alabama at Birmingham, Alabama

About the Editors

BOYD L. O'DELL is a Professor Emeritus at the University of Missouri, Columbia. A Fellow of the American Institute of Nutrition and a member of the American Society of Biochemistry and Molecular Biology, the American Chemical Society, and the Society for Experimental Biology and Medicine, he is the author or coauthor of over 200 professional papers. Dr. O'Dell received the A.B. degree (1940) in chemistry and the Ph.D. degree (1943) in biochemistry from the University of Missouri, Columbia.

ROGER A. SUNDE is Food for the 21st Century Nutrition Cluster Leader, Chair of the Graduate Nutritional Sciences Program, and a member of the Department of Biochemistry and the Department of Food Sciences and Human Nutrition at the University of Missouri, Columbia. The author or coauthor of more than 100 professional papers and abstracts that reflect his research interests in the nutritional biochemistry and molecular biology of trace elements, he is a member of the American Society for Nutritional Sciences and the American Society for Biochemistry and Molecular Biology. Dr. Sunde received the B.S. (1972) and Ph.D. (1980) degrees in biochemistry from the University of Wisconsin—Madison.

1

Introduction

BOYD L. O'DELL AND ROGER A. SUNDE
University of Missouri, Columbia, Missouri

The term *mineral element* refers to elements that are not normally volatilized when their organic matrix is ashed to remove the carbonaceous material. *Elements* are substances that cannot be decomposed to simpler substances nor formed by chemical union. The definition of essentiality is more elusive, but in the broad sense, *a nutritionally essential element* is required in the diet of animals and humans in order to allow completion of the life cycle.

I. DISCOVERY OF MINERAL ELEMENT ESSENTIALITY

In 1874 Forster [referenced in (1)] observed that the minerals in the ash of tissues are required to support animal life. This observation established the dietary essentiality of mineral elements. This requirement was distinct and beyond that recognized for carbon, hydrogen, oxygen and sulfur, the elements supplied by water, carbohydrate, fat, and protein. Except for vitamin B_{12}, the dietary requirement for mineral elements is also distinct from that of the vitamins. This Handbook is concerned primarily with the metabolism and metabolic function of these elements in humans and other animals.

The discovery of mineral element essentiality and function has proceeded along multiple routes, employing techniques and observations such as (a) use of purified diets composed of known ingredients, (b) the result of parenteral nutrition, i.e., intravenous infusion of highly purified nutrients, (c) study of animals and people living in ecological niches deficient in specific elements, and (d) determination of the basis of certain genetic diseases. Perhaps the most important tool in the discovery of all essential nutrients, including the mineral elements, has been the purified diet. Total parenteral nutrition is an extension of the purified diet concept, but the discoveries made in the course of its use were

1

accidental in that the elements were not deliberately omitted, but were found to be deficient in the original formulations. Deficiencies of some elements, such as those of iodine, fluorine, cobalt, and copper, were observed first because the soil, water, or plants in a particular area were deficient in the specific element. Other deficiencies have occurred because the essential element was made biologically unavailable by other dietary constituents. Some genetic diseases result from deficiency of an essential element caused by gene mutations. Such mutations may prevent the production of the proteins required to absorb or metabolize the element in the normal manner. Examples of such genetic diseases in humans include Menkes' disease, which leads to copper deficiency, and acrodermatitis enteropathica, which gives rise to zinc deficiency. Lack of these elements commonly results in defective enzymes whose activities are dependent on the element; e.g., molybdenum deficiency induced by a gene mutation impairs sulfite oxidase activity.

Recognition of the physiologic significance of the mineral elements has developed over a period of some 300 years, but the importance of most of the essential elements has been recognized only during the twentieth century. Table 1 lists chronologically some major observations that have led to the recognition of the essential mineral elements. Many of these observations have stood the test of time, having been confirmed repeatedly by other investigators. The conclusions suggested by some observations may be modified with time, and other elements may be added to the list. More detailed history of each element will be found in the respective chapters.

II. DEFINITION OF ESSENTIALITY

An *essential element* is one that is required to support adequate growth, reproduction and health throughout the life cycle, when all other nutrients are optimal. The difficulty with this definition arises in the interpretation of the word *adequate*. Under normal circumstances, an element is clearly essential if a distinct pathology results when it is omitted from the diet. Essentiality is less clearly defined when there is only a small change in the rate of growth, when the environment is suboptimal, or when there is a microbial infection. Observed improvements in performance upon supplementation with an element may be due to changes in the intestinal microflora, to a pharmacologic effect, or to interaction with another element. Conceivably, a nonessential element might provide temporary improvement in a critical physiologic parameter by releasing a similar but essential element from a less critical site and thus making it available. However, if an element exerts a catalytic or regulatory role in a critical biochemical pathway, there is little or no doubt about its essentiality.

A list of the essential mineral elements is presented in Table 2. For convenience and historical reasons, the elements are divided into two groups, the *macro elements* and the *micro elements*. The requirement for macro elements is in the range of grams per kilogram of diet, while that for the micro elements is in the range of milligrams, or even micrograms, per kilogram. In the case of adult humans, the same distinguishing units apply when expressed as intake per day. The micro elements are also referred to as *trace elements* because the early analytical methods did not allow their quantitation, and they were reported simply as a "trace." For this reason and the lack of sufficiently pure dietary ingredients, the essentiality of most of the micro elements was discovered considerably later than that of the macro elements. The list of essential mineral elements in Table 2 is divided into two categories: those whose essentiality has been confirmed by evidence for an essential biochemical mechanism, involving the element in a catalytic or regulatory role; and those whose essentiality is suggested by impairment of physiological function only.

TABLE 1 Chronological Observations Providing Evidence of Mineral Element Essentiality[a]

Year	Element	Laboratory and reference	Observation
1664	Iron	Sydenham (1)	Iron salts restored skin color in anemic patients.
1747	Iron	Menghini (1)	Blood contains iron.
1842	Calcium	Chossat (2)	$CaCO_3$ prevented fragile bones in pigeons.
1847	Sodium and potassium	Liebig (2)	Tissues contain primarily K, and blood and lymph contain primarily Na.
1849	Sodium	Boussingalt (1)	Oxen fed low Na became depressed, unthrifty, and showed loss of hair.
1881	Sodium and potassium	Ringer (2)	Na and K are essential for maintenance of tissues and organs in vitro.
1908	Iodine	Marine (1)	Goiter in pups can be prevented by giving iodine to dams.
1909	Phosphorus	Huebner (2)	Low-P diet produced rickets in dogs.
1918	Phosphorus	Osborne and Mendel (1)	P restriction in rats retarded growth.
1921	Calcium and phosphorus	Sherman (1)	Ca:P ratio is important for bone formation in rats.
1928	Copper	Hart (1)	Cu as well as Fe is required for prevention of anemia in rats fed milk-based diet.
1931	Magnesium	McCollum (1)	Rats fed low Mg developed dilatation of vessels, extreme hyperirratibility.
1931	Manganese	Hart (1); McCollum (1)	Mice failed to grow and ovulate; rats failed to suckle and survive.
1934	Zinc	Hart (1)	Rats fed low Zn showed growth retardation and hair loss.
1935	Cobalt	Underwood (1); Marston (1)	Co prevented loss of appetite, anemia, and lethargy in sheep.
1937	Chloride	Orent-Keiles (1)	Low Cl caused growth retardation and hypersensitivity; low Na caused "fatigue" and dehydration in rats.
1938	Fluoride	Dean (1)	Dental caries is lower in children who drink water with 1.9 than with 0.2 ppm F.
1953	Molybdenum	Richert and Westerfeld (3)	Mo is a component of xanthine oxidase.
1957	Selenium	Schwarz (4)	Se (Factor3) prevents liver necrosis in rats.
1959	Chromium	Mertz (5)	Cr(III) is the factor involved in maintenance of glucose tolerance (GTF).
1972	Silicon	Carlisle (7); Schwarz (8)	Retarded growth in chicks, rats.
1975	Nickel	Nielsen (9)	Ni deprivation increased perinatal mortality, depressed growth and hematocrit.
1976	Arsenic	Anke (10)	Low (50 ppb) As decreased fertility, birth weight, and survival of goats and minipigs.
1981	Lithium	Anke (11)	Low (1.9 ppm) Li decreased fertility and birth weights of goats.
1981	Lead	Kirchgessner (12)	Low (20 ppb) Pb produced anemia and decreased growth in second-generation rats.
1981	Boron	Nielsen (13)	B added to low (0.3 ppm)-B diet stimulated growth and prevented leg abnormalities in chicks fed diets low in cholecalciferol.

[a]This table lists pertinent observations that led to the discovery of the essential elements, but it is not complete and is not meant to establish priority of discovery. The history of the early literature came from Refs. 1 and 2.

TABLE 2 Essential Mineral Elements

Essentiality confirmed by biochemical mechanism(s)		Essentiality suggested by physiologic impairment	
Macro elements			
Calcium	Chloride		
Phosphorus	Potassium		
Sodium	Magnesium		
Micro elements			
Iron	Cobalt	Fluoride	Arsenic
Iodine	Molybdenum	Chromium	Lithium
Copper	Selenium	Vanadium	Lead
Manganese	Zinc	Silicon	Boron
		Nickel	

While these categories are somewhat arbitrary, they are presented to provide a measure of the validity of their assessment as being essential. It is anticipated that future research will move several elements from the latter list into the confirmed list.

While the macro and micro classes of essential elements tend to differ in function, there is considerable overlap. There are three general physiologic roles for the elements in biology: *structural, catalytic,* and *signal transduction.* Of the six macro elements, calcium and phosphorus play important roles in the *skeletal structure* of vertebrates. Phosphorus is also an important component of phospholipids, phosphoproteins, and nucleic acids. Sodium, potassium, and chloride perform major roles in the maintenance of osmotic pressure, water balance, and membrane potentials. Magnesium lies on the border between the macro and micro elements. It is primarily an intracellular element, and it exerts regulatory and catalytic roles in numerous biochemical systems. While the macro elements perform largely structural functions, some also perform regulatory functions involving low or catalytic concentrations. For example, calcium plays a key regulatory role as a messenger in *signal transduction,* notably in nerve and muscle cells. Phosphorus, by way of the phosphorylation–dephosphorylation cycle, exerts a highly important function in the regulation of enzyme activity by changing protein conformation or tertiary structure. Sodium, potassium, and chloride ions are of importance in the function of all cells in the maintenance of water balance. Micro quantities of these elements are important in the function of the nervous system through development of the action potential.

As expected by the low concentrations required, the micro elements serve primarily *catalytic* functions in cells and organisms. Iron performs both major and minor functions. Its deficiency causes anemia, providing clear evidence of iron essentiality, but it is also a component of numerous proteins that exert critical roles in energy metabolism, notably the cytochromes and the enzymes that participate in the electron transport system. Iodine deficiency causes goiter and cretinism, and it is a known component of the important thyroid hormones. Copper deficiency gives rise to many distinct aspects of pathology that can be identified with specific cuproenzymes, e.g., depigmentation and low tyrosinase activity, or aortic rupture and low lysyl oxidase activity. Manganese deficiency results in distinct pathology, including reproductive failure, skeletal defects, and ataxia; the manganese ion is a component of several enzymes, including mitochondrial superoxide dismutase, pyruvate carboxylase, and arginase, although these enzymes may not be related directly to the observed pathology of manganese deficiency. A similar situation exists in the case if zinc, whose deficiency pathology includes stunted growth, skin lesions, and reproductive difficulties. While zinc is a component of enzymes that catalyze more than 50 different biochemical reactions as well as a component of proteins involved in gene expression, none of these proteins or enzymes has been identified with specific zinc deficiency pathology. Besides its catalytic role in some enzymes, zinc exerts a *structural* role in proteins, particularly in the zinc finger proteins involved in gene transcription. Cobalt is a component of vitamin B_{12} and is thus classed as an essential element, but there is no evidence that the cobalt ion has any other biochemical function. The fact that molybdenum is a component of enzymes, such as xanthine oxidase and sulfite oxidase, provides stronger evidence of its essentiality than does the physiologic response of animals to dietary molybdenum deprivation. Not only does selenium deficiency result in severe pathology, including cardiomyopathy and skeletal muscle defects, it is also a component of several proteins, including the glutathione peroxidases and the iodothyronine-5'-deiodinases. The fact that a biochemical as well as a physiologic function has been established for some elements adds materially to the validity of their classification as essential.

III. MECHANISMS BY WHICH MINERAL ELEMENTS EXERT FUNCTION

Biochemical functions have been established for the macro elements and at least eight of the micro elements listed in Table 2. An obvious challenge for future research is to establish biochemical mechanisms that depend on the other elements listed. Fluoride is probably unique among the essential micro elements in the sense that its function appears to be more protective than catalytic. Low fluoride intake often results in dental caries, but it is not essential to prevent caries under all conditions. Sugar consumption plays a major role in the incidence of caries, because of its effect on the microflora associated with teeth. Fluoride is a structural component of bones and teeth, but there is no evidence that it exerts a specific biochemical function.

Of the eight micro elements whose biochemical functions have been identified, at least in part, six are metals and two, iodine and selenium, are nonmetals. The essential metal ions, which belong to the first two transition series of the Periodic Table, generally function as cations complexed with organic ligands or chelators. Proteins are the most common naturally occurring chelators, but there are many other biochemically important chelators, such as the porphyrins and corrins. Molybdenum differs from most of the other metals in that it commonly exists as an anion containing oxygen (MoO_4^{2-}), or analogous anions in which part or all of the oxygen is replaced with sulfur. In biological cofactors the oxygen and sulfur may be provided by organic molecules. The divalent cations in the first transition series have unfilled d orbitals and may be designated by the number of electrons present, e.g., Mn^{d5}, Fe^{d6}, Co^{d7}, and Cu^{d9}. While Zn^{2+} (Zn^{d10}) is not strictly a transition element, because its d orbitals are filled, its atomic structure is similar, and it readily forms complexes analogous to those formed by the transition metal ions. All of the transition metal ions form coordinate covalent bonds with ligands that contain the electron-donor atoms N, O, and S, which are found extensively in proteins. There is a degree of selectivity of metal ions for electron-donor atoms—zinc tends to prefer sulfur, and copper prefers nitrogen—but several different donor atoms will complex with each metal ion. The amino acid residues in proteins serve as rich sources of electron-donor atoms; for example, the imidazole group of histidine supplies nitrogen, the carboxyl groups of aspartic and glutamic acids supply oxygen, and the sulfhydryl group of cysteine supplies sulfur for complexation. Besides proteins that form chelates with the micro elements, porphyrins chelate iron and the corrins chelate cobalt to form specialized enzyme cofactors. The essential micro elements prefer coordination numbers of 4 or 6; i.e., they complex with four or six ligands. Copper and zinc have coordination numbers of 4 and generally form square planar and tetrahedral complexes, respectively. The other cations have coordination numbers of 6 and prefer octahedral complexes. The metal ions complex with chelators with greatly different degrees of affinity. The relative affinities are characterized by thermodynamic dissociation constants that are specific for the ion and the chelator. In general, the stability of a complex is greater if all ligands are present in a single organic molecule, depending on how well their arrangement fits the preferred configuration of the metal ion.

The biologically active molecules that contain the essential nonmetal elements differ distinctly from the metallocompounds. Compounds containing nonmetal elements, such as the iodinated thyroid hormones and the selenoenzymes, bond the respective elements covalently. Thus, the elements in these compounds do not dissociate from the organic moiety and are not in equilibrium with a free ion as in the case of metal ions. The metal ions can associate with preformed apo-proteins, while selenium, for example, is incorporated into proteins as a selenoamino acid at the time of synthesis. Iodine is incorporated into protein posttranslationally, being covalently linked to thyroglobulin after protein synthesis.

IV. QUANTITATIVE INTAKE AND THE PHYSIOLOGIC RESPONSE

As in the case of other essential nutrients, the physiologic effects of the essential mineral elements depend on the level of intake. This concept, based on that of Schulz as proposed in 1888 [referenced in (14)], is depicted in Figure 1. There is a range of intake, the so-called safe and adequate range, which provides optimal function. At intakes progressively below this range there is graded decrease in function until overt signs of deficiency appear. At the same low dietary intake of an element, some organs and functions are affected before others, depending on species and other conditions. For example, copper deficiency adversely affects the cardiovascular system in the pig and chicken before it affects the central nervous system, while in the sheep the nervous system is affected while little or no damage

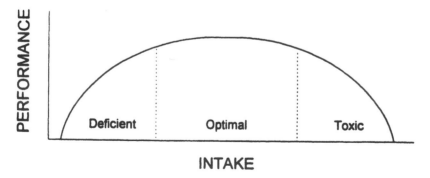

FIGURE 1   Theoretical dose–response curve. The physiologic effect of an essential mineral element is dependent on diet concentration, ranging from deficiency at low intake to toxicity at extremely high intake. The aim of nutritional science is to achieve intakes at safe and adequate levels.

occurs in the vascular system. Zinc deficiency has a more dramatic effect on the nervous system in the guinea pig than it does in the rat. Similar examples can be cited for selenium and other elements. Presumably, these differences occur due to a summation of several factors, including the relative affinities of biologically active proteins for specific metal ions and the relative concentrations and activities of the protein in the different species. The relative rates of expression of critical proteins, the prevalence of alternative protective pathways, as well as the relative rates of generation of substrates could also contribute to the differences.

Signs of toxicity begin to appear when intake exceeds the safe and adequate range. For example, fluoride, selenium, arsenic, and lead have long been considered to be "toxic" elements. As a matter of fact, all of the essential elements are toxic if consumed or administered in excess, although the concentration at which toxicity occurs varies widely. Although it is not valid to arbitrarily classify elements as toxic or nontoxic, the ratio of the minimal toxic level to the minimal adequate level may be a useful index of relative toxicity. For example, although the physiologic significance of selenium was first recognized because of its toxicity in livestock, the ratio of selenium's toxic to its required level is not substantially less than that of many other essential elements, e.g., iron (see Table 3). At concentrations between the safe and toxic levels, there may be a pharmacologic effect of the element. A question that needs to be addressed is, at what levels, if any, do the essential elements act as pharmacologic rather than essential or toxic agents.

Other dietary factors can affect both the requirement and toxicity levels of an element, although the effects on requirement have received the most research attention. Other dietary constituents can increase or decrease the bioavailability of an essential element. By the same token, other dietary components can affect the level of toxicity of both essential and nonessential elements. Relative bioavailability is defined as the proportion of an element in a food that can be absorbed and utilized, compared to a pure standard. Bioavailability of an element is most commonly decreased by its chelation in the gut to form a strong or insoluble complex, or by the presence of a competitive antagonist. For example, phytate, found in seeds, chelates and decreases the bioavailability of zinc; an excess of zinc antagonizes the absorption and utilization of copper. One would expect chelators and antagonists of toxic elements to have an analogous effect on bioavailability of toxic elements. The physiologic effects of the essential elements are concentration-

TABLE 3 Estimated Toxicity: Requirement Ratios of Selected Mineral Nutrients

Element	Highest recommended daily intake (mg)	Estimated minimal toxic daily dose (mg)	Ratio
Calcium	1,200	12,000	10
Phosphorus	1,200	12,000	10
Magnesium	400	6,000	15
Iron	18	100	6
Zinc	15	500	33
Copper	3	100	33
Iodine	0.15	2	13
Selenium	0.2	1	5

Source: Adapted from Ref. 15.

dependent. While the major thrust of this Handbook relates to biological functions of the various elements, generally each chapter gives a brief treatment of the quantitative aspects of requirements and toxicity.

V. MOLECULAR BIOLOGY IN ESSENTIAL MINERAL ELEMENT NUTRITION

A. A New Paradigm for Research

Listed above are four experimental approaches or routes that have been employed successfully to identify and to understand the essential mineral elements. A new paradigm—molecular biology methods of analysis—has emerged in the last decade, and the current and future techniques employing this intellectual base will undoubtedly revolutionize our ability to understand nutrition of the essential elements.

The use of the purified diet in nutrition research was a clever method of analysis that allowed meaningful study of nutrition with little or no knowledge about the underlying processes. Early criteria such as animal survival were subsequently replaced by growth, reproduction, and protection against a specific disease or pathology (16). Later, analytical methods progressed to permit determination of maintenance (balance) of tissue mineral levels. Later still, measurement of biochemical markers, such as circulating alkaline phosphatase or glutamic-oxaloacetic transaminase, or element-specific biochemical markers, such as glutathione peroxidase, angiotensin-converting enzyme, or serum ferritin, gave increasing sophistication to our assessment of mineral requirements. At each increased level of sophistication, additional important knowledge was obtained to help us understand the nutritional biochemistry of the essential elements. These procedures, however, were all dependent on appropriate choice of the parameter on which to make the measurement, and the conclusions were perhaps more dependent on the observer than on the subject of the study. The number of publications in the two decades from 1970 to 1990, reporting discovery of a function for an identified metalloprotein, or of looking for a biochemical mechanisms for an impaired physiologic function (see Table 2), is tremendous. In the late 1980s, the new molecular biology paradigm began to offer exciting routine potential for bridging the gap between a protein and a function. The following examples illustrate this potential.

The ability to sequence proteins, cDNAs, and genes, rapidly and accurately, in combination with the technological revolution that allows rapid searching of the resulting databases, now allows rapid interconversion of information among these three tiers of gene expression. What previously was a seeming miracle of serendipity that married a function and a protein, such as the marriage of hemocuprein and copper, zinc-superoxide dismutase (17), can now be done routinely: for example, the convergent identification of cytosolic aconitase as the iron-regulatory element (IRE)-binding protein (18). In contrast to the hemocuprein story, this regulatory protein is found in trace amounts and would likely not have been detected without the advent of molecular biology.

A second important area is the ability to discern changes in the regulation of protein expression, not only by use of antibodies, but also by use of Northern blotting techniques to monitor changes in mRNA levels, and using footprinting techniques or gel retardation/mobility shift assays to determine interaction of regulatory proteins with nucleic acids. This permits a refinement of our ability to determine the impact of small changes in nutritional status on gene expression and to determine the mechanism of this process at a molecular level. An exciting recent development, employing variations on the polymerase chain reaction techniques, uses an approach called differential display; without any knowledge of what one is looking for or of the processes involved, one can compare gene expression under two conditions, such as nutrient deficiency versus adequacy, or disease versus health. And the outcome is to identify a series of cDNAs of genes that are potentially regulated differentially under these two conditions.

A third powerful approach is the use of heterologous expression systems, such as the xenopus oocyte (frog), baculovirus (insect), yeast or baby kidney hamster cell systems, to clone, characterize, and identify an animal or human gene from a library. The host system is typically devoid or low in native expression, so modest restoration of activity can be detected when the cells are transfected with a sample containing a gene for the activity of interest. With these heterologous expression techniques, we have powerful ability to identify the proteins and the genes for critical regulatory steps in metabolic pathways which may only be present at the level of a few copies per cell. Because mineral elements were likely critical components of metabolic pathways at the earliest stages of evolution as well as being fundamentally important for maintenance of a constant intracellular environment, these nutrients are emerging as important effectors in gene regulation. The recent identification of a molecular role for copper in iron uptake in yeast, for instance (19), shows the power of this approach in answering long-standing nutritional questions. The identified mechanisms are also likely to play important roles in how nutrition modulates health.

The last general molecular biology technique that we would like to highlight briefly is the powerful technique of producing transgenic and knockout animals. Spontaneous inborn errors of metabolism, such as sulfite oxidase deficiency, have provided tremendous insight into the identification of essential elements, such as molybdenum, that were not readily identified using the purified-diet approach. Today, researchers not only can delete or add a specific gene in a single-celled experimental model, they can also readily create mice with three or four copies of a specific gene, or strains of mice lacking one or more genes. For instance, production of mice lacking both metallothionein I and metallothionein II is helping to specifically identify the essential biochemical function of this regulated copper/zinc/cadmium protein (20).

B. Molecular Biology and Determination of Requirements

The reader will find that most if not all of the nutrient requirements described in the subsequent chapters were established under rather specific conditions, including age, diet, and choice of indicating parameter. Often times, the results were less than clear-cut, and required corollary support from experiments with other species and other methods of requirement determination. Several aspects lie at the heart of this problem. The first is that the easiest, least invasive parameter to be measured may not be a meaningful endpoint, or it may be adversely affected by a number of quite common situations, such as disease, stress, pregnancy, etc. The second is that it is increasingly clear that homeostasis protects organisms from deficiency or excess of a nutrient; this tends to obscure modest or even relatively large changes in nutrient status. Third, attempts to correct for genetic variation, or to provide a margin of safety, further confuse this situation. The emergence of molecular biology techniques and knowledge offers the first true promise for an alternative approach to the determination of biological dietary requirements.

This premise is based on the idea that the status of each mineral element is regulated both intracellularly and at the level of the whole organism. Molecular biology offers the potential of identifying the specific biochemical mechanism, and it offers the potential to monitor these changes in a meaningful way. A sensor or thermostat, which senses and reacts to changes in the nutrient status, is at the heart of both mechanical and biological feedback systems. Today, work identifying the integrated process for regulating intercellular iron storage (ferritin) and iron uptake (transferrin receptor) via the iron regulatory protein (formally called IRE-binding protein and cytosolic aconitase) suggests that we are close to understanding the specific feedback regulatory mechanism used to control iron status within an individual cell. Similar mechanisms are likely to be obtained in the next decade for zinc, selenium, and many other trace elements.

Equally exciting will be the characterization of these molecular feedback systems. Evolution has undoubtedly refined these sensors to place them at an optimal range for survival; the sensor is neither set so low that it makes the organism prone to deficiency nor so high as to make the organism prone to toxicity. The molecular basis of a specific biological setpoint remains obscure for virtually all nutrient feedback systems, but one can envision an altered three-dimensional protein structure or replacement of an amino acid ligand as mechanisms to modulate the binding constant of a sensor protein for its nutrient target. For instance, replacement of a cysteine with a histidine undoubtedly would have changed the affinity of a regulatory factor for zinc. In just this way, evolution may have adjusted the regulatory factor that maintains intercellular concentrations of elements and or circulating levels of elements at their optimal levels. The use of molecular biology techniques should permit us to determine what nutritional levels correspond to the saturation point of these sensors. For instance, comparison of the minimum dietary selenium requirement for maximum expression of enzyme activity or mRNA level for two distinct intracellular glutathione peroxidase yields dramatic differences (21). The exciting aspect of this fact is not that we can use molecular biology to determine nutrient requirements under the usual conditions that have been used in the past, such as in the rapidly growing animal, but because it will give us the ability to determine optimal nutrient requirements under less than ideal conditions such as during infection, old age, or chronic disease. If the homeostatic mechanisms is still operating, these new techniques will let us determine potentially where the thermostat is set. Equally exciting, we may well be able to determine individual genetic differences for a nutrient. For example, a recent report by Morrison et al. (22) found that the wrong two alleles of the vitamin-D receptor have dramatic impact on bone density, suggesting that a genetic approach has the potential to become, first, an important experimental tool, and second, an important component in the determination of individual nutrient requirements.

The implications of this concept are even greater. It is likely that there will be a gap between saturation of the regulatory thermostat protein and the effector protein that responds to the regulatory protein. Here, too, evolution may have changed the relative affinities of these two proteins to provide optimal survival advantage under typical conditions. The dietary difference between nutrient intakes that trigger the sensor protein and the nutrient intakes that maximize responding protein could be called an evolutionary-derived margin of safety; the gap between the level of dietary selenium necessary for maximal glutathione peroxidase mRNA expression and for maximal glutathione peroxidase activity may be such a margin of safety (23). The point is that careful determination of the molecular mechanism may, for the first time, give us true insight into where evolution has set the nutrient requirements; with this information the nutrient requirement could be based on the intercellular and/or the organism setpoint. Second, we could determine how this setpoint is changed depending on genetic variation, and third, we might no longer have to determine arbitrarily what margin of safety is necessary. For the mineral nutritionist willing to use molecular biology techniques, the opportunity to unravel these processes is unlimited.

C. Pharmacologic or Conditional Levels of Essential Elements

We are likely, however, to need to contain our excitement about the potential for molecular biology to solve all of the nutrition questions related to nutrient requirements. Numerous epidemiologic studies and prospective studies are identifying conditions that require nutrient intakes outside the usual nutritional realm, and thus outside the formative evolutionary pressures that may have shaped and refined the biochemical requirement setpoints. Examples outside the essential element area include supernutritional levels of vitamin E for prevention of cardiovascular disease; and potential benefit of a synthetic compound, aspirin, to prevent the development of overt cardiovascular disease in middle-aged men and perhaps women. One long-standing nutritional example is fluoride, which may not have a prescribed biochemical role, but which appears to have a defined level in the diet that protects teeth against decay and bones against premature calcium loss. Another example might well be the antitumorigenic effect of selenium at levels well above nutritional levels required to maximize glutathione peroxidase expression. In both of these cases, maximum protective levels may occur just at the onset of apparent toxicity. Second, these effects may be antagonized by normal mechanisms that protect animals against toxicity.

In summary, sophisticated molecular nutrition techniques will be called upon in exciting new ways to set safe and adequate levels of these conditionally essential nutrients. Importantly, the protective regulatory and homeostatic mechanisms on which we have relied to provide protection against day-to-day variation and against drift in requirements due to disease state, health, stress, and age, are likely not to be in effect for these conditional nutrients. Identification of proper reporter markers for setting these requirements is likely to be an important area of nutrition research in the future.

REFERENCES

1. McCollum EV. A History of Nutrition. Boston: Houghton Mifflin Company, 1957.
2. McCay CM. Notes on the History of Nutrition Research, Verzar F, ed. Berne: Hans Huber, 1973.
3. Richert DA, Westerfeld WW. Isolation and identification of the xanthine oxidase factor as molybdenum. J. Biol Chem 1953; 203:915–923.
4. Schwarz K, Foltz CM. Selenium as an integral part of Factor 3 against dietary necrotic liver degeneration. J Am. Chem Soc 1957; 79:3292–3293.
5. Schwarz K, Mertz W. Chromium(III) and the glucose tolerance factor. Arch Biochem Biophys 1959; 85:292–295.
6. Schwarz K, Milne DB. Growth effects of vanadium in the rat. Science 1971; 174:426–428.
7. Carlisle EM. Silicon: an essential element for the chick. Science 1972; 178:619–621.
8. Schwarz K, Milne DB. Growth-promoting effects of silicon in rats. Nature 1972; 239:333–334.
9. Nielsen FH, Myron DR, Givand SH, Ollerich DA. Nickel deficiency in rats. J Nutr 1975; 105:1620–1630.
10. Anke M, Gruen M, Partschefeld M. The essentiality of arsenic for animals. In: Hemphill DD, ed. Trace Elements in Environmental Health—10. Columbia, MO: University of Missouri, 1976:403–409.
11. Anke M, Gruen M, Groppel B, Kronemann H. The biological importance of lithium. Mengen- und Spurenelemente 1981; 1:217– 239.

12. Reichlmayr-Lais AM, Kirchgessner M. Haematologische veraenerungen bei alimentaerem Bleimangel. Ann Nutr Metabol 1981; 25:281–288.

13. Hunt CD, Nielsen FH. Interaction between boron and cholecalciferol in the chick. In: Howell JMcC, Gawthorne JM, White CL, eds. Trace Element Metabolism in Man and Animals (TEMA-4). Canberra: Australian Academy of Science, 1981:597–600.

14. Underwood EJ, Mertz W. Introduction. In: Mertz W, ed. Trace Elements in Human and Animal Nutrition. Vol. 1. New York: Academic Press, 1986:1–19.

15. Committee on Diet and Health, Food and Nutrition Board. Diet and Health. Washington, DC: National Academy Press, 1989:518.

16. Schneider HA. Rats, fats, and history. In: Perspectives in Biology and Medicine. Chicago: University of Chicago Press, 1986; 29:392–406.

17. McCord JM, Fridovich I. Superoxide dismutase. An enzymatic function for erythrocuprein (hemocuprein). J Biol Chem 1969; 244:6049–6055.

18. Kaptain S, Downey WE, Tang CC, et al. A regulated RNA binding protein also possesses aconitase activity. Proc Natl Acad Sci (USA) 1991; 88:10109–10113.

19. Dancis A, Yuan DS, Haile D, et al. Molecular characterization of a copper transport protein in *S. cerevisiae*: an unexpected role for copper in iron transport. Cell 1994; 76:393–402.

20. Masters BA, Kelly EJ, Quaife CJ, Brinster RL, Palmiter RD. Targeted disruption of metallothionein I and II genes increases sensitivity to cadmium. Proc Natl Acad Sci (USA) 1994; 91: 584–588.

21. Lei XG, Evenson JK, Thompson KM, Sunde RA. Glutathione peroxidase and phospholipid hydroperoxide glutathione peroxidase are differentially regulated by dietary selenium. J Nutr 1995; 125:1438–1446.

22. Morrison NA, Qi JC, Tokita A, et al. Prediction of bone density from vitamin D receptor alleles. Nature 1994; 367:284–287.

23. Sunde RA. Intracellular glutathione peroxidases—structure, regulation and function. In: Burke RF, ed. Selenium in Biology and Human Health. Vol. 5 45–47, New York: Springer-Verlag, 1994:45–57.

2
Calcium

FELIX BRONNER

University of Connecticut Health Center, Farmington, Connecticut

I. INTRODUCTION

A. Distribution of Calcium in Nature

Calcium is the fifth most abundant element of the globe. It is found in a variety of rocks, such as aragonite or dolomite, and throughout most waters. The concentration of calcium in seawater varies from 1 to 10 mM (1); concentrations of calcium ion in fresh waters tend to be one to two orders of magnitude lower than in the oceans, but may reach the higher concentrations found in the ocean if the ground waters come from reservoirs in limestone. The latter are typically known as "hard" waters and are usually also high in magnesium. The average calcium concentration of the crust of the earth is almost 1 mol/kg, with more than 80% of the calcium found there occurring in the form of limestone ($CaCO_3$) deposits, which therefore constitute the principal forms of calcium in the earth. Kretsinger (1), in discussing these relationships, has called attention to the close link between carbon and calcium in living organisms. Moreover, since calcium phosphate is fairly insoluble and since phosphates and phosphorylation serve cells in a variety of ways (1)—to assure hydrophilicity for metabolites, as leaving groups in nucleophilic displacement reactions, as significant forms of energy storage (ATP), to link RNA and DNA—cells have to find ways to keep calcium from tying up phosphate and preventing its utilization.

As cells evolved, they learned to get rid of excess calcium, adapting calcium extrusion to a variety of cellular processes—protein secretion, intracellular signaling, and the many calcium-dependent processes that have come to light in recent years. Thus the conquest of the ocean by living systems, uni- and multicellular, was paralleled by their ability to deal with the calcium in their surroundings. When organisms began to leave the ocean to conquer the land, they required mechanisms of support and developed external and ultimately internal skeletons, calcium deposits which also served as storage depots, i.e., for the accumulation and release of calcium, thereby maintaining the plasma calcium concentration constant, typically 2.5 mM.

B. Distribution of Calcium in the Body

The adult human body contains easily 1 kg of Ca, with less than 1% of that amount found outside the skeleton. The body's calcium traffic, which will be described in detail later, involves multiple gradients of calcium concentration and changes in state from solid to liquid and back. Thus an individual may ingest 1 g of Ca daily, of which perhaps two-thirds is in solution (as in milk) or readily solubilized, as from cheese. The remainder may be ingested in solid form and require both digestion and solubilization before it moves across the intestinal epithelium. The calcium concentration in the luminal fluid of the intestine can readily reach 10 mM or higher, whereas the free calcium concentration of lymph and blood is maintained at 0.5 and ~1 mM, respectively. Calcium enters bone from blood and is precipitated in the form of various calcium phosphate phases, e.g., whitlockite, carbonate, phosphate, hydroxyapatite.

When calcium is mobilized from bone, it changes its state from solid to solution and returns to the circulation. Excretion in the urine involves a change in concentration, from 0.5 to 3 mM. Excretion in sweat and in the stool as endogenous fecal calcium (see below) probably involves no change in concentration as the calcium passes through the skin or into the intestinal lumen, but evaporation of sweat and water reabsorption in the intestine markedly change the calcium concentration of the final product.

Total cellular calcium varies between 1 and 5 mmol/kg, but the free intracellular calcium is ~100 nmol/L in most cells. Thus there is a very large gradient between free and bound intracellular calcium, the latter accounting for nearly the entire cellular calcium. It is undoubtedly this huge gradient that has made it possible for calcium to be such an effective intracellular signal. The requirement for separation of calcium and phosphate signifies that entry into the cell must be severely restricted, while cellular calcium extrusion must be at a maximum. How these characteristics affect transcellular calcium transport and bone calcium deposition and removal will be discussed in the relevant sections on transport and bone calcium.

C. Calcium Movement in the Body

Figure 1 summarizes in schematic form the pathways that calcium follows as it is ingested, absorbed, transported to and from the skeleton, and excreted from the body. Details of the processes involved will be presented in the appropriate sections.

II. CALCIUM IN FOOD AND DIET

If one classifies foods on the basis of their calcium content, then foods that contain more than 2.0 mmol per portion include (2) milk, cheese, ice cream, broccoli, cheese pizza, custard, Cream of Wheat, a whole orange (but not orange juice). Block et al. (3) have done a detailed study of the dietary sources of calcium in the second U.S. National Health and Nutrition Examination Survey (1976–1980) and found that dairy products contributed about 55% of dietary calcium. However, if one considers that most calcium in white bread, in many flours, and in other foods is contributed by the addition of milk powder, one can estimate that calcium derived from dairy products constitutes about 70% of the calcium

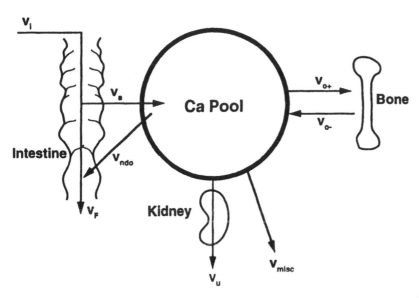

FIGURE 1 Schematic diagram of the flow of calcium through the body. The Ca pool includes calcium in solution in blood plasma, in the extracellular fluid, and in, or associated with, bone, described in units of mass, e.g., mmol. v_i = Ca ingested in food; v_a = Ca absorbed from food; v_{ndo} = endogenous Ca lost in stool; v_u = Ca excreted in urine; v_F = Ca excreted in stool; v_{misc} = Ca lost from the body via sweat, semen, menstrual fluid, milk; v_{o+} = Ca deposited in bone; v_{o-} = Ca resorbed from bone, described in units of mass per unit time, e.g., mmol/day. v_T = rate at which Ca enters or leaves the pool, i.e., = $v_a + v_{o-} = v_u + v_{ndo} + v_{o+} + v_{misc}$; In a nonlactating organism, v_{misc} is generally negligibly small. For illustrative numbers of the various parameters, see Table 4.

intake, not very different from an earlier estimate (4). In 1984, U.S. women 35–50 years old consumed on average 13.3 mmol of calcium, a mean value not much lower than what was reported in 1959 (5). Both values are significantly lower, however, than the daily recommended dietary allowance (RDA) for women of 20 mmol (6).

Men aged 19–50 years, on the other hand, consumed 125% of their RDA for calcium when surveyed for one summer day in 1985 (7).

Increasingly, the diet of people in industrialized countries is made up of foods that have undergone substantial processing. While processing of foods may alter their vitamin content, the nature of their proteins, or cause the loss of trace minerals (8), the calcium content of these foods is less likely to be affected. Moreover, processing may render a given food more digestible, and fortification with nonfat dry milk powder enriches the food's calcium content.

III. CALCIUM ABSORPTION

A. Digestion and Solubilization

Calcium becomes absorbed when it moves across the intestinal epithelium. Obviously, only calcium that is in solution in the intestinal lumen can undergo absorption. Calcium may already be in solution in a food before it is ingested, as in milk, or it may become solubilized as the result of the combined actions of gastric acid and intestinal enzymes and of intestinal contractions and peristalsis, all of which act to bring about digestion and solubilization.

One aspect of the bioavailability of calcium is the degree to which it can be solubilized from a given food. Clearly, the more completely a given food is digested, the larger the fraction of its calcium that becomes available for absorption.

Consider the situation when $CaCO_3$ is fed as a salt and is the only calcium source in the diet. In an individual with normal acid production in the stomach, the chyme as it leaves the stomach will have a fairly low pH and—unless the quantity of $CaCO_3$ that has been ingested is very large—all the calcium will be in ionic form. Some will then undergo absorption in the duodenum. As the chyme travels caudad, its pH will go up and, depending on the amount of calcium still in solution, some of the calcium may in fact precipitate. At the neutral or slightly alkaline pH found in the lower intestine, no more than about 4 mmol of $CaCO_3$ will dissolve per liter (9), and that is the maximum available for absorption in that portion of the intestine. To be sure, as calcium is absorbed from the lumen, precipitated calcium goes into solution. Hence the rate of absorption and the length of the time that the chyme remains in a given intestinal segment will determine the amount absorbed.

If more than one calcium salt is present—e.g., carbonate and phosphate—the ratio of the respective solubility products for each salt will determine how much calcium, derived from each salt, will be in solution. In the case of monobasic calcium phosphate and calcium carbonate, virtually all of the calcium in solution will be due to the phosphate, because the phosphate is 18 times more soluble than $CaCO_3$. In other words, the availability of calcium from $CaCO_3$ is markedly reduced if other sources of calcium are present in addition to the carbonate. In terms of overall availability of calcium, the fact that only a tiny faction of the absorbed calcium is derived from carbonate, with most coming from other sources, is of course of no practical significance, provided enough calcium is present in the lumen for calcium absorption to proceed throughout the period the chyme remains in the intestinal lumen. In the rat this is typically 3–4 h (10,11).

B. Transcellular Movement

Calcium moves across the intestinal epithelium by two routes (12): through the cell, i.e., transcellularly; and between cells, i.e., paracellularly. The transcellular movement is saturable, regulated (largely by vitamin D; see Sec. VIII.A), and takes place in the proximal intestine, mostly the duodenum (Fig. 2). Paracellular transport occurs throughout the intestine and does not appear to be subject to acute regulation.

Transcellular movement of calcium is a metabolically active process, requiring oxygen, and is against a chemical gradient. It is experimentally demonstrated by means of everted intestinal sacs (13,14), filled with and immersed in the same calcium-containing buffer (15). When the outside solution of such a preparation is oxygenated, the tissue accumulates calcium on the inside of the everted sac. Only sacs from the proximal intestine transport calcium actively (12,15).

Intestinal loops can be prepared from all three segments of the intestine. As shown in Figure 3, calcium absorption in the duodenum and upper jejunum, when evaluated by the in-situ intestinal loop procedure (16), involves the sum of two processes, saturable and nonsaturable, whereas no saturable step is observed in the ileum. Figure 4 shows the time course of duodenal calcium transport, as evaluated by in-situ loops. As can be seen, completion of absorption is concentration-dependent; i.e., it is completed by 30 min when the instilled solution contains 10 mM Ca, whereas it is only half complete at 2.5 h when the concentration of the instilled solution is 150 mM. If absorption were due to simple diffusion

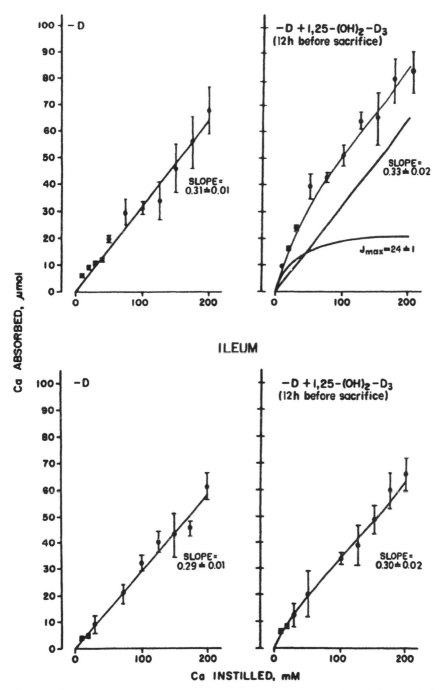

FIGURE 2 Calcium absorption in duodenum and ileum of vitamin D-deficient rats before and after treatment with 1,25-dihydroxyvitamin D_3. Male weanling Sprague-Dawley rats were fed a vitamin D-deficient diet (1.5% calcium, 1.5% phosphorus) and about 4 weeks later, when they weighed 116 $\pm$ 4 g and their mean plasma calcium level was 5.6 $\pm$ 0.1 mg/dL, calcium absorption studies by the in-situ loop procedure were initiated. The left panels show calcium absorption of the duodenum and ileum of the vitamin D-depleted animals ($n = 72$); the right panels show calcium absorption in the duodenum and ileum of vitamin D-deficient animals that had received 3 ng of 1,25-(OH)$_2$-D$_3$ by i.p. injection 12 h before sacrifice. (Reproduced by permission from Ref. 16.)

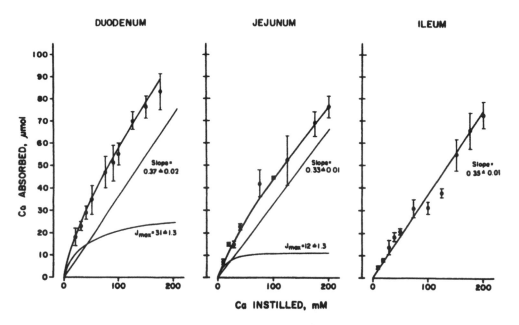

FIGURE 3   Calcium absorption in three intestinal segments of rats. Seventy male weanling rats were fed a high-Ca diet (1.5% Ca, 1.5% P) for 10 days. When their body weight averaged 77 ± 1.2 (SE) g, calcium absorption was analyzed by an in-situ loop procedure. J_{max} (equivalent to V_m) (μmol), and slope P are given as mean values ± SE. The experiment lasted 150 min, so the slope averaged 0.14 h^{-1}. (Reproduced with permission from Ref. 16.)

alone, the extraction rate would be identical at all concentrations. Hence a saturable process is involved.

The simplest description of a saturable process is the Michaelis-Menten relationship:

$$a = \frac{-d[Ca]_L}{dt} = \frac{V_m[Ca]_L}{K_m + [Ca]_L} \tag{1}$$

where v_a = initial rate and V_m = maximum rate of luminal Ca ($[Ca]_L$) efflux or rate of uptake, and K_m = that concentration of calcium in the lumen, $[Ca]_L$, when $v_i = V_m/2$. Integration of Eq. 1 between the limits $[Ca]_0$ at time = 0 and $[Ca]_t$ at time = t yields

$$\ln\frac{[Ca]_t}{[Ca]_0} + \frac{[Ca]_t - [Ca]_0}{K_m} = \frac{-V_m t}{K_m} \tag{2}$$

When K_m is large compared to $[Ca]_t - [Ca]_0$, the second term of Eq. 2 becomes negligible. Figure 5 is a plot of $\ln [Ca]_t/[Ca]_0$ against t. At low calcium concentrations (5 and 10 mM), a straight line, with slope V_m/K_m, describes the data well. At a calcium concentration of 25 mM, the function is clearly curvilinear and the value of K_m must be markedly smaller than the prevailing calcium concentrations. It has been shown (12) that the function that fits the loop data at 25 mM has a V_m of 23 μmol/g/h and a K_m of 3.9 mM; with the aid of these values, theoretical time courses were calculated for calcium efflux at concentrations from 50 to 150 mM (Fig. 5). At the highest concentration, the theoretical time course no longer fitted the data, which diverged widely from the theoretical curve. This can only mean that

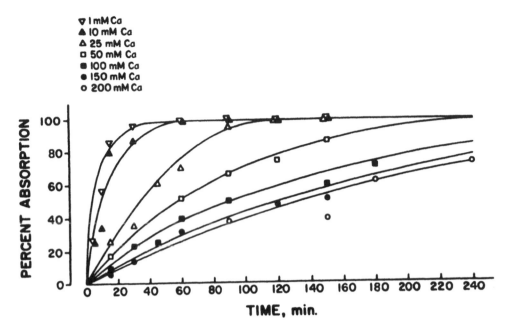

FIGURE 4 Time course of calcium efflux from in-situ duodenal loops. Male Sprague-Dawley rats, 40–50 days of age and 120–160 g body weight, were fed a semisynthetic diet containing 1.5% calcium and 1.5% phosphate for approximately 10 days. Two days before experiment, animals were fed a low-Ca diet (0.05% Ca, 0.2% P). Calcium at various concentrations, shown in the figure, was instilled in the intestinal lumen. Efflux, estimated from the amount of ^{45}Ca lost in the indicated time period, is shown as percent absorbed. Each point represents a mean estimate of 2–6 loops; average SE is 7%. (Reproduced by permission from Ref. 12.)

at high calcium concentrations, efflux from the loop was substantially augmented by a process other than that which saturates at low calcium concentrations (12).

Transcellular movement of calcium involves three sequential steps: entry across the brush border membrane; intracellular movement from one to the other pole of the cell; and extrusion at the basolateral cell membrane. For each of these steps one can ask at what rate and by what mechanism each takes place.

1. Calcium Entry

Calcium enters intestinal cells through the brush border membrane. It travels down an electrochemical gradient, inasmuch as the luminal calcium concentration is in the millimolar range, whereas the free intracellular calcium concentration is approximately 100 nM. Also, the intracellular content is electronegative with respect to the intestinal lumen. In principle, one can envision one of two possible modes of calcium entry into the cell: via a channel or via facilitated diffusion, utilizing a transport molecule. Calcium uptake by isolated brush border vesicles that have been sheared off the intestinal cells is appropriately described by a curvilinear function. The latter has been interpreted as being due to a transmembrane flux that is linear, followed by binding to the inside of the vesicle membrane (17,18). Others (19–21) have analyzed the curvilinear function in terms of a linear and a saturable component, interpreting the existence of the latter as evidence for mediated

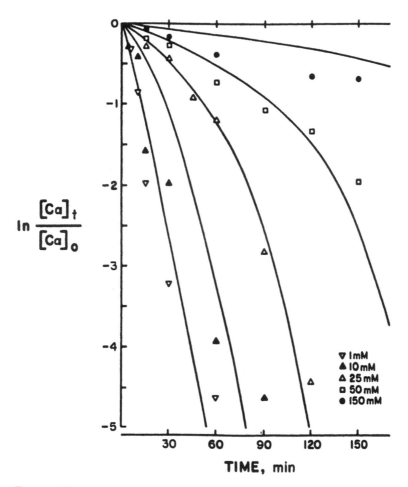

Figure 5 A plot of $\ln[Ca_t/[Ca]_0$ against time, using the data of Figure 4. Lines shown are calculated with use of Eq. 2, with $V_m = 22.25$ μmol/h/loop and $K_m = 3.85$ mM, with $[Ca]_0 = 1, 10, 25, 50,$ and 150 mM (left to right). (Reproduced by permission from Ref. 12.)

transport, i.e., a transporter. While current evidence is insufficient to reject the possibility of a brush border transporter—an idea first advanced by Holdsworth (22)—calcium movement is down an electrochemical gradient and calcium would flood the cell if there existed no barrier to its entry (23). Consequently, the existence of a transporter seems unlikely. Additional arguments against the existence of a transporter include the only modest effect of vitamin D on calcium entry (17), even though vitamin D is the major regulator of active, transcellular calcium transport (Fig. 2).

    The ubiquitous presence of calcium channels makes it likely that entry into the cell is in fact mediated by such channels. Both the nature and the number of channels in the intestinal cell are as yet unknown. No report has appeared detailing the location of calcium channels on the brush borders of intestinal cells; the existence of calcium channels on the basolateral pole of ileal cells has been reported (24). In the colon, tension development depends on extracellular calcium influx, mediated in turn by potential-dependent calcium channels (25). Such channels have also been observed in the rabbit nephron (26). Based on analogy with calcium channels in guinea pig ventricular cells (27), a rat duodenal cell has been estimated to contain 873 channels (12), a reasonable number. Functional evidence for the existence of calcium channels in clonal rat osteosarcoma cells has been reported (28,29). These cells have osteoblastlike characteristics and respond within seconds to 1,25-dihydroxyvitamin D_3 with a 50–100% increase in intracellular free calcium (29,30). Conceivably, the enhanced calcium uptake by stimulated intestinal cells (31) and by brush border membranes isolated from vitamin D-repleted rats (17) utilizes a similar mechanism, i.e., a calcium channel that contains a vitamin D-sensitive element. A large, brush border membrane-related particulate complex, a part of which is vitamin D-dependent, has been identified (32) and assigned a transport role (33). Miller and colleagues (34) have identified a membrane-bound, vitamin D-dependent calcium-binding protein from the brush border which differs importantly from the cytosolic calbindin (CaBP, see below) and which may represent the monomer of the larger protein of Kowarski and Schachter (32).

In summary, it is probable that calcium enters the duodenal cell through calcium channels which may contain a vitamin D-dependent calcium-binding component. Entry is down an electrochemical gradient at a rate that is probably not limiting for transcellular calcium transport.

2. Intracellular Diffusion

Once calcium has entered the cell, it must diffuse through the cell interior to the basolateral membrane where extrusion takes place. The rate at which a calcium ion diffuses through the interior of an intestinal cell is given by Fick's law, which may be written as

$$F = \frac{AD_{Ca}}{L}([Ca]_1 - [Ca]_2) \tag{3}$$

where

F = transcellular flux rate of the calcium ion
A = cross-sectional area of the intestinal cell
D_{Ca} = diffusion coefficient for calcium ion in the cell sap at 37°C
$[Ca]_1$ = calcium concentration at the brush border pole of the cell
$[Ca]_2$ = calcium concentration at the basolateral pole of the cell
L = Length of the diffusion path, i.e., length of the intestinal cell

For a rat intestinal cell, $A = 80 \mu m^2$, $L = 10 \mu m$, and the difference in calcium concentration between the two poles can be reasonably estimated at 200 nM, since the average free intracellular calcium ion concentration is typically 100 nM. With $D = 3 \times 10^{-3}$ cm²/min (35), F becomes 96×10^{-18} mol/min/intestinal cell. When the experimental value for the V_m of transcellular calcium flux is expressed on a cell basis, however, its value is some 70 times greater than the calculated self-diffusion rate of calcium. This means that, in the duodenal cell, calcium moves transcellularly at a rate some 70 times greater than the rate at which the ion alone can diffuse. This implies that in the calcium-transporting duodenal cell there must exist a mechanism that significantly and markedly enhances the self-diffusion of the calcium ion. This is accomplished by the presence in the cell of a calcium-binding protein, calbindin D-9K ($M_r \approx 9$ kDa).

This molecule, discovered by Wasserman and colleagues (36–38), whose biosynthesis is totally dependent on vitamin D (39–41), contains two calcium-binding sites, has a quaternary structure resembling an E–F hand (42), a pI of 4.3, and K_d for calcium of about 0.3 μM (43,44). Under conditions of maximum V_m (Fig. 6), the calbindin (CaBP)

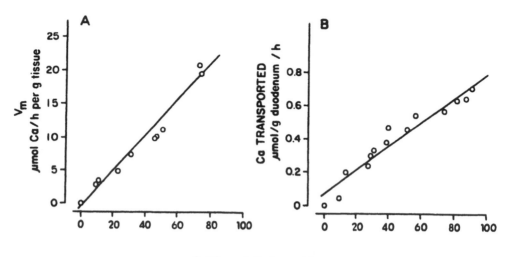

FIGURE 6 Relation between intestinal calcium transport and calbindin (CaBP) content. A. V_m, calculated from in-situ duodenal, jejunal, and ileal loop experiments, shown as a function of CaBP content. Equation describing the relationship is $V_m = 0.59 + 0.26$ CaBP, units as shown, $n = 10$, $r = 0.98$. B. Calcium transport, as evaluated from everted duodenal sac experiments (90 min incubation, 0.25 mM calcium), shown as a function of CaBP content. Equation describing relationship is Ca transport $= 0.070 + 0.00714$CaBP, units as shown, $n = 14$, $r = 0.97$. Data from male Sprague-Dawley or Wistar rats, 70 to 150 g body weight, fed a semisynthetic, high-calcium regimen (1.5% calcium and 1.5% phosphate), with or without vitamin D. (Reproduced by permission from Ref. 12.)

concentration in the cell is 0.2–0.4 mM (45), a concentration sufficient to augment the diffusion rate of calcium to the required value.

Stein (23) has shown how Eq. 3 can be transformed to yield an expression that predicts the augmentation factor for calcium diffusion in the cell:

$$\text{AUG} = \frac{D_{\text{CaBP}} \times \text{Tot CaBP} \times K_{\text{CaBP}}}{D_{\text{Ca}} \times (K_{\text{CaBP}} + [\text{Ca}]_1)\,(K_{\text{CaBP}} + [\text{Ca}]_2)} \tag{4}$$

where

AUG = augmentation of calcium flux, i.e., the ratio of calcium flow due to calbindin compared with calcium flow in the absence of calbindin
D_{CaBP} = diffusion coefficient of calbindin
Tot CaBP = total calbindin concentration
K_{CaBP} = dissociation constant of calbindin with calcium
$[\text{Ca}]_1$, $[\text{Ca}]_2$ = Ca^{2+} concentrations at the two poles of the cell

As predicted (12,23) and found experimentally (Fig. 6), Feher et al. (46) report in their in-vitro studies that "the enhancement of transcellular [calcium] transport was nearly linearly dependent on calbindin-D9K concentration."

Stein (23) has shown that the augmentation factor predicted from Eq. 4 equals the amplification needed, i.e., some 70-fold, and called attention to the three components of Eq. 4 that contribute most to the efficiency of the transcellular transport systems: (1) a high ratio of calbindin to the free calcium ion concentration [$(2 \times 10^{-4}$ M$)/10^{-7}$ M]; (2) a high ratio of the diffusion coefficient of the bound to that of the free substrate (It should be borne in mind, however, that the bound calcium, being attached to a large carrier molecule, will always diffuse more slowly than the free calcium ion.); (3) an optimal value for the dissociation constant of the substrate-carrier complex. Feher et al. (46) have shown that the experimental value of the K_d of calbindin obtained in the presence of 0.1 M KCl, a situation similar to what prevails in the cell sap, is optimum for enhancing transport. The value they utilized, 4.3×10^{-7} M (46,47), was also used by Stein (23).

We thus see that intracellular calcium diffusion, the second of the three steps making up transcellular calcium transport, is assured by and is in direct proportion to the quantity of the intracellular calcium-binding potein, calbindin-D9K, whose action may be compared to that of an intracellular ferry. It should be pointed out that this process is "exactly equivalent to the process postulated to occur within the muscle cell (48), where myoglobin is thought to ferry oxygen across the cell, thus speeding up the loading and unloading of oxygen from and to the tissue" (23).

3. Calcium Extrusion

The intracellular free calcium concentration is in the 100-nM range, whereas the concentration of calcium in the extracellular fluids is in the millimolar range; calcium extrusion therefore is necessarily against a chemical gradient. Since, moreover, the cell interior is electronegative with respect to the outside of the cell, calcium extrusion is also against an electrical gradient. It is effected by Ca-ATPase, a large, membrane-spanning molecule ($M_r \approx 123$ kDa) that "couples the hydrolysis of ATP to the transport of Ca^{2+}" (49). Available information, based on the primary structure of the pump molecule from a cDNA isolated from a human teratoma library (50), indicates that on the cytoplasmic side of the membrane there is a calmodulin-binding domain and a cAMP-dependent phosphorylation site. The latter is located near the carboxyl terminus. Also on the cytoplasmic side is a putative calcium-binding domain somewhat nearer the N terminus, and a "hinge region," thought to bring about the conformational change in the transmembrane elements. This change would then propel the calcium through the channel-like transmembrane elements to the outside of the cell. The conformational change is thought to be the sequel to a phosphorylation step, and the site on the molecule that is thought to undergo phosphorylation has been identified (51). While the general aspects of the molecular structure and pump action are likely to apply to all Ca-ATPases, it should be emphasized that no detailed structure of the intestinal Ca-ATPase has been published. Until specific information is available, the picture of how the enzyme works must be regarded as speculative.

An important question with respect to the enzyme is whether pump activity is sufficient to cope with transcellular calcium traffic. All cells are probably equipped with a calcium extrusion mechanism, but is its capacity sufficient to meet the needs of the duodenal cell? Ghijsen et al. (52) have estimated the V_m of isolated basolateral membrane vesicles from rat intestine to be about 8.5 nM Ca/min/mg protein, a number subsequently confirmed by Wasserman et al. (53). Inasmuch as only inside-out vesicles can dephosphorylate ATP that is added to a vesicle preparation and only about half of the vesicles are likely to be inside-out, the actual V_m of Ca transport by these vesicles and therefore by the basolateral membrane is more likely to be near 20 nM Ca/min/mg protein. Carafoli (54) has estimated the V_m of the general plasma membrane Ca-ATPase to be about 30 nM Ca/min/mg protein. The enzyme therefore seems capable of handling maximum loads. Nevertheless, membrane preparations from vitamin D-replete animals seem to have maximum transport capacities that exceed those of preparations from vitamin D-deficient animals by a factor of two to three (12,53,55), with no apparent change in the K_m (53). This suggests that vitamin D acts to increase the number of pumps per cell, but the mechanism by which this occurs is not known.

In addition to a Ca-ATPase, many cells contain a Na/Ca exchanger, but this enzyme is less widely distributed than is the Ca-ATPase (56). Na^+/Ca^{2+} exchange is an antiport system, i.e., the translocation of calcium is coupled to sodium movement in the opposite direction. Sodium enters the cell via the Na/K-ATPase, and the inward concentration gradient thus established for sodium provides the energy for calcium extrusion (56). In intestinal cells, Na/Ca exchange does not appear to play a significant role in calcium extrusion (57), in contrast with Ca-ATPase which is the major mechanism for Ca extrusion from duodenal cells.

C. Paracellular Movement

As pointed out above (Fig. 2), the nonsaturable component of transepithelial calcium transport is found throughout the small intestine, with the rate of calcium movement independent of the calcium concentration. This is evident from the fact that the slope of calcium absorption, when plotted as a function of the calcium concentration of the instilled solution (Fig. 2), is relatively constant throughout the intestine.

A compilation of in-situ loop experiments (58) showed that the average rate of nonsaturable transepithelial movement of calcium was 0.16 h^{-1}. In other words, approximately 16% of the luminal calcium concentration was being moved per hour spent in intestinal sojourn. This was verified in subsequent experiments (59), where the rate of nonsaturable calcium movement was compared to the rate with which phenol red moved transepithelially. Phenol red does not enter cells (60). The overall rate of transmucosal movement of the ion and the dye were the same, $16\% \text{ h}^{-1}$.

Scattered through the literature are reports on changes in calcium absorption that in all likelihood have resulted from a modification of the paracellular flow rate. Thus, Pansu et al. (61) showed that the addition of either glucose or xylose to a solution instilled in a jejunal loop—where active calcium transport is quite limited (Fig. 3)—doubled the rate. Presumably this resulted from the fact that the solution was hyperosmolar so that body fluid entered the lumen and distended the tissue, thereby increasing fluid transport out of the lumen (62) and raising the net absorption of calcium. The same explanation is likely to apply to the enhancement of calcium absorption in the ileum by various carbohydrates (63,64).

Lactose has long been known to enhance calcium absorption, but the mechanism has been uncertain (63–65). That lactose must act, as other sugars do, by enhancing paracellular transport of calcium, presumably due to hyperosmolar distention of the extracellular passage, was shown (66) in experiments where rats were fed 30% lactose in their diet. Their total calcium absorption increased, their fractional absorption decreased, and the active CaBP-related transport was downregulated. Thus adding lactose in sufficient concentrations to the diet caused the net level of calcium absorption to increase in a manner equivalent to increasing the calcium content of the regimen from 0.4% to 0.7% (67). As pointed out above, CaBP and active calcium transport vary inversely with calcium intake, whereas net absorption varies linearly with intake (66,67).

Other substances whose effect on calcium absorption may be mediated by their effect on paracellular transport are amino acids such as L-lysine (68) or medium-chain tri-glycerides (69). In neither of these cases does it seem probable that the active transport process is modified; rather, modification of the intercellular pathway seems more probable. Some detergents and bile salts may similarly enhance calcium absorption (69) by acting on the paracellular pathway.

D. In Vivo Applications

As is evident from the above discussion and as was formulated many years ago by Wasserman and Taylor (64), calcium absorption is the sum of a saturable and a nonsaturable process which may be formulated as follows:

$$v_a = \frac{V_m \times [Ca]_L}{K_m + [Ca]_L} + b[Ca]_L$$ (5)

where

v_a = amount of calcium absorbed per unit time e.g., mmol/h of mg/d
V_m = maximum amount transported by the saturable component
$[Ca]_L$ = calcium concentration of the luminal fluid
K_m = concentration of $[Ca]_L$ when $V_m/2$ has been attained
b = an apparent permeability constant, e.g., 0.16 h^{-1} in the rat (58)

Under normal conditions, $[Ca]_L$ is proportional to the calcium intake, v_i, so that one can substitute v_i for $[Ca]_L$ in Eq. 5. If, however, the ingested calcium is highly insoluble, as when $CaCO_3$ constitutes the only source, then raising intake beyond the solubility of calcium in the intestinal fluid will lead to no further absorption (70).

To apply Eq. 5 to what happens in vivo necessitates taking into account the functional history of the organism under study, inasmuch as the value of V_m at any time is the result of prior calcium intake, vitamin D status, sex, age, and reproductive status. Figure 7 shows how, in a group of male rats fed a high-calcium diet from weaning, V_m and CaBP (= calbindin-D9K) varied in the course of development, whereas the passive component of transepithelial calcium transport remained invariant after about 28 days of age. Absolute values of V_m and CaBP would be higher in rats raised on a low-calcium intake (67), and active calcium transport seems to be downregulated with age (71,72).

Active calcium transport being totally vitamin D-dependent, it proved possible (12) to estimate the value of V_m from experiments (73) with vitamin D-replete rats whose calcium intake (v_i) ranged from 45 to 115 mg/day, and vitamin D-deficient rats, whose calcium intake ranged from 18 to 85 mg/day.

The values arrived at (12) were V_m = 12 mg Ca/day and K_m = 9.5 mg Ca/day. Inserting these in Eq. 5 and using the experimentally derived mean value of 0.53 for the fraction of calcium absorbed by these rats by the nonsaturable route in a 24-h period yields

$$v_a = \frac{12 \times v_i}{9.5 + v_i} + 0.53v_i$$ (6)

The values predicted for v_a on the basis of Eq. 6 have been shown (70) to agree well with experimental ones, if one takes into account that the numerical values for V_m and K_m

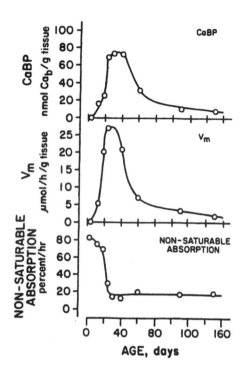

FIGURE 7 The developmental course in rats of calbindin (CaBP), active calcium transport (V_m), and nonsaturable absorption, i.e., of the paracellular route. Data obtained from experiments with male rats fed a high-Ca diet (1.5% Ca, 1.5% P) from weaning. (Adapted from Ref. 206.)

are only approximate. An even better fit is likely if the value for V_m is derived from the relationship between V_m and calbindin, following experimental determination of the calbindin content in a given study. This relationship, derived from Figure 6, is

$$V_m = -0.59 + 0.52 \; \text{CaBP} \tag{7}$$

where

V_m = μmol Ca transported/h/g
CaBP = nmol calbindin/g

(Note: 1 nmol calbindin = 2 nmol Ca_{bound}.)

On the basis of the above analysis, it is evident that the most efficient way of increasing the amount of calcium that is absorbed is to increase intake of calcium in a form that is readily digested and solubilized. Increased intake will, with time, lead to diminished absorption by the active route. The amount transported by the passive route, on the other hand, increases with increased intake. Because of the downregulation of the active transport route with increased calcium intake, the relative role played by the active transport route also decreases as calcium intake increases. This is readily appreciated by inspecting Eq. 5, whose first term approaches V_m as the luminal calcium concentration, $[\text{Ca}]_L$, which normally varies with intake, v_i, becomes large in relation to K_m. As a result, the proportion of v_a contributed by the second term of Eq. 5, i.e., by the paracellular route, becomes dominant, particularly as V_m goes down with increased calcium intake (67). In the vitamin D-replete rat on a high-calcium intake, CaBP and presumably V_m respond very rapidly to exogenous

1,25-dihydroxyvitamin D_3, increasing within 1 h of the injection of the metabolite (74). Vitamin D-deficient rats take several hours to increase CaBP levels in response to exogenous 1,25-$(OH)_2$-D_3 (40,74). Since dietary manipulation leads to relatively rapid changes in the serum levels of 1,25-$(OH)_2$-D_3, up- and downregulation of the active transport component will happen relatively quickly—within 24 h in the rat—so that dietary manipulation of calcium intake is an effective and safe procedure. Administration of vitamin D will, to be sure, enhance the active component of calcium transport, but it needs medical supervision and may lead to other complications, such as hypercalcemia, hypercalciuria, and depressed bone turnover (75).

IV. CALCIUM IN BLOOD

A. Biological Description

Virtually all blood calcium is found in the plasma, so the plasma calcium content, 2.5 mM, is the parameter dealt with in biology and medicine. The plasma calcium concentration is closely regulated in vertebrates. It has about the same value in all species and varies little with age and physiological status. A notable exception is the laying hen, whose total plasma calcium level may reach 5 mM, but whose dialyzable free plasma calcium concentration, like that of all other vertebrates, lies between 1 and 1.5 mM. The major calcium-binding protein that is responsible for the high calcium concentration of chicken plasma during the egg-laying cycle is vitellin.

Table 1 lists the compounds and forms of calcium in human blood, typical of mammalian blood. As shown in Table 1, somewhat less than half of the total plasma calcium is bound to protein, albumin being the major component. Somewhat more than half of the plasma calcium is not bound to protein, mostly in the form of the free ion, and a small portion, ~ 6%, is bound to citrate, phosphate, and other complexes. Although dissociation constants between calcium and its ligands in the plasma vary, the rate at which equilibrium is established with albumin is so rapid (<5 s; 77) that total and ionized calcium concentrations will give equivalent functional information under nearly all circumstances, even though it is the ionized calcium concentration that is the relevant functional variable. Automated methods for measuring ionized calcium in plasma now exist, but in general still seem to be less reliable than automated methods for measuring total plasma calcium. In any event, current data support the older literature that the ionized calcium concentration in human plasma is between 1.1 and 1.2 mM (for further discussion, see Ref. 78).

TABLE 1 Distribution of Calcium in Normal Human Plasma

Form	mM	Percent of total
Ionized	1.18	47.5
Protein-bound	1.14	46.0
Phosphate	0.04	1.6
Citrate	0.04	1.7
Other complexes	0.08	3.2
Total	2.48	100.0

Reproduced from Ref. 76.

Plasma calcium levels tend to be higher in men than in women (79) and to decrease with age (79–81). As will be shown later, the age-dependent decrease in plasma calcium is related to the increasing proportion of hydroxyapatite as bone mineral matures. As a result the average calcium-binding sites in the skeleton have a higher affinity for calcium, causing the plasma calcium to drop.

The plasma calcium is in extremely rapid, dynamic equilibrium with calcium in the extracellular fluid, plasma constituting about 17% of the extracellular fluid volume (82,83). Evidence for this comes from experiments in which calcium was injected intravenously or intraperitoneally, and the plasma concentration dropped with a $t_{1/2}$ of <1 min to about one-sixth of what it would have been if none of the injected calcium had left the plasma compartment (84,85). Following this initial expansion, the calcium load is disposed of in a strictly exponential manner; in other words, the plasma calcium concentration, elevated due to a positive load or depressed due to a "negative" load—e.g. intravenous injection of a calcium chelator such as EDTA (86)—returns to the pretreatment (baseline) value with a $t_{1/2}$ that approximates the time it would take for the plasma to be cleared of half of its positive or negative load in about 27 circulations (87). This value was arrived at because, in the dog, approximately 5% of the cardiac output goes to the skeleton (88). Moreover, 50% of the ^{45}Ca that enters the circulation of a dog's femur is extracted from the blood (89). If one assumes that this figure also applies to the reduction of calcium load, then 2.5% of the plasma calcium would be cleared by bone in one circulation and it would take 27 circulations (ln 0.5/ln 0.975) to clear the blood of half of its circulating (positive or negative) load. Circulation times multiplied by 27 should then represent the $t_{1/2}$ of load reduction in various species.

In addition to bone, the other major gateways for calcium entry to and exit from the circulation are the gut and the kidney. The latter in particular has often been implicated as a significant regulator of blood calcium (90). If, however, one calculates the time required for a load to be cleared by the kidney or the gut, it is apparent (87) that neither of these organs can compete effectively with bone.

The initial pool of virtual distribution of calcium, i.e., what is likely to represent the extracellular water, seems to be largely independent of the functional state of the organism. In other words, a calcium load will be diluted approximately sixfold, whatever the state of the organism. On the other hand, as evident from Table 2, the rate at which the blood is cleared by the skeleton of its calcium load is very much dependent on the endocrine status and the age of the individual. Thus, as Table 2 shows, the rate of clearance—i.e., the rate at which the error in the plasma calcium is being corrected—is much faster in young than in old dogs and much faster in euparathyroid than parathyroidectomized rats.

B. Regulatory Model

To explain how bone can overcome a calcium load, it is first necessary to analyze the nature of the interaction of plasma calcium with bone. As shown by Table 2, the time of return of the plasma calcium to the preload level is the same whether the load is positive or negative. It therefore appears that each time the blood plasma courses over bone, half of the positive or negative difference between the concentration of the plasma calcium as it enters and leaves the bone is abolished. Consequently, the plasma calcium seems to be in rapid, dynamic equilibrium with calcium-binding sites in bone.

The concept of a dynamic equilibrium derives support from the analysis of plasma disappearance curves following the intravenous administration of tracer calcium. When

TABLE 2 Response Times to Calcium Loads

Species	Hormonal status[a]	Ca load and route[b]	$t_{1/2}$ (min)
Rat	N	3.8 mg/animal, i.v.	14
	N	2–18 mg/animal, i.p.	22.5 ± 2.0
	−D	2–15 mg/animal, i.p.	51.0 ± 2.5
	PTX	8 mg/animal, i.p.	53
	CTX	8 mg/animal, i.p.	41
Dog	N	10 mg/kg, i.v. infusion	58
	N	−10 mg/kg, i.v. infusion	80
	N (young)	not given	23.0 ± 0.8
	N (mature)	−4.3 to −8.3 mg/kg, i.v. infusion	78.0 ± 12

[a]N = normal; −D = vitamin D-deficient; PTX = parathyroidectomized; CTX = endogenous thyrocalcitonin supply excised.
[b]A negative sign before the load indicates that a calcium chelator was given to depress the plasma calcium to the same extent to which a positive load would have raised it; i.v. = intravenous route; i.p. = intraperitoneal route.
Reproduced from Ref. 87 with permission.

analyzed in terms of a four-termed exponential expression (91,92), the first term, with a half-time of less than 1 min, represents dilution into the extracellular fluid, as described above, whereas the second term, with a half-time in terms of minutes, is the equivalent of the clearance of calcium by bone (93–95). The later terms of the disappearance equation have been taken to represent losses from the calcium pool due to excretion and long-term bone calcium deposition (91,92,96).

The qualitative and quantitative similarity between results obtained with the use of calcium loads and isotopic calcium gives special significance to the observation (89), already referred to, that about half of the tracer calcium is extracted in a single passage of the circulation that enters bone, yet the total calcium concentration of blood that enters and leaves bone is unchanged. Bone must therefore contain calcium-binding sites that are in rapid and dynamic equilibrium with the plasma calcium.

Such a dynamic equilibrium is generally considered in terms of the solubility product of ionic calcium and phosphate in the blood. However, the equilibrium for bone calcium-binding sites can be equally well described in terms of an apparent half-concentration, K_m. When there is no net gain or loss of calcium from the plasma, the free energy of calcium binding must be zero. Consequently, the plasma calcium level $[Ca_s]$ must equal the mean K_m of the bone calcium-binding sites. In other words, $K_m = [Ca_s]$.

The rapidity with which the equilibrium between blood and bone is established can be assessed by calculating the apparent permeability constant P for a dog of 10 kg whose trabecular bone surface area, A, is 1.6×10^4 cm^2 (97). $P = (0.693V)/At_{1/2}$, where V is the volume of plasma cleared. With a circulation time of 40 s (99), the value of P is 0.5×10^{-5} cm^{-1} (87). This value is comparable to what can be conservatively calculated for the vitamin D-deficient rat duodenum (12), where calcium moves paracellularly, but not transcellularly. As pointed out earlier (Sec. III.B), it is the presence of the intracellular, vitamin D-dependent calbindin-D9K that assures transcellular calcium transport at a rate compatible with the experimental V_m (Fig. 6). It is as yet uncertain whether bone cells contain any calbindin, but its concentration in bone cells is at best 1% of that in the vitamin D-replete duodenal cell (45). The low calbindin content of bone cells, combined with the relatively high apparent permeability of bone for calcium, makes it unlikely that calcium enters bone by fluxing through bone cells. Rather, calcium must move between bone cells, with the calcium-binding sites therefore located on (or in) the bone mineral itself.

The nature and type of calcium-binding sites in bone mineral have not been described as such. However, at least five phases of calcium phosphate are likely to occur in bone (Table 3). Inasmuch as calcium-binding affinity varies inversely with solubility, then the K_m must also. Because the calcium phosphate phases with the highest calcium-to-phosphorus ratio are least soluble, they must have the lowest K_m. Moreover, the average K_m of a given section of bone will depend on the relative content of the various bone salts. Mature bone, having a high content of hydroxyapatite, would therefore be associated with a low K_m and a relatively depressed plasma calcium level, whereas in newly forming bone the bone salt would be less mature and its average K_m and the associated plasma calcium level would be relatively high. Shifts in the mean K_m and associated plasma calcium level would then be brought about by shifts in the proportions of calcium-binding sites in bone.

The question then arises how those rapid shifts in the proportion of calcium-binding sites, leading to a change in the K_m, can be brought about. To illustrate the speed with which plasma calcium changes, it is only necessary to recall that, following parathyroidectomy, the plasma calcium drops with a $t_{1/2} < 2$ h (86) from the normal or reference level of 2.5 mM to approximately 1.5 mM. This means that the average K_m of calcium-binding sites in bone has changed. Conversely, if parathyroid hormone (PTH) is administered, the well-documented rise in plasma calcium that follows must parallel a comparable rise in the average K_m. Calcitonin injection leads to a rapid ($t_{1/2} < 15$ min) transient drop in plasma calcium (100), which would result from the postulated drop in the average K_m of the binding sites.

The model of regulation that has been proposed (87) is based on the rapid changes in shape that bone cells have been observed to undergo (101,102). Osteoblasts and osteo-clasts, together with the bone-lining cells and osteocytes, constitute the cell population of the mammalian skeleton, but only osteoblasts and osteoclasts are metabolically active (103) and are the cells that primarily regulate bone growth and turnover.

Osteoblasts possess receptors (102) for PTH and 1,25-dihydroxyvitamin D_3, 1,25-$(OH)_2$-D_3, whereas only osteoclasts possess receptors for calcitonin (102,104,105), the third of the three major calcitropic hormones (see Sec. VIII). A very early response of osteoblasts to PTH (101) or 1,25-$(OH)_2$-D_3 (102) is to round up, followed by a cascade of

TABLE 3 Solid Phases of Calcium Phosphate Linked to Biological Calcification[a]

Name	Formula	Molar ratio of Ca to P
Hydroxyapatite	$Ca_{10}(PO_4)_6(OH)_2$	1.66
Whitlockite	$(Ca,Mg)_3(PO_4)_2$	1.50
Amorphous CaXPO$_4$	$Ca_9(PO_4)_6$(variable)	1.30–1.50
Octacalcium phosphate	$Ca_8H_2(PO_4)_6 \cdot 5H_2O$	1.33
Brushite	$CaHPO_4 \cdot (2H_2O)$	1.00

[a]Listed in order of increasing acidity, solubility, and, by inference, increasing K_m, i.e., decreasing calcium-binding affinity.

Note: At least 90% of the cystalline solid is hydroxyapatite, based on X-ray diffraction analysis (98).

Reproduced by permission from Ref. 98.

events such as inhibition of collagen synthesis (106,107), characteristic either of an arrest or a marked slowing of metabolic activity. Calcitonin, on the other hand, induces a rounding up of osteoclasts and inhibition of their metabolic activity (102,104).

The rounding up of osteoblasts is thought to lead to an opposite shape change in osteoclasts, i.e., their spreading out and extending apposition to the bone surface (108). Contrariwise, the rounding up of osteoclasts, as under the influence of calcitonin, allows osteoblasts to extend and to enhance their metabolic activity. For example, calcium repletion of calcium-deficient rats, whose PTH levels are high (109), has led to lowering of PTH levels and to rapid positional changes in osteoclasts, these cells clearly lifting off the bone surfaces (110).

Shape changes of bone cells may be thought to be associated with changes in the average calcium-binding affinity of bones by causing a change in the relative proportion of high- and low-affinity calcium-binding sites. It is therefore hypothesized (87) that osteoblasts, when extended and apposed to bone, block the low-affinity extremes of the population of calcium-binding sites (Fig. 8A). But when osteoblasts retract under the action of PTH or $1,25-(OH)_2-D_3$, they expose these low-affinity sites (Fig. 8B).

Conversely, osteoclasts may be thought to be associated with binding sites that have high affinity for calcium. Thus, when osteoclasts are caused to contract, as under the action of calcitonin (Fig. 8C), high-affinity calcium-binding sites are exposed.

When osteoblasts contract, the proportion of low-affinity binding sites goes up for two reasons: More are exposed as a result of the contraction of osteoblasts; and osteoclasts, which are associated with binding sites that have a higher calcium-binding affinity, tend to spread out over the bone surface, covering up high-affinity binding sites. The result is a rise in K_m and in the plasma calcium.

When osteoclasts contract, the proportion of high-affinity calcium-binding sites goes up because high-affinity binding sites are exposed and because osteoblasts, in extending over the bone surface, now cover more low-affinity binding sites. Consequently, the proportion of high-affinity sites increases, the K_m goes down, and the plasma calcium falls.

That osteoclasts and osteoblasts are associated with bone surfaces that differ in calcium-binding capacity can be inferred from studies using biphosphonates (111) and gallium (112,113). Both of these substances inhibit osteoclastic action specifically, presumably by becoming associated with bone salt sites that would normally be attacked by osteoclasts.

Changes in the rate of ^{45}Ca movement into and out of bone have been shown to be quite rapid after hormone addition. In chicks and rats, calcium uptake by the femur was reduced to nearly half within 3 min of PTH injection (94). In chicks, following the injection of 16,16-dimethyl prostaglandin E2, calcium uptake by bone was markedly reduced, whereas cAMP levels in the bone cells increased in parallel (114). These responses are too rapid to be accounted for by changes in the synthesis or degradation of proteins that regulate calcium deposition or removal. They are of the right time scale, however, to have resulted from changes in cell shape, presumably involving such hormonally induced biochemical signals as changes in ion channel permeability (115) and in cAMP (116).

Shape changes of osteoblasts and osteoclasts need not constitute the sole mechanism for changes in binding-site affinity. Cell-mediated changes in the pH of the immediate surroundings of a calcium-binding site or liberation of protein factors may contribute to affinity changes. Moreover, shape changes are only a first step in the cascade of events that lead to long-term bone deposition and remodeling.

Four factors play major roles in determining the rate at which the skeleton responds to a calcium load: (a) circulation time, which increases with age (117); (b) the fraction

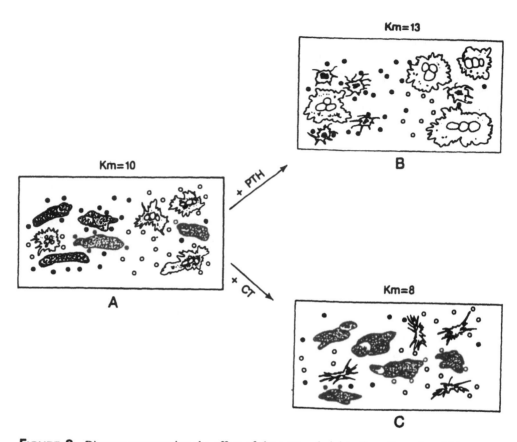

FIGURE 8 Diagram representing the effect of the acute administration of parathyroid hormone (PTH) or calcitonin (CT) on the spatial relationships of osteoblasts and osteoclasts on a bone surface. The open and closed circles represent, respectively, the K_m values of high-affinity and low-affinity bone calcium-binding sites. Diagram A represents a normocalcemic situation, with an equal number of high- and low-affinity sites. Diagram B represents the result of PTH administration, where the shrinkage of osteoblasts has exposed low-affinity sites and the associated expansion of osteoclasts has blocked high-affinity sites, leading to an average K_m of 13 and hypercalcemia. Diagram C represents the result of CT administration, where the shrinkage of osteoclasts has exposed high-affinity sites and the consequent expansion of osteoblasts has blocked low-affinity sites, leading to an average K_m of 8 and hypocalcemia. *Note*: High-affinity sites are considered to have an apparent K_m of 5 mg Ca/dL, and low-affinity sites an apparent K_m of 15 mg Ca/dL. For the sake of convenience, the K_m's refer to total plasma calcium, rather than the theoretically correct ionic calcium concentration, approximately half of the total. Bone mineral with a high Ca/P ratio is considered to have a relatively higher affinity for calcium binding than bone mineral with a low Ca/P ratio (see text and Table 3). (Reproduced with permission from Ref. 87.)

of cardiac output that goes to bone, which decreases with age (118); (c) the nature of the bone mineral, which affects the extraction rate; and (d) the driving force, i.e., the differential between the plasma calcium level as it enters the skeleton and the mean K_m of the bone calcium-binding sites.

Factors (a), (b), and (c) may be considered responsible for the slowing of the rate of return (or reduction of the error correction rate) that differentiates young and old dogs

(Table 2). The absolute plasma calcium level of young and old dogs is similar, hence their mean K_m—i.e., the proportion of high- to low-affinity bone calcium-binding sites—must be similar. The difference in the error correction rate would arise therefore from a slower circulation rate, a smaller fraction of the cardiac output going to bone, and perhaps a smaller extraction rate.

Rats deprived of their endogenous calcitonin have a slower error correction rate than normal animals (Table 2), yet their skeletons are neither smaller nor less well mineralized than those of controls (100), their plasma calcium is the same as that of controls (100), and there is no reason to believe that cardiac output or circulation time is altered. Hence factors (a), (b), and (c) would not come into play. Instead, a difference in driving force can be postulated, as follows. In normal mammals, calcitonin is released when plasma calcium rises acutely (119), acting directly on osteoclasts (104). This leads to osteoclast retraction and the exposure of high-affinity binding sites. In turn, this results in a greater driving force for calcium deposition and an increase in the rate at which normocalcemia is restored. In animals without calcitonin, this response cannot occur and the half-time of error correction is correspondingly lengthened.

A difference in driving force can also explain why parathyroidectomized (PTX) animals require more time to overcome a positive calcium load (see Ref. 87 for details).

The explanation involving a driving force cannot apply to vitamin D deficiency, which in some ways resembles parathyroidectomy, yet vitamin D-deficient rats have maximum levels of circulating PTH (109). It is the low absolute amounts of bone in vitamin D deficiency (73) that are likely to cause calcium extraction to be reduced [factor (c)], hence leading to a lengthening of $t_{1/2}$ of the error reduction rate.

The preceding discussion makes it obvious that ablation of hormonal control, due to PTH, calcitonin, or vitamin D, reduces the rate at which an error in plasma calcium is overcome by bone. It is bone, however, whether or not under hormonal control, that is the principal regulator of the plasma calcium and that is responsible for causing the plasma calcium to return to its preload level and to maintain it at that level.

V. INTRACELLULAR CALCIUM

Three mechanisms contribute to maintaining a low intracellular calcium concentration: (a) a limited entry rate, governed by a limited number of plasma calcium channels, probably less than 1000/cell (12); (b) a significant intracellular store of calcium-binding sites, found in the various cell membranes, the endoplasmic reticulum, in and on the various organelles, with mitochondria playing a major role; and (c) efficient extrusion mechanisms, i.e., Ca-ATPase and Na/Ca exchanger.

Entry and extrusion mechanisms have already been described in the relevant sections on transcellular calcium transport (Sec. III.B). Different cells and tissues may have specific entry and extrusion mechanisms that differ in structural and/or functional details from the general model. For example, the vitamin D-dependent protein (32,33) or peptide (34) that occurs in intestinal cells, and that may play a role in modulating calcium entry into the intestinal cell, may be specific to that cell, as there is no logical requirement that calcium entry into cells which do not transport calcium be enhanced by vitamin D. Similarly, while vanadate is an effective inhibitor of the plasma membrane Ca-ATPase, it has little effect on the renal Ca-ATPase (120). Whereas calmodulin modulates the activity of the Ca-ATPase of plasma membrane or cardiac sarcoplasmic reticulum, it does not seem to do so in the case of the liver plasma membrane enzyme (121).

In resting liver cells, as in most cells, the free intracellular Ca^{2+} concentration is in the 100-nM range. In stimulated hepatocytes, the intracellular free calcium concentration reaches 600 nM and, when the cells are under oxidative stress, intracellular calcium may reach micromolar concentrations. Moreover, total cytosolic calcium of liver cells is 3–4 mmol/kg dry weight. It is obvious, therefore, that liver cells, like other cells, have significant cellular calcium stores. These include the rough and smooth endoplasmic reticulum, the Golgi complex, mitochondria, inner and outer leaflets of the plasma membrane, lysosomes, and possibly secretory granules. (For documentation and further discussion of the liver cell, see Ref. 122.) The endoplasmic reticulum probably contains the largest fraction of intracellular calcium, perhaps a quarter of the total (123)—easily four times that found in the mitochondria. This quantitative disparity would not necessarily make it unlikely for mitochondria to play a major role in intracellular calcium regulation, as proposed by Lehninger et al. (124), since mitochondrial calcium might turnover more rapidly than that of other organelles, but more recent analyses have made it less likely that mitochondria play a significant regulatory role (125).

External signals to cells, such as hormones, neurotransmitters, or growth hormones, are detected by receptors located on the outer aspect of the plasma membrane and transmitted to the cell interior by second messengers. 1,2-Diacyl glycerol and myo-inositol 1,4,5-trisphosphate (Ins 1,4,5-P_3) are two major messenger molecules (122). Ins 1,4,5-P_3 causes calcium to be released reversibly from intracellular calcium stores, typically the endoplasmic reticulum; the released calcium is the "calcium signal" or "second messenger." The released calcium travels to various intracellular locations and, depending on the cell in question, induces a calcium-dependent reaction. Since the discovery of these events in 1983 (126; for more details see 127) a very large number of cellular events have been shown to involve and/or be mediated by calcium signaling. Typical examples include cell volume regulation (128), egg activation (129) and fertilization (130), growth factor-induced changes in cell proliferation (131), secretion, as in adrenal chromaffin cells (132), transmitter secretion from presynaptic nerve terminals (133), and platelet activation (134), to name just some of the many processes that seem to involve calcium signaling.

While Ins 1,4,5-P_3 is involved in all instances in the release of the calcium signal from an internal source, it is less certain whether this inositol molecule is also involved in calcium gating and/or the uptake of calcium from the extracellular milieu (127). The quantity of calcium released for signaling is generally so low that this alone would not necessarily lead to increased calcium influx. In other words, whether calcium channels, the entry ports for calcium, are closely linked to or regulated by phosphatidyl-inositol turnover is not established. Moreover, while Ins 1,4,5-P_3 plays a key role in mediating intracellular release of calcium, it has not yet been demonstrated that this molecule is formed fast enough to account for the very rapid release of Ca^{2+} (250 ms, Ref. 134). Protein kinase C and elevation of cAMP inhibit calcium mobilization (134) and may therefore inhibit processes stimulated by the calcium signal, e.g., secretion, contraction, or changes in conductivity.

An interesting but as yet incompletely understood phenomenon of calcium signaling—or intracellular calcium movement—involves discrete transients or oscillations (135). Oscillations may result from fluxes across the plasma membrane or from fluxes across intracellular membranes. In hepatocytes (136) agonists that act via Ins 1,4,5-P_3 provoke dose-dependent increases in intracellular free calcium, with oscillation frequency increasing, the latency period decreasing, but the amplitude of the oscillations remaining constant.

In the case of the hepatocytes, the changes in intracellular calcium concentrations are initiated at a specific subcellular domain, adjacent to the plasma membrane, and are then propagated through the cell in the form of a wave. The most reasonable explanation of this phenomenon at present is a calcium-induced calcium release. Something like this is also thought to occur in the muscle cell of the heart (137; see also below). Thomas and Renard (136) propose that the oscillating calcium signal may function to allow all parts of the cell to respond to the stimulus.

The muscle cell is probably where intracellular calcium traffic is most elaborate and tied most closely to its function. Langer (137) has reviewed the sequence of calcium movements in the muscle cell in the course of a contraction cycle. When the cell becomes depolarized, calcium enters via L-type calcium channels, the best characterized voltage-sensitive calcium channels (for further description, see Ref. 138). Entry occurs during the plateau phase of the action potential and induces calcium release via the "feet," i.e., the connection between the sarcoplasmic reticulum and the sarcolemma. Calcium that is released is the major source of the calcium-activating contraction. As calcium enters the narrow subsarcolemmal space, calcium concentration of the space goes up transiently, thereby activating the Na/Ca exchanger, which then extrudes calcium even as the myofilaments are being activated. The rate of calcium efflux is such as to maintain the cellular calcium at a steady state.

As the myocardial cell repolarizes, calcium is pumped into the longitudinal sarcoplasmic reticulum, at the same time diffusing into the cistern. Calcium extrusion via the exchanger continues and calcium is pumped out through the diastole by the calcium pump of the sarcolemma, the pump being a Ca-ATPase (139).

In summary, it appears that intracellular calcium is very closely controlled, with rises in intracellular calcium, when due to external signals such as hormones or neurotransmitters, serving as intracellular signals which in turn elicit calcium-dependent processes such as secretion, contraction, etc. Transient rises in intracellular free calcium are readily overcome by calcium becoming bound to a large number of organelles. Calcium entry is via channels, and calcium extrusion is via the Na/Ca exchanger and the Ca-ATPase. In specialized cells such as muscle cells, intracellular calcium is shuttled back and forth via intracellular pumps.

VI. CALCIUM IN BONE

Calcium, along with phosphate, constitutes the principal structural substance of the skeleton that gives vertebrates their internal support and, in the case of people, allows them to be erect. The skeleton constitutes about 16% of an adult's body weight. Forty-seven percent of the skeletal weight is dry, fat-free bone, and 26% of the latter is calcium (140). Table 3 lists the various phases in which calcium phosphate occurs in bone. The precise order in which calcium is precipitated and the path it follows as calcium salts mature and become increasingly less soluble is not yet known. The final calcium salt is a carbanato-hydroxyapatite, i.e., an apatitic type of calcium phosphate that also contains, at least on the surface, calcium carbonate. The mechanism of calcification, many years of study notwithstanding, is not fully known. The initial calcium phosphate is deposited on or inside collagen fibrils that have formed extracellularly from collagen molecules that had been extruded by osteoblasts, the bone-forming cells. Once the calcium phosphate molecule is in place, additional calcium phosphate is deposited by accretion so that the calcium salt is arranged in a very orderly fashion. The crystals are platelike, with a long axis that is 30–70 nm, and a short axis that is 10–25 nm (98). The surface layers of the bone crystals constitute 50% of the newly formed crystals, but ultimately, in the fully mature crystal, they constitute only about 25% of the fully mature crystal volume (98).

The principal function of the metabolically active osteoblast is to produce the collagen which represents the major component of the extracellular matrix on which calcium phosphate precipitates. Depending on species, age, and type of bone, osteoblasts cover some 5–10% of the bone surface. They are more numerous in trabecular than in cortical bone, more numerous in young than in mature bone, and their capacity to respond to fracture—i.e., the ability of connective tissue cells to respond to the osteoinductive stimulus that results from fracture—is diminished with age. Osteoblastic activity also diminishes with age (98). From Eriksen's data, as tabulated by Simmons and Grynpas (98), bone remodeling by osteoblasts and osteoclasts takes around 10 days in humans, but mineralization of sites laid down by osteoblasts takes an order of magnitude longer, i.e., some 100+ days. The extracellular matrix in which mineralization takes place also contains numerous molecules; some bind calcium, all in some way seem to aid in bone formation and mineralization, even though in many instances specific functions are not known. For a more detailed review of these molecules, see Refs. 141–143.

Calcium exists in bone in two forms: in solution, as part of the fluid that surrounds and exists in bone, and in a solid state, as the phases of calcium phosphate described above and listed in Table 3. The bone calcium pool contains five to six times more calcium than is found in the extracellular fluid, but constitutes only a small fraction of the total body calcium. For example, in a 220-g male rat, the extracellular calcium amounts to 0.67 mmol of Ca, the bone calcium pool contains about 3.45 mmol of Ca, whereas the total skeletal calcium amounts to about 120 mmol of Ca (144).

The bone calcium pool serves two functions: as the source of calcium that becomes deposited as bone salt, and as the source of exchangeable calcium, i.e., the calcium that leaves and reenters blood, with the concentration of blood plasma calcium determined by the average calcium-binding capacity of the bone salt.

In the example of the male rat quoted above, the bone calcium pool turns over about 1.3 times per day, with bone calcium deposition constituting about 43% of the total calcium flow into the bone calcium pool. The fraction of calcium entering the bone calcium pool that then undergoes a phase transformation to become bone salt diminishes with age more than does the total flow of calcium into the bone calcium pool (Table 4).

Bone calcium resorption, i.e., the phase transformation of solid to solution and the return of that calcium into the circulation, also decreases with age, but somewhat less rapidly than does the bone calcium deposition rate. As a result, the individual goes into negative bone calcium balance; i.e., the bone mass decreases. This is illustrated in Table 4. Note in particular in Table 4 how the bone calcium deposition rate decreases with age and sex in humans and rats, with corresponding decreases in the calcium balance.

Modeling and remodeling of bone also involve structural changes, i.e., osteoclast-mediated dissolution of calcium and partial or total degradation of the extracellular matrix from which the bone salt has been removed. These structural changes proceed necessarily more slowly than the initial steps which involve calcium binding and release by the bone salt.

Thus bone formation and bone resorption are terms, each of which designates a cascade of events, with calcium constituting the principal cation of bone salt, the major product of the osteoblasts.

TABLE 4 Parameters of Calcium Metabolism in People and Rats

	Young male human	Postmenopausal female human	Young male rat	Young female rat	Old female rat
Body wt (kg)	76	55	0.23	0.17	0.30
Age (yr)	17	62	0.19	0.33	0.83
Plasma calcium (mg/dL)	10.3	9.9	11.0	9.5	n.d.
Calcium pool (mg)	6100	3500	165	148	42
Pool turnover (mg/day)	1500	650	84	71	31
v_i = calcium intake (mg/day)	1160	625	70	51	n.d.
v_u = urinary calcium output (mg/day)	250	100	1	1	n.d.
v_{ndo} = fecal endogenous output (mg/day)	150	75	5	9	n.d.
v_F = total fecal Ca (mg/day)	860	550	34	20	n.d.
Δ = calcium balance (mg/day)	+50	−25	35	30	n.d.
v_a = calcium absorbed (mg/day)	450	150	41	30	n.d.
Percent calcium absorption	39	24	59	59	n.d.
v_{o+} = bone calcium deposition (mg/day)	1100	475	78	61	15
v_{o-} = bone calcium removal (mg/day)	1050	500	43	31	n.d.
Fraction to bone, v_{o+}/v_T	0.73	0.73	0.93	0.86	0.50
Fraction excreted, $v_u + v_{ndo}/v_T$	0.27	0.27	0.07	0.14	0.50

The plasma calcium is part of the calcium pool (Fig. 1).
Pool turnover, $v_T = v_a + v_{o-} = v_{o+} + v_u + v_{ndo}$
n.d. = not determined.
40 mg Ca = 1 mmol.
Data based on reports in Refs. 75, 109, 144–146.

VII. CALCIUM EXCRETION

A. Urine

Of the calcium circulating in the blood, less than 0.1% is typically excreted in the urine. Thus, in an adult man of 70 kg, the plasma volume is about 2.5 L and contains about 6 mmol calcium. Cardiac output would be 5.1 L/min (99), with 20–25% of the cardiac output being presented to the kidney and half of that amount filtered at the glomerulus. Thus the nephron handles approximately 1.5 mmol of Ca per minute or some 2100 mmol of Ca/day. The urinary calcium output of the typical 70-kg man might be 7 mmol/day, or 0.3% of the filtered load. Actual calcium excretion in the urine is a complicated function of an individual's prior calcium intake, vitamin D and nutritional status, sex, reproductive status (if female), as well as age and therefore skeletal maturity.

Calcium in the lumen of the nephron is subject to two transport processes (147): A paracellular, concentration-dependent transepithelial movement, and a transcellular movement that constitutes active transport against an electrochemical gradient. Calcium is reabsorbed, i.e., moves transepithelially, in the proximal tubule (straight and convoluted), mostly by a passive mechanism, although some movement may be transcellular and involve entry via calcium channels and extrusion via Ca-ATPase (148). Very little calcium is reabsorbed as the luminal fluid passes through the thin limbs of Henle. As the fluid enters the thick ascending limb of the nephron, calcium reabsorption is resumed, largely by a passive process. Active transepithelial calcium transport occurs principally in the distal convoluted tubule (DCT; 147,148). Once the luminal fluid has passed the region of the DCT, it enters those regions of the nephron designated as connecting and collecting ducts, where transport is essentially by a paracellular route.

Active calcium transport in the DCT, as across the duodenal cell, involves three steps: entry across the brush border region of the cells lining the lumen of the DCT, intracellular diffusion, and extrusion across the basolateral pole of the renal cell. Entry is likely to be via calcium channels, the existence of which in the kidney has been documented (26).

Intracellular self-diffusion of the calcium ion through the DCT cell has been estimated as nearly two orders of magnitude too slow (149), compared with the experimentally determined V_m (150). In other words, transcellular calcium transport in the kidney, i.e., in the DCT, requires the same kind of amplification that is provided in the duodenal cell by the intestinal calbindin. Indeed, there exists a vitamin D-dependent, intracellular calcium-binding protein, termed calbindin D28K, found almost exclusively in the kidney (151,152). It is a separate gene product from calbindin D9K. Both calbindin D9K and calbindin D28K are found in the embryonic kidney, but as development proceeds, expression of calbindin D9K is repressed and calbindin D28K remains as the only calcium-binding protein with an E-F hand. Calbindin D28K has a molecular weight of 28,000 Da, has four calcium-binding sites, and has $K_D = 2 \times 10^{-6}$ M. It occurs principally in the DCT (153) and therefore may serve as a calcium ferry. It has been calculated (149) that the amplification provided by the renal calbindin is similar to that due to the intestinal calbindin, i.e., about 76-fold, if its concentration in the DCT is similar to that in the duodenal cell, a reasonable possibility. All available evidence thus indicates that the renal calbindin fulfills the same kind of ferrying role in the DCT as does the intestinal calbindin, thus providing the molecular basis for calcium reabsorption in the DCT.

Calcium extrusion from the renal cell is against an electrochemical gradient and is effected by the Ca-ATPase in the basolateral membrane and perhaps also by the Na/Ca exchanger. The nature and characteristics of the renal Ca-ATPase are likely to be similar to those of the intestinal Ca-ATPase, but no detailed report on the renal Ca-ATPase has come to this reviewer's attention.

Whereas in the intestine the Na/Ca exchanger appears to play no role in calcium extrusion (57), this may not be true in the kidney. However, it is not clear whether the exchanger's principal role is calcium extrusion or whether it is even involved in calcium traffic. There exists in the renal proximal tubule a reciprocal relationship between sodium reabsorption and intracellular calcium concentration, a rise in calcium depressing sodium reabsorption (154). The Na/Ca exchanger may regulate sodium channels indirectly, inasmuch as channel activity is diminished as intracellular calcium rises (155). Whether these observations also apply to the DCT and how sodium metabolism modulates active calcium transport is not clear. It is probable, however, that a disturbance of sodium metabolism of the renal cell—or, for that matter, of the duodenal cell—will play havoc with calcium transport (14).

Paracellular calcium transport accounts for most of the calcium reabsorption in the kidney. The mechanisms by which this occurs have not been fully clarified.

In addition to vitamin D, the major regulator of urinary calcium excretion is parathyroid hormone (PTH), causing increased reabsorption of calcium from the renal tubule, while phosphate excretion is simultaneously increased. The mechanism by which PTH enhances calcium reabsorption is unclear. PTH causes a rise in 1,25-dihydroxyvitamin D_3 (1,25-OH_2-D_3), so that increased calcium reabsorption due to elevated PTH levels may have resulted from an increased level of the renal calbindin. However, the initial response to PTH seems faster (156) than if only a biosynthetic pathway were involved. Whether PTH acts on the entry or extrusion steps of transcellular transport or causes changes in the configuration of the tight junctions via a cAMP-mediated intracellular event has not been clarified.

In summary, urinary calcium excretion represents significantly less than 1% of the calcium that is circulated to the kidney. Most of the calcium filtered by the kidney is reclaimed by the body by passive transport, with active transport, mediated by the renal calbindin ($M_r \sim 28,000$ Da), occurring largely in the distal convoluted tubule.

B. Stool

Calcium in the stool has two sources: unabsorbed food calcium and unreabsorbed "body" calcium, i.e., calcium that entered the intestinal lumen with the various body fluids such as bile, succus entericus, etc., but that was not reabsorbed. One can therefore write

$$v_F = v_i - v_a + v_{ndo} \tag{8}$$

where

v_F = fecal calcium excretion rate
v_i = calcium ingestion rate
v_a = rate of calcium absorption
v_{ndo} = endogenous fecal calcium excretion rate
units = mg Ca/day

To determine the rates in Eq. 8, it is necessary to differentiate between $(v_i - v_a)$, on the one hand, and v_{ndo}, on the other hand. Otherwise all that can be measured is S_i, net absorption, that is, $v_i - v_F$. In either case, whether measuring S_i or v_a and v_{ndo}, it is necessary to use fecal markers to take into account the time delay between ingestion and excretion. The simplest way to resolve Eq. 8 is to administer a calcium tracer intravenously at about the time the intestinal balance measurement is initiated. The amount of tracer collected in the stool during the intestinal balance period can be converted to v_{ndo} by simultaneously estimating the area under the plasma tracer curve during the same period and dividing that area into the amount of fecal tracer collected between fecal markers. Thus, combining an intestinal mass balance with a tracer study will yield numerical values for v_F, v_i, and v_{ndo} in Eq. 8, so that all four values are determined. See Refs. (58) and (91) for equations and practical details.

Concerning the endogenous fecal calcium, v_{ndo}, one can ask whether it plays a regulatory role in calcium metabolism. The origin of endogenous fecal calcium is calcium secreted into the intestine in bile juices, pancreatic juices, the *succus entericus*, and calcium from cellular debris.

It seems unlikely that bile juices are secreted in response to the body's calcium needs. Moreover, over 90% of bile fluids are reabsorbed as hepatic circulation (157). Pancreatic juices and the various secretions that are poured into the intestinal lumen appear to function mostly in facilitating digestion and absorption, with the bulk of the fluid presented to the entire intestine being reabsorbed (158). The calcium content of these fluids is not well known, but they form largely by osmotic equilibration in response to the contents of the upper intestine. Therefore their calcium content, like their monovalent ion content, probably simply reflects the body fluid composition (158). On the basis of these considerations, a direct regulatory role of v_{ndo} in calcium metabolism seems unlikely.

In summary, fecal calcium excretion consists of unabsorbed food calcium and endogenous calcium that has not been reabsorbed. In human subjects, the latter is approximately equal in amount to the urinary calcium. In rats, it is 10 times greater than the calcium lost from the body in urine. There is no indication, however, that endogenous fecal calcium is subject to regulation or plays a regulatory role in calcium metabolism.

VIII. REGULATORS OF CALCIUM METABOLISM

A. Calcitropic Hormones*

Three systemic hormones are involved in the regulation of calcium metabolism: parathyroid hormone (PTH), vitamin D, and calcitonin (CT). PTH and CT are both peptides; vitamin D is a secosterol whose hormonelike action was recognized less than 30 years ago. PTH and CT interact with plasma membrane receptors on their target cells, whereas vitamin D, after a two-step transformation in liver and kidney to 1,25-dihydroxyvitamin D, acts on target cells via a gene-mediated mechanism. As a result, PTH and CT have quite rapid effects, whereas the vitamin D-mediated responses tend to be somewhat slower (102). One target of vitamin D is the parathyroid cell (159); consequently, there exists some interaction between vitamin D and PTH, but most responses associated with one hormone occur independently of the action of the other two.

1.   Parathyroid Hormone

Chemistry, Biosynthesis, and Metabolism

PTH is a protein of 84 amino acids (Fig. 9). It is synthesized in the form of a precursor, termed for historical reasons the "prepro PTH," a protein of 115 amino acids. The "pre" sequence of 25 amino acids is thought to be a signal sequence that permits establishing a polyribosomal/membrane junction in the rough endoplasmic reticulum. The second cleavage, i.e., the removal at the amino terminal of the six-amino acid sequence that constitutes the "pro" segment, occurs in the Golgi complex about 15 min after the signal sequence has been cleaved off. The hormone molecule, i.e., the 84-amino acid polypeptide, is then extruded, probably by means of exocytosis. It is thought that the hormone is located inside a vesicle or granule whose limiting membrane fuses with the plasma membrane. This step is followed by lysis of the membrane and eventual extrusion or release of the hormone molecule into the circulation (161).

The circulating PTH is transported to its target tissues, bone and kidney, as well as to the liver. In the liver, the molecule undergoes further cleavage, either between residues 33 and 34 or at several other sites that are near the 33/34 site; it is also cleaved near the middle of the molecule. Whether this cleavage has functional significance is not known, but it may yield a fragment that still can exert PTH action. Other fragments also result from this and

---

*The literature on the endocrine aspects of calcium metabolism is very extensive, and appropriate treatment would far exceed the confines of this chapter. For this reason, the text of Section VIII has been adapted from Ref. 159. Where references to a particular phenomenon are multiple, the reader is referred to appropriate reviews. As a result, cited references are not exhaustive and may not reflect all publications that document a point or conclusion.

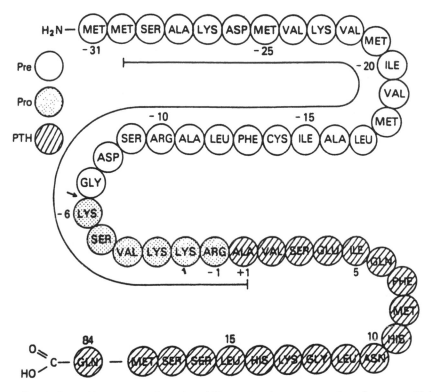

FIGURE 9 Amino acid sequence of parathyroid hormone, the prepro- and pro-hormone. (Adapted from Ref. 160.)

other cleavages. Most fragments, except the 1–34 amino-terminal sequence, have no or only limited biological activity. The 1–34 fragment has biological activity that appears to be identical, both qualitatively and quantitatively, to that of the intact hormone. The functional significance of the 35–84 sequence of the intact hormone is not known.

The genes of murine, bovine, and human PTH have been cloned (162). The human and bovine gene, like their hormone products, are more alike, while the rat gene (and hormone) exhibits fewer homologies with the human gene (and hormone). The human gene is located near the end of the short arm of chromosome 11, close to the genes encoding the hormones calcitonin and insulin. Transfection studies in which the PTH gene has been inserted in lines of cells that do not normally express PTH are under way and should yield information on gene activation, transcription, and translation.

When PTH interacts with the receptor site on the plasma membrane of kidney or bone cells, there results a stimulation of the adenyl cyclase system leading to increased production of 3′,5′-cAMP (162,163). This is a specific test for PTH, inasmuch as only target cells respond to PTH by an increase in their adenyl cyclase activity and their cAMP content.

One of the earliest responses of the osteoblast, the bone cell that is equipped with PTH receptors, is a shape change, i.e., a retraction of peripheral lamellipodia (101,102), probably modulated via cAMP. The change in shape would then be the first step in the cascade of steps that ultimately leads to increased bone resorption, mediated by the osteoclast.

Function

The principal function of PTH is to regulate the calcium concentration of extracellular fluid. This is accomplished by altering the transfer of calcium from and into bone (144), by changes in renal calcium reabsorption (147), and by indirectly inducing changes in intestinal calcium absorption (164).

In the normal mammalian organism, major regulation of the bone calcium balance is effected by modulation of bone calcium resorption. Figure 10 shows that in the parathyroidectomized animal, the relationship between bone calcium deposition and resorption rates is altered both quantitatively and qualitatively. In the normal organism, the rate of bone calcium deposition is virtually constant, regardless of how much calcium enters the body via the gut. Bone resorption drops in direct proportion to the amount of calcium absorbed. In the organism without functioning parathyroid glands, on the other hand, the intensity of both parameters is reduced to nearly one-half. Moreover, as calcium comes in from the gut, bone resorption goes down, but at a lesser rate than in the normal animal (165). At the same time, the rate of bone calcium deposition goes up, at a rate that is almost twice as fast as in the normal animal (144). In other words, in the presence of PTH, regulation of calcium flow to the skeleton is exerted almost exclusively by means of the resorptive processes, whereas in the absence of PTH, the regulatory action of bone calcium resorption, although still dominant, is lessened.

These effects, observed some years ago (144), may now be explained as having resulted from the complementary behavior of osteoblasts and osteoclasts. When PTH is released from the parathyroid glands, in response to a drop in the plasma calcium, osteoblasts assume their contracted state and their metabolic activities such as collagen synthesis and secretion are largely arrested. Osteoclasts in turn spread out, occupying some of the space freed up by osteoblastic retraction, and their metabolic action is intensified,

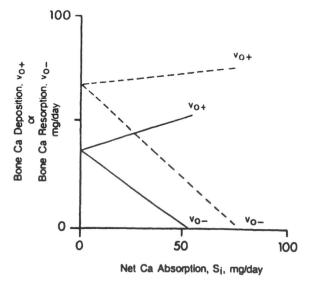

FIGURE 10   Effect of parathyroidectomy on bone calcium deposition and resorption in rats. Dashed line, euparathyroid; solid line, parathyroidectomized animals. The experimental points have been omitted for the sake of clarity. (Adapted from Ref. 144.)

leading to resorption of bone mineral and degradation of the extracellular matrix and collagen fibers (Sec. VI).

The second organ that responds to PTH is the kidney. One response involves the release into the urine of cAMP (166), about half of which is of renal origin. It is the latter that is significantly increased as a result of an infusion of PTH, and the increase in nephrogenous cAMP may be used to assess the amount of circulating PTH (163). The hormone also causes a marked phosphaturia; this is the best-known clinical effect. Finally, PTH leads to an increase in the glomerular clearance of calcium, i.e., the amount of calcium that is cleared from the luminal fluid and returned to the plasma (167).

The mechanisms by which PTH causes increased phosphate excretion and diminished calcium excretion have not been fully clarified. The phosphaturic effect of PTH may be due to a direct effect of PTH on phosphate transport and/or to its effect on sodium or bicarbonate reabsorption (168). The effect of PTH on calcium reabsorption may involve a modulation by the hormone of the intercellular space and a resultant increase in paracellular calcium flux (147).

The indirect effect of PTH on calcium absorption is mediated by 1,25-dihydroxy-vitamin D_3, 1,25-$(OH)_2$-D_3, the active metabolite of vitamin D, the renal hydroxylation of which is stimulated by PTH (168). The mechanism by which PTH acts to enhance either the rate of hydroxylation of 25-$(OH)D_3$ or the amount that becomes converted to the dihydroxylated form is not known. The increase in 1,25-$(OH)_2$-D_3 leads to increased synthesis of intestinal calbindin (CaBP) (164). Shifting animals to a low-calcium diet leads to a rise in intestinal CaBP, whether or not the animals are parathyroidectomized; however, the response in the parathyroidectomized animal seems smaller (164).

The normal plasma calcium level is quite invariant at 2.5 mM (Sec. IV). Following parathyroidectomy, plasma calcium drops to about 1.5 mM and remains much less constant. Diurnal variations, due partly to variations in intake, which are small in the normal state, are greatly magnified, as is the increase in plasma calcium in response to higher intakes (144). This increase in the euparathyroid state is about 2%, but is about 30% in the parathyroidectomized state. Thus, the ability to maintain the plasma calcium steady is markedly impaired in the parathyroidectomized or parathyroprivic state. In the euparathyroid animal, the presence of the hormone permits inflow of calcium from bone during periods when inflow from the gut is nil or low, as in nonfeeding periods (165). This compensatory mechanism is absent in the parathyroidectomized animal and partly accounts for the greater diurnal variability of the plasma calcium. In addition, as calcium turnover in bone is much slower in animals without parathyroids (73), the calcium pool expands more when calcium enters it from the gut, even if most of the incoming calcium is absorbed by the paracellular route only (Sec. III).

PTH is released from the gland when the extracellular calcium level drops, and its release is inhibited when extracellular calcium rises. The extracellular changes in calcium concentration are paralleled by changes in intracellular calcium, but the mechanism by which intracellular calcium alters hormone release and directly or indirectly affects hormone synthesis is not known.

2. Calcitonin

Chemistry and Biosynthesis

Calcitonin is a 32-amino acid polypeptide (Fig. 11) that is synthesized in the parafollicular cells, also known as "C," or "clear" cells of the thyroid gland. These cells arise embry-

(A)

```
              1            5              10              15
            Cys-Gly-Asn-Leu-Ser-Thr-Cys-Met-Leu-Gly-Thr-Tyr-Thr-Gln-Asp-
```

<u>Human</u>   20   25   30
<u>Calcitonin</u>   -Ph-Asn-Lys-Phe-His-Thr-Phe-Pro-Gln-Thr-Ala-Ile-Gly-Val-Gly-

            -Ala-Pro-NH2

```
                          S
<u>Human</u>       1  ┌──────────────┐        10              15
<u>CGRP</u>      Ser-Cys-Asn-Thr-Ala-Thr-Cys-Val-Thr-His-Arg-Leu-Ala-Gly-Leu-
```

                    20   25   30
        -Leu-Ser-Arg-Ser-Gly-Gly-Val-Val-Lys-Asp-Asn-Phe-Val-Pro-Thr-

                    35
        -Asn-Val-Gly-Ser-Glu-Ala-Phe-amide

(B)

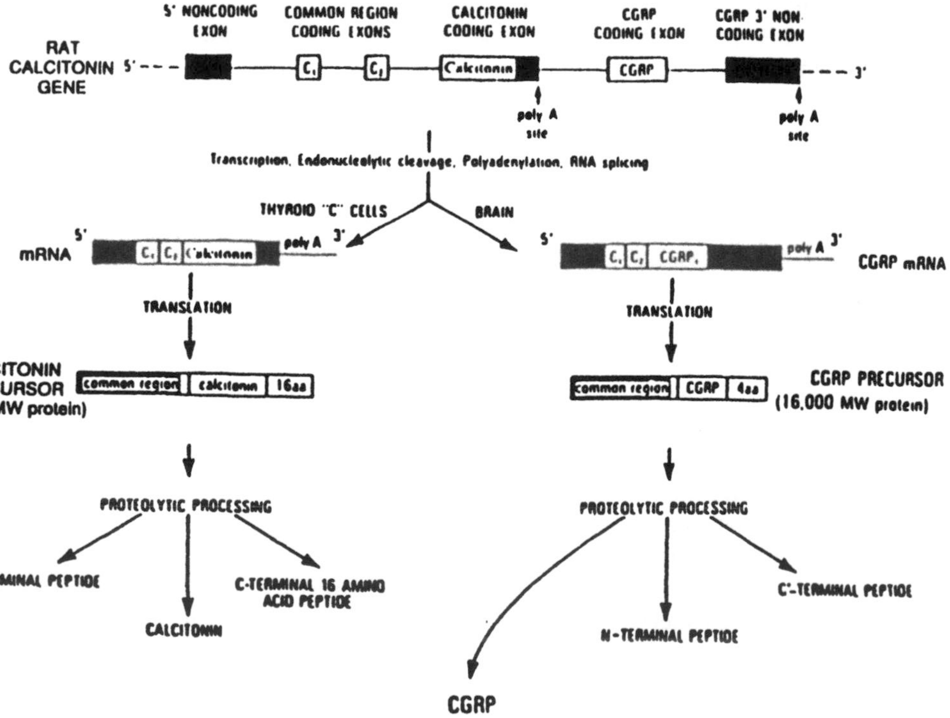

FIGURE 11   A. Amino acid sequence of calcitonin and CGRP. B. Transcription of calcitonin gene, translation of calcitonin and CGRP. (Reproduced by permission from Ref. 159.)

ologically from the fifth branchial pouch and migrate into the thyroid gland in mammals, but in fish they form the ultimobranchial body, a distinct entity (for review, see Ref. 169). Remarkably, there is considerable similarity between calcitonin from fish and mammals, and the bovine and human molecules are more distinct than human and salmon calcitonin. The latter exists in three forms, one of which is the most potent, biologically speaking, of all calcitonins that have been sequenced (163).

Calcitonin was one of the first hormones to be sequenced, but its function has remained a mystery. It has a pronounced, transient hypocalcemic effect; it is this effect that was utilized to purify and determine its structure. However, its role in calcium metabolism is unclear.

Studies of the calcitonin gene have shown that it gives rise by differential splicing (Fig. 11B) to two products, calcitonin and another protein, called the calcitonin gene-related peptide (CGRP; Fig. 11B). Whereas calcitonin is expressed in the C cells of the thyroid, different controls lead to the expression of CGRP, largely in the central nervous system. As is true for many gene products, the messenger RNA for calcitonin is translated into a precursor molecule of 136 amino acids (in the rat), which is then cleaved into three fragments, one of which is the hormone (163). In the case of the messenger RNA for CGRP, the precursor is again split into three peptides, one of which is CGRP.

The function of CGRP is unknown. Systemic and local administration of CGRP increase the rate and force of contraction of the isolated atrium of the heart (170). Administration of CGRP to normal human subjects leads to vasodilatation and to flushing of the face. Some of these effects can also be induced by calcitonin, but require much greater doses. This can be explained by cross-reaction of receptor binding, plus the existing homology of these two products of a single gene. CGRP is a 37-amino acid polypeptide.

Function

Calcitonin interacts with a receptor located on the plasma membrane of osteoclasts (104,105). This interaction leads to a stimulation of the adenyl cyclase system, with increased accumulation of cAMP. The interaction of calcitonin with the osteoclast causes the latter to stop its searching action, expressed by the movement of pseudopodlike extensions that move over the extracellular bone surface and presumably precede the release of lysosomes and dissolution of bone (171,172). Osteoblasts do not have receptors for calcitonin.

At the level of the whole organism, the function of calcitonin is not understood. When calcitonin was first discovered, it was thought to function in a push–pull fashion with PTH, PTH causing bone resorption to be enhanced, while calcitonin inhibited bone resorption. However, extensive studies of animals deprived of endogenous calcitonin have failed to reveal major changes in bone metabolism (100,169). Animals that have been deprived of their C cells exhibit no change in their steady-state plasma calcium level and the rates of bone calcium deposition and resorption are unchanged, as are their urinary calcium and endogenous fecal calcium excretions. Calcium absorption is also unchanged. Patients with medullary thyroid carcinoma and excess amounts of circulating calcitonin also seem to have no obvious disturbance of calcium metabolism (173).

The major effect of a deficiency in calcitonin is the inability to overcome a hypercalcemic challenge as readily as when calcitonin can be released normally. When a large amount of calcium is given so as to expand the calcium pool, the rate at which the expanded pool returns to the preinjection value in a calcitonin-deficient organism is about half what it would be normally (Table 2; Ref. 84).

3. Vitamin D

In contrast with the peptides, PTH, and calcitonin, vitamin D is a secosteroid, a cyclo-pentanoperhydrophenanthrene-related structure. The amount of the vitamin that the body can produce from precursors in the absence of sunlight is insufficient to meet the need for this compound, especially in growing infants and children living in northern climates. When it was identified in the early 1920s, the compound was classified as a vitamin, i.e., as an essential micronutrient. About 40 years after its identification, as the metabolism of vitamin D became known, it became clear that the mode of action of the biologically active metabolite derived from vitamin D was close to that of steroid hormones, that is, the genomic induction of specific proteins.

Chemistry and Metabolism*

Cholesterol is the precursor compound that, in a series of steps, becomes converted to 7-dehydrocholesterol, the provitamin D. The latter accumulates in the skin and, under the action of ultraviolet light, is converted to vitamin D in two steps. In the first step, one of the rings (B) is opened up, yielding the secosteroid structure typical of the vitamin. The second step involves a rearrangement of the "previtamin D" to vitamin D. Neither of these will take place in the absence of sunlight (or ultraviolet light), hence the need for ingesting preformed vitamin D in the absence of sunlight.

Vitamin D undergoes two sequential hydroxylations, one in the liver, the other in the kidney. In the liver cell, vitamin D undergoes hydroxylation at carbon 25. In the kidney cell, 25-hydroxyvitamin D_3 is further hydroxylated to 1,25-dihydroxyvitamin D_3, 1,25-$(OH)_2D_3$, biologically the most active vitamin D metabolite. Alternatively, 25-hydroxyvitamin D_3 can be hydroxylated at the 24-carbon, to form 24,25-$(OH)_2D_3$.

From the regulatory viewpoint, the relative amount of 1,25-$(OH)_2$-D or 24,25-$(OH)_2$D plays a key role, as the major functions of vitamin D in kidney, intestine, and bone are associated with the effects due to 1,25-$(OH)_2$-D. Thus, under conditions of calcium deficiency, production of 1,25-$(OH)_2$-D is increased leading to an increase in the active step of intestinal calcium absorption (67,74), enhanced renal reabsorption (109,147), and stimulation of bone metabolism (73). Under conditions of calcium excess, the production of 1,25-$(OH)_2$-D is downregulated and larger amounts of 24,25-$(OH)_2$D are produced. How the renal enzyme systems respond to what must be changes in intracellular calcium concentrations so as to favor production of one or the other vitamin D metabolite is not known.

Function

The major functions of vitamin D are to enhance active calcium transport in intestine and kidney and to enable bone cells to function at a suitably high level of intensity. In addition, vitamin D appears to have a series of pleiotropic functions related to development and cell differentiation (174).

Intestine: Table 5 summarizes the quantitative and qualitative effects of vitamin D on the various steps of transcellular calcium transport. Calcium entry is moderately enhanced as a result of the action of the vitamin (17). This may involve a vitamin D-dependent gating molecule that either regulates or amplifies the putative calcium channel (32–34).

---

*For greater detail and additional references, see Ref. 174.

TABLE 5 Effects of Vitamin D on Transcellular Calcium Transport in the Intestine

Step	Mechanism or structure	Effect of vitamin D	Mechanism
Entry across brush border	Down chemical gradient (via channel?)	Enhances 20–30% (17)	Possibly via integral Ca-binding protein (32–34)
Binding to fixed cellular sites (buffering)	Golgi apparatus, RER,[a] mitochondria	Enhances 100% (175)	Unknown
Intracellular movement	Diffusion	Facilitates in direct proportion (≈ 100-fold) (15)	Biosynthesis of soluble CaBP (M_r 8800 in mammals, 28,000 in birds), which acts as Ca ferry (12,46,205)
Extrusion	Pumping against a gradient, Ca-ATPase, Na/Ca exchange	Increases action Ca-ATPase 200–300% (12,53)	Unknown

[a]Rough endoplasmic reticulum.
Adapted from Ref. 12. Numbers in parentheses refer to reference citations.

Once calcium enters the cell, it encounters a series of calcium-binding sites associated with either mobile or fixed molecules or organelles. Vitamin D seems to increase the number of these calcium-binding sites in the Golgi apparatus and endoplasmic reticulum (175). The synthesis of the intestinal calbindin (CaBP) is totally dependent on vitamin D. As explained in Section III, active calcium transport varies directly and proportionately with the cellular content of CaBP. The latter molecule acts as a ferry, effectively shuttling calcium from the luminal to the serosal pole of the intestinal cell at a rate directly proportional to the amount of CaBP (Fig. 6).

Calcium extrusion is also enhanced by vitamin D. The number of pump molecules is increased (53), although the mechanism may be indirect, as most Ca-ATPases are not—and would not be expected to be—vitamin D-dependent.

Quantitatively speaking, as also shown in Table 5, the major effect of vitamin D is on the intestinal CaBP, which in turn varies linearly and directly with the V_m of active transport (Fig. 6). The enhancing effect on calcium entry is only some 30%. Calcium extrusion and binding to fixed sites are enhanced twofold to threefold. It has been estimated (12) that neither entry, nor extrusion, nor binding to fixed intracellular sites is the limiting rate; only intracellular diffusion in the absence of the cellular CaBP is severely limiting.

Kidney: The action of vitamin D in the kidney is to increase calcium reabsorption (Sec. VII). Vitamin D regulates transcellular calcium movement in the distal convoluted tubule (DCT) in a manner analogous with what it does in the intestine. The biosynthesis of the renal calcium-binding protein (CaBP$_r$, calbindin D28k, M_r 28 kDa) is totally dependent on vitamin D (176). The protein is thought to function in the DCT by amplifying transcellular transport of calcium by a factor of about 70 (149). To what extent vitamin D also plays a role in the entry or extrusion processes in the DCT cell is not known, but it may do so, in analogy with what is known in the intestine.

Bone: The effect of vitamin D on bone is to increase the rates of bone formation and resorption (73). Receptors for 1,25-$(OH)_2$-D have been found only in osteoblasts (102), so the effect of vitamin D on bone resorption is likely to be indirect, i.e., via the osteoblast. The principal molecular effect of 1,25-$(OH)_2$-D on osteoblasts is to increase their production of the extracellular matrix molecule, the Gla protein (also known as osteocalcin; 177). Treatment of osteoblasts in culture leads to a state equivalent to enhanced differentiation— that is, a higher level of alkaline phosphatase and shape changes—but the relationship of these observations to the in vivo effect of vitamin D has not been clarified.

The role of vitamin D in mineralization is problematical from the viewpoint of mechanisms. Soft bones and the clinical signs associated with rickets are well known, but many of these can be attributed to a phosphate deficiency that is aggravated by the lack of vitamin D (178).

Experimental vitamin D deficiency leads to minor bone changes in rats (73,109). Hypocalcemia due to vitamin D deficiency is not generally associated with obvious skeletal changes visible on radiographic examination. Moreover, it has been reported that in some animals the provision of abundant minerals, either in the diet or systemically, can overcome the skeletal defects associated with vitamin D deficiency. While it seems probable that vitamin D plays a hormonelike role in bone cells, as it does in cells of duodenum and the DCT of the kidney, the nature of this role and its relationship to mineralization are not yet clarified. There is little doubt, however, that bone turnover of calcium is diminished in vitamin D deficiency (109).

B.   Other Systemic Hormones

Parathyroid hormone, calcitonin, and vitamin D are considered the primary hormones that regulate calcium metabolism, as discussed earlier. Other hormones that act directly or indirectly on calcium fluxes or bone include the gonadal steroids, the adrenal glucocorticoids, the thyroid hormones, growth hormone and somatomedin, and insulin and glucagon. A general discussion of these hormones is beyond this chapter's scope, but their specific roles in calcium metabolism will now be discussed briefly.

1.   Gonadal Steroids (168)

Mineral metabolism and bones and cartilage are profoundly affected in conditions of excess or deficiency of the gonadal steroids. Osteoblasts have receptors that respond equally to estrogens (179) or testosterone (180). The existence of gonadal hormone receptors in osteoclasts is less certain. Avian osteoclasts may possess such receptors (181), and in-vitro studies (182) suggest that mammalian osteoclast development may be enhanced by the absence of estrogens; in other words, estrogens may, perhaps by action on precursor cells via cytokines, inhibit osteoclast development and/or differentiation. It has also been shown that the inhibitory effect exerted by parathyroid hormone on osteoblasts (Sec. VI) is diminished when estrogen or androgen is added to an osteoblast culture (183,184).

Estrogen administration leads to diminished urinary calcium output (185). Estrogens probably do not affect intestinal calcium absorption directly (185).

Testosterone seems to have mechanisms of action that are similar to those of estrogen. At one time, testosterone was used to treat women with postmenopausal osteoporosis, partly because testosterone administration leads to significant improvement in the nitrogen balance (186). However, because of the undesirable masculinizing effect, it is rarely used today.

2. Corticosteroids

Cortisol, corticosterone, and deoxycorticosterone are the major products of the zona fasciculata of the human adrenal gland and represent the chemical response of the body to stress. They have a pronounced effect on bone metabolism, inhibiting cartilage growth and development, impairing synthesis of the bone matrix, and inhibiting bone formation. These antianabolic actions of the corticosteroids may be the result of their inhibition of protein synthesis. As a result, bone absorption is stimulated.

Glucocorticoids seem to have no acute effect on urinary calcium excretion (187). Chronic administration causes calcium excretion to rise (185). Long-term administration of glucocorticoids or glucocorticoid excess may induce excess calcium mobilization from the skeleton and thus lead to hypercalciuria. The major metabolic effect of glucocorticoids is on bone. An excess of these hormones, as in Cushing's disease, or when administered exogenously, is associated with decreased bone growth in children, loss of bone volume in adults, and the impairment of fracture healing (185). Glucocorticoids inhibit incorporation of sulfate into cartilage (188) and of amino acids into cartilage collagen (189); thus, they have an antianabolic effect. Glucocorticoid insufficiency, if untreated, is life-threatening. It is associated with hypercalcemia, which may be the result of excessive osteoclastic activity that would normally be modulated by these hormones (185).

3. Thyroid Hormones

The two principal thyroid hormones are triiodothyronine and thyroxine, the latter containing four atoms of iodine. Even though they are peptides and not steroids, the most probable mechanism of action of the thyroid hormones involves nuclear localization and genomic activation by a ligand-receptor complex. This in turn leads to selective synthesis of specific proteins. Consequently, the action of the thyroid hormones can be likened to that of steroid hormones (168).

Both thyroid hormone excess and hypothyroidism have significant effects on bone metabolism. Hyperthyroidism is associated with a marked increase in bone resorption, particularly in cortical bone, caused mainly by increased osteoclastic activity (185). At the same time, bone turnover is increased. However, the stimulation to bone calcium resorption seems greater than that of bone calcium deposition. As a result, the bone calcium balance, especially in cortical bone, is diminished. Biochemically, hyperthyroidism is often associated with an increase in hydroxyproline excretion in urine and sometimes with increased hydroxyproline levels in serum, indications of heightened collagen turnover (190). Alkaline phosphatase levels are increased in hyperthyroidism, the enzyme presumably originating in the skeleton (185). Thyroid hormones appear to have a direct effect on osteoclasts, as enhanced radiocalcium release from labeled bones can be demonstrated in bone organ cultures (191). Hyperthyroidism is associated with hypercalcemia, hyperphosphaturia, and hypercalciuria. Calcium absorption from the intestine tends to be diminished in conditions of excess thyroid hormone (185). This appears to be due to a diminution of the production of intestinal calbindin, mediated by a diminution of $1,25\text{-}(OH)_2\text{-}D_3$ production consequent to the hypercalcemia.

In hypothyroidism, the effects on calcium metabolism are the obverse of what occurs in the case of thyroid hormone excess. Bone turnover is slowed, hydroxyproline excretion is diminished, and there is a tendency to mild hypocalcemia and diminished serum phosphate levels. Hence, urinary calcium and phosphate excretion are also lower than normal. The bone calcium pool is diminished.

Thyroid hormone promotes skeletal growth in prepubertal children by acting on cartilage growth directly and by stimulating the growth hormone–somatomedin pathway. Therefore, hypothyroidism in children is associated with diminished skeletal growth and an increase in density in the zone of provisional calcification and delayed appearance of the centers of epiphyseal ossification (192).

4.   Growth Hormone and Somatomedin

The growth hormone molecule is a large protein consisting of 191 amino acids, the active core of which involves the N-terminal two-thirds of the sequence, while the remainder, the C-terminal one-third, is thought to stabilize the molecular structure (168). Growth hormone is the major hormonal growth factor, acting on bone and cartilage. The hormone promotes growth through the somatomedins, low molecular weight (~7000 Da) peptides synthesized in the liver. Somatomedin receptors have been found in adipocytes, hepatocytes, lymphocytes, and bone cells. Of the three human somatomedins—A, B, and C—the latter, C, is identical with the insulin-like growth factor.

Growth hormone is essential for normal growth and development (185). One form of human dwarfism is caused by defective production of growth hormone, an autosomal recessive characteristic. Growth hormone is essential for somatomedin synthesis (168). Patients with acromegaly, i.e., enlarged stature due to excess growth hormone production, exhibit increased rates of calcium uptake and release by the skeleton, with formation stimulated more than resorption (185). Acromegaly is associated with hypercalciuria and, in some patients, with increased calcium absorption from the intestine. The mechanism(s) by which growth hormone and/or somatomedin act on these processes is unknown; direct action on transcellular calcium transport seems unlikely.

5.   Insulin and Glucagon (168,185)

It seems probable that bone cells are a direct target of the action of insulin, although other tissues—adipose, muscle, and liver—are generally considered major targets.

Insulin deficiency leads to a diminution of bone turnover, with bone calcium removal markedly enhanced in insulin-deprived animals. Insulin-deprived rats in the growth phase are only slightly hypocalcemic, but have stopped adding calcium to their skeletons. In other words, their bone balance, instead of being positive, is zero or slightly negative (193). Insulin deficiency is associated with a drop in active calcium absorption in the intestine and a rise in urinary calcium output; this suggests a diminution of the calcium-conserving capacity of the kidney (193).

Glucagon administration produces transient hypocalcemia in several mammalian species, including humans, presumably by direct interaction with the skeleton (185). There is evidence that glucagon inhibits parathyroid-stimulated osteoclastic action, but probably has no effect in unstimulated bone cells (194,195).

IX.   OSTEOPOROSIS—AN INTEGRATIVE VIEW

Osteoporosis may be defined as a condition in which the mass of bone per unit volume is significantly decreased, to the point where the risk of fracture is high. While the disorder is clinically relevant only when a fracture has occurred—typically a vertebral or hip fracture—it is prevention rather than treatment of the fracture that seems the more effective approach (196).

As shown in Figure 12, bone mass increases from infancy until the late teens, thereafter remains at a plateau until the mid-thirties, and then begins to decline. In women

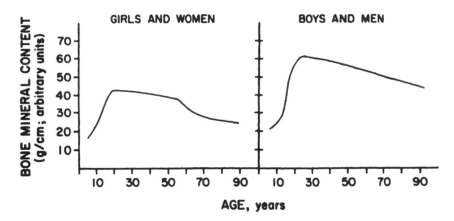

FIGURE 12 Bone mineral content as a function of age, determined by photon absorptiometry. (Unpublished data provided by C. Christiansen, Denmark.)

there occurs a rather drastic decline in the years following the menopause, whereas in men the decline is more gradual. Some 10 years after the menopause, the rate of decline of bone mass in women parallels that in men. Total bone mass is lower in women than in men.

Bone mass in a given individual is genetically programmed, but the final expression is modulated both qualitatively and quantitatively by environmental factors. Thus, in the absence or with reduced availability of the bone minerals, calcium and phosphate, the genetically determined optimum expression of the skeleton is diminished; bone then is thinner and therefore weaker at any age, and the risk of fracture is greater. This is illustrated by the now classical study of Matkovic and colleagues (197), who reported a higher and earlier incidence of certain fractures in a Yugoslav population consuming by custom low quantities of calcium, as compared to a presumably comparable population, genetically speaking, that by custom ingested large quantities of calcium. Similarly, the Japanese, who before World War II were largely vegetarian and consumed only about 10 mmol of Ca per day (91), are now, two generations later, closer to a Western diet in terms of calcium and protein intake and are now also taller.

While the attained bone mass can be modified by calcium intake, the question arises whether the age- and hormone-dependent drop in bone mass can be altered by a change in calcium intake (and absorption). There can be little doubt that a negative calcium balance will increase the rate at which bone mass is lost. The reverse, however, is far from obvious. There is reasonable evidence that the rate of cortical bone loss is similar in individuals of different statures (198), and that this rate is relatively independent of calcium intake. It is therefore not surprising that increased calcium intake in women with postmenopausal osteoporosis had virtually no effect on their rate of bone loss (199), whereas estrogen replacement therapy (200), accompanied by a nutritionally adequate intake of calcium, arrested the loss of trabecular bone characteristic of the menopause (201) or of oophorectomy (202).

The mechanism by which gonadal hormones stimulate bone cells is not well understood. Both male and female gonadal hormones interact with receptors on the osteoblast, causing these cells to increase in activity and number. Part of the responses of osteoblasts seems to involve a reduced release of cytokines, leading in turn to diminished osteoclastic activity and number (203). Osteoclasts, when relieved of the repression exerted by the gonadal hormones—whether directly or indirectly—become more active, with the result that bone resorption exceeds bone formation.

Of the two general classes of bone, trabecular and cortical, it is the former that undergoes more rapid turnover and is the site of the majority of osteoblasts and osteoclasts (97). Consequently, in the menopause, with gonadal hormone function ceasing abruptly, it is trabecular bone that is more particularly affected. When elements of trabecular bone, the trabeculae, are destroyed, rebuilding seems no longer to be possible. Lost cortical bone can be replaced more readily. In males, gonadal hormone loss, or at least loss of function, is more gradual, as is loss of bone mass in aging men (Fig. 12).

To combat osteoporosis thus involves several approaches: (a) assuring optimum genetic expression of skeletal size and strength by providing the needed nutrients, calcium in particular. This is of especial importance for girls and young women, whose average calcium intake tends to be half of what appears to be needed (204); (b) replacing, under suitable medical supervision, the gonadal hormones whose concentration drops abruptly at the menopause or gradually with aging; (c) assuring an adequate calcium intake throughout life; (d) recognition of the age-dependent drop of active calcium absorption from the intestine with maturity of the skeleton and compensation therefor by increased intake; (e) recognition that slowing the rate of bone loss, preferably by stimulating bone formation, can have long-term benefits in the decrease, and perhaps the severity, of fractures.

X. OUTLOOK

The past two generations have seen significant advances in the understanding of extracellular calcium metabolism and its regulation. The molecular nature of hormones, their receptors, and intracellular events that occur in response to hormonal stimuli are being studied intensively, and many significant factors are bound to be uncovered in coming years. What is less well understood at present is the relationship between intracellular and extracellular calcium homeostasis. The constancy of the free calcium concentration, now recognized to prevail inside essentially all cells, raises the question of why it is necessary for both intra- and extracellular calcium concentrations to be so exquisitely regulated, and whether and how maintenance of the calcium concentration of the two milieus is related or interconnected. The discovery of calcium-responsive proteins in cell membranes will contribute to that understanding, as will analysis of their evolution in relation to the fundamental cellular task of separating calcium from phosphate (1).

Another aspect of calcium metabolism that needs substantial development is the construction of quantitative schemes of extracellular calcium metabolism. The transformation of qualitative into quantitative information, the development of hierarchical relationships between various cellular and tissue events, and the ability to predict quantitatively how changes in, say, calcium intake will affect bone metabolism both acutely and over the long-term are needed if calcium research is to yield information that has both theoretical and practical importance for human and animal health. Ultimately, such information will also permit effective planning of the cultivation and distribution of food supplies, thereby contributing in turn to the betterment of population health.

REFERENCES

1. Kretsinger RH. Why cells must export calcium. In: Bronner F, ed. Intracellular Calcium Regulation. New York: Wiley-Liss, 1990: 439–457.

2. Latham MC, McGandy RB, McCann M, Stare FJ, eds. Scope Manual on Nutrition. Kala-mazoo, MI: Upjohn Co, 1972: Table B, Appendix.

3. Block G, Dresser CM, Hartman AM, Carroll MD. Nutrient sources in the American diet: quantitative data from the NHANES II Survey. I. Vitamins and minerals. Am J Epidemiol 1985; 122: 13–26.

4. Eckelman R, Kulp J, Schubert AR. Strontium-90 in man. II. Science 1958; 127: 266–274.

5. Morgan AF, ed. Nutritional status USA. Calif Agr Bull 769, 1959.

6. Recommended Dietary Allowances, 10th ed. Washington, DC: National Academy Press, 1989: 284.

7. U.S. Department of Agriculture. CSF II. Nationwide food consumption survey. Continuing survey of food intakes by individuals. Men 19–50 years, 1 day, 1985. NFCS, CSFII, 85-3, November 1986. Hyattsville, MD: USDA.

8. American Medical Association. Nutrients in Processed Foods—Proteins; Vitamins, Minerals; Fat, Carbohydrates. Acton, MA: Publishing Sciences Group, 1974.

9. Washburn EW, ed. International Critical Tables of Numerical Data, Physics, Chemistry and Technology. Vol. 3. New York: McGraw-Hill, 1928: 377.

10. Cramer CF, Copp DH. Progress and rate of absorption of radiostrontium through intestinal tracts of rats. Proc Soc Exp Biol Med 1959; 102: 514–517.

11. Marcus CS, Lengemann FW. Absorption of Ca^{45} and Sr^{85} from solid and liquid food at various levels of the alimentary tract of the rat. J Nutr 1962; 77: 155–160.

12. Bronner F, Pansu D, Stein WD. An analysis of intestinal calcium transport across the rat intestine. Am J Physiol 1986; 250 (Gastrointest Liver Physiol 13): G562–G569.

13. Schachter D, Dowdle EB, Schenker H. Active transport of calcium by the small intestine of the rat. Am J Physiol 1960; 198: 263–268.

14. Martin DL, DeLuca HF. Influence of sodium on calcium transport by the rat small intestine. Am J Physiol 1969; 216: 1351–1359.

15. Roche C, Bellaton C, Pansu D, Miller A III, Bronner F. Localization of vitamin D-dependent active Ca^{2+} transport in rat duodenum and relation to CaBP. Am J Physiol 1986; 251 (Gastrointest Liver Physiol 14): G314–G320.

16. Pansu D, Bellaton C, Roche C, Bronner F. Duodenal and ileal calcium absorption in the rat and effects of vitamin D. Am J Physiol 1983; 244 (Gastrointest Liver Physiol 7): G695–G700.

17. Miller A III, Bronner F. Calcium uptake in isolated brush-border vesicles from rat small intestine. Biochem J 1981; 196: 391–401.

18. Miller A III, Li ST, Bronner F. Characterization of calcium binding to brush border membranes from rat duodenum. Biochem J 1982; 208: 773–782.

19. Schedl HP, Wilson HD. Calcium uptake by intestinal brush border membrane vesicles. Comparison with in vivo calcium transport. J Clin Invest 1985; 76: 1871–1878.

20. Wilson HD, Schedl HP, Christensen K. Calcium uptake by brush-border membrane vesicles from the rat intestine. Am J Physiol 1989; 257 (Renal Fluid Electrolyte Physiol 26): F446–F453.

21. Takito J, Shinki T, Sasaki T, Suda T. Calcium uptake by brush-border and basolateral membrane vesicles in chick duodenum. Am J Physiol 1990; 258 (Gastrointest Liver Physiol 21): G16–G23.

22. Holdsworth ES. Vitamin D_3 and calcium absorption in the chick. Biochem J 1965; 96: 475–483.

23. Stein WD. Facilitated diffusion of calcium across the intestinal epithelial cell. J Nutrition 1992; 122: 651–656.

24. Homaidan FR, Donowitz M, Weiland GA, Sharp GWG. Two calcium channels in basolateral membranes of rabbit ileal epithelial cells. Am J Physiol 1989; 257 (Gastrointest Liver Physiol 20): G86–G93.

25. Butler DJ, Hillier K. Calcium and human large-bowel motility. Ann NY Acad Sci 1989; 560: 447–450.

26. Saunders JCJ, Isaacson LC. Patch clamp study of Ca channels in isolated renal tubule

segments. In: Pansu D, Bronner F, eds. Calcium Transport and Intracellular Calcium Homeo-stasis. Heidelberg: Springer, 1990: 27–34.

27. Hess P, Tsien RW. Mechanism of ion permeation through calcium channels. Nature 1984; 309: 453–458.

28. Guggino SE, Lajeunesse D, Wagner JA, Snyder SH. Bone remodeling signaled by a dihydropyridine-and phenylalkylamine-sensitive calcium channel. Proc Natl Acad Sci USA 1989; 86: 2957–2960.

29. Caffrey JM, Farach-Carson MC. Vitamin D_3 metabolites modulate dihydropyridine-sensitive calcium currents in clonal rat osteosarcoma cells. J Biol Chem 1989; 264: 20265–20274.

30. Lieberherr M. Effects of vitamin D_3 metabolites on cytosolic free calcium in confluent mouse osteoblasts. J Biol Chem 1987; 262: 13168–13173.

31. Bronner F, Pansu D, Bosshard A, Lipton LH. Calcium uptake by isolated rat intestinal cells. J Cell Physiol 1983; 116: 322–328.

32. Kowarski S, Schachter D. Intestinal membrane calcium-binding protein: vitamin D-dependent membrane component of the intestinal calcium transport mechanism. J Biol Chem 1980; 255: 10834–10840.

33. Schachter D, Kowarski S. Isolation of the protein 1M Cal, a vitamin D-dependent membrane component of the intestinal transport mechanism for calcium. Fed Proc 1982; 41: 84–87.

34. Miller A III, Ueng TH, Bronner F. Isolation of a vitamin D-dependent, calcium-binding protein from brush borders of rat duodenal mucosa. FEBS Lett 1979; 103: 319–322.

35. Washburn WE, ed. International Critical Tables of Numerical Data, Physics, Chemistry and Technology. Vol. 5. New York: McGraw-Hill, 1929; 66.

36. Wasserman RH, Corradino RA, Taylor AN. Vitamin D-dependent calcium binding protein: purification and some properties. J Biol Chem 1968; 243: 3978–3986.

37. Wasserman RH, Feher JJ. Vitamin D-dependent calcium-binding proteins. In: Wasserman RH, Corradino RA, Carafoli E, Kretsinger RH, MacLennan DH, Siegel FL, eds. Calcium Binding Proteins and Calcium Function. New York: Elsevier-North Holland, 1977: 293–302.

38. Wasserman RH, Fullmer CS, Taylor AN. The vitamin D-dependent calcium binding proteins. In: Lawson DEM, ed. Vitamin D. London: Academic Press, 1978: 133–166.

39. Thomasset M, Desplan C, Parkes O. Rat vitamin D-dependent calcium-binding proteins. Specificity of mRNAs coding for the 7500-Mr protein from duodenum and the 28000-Mr protein from kidney and cerebellum. Eur J Biochem 1983; 129: 519–524.

40. Perret C, Desplan C, Thomasset M. Cholecalcin (a 9-kDa cholecalciferol-induced calcium-binding protein) messenger RNA. Distribution and induction by calcitriol in the rat digestive tract. Eur J Biochem 1985; 150: 211–217.

41. Perret C, Lomri N, Gouhier N, Auffray C, Thomasset M. The rat vitamin D-dependent calcium-binding protein (9-kDa CaBP) gene. Complete nucleotide sequence and structural organization. Eur J Biochem 1988; 172: 43–51.

42. Kretsinger RH. Calcium-binding proteins. Annu Rev Biochem 1976; 45: 239–266.

43. Ueng TH, Golub EE, Bronner F. The effect of age and 1,25-dihydroxyvitamin D_3 treatment on the intestinal calcium-binding protein of suckling rats. Arch Biochem Biophys 1979; 196: 624–630.

44. Ueng TH, Bronner F. Cellular and luminal forms of rat intestinal calcium binding protein as studied by counter ion electrophoresis. Arch Biochem Biophys 1979; 197: 205–217.

45. Thomasset M, Parkes CO, Cuisinier-Gleizes P. Rat calcium-binding proteins: distribution, development and vitamin D-dependence. Am J Physiol 1982; 243 (Endocrinol Met 6): E483–E488.

46. Feher JJ, Fullmer CS, Wasserman RH. Role of facilitated diffusion of calcium by calbindin in intestinal calcium absorption. Am J Physiol 1992; 262 (Cell Physiol 31): C517–C526.

47. Martin SR, Linse S, Johnson C, Bayley PM, Forsen S. Protein surface changes and Ca^{2+} binding to individual sites in calbindin D_{9k}: stopped flow studies. Biochemistry 1990; 29: 4188–4193.

48. Wyman J. Facilitated diffusion and the possible role of myoglobin as a transport molecule. J Biol Chem 1966; 241: 115–121.

49. Garrahan PJ, Rega AF. Plasma membrane calcium pump. In: Bronner F, ed. Intracellular Calcium Regulation. New York: Wiley-Liss, 1990; 271–303.

50. Verma AK, Filoteo AG, Stanford DR, et al. Complete primary structure of a human plasma membrane Ca^{2+} pump. J Biol Chem 1988; 263: 14152–14159.

51. Carafoli E, James P, Strehler EE. Structure-function relationships in the calcium pump of plasma membranes. In: Peterlik M, Bronner F, eds. Molecular and Cellular Regulation of Calcium and Phosphate Metabolism. New York: Wiley-Liss, 1990: 181–193.

52. Ghijsen WEJM, Van Os CH, Heizmann CW, Murer H. Regulation of duodenal Ca^{2+} pump by calmodulin and vitamin D-dependent Ca^{2+}-binding protein. Am J Physiol 1986; 251 (Gastrointest Liver Physiol 14): G223–G229.

53. Wasserman RH, Chandler JS, Meyer SA, et al. Intestinal calcium transport and calcium extrusion processes at the basolateral membrane. J Nutr 1992; 122: 662–671.

54. Carafoli E. Membrane transport of calcium: an overview. Meth Enzymol 1988; 157(Q): 3–11.

55. Van Os CH. Transcellular calcium transport in intestine and renal epithelial cells. Biochim Biophys Acta 1987; 906: 195–222.

56. Reeves JP. Sodium-calcium exchange. In: Bronner F, ed. Intracellular Calcium Regulation. New York: Wiley-Liss, 1990: 305–347.

57. Nellans HN, Popovitch JR. Role of sodium in intestinal calcium transport. In: Bronner F, Peterlik M, eds. Epithelial Calcium and Phosphate Transport: Molecular and Cellular Aspects. New York: Alan R. Liss, 1984: 301–306.

58. Bronner F. Calcium absorption. In: Johnson LR, Christensen J, Jacobson ED, Jackson MJ, Walsh JH, eds. Physiology of the Gastrointestinal Tract. 2d ed. Vol. 2. New York: Raven Press, 1987: 1419–1433.

59. Bronner F, Spence K. Non-saturable Ca transport in the rat intestine is via the paracellular pathway. In: Bronner F, Peterlik M, eds. Cellular Calcium and Phosphate Transport in Health and Disease. New York: Alan R. Liss, 1988: 277–285.

60. Cassidy MM, Tidball CS. Cellular mechanisms of intestinal permeability alterations produced by chelation depletion. J Cell Biol 1967; 32: 685–698.

61. Pansu D, Chapuy MC, Milani M, Bellaton C. Transepithelial calcium transport enhanced by xylose and glucose in the rat jejunal ligated loop. Calcif Tiss Res 1976; 21: 45–52.

62. Diamond J, Tormey JM. Role of long extracellular channels in fluid transport across epithelia. Nature 1966; 210: 817–820.

63. Vaughn DW, Filer LJ. The enhancing action of certain carbohydrates on the intestinal absorption of calcium in the rat. J Nutr 1960; 71: 10–14.

64. Wasserman RH, Taylor AN. Some aspects of the intestinal absorption of calcium, with special reference to vitamin D. In: Comar CL, Bronner F, eds. Mineral Metabolism—An Advanced Treatise. Vol. 3. New York and London: Academic Press, 1969: 321.

65. Armbrecht HJ. Effect of age and the milk sugar lactose on calcium absorption by the small intestine. Adv Exp Med Biol 1989; 249: 185–192.

66. Pansu D, Bellaton C, Bronner F. Effect of lactose on duodenal calcium-binding protein and calcium absorption. J Nutr 1979; 109: 509–512.

67. Pansu D, Bellaton C, Bronner F. The effect of calcium intake on the saturable and non-saturable components of duodenal calcium transport. Am J Physiol 1981; 240 (Gastrointest Liver Physiol 8): G32–G37.

68. Wasserman RH, Comar CL, Nold MM. The influence of amino acids and other organic compounds on the gastrointestinal absorption of calcium[45] and strontium[89] in the rat. J Nutr 1956; 59: 371–383.

69. Kehayoglou CK, Williams HS, Whimster WF, Holdsworth C. Calcium absorption in the normal, bile duct ligated and cirrhotic rat, with observations on the effect of long- and medium-chain triglycerides. Gut 1968; 9: 597–603.

70. Pansu D, Duflos C, Bellaton C, Bronner F. Solubility and intestinal transit time limit calcium absorption in rats. J Nutr 1993; 123: 1396–1404.

71. Armbrecht HJ, Zenser TV, Bruns MEH, Davis BB. Effect of age on intestinal calcium absorption and adaptation to dietary calcium. Am J Physiol 1979; 236 (Endocrinol Metab Gastrointest Physiol 5): E769–E774.

72. Armbrecht HJ, Zenser TV, Davis BB. Effect of vitamin D metabolites on intestinal calcium absorption and calcium-binding protein in young and adult rats. Endocrinology 1980; 106: 469–475.

73. Hurwitz S, Stacey RE, Bronner F. Role of vitamin D in plasma calcium regulation. Am J Physiol 1969; 216: 254–262.

74. Buckley M, Bronner F. Calcium-binding protein biosynthesis in the rat: regulation by calcium and 1,25-dihydroxyvitamin D_3. Arch Biochem Biophys 1980; 202: 235–241.

75. Hall BD, MacMillan DR, Bronner F. Vitamin D-resistant rickets associated with high fecal endogenous calcium output. A report of two cases. Am J Clin Nutr 1969; 22: 448–457.

76. Walser M. Ion association VI. Interaction between calcium, magnesium, inorganic phosphate, citrate and protein in normal human plasma. J Clin Invest 1961; 40: 723–730.

77. Carr CW. Studies on the binding of small ions in protein solutions with the use of membrane electrodes II. The binding of calcium ions in solutions of bovine serum albumin. Arch Biochem Biophys 1953; 43: 147–156.

78. Bronner F. Calcium homeostasis. In: Bronner F, Coburn JW, eds. Disorders of Mineral Metabolism. Vol. 2. New York: Academic Press, 1982: 43–102.

79. Roof BS, Piel CF, Hansen J, Fudenberg HH. Serum parathyroid hormone levels and serum calcium levels from birth to senescence. Mech Ageing Develop 1976; 5: 289–304.

80. Ryckewaert A, Ricket G, Lemaire V, Begue MC, Fenelon JP. Etude de la calcémie dans une population de 6048 hommes. Variation avec l'age. Correlations avec d'autres valeurs biologiques. Rev Rheumat 1974; 41: 473–478.

81. Franke H, Gall L, Gross W, Mull E, Weisshaar D. Klinisch-chemische Befunde bei 41 Hundertjährigen und Vergleich mit jüngeren Altersstufen. Klin Wchschr 1973; 51: 183–190.

82. Edelman IS, Leibman J. Anatomy of body water and electrolytes. Am J Med 1959; 27: 256–277.

83. Robinson RA. Observations regarding compartments for tracer calcium in the body. In: Frost HM, ed. Bone Biodynamics. Boston: Little Brown, 1964: 423–439.

84. Bronner F, Sammon PJ, Nichols C, Stacey RE, Shah BG. Thyrocalcitonin and plasma calcium homeostasis in the rat. In: Talmage RV, Belanger LF, eds. Parathyroid Hormone and Thyrocalcitonin. Amsterdam and New York: Excerpta Medica, 1968: 353–369.

85. Bronner F, Bosco JJ, Stein WD. Acute plasma calcium regulation in rats: effect of vitamin D deficiency. Bone and Mineral 1989; 6: 141–154.

86. Copp DH, Moghadam H, Mensen ED, McPherson GD. The parathyroids and calcium homeostasis. In: Greep RO, Talmage RV, eds. The Parathyroids. Springfield, IL: C C Thomas, 1961: 203–219.

87. Bronner F, Stein WD. Modulation of bone calcium-binding sites regulates plasma calcium: an hypothesis. Calcif Tissue Int 1992; 50: 483–489.

88. Ray RD, Kawabata M, Galante J. Experimental studies of peripheral circulation and bone growth. Clin Orthop & Rel Res 1967; 54: 175–185.

89. Ray RD. Circulation and bone. In: Bourne GH, ed. The Biochemistry and Physiology of Bone. Vol. IV. New York: Academic Press 1976: 385–402.

90. Peacock M. Renal excretion of calcium. In: Nordin BEC, ed. Calcium in Human Biology. London & Berlin: Springer Verlag, 1988: 125–169.

91. Bronner F. Dynamics and function of calcium. In: Comar CL, Bronner F, eds. Mineral Metabolism—An Advanced Treatise. Vol. 2A. New York: Academic Press, 1964: 341–444.

92. Aubert JP, Milhaud G. Méthode de mesure des principales voies du métabolisme calcique chez l'homme. Biochim Biophys Acta 1960; 39: 112–139.

93. Thomas RO, Litovitz TA, Rubin MI, Geschickter CF. Dynamics of calcium metabolism. Time distribution of intravenously administered radiocalcium. Am J Physiol 1952; 169: 568–575.

94. Dacke CG, Shaw AJ. Studies of the rapid effects of parathyroid hormone and prostaglandins on ^{45}Ca uptake into chick and rat bone *in vivo*. J Endocrinol 1987; 115: 369–377.

95. Bronner F. Disposition of intraperitoneally injected calcium-45 in suckling rats. J Gen Physiol 1958; 41: 767–782.

96. Heaney RP. Calcium kinetics in plasma: as they apply to the measurements of bone formation and resorption rates. In: Bourne GH, ed. The Biochemistry and Physiology of Bone. Vol. IV. New York: Academic Press. 1976: 105–133.

97. Polig E, Jee WSS. Bone structural parameters, dosimetry and relative radiation risk in the beagle skeleton. Rad Res 1989; 120: 83–101.

98. Simmons DJ, Grynpas MD. Mechanisms of bone formation *in vivo*. In: Hall BK, ed. Bone: The Osteoblast and Osteocyte. Vol. 1, NJ: Telford Press, 1990: 193–302.

99. Spector WS, ed. Handbook of Biological Data. Philadelphia: Saunders, 1956: 584.

100. Sammon PJ, Stacey RE, Bronner F. Further studies on the role of thyrocalcitonin in calcium homeostasis and metabolism. Biochem Med 1969; 3: 252–270.

101. Miller SS, Wolf AM, Arnaud CD. Bone cells in culture: morphologic transformation by hormones. Science 1976; 192: 1340–1342.

102. Sato M, Rodan GA. Bone cell shape and function. In: Stein WD, Bronner F, eds. Cell Shape Determinants, Regulation and Regulatory Role. New York: Academic Press, 1989: 329–362.

103. Jee WSS. Introduction to skeletal function: structural and metabolic aspects. In: Bronner F, Worrell RV, eds. A Basic Science Primer in Orthopaedics. Baltimore: Williams & Wilkins, 1991: 3–34.

104. Chambers TJ, McSheehy PMJ, Thompson BM, Fuller K. The effect of calcium regulating hormones and prostaglandins on bone resorption by osteoclasts disaggregated from neonatal rabbit bones. Endocrinology 1985; 60: 234–239.

105. Boyde A, Jones SJ. Early scanning electron microscopic studies of hard tissue resorption: their relation to current concepts reviewed. Scanning Microsc 1987; 1: 369–381.

106. Kream BE, Rowe DW, Givorek SC, Raisz LG. Parathyroid hormone alters collagen synthesis and procollagen mRNA levels in fetal rat calvaria. Proc Natl Acad Sci (USA) 1980; 77: 5654–5658.

107. Raisz LG, Kream BE, Smith M, Simmons HA. Comparison of the effects of vitamin D metabolites on collagen synthesis and resorption of fetal rat bone in organ culture. Calcif Tissue Int 1980; 32: 135–138.

108. Rodan GA, Martin TJ. Role of osteoblasts in hormonal control of bone resorption—a hypothesis. Calcif Tissue Int 1981; 33: 349–351.

109. Bronner F, Golub EE, Fischer JA. The effect of vitamin D on renal calcium clearance. In: Fleisch H, Robertson WG, Smith LH, Vahlensieck W, eds. Urolithiasis Research. New York: Plenum, 1976: 383–388.

110. McMillan PJ, Dewri RA, Joseph EE, Schultz RL, Deftos LJ. Rapid changes of light microscopic indices of osteoclast-bone relationships correlated with electron microscopy. Calcif Tissue Int 1989; 44: 399–405.

111. Thompson DD, Seedor JG, Weinreb M, Rosini S, Rodan GA. Aminohydroxybutane biphosphonate inhibits bone loss due to immobilization in rats. J Bone and Mineral Res 1990; 5: 279–286.

112. Bockman RS, Repo MA, Worrell RP Jr, et al. Distribution of trace levels of therapeutic gallium in bone as mapped by synchrotron x-ray microscopy. Proc Natl Acad Sci (USA) 1990; 87: 4149–4153.

113. Hall TJ, Chambers TJ. Gallium inhibits bone resorption by a direct effect on osteoclasts. Bone and Mineral 1990; 8: 211–216.

114. Shaw AJ, Dacke CG. Cyclic nucleotides and the rapid inhibitions of bone ^{45}Ca uptake in response to bovine parathyroid hormone and 16,16-dimethyl prostaglandin E_2 in chicks. Calcif Tissue Int 1989; 44: 209–213.

115. Sachs F. Ion channels as mechanical transducers. In: Stein WD, Bronner F, eds. Cell Shape. Determinants, Regulation and Regulatory Role. San Diego, CA: Academic Press, 1989: 63–92.

116. Rodan GA, Bourret LA, Harvey A, Mensi T. 3′,5′-cyclic AMP and 3′,5′-cyclic GMP: mediators of the mechanical effects on bone remodeling. Science 1975; 189: 467–469.

117. Weinman DT, Kelly PJ, Owen CA, Orvis AL. Skeletal clearance of Ca^{47} and Sr^{85} and skeletal blood flow in dogs. Proc Staff Meetings, Mayo Clin 1963; 38: 559–570.

118. Brandfonbrener M, Landowne M, Shock NW. Changes in cardiac output with age. Circulation 1955; 12: 559–570.

119. Care AD, Cooper CW, Duncan J, Orimo H. A study of thyrocalcitonin secretion by direct measurement of in vivo secretion rates in pigs. Endocrinology 1986; 83: 161–169.

120. Tsukamoto Y, Suki WN, Liang CT, Sacktor B. Ca^{2+}-dependent ATPases in the basolateral membranes of rat kidney cortex. J Biol Chem 1986; 261: 2718–2724.

121. Lin HS, Fain JN. Ca^{2+}-Mg^{2+}-ATPase in rat hepatocyte plasma membranes: inhibition by vasopressin and purification of the enzyme. In: Bronner F, Peterlik M, eds. Epithelial Calcium and Phosphate Transport: Molecular and Cellular Aspects. New York: Liss, 1984: 25–31.

122. Gerok W, Helmann C, Spamer C. Regulation of intracellular calcium by endoplasmic reticulum of hepatocytes. In: Bronner F, ed. Intracellular Calcium Regulation. New York: Liss, 1990: 139.

123. Somylo AP, Bond M, Somlyo AV. Calcium content of mitochondria and endoplasmic reticulum in liver frozen rapidly in vivo. Nature 1985; 314: 622–625.

124. Lehninger AL, Fiskum G, Vercesi A, Tew W. Ca^{2+} transport by mitochondria: a survey. In: Bronner F, Peterlik M, eds. Calcium and Phosphate Transport Across Biomembranes. New York: Academic Press, 1981: 73–82.

125. Crompton M. Role of mitochondria in intracellular calcium regulation. In: Bronner F, ed. Intracellular Calcium Regulation. New York: Wiley-Liss, 1990: 181–209.

126. Streb H, Irvine RF, Berridge MJ, Schultz J. Release of Ca^{2+} from a non-mitochondrial intracellular store in pancreatic acinar cells by inositol-1,4,5-triphosphate. Nature 1983; 306: 67–69.

127. Petersen OH. Regulation of calcium entry in cells that do not fire action potentials. In: Bronner F, ed. Intracellular Calcium Regulation. New York: Wiley-Liss, 1990: 77–96.

128. McCarty NA, O'Neill RG. Calcium signaling in cell volume regulation. Physiol Rev 1992; 72: 1037–1061.

129. Bement WM. Signal transduction by calcium and protein kinase C during egg activation. J Exp Zool 1992; 263: 382–391.

130. Shen SS. Calcium signaling at fertilization. Curr Opin Genet Devel 1992; 2: 642–646.

131. Villereal ML. Calcium signals in growth factor signal transduction. Rev Physiol, Biochem, Pharmacol 1992; 119: 67–121.

132. Cheek TR. Calcium signalling and the triggering of secretion in adrenal chromaffin cells. Pharmacol Therapeut 1991; 52: 173–189.

133. Augustine GJ, Adler EM, Charlton MP. The calcium signal for transmitter secretion from presynaptic nerve terminals. Ann NY Acad Sci 1991; 635: 365–381.

134. Rink TJ, Sage SO. Calcium signaling in human platelets. Annu Rev Physiol 1990; 52: 431–449.

135. Muallem S. Calcium transport by resting and stimulated cells. In: Bronner F, ed. Intracellular Calcium Regulation. New York: Wiley-Liss, 1989: 349–380.

136. Thomas AP, Renard DC. Spatial and temporal organization of calcium signalling in hepatocytes. Cell Calcium 1991; 12: 111–126.

137. Langer GA. Calcium and the heart: exchange at the tissue, cell, and organelle levels. FASEB J 1992; 6: 893–902.

138. Miller RJ, Fox AP. Voltage-positive calcium channels. In: Bronner F, ed. Intracellular Calcium Regulation. New York: Wiley-Liss, 1990: 97–138.

139. Carafoli E. Sarcolemmal calcium pump. In: Langer GA, ed. Calcium and the Heart. New York: Raven Press, 1990: 109–126.

140. Bronner F, Lemaire R. Comparison of calcium kinetics in man and the rat. Calcif Tiss Res 1969; 3: 238–248.

141. vander Rest M. The collagens of bone. In: Hall BK, ed. Bone. Vol. 3. Bone Matrix and Bone Specific Products. Boca Raton, FL: CRC Press, 1991: 187–237.

142. Cole DEC, Hanley DA. Osteocalcin. In: Hall BK, ed. Bone. Vol. 3. Bone Matrix and Bone Specific Products. Boca Raton, FL: CRC Press, 1991: 239–294.

143. Tracy RP, Mann KG. Osteonectin. In: Hall BK, ed. Bone. Vol. 3. Bone Matrix and Bone Specific Products. Boca Raton, FL: CRC Press, 1991: 295–319.

144. Sammon PJ, Stacey RE, Bronner F. Role of parathyroid hormone in calcium homeostasis and metabolism. Am J Physiol 1970; 218: 479–485.

145. Bronner F, Richelle LJ, Saville PD, Nicholas JA, Cobb JR. Quantitation of calcium metabolism in postmenopausal osteoporosis and in scoliosis. J Clin Invest 1963; 42: 898–905.

146. Lemaire RG, Lance EM. Etude cinétique du métabolisme calcique chez des rats parathyroidectomisés, porteurs d'implants thyroparathyroidiens autologues ou homologues. In: Richelle LJ, Dallemagne MJ, Blackwood HJJ, Lloyd E, Dulce HJ, eds. Calcified Tissues. Proceedings of the Second European Symposium. Coll des Colloques de l'Universite de Liege, 1965: 417–429.

147. Bronner F. Renal calcium transport: mechanisms and regulation—an overview. Am J Physiol 1989; 257 (Renal Fluid Electrolyte Physiol 126): F707–F711.

148. Ullrich KJ, Rumrick G, Kloss S. Acute Ca^{2+} reabsorption in the proximal tubule of the rat kidney. Dependence on sodium- and buffer transport. Pflüger's Arch 1976; 364: 223–228.

149. Bronner F, Stein WD. CaBPr facilitates intracellular diffusion for Ca pumping in distal convoluted tubule. Am J Physiol 1988; 255 (Renal Fluid Electrolyte Physiol 24): F558–F562.

150. Costanzo LS, Windhager EE. Calcium and sodium transport by the distal convoluted tubule of the rat. Am J Physiol 1978; 235 (Renal Fluid Electrolyte Physiol 4): F492–F506.

151. Taylor AN, McIntosh JE, Bourdeau JE. Immunocytochemical localization of vitamin D-dependent calcium-binding protein in renal tubules of rabbit, rat and chick. Kidney Int 1982; 21: 765–773.

152. Christakos S, Iacobino AM, Li H, Lee S, Gill R. Regulation of calbindin-D_{28K} gene expression. In: Pansu D, Bronner F, eds. Calcium Transport and Intracellular Calcium Homeostasis. Berlin: Springer Verlag, 1990: 339–346.

153. Christakos S, Brunette MG, Norman AW. Localization of immunoreactive vitamin D-dependent calcium-binding protein in chick nephron. Endocrinology 1981; 109: 322–324.

154. Yang JM, Lee CO, Windhager EE. Regulation of cytosolic free calcium in isolated perfused proximal tubules of *Necturus*. Am J Physiol 1988; 255 (Renal Fluid Electrolyte Physiol 24): F787–F799.

155. Palmer LG, Frindt G. Effects of cell Ca and pH on Na channels from rat cortical collecting tubules. Am J Physiol 1987; 253 (Renal Fluid Electrolyte Physiol 22): F333–F339.

156. Yates AJP, Gutierrez GE, Smoleus P, et al. Effects of synthetic peptide of a parathyroid hormone-related protein on calcium homeostasis, renal tubular calcium reabsorption, and bone metabolism in vivo and in vitro in rodents. J Clin Invest 1988; 81: 932–938.

157. Erlinger S. Physiology of bile secretion and enterohepatic circulation. In: Johnson LR, Christensen J, Jacobson ED, Jackson MJ, Walsh, JHW, eds. Physiology of the Gastrointestinal Tract. 2d ed. Vol. 2. New York: Raven Press, 1987: 1557–1580.

158. Powell D. Intestinal water and electrolyte transport. In: Johnson LR, Christensen J, Jacobson ED, Jackson MJ, Walsh JHW, eds. Physiology of the Gastrointestinal Tract. Vol. 2 2d ed. New York: Raven Press, 1987: 1267–1305.

159. Bronner F. The calcitropic hormones: parathyroid hormone, calcitonin and vitamin D. In: Bronner F, Worrell RV, eds. A Basic Science Primer in Orthopaedics. Baltimore: Williams & Wilkins, 1991: 91–103.

160. Fischer JA. Parathyroid hormone. In: Bronner F, Coburn J, eds. Disorders of Mineral Metabolism. Vol. 2. New York: Academic Press, 1982: 271–358.

161. Habener JF. Regulation of parathyroid hormone secretion and biosynthesis. Annu Rev Physiol 1981; 43: 211–223.

162. Habener JF, Potts JT Jr. Fundamental considerations in the physiology, biology and biochemistry of parathyroid hormone. In: Avioli LV, Krane SM, eds. Metabolic Bone Disease and Clinically Related Disorders. Philadelphia: Saunders, 1990: 69–130.

163. Aurbach GD. Calcium-regulating hormones: parathyroid hormone and calcitonin. In: Nordin B, ed. Calcium in Human Biology. Berlin: Springer Verlag, 1988: 43–68.

164. Thomasset M, Cuisinier-Gleizes P, Mathieu H, Golub EE, Bronner F. Regulation of intestinal calcium-binding protein in rats: role of parathyroid hormone. Calcif Tissue Int 1979; 29: 141–145.

165. Wong KM, Klein L. Circadian variations in contributions of bone and intestine to plasma calcium in dogs. Am J Physiol 1984; 246 (Regulat Integrative Comp Physiol 15): R688–R692.

166. Chase LR, Aurbach GD. Parathyroid function and the renal excretion of 3',5'-adenylic acid. Proc Natl Acad Sci (USA) 1967; 58: 518–525.

167. Massry SG. Renal handing of calcium. In: Bronner F, Coburn J, eds. Disorders of Mineral Metabolism. Vol. 2. New York: Academic Press, 1982: 189–235.

168. Norman AW, Litwack G. Hormones. Orlando, FL: Academic Press, 1987.

169. Deftos LJ. Calcitonin Secretion. In: Bronner F, Coburn JW, eds. Disorders of Mineral Metabolism. Vol. 2. New York: Academic Press, 1982: 433–479.

170. Brain SD, Williams TJ, Tippins JR. Calcitonin-gene related peptide is a potent dilator. Nature 1985; 313: 54–56.

171. Malgaroli A, Medolesi J, Zambonin Zallone A, Teti A. Control of cytosolic free calcium in rat and chicken osteoclasts. The role of extracellular calcium and calcitonin. J Biol Chem 1989; 264: 14342–14347.

172. Teti A, Zambonin Zallone A. Control of cytosolic calcium in osteoclasts in vitro. In: Bronner F, Peterlik M, eds. Extra- and Intracellular Calcium Regulation: From Basic Research to Clinical Medicine. Boca Raton, FL: CRC Press, 1992: 113–118.

173. Melvin KEW, Tashjian AH, Bordier P. The metabolic significance of calcitonin-secreting thyroid carcinoma. In: Frame B, Parfitt AM, Duncan H, eds. Clinical Aspects of Metabolic Bone Disease. Excerpta Medica, Amsterdam, 1973: 193–201.

174. Collins ED, Norman AW. Vitamin D. In: Machlin LG, ed. Handbook of Vitamins. New York: Dekker, 1991: 59–98.

175. Weiser MM, Bloor JH, Dasmahapatra A, Freedman RA, Maclaughlin JA. Vitamin D-dependent rat intestinal Ca^{2+} transport. Ca^{2+} uptake by Golgi membranes and early nuclear events. In: Bronner F, Peterlik M, eds. Calcium and Phosphate Transport Across Biomembranes. New York: Academic Press, 1981: 264–273.

176. Christakos S, Gill R, Lee S, Li H. Molecular aspects of the calbindins. J Nutr 1992; 122: 678–682.

177. Price PA. GLA-containing proteins of mineralized tissues. In: Slavkin H, Price P, eds. Chemistry and Biology of Mineralized Tissues. Amsterdam: Excerpta Medica, 1992: 169–176.

178. Bronner F. Vitamin D deficiency and rickets. Am J Clin Nutr 1976; 29: 1307–1314.

179. Ernst M, Schmid CH, Froesch ER. Enhanced osteoblast proliferation and collagen gene expression by estradiol. Proc Natl Acad Sci (USA) 1988; 85: 2307–2310.

180. Colvard DS, Eriksen EF, Keeting PE, et al. Identification of androgen receptors in normal human osteoblast-like cells. Proc Natl Acad Sci (USA) 1989; 86: 854–857.

181. Oursler MJ, Osdoby P, Pyfferoen J, Riggs BL, Spelsberg TC. Avian osteoclasts as estrogen target cells. Proc Natl Acad Sci (USA) 1991; 88: 6613–6617.

182. Jilka RL, Hangoc G, Girasole G, et al. Increased osteoclast development after estrogen loss: mediation by interleukin-6. Science 1992; 257: 88–91.

183. Fukayama S, Tashjian AH, Jr. Direct modulation by estradiol of the response of human bone cells (SaOS-2) to human parathyroid hormone and PTH-related protein. Endocrinology 1989; 124: 397–401.

184. Fukayama S, Tashjian AH Jr. Direct modulation by androgens of the response of human bone cells (SaOS-2) to human parathyroid hormone (PTH) and PTH-related proteins. Endocrinology 1989; 125: 1789–1794.

185. Rude R, Singer F. Hormonal modifiers of mineral metabolism other than parathyroid hormone, vitamin D and calcitonin. In: Bronner F, Coburn JW, eds. Disorders of Mineral Metabolism. Vol. 2. New York: Academic Press, 1982: 481–556.

186. Albright F, Reifenstein EC. The parathyroid glands and metabolic bone disease. Selected studies. Baltimore: Williams & Wilkins, 1948.

187. Massry SG, Coburn JW. The hormonal and non-hormonal control of renal excretion of calcium and magnesium. Nephron 1973; 10: 66–112.

188. Schryver HF. The effect of hydrocortisone on chondroitin sulfate production and loss by embryonic chick tibiotarsi in organ culture. Exp Cell Res 1965; 40:610–618.

189. Doughaday WH, Mariz IK. Conversion of proline-U-C^{14} to labelled hydroxyproline by rat cartilage in vitro: effects of hypophysectomy, growth hormone, and cortisol. J Lab Clin Med 1962; 59: 741–751.

190. Kivirikko KI, Laitenen O, Lamberg BA. Value of urine and serum hydroxyproline in the diagnosis of thyroid disease. J Clin Endocrinol Metab 1965; 25: 1347–1352.

191. Mundy GR, Shapiro JL, Baudelin JG, Canalis EM, Raisz LG. Direct stimulation of bone resorption by thyroid hormones. J Clin Invest 1976; 58: 529–534.

192. Krane SM, Goldring SR. Hypothyroidism. Skeletal system. In: Werner SC, Ingbar SH, eds. The Thyroid. Hagerstown, MD: Harper & Row 1978: 892–900.

193. Wood RJ, Allen LH, Bronner F. Regulation of calcium metabolism in streptozotocin-induced diabetes. Am J Physiol 1984; 247 (Regulatory Integrative Comp Physiol): R120–R123.

194. Stern PH, Bell NH. Effect of glucagon on serum calcium in the rat and on bone resorption *in vitro*. J Pharmacol Exp Therapeut 1970; 168: 211–217.

195. Kahn DN, Hillyard C, Foster GV. Effect of glucagon on bone collagen metabolism in the rat. J Endocrinol 1972; 55: 245–252.

196. Avioli LV. Epidemiology of osteoporosis and its complications. In: Peck WA, ed. Prevention of Postmenopausal Osteoporosis—Dream or Reality? Park Ridge, NJ: Parthenon, 1990: 11–19.

197. Matkovic V, Kostial K, Simonovic I, Buzina R, Brodarec A, Nordin BEC. Bone status and fracture rate in two regions of Yugoslavia. Am J Clin Nutr 1979; 32: 540–549.

198. Garn SM. The earlier gain and later loss of cortical bone in nutritional perspective. Springfield, IL: C C Thomas, 1970.

199. Riis B, Thomsen K, Christiansen C. Does calcium supplementation prevent postmenopausal bone loss? N Engl J Med 1987; 316: 173–177.

200. Lindsay R, Cosman F. Estrogen therapy: benefits and risks in osteoporosis therapy. In: Peck WA, ed. Prevention of Postmenopausal Osteoporosis—Dream or Reality? Park Ridge, NJ: Parthenon, 1990: 29–42.

201. Nilas L, Christiansen C. Rates of bone loss in normal women: evidence of accelerated trabecular bone loss after the menopause. Eur J Clin Invest 1988; 18: 529–534.

202. Aitkeen JM, Hart DM, Anderson JB, Lindsay R, Smith DA. Osteoporosis after oophorectomy for non-malignant disease. Br Med J 1973; 1: 325–328.

203. Horowitz MC. Cytokines and estrogen in bone: antiosteoporotic effect. Science 1993; 260: 626–628.

204. Heaney RP, Recker RR, Saville PD. Menopausal changes in calcium balance performance. J Lab Clin Med 1978; 92: 953–963.

205. Bronner F. Calcium transport across epithelia. Int Rev Cytol 1991; 131: 169–212.

206. Pansu D, Bellaton C, Bronner F. Developmental changes in the mechanisms of duodenal calcium transport in the rat. Am J Physiol 1983; 244 (Gastrointest Liver Physiol 7): G20–G26.

3

Phosphorus

YITSHAL N. BERNER
Harzfeld Geriatric Hospital, Kaplan Medical Center, Gedera, Israel

Phosphorus is the sixth most abundant element in the human body, amounting to 500–700 g in the human body. Most of the phosphorus in nature is combined with oxygen in the form of phosphate. Phosphate in the form of a structural crystal gives strength to the bones. Combined with glycerol, fatty acids, and certain amines, in the form of phospholipids, it provides structural substance for the cell membrane, providing a barrier between two media. Phosphate in the form of nucleotides serves as a source of a high free-energy bond and performs an important function in conserving and providing bursts of metabolic energy. It is involved in many metabolic pathways, including particularly those involved in energy transformation and those involved in transcription and transduction of the genetic information. It is commonly a component of the enzyme cofactors derived from water-soluble vitamins. A summary of the types of biologically important phosphorus compounds is presented in Table 1. The regulation of phosphate homeostasis in the human body depends on many metabolic pathways. A special regulatory mechanism, the parathyroid hormone–vitamin D-thyrocalcitonin axis, is involved in the control of both calcium and phosphorus balance. This hormonal axis controls the absorption rate in the gut, the excretion rate in the kidney, and the storage capacity of bones. Therefore, phosphorus is involved in a multitude of process in the entire life cycle, serving both structural and catalytic functions.

I. CHEMISTRY

The element phosphorus (P) has an atomic number of 15 and an atomic weight of 30.97; in nature it has valencies of 3 and 5 and exists as only one isotope, ^{31}P. Only valence-5 phosphorus, phosphate, is commonly found in the body. The element was named according

TABLE 1 Types of Biologically Important Compounds

Type	Example	Function
Nucleic acids	DNA	Storage of genetic information
	RNA	Transcription of DNA and protein synthesis
Phospholipid	Phosphatidyl choline	Structural component of membranes
Bone salt	Hydroxyapatite	Bone structure and function
Phosphoprotein	Casein	Nutrient storage
Sugar phosphate	Glucose-6-P	Glycolysis
Nucleotides	ATP	Energy transformations, molecular activation
	cAMP	Second messenger
	Uridine di-P glucose	Glycogen synthesis

to its appearance; in ancient Greek it means "light bearing." It was also the ancient name for the planet Venus when it appeared before sunrise. Phosphorus exists in several different allotropic forms: white, with a melting point of 44.1°C, a boiling point of 280°C, and a specific gravity of 1.82 g/cm^3; red and black, which are heavier, with specific gravities of 2.2 and 2.69, respectively (1). Ordinary P is a white solid, soluble in carbon disulfide but insoluble in water. When exposed to ultraviolet light or heated to its own vapor at 250°C, it is converted to the red variety which does not phosphoresce in air and is fairly stable. Elemental phosphorus is not found free in nature, but is combined with various other elements in the form of inorganic minerals or as components of organic compounds.

Of the five outermost electrons of the P atom, which determine valence, two occupy an s orbital and three unpaired electrons occupy p orbitals. Phosphorus can give rise to trivalent compounds, but the biologically most important form is the pentavalent oxygen compound, phosphate (PO_4^{3-}).

A. Organic Phosphates

Organic phosphate compounds are typically colorless liquids or solids. Those that play a major role in biology are phosphate esters, $RO\text{-}PO(OH)_2$, and their salts. Phosphate occurs in the form of mono-, di-, and triphosphoesters. For example, the genetic code is carried by a diester, DNA, which is based on a phosphate ester backbone with deoxyribose. Nucleoside triphosphates, such as adenosine triphosphate, are crucial to phosphate transfer-phosphorylation, a key reaction for the transfer of energy from food to useful work. Each form has specific chemical properties leading to different biologic function.

B. Determination and Measurement

Although phosphorus exists in the body as phosphate, historically its concentration has been expressed as elemental phosphorus. Determination of the P concentration in plasma and other body fluids is the most common way to evaluate physiological status. Urinary concentrations determine mainly how the kidneys handle phosphate. In all of these methods the phosphate concentration is measured by the Fiske-Subbarow colorimetric method (63). Commonly the results have been reported as the concentration of the element in units of mass per volume, but moles per volume is preferable. Although extracellular fluid phosphate concentration is the most common phosphate status evaluation, it represents only 1% of the total body phosphorus.

The only way in the past to determine P content in different tissues was to ash them, and then to use one of the analytical methods. Since the advent of body-imaging systems based on nuclear magnetic resonance measurement, it is possible to detect phosphate in different tissues in vivo and determine changes with time under different conditions. This method is now being studied mainly with the human liver and heart. It will likely supply much data in the future on biochemical and physiologic processes. These methods open the most fascinating horizons for understanding the role of phosphorus in different metabolic pathways.

II. TISSUE CONCENTRATIONS AND METABOLISM

Phosphorus makes up approximately 1% of body weight. As illustrated in Figure 1, approximately 85% is in hard tissue, bone. This serves as the main body reservoir of P as well as a structural function, mainly in the form of hydroxyapatite crystals. Approximately 14% of the P is found in soft tissue, where it serves both structural and metabolic roles. Only 1% is found in the extracellular fluids, the only readily accessible source for P analysis and assessment of physiologic status.

The widespread structural and metabolic functions of phosphate makes it essential for the utilization of other nutrients, particularly N in all of its forms. Tissues contain relatively constant ratios of N and other elements; however, in adult nonskeletal tissue, the N:P:Na:K:Cl ratio is 1:0.06:1.2:3.0:0.72 (3), while in the muscle it is 1:2.03:0.93:3.2:0.69 (4). An adequate supply of N without adequate phosphate results in suboptimal utilization of N (3). We have previously described the distribution of P in the human body (5).

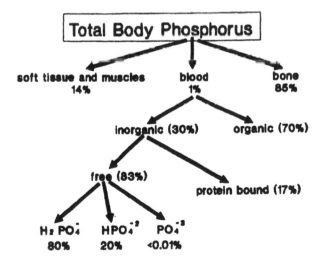

FIGURE 1 Distribution of phosphorus in the human body. Of the 500–700 g of total phosphorus, most occurs in hard tissues and only 1% in blood. Approximately 30% of the latter (0.3%) exists as inorganic phosphate ions, the component most commonly sampled for diagnosis.

A. Bone

In bone, phosphate is a constituent of crystalline hydroxyapatite, $Ca_{10}(PO_4)_6(OH)_2$, which is deposited in the organic matrix during the mineralization process and gives bone its strength. Its crystal structure is depicted in Figure 2. Phosphorus is essential for bone mineralization; a deficiency interrupts this process and results in osteomalacia. The ratio of P to Ca in the bone is normally 1:2 (6). Crystalline hydroxyapatite, as a hexagonal plate, has an extremely small crystal size, about 500 Å, and provides a large surface area, 100 m^2 per gram. The unique properties of the crystal are due to its structure. It is built from columns of calcium ions and the oxygen atoms of the phosphate molecule. These substances form the walls of the channels which run parallel to the hexagonal axis. Hydroxyl groups lie inside the channels (Fig. 2).

B. Soft Tissues

In soft tissues phosphate plays various roles, as a structural component, as a factor in intermediate metabolism, and as a component of genetic material. Phospholipids are major constituents of cell membranes and intracellular organelles. The most common phospholipid is phosphatidylcholine, previously termed lecithin. Its hydrophilic–hydrophobic poles, as it exists in cell membranes, makes it an excellent compound for separation of various aqueous media (Fig. 3). The specific role of some other phospholipids has been described; phosphatidylethanolamine and phosphatidylcholine are important ones, with crucial roles in the cellular immune response. Table 1 provides examples of the wide distribution of phosphorus containing compounds in living sustems and their many different functions.

C. Absorption

Phosphate is absorbed all along the intestinal tract, with the jejunum being the most active absorptive site (43,44). Approximately 200 mg/day is excreted into the gastrointestinal (GI) tract with the digestive juices (45), and about two-thirds of this is reabsorbed (46). Saliva and bile acids are the most important GI secretory fluids of phosphate (47). Studies in both

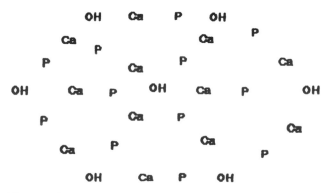

FIGURE 2 Schematic structure of hydroxyapatite. The hydroxyapatite crystal is a hexagonal plate and the lattice is built from columns of calcium ions (Ca) and the oxygen atoms of the phosphate anion (P). These ions form channels which contain the hydroxyl ions (OH) and run parallel to the axis of the crystal. This structure provides the unique properties of the crystal, small size and large surface area.

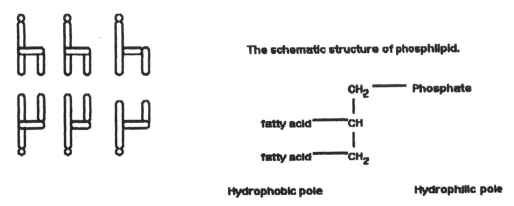

The schematic structure of phospholipid.

Hydrophobic pole   Hydrophilic pole

FIGURE 3 Orientation of phospholipids in membranes. The bilayer structure of cellular membranes is depicted on the left and the structure of a diacylglycerol phosphate on the right. For example, the hydrophilic pole, i.e., the phosphate and organic bases, is on the inside and the hydrophobic pole is on the outside of the plasma membrane. This provides a barrier between the aqueous media inside and outside the cell.

animals and humans suggest two mechanisms for intestinal absorption of phosphate. The first, which takes place mainly in the proximal intestine, is a sodium-dependent, active transport and can be blocked by arsenate, diphosphonate, mercury (48), and calcitonin (49,50). This active transport can be enhanced by $1,25(OH)_2D_3$ and is linearly related to the Na concentration in the GI lumen (48). The second mechanism operates mainly in the jejunum and ileum and is linearly related to the phosphate concentration in the intestinal lumen (48). When the oral phosphate intake is low, the reduced intraluminal phosphate concentration does not allow passive diffusion, and active absorption in the proximal small bowel becomes the main absorptive mechanism. Studies with lambs showed that the fecal P excretion is significanlty decreased on very low phosphate diets with high Ca content (51).

The intestinal absorption of phosphate is influenced by the endocrine system and by interaction with other substances in the intestinal lumen. Vitamin D enhances phosphate absorption independently of its effect on Ca absorption. Of the vitamin D metabolites, $1,25-(OH)_2D_3$ seems to be the most active in enhancing phosphate intestinal absorption (52–55). Other forms of vitamin D, such as $24,25-(OH)_2D_3$, were not found to be active in phosphate absorption in the rat jejunum (56). Parathyroid hormone indirectly enhances intestinal phosphate absorption by stimulating the synthesis of $1,25-(OH)_2D_3$ in the kidney. Calcium has both direct and indirect effects on intestinal phosphate absorption: The direct effect is mediated through formation of insoluble complexes with phosphate in the intestinal lumen, thus decreasing the bioavailability and absorption of both phosphate and Ca (57); the indirect effect is mediated through the effect of Ca on vitamin D metabolism. The synthesis of $1,25-(OH)_2D_3$ is inversely related to the serum Ca concentration (42,58) and is independent of PTH (59). As noted above, $1,25-(OH)_2D_3$ enhances intestinal phosphate absorption. An overabundance of Ca in the GI tract, with a Ca:P ratio greater than 3, can result in decreased phosphate absorption and deficiency (60,61).

The P in foods originating from plants is mainly in the form of phytic acid (120), and P absorption requires the presence of the enzyme phytase in the gut; the activity of this enzyme rises with increased phytate consumption. Phosphorus from animal food sources is more available.

D. Transport

The normal plasma levels of phosphate in the adult range between 2.2 and 4.4 mg/dL (0.7–1.4 mmol/L), with values approximately 50% higher in babies and 30% higher in children (64,65); these higher levels in the pediatric group are considered to be secondary to the effects of growth hormone (28,46). Plasma phosphate serves as an exchange pool between the various phosphate-containing and -regulating organs (intestines, bones, kidneys); cellular phosphates also serve as buffers due to their buffering capacity, derived from the $HPO_4^{2-}/H_2PO_4^-$ balance according to the Henderson-Hasselbach equation. These ions account for about 5% of the nonbicarbonate buffer capacity of plasma.

   Approximately 70% of blood phosphate is present as a constituent of phospholipids; the remaining 30% is inorganic phosphate (orthophosphate). At physiologic pH, approximately 80% of the free phosphate circulates in the form of HPO_4^{2-}, 20% as H_2PO4^-, with less than 0.01% actually as PO_4^{3-}. These anions are associated with counterions, Na, Ca, and Mg (46,62,63).

E. Excretion

The kidney is the main regulatory organ for maintenance of phosphate balance. In the healthy human, the kidney excretes phosphate in an amount equal to the net phosphate absorption in the gut (defined as the amount absorbed minus the endogenous excreted in the feces), thus maintaining a zero balance. The urinary phosphate excretion of individuals consuming an average American diet is 600–800 mg/day (11). In states of phosphate depletion, the kidney responds by reducing excretion virtually to zero, thus conserving body phosphate (71,73). Approximately 90% of the plasma phosphate is filtered at the glomerulus (74). No phosphate is excreted into the renal tubules (47). Renal phosphate reabsorption occurs mainly in the proximal tubule through an active process. This process is reduced with body water volume expansion (76).

   The fractional urinary excretion can vary between 0.1 and 20% (Fig. 4) and thus serves as a powerful homeostatic mechanism (77–79). The precise details of the tight regulation of phosphate reabsorption in the renal tubules have not been fully elucidated. It is known that the primary regulatory factors are the serum phosphate and, to a lesser degree, PTH (11). Increased serum phosphate enhances urinary excretion, while PTH reduces it.

III. REGULATION OF METABOLISM

Intestines, bones, and kidneys are the main organs involved in the maintenance of phosphate balance: The intestinal tract is the absorption organ; the kidneys are the most important excretion organ; and the bones serve as a reservoir of phosphate. The plasma levels of phosphate are not so closely controlled as those of Ca, although both share the same homeostatic hormones and are mostly stored in the same crystal in the bone (66).

   Phosphate metabolism is regulated by three different hormones, PTH, 1,25-$(OH)_2D_3$, and calcitonin. Vitamin D, and particularly its metabolite 1,25-$(OH)_2D_3$, is an important hormonal regulator of both Ca and phosphate levels in the blood. The activity of 1,25-$(OH)_2D_3$ is mediated by intracellular proteins. Vitamin D affects phosphate homeostasis and balance by the following mechanisms:

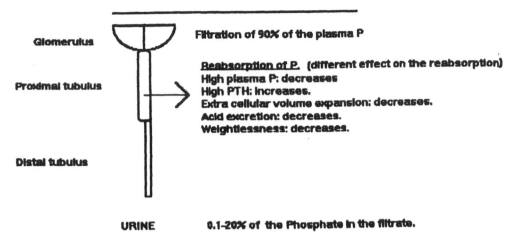

FIGURE 4 Kidney structure and the urinary excretion of phosphate. Approximately 90% of plasma phosphate is filtered at the glomerulus, and reabsorption occurs mainly in the proximal tubules by an active process. Factors that regulate reabsorption are listed. Depending on physiologic conditions, 0.1–20% of the glomerular filtrate appears in the urine.

1. Direct stimulation of intestinal absorption of phosphate (43,54,56).
2. Enhancement of bone resorption by mobilization of Ca and phosphate (38,43) into the plasma; this effect is independent of PTH. The metabolite 24,25-$(OH)_2D_3$ is thought to enhance bone mineralization (6,53,67–70) and thus removal of phosphate from the plasma into the bone.
3. The effect of vitamin D on the renal handling of phosphate is thought to be indirect: The increase in serum Ca mediated by 1,25-$(OH)_2D_3$ suppresses PTH secretion, and thus enhances phosphate reabsorption in the tubules (71,72).

The parathyroid hormone exerts its regulation primarily by way of the kidney, exerting a phosphaturic effect through cyclic adenosine 3′,5′-monophosphate (cAMP) in the tubular cells. It has been suggested (87) that cAMP, which stimulates protein kinase A, enhances gluconeogenesis. In the process, NAD^+ is produced, and this inhibits phosphate uptake across the brush borders of the tubular cells (87). The parathyroid hormone increases the activity of adenylate cyclase 10-fold in the proximal tubules (88), an effect which is not changed with low phosphate intake. Low phosphate intake increases significantly the phosphodiesterase activity and thus the tubular cAMP content (88). Propranolol was shown to restore the phosphaturic effect of PTH in short-term phosphate deprivation (89).

The conservation of phosphate by the kidney in phosphate-deprived animals does not depend on PTH (80,81) or vitamin D (67). During phosphate deprivation for a period as short as 2 days, transport of phosphate across the proximal tubules increases (82,83); with prolonged phosphate deprivation, the whole nephron conserves phosphate. In states of phosphate depletion, resistance develops to the phosphaturic effects of exogenous PTH (80,83–85). Thus, low serum level phosphate is the most potent regulator of phosphate conservation, acting both by enhancing the reabsorption in the tubules and by desensitizing the latter to the hyperphosphaturic effect of PTH and control of vitamin D hydroxylation (86). Decreased renal phosphate reabsorption also occurs as a result of increased plasma levels of phosphate, steroid hormones (90,91) and calcitonin (78), and of acute respiratory and metabolic acidosis (92–94).

Other factors also play a role in regulation. Recently, human studies showed that changes in titratable acid excretion were significantly correlated with the renal excretion of phosphate, and that this capacity decreased with aging (95). Phosphate-dependent Na-K transport also decreases with aging (96). Impaired phosphate excretion is manifested postprandially in patients with idiopathic calciuria and is responsible for transient idiopathic calciuria (97). Factors that increase phosphate reabsorption in the renal tubules include reduced dietary intake, insulin (98,99), thyroid hormone (100–103), growth hormone (104), glucagon (105), and metabolic (94,106) and respiratory (92) alkalosis. Extracellular volume expansion is associated with inhibition of phosphate reabsorption in the proximal tubule (76–78), while volume contraction enhances it (77,78,107,108). Diuretics have a phosphaturic effect which is mediated by different mechanisms. Furosemide increases urinary phosphate excretion indirectly; its calciuric effect enhances PTH secretion, which in turn inhibits tubular phosphate reabsorption (11,109,110). The carbonic anhydrase inhibitor Diamox diminishes phosphate reabsorption in the proximal tubules independently of the effect of PTH (111,112). Hypokalemia decreases the sensitivity of PTH receptors to the hormone (113–115), and this reduces phosphate urinary excretion. The atrial natriuretic factor (ANF) inhibits phosphate transport in rat kidney cells (116). Blockage of the dopamine I receptor significantly blunts the influence of ANF on urinary phosphate excretion (117). Studies of humans with cirrhosis demonstrated no effect of ANF on urinary phosphate excretion (118). Weightlessness in space flight is associated with increased phosphate excretion (119).

IV. DIETARY CONSIDERATIONS

The dietary intake of P can vary substantially with the types of foods consumed. Studies of the American diet reveal that the amount of ingested P has been stable since the beginning of this century, and averages approximately 800–1500 mg/day (121,122). Diets that provide sufficient protein and calories also contain P in adequate amounts, regardless of the source of protein, carbohydrates, and fat. Milk and diary products are the richest source of P in the diet, but P is widely available in other foods. Thus, hypophosphatemia and phosphate depletion secondary to inadequate dietary intake are extremely rare. However, the interaction of dietary P with other nutrients may affect the P status. A high-protein diet is associated with increased urinary excretion of calcium, sulfur, ammonia, and phosphate (123). Proper utilization of N requires an adequate supply of P (3). Wheat bran is known to affect the absorption of certain minerals, such as Ca and Fe, but does not affect P (124), while P may impair Fe absorption (125). Not all the P in our diet is of natural origin. Polyphosphates, which are created by heating orthophosphate, are popular additives (at concentrations up to 0.1–0.3%) in many meat products. They enhance the water-binding properties of the meat proteins. The dietary content of P was shown to regulate physiologically the serum concentration of PTH (126), and thus indirectly the phosphate homeostasis.

V. METABOLIC FUNCTIONS

A. Genetic Material

Phosphate is an essential part of the nucleic acids, DNA and RNA, although there is no evidence that it is ever limiting for their formation. However, the rate of protein phosphorylation, particularly of transcription factors, affects the rate of transcription and translation, thus protein production (7,231). In yeasts it has been shown that during the G_1 phase, phosphorylation occurs mainly on serine residues, and during the G_2 phase phosphorylation and dephosphorylation of threonine and tyrosine residues precede the cell's entry into mitosis (8). In bacteria (*Escherichia coli*), phosphotransacetylase and acetylphosphate synthesis are involved in the regulation of the genetic material expression (9).

B. High-Energy Compounds

Phosphate is a constituent of numerous highly active intracellular compounds. Release of free energy by hydrolysis of adenosine triphosphate (ATP) provides the main energy source for various metabolic processes and for muscle contraction. Table 2 lists the free energy of hydrolysis of phosphate bonds in several compounds involved in metabolism. Acetyl CoA, a nucleotide-containing thioester, is included for comparison with the "high-energy" phosphate ester bonds found in ATP.

In the frog muscle during resting conditions, approximately 0.09 kcal/g muscle is ready to use in the form of ATP, and 0.23 kcal/g muscle is stored in the form of creatine phosphate. Both of these compounds are refueled by the high-energy P bonds from the aerobic and anaerobic glycolytic pathways, which provide approximately 30–60 kcal/g and 1.2 kcal/g muscle, respectively (10). With the increase in the net O_2 consumption (VO_2), there is a reduction in the muscular creatine phosphate content, but the ATP and adenosine diphosphate (ADP) levels remain constant (10).

Intracellular phosphate is a regulator of enzymes in the glycolytic pathway (11,12). Within the erythrocyte, the concentration of 2,3-diphosphoglycerate (2,3-DPG) is of crucial importance in oxygen availability to the tissues. In phosphate deficiency, synthesis of 2,3-DPG is decreased, a condition with leads to greater affinity of oxygen to hemoglobin and thus reduces the amount of oxygen released to the tissues (13–15). Consequently, ATP production is decreased. In addition, there is irreversible degradation of AMP to inosine monophosphate (16), which creates a shortage of this ATP precursor. Phosphate has been shown to maintain ATP levels in stored red blood cells in vitro (17). The activity of Na,K-ATPase, which controls the intracellular concentrations of these major electrolytes, is affected by the type of amino acid at position 480, with in turn affects the kinetics of

TABLE 2 Free Energy of Hydrolysis

Compound	Energy (cal/mol)
Phosphoenolpyruvate	−14,800
1,3-Diphosphoglycerate	−11,800
Phosphocreatine	−10,300
ATP = AMP + PP	−8,600
Uridine diphosphate-glucose	−7,600
Acetyl CoA	−7,500
ATP = ADP + P	−7,300
ADP = AMP + P	−6,500
Glucose-1-P	−5,000
Fructose-6-P	−3,800
Glucose-6-P	−3,300
Glycerol-3-P	−2,200

phosphorylation and thus the enzyme activity (18). A rapid phosphate-dependent pathway is one of two pathways of adenine nucleotide loss from cells during ischemia (19). Phosphate high-energy bonds are reduced in ischemia and can be restored partially by the free-radical scavenger, superoxide dismutase (SOD) (20).

In the mitochondrion, phosphate-containing proteins play essential roles in the electron transport system. This process provides most of the metabolically useful energy from carbohydrates and lipids. The structure of the mitochondrial phosphate carrier protein was described recently (21); it consists of 312 amino acids. Like other mitochondrial transport proteins, the human phosphate carrier has a tripartite structure. Each of the three repeats contains hydrophobic regions which presumably span the membrane in the form of alpha helices. Figure 5 depicts the structure and its relation to the mitochondrial membrane.

The cardiac mitochondrial phosphate carrier in rats is modified with age (22). There is no difference in the respiratory control and ADP/O_2 ratio between young and old animals. The kinetic changes in the process occur only in the V_{max} but not in the K_m of the transport reaction (23). These phenomena are partially restored in rats by the addition of L-carnitine (24).

C. Phosphorylation and Catalytic Activity

Phosphorylation and dephosphorylation regulate many activities within cells, including the function of enzymes, hormones, and the transcription of genetic information. These reactions are catalyzed by phosphorylases (kinases) and phosphatases, respectively. The first enzyme whose activity was observed (25) to undergo phosphorylation and dephosphorylation was glycogen phosphorylase, the key enzyme that catalyzes the initial step in the breakdown of tissue glycogen to glucose 1-phosphate. This process, which requires the active form of phosphorylase (a), occurs in muscle cells stimulated with epinephrine and in liver cells stimulated with glucagon. Activation of phosphorylate b to phosphorylase a may be depicted by the following cascade of reactions:

Phosphorylase kinase + ATP ————————————→ Phosphorylase kinase(+P) + ADP
  cAMP-protein kinase

Phosphorylase b + ATP ————————————→ Phosphorylase a(+P) + ADP
  Phosphorylase kinase(+P)

The inactive (unphosphorylated) form of phosphorylase kinase has a high K_d for calcium, an ion that is essential for the reaction. Phosphorylase b is also inactive until phosphorylated. The enzymes are returned to the inactive or resting state by dephosphorylation

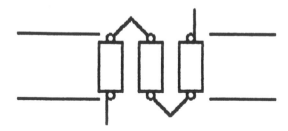

FIGURE 5 Schematic of the mitochondrial phosphate carrier. This 312-amino acid protein has a tripartite structure. Each of the three repeats contains two hydrophilic regions (symbolized with circles) and a hydrophobic region of alpha helices (rectangles) that spans the membrane.

reactions catalyzed by the respective phosphatases. The initial phosphorylation is catalyzed by a protein kinase that is activated by cAMP, the second messenger of several hormones. cAMP, whose formation from ATP is catalyzed by adenylate cyclase, was discovered by the late Earl Sutherland.

Other hormones whose activity is mediated by cAMP include the parathyroid hormone (PTH) and the antidiuretic hormone (ADH). Protein activity and concentration in the collecting ducts of the dog kidney affect adenylate cyclase activity (26). These changes are also correlated with acidosis (26) and thus influence the efficiency of PTH activity in various metabolic situations.

Phosphorylation plays a role in gene expression by increasing the function of transcription factors. For example, the phosphorylated form of Egr-1 (Early growth response-1) is bound more efficiently to its DNA binding element (231).

D. Growth Factors

Growth factors or cytokines are proteins that influence intracellular activities to induce mitosis, in some cases via activation of the enzyme tyrosine kinase.

Insulinlike growth factors stimulate Na-dependent phosphate transport in tissue cultures (27). The same effect was manifested with the growth hormone (GH) in a study of 16 children with GH deficiency (28). Thus, growth factors, in addition to acting through kinases, may influence phosphate metabolism. Oncogenes influence intracellular activity through the tyrosine kinase mechanism. P53 gene mutation with chromosome 17 deletion is common in colon carcinoma and breast cancer (29). The oncogenic activity induces the production of erg-1 mRNA (also known as NGFI-A, Zif/268 and Kro ×24). This phosphoprotein contains three Zn fingers and is rapidly and transiently induced by many growth factors (30). Another phosphoprotein-regulating gene expression is the tumor-suppressor gene RB (31), which is regulated by histone kinase. Estrogen binding to its response element (ERE) is affected by the sugar phosphate backbone of the ERE; the effect is achieved by electrostatic changes (32).

E. Phosphoproteins

Many other less well characterized phosphoproteins have been described. A partial list is presented in Table 3. Stathmin is involved in the regulation of cell proliferation, differentiation, and other functions (33). It is also suggested to play a general role as an intracellular relayer, integrating diverse regulating signals of the cell (34). GAP-43 (calmodulin) is a calcium-binding protein whose amino acid sites 41, 110, and 122 are occupied by serine. A

TABLE 3 Phosphoproteins

Substance	Function	Ref.
Stathmin	Cell proliferation and differentiation	33,34
Calmodulin	Intracellular calcium concentration	35
Synapsin, ARPP	Basal ganglia dopamine metabolism	36,37,38
Phosducsin	Bovine photoreceptor function	39
hsp90	Adaptation to stress	40
Glutaminase	NH_3 production; acid–base regulation	41,16

phosphorylated mutation at the 41 may affect the activity of the protein, as an activator of protein kinase (35).

Certain special phosphoproteins in the brain have been described. Synapsin (36) and the ARPP group of phosphoproteins (consisting of ARPP-16, ARPP-19, and ARPP-21) are located in the basal ganglia and other dopamine-innervated brain regions. They are rich in phosphate and are cAMP-regulated (37,38). Phosducsin is a soluble phosphoprotein isolated from bovine photoreceptor cells (39). The heat shock protein (hsp90) is responsible for the adaptation of animals to stress (40). This phosphoprotein acts to enhance the phosphorylation and dephosphorylation activities of different enzymes (40). Glutaminase is a phosphate-dependent enzyme located in the kidney (41), the brain—mainly in the cerebellum, hippocampus, and striatum (42)—and the heart (16). In the rat, acidosis enhances renal glutaminase activity (41). Glutaminase is activated through the cAMP mechanism stimulated by PTH. Thus, phosphate levels and balance influence the entire spectra of energy utilization and protein production enzymes.

VI. PHOSPHORUS DEFICIENCY OR IMBALANCE

The significance of hypophosphatemia is related to the clinical setting in which it occurs. It can be a manifestation of total body phosphate deficiency, resulting in the potentially lethal phosphate deficiency syndrome. It can also be a result of acute phosphate shifts from the serum into the cells; as long as such shifts occur without prior intracellular phosphate depletion, the condition is usually benign and not associated with significant intracellular metabolic alterations. As noted previously, less than 1% of body phosphate is found in the extracellular space. Consequently, even small shifts of less than 200 mg of phosphate from the extracellular fluids into the cells can induce significant changes in the serum phosphate level.

A. Hypophosphatemia Without Cellular Phosphate Depletion

Administration of glucose or fructose, and excessive feeding after starvation, are the main causes of shifts of large amounts of phosphate from the extracellular fluid into the cells (34,63,127). The phosphate is needed inside the cells for phosphorylation of glucose and fructose and for ATP synthesis. It is well established that glucose load (as in the glucose tolerance test) induces a transient reduction in the serum phosphate levels (127,128). In poststarvation feeding, hypophosphatemia can occur if insufficient phosphate is given. Again, the carbohydrate load given during feeding causes phosphate shifts into the cells, resulting in hypophosphatemia. The degree of prior starvation and phosphate losses determines whether the hypophosphatemia associated with feeding will be benign or associated with the phosphate depletion syndrome. Respiratory alkalosis of any cause can induce hypophosphatemia by enhancing phosphate shifts into the cells (105). The mechanism is thought to be secondary to an increase in the glycolytic pathway induced by the alkalotic milieu of the cells. Glycolysis enhances utilization of phosphate and thus induces shifts from the extracellular fluid into the cell. Hypophosphatemia seen in a variety of clinical settings such as sepsis, salicylate poisoning, acute gout, hepatic coma, and hyperventilation can be explained by the associated respiratory alkalosis. A diagnosis of hypophosphatemia is based on the clinical setting in which it occurs, and by ruling out the phosphate deficiency syndrome. It is usually benign and does not require specific treatment (5).

B. The Phosphate Deficiency Syndrome

The phosphate deficiency syndrome (PDS) occurs usually when hypophosphatemia is present in association with a decrease in the cellular phosphate concentration. This syndrome has a wide range of clinical and metabolic manifestations, which are the consequences of intracellular depletions.

The PDS is usually a chronic condition, with a gradual onset of symptoms seen in a situation of long-standing negative phosphate balance due to decreased GI phosphate influx or increased urinary losses. A more acute form of the syndrome can be seen when a patient with preexisting phosphate depletion is given intensive alimentation (enterally or parenterally) without adequate amounts of phosphate. In such cases, the a-priori depleted cell quickly utilizes its remaining phosphate, and there is a rapid shift of plasma phosphate into the cells. However, this process does not provide all the phosphate required for cellular metabolism, and a life-threatening syndrome develops, with severe hypophosphatemia and intracellular phosphate deficiency.

1. Starvation and Refeeding Syndrome

Tissue breakdown in starvation releases various minerals (P, K, Zn) into the plasma, with subsequent losses in the urine. Thus, gradual total body depletion of these minerals may occur. The plasma levels of phosphate in starvation may be maintained in the normal range through the continuous release of phosphate from tissue catabolism. This is an important point to consider when nutritional repletion is undertaken, since the normal plasma phosphate may not reflect the body phosphate depletion. Adequate amounts of phosphate in the diet or formula given after starvation must be provided to prevent acute intracellular phosphate depletion.

Nutritional repletion of the malnourished patient implies the provision of sufficient calories, protein, and other nutrients to allow accelerated tissue accretion. In the course of this process, cellular uptake and utilization of phosphate increase. When insufficient amounts of phosphate are provided, an acute state of severe hypophosphatemia and intracellular phosphate depletion with serious clinical and metabolic consequences can occur. This chain of events has been well described in experimental animal studies (132) and has been proposed as one of the mechanisms of the refeeding syndrome observed in starved prisoners of war fed overzealously, particularly with carbohydrates (133,134). The morbidity of feeding malnourished prisoners decreased with the consumption of milk, which provides large amounts of potassium and phosphorus (121,133).

The introduction of total parenteral nutrition (TPN) facilitated studies of the metabolism of various nutrients and of the clinical and metabolic consequences of their deficiency. In TPN, the exact composition of the administered solutions is known and can be controlled effectively. With the introduction of synthetic amino acid solutions as the nitrogen source, reports of TPN-induced hypophosphatemia with a wide spectrum of manifestations appeared in the literature (13,15,135,136). The observations on hypophosphatemia following glucose infusions (137,138) suggest that TPN-induced hypophosphatemia and PDS are due to the large glucose load administered in TPN. Other mechanisms include increased urinary losses of phosphate with excretion of amino acids (139), and impaired calcium and phosphate accretion in the bone (140–142).

In detailed balance studies, Rudman et al. (3) determined P requirements in TPN and the effect of P balance on the accretion of other nutrients. They showed that in malnourished patients maintained on parenteral nutrition, daily P requirements amount to 0.018

g/kg ideal body weight (1.25 g is the average for a 70-kg patient). They reported that P-deficient TPN solutions impaired the retention of N, K, and Cl. Even in the presence of zero or negligible phosphate accretion, patients continued to gain weight, but the increments in weight consisted mainly of adipose tissue with little or no increase in protoplasm or extracellular fluids. Thus, the inclusion of sufficient amounts of phosphate in TPN solutions is essential to prevent the PDS, achieve optimal utilization of other nutrients, and ensure appropriate composition of the weight gained.

This is another example of the nutritional conclusions which can be drawn from the TPN experience. Here, the essential role of P as an independent component, and as a crucial component for the utilization of other nutritional components, was understood from the experience with TPN, and consequently was able to explain various other observations (121,133).

2.   Gastrointestinal Malabsorption

Diseases leading to GI malabsorption can cause hypophosphatemia and phosphate depletion through different mechanisms, which include (56,143): (a) phosphate malabsorption secondary to decreased absorptive capacity of the intestines, a situation which occurs in diseases that affect large areas of the small bowel, such as Crohn's disease, celiac disease, short bowel syndrome, and radiation enteritis; (b) malabsorption of vitamin D, which, as noted above, plays a role in phosphate intestinal absorption; and (c) increased urinary losses due to secondary hyperparathyroidism induced by calcium malabsorption.

Antacids, widely used for the treatment of peptic ulcers, contain magnesium and aluminum, both of which bind phosphate and form insoluble complexes in the intestines and thus prevent phosphate absorption. There are 10 well-documented cases in the literature of antacid-induced PDS (14,144–153). Interestingly, one of the reported cases had hypophosphatemia despite renal failure. The duration of antacid therapy in patients with this syndrome ranged between 2 and 12 years prior to diagnosis, by which time widespread clinical and metabolic manifestations of the phosphate depletion had appeared.

3.   Diabetes Mellitus

Patients with well-controlled diabetes mellitus do not suffer excessive losses of phosphate. However, abnormalities in postprandial glucose metabolism were described accompanying renal phosphate leak (106). In the presence of hyperglycemia, especially when accompanied by polyuria and acidosis, phosphate is lost through the urine in excessive amounts of up to 7.5 mg/kg body weight daily (81,154–156). In ketoacidosis, intracellular organic components tend to be broken down, releasing large amounts of phosphate into the plasma, which is subsequently lost in the urine (155,157). This process, combined with the enhanced osmotic phosphate diuresis that is secondary to glycosuria, ketonuria, and polyuria, causes large urinary losses and subsequent depletion of phosphate. The plasma phosphate is usually normal or slightly elevated in the ketotic patient, in spite of the excessive urinary losses, because of the continuous large shift of phosphate from the cells into the plasma. In the corrective treatment of ketoacidosis, administration of fluids and insulin induces large shifts of phosphate back into the cells, with ensuing hypophosphatemia. Thus, within a few hours of treatment of ketoacidosis, a state of severe hypophosphatemia may develop unless large amounts of phosphate are administered (154,156).

4.   Alcoholism

There are multiple causes of phosphate depletion in the chronic alcoholic, including decreased dietary intake, malabsorption, increased urinary losses (158,159), hypomagnesemia, hypokalemia (113,160), and secondary hyperparathyroidism. It is unclear whether alcohol directly increases urinary loses of phosphate. In one study (161), significant amounts of phosphate were excreted in the urine following alcohol infusion. In other studies of normals and chronic alcoholics, no such effect of alcohol was found (162,163). It should be noted that chronic alcoholism results in widespread metabolic abnormalities, which may indirectly mediate the effect of alcohol on phosphate metabolism. Thus, alcohol-induced hypomagnesemia and hypokalemia can result in urinary phosphate wasting, while dehydration and impaired urinary function may cause the opposite.

5. Increased Urinary Losses

The kidney plays an essential role in phosphate conservation. Disruption of this function can cause large urinary losses with subsequent phosphate depletion and hypophosphatemia. Abnormalities in tubular handling of phosphate have been implicated in the genesis of hypophosphatemia induced by hypokalemia (113–115), hypomagnesemia (160,167), renal tubular acidosis, systemic acidosis (80), acute gout (168), paraneoplastic syndrome (169,170), and hypothyroidism (102,103). During the recovery phase from severe burns, hypophosphatemia may occur secondary to massive diuresis with phosphaturia, and an increase in phosphate utilization during tissue reconstruction (158). A similar phenomenon was noted in the course of treatment of hypothermia (171). In the rare genetic disorder X-linked hypophosphatemic rickets, there is a renal tubular defect that impairs phosphate reabsorption and results in excessive urinary phosphate losses and subsequent phosphate depletion (172,173). It is unclear whether the renal tubular defect in this disease is primary or secondary to a hormonal disorder (174,175).

C. Clinical Manifestations of Hypophosphatemia

Hypophosphatemia can result in tissue hypoxia secondary to the decrease in red blood cell (2,3-DPG) and in impairment in the generation of ATP. The central role of oxygen and ATP in cellular metabolism explains the widespread clinical and metabolic manifestations of phosphate depletion and hypophosphatemia. Constitutional symptoms such as anorexia, malaise, debility, lethargy, and joint stiffness have been described in association with hypophosphatemia (148). These symptoms can be present in addition to the specific manifestations described below (Table 4).

1. Nervous System

Abnormalities occur both in the central nervous system and in peripheral nerves. Central nervous system damage may be manifested as a range of clinical pictures, including altered sensorium (135,178), convulsions, confusion, delirium, stupor, and coma (179–181). There are several reports of EEG abnormalities (15,177) that characterize metabolic damage to the CNS. Peripheral nerve dysfunctions due to phosphate depletion are manifested as parasthesias and a decrease in the nerve conduction velocity (182). Recently, sensory neural hearing loss was found in three adult patients with hypophosphatemic bone disease (183).

2. Blood Cells

The red blood cell (RBC) derives its high-energy compounds through the glycolytic pathway. Low intracorpuscular phosphate levels impair the activity and regulation of the glycolytic enzymes, glyceraldehyde-3-phosphate dehydrogenese, hexokinase, and phosphofructokinase, resulting in low levels of ATP and 2,3-DPG (14,16,184,185). When the

TABLE 4 Clinical Signs of Hypophosphatemia

System	Manifestations	Ref.
CNS	Confusion, stupor, coma	179–181
	EEG abnormality	177
	paresthesia	135,178
	Decreased nerve conduction	182
	Neural hearing loss	183
Blood	Hemolysis	13,186
	Impaired oxygen transport	186,190
	Impaired leukocytes function	187
	Impaired clot formation	182,185
GI tract	Dysphagia	189,190
Muscles	Myalgia	177,191,193
	Weakness	177,191,192
	Diaphragm: respiratory failure	195
	Heart muscle: cardiac failure	192,196
	Myopathy	194,153
	Rhabdomyolysis	158,178
Bones	Osteomalacia	148,174,198
Kidney	Renal tubular acidosis	205
	Glycosuria	207
	Magnesuria	208,209

ATP levels drop, the erythrocyte becomes rigid and is entrapped in the spleen. Further reduction in the ATP levels to less than 50% of the normal, usually when serum phosphate is lower than 0.2 mg/dL (13,14), is associated with hemolysis (13,186). The erythrocyte ATP concentrations are closely correlated with serum phosphate (14). The blood smear of the phosphate-depleted patient shows fragmented erythrocytes and microspherocytes. Functionally, the RBCs have increased osmotic fragility (13), a manifestation of membrane dysfunction. In addition to the damage to the RBC itself, phosphate depletion decreases its ability to deliver oxygen to the tissues. The production of 2,3-DPG is reduced, thereby increasing oxygen affinity to hemoglobin and, subsequently, causing tissue hypoxia. The consequences of hypophosphatemia to the RBC can be reversed with adequate phosphate supplementation (13,76,84,186). Reduction in leukocyte ATP content is associated with reduced phagocytic, chemotactic, and bactericidal activity, abnormalities which can result in increased susceptibility to infection. The defect in the leukocyte function is reversible either by correcting the hypophosphatemia or by incubating the leukocyte with adenosine and phosphate (187).

Hypophosphatemia is also associated with reduced ATP in platelets. When the level falls below 50% of the normal, clot retraction becomes impaired (182), and with further reductions there occur thrombocytopathia, hemorrhages, and a decrease in platelet survival (185,187). The bone marrow reacts by increasing the number of megakaryocytes and the production of platelets.

3. Gastrointestinal System

Hypophosphatemia affects the GI tract mainly by disrupting the contractility of the smooth muscles of the intestines. This can lead to dysphagia, gastric atony, and ileus. Patients with chronic hepatic failure due to cirrhosis have greater impairment of their hepatic function when they are hypophosphatemic (185,188). Hepatic oxygen extraction is worse in malnourished hypophosphatemic cirrhotic patients than in normophosphatemic patients (189). It is suggested that the lower levels of 2,3-DPG and ATP in the erythrocytes are responsible for the greater hepatic hypoxemia in the hypophosphatemic patient (190).

4. Muscles and Bones

Muscles require the production of large amounts of high-free-energy compounds (ATP, creatine phosphate) and oxygen for contraction, maintenance of membrane potential, and other functions. Phosphate deprivation (alone or in conjunction with starvation) induces muscle cell injury characterized by a decrease in intracellular phosphate and an increase in water, sodium, and chloride (178). The muscular clinical manifestations of the PDS include myalgia (177,191,193), objective weakness (145,177,191,192), and myopathy with histopathologic and electromyographic changes (153,194). The most severe form of phosphate depletion-induced myopathy is rhabdomyolysis, which can lead to renal failure. This disease usually develops in patients with preexisting phosphate deficiency who manifest acute hypophosphatemia. It has been described in alcoholics with preexisting subclinical myopathy (132,158,178), following infusion of large amounts of carbohydrates (178,194), and in the course of treatment of diabetic ketoacidosis (178). Hypophosphatemia can decrease muscle contractility in the diaphragm, leading to respiratory failure (195), and in the heart, leading to decreased cardiac output and cardiac failure (196,197).

Hypophosphatemia may lead to osteomalacia and rickets. Skeletal defects have been reported in association with phosphate depletion of different causes: dietary deprivation in experimental animals (198,199), prolonged use of antacids (60,145,146,148), hemodialysis (173,174), and vitamin D-resistant rickets (173,174,200,201). Both mineralization defects and bone resorption have been demonstrated in conjunction with phosphate depletion. The mechanism of the mineralization defect has not been elucidated (202). Hypophosphatemia was proposed to result in a decreased calcium and phosphate multiplication product at the mineralization front (203), with a decrease in the precipitation of hydroxyapatite crystals in the bone matrix. This mechanism has been disputed because of the low equilibrium constant (K_p) of the reaction that produces apatite (A. Boskey, personal communication, 1986). The enhanced bone resorption of the PDS does not seem to be PTH-mediated (174), since plasma PTH is increased during hypophosphatemia. Increased serum levels of 1,25-(OH)2D, which may accompany hypophosphatemia, could enhance bone resorption. However, elevated levels of 1,25-$(OH)_2D_3$ have not been observed consistently in patients with phosphate depletion and bone abnormalities (153).

The role that vitamin D metabolites play in the mineralization defects of the PDS is controversial. It is highly unlikely that 1,25-$(OH)_2D_3$ deficiency is the cause, since synthesis of this metabolite is enhanced in hypophosphatemia. It has not been established whether generation of other vitamin D metabolites, such as 24,25-$(OH)_2D_3$, is impaired secondary to hypophosphatemia. Vitamin D supplementation does not protect against osteomalacia of dietary phosphate deficiency (165,204).

5. Kidney

Impaired tubular function and abnormalities in the handling of acid in the kidney are the main renal manifestations of hypophosphatemia. Phosphate acts as a proton trap in the kidney by converting HPO_4^{2-} to $H_2PO_4^{-}$, which is excreted in the urine. Decrease in filterable acid phosphate may lead to renal tubular acidosis (205). Subsequent systemic acidosis rarely occurs, because of the bicarbonatemia (205,206). However, in children with the refeeding syndrome, systemic acidosis has been described (64). Glycosuria (207) and magnesuria (208,209) have been reported secondary to hypophosphatemia-induced disturbance in tubular function.

D. Treatment of Hypophosphatemia and Phosphate Depletion

The appropriate management of hypophosphatemia and phosphate depletion require identification of the underlying causes, treatment with supplemental phosphate when necessary, and prevention of recurrence of the problem by correcting the underlying causes. Phosphate can be administered orally, intravenously, rectally, and in dialysis fluids. Phosphate supplementation is essential in patients with profound hypophosphatemia and in those who become symptomatic. The symptoms and signs of phosphate depletion can vary, are nonspecific, and are usually seen in patients with multiple problems. This makes it difficult to identify phosphate depletion as the cause of the clinical manifestations. Oral phosphate can be given in the form of skim milk (which contains 0.9–1.0 mg elemental P/mL or of Neutraphos tablets (which contain 250 mg P per tablet, as a Na or K salt). The dose or oral phosphate in mild hypophosphatemia is up to 3 g/day. Serum phosphate levels rise by as much as 15 mg/L 60 to 120 min after ingestion of 1000 mg P (212).

Severe hypophosphatemia with serum levels lower than 0.15 mmol/L needs replacement therapy. Treatment can be initiated with a dose of 2 mg/kg body weight over a period of 6 h (213). This dose is effective in restoring serum levels to above 0.5 mmol/L within 36 h. There have been reports of intravenous therapy with doses as high as 7.5 mg/kg over 6 h (214).

E. Hyperphosphatemia

1. Etiology

The healthy kidney can excrete a high phosphate load and thus prevent hyperphosphatemia. The amount excreted is determined by the difference between the amount filtered in the glomerulus and that reabsorbed in the tubules. Hyperphosphatemia usually occurs as a result of renal failure and reduced ability of the kidney to excrete a phosphate load. A large influx of phosphates from the cell into the plasma can also result in hyperphosphatemia, particularly in the presence of reduced renal function. Such an influx occurs most commonly in severe hemolysis, tumor lysis syndrome, and rhabdomyolysis. In hemolysis, the disintegrating RBCs release phosphate into the plasma. The most common tumors associated with hyperphosphatemia induced by the tumor lysis syndrome are lymphomas and lymphocytic leukemia, because of the high phosphate content of the lymphocytes (215). Large amounts of phosphates are released into the plasma either because of primary cell destruction (216–218) or as a result of chemotherapy (219). In rhabdomyolysis the damaged muscle releases large amounts of phosphate or phosphate-containing compounds into the plasma. The large amounts of myoglobin released during rhabdomyolysis often precipitate acute renal failure, which thus limits the ability of the kidneys to excrete the excess phosphate. False hyperphosphatemia is described in multiple myeloma (220) and hyperproteinemia (221).

Phosphate loading through the GI tract and resulting in hyperphosphatemia can occur through enemas (222) and phosphate-containing laxatives (223,224), particularly in the presence of some degree of renal failure.

Hypoparathyroidism, either primary or secondary, can be associated with hyperphosphatemia in the patient with normal renal function. Mild hyperphosphatemia can be seen in acromegaly (225). This is secondary to growth hormone-induced enhancement of tubular reabsorption of phosphate. In severe hyperthyroidism up to 30% of patients may have hyperphosphatemia due to increased renal retention (100) as well as bone resorption (226). The hyperphosphatemia resolves itself with the return of normal thyroid function.

2. Etopic Calcification

Prolonged hyperphosphatemia may be accompanied by ectopic calcification arising from the precipitation of calcium phosphate crystals in different tissues. This happens usually when the Ca-P multiplication product is >60 (216). The anatomic distribution of calcification depends on local tissue factors, particularly necrosis (227). There is a predisposition for tissue calcinosis, especially in the periarticular region of large joints (223,228). It happens only due to metabolic derangements. The syndrome of tumoral calcinosis, first described by Duret in 1899 (cited in 99), is characterized by mild hypophosphatemia without renal failure. It is usually of juvenile onset. PTH levels were found to be at the low end of normal in these patients (229,230). Diamox, which inhibits proximal tubular reabsorption of phosphate, induces phosphaturia in these patients (221).

VII. FUTURE RESEARCH NEEDS

Although phosphate is not commonly a limiting nutrient, it plays many different physiological roles; one can hardly find a metabolic process in which phosphate is not a participant. Much more attention needs to be paid to the affinity of phosphorus to different proteins and other organic compounds. Its effect on the activation, deactivation, and signaling systems requires further study. The role of phosphorus in many new biological systems has been described, and more are likely to be described and evaluated. Understanding more about the physical properties is crucial for the explanation of many biological activities. The use of nuclear techniques in biochemical and biological research has opened new dimensions. Nuclear magnetic resonance, isotope studies, and a whole body of neutron activation scanning techniques enable scientists to combine quantitative chemical information on the molecular level with mapping of where these reactions occur in different clinical conditions. The biochemical study of kinetics and structure, using genetic technologies, can give and are already giving us much information about substances and processes in which phosphate compounds participate.

There is need for research on the molecular basis of phosphorus homeostasis, absorption, and excretion, and the mechanisms involved in the regulation of these processes. What role does phosphate play in the process of gene expression, and in the regulation of its own metabolism?

Finally, observation of natural phenomena as well as clinical inspections were and still remain the essential tools for any scientist, despite the progress in technology. It has to be remembered that only 20 years ago did clinical observation of patients on total parenteral nutrition indicate how essential phosphorus is as a nutrient (135).

VIII. SUMMARY

Phosphorus is the sixth most abundant element in the body, after oxygen, hydrogen, carbon, nitrogen, and calcium; it accounts for approximately 1% of the total body weight of humans. Altogether, 85% of it is stored in the bone in the form of hydroxyapatite crystal; 14% in the soft tissues in the form of energy-storing bonds with nucleotides (ATP, GTP), nucleic acids in chromosomes and ribosome, 2,3-DPG in the RBCs, phosphoproteins which take part in many metabolic activities, and phospholipids in the cells' membranes; less than 1% is found in the extracellular fluids.

Phosphate balance is maintained by numerous systems. The gut is responsible for the absorption of two-thirds of the daily intake of 4–30 mg/kg body weight. Absorption sites exist all along the gut, the most active site in humans being the jejunum. The kidney filters 90% of the plasma phosphate and reabsorbs it in the tubules. In states of hypophosphatemia the kidney can reabsorb the filtered phosphates very efficiently, reducing the amount excreted in the urine virtually to zero. The healthy kidney can excrete high loads of P and rid the body of P overload. Through the vitamin D-PTH axis, the endocrine system regulates the phosphate balance by influencing the kidney, gut, and bone. Other hormones, including thyroid, insulin, glucagon, glucocorticosteroid, and thyrocalcitonin, play a lesser role in the regulation of phosphate metabolism.

Hypophosphatemia is a severe metabolic disturbance which leads to the failure of many systems and organs: the nervous system, kidney, bone and muscles, the GI tract, blood cells, and the immune system. Nutrition is an important factor in the prevention as well as management of this disturbance.

REFERENCES

1. Handbook of Chemistry and Physics. 70th ed. Boca Raton, FL: CRC Press, 1990.
2. Politi L, Chiaraluce R, Consalvi V, Cerulli N, Scandurra R. Oxalate, phosphate and sulphate determination in serum and urine by ion chromatography. Clin Chim Acta 1989; 184(2): 155–165.
3. Rudman D, Millikan WJ, Richardson TJ, et al. Elemental balances during intravenous hyperalimentation of underweight adult subjects. J Clin Invest 1975; 55: 94–104.
4. Dickerson JWT, Widdowson EM. Chemical changes in skeletal muscles with development. Biochem J 1960; 74: 247–257.
5. Berner YN, Shike M. Consequences of phosphate imbalance. Annu Rev Nutr 1988; 8: 121–148.
6. Hegsted DM. In: Goodhardt RS, Shils ME, eds. Modern Nutrition in Health and Disease. Philadelphia: Lea & Febiger, 1973; 268–286.
7. Hershey JW. Protein phosphorylation controls translation rates. J Biol Chem 1989; 264(35): 208–236.
8. Wanner BL, Wilmes-Riesenberg MR. Involvement of phosphotransacetylase, acetate kinase, and acetyl phosphate synthesis in control of the phosphate regulon in *Escherichia coli*. J Bacteriol 1992; 174(7)1: 2124–2130.
9. Norbury C, Nurse P. Controls of cell proliferation in yeast and animals. Ciba Found Symp 1990; 150: 168–177, discussion 150: 177–183.
10. Stegemann J. Exercise Physiology. Stuttgart: George Thieme Verlag, 1981: chap 1.7.
11. Lau K. Phosphate disorders. In: Kokko JP, Tannen RL, eds. Fluids and Electrolytes. Philadelphia/London: Saunders, 1986: 398–470.
12. Tsuboi KK, Fukunaga K. Inorganic phosphate and enhanced glucose, degradation by the intact erythrocyte. J Biol Chem 1965; 240: 2806–2810.

13. Jacob HS, Amsden T. Acute hemolytic anemia with rigid cells in hypophosphatemia. N Engl J Med 1971; 285: 1446–1450.

14. Lichtman MA, Miller DR, Cohen J. Reduced red cell glycolysis. 1,2-Diphosphoglycerate and adenosine triphosphate concentration and increased hemoglobin-oxygen affinity caused by hypophosphatemia. Ann Int Med 1971; 74: 562–568.

15. Trechsel U, Eisman JA, Fischer JA, Bonjour JP, Fleisch H. Calcium-dependent, parathyroid hormone-independent regulation of 1,25-dihydroxyvitamin D. Am J Physiol 1980; 239: E119–124.

16. Farber E. ATP and cell integrity. Fed Proc 1973; 32: 1534–1539.

17. Kay A, Beutler E. The effect of ammonium, phosphate, potassium, and hypotonicity on stored red cells. Transfusion 1992; 32(1): 37–41.

18. Wang K, Farley RA. Lysine 480 is not an essential residue for ATP binding or hydrolysis by Na,K-ATPase. J Biol Chem 1992; 267(6): 3577–3580.

19. Sandhu GS, Asimakis GK. Mechanism of loss of adenine nucleotides from mitochondria during myocardial ischemia. J Mol Cell Cardiol 1991; 23(12): 1423–1435.

20. Ambrosio G, Zweier JL, Flaherty JT. The relationship between oxygen radical generation and impairment of myocardial energy metabolism following post-ischemic reperfusion. J Mol Cell Cardiol 1991; 23(12): 1359–1374.

21. Dolce V, Fiermonte G, Messina A, Palmieri F. Nucleotide sequence of a human heart CDNA encoding the mitochondrial phosphate carrier. DNA Seq 1991; 2(2): 133–135.

22. Parodies G, Ruggiero FM, Dinoi P. Decreased activity of the phosphate carrier and modification of lipids in cardiac mitochondria from senescent rats. Int J Biochem 1992; 24(5): 783–787.

23. Nelson D, Rumsey WL, Erecinska M. Glutamine catabolism by heart muscle. Properties of phosphate-activated glutaminase. Biochem J 1992; 282(2): 559–564.

24. Parodies G, Ruggiero FM, Gadaleta MN, Quagliariello E. The effect of aging and acetyl-L-carnitine on the activity of the phosphate conier and on the phospholipid composition in rat heart mitochondria. Biochim Biophys Acta 1992; 1103(2): 324–326.

25. Krebs EG. The Albert Lasker Medical Awards. Role of the cyclic AMP-dependent protein kinase in signal transduction. JAMA 1989; 262(13): 1815–1818.

26. BeHorin-Font E, Starosta R, NElanes CL, et al. Effect of acidosis on PTH-dependent renal adenylate cyclase in phosphorus deprivation:role of G proteins. Am J Physiol 1990; 258(6, pt 2): FI 640–1649.

27. Caverzasio J, Bonjour JP. Insulin-like growth factor I stimulates Na-dependent Pi transport in cultured kidney cells. Am J Physiol 1989; 257(5, pt 2): F712–F717.

28. Harbison MD, Germer JM. Permissive action of growth hormone on the renal response to dietary phosphorus deprivation. J Clin Endocrinol Metab 1990; 70(4): 1035–1040.

29. Bartek J, Iggo R, Gannon J, Lane DP. Genetic and immunochemical analysis of mutant p53 in human breast cancer cell lines. Oncogene 1990; 5(6): 893–899.

30. Waters CM, Hancock DC, Evan GI. Identification and characterisation of the erg-I gene product as an inducible, short-lived, nuclear phosphoprotein. Oncogene 1990; 5(5): 669–674.

31. Taya Y, Yasuda H, Kamijo M, et al. In vitro phosphorylation of the tumor suppressor gene RB protein by mitosis-specific histone H1 kinase. Biochem Biophys Res Commun 1989; 164(1): 580–586.

32. Koszewski NJ, Notides AC. Phosphate-sensitive binding of the estrogen receptor to its response elements. Mol Endocrinol 1991; 5(8): 1129–1136.

33. Koppel J, Boutterin MC, Doye V, Peyro-Saint-Paul H, Sobel A. Developmental tissue expression and phylogenetic conservation of stathmin, a phosphoprotein associated with cell regulations. J Biol Chem 1990; 265(7): 3703–3707.

34. Maucuer A, Doye V, Sobel A. A single amino acid difference distinguishes the human and the rat sequences of stathmin, an ubiquitous intracellular phosphoprotein associated with cell regulations. FEBS Lett 1990; 264(2): 275–278.

35. Nielander HB, Schrama LH, van Rozen AJ, et al. Mutation of semine 41 in the neuron-specific protein B-50 (GAP43) prohibits phosphorylation by protein kinase C. J Neurochem 1990; 55(4): 1442–1445.

36. Thiel G, Sudhof TC, Greengard P. Synapsin II. Mapping of a domain in the NH2-terminal region which binds to small synaptic vesicles. J Biol Chem 1990; 265(27): 16527–16533.

37. Horiuchi A, Williams KR, Kurihara T, Naim AC, Greengard P. Purification and CDNA cloning of ARPP-16, a cAMP-regulated phosphoprotein enriched in basal ganglia, and of a related phosphoprotein, ARPP-19. J Biol Chem 1990; 265(16): 9476–9484.

38. Williams KR, Hemmings HC Jr, LoPresti MB, Greengard P. ARPP-21, a cyclic AMP-regulated phosphoprotein enriched in dopamine-innervated brain regions. I. Amino acid sequence of ARPP-2IB from bovine caudate nucleus. J Neurosci 1989; 9(10): 3631–3637.

39. Lee RH, Fowler A, McGimis JF, Lolley RN, Craft CM. Amino acid and CDNA sequence of bovine phosducin, a soluble phosphoprotein from photoreceptor cells. J Biol Chem 1990; 265(26): 15867–15873.

40. Legagneux V, Morange M, Bensaude O. Heat shock increases turnover of 90 kDA heat shock protein phosphate groups in HeLa cells. FEBS Lett 1991; 291(2):359–362.

41. Hortelano P, Garcia-Salguero L, Lupianez JA, Alleyne GA. Influence of acute metabolic acidosis on the monomer and polymer forms of renal phosphate-dependent glutaminase. Life Sci 1990; 46(26): 1903–1912.

42. Lellos V, Moraitou M, Tselentis V, Philippidis H, Palaiologos G. Effect of starvation or streptozotocin-diabetes on phosphate-activated glutaminase of different rat brain regions. Neurochem Res 1992; 17(2): 141–145.

43. Kowarski S, Schachter D. Effects of vitamin D on phosphate transport and incorporation into mucosal constituents of rat intestinal mucosa. J Biol Chem 1969; 244: 211–217.

44. Walling MW. Intestinal inorganic phosphate transport. Adv Exp Med Biol 1977; 103: 131–147.

45. Wheeler TJ, Lowenstein JM. Adenylate deaminase from rat muscle: regulation of purine nucleotides and orthophosphate in the presence of 150 MM KCl. J Biol Chem 1979; 254: 8994–8999.

46. Robertson WG. Plasma phosphate homeostasis. In: Nordin BEC, ed. Calcium, Phosphorus and Magnesium Metabolism. London: Churchill Livingstone, 1976: 217–219.

47. Wilkinson R. Absorption of calcium, phosphorus and magnesium. In: Nordin BEC, ed. Calcium, Phosphorus and Magnesium Metabolism. London: Churchill Livingstone, 1976: 36–113.

48. Danisi G, Straub RW. Unidirectional influx of phosphate across the mucosal membrane of rabbit small intestine. Pflugers Arch 1980; 385: 117–122.

49. Caniggia A, Gennari C, Palazzuoli V. Influenza della thirocalcitonina sul asorbinento intestinale del radiocalcio (Ca 47) nell nona. Boll Soc Ital Biol Sper 1968; 44: 458–460.

50. Juan D, Liptak P, Gray TK. Absorption of inorganic phosphate in the human jejunum and its inhibition by salmon calcitonin. J Clin Endocrinol Metab 1976; 43: 517–522.

51. Meschy F, Gueguen L. Minimal requirement of phosphorus for maintenance in lambs. Reprod Nutr Dev Suppl 1990; 2: 189s–190s.

52. Birge SJ, Avioli RC. Intestinal phosphate transport and alkaline phosphatase activity in the chick. Am J Physiol 1981; 240: E384–E390.

53. Boyle IT, Omdahl JL, Gray RW, DeLuca HF. The biological activity and metabolism of 24, 25 vitamin D. J Biol Chem 1973; 248: 4174–4180.

54. Kabakoff B, Kendrick NC, DeLuca HF. 1,25-Dihydroxyvitamin D3 stimulated active uptake of phosphate by rat jejunum. Am J Physiol 1982; 243: E470–E475.

55. Peterlik M, Wasserman RH. Effect of vitamin D on transepithelial phosphate transport in chick intestine. Am J Physiol 1978; 234: E379–388.

56. Chen TC, Castilla L, Korycka-Dahl M, DeLuca HF. Role of vitamin D metabolites in phosphate transport of rat intestine. J Nutr 1974; 104: 1056–1060.

57. Claric I. Importance of dietary Ca:PO$_4$ ratios on skeletal Ca, Mg and PO$_4$ metabolism. Am J Physiol 1969; 217: 865–870.
58. HoRick MF, Clark MB. The photobiogenesis and metabolism of vitamin D. Fed Proc 1978; 37: 2567–2570.
59. Travis SJ, Sugerman MJ, Ruberg RL, et al. Alteration of red-cell glycolytic intermediates and oxygen transport as a consequence of hypophosphatemia in patients receiving intravenous hyperalimentation. N Engl J Med 1971; 285: 763–769.
60. Cooke N, Teitelbaum S, Avioli LV. Antacid-induced osteomalacia and nephrolithiasis. Arch Intern Med 1979; 138: 1007–1009.
61. Lau K, Chen S, Eby B. Evidence for the iole of PO4 deficiency in antihypertensive action of a high-Ca diet. Am J Physiol 1984; 246: H324–H331.
62. Marshall W. Plasma fractions. In: Nordin BEC, ed. Calcium, Phosphate and Magnesium Metabolism. London: Churchill Livingstone, 1976: 162–185.
63. Tietz NW. Electrolytes. In: Tietz NW, Carraway WT, Freier EF, Kachmar JF, Rawnsely HM, eds. Fundamentals of Clinical Chemistry. Philadelphia: Saunders, 1976.
64. Parfitt AM, Kleerekoper M. Clinical disorders of calcium, phosphorus and magnesium metabolism. In: Maxwell MH, Kleeman CR, eds. Clinical Disorders of Fluid and Electrolyte Metabolism. 3d ed. New York: McGraw-Hill, 1980: 947–1151.
65. Harrison HE. Phosphorus. In: Present Knowledge in Nutrition. 5th ed. Washington, DC: Nutr Found, 1984: 413–420.
66. Staff JS. Phosphate homeostasis and hypophosphatemia. Am J Med 1982; 72: 489–495.
67. Brautbar N, Walling MW, Cobum JW. Interactions between vitamin D deficiency and phosphorus depletion in the rat. J Clin Invest 1979; 63: 335–341.
68. Carlson A. A tracer experiment on the effect of vitamin D on the skeletal metabolism of calcium and phosphorus. Acta Physiol Scand 1952; 26: 212–220.
69. DeLuca HF. The kidney as an endociine organ for the production of 1,25-dihydroxyvitamin D3'a calcium mobilizing hormone. N Engl J Med 1973; 289: 359–364.
70. Omoy A. 24,25-Dihydroxyvitamin D is a metabolite of vitamin D essential for bone fonnation. Nature 1978; 276: 517–518.
71. Dominguez JH, Gray RW, Seean J Jr. Dietary phosphate deprivation in women and men: effect on mineral and acid balances, parathyroid hormone, and the metabolism of 25-OH-vitamin D. J. Clin Endocrinol Metab 1976; 43: 1056–1068.
72. Amiel C, Kuntziger H, Richet G. Micropuncture study of handling of phosphate by proximal and distal nephron in normal and parathyroidectomized rats. Evidence for distal reabsorption. Pflugers Arch 1970; 317: 93–109.
73. Sheldon GF, Grzyb S. Phosphate depletion and replation. Relation to parenteral nutrition and oxygen transport. Am Surg 1975; 182: 683–687.
74. Harris CA, Barr PG, Chirito E, Dirics JH. Composition of mammalian glomerular filtrate. Am J Physiol 1974; 227: 972–976.
75. Popovtzer MM, Knochel JP. Disorders of calcium, phosphorus, vitamin D and parathyroid hormone activity. In: Schrier R, ed. Renal and Electrolyte Disorders. Boston: Little, Brown, 1986: 235.
76. Liput J, Rose M, Galya C, Chen TC, Puschett JB. Inhibition by volume expansion of phosphate uptake by the renal proximal tubule brush border membrane. Biochem Phamiacol 1989; 38(2): 321–325.
77. Knox FG, Oswald H, Marchand GR, et al. Editorial review: phosphate transport along the nephron. Am J Physiol 1977; 233: F261–F268.
78. Lang F, Greger R, Knox FG. Editorial review: factors modulating the renal handling of phosphate. Renal Physiol 1981; 4: 1–16.
79. Lelievre-Pegoner M, Merlet-Benichou C, Roinel N, De Rouffignac C. Developmental pattern of water and electrolyte transport in rat superficial nephrons. Am J Physiol 1983; 245: F15–F21.

80. Giasson SD, Brunette MG, Danan G, Vigneault N, Carriers S. Micropuncture study of renal phosphorus transport in hypophosphatemic vitamin D-resistant rickets mice. Pflugers Arch 1977; 371: 33–38.

81. Nabarro JDN, Spencer AG, Stowers JM. Metabolic studies in severe diabetic ketosis. Q J Med 1952; 21: 225–243.

82. Muhlbauer RC, Bonjour JP, Fleisch H. Tubular localization of adaptation to dietary phosphate in rats. Am J Physiol 1977; 233: F342–F348.

83. Pastoriza-Munoz E, Mishler DR, Lechene C. Effect of phosphate deprivation on phosphate reabsorption in rat nephron: role of PTH. Am J Physiol 1983; 244: FI40–FI49.

84. Steele TH. Renal resistance to parathyroid hormone during phosphorus deprivation. J Clin Invest 1976; 58: 1461–1464.

85. Suttle NF, Field AC. Studies on magnesium in ruminant nutrition: VIII. Effect of increased intakes of potassium and water on the metabolism of magnesium, phosphorus, sodium, potassium and calcium in sheep. Br J Nutr 1967; 21: 819–831.

86. Tanaka Y, DeLuca HF. The control of 25-hydroxyvitamin D metabolism by inorganic phosphorus. Arch Biochem Biophys 1973; 154: 566–570.

87. Dousa TP. Possible relationship of gluconeogenesis to modulation of phosphate transport in the proximal tubule. Adv Exp Med Biol; 151: 55–64.

88. Bemdt TJ, Homma S, Yusufi AN, Dousa TP, Knox FG. Effect of phosphate deprivation on enzymes of the cyclic adenosine monophosphate metabolism in rat proximal convoluted and proximal straight tubules. Renal Physiol Biochem 1990; 13(5): 241–247.

89. Rybczynska A, Hoppe A, Knox FG. Propranolol restores phosphaturic effect of PTH in short-term phosphate deprivation. Am J Physiol 1990; 258(1, pt 2): RI20–RI23.

90. Bunim JJ, Black RL, Lutwak L, et al. Studies on dexamethasone, a new preliminary report. Arthritis Rheum 1958; 1: 313–331.

91. Eby B, Gutnupalli J, Lau K. Evidence that glucocorticoid exerts a direct inhibitory effect on renal PO_4, reabsorption (abstr). Proc Am Soc Nephrol, 13th Annu Meet, Washington, DC, p 5A.

92. Barker ES. The renal response in man to acute experimental respiratory alkalosis and acidosis. J Clin Invest 1957; 36: 515–529.

93. Zilenovski AM, Kuroda S, Bhat S, Bank DE, Bank N. Effect of sodium bicarbonate on phosphate excretion in acute and chronic PX rats. Am J Physiol 1979; 236: F184–F191.

94. Ulfich KJ, Rumfich G, Kloss S. Phosphate transport in the proximal convolution of the rat kidney. III. Effect of the extracellular and intracellular pH. Pflugers Arch 1978; 377: 33–42.

95. Schuck O, Nadvomikova H, Teplan V. Acidification capacity of the kidneys and aging. Physiol Bohemoslov 1989; 38(2): 117–125.

96. Adragna NC. Cation transport in vascular endothelial cans and aging. J Membr Biol 1991; 124(3): 285–291.

97. Schwille PO, Rumenapf G, Kohler R. Blood levels of glucometabolic hormones and urinary saturation with stone forming phases after an oral test meal in male patients with recurrent idiopathic calcium urolithiasis and in healthy controls. J Am Coll Nutr 1989; 8(6): 557–566.

98. DeFronzo RA, Goldberg M, Agus ZS. The effect of glucose and insulin on the renal and electrolyte transport. J Clin Invest 1976; 58: 83–90.

99. Lau K, GutnupaUi J, Eby B. Effects of somatostatin on phosphate, transport evidence for the role of basal insulin. Kidney Int 1983; 2: 10–15.

100. Bommer J, Bonjour JP, Ritz E, Fleisch H. Parathyroid-independent changes in renal handling of phosphate in hyperthyroid rats. Kidney Int 1979; 15: 325–332.

101. Espinosa RE, Keller MJ, Yusufi ANK, Dousa TP. Effect of thyroxine administration on phosphate transport across renal cortical brush border membrane. Am J Physiol 1984; 246: FI33–FI39.

102. Menezel J, Rachmani R, Chowers I. Effect of triodothyronine on calcium and phosphorus metabolism in hypothyroidism. Isr J Med Sci 1967; 3: 761–764.

103. Robertson JD. Calcium and phosphorus studies in myxedema. 1941; Lancet 2: 216–218.
104. Corvilain J, Abramou M. Some effects of human growth hormone on renal hemodynamics. J Clin Invest 1962; 41: 1230–1235.
105. Eby B, Lau K. Effects of glucagon on tubular P transport: contrast with nicotinaminde (abstr). Kidney Int 1982; 21: 132.
106. Mostellr ME, Tuttle EP. Effects of alkalosis on plasma concentration and urinary excretion of inorganic phosphate in man. J Clin Invest 1964; 43: 138–149.
107. Kuntziger H, Amiel C, Guaderbout C. Phosphate handling by the rat nephron during saline diuresis. Kidney Int 1972; 2: 318–323.
108. Dennis VW, Stead WW, Myers JL. Renal handling of phosphate and calcium. Ann Rev Physiol 1979; 41: 257–271.
109. Briscoe AM, Ragan C. Diurnal variations in calcium and magnesium excretion in man. Metabolism 1966; 15: 1002–1010.
110. Lau K, Agus ZS, Goldberg M, Goldfarb S. Renal tubular site of altered calcium transport in phosphate-depleted rats. J Clin Invest 1979; 64: 1681–1687.
111. Beck LH, Goldberg C. Effect of acetazolamide and parathyroidectomy on renal transport of sodium, calcium, and phosphate. Am J Physiol 1973; 22: 1136–1142.
112. Knox FG, Haas JA, Lechene CP. Effect of parathyroid hormone on phosphate reabsorption in the presence of acetazolamide. Kidney Int 1976; 10: 216–220.
113. Anderson DC, Peter TJ, Stewart WK. Association of hypokalaemia and hypophosphatemia. Br Med J 1969; 4: 402.
114. Beck N, Davis BB. Impaired renal response to parathyroid hormone in potassium depletion. Am J Physiol 1975; 228: 179–183.
115. Vianna NJ. Severe hypophosphatemia due to hypokalemia. JAMA 1971; 215: 1497–1498.
116. Yusufi AN, Berndt TJ, Moltaji H, Donovan V, Dousa TP, Knox FG. Rat atzial natriuretic factor (ANF-III) inhibits phosphate transport in brush border membrane from superficial and juxta-medullary cortex. Proc Soc Exp Biol Med 1989; 190(1): 87–90.
117. Ortola FV, Seri I, Downes S, Brenner BM, BaRermann BJ. Dopamine-receptorblockade inhibits ANP-induced phosphaturia and calciuria in rats. Am J Physiol 1990; 259(1, pt 2): FI38–FI46.
118. Fried T, Aronoff GR, Benabe JE, et al. Renal and hemodynamic effects of atrial natriuretic peptide in patients with cirrhosis. Am J Med Sci 1990; 299(1): 2–9.
119. Pak CY, Hill K, Cintron NM, Huntoon C. Assessing applicants to the NASA flight program for their renal stone-forming potential. Aviat Space Environ Med 1989; 60(2): 157–161.
120. Coultate TP. Food: The Chemistry of Its Components. 2d ed. London: Royal Society of Chemistry, 1988: 280–282.
121. DeFronzo RA, Lang R. Hypophosphatemia and glucose intolerance: evidence for tissue insensitivity to insulin. N Engl J Med 1980; 303: 1259–1263.
122. Recommended Dietary Allowances. Washington, DC: National Academy of Sciences, 1989.
123. Kaneko K, Masaki U, Aikyo M, et al. Urinary calcium and calcium balance in young women affected by high protein diet of soy protein isolate and adding sulfur-containing amino acids and/or potassium. J Nutr Sci Vitaminol, Tokyo, 1990; 36(2): 105–116.
124. Tizzani A, Casetta G, Piana P, Vercelli D. Wheat bran in the selective therapy of absorptive hypercalciuria: a study performed on IS litwastic patients. J Urol 1989; 142(4): 1018–1020.
125. Brune M, Rossander-Hulten L, Hallberg L, Gleerup A, Sandberg AS. Iron absorption from bread in humans: inhibiting effects of cereal fiber, phytate and inositol phosphates with different numbers of phosphate groups. J Nutr 1992; 122(3): 442–449.
126. Portale AA, Halloran BP, Morris RC Jr. Physiologic regulation of the serum concentration of 1,25-dihydroxyvitamin D by phosphorus in normal men. J Clin Invest 1989; 83(5): 1494–1499.
127. Juan D, Elrazak M. Hypophosphatemia in hospitalized patients. JAMA 1979; 242: 163–164.
128. Zhang XY. Perioperative hypophosphatemia in general surgery. Chung Hua Wai Ko Tsa Chih 1990; 28(4): 225–227, 253.

129. George R, Shin MH. Hypophosphatemia after major hepatic resection. Surgery 1992; 111(3): 281–286.

130. Laaban JP, Grateau G, Psychoyos I, Laromiguiere M, Vuong TK, Rochemaure J. Hypophosphatemia induced by mechanical ventilation in patients with chronic obstructive pulmonary disease. Crit Care Med 1989; 17(11): 1115–1120.

131. Popelier M, JoRivet B, Fouquet B, et al. Phosphorus-calcium metabolism in hyperthyroidism. Presse-Med 1990; 19(15): 705–708.

132. Smith GS, Smith JL, Mameesh MS, Simon J, Comor-Johnson B. Hypertension and cardiovascular abnormalities in starved-refed swine. J Nutr 1964; 82: 172–182.

133. Schnitker MA, Mattman P, Bliss TL. A clinical study of malnutrition in Japanese prisoners of war. Ann Intern Med 1951; 35: 69–95.

134. Evans G. Physiology and treatment of starvation: experiences in war-starved Europe. Br Med J 1945; 1: 818–820.

135. Silvis SE, Paragas PD Jr. Paresthesias, weakness, seizures, and hypophosphatemia in patients receiving hyperalimentation. Gastroenterology 1972; 62: 513–517.

136. Weinsier RL, Krumdieck CL. Death resulting from overzealous TPN: The refeeding syndrome revisited. Am J Clin Nutr 1981; 34: 393–399.

137. Betro MG, Pain PW. Hyperphosphatemia and hypophosphatemia in a hospital population. Br Med J 1972; 1: 273–276.

138. Gufllou PS, Morgan DB, Hill GL. Hypophosphatemia: a complication of "innocuous dextrose-saline." Lancet 1976; 2: 710–712.

139. Metzger R, Bruke P, Thompson A, Lordon R, Frimpter GW. Hypophosphatemia and hypouricemia during parenteral hyperalimentation with an amino acid glucose preparation (abstr). J Clin Invest 1971; 50: 219.

140. Shike M, Harrison JE, Sturnidge WC, et al. Metabolic bone disease in patients receiving long-term total parenteral nutrition. Ann Intern Med 1980; 92: 343–350.

141. Shike M, Shils ME, Heller A, et al. Bone disease in prolonged parenteral nutrition: osteopenia without mineralization defect. Am J Clin Nutr 1986; 44: 89–98.

142. Shike M, Sturtridge WC, Tam CS, et al. A possible role of vitamin D in the genesis of parenteral nutation-induced metabolic bone disease. Ann Intern Med 1981; 95: 560–568.

143. Sitrin M, Meredith S, Rosenberg JH. Vitamin D deficiency and bone disease in gastrointestinal disorder. Arch Intern Med 1978; 138: 886–888.

144. Ahmed KY, Wills MR, Skinner RK, et al. Persistent hypophosphatemia and osteomalacia in dialysis patients not on oral phosphate binders: response to DHT. Lancet 1976; 2: 439–442.

145. Baker LRJ, Ackrill P, Cattell WR, Stamp TCB, Watson L. Iatrogenic osteomalacia and myopathy due to phosphate depletion. Br Med J 1974; 3: 150–153.

146. Bloom WL, Flinchum D. Osteomalacia with pseudofractures caused by the ingestion of aluminum hydroxide. JAMA 1960; 174: 1327–1331.

147. Carmichael RA, Fallon MD, Dalinka M, Kaplan MS, Axel R, Haddad J. Osteomalacia and osteitis fibrosa cystica in a man ingesting aluminum hydroxide antacid. Am J Med 1984; 76: 1137–1143.

148. Dent CE, Winter WS. Osteomalacia due to phosphate depletion from excessive aluminum hydroxide ingestion. Br Med J 1974; 1: 551–552.

149. Godsall JW, Baron R, Insogna KL. Vitamin D metabolism and bone histomorphometry in a patient with antacid-induced osteomalacia. Am J Med 1984; 77: 747–750.

150. Insogna KL, Bordley DR, Caro JF, Lockwood DH. Osteomalacia and weakness from excessive antacid ingestion. JAMA 1980; 244: 2544–2546.

151. Lotz M, Ney R, Banter FC. Osteomalacia and debility resulting from phosphorus depletion. Trans Assoc Am Physicians 1964; 77: 281–295.

152. Ludvig GD, Kyle GC, DeBlanco M. "Tertiary" hyperparathyroidism induced by osteomalacia resulting from phosphate depletion. Am J Med; 43: 409–515.

153. Levy Y, Majula B, Ackson DA, SWke M. Antacid-induced phosphate depletion syndrome. J Parenteral Enteral Nutr 1988; 12: 313–317.

154. Atchley DW, Loeb RF, Richards DW Jr. On diabetic acidosis: a detailed study of electrolyte balances following withdrawal and reestablishment of insulin therapy. J Clin Invest 1933; 12: 297–326.

155. Kanter Y, Gerson JR, Bessman AN. 2,3-Diphosphoglycerate, nucleotide phosphate and organic phosphate levels during the early phases of diabetic ketacidosis. Diabetes 1977; 26: 429–433.

156. Martin HE, Smith K, Wilson ML. The fluid and electrolyte therapy of severe diabetic acidosis and ketosis: a study of twenty-nine episodes (twenty-six patients). Am J Med 1958; 24: 376–389.

157. Franks M, Berris RF, Kaplan NO, Myers GB. Diabetic acidosis. Arch Intern Med 1948; 81: 42–55.

158. Knochel JP. The pathophysiology and clinical characteristics of severe hypophosphatemia. Arch Intern Med 1977; 137: 203–220.

159. Matter BJ, Worona M, Donat P, Smith WO, Ginn HE. Effect of ethanol on phosphate excretion in man (abstr). Clin Res 1964; 12: 255.

160. Wen SF, Boynar JW Jr, Stoll RW. Effect of phosphate deprivation on renal phosphate transport in the dog. Am J Physiol 1978; 234: F199–F206.

161. Markkanen T, Nanto V. The effect of ethanol infusion on the calcium phosphorus balance in man. Experientia 1966; 22: 753–754.

162. Kalbfleisch JM, Lindeman RD, Ginn HE, Smith WO. The effect of ethanol administration on urinary excretion of magnesium and other electrolytes in alcoholics and normal subjects. J Clin Invest 1963; 42: 1471–1475.

163. Knochel JP, Bilbrey GL, Fuller TJ, Carter NW. The muscle cell in chronic alcoholism: the possible role of phosphate depletion in alcoholic myopathy. Ann NY Acad Sci 1975; 252: 274–291.

164. Quamme GA, Wong NLM. Phosphate transport in the proximal convoluted tubule: effect of intraluminal pH. Am J Physiol 1984; 246: F323–333.

165. Straus NB, Rosenbaum JD, Nelson WP III. The effect of alcohol on the renal excretion of water and electrolytes. J Clin Invest 1950; 29: 1053–1058.

166. Territo MC, Tanaka KR. Hypophosphatemia in chronic alcoholism. Arch Intern Med 1974; 134: 445–447.

167. Shils ME. Experimental production of magnesium deficiency in men. Ann NY Acad Sci 1969; 162: 846–855.

168. DeOliveira HL, Laus-Filho JA. Hypophosphatemia in gout. Lancet 1961; 2: 215.

169. Olefsky J, Kempson R, Jones H, Reaven G. Tertiary "hyperparathyroidism" and "apparent cure" of vitamin D-resistant rickets after removal of an ossifying mesenchymal tumor of the pharynx. N Engl J Med 1972; 286: 740–745.

170. Salassa RM, Jowsey J, Amaud CD. Hypophosphatemic osteomalacia associated with non-endocrine tumors. N Engl J Med 1970; 283: 65–73.

171. Levy LA. Severe hypophosphatemia as a complication of treatment of hypothermia. Arch Intern Med 1980; 140: 128–129.

172. Short EM, Binder HJ, Rosenberg LE. Familial hypophosphatemic rickets: defective transport of inorganic phosphates by intestinal mucosa. Science 1973; 179: 700–702.

173. Wison DR, York SE, Jaworski ZF, Yendt ER. Studies in hypophosphatemic vitamin D-refractory osteomalacia in adults. Medicine 1965; 44: 99–134.

174. Reitz RE, Weinstein RL. Paraihyroid hormone secretion in familial vitamin D-resistant rickets. N Engl J Med 1973; 289: 941–948.

175. Scriver CR, Reade TM, DeLuca HF, Hamstra AJ. Serum 1,25-dihydroxyvitamin D levels in normal subjects and in patients with hereditary rickets or bone disease. N Engl J Med 1978; 299: 976–979.

176. Abrams DE, Silcott RB, Terry R, Beme TV, Barbour BH. Antacid induction of phosphate depletion syndrome in renal failure. West J Med 1974; 120: 157–161.

177. Boelens PA, Howard W, KjeUstrand C, Brown DM. Hypophosphatemia with muscle weakness due to antacids and hemodialysis. Am J Dis Child 1970; 120: 350–353.

178. Knochel JP. Neuromuscular manifestation of electrolytes disorders. Am J Med 1982; 72: 521–535.

179. Allen TR, Ruberg RL, Dudrick SJ, Long JM, Steiger E. 1971. Hypophosphatemia occurring in a patient receiving total parenteral hyperalimentation 1971 (abstr 2154). Fed Proc 1971; 30: 580.

180. Prins JG, Schrijver H, Staghouwre JH. Hyperalimentation, hypophosphatemia and coma. Lancet 1973; 1: 1253–1254.

181. Yawata Y, Craddock P, Hebbel R, Howe R, Silvis S, Jacob H. Hypophosphatemia: hematologic neurologic dysfimction due to ATP depletion (abstr). Clin Res 1973; 21: 729.

182. Weintraub M. Hypophosphatemia mimicking acute Guillian-Barré Syndrome. JAMA 1976; 235: 1040–1041.

183. Maister M, Johnson A, Kim GS, Popelka GR, Whyte MP. Audiologic finding in young patients with hypophosphatemic bone disease. Ann Otol Rhinol Laryngol 1986; 95: 415–420.

184. Wargovich MJ, Eng VWS, Newmark HL, Bruce WR. Calcium ameloriates the toxic effect of deoxycholic acid on colonic epithelium. Carcinogenesis 1983; 4: 1205–1207.

185. Yawata Y, Hebbel RP, Silvis S, Howe R, Jacob H. Blood cell abnormalities complicating the hypophosphatemia of hyperalimentation: erythrocyte and platelet AT deficiency associated with hemolytic anemia and bleeding in hyperalimented dogs. J Lab Clin Med 1974; 84: 643.

186. Klock JC, Williams HE, Mentzer WC. Hemolytic anemia and somatic cell dysfunction in severe hypophosphatemia. Arch Intern Med 1974; 134: 360–364.

187. Craddock PR, Yawata Y, Van Santen L, Gilberstadt S, Silvis S, Jacob HS. Acquired phagocyte dysfunction: a complication of hyperalimentation. N Engl J Med 1974; 290: 1403–1407.

188. Frank BW, Keon F Jr. Serum inorganic phosphorus during hepatic coma. Arch Intern Med 1962; 110: 865–871.

189. Rajan KS, Levinson R, Leevy CM. Hepatic hypoxia secondary to hypophosphatemia. Clin Res 1973; 21: 521.

190. Hurt GA, Chanutin A. Organic phosphate compounds of erythrocytes from individuals with cirrhosis of the liver. Proc Soc Exp Biol Med 1965; 118: 167–169.

191. Lotz M, Zisman E, Banter FC. Evidence for a phosphorus depletion syndrome in man. N Engl J Med 1968; 276: 409–415.

192. Bollaert PE, Gimenez M, Robin-Lherbier B, et al. Respective effects of malnutrition and phosphate depletion on endurance swimming and muscle metabolism in rats. Acta Physiol Scand 1992; 144(1): 1–7.

193. Moser CR, Fesser WJ. Rheumatic manifestations of hypophosphatemia. Arch Intern Med 1974; 13: 674–677.

194. Knochel JP, Barcenas C, Cotton JR, Fuller TJ, Haller R. Hypophosphatemia and rhabdomyolysis. J Clin Invest 1978; 62: 1240–1246.

195. Newman JH, Neff TA, Ziporin P. Acute respiratory failure associated with hypophosphatemia. N Engl J Med 1977; 308: 1101–1103.

196. O'Conner LR, Wheeler WS, Bethune JE. Effect of hypophosphatemia on myocardial performance in man. N Engl J Med 1977; 297: 901–903.

197. Darsee JR, Nutter DOP. Reversible severe congestive cardiomyopathy in three cases of hypophosphatemia. Ann Intern Med 1978; 89: 861–867.

198. Baylink D, Wergedal J, Stauffer M. Formation, mineralization and resorption of bone in hypophosphatemic rats. J Clin Invest 1971; 50: 2519–2530.

199. Freeman S, McLean HC. Experimental rickets: blood and tissue changes in puppies receiving a diet very low in phosphorus with and without vitamin D. Arch Pathol 1941; 32: 387–408.

200. Evans DJ, Azzopardi JG. Distinctive tumours of bone and soft tissue causing acquire vitamin D-resistant osteomalacia. Lancet 1972; 1: 353–360.

201. Stickler GB, Beabout JW, Riggs BL. Vitamin D-resistant rickets: clinical experience with 41

typical familial hypophosphatemia patients and two atypical nonfamilial cases. Mayo Clin Proc 1970; 45: 197–218.

202. Bruin WJ, Baylink DJ, Wergedal JE. Acute inhibition of mineralization and stimulation of bone resorption mediated by hypophosphatemia. Endocrinology 1975; 96: 394–398.

203. Coburn JW, Massey SG. Changes in serum and urinary calcium during phosphate depletion: studies on mechanisms. J Clin Invest 1970; 49: 1073–1087.

204. Lyles KW, Harrelson JM, Drezner MK. The efficacy of vitamin D₂ and oral phosphorus therapy in X-linked hypophosphatemic rickets and osteomalacia. J Clin Endocrinol Metab 1982; 54: 307–315.

205. Emmett M, Goldfarb S, Agus ZS, Narins RG. The pathophysiology of acid-base changes in chronically phosphate-depleted rats: bone kidney interactions. J Clin Invest 1977; 59: 291–298.

206. Gold LM, Massey SG, Arieff AL, Coburn JW. Renal bicarbonate wasting during phosphate depletion: a possible cause of altered acid-base homeostasis in hyperparathyroidism. J Clin Invest 1973; 52: 2556–2562.

207. Gold LM et al. Effect of phosphate depletion on renal tubular reabsorption of glucose. J Lab Clin Med 1977; 89: 554–559.

208. Massey SG. The clinical syndrome of phosphate depletion. Adv Exp Med Biol 1978; 103: 301–312.

209. Whang R, Welt LG. Observation in experimental magnesium deficiency. J Clin Invest 1963; 42: 305–313.

210. Lee DBN, Brautbar N, Walling MW, Sills V, Coburn JW, Kleeman CR. Effect of phosphorus depletion on intestinal calcium and phosphorus absorption. Am J Physiol 1979; 236: E451–E457.

211. Kleeman CR. Should hypophosphatemia be treated? Adv Exp Med Biol 1982; 151: 309–316.

212. Lau K, Wolf C, Nussbaum P, et al. Differing effects of acid versus neutral phosphate therapy of hypercalciuria. Kidney Int 1979; 16: 736–742.

213. Vannatta JB, Whang R, Papper S. Efficacy of intravenous phosphorus therapy in the severely hypophosphatemic patient. Arch Intern Med 1981; 141: 885–887.

214. Lenz DR, Brown DM, Kjellstrand CM. Treatment of severe hypophosphatemia. Ann Intern Med 1978; 89: 941–944.

215. Rigas DA, Duerst ML, Junp ME, Osgood EE. The nucleic acids and other phosphorus compounds of human leukemic leucocytes: relation to cell maturity. J Lab Clin Med 1956; 48: 356–361.

216. Walser M. The separate effects of hyperparathyroidism, hypercalcemia of malignancy, renal failure, and acidosis on the state of calcium, phosphate and other ions in plasma. J Clin Invest 1962; 41: 1554–1565.

217. Zusman J, Brown DM, Nesbit ME. Hyperphosphatemia, hyperphosphaturia, and hypocalcemia. Acute lymphoblastic leukemia. N Engl J Med 1973; 289: 1335–1340.

218. Cardman EC, Lundberg WB, Bertino JR. Hyperphosphatemia and hypocalcemia accompanying rapid cell lysis in a patient with Burkitt's lymphoma and Burkitt cell leukemia. Am J Med 1977; 62: 283–290.

219. Brerton HD, Anderson T, Johnson RE, Schein SP. Hyperphosphatemia and hypocalcemia in Burkitt's lymphoma. Complications of chemotherapy. Arch Intern Med 1975; 135: 307–309.

220. Lorcerie B, Besancenot JF, Maillefert F, et al. False hyperphosphoremia in multiple myeloma. Interference of monoclonal immunoglobulin G with the determination of blood phosphorus level. Rev Med Interne 1991; 12(4): 262–264.

221. Dugre V, Levillain P, Lemonnier A. Hypeiphosphatemia in cases of abnormal proteinemia (letter). Presse Med 1990; 19(7): 338.

222. Ilberg JJ, Turner GG, Nuttall FQ. Effect of phosphate or magnesium cathartics on serum calcium. Arch Intern Med 1978; 138: 1114–1116.

223. Jimenez, RAH, Larson EB. Case report. Tumoral calcinosis: an unusual complication of the laxative abuse syndrome. Am J Med Sci 1981; 282: 141–147.

224. McConnell TH. Fatal hypocalcemia from phosphate absorption from laxative preparation. JAMA 1971; 216: 147–148.
225. Albright F, Reifenstein EC Jr, eds. The Parathyroid Glands and Metabolic Bone Disease. Baltimore: Williams & Wilkins, 14.
226. Krane SM, Brownell GL, Stanbury JB, Conigan H. The effect of thyroid disease on calcium metabolism in man. J Clin Invest 1956; 35: 874–881.
227. Alfrey AC, Solomons CC. Bone pyrophosphate in uremia and its associations with extra-osseous calcification. J Clin Invest 1976; 57: 700–705.
228. Palmer PES. Tumoral calcinosis. Br J Radiol 1966; 39: 518–525.
229. Mitnick PD, Goldfarb S, Slatopolsky E, et al. Calcium and phosphate metabolism in tumoral calcinosis. Ann Intern Med 1980; 92: 482–487.
230. Lufkin EG, Wilson DM, Smith LH, et al. Phosphorus excretion in tumoral calcinosis: responses to parathyroid hormone and acetazolamide. J Clin Endocrinol Metab 1980; 50: 648–653.
231. Huang RP, Adamson ED. The phosphorylated forms of the transcription factor, Egr-1, bind to DNA more efficiently than non-phosphorylated. Biochem Biophys Res Commun 1994; 200: 1271–1276.

4

Sodium and Chloride in Nutrition

MARY-ELLEN HARPER
University of Ottawa, Ottawa, Ontario, Canada

JOHN S. WILLIS
University of Georgia, Athens, Georgia

JOHN PATRICK
University of Ottawa, Ottawa, Ontario, Canada

I. INTRODUCTION

After water, sodium and chloride are the two nutrients whose deficiency leads most acutely and frequently to premature death, usually from circulatory failure secondary to diarrhea and often complicated by disorders of osmolality. Their physiology is consequently characterized by multiple control mechanisms to conserve their content and control their concentration within the body.

Excessive intake of sodium and chloride can also be an important aggravating factor in several diseases. Inadvertent excessive administration, without sufficient water, to patients unable to complain of thirst has caused deaths, most notably in infants. When thirst mechanisms are operative and the subject is able to get or demand water, excessive salt intake is not an acute problem and salt loads are largely excreted in slightly more than 24 h. Body weight can be permanently changed by about 1 kg with large changes in habitual salt intake.

The early humans were mainly carnivorous. Their diets therefore contained adequate amounts of sodium and chloride. As societies became agriculturally orientated and the consumption of vegetables and grains increased, the addition of salt to the diet became important. For that reason, control over the supply of salt has been frequently of political importance in world history. Wars have been fought over salt deposits. In India, Gandhi used disobedience over the salt tax to oppose the British. In our everyday speech, an echo of the importance of salt remains in the word "salary," which is derived from the allowance of salt made to officers in the Roman army—*salarium*. Salt production worldwide is in excess of 150 million tons.

Sodium ion and chloride are the chief extracellular ions, and they play key roles in the maintenance of water balance. Their intracellular concentrations are less than 10% of the extracellular concentrations. Maintenance of this gradient and the related membrane potential requires major expenditure of energy. It is essential for the function of excitable cells and is critical to nerve and muscle function. The co-transport of sodium across this gradient plays a key role in the absorption of other nutrients such as glucose and amino acids. Chloride exerts an important function in pH regulation and CO_2 transport. The mechanisms by which sodium and chloride exert these functions will be discussed.

II. CHEMISTRY AND ANALYSIS

A. Chemistry

Sodium occurs in high abundance (2.6%) in the lithosphere. It is an alkali metal that readily loses one electron, its only oxidation state. The chemistry of sodium in the body is almost entirely that of a strong monovalent cation. It hardly forms covalent bonds except in bone. In solution the Na^+ attracts a fairly large shell of water molecules. Although the anhydrous Na^+ ion is smaller than that of K^+, the common hydrated form is larger than that of K^+. The greater permeability of cell membranes to potassium over sodium may be due to the different hydration shells, because although sodium is smaller in the dehydrated form, thought to be required for passage through membranes, it would require more energy to shed its hydration shell.

Chloride derives from chlorine, a member of the halogen family. These elements readily gain an electron, and their chemistry is entirely nonmetallic. Chlorine exists in nature mainly as sodium chloride. The hydrated chloride ion is similar in size to that of potassium, and it moves readily across membranes.

B. Analytical Methods for Sodium and Chloride

The methods for measurement of these ions are well established and validated (1). Flame photometry, atomic absorption, and ion-sensitive electrodes are used to determine sodium, and electrometric methods to measure chloride. The difference between the concentration and activity of sodium and chloride in extracellular fluid is sometimes of importance in clinical practice. The difference is often not appreciated and thus a brief review of the relevant terms follows.

The concentration of a substance in a biological fluid is still expressed in many clinics and hospitals as combining equivalents (mEq/L). The introduction of the SI unit, mmol/L, has been rather slow but will eventually lead to the replacement of combining equivalents. Because the concept of the combining equivalent is useful in that it relates the ionic weight of an electrolyte to the number of charges that it carries, the use of combining equivalents for some ions will continue to be necessary. The term *activity* refers to the contribution of the particular ion or substance to the osmotic activity of the solution in which it is suspended. The osmotic activity of a solution is usually determined by measuring the degree to which the freezing point is altered. For substances that do not dissociate, such as glucose, the number of osmotically active particles is equal to the number of molecules and therefore 1 mmol/L is equal to 1 mosmol/L. For sodium chloride, which dissociates into the sodium cation and the chloride anion, 1 mmol of NaCl will result in approximately 2 mosmol in solution. Frequently it is wrongly assumed that NaCl dissociates completely. However, sodium chloride has a osmotic coefficient of 0.9 and thus dissociation is only 90% complete. This will vary slightly depending on the concentration of the solution. The term *osmolality* refers to the concentration of active particles in a kilogram of water, and *osmolarity* refers to the concentration of active particles in a liter of solution. Because osmotic activity depends on the concentration of active particles per kilogram of water, the term *osmolality* is the correct one to use, although practically the differences are small.

Falsely low values for sodium are an important occasional phenomenon in clinical medicine. Normally the concentration of solids in plasma is so constant that the relationship between true concentration in plasma water and the concentration in whole plasma is essentially constant and the difference is so small that clinicians treat them as identical. But if urea, glucose, or most particularly, lipids increase dramatically, then the concentration of sodium in plasma can fall as much as 50 mmol/L below that in plasma water. Clinical chemistry is performed on samples of plasma, not plasma water. Failure to recognize this phenomenon can lead to inappropriate treatment. The lack of agreement between the apparent sodium value and a measurement of osmolality by freezing-point depression can be used to quickly calculate the true concentration in plasma water (20).

Another term that relates to the importance of sodium and chloride in biological fluids is tonicity. *Tonicity* refers to the effective osmolality of a solution. Solutions that have the same effective osmolality as serum are referred to as *isotonic*, while solutions that have lower and higher osmolalities than plasma are referred to as *hypotonic* and *hypertonic*, respectively. Thus a solution of isotonic sodium chloride is approximately 285 mosmolal and is provided by a solution of 154 mM sodium chloride. The terms *normal saline* and *physiological saline* are obsolete but were used in the past (and are sometimes used today) to describe isotonic sodium chloride. A useful reference for a description of the basics of fluid and electrolyte balance was provided by Smith (3).

III. METABOLISM

A. Body Distribution

The major sodium-containing compartment in the body is the extracellular space (Table 1), with a normal sodium concentration of 135–145 mmol/L. Chloride is the major accompanying anion, with an extracellular concentration of 100–110 mmol/L. Extracellular water accounts for approximately half of total body water in the newborn, falling to nearer 30% by the end of the first year. About 20% of body sodium is in bone, where it only slowly exchanges with the rest of the extracellular pool. Intracellular sodium concentrations vary from tissue to tissue but are commonly close to 10 mmol/L and rarely more than 30 mmol/L cell water in the absence of disease.

B. Absorption

There appears to be no control on the absorption of dietary sodium and chloride, with virtually all being absorbed, provided glucose is available for transport processes. Sodium and chloride absorption occur by several mechanisms, of which electroneutral co-transport systems account for about 20%, diffusion possibly up to 50%, and other transport processes, many of which are dependent at least in part on electrogenic forces, for the rest.

TABLE 1   Distribution of Sodium in the Body as a Percentage
of Total Body Sodium and as mEq/kg Body Weight

	Percent total body sodium	mEq/kg
Total body sodium	100	58
Exchangeable body sodium	71	41
Total intracellular	9	5
Total extracellular	91	53
Interstitial fluid	29	17
Plasma	11	7
Connective tissue and cartilage	12	7
Bone		
Exchangeable	11	6
Nonexchangeable	26	15
Transcellular	3	2

From Ref. 4.

Sodium-glucose and sodium-amino acid cotransporters exist in the apical membranes of enterocytes and mediate sodium uptake coupled to glucose or amino acid uptake. Thus the absorption of glucose and some amino acids is dependent on sodium uptake. There are always simultaneous absorptive and secretory processes operative, thus increased secretion or decreased absorption may produce similar overall results. In the absence of glucose, infusion of saline via a nasogastric tube at high flow rates induces an osmotic diarrhea which is therapeutically useful in conditions such as cystic fibrosis and severe constipation, where fecal obstruction is often beyond the reach of enemata (5). Physiologic controls on whole-body sodium are mediated through the kidney, but each cell membrane contains the means to regulate intracellular sodium and chloride. Hypothalamic mechanisms are the major determinants of plasma concentration, modifying renal function by way of antidiuretic hormone. Figure 1 shows the important mechanisms involved in the intestinal absorption of sodium and chloride.

C. Control Mechanisms

1. Renal and Hormonal

Sodium, chloride, and bicarbonate, the three major osmotically active particles in the extracellular fluid, are freely filtered at the glomerulus. Thus, knowing the glomerular filtration rate, it is easy to calculate the filtered load and the fractional excretion, but because this is a small number derived from subtraction of two large numbers, it is highly vulnerable to methodological errors. The efficiency with which these three ions are reabsorbed from the filtered load is remarkable. Each day, for a healthy adult consuming a normal diet, approximately 25 mol of sodium, 18 mol of chloride, and 5 mol of bicarbonate are filtered. With only 100 mmol each of sodium and chloride and no bicarbonate being excreted each day, the efficiency (or percentage reabsorbed) is greater than 99.5% in all cases.

As shown in Figure 2, approximately 65% of the filtered load of sodium is reabsorbed in the proximal tubule. The process is mediated by active sodium transport and also modulated by alterations in luminal surface permeability. Chloride, which is passively reabsorbed, accompanies the actively transported sodium and is the major ion transported

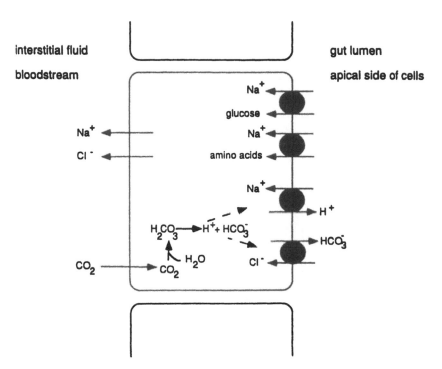

FIGURE 1 Important mechanisms in the intestinal absorption of sodium and chloride. Na^+ uptake is coupled to glucose and amino acid uptake by cotransporters, and to H^+ extrusion by the Na-H antiporter. Intracellular H^+ is generated by carbonic anhydrase. The other product of carbonic anhydrase, HCO_3^-, is extruded into the lumen of the gut in exchange for Cl^-. Na^+ and Cl^- then leave the enterocyte through channels in the basolateral membrane.

to balance the electrochemical gradient that is established by the activity of the Na–K pump in the proximal tubule. About 25% of the filtered load of sodium chloride is reabsorbed in the loop of Henle. The countercurrent system for the reabsorption of water is dependent in part on the reabsorption of sodium chloride in the loop of Henle. In this section of the nephron, sodium is reabsorbed passively; it balances the movement of chloride, which is actively transported by a chloride pump. It is in the loop of Henle where the "loop" diuretics such as furosemide act. In most physiologic conditions this proportion of sodium reabsorption remains constant. Approximately 10% of the filtered load is reabsorbed from the distal tubule and the proximal part of the collecting duct. The reabsorption process here is similar to that in the proximal tubule except that active sodium reabsorption is more closely coupled to the excretion of potassium and hydrogen and less closely coupled to the reabsorption of chloride. It is in this part of the nephron where the "fine-tuning" mechanisms for reabsorption occur.

The interactions among the various systems known to be involved in the maintenance of sodium balance are a continuing challenge to the clinician. Even a simple listing of these systems indicates how great the ramifications are:

1. Renin, angiotensin, and aldosterone
2. Renal blood flow (RBF) and glomerular filtration rate (GFR)
3. Plasma sodium concentration

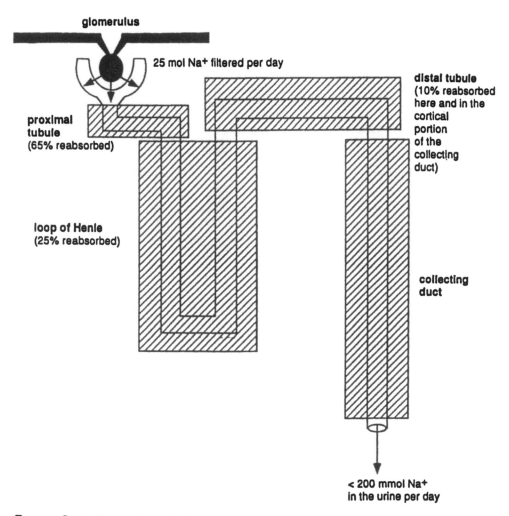

FIGURE 2 Sodium reabsorption in the nephron. In a healthy adult consuming a normal diet, approximately 25 mol of sodium is filtered per day from the glomeruli. About 16 mol (65% of the filtered load) is reabsorbed in the proximal tubule. About 6 mol is reabsorbed in the loop of Henle and approximately 3 mol is reabsorbed in the distal tubule and cortical part of the collecting duct. Only a very small proportion of the filtered load (< 1%) is excreted in the urine.

4. Antidiuretic hormone
5. Adrenal hormone secretion other than aldosterone
6. Atrial natriuretic peptide
7. Plasma oncotic pressure interacting with RBF
8. Intrarenal distribution of blood flow

The last seven systems interact with the renin angiotensin axis, which is the primary control system on overall sodium balance. However, under particular pathophysiologic conditions, each can become the dominant factor.

These systems have been extensively reviewed (6–8). For the nutritionist it is important to realize that in the event of one system malfunctioning or in the context of very unusual salt intakes, the proportion of sodium balance attributable to each mechanism may be statistically very unusual without any necessary problem with salt balance. The Yanamamo people of the Amazon Basin, for example, have extremely high renin levels without any untoward effects. Presumably this reflects a physiologic response to their extremely low intake of salt.

2. Cellular

The cellular aspect of sodium balance is far from being completely known, but it is of particular interest to nutritionists for several reasons: first, because of its implications for energy expenditure; second, because other dietary constituents such as fats may alter membrane transport indirectly; and finally, because sodium transport is abnormal in a range of diseases, many of which have malnutrition as the common element.

There are three fundamental principles which must be borne in mind when discussing sodium and its transport systems. First, the sodium gradient can be exploited as an energy source for the uphill transport of solutes into the cell by cotransporting on common carriers (e.g., amino acids) or by countertransport on exchange carriers (e.g., Ca^{2+}, Mg^{2+}, H^+). Second, many channels and carriers are regulated which is particularly important for the regulation of cell volume. Finally, the mechanisms involved in the regulation of the ionic content of cells are closely analogous to those used by epithelial tissues to regulate whole-body content.

Numerous studies in the 1960s (9–11) demonstrated the energetic costs of the maintenance of a low intracellular sodium. Necessarily these conclusions were based on studies of isolated cells and tissue slices. Of the oxygen utilization by brain and renal slices, 40% was inhibited by ouabain, whose primary molecular target is the Na-K pump. Sodium removal had the same effect, and reintroduction of sodium activated transport and raised oxygen consumption.

Because of the substantial proportion of resting energy expenditure of cells that is proposed to be due to Na-K pump activity, attempts to find evidence of adapted sodium transport in starvation followed. Two models have been used: laboratory rats and hibernating black bears. In rats, fasting to 75% of starting weight caused a reduction in red cell ouabain-sensitive potassium influx, associated with a parallel change in the ouabain-insensitive leak. However, in studies of other tissues, comparable results were not obtained. It appears that adaptational effects are seen only in severe fasting and perhaps only in some tissues. In black bears, amiloride-sensitive sodium influx (the Na–H exchanger) declined in some cases by 80% in late January, after 2 months of fasting. It rose with springtime feeding.

The most cogent argument in favor of the Na-K pump accounting for a substantial proportion of energy expenditure remains the known stoichiometry of ATP consumption to sodium transport.

The action of the Na-K pump is controlled primarily by the intra- and extracellular concentrations of Na^+ and K^+. Other nutrients have also been shown to modify cell membrane transport; particularly important are lipids and minerals. There are several good reviews (12–14). Cholesterol has been studied most extensively; an increase in membrane cholesterol is thought to stiffen the membrane and make it less permeable, while the opposite occurs with cholesterol depletion. There is a clinical correlate of cholesterol excess, which produces characteristic morphological changes in red cells and is called spur cell anemia. Red cell sodium concentration is increased in this condition. Changes in fatty acids have only minor effects on cell membrane transport of sodium and potassium but more marked effects on mitochondrial membranes. Some tissues have unique sensitivities; e.g., white cell membrane sodium transport is extremely sensitive to the effects of zinc (15). Presumably this effect has some relevance to the relationship between zinc and immune function, but the linkage has not been elucidated.

3. Biochemical Regulation

The entire biochemistry of sodium revolves around its passage across cell membranes through channels, on selective saturable carriers or via the Na-K pump. To the extent that chlorine occurs as chloride ion, the same may be said of it. This is a large and rapidly expanding subject; what follows is only a brief catalog of a few of the relevant generic pathways. Figure 3 depicts the major ion transporters and channels of cell membranes and the normal concentrations of the principal ions in the intracellular and extracellular spaces.

1.   The *Na-K pump* (*Na-K ATPase*) is a ubiquitous, highly conserved mechanism among animal cells. Its structure comprises two subunits, the 100-kDa alpha subunit, which is the catalytic component that binds ATP, Na^+, K^+, and the inhibitor ouabain (or other cardiac glycosides), and the 35-kDa beta subunit, a glycoprotein that accompanies the alpha subunit in its deployment to the plasma membrane but that has no other recognized role. Both molecules have been cloned and sequenced; to date, three tissue-specific isoforms of alpha and two principal isoforms of beta have been identified (16). The pump operates to extrude three ions of Na^+ and take in two ions of K^+ for each molecule of ATP hydrolyzed. This stoichiometry can be altered artificially, but it is not clear if it can vary in physiologic circumstances. The mechanism of action of the Na-K pump is shown in Figure 4. Based on ouabain binding, the number of pump sites on a cell may range from as large as 250,000 to as few as 250, and may vary according to physiologic conditions. Pump synthesis is promoted by aldosterone and thyroid hormone. The most potent activators of the pump are its ligands, intracellular Na^+ and Mg^{2+}. Endogenous ouabain-like inhibitors of the Na-K pump are found in the circulation and may be produced in the adrenal cortex and elsewhere (17,18). In transporting epithelial cells the Na-K pump is believed to be restricted to the basolateral face of the cell, and in conjunction with other carrier or channel pathways to be the ultimate determinant of transcellular translocation of Na^+, K^+, and Cl^- ions, but not of Ca^{2+} or H^+ ions.

2.   The *Na–H exchanger* is a widespread mechanism that plays several cellular roles, most commonly cell alkalinization and cell swelling following shrinkage (so-called regulatory volume increase; see further discussion below). Among various transporting epithelial cells (e.g., small intestine, stomach), it plays several roles such as promoting Na^+ entry into cells, allowing absorption and regulation of extracellular pH. One isoform, NHE1, seems to be virtually ubiquitous; at least four other isoforms have been identified in specific tissues, with presumably specialized roles (19). NHE1 is inhibited by amiloride and its derivatives; some of the isoforms are less sensitive to these inhibitors. It possesses a cytoplasmic regulatory site, and at least the more familiar mechanisms of activation of this carrier (mitogens, cell shrinkage) are thought to operate through altering the sensitivity of this site to cytoplasmic H^+. The carrier is also the substrate for kinase activation, which may operate either through or independently of the H^+ activator site (19).

3.   The *Na-K-Cl cotransporters* transport Na^+, K^+, and Cl^- electroneutrally into and out of cells with a usual stoichiometry of 1Na:1K:2Cl. They are widely distributed in cells and tissues including reabsorptive and secretory epithelia, muscle and nerve cells,

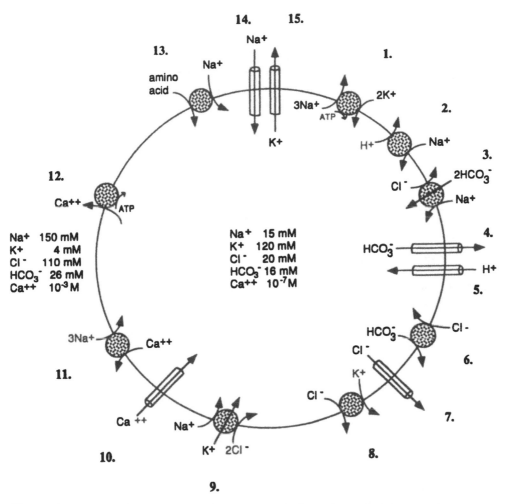

FIGURE 3 The major ion transporters and channels of cell membranes and the normal concentrations of the principal ions in the intracellular and extracellular spaces. The following transport pathways correspond to the numbers identifying the pathways: 1, Na-K pump; 2, Na-H antiporter; 3, Na-HCO$_3$-Cl cotransporter; 4, HCO$_3^-$ uniport (outward directed); 5, H$^+$ uniport (inward directed); 6, HCO$_3$-Cl antiporter; 7, Cl$^-$ channel; 8, K-Cl cotransporter; 9, Na-K-Cl cotransporter; 10, Ca^{2+} channel; 11, Na–Ca exchanger; 12, Ca^{2+} pump; 13, Na$^+$-amino acid cotransporter; 14, Na$^+$ channel; 15, K$^+$ channel.

endothelial cells, fibroblasts, and blood cells. Na-K-Cl cotransporters are important in renal salt reabsorption and in salt secretion by intestinal, airway, salivary gland, and other secretory epithelia. They also operate to reswell cells following osmotic shrinkage. In some epithelial cells (e.g., colonic crypt cells, pancreatic acinar cells, parotid glands, tracheal epithelium), they also promote Cl$^-$ entry as an essential step in transepithelial chloride transport (20). Both the kidney-specific and the secretory isoforms of the epithelial Na-K-Cl cotransporters have been identified by cDNA cloning and sequencing and Northern blot analyses. The proposed model of the shark rectal gland Na-K-Cl cotransporter, based on its cDNA sequence and hydropathy plot analysis, has 12 transmembrane segments and

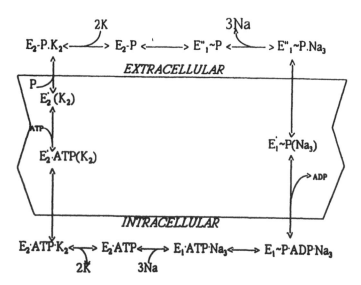

FIGURE 4 Mechanistic model of the Na-K pump. The model is as described in a recent review by Skou (14). The symbols E_1, E'_1, E''_1, E_2, and E'_2 refer to the different conformations of the enzyme, Na-K ATPase. Note that E_1 has three monovalent cation binding sites, while E_2 has two binding sites. Phosphoenzymes are represented as E-P. To indicate that the cations are occluded in the membrane phase, brackets surround the cations. The binding sites for ATP, phosphate, and Na are on the intracellular side of the membrane, while the binding site for K is on the extracellular side of the membrane.

two large cytoplasmic domains that include multiple phosphorylation consensus sequences. The activity of the carrier is mediated by adenosine 3',5'-cyclic monophosphate (cAMP) and kinase A (e.g., in response to ligands such as catecholamines, vasointestinal peptide, and adenosine) (21), but the activation by shrinkage appears to operate through a different route. It is powerfully inhibited by loop diuretics (e.g., bumetanide and furosemide), whose binding increases dramatically with activation of the pathway. An excellent review of the Na-K-Cl cotransporters has been written recently by Haas (20).

A separate cotransporter for K^+ and Cl^- that is also inhibited by loop diuretics (furosemide) has been identified mainly in red blood cells. It is activated by cell swelling, by oxidizing agents, and by mild warming. Its response to swelling, and possibly to warming, is thought to restore cell volume by causing KCl dumping (22,23). It is implicated in the sickling phenomenon of red cells in persons with sickle cell anemia and is believed to be present in other types of cells (e.g., kidney). Its role in other tissues has not yet been determined.

4. While the *Na–Ca exchanger* was originally identified in squid giant axons, it is now recognized to be of paramount importance in determining Ca^{2+} concentrations of cytoplasm and cytoplasmic structures in cardiac muscle, smooth muscle cells, and nerve endings (24). It is a low-affinity, high-velocity pathway that works in parallel with Ca-ATPases to maintain low cell Ca^{2+} between episodes of electrical activity. It may also supplement voltage-activated Ca^{2+} channels in promoting Ca^{2+} entry during excitation. Its stoichiometry of $3Na^+:1Ca^{2+}$ renders it an electrogenic pathway sensitive to membrane

potential (depolarization causes reversal from the "forward" mode, Ca^{2+} out for Na^+ in, to the "reverse" mode, Na^+ out for Ca^{2+} in). It is activated by cytoplasmic Ca^{2+} and by phosphorylation by ATP (kinase not identified). It has recently been cloned and at least partially sequenced; the sequenced amino acids account for about 108 of its 160-kDa molecular weight. It is purported to have 12 transmembrane sequences and one large cytoplasmic domain with putative phosphorylation and calmodulin-binding sites.

5.   *Other Na^+ carriers*: Na^+-Mg^{2+} exchangers have been described in mammalian and avian erythrocytes. Their properties vary somewhat depending on source, but most of them are inhibited by amiloride and dependent on cytoplasmic ATP (25,26). Assuming that they represent one family of carriers, the published data are not fully consistent with their being an ATP-dependent pump or a simple exchanger. Possibly more than one type of mechanism is represented. There are numerous distinct cotransporters for Na^+ and amino acids, organic acids, and phosphate in various mammalian cell types.

6.   The voltage-gated Na^+ *channel* is widespread in the animal kingdom among excitable nerve and muscle cells and is familiar at some level to every student of physiology. It is peculiar in being opened and closed by depolarization. The alpha subunit of the channel has been cloned and sequenced, and it is characterized by having four repeated sequences each of which contains six hydrophobic segments. Much progress has been made in identifying parts of the molecule with specific properties of the channel: The fourth transmembrane segment in each of the repeated sequences is associated with voltage sensitivity and opening; the cytoplasmic domain, linking the third and fourth repeated sequence, is thought to correspond to the "gate" that shuts during inactivation (27).

Epithelial cells often contain Na^+ channels at their apical surface. When present, these allow the Na^+ to enter the cell, from which it is pumped out of the basolateral side of the cell by the Na-K pump. (In some cells Na^+ may enter via Na–H exchange or Na-K-Cl cotransport.) These channels are characterized by sensitivity to the drug, amiloride, at concentrations (e.g., $< 1\ \mu M$) far less than those required to inhibit the Na–H exchanger (28). Na^+ permeation through these pathways may be increased in various ways, such as mobilization (increase in number) from subcellular pools of membrane or activation by phosphorylation mediated by protein kinase A in response to an activating ligand (e.g., vasopressin in renal collecting duct) (29).

Chloride transport is similarly characterized by various carriers, apart from those described above, and by channels. Intracellular chloride levels are maintained at concentrations that are much lower than those in the extracellular fluid. If chloride were transported exclusively through passive processes across the plasma membrane, which typically has a potential of approximately 60 mV, then the intracellular concentration of chloride would be about one-tenth of that in the extracellular fluid. However, the fact that intracellular concentrations are about 20% of the extracellular chloride concentrations indicates that uphill net uptake occurs. This is likely energized by the downhill entry of Na^+ into the cell, such as, for example, that through the Na-K-Cl cotransporter (see above), and thus is ultimately dependent on ATP hydrolysis by the Na-K pump.

Most cells are able to counteract perturbations in cell volume. Swollen cells tend to reduce their volume to basal levels by the loss of KCl and the synchronous loss of water; this is referred to as regulatory volume decrease. Ion transport systems proposed to be activated during regulatory volume decrease in various cell types include conductive K^+ and Cl^- channels and K-Cl cotransport (30). Cell shrinkage often results in increased cell volume toward basal levels by the net uptake of K^+ and Cl^- and the ensuing regulatory volume increase. The transport systems thought to be involved include Na-K-2Cl cotransport and functionally coupled Na-H and Cl-HCO$_3$ exchange (20). These same pathways are involved in the regulation of intracellular pH in many cells.

Some of the better-recognized chloride transport pathways, not already discussed, are outlined below.

1. The *Cl-HCO$_3$ exchangers* are principally involved in the regulation of pH$_i$. There are two known exchangers, both of which are electroneutral, a Na-independent Cl-HCO$_3$ exchanger and a Na-dependent Cl-HCO$_3$ exchanger. The latter, like the Na–H antiporter, defends against cell acidification by activating as a pathway for HCO$_3^-$ entry in exchange for intracellular Cl$^-$. The former operates to extrude HCO$_3^-$ in exchange for external Cl$^-$. Both are inhibited by cyclic nucleotides and by stilbene derivatives such as 4,4'-diisothiocyanostilbene-2,2'-disulfonic acid (DIDS) (31).

2. *Cystic fibrosis transmembrane conductance regulator (CFTR)*: A genetic disease related to chloride metabolism that is of particular concern to nutritionists is cystic fibrosis (CF). CF is caused by mutations in the gene product CF transmembrane conductance regulator (CFTR), a 180-kDa glycoprotein that functions as an cAMP-regulated Cl$^-$ channel. The cAMP-activated Cl$^-$ currents associated with CFTR are voltage and time independent, sensitive to the inhibitors glibenclamide and diphenylamine carboxylic acid (DPC), but unaltered by the stilbene derivatives including DIDS (32). This protein is defective in cystic fibrosis; the most common mutation is the deletion of phenylalanine at residue 508. It has been proposed that the defect in CF is not in the potential function of the channel but in the intracellular processing involved in the transport of the CFTR to the apical membrane (33). Moreover, it has recently been shown that the CFTR not only functions as a cAMP-regulated Cl$^-$ channel in epithelial cells, it also controls the regulation of protein kinase A-stimulated outwardly rectifying Cl$^-$ channels (34). The CFTR has been reviewed recently (35).

3. *Calcium-activated chloride channels*: Another important type of chloride channel is activated by intracellular calcium. Calcium acts either directly through binding to the channel protein or indirectly by inducing the phosphorylation of proteins. None of the calcium-activated chloride channels has been cloned, and there is little biochemical data for this type of channel.

4. *Voltage-sensitive chloride channels*: Most ion channels exhibit some degree of membrane voltage dependence. If the dependence is strong or is the primary mechanism of channel regulation, then they are termed voltage-sensitive channels. Voltage-sensitive chloride channels are widely distributed and involved in various important physiological processes such as central neural inhibition, the shaping of action potentials of excitable cells and of the synaptic currents of muscular and neuronal preparations, as well as the regulation of cellular osmolality (36). Many voltage-sensitive chloride channels have been identified and include, among others, the major skeletal muscle chloride channel, the outwardly rectifying channels in epithelial cells, and the hyperpolarized-activated channels found in Leydig cells and in the mandibular gland. The molecular physiology of voltage-dependent chloride channels has recently been reviewed by Pusch and Jentsch (37).

5. *Mechanically (or "stretch-") activated chloride channels*: Volume-sensitive ion channels permeable to K$^+$ and Cl$^-$ or nonselective cation channels have been described in various nonexcitable cells in which they are thought to play an important role in volume regulation (see Ref. 37). In some cells (e.g., fibroblasts and endothelial cells), components of the cytoskeleton respond to changes in mechanical events (e.g., shear stress and stretch)

and trigger the opening of Cl^- channels. The mechanisms are not well understood but may include a G-protein-mediated second messenger and the activation of a plasma membrane P-glycoprotein (38). These volume-activated currents are fundamentally different from the Ca^{2+}-dependent Cl^- channels that are also characteristic of endothelial cells.

D. Response to Intake

Nutritionists are accustomed to think about nutrient requirements in terms of recommended intakes. However, for elements such as sodium, potassium, and chloride, which are richly endowed with physiologic control mechanisms, this is not the most meaningful or useful approach. A more rational approach is to think in terms of maximal conservation capacity and maximal excretory capacity together with an assessment of the particular renal, hormonal, and membrane responses underlying overall balance for these nutrients. Sometimes, as in cardiac failure, the kidney becomes inappropriately sodium retentive. In these circumstances, where it is often difficult to modify renal function, it is possible to modify the diet to match the renal aberration by restriction to an extremely low sodium intake.

Sodium and chloride intakes can vary tremendously within human populations. The range of habitual daily intakes of salt compatible with a normal lifespan is from less than 2 g (Yanamamo Indians of the Amazon Basin) to 35 g (N. Island of Japan). There are subsets of people for whom either of the extremes of intake would be dangerous, but the problem lies primarily with the limitations of their homeostatic mechanisms rather than any intrinsic property of salt. Thus, some children with cystic fibrosis whose maximal capacity to conserve salt is limited will not survive on a low salt intake, and some individuals with salt-sensitive hypertension will die prematurely on a high intake.

The nutritionist needs also to be sophisticated in consideration of changes in the concentrations of these ions in the blood, not being seduced into simplistic interpretations of acute changes in concentration but rather attendant to the total body content of the ions and their role in the control of extracellular volume and therefore body weight. Weight gain or loss without concurrent changes in energy balance sufficient to explain the alteration in weight should always be taken as evidence of a problem with the control of salt and water.

McCance's classic experiment in the 1930s, in which he depleted himself of 758 mmol of sodium, documented the normal human renal adaptation to salt depletion: the progressive fall in urinary sodium, the rather modest changes in plasma sodium and renal function, and the dramatic reduction in work capacity and psychologic function (39).

Subsequent studies of the rate of change of sodium excretion with dietary changes of intake have shown that it is an exponential function such that switching to a zero sodium intake will cause the 24-h sodium excretion to fall by approximately 50% each 24 h until balance is achieved. Ultimately, urine can become almost sodium free at <1 mmol/day. Strauss et al. (40) investigated elegantly the rates of response of the kidney to salt surfeit and deficit and showed that with a normal eating pattern, a salt intake of 60 mmol will be largely excreted in about 6 h except at night, when the rate is much slower. They showed that the response is inhibited by overall sodium deficit and that it returns rather precisely when the deficit is replaced. The effects were clearly volume rather than concentration dependent and not entirely explained by renal hemodynamics or the renin angiotensin axis. Thus they anticipated modern discoveries over 35 years ago.

It is important to appreciate that other factors, particularly osmotic loads, can dramatically override the normal responses and increase sodium and chloride output acutely

(41) and inappropriately, as with the osmotic diuresis that occurs with an acute onset of insulin-dependent diabetes mellitus. An established osmotic diuresis usually produces a urinary sodium concentration of around 40–50 mmol/L, with flow rates up to 1.5 L per hour. Thus if the osmotic agent is entirely sodium free, desalination can occur very rapidly indeed. Use of mannitol in head injury is one situation where this problem can occur.

One interesting logical corollary of the normal exponential response of renal and sweat sodium concentrations to sodium deficit is that the appropriate diet for hot climates is a low-salt diet, because the sodium content of sweat becomes very low (<10 mmol/L). Consequently, the large volumes of water lost by evaporation to maintain thermal regulation do not lead to such large sodium and chloride losses as would occur on a normal salt diet, where sweat sodium could be 50 mmol/L.

Because of the exponential relationship between renal excretion of sodium and oral intake, the measurement of 24-h sodium intake does not relate directly to the current day's intake except where dietary intake is held constant for some days. (The literature is somewhat confusing on this point, with some authors maintaining that urinary sodium is not sufficiently closely related to intake to be at all useful.) However, if one compares intake and output in clinical situations where the input is often known precisely, then observation of the trends in excretory patterns can be exceedingly useful for the prediction of inappropriate renal loss or inappropriate retention.

Dietary assessment of sodium and chloride intake by means of dietary histories produces neither precise nor accurate data. Because sodium and chloride are nutrients that are found in high concentrations in relatively few foods, both inter- and intraperson variation are high, and it is difficult to obtain precise estimates of usual intakes. Moreover, the major portion of salt intake in the Western diet, approximately 80%, is "hidden" in processed foods. The best dietary assessment methods for a *qualitative* estimate of the *usual* intake of sodium and chloride include month-long dietary histories and modified food frequency questionnaires. However, the dietary history method is very labor intensive, and the quality of the results depends on the skill of the interviewers. The advantages, limitations, and applications of these methods and others are described in detail by Gibson (42). Total daily urinary sodium excretion is also not necessarily an accurate estimate of concurrent intake (43,44). Methods for tracking added sodium using a lithium marker have been described (45).

IV. PHYSIOLOGIC FUNCTION

A. Alterations in Extracellular Sodium

A consideration of body composition is of fundamental importance to a rational approach to alterations in sodium concentration. The major determinant of extracellular volume (ECV) is total exchangeable body sodium (Na^+_e) and of intracellular volume (ICV) − potassium (K^+_e). So close is this relationship that for practical purposes a change in total body sodium is directly proportional to a change in extracellular volume.

Because total body water (TBW) is the sum of ECV and ICV, the sum of K^+_e and Na^+_e multiplied by a constant must be equal to TBW. Edelman's experimentally derived equation (46) is therefore in one sense a tautology, but an extremely useful one because it reminds us to consider all the possibilities for any alteration in plasma sodium concentration, an alteration in Na^+_e, K^+_e, or TBW, or any combination of the three. The most frequently forgotten cause of hyponatremia is potassium deficiency. The range over which

Edelman's equation was shown to apply empirically was from 109 to 192 mmol/L, i.e., almost the total range compatible with life.

Hyponatremia is most frequently caused by water intoxication in the adult and by salt depletion secondary to gastroenteritis in children, provided water continues to be given. In the absence of adequate water, hypernatremic dehydration occurs.

About 1 kg of body weight is dietary salt dependent, a fact often unethically exploited by weight-loss programs.

Hypernatremia was extensively investigated after several children died as a result of a tragic accident in which salt was accidentally substituted for sugar in an infant nursery. Death was associated with convulsions, and at postmortem there was a shrunken brain with multiple petechial hemorrhages. Subsequently it was shown that rapid correction of hypernatremia was also dangerous, because children so treated also died but this time with edematous brains. The results suggest that there is a normal osmotic mechanism from resisting brain shrinkage which must be allowed to switch off before aggressive attempts are made to correct the hypernatremia.

B. Alterations in Intracellular Sodium

Over the last 20 years it has become apparent that many diseases states, including uremia, hyperthyroidism, hypertension, and malnutrition, are associated with increased concentrations of intracellular sodium. This evidence has been almost entirely derived from studies of isolated cells and has not been consistently demonstrated by isotope dilution studies and whole tissue samples. The reason for this is still not widely appreciated by nutritionists. We cannot accurately measure extracellular space in disease states, and therefore we cannot accurately determine intracellular sodium except where, as in isolated cells, adequate and rapid washing of cells can be achieved. The extracellular space is estimated by a variety of agents which give figures in healthy subjects which vary from 14% to 28% of body weight (47). In disease states the permeability of cell membranes to these putative extracellular space markers can increase very dramatically, as in malaria, where thiocyanate space has been reported to approach the volume of total body water (48). The use of chloride spaces to measure extracellular space in malnourished children has led to the reporting of negative values for intracellular sodium (49). This is a clear indication that the assumption underlying the use of chloride, namely, a normal membrane potential, is not valid in all cases.

C. Alterations in Membrane Transport with Alterations in Nutritional State

Sodium transport has been reported to be abnormal in the red cells and in leukocytes obtained from malnourished children. Those with kwashiorkor (abnormal sodium retention) have increased rates of unidirectional sodium flux, and those with marasmus have reduced rates. Intracellular sodium is elevated in both groups (50–53).

Another interesting finding emerged from these studies, namely, that it was possible to identify those children who were at risk of sudden death when they were placed in positive energy balance. Leukocyte sodium transport data obtained upon admission to hospital suggested an abnormality of sodium transport that would theoretically respond to digoxin, and this proved to be so (54). This is of practical importance, since the syndrome described can be recognized without need for the transport measurements. The major features were the sudden onset of tachypnea, tachycardia, increased venous pressure, and sometimes diarrhea at the point where energy intake significantly exceeded maintenance requirements. Finally, as a result of observations that leukocyte sodium transport in malnourished children was altered by small oral supplements of zinc (55), it was found that skin sensitivity to antigens was restored by cutaneous zinc (56). Normal leukocyte sodium transport is also sensitive to extracellular zinc concentration (57). However, in protein energy malnutrition that is secondary to severe cerebral palsy in children, erythrocyte Na-K-pump-mediated K^+ influx is increased compared with that of well-nourished children with cerebral palsy (58). Thus the effects of undernutrition on erythrocyte Na^+-K^+ pump activity in children with severe cerebral palsy are distinct from the effects observed in children with protein energy malnutrition in developing countries. No mechanism has been described to explain this difference.

V. RELATION TO DISEASE

A. Hypertension

The major disease clearly linked with disordered sodium homeostasis is hypertension, but the linkage to dietary sodium is much less clear. There is still no overall agreement about the fundamental mechanisms underlying hypertension. The undisputed facts are that there are human populations with very low salt intakes and very low prevalences of hypertension, whose presumably normal renin levels would alarm a Western physician (e.g., a mean for renin activity of 13 ng/ml/h). Some of these people even fail to show the "normal" Western increase in blood pressure with age (59). Between-country comparisons of sodium intake and blood pressure also show a correlation between sodium intake and blood pressure such that for every 100 mmol increase in daily sodium intake, systolic blood pressure increased by 5–10 mmHg, with the lower figure typical of the young and the higher of the elderly. There are many potentially confounding factors such as coincidental intakes of potassium and calcium. Clear relationships within communities were demonstrated in only 7 out of 52 communities in the Intersalt study (60). Thus, although a very low salt intake will inevitably lower blood pressure at some point through dangerous reduction in extracellular volume, that does not mean that excess dietary salt is the cause of hypertension.

Dahl originally demonstrated in rats the existence of the salt-sensitive phenotype; subsequent studies have demonstrated in humans that some people are salt sensitive. This phenomenon is more common in diabetics, and this appears to be related to a change in insulin sensitivity and an increase in circulating free fatty acids which occurs with high salt intakes (61).

B. Cystic Fibrosis

Cystic fibrosis is a genetically determined defect in a chloride channel. This leads to the secretion of sweat with high chloride and sodium concentrations which are not reduced by aldosterone. In hot weather CF patients will collapse from salt depletion if not given salt supplements. This is only a minor aspect of cystic fibrosis. The major effects caused by the CFTR (cystic fibrosis transmembrane conductance regulator) gene seem to be due to the fact that because of the defect in chloride transport, less ions are secreted into critical fluids and are not therefore available to keep water in the secretions of the pancreas, lung, and other exocrine glands. The pathology is a consequence of the inevitable blockage which occurs with highly viscid secretions. The effects of the description of the fundamental defects of CF on the understanding and management of the disease have been recently reviewed (62).

C. Hyperthyroidism

In the past it has been claimed that almost all of the excess energy expenditure associated with hyperthyroidism is accounted for by increased ATP turnover by Na-K ATPase. The quantitative contribution of Na-K ATPase activity toward the increase in respiration rate is indeed controversial. Estimates of the contribution of Na-K ATPase to the increased respiration rates of cells and tissues during hyperthyroidism range from less than 10% (63) to 85–90% (64,65).

Estimates of the proportion of respiration rate that is due to Na-K ATPase activity are usually made using the specific inhibitor of the enzyme, ouabain. However, many of these determinations have been made without considering the secondary effects of ouabain which occur following prolonged incubations in its presence. Ouabain rapidly binds to and inhibits Na-K ATPase, but with extended incubation times it alters Na^+ and K^+ fluxes and results in K^+ depletion, which then can result in decreased oxygen consumption (66). Moreover, these estimates have been conducted in many different types of tissue preparations using varied protocols. It is thus not surprising that the estimates vary and that some are erroneously high.

Recently, a quantitative approach which is referred to as top-down elasticity analysis (67) has been used to identify the important sites of action of thyroid hormones on oxidative phosphorylation in isolated hepatocytes from rats. The results showed that approximately 50% of the difference in respiration rates was attributable to changes in the rate of the leak of protons across the mitochondrial inner membrane in hepatocytes from both hyperthyroid and hypothyroid rats compared with euthyroid control data. Because the mitochondrial proton leak dissipates the mitochondrial electrochemical potential, the respiratory chain is driven faster in an attempt to maintain the membrane potential and thus oxygen consumption is increased. The remaining 50% of the increase in respiration rate during hyperthyroidism was due to an increase in ATP-consuming reactions such as Na-K ATPase, Ca ATPase, and the ATP turnover involved in gluconeogenesis and ureogenesis. All four mechanisms are known to increase with hyperthyroidism (68,69). With regard to the importance of Na-K ATPase in hepatocytes toward the thyroid hormone-induced increase in respiration rate, Nobes et al. (70) obtained a value of 29% based on their studies of rat hepatocytes that were incubated for a few minutes in the presence of ouabain. Thus, with this limited amount of data it seems that alterations in the activity of the Na-K ATPase are important in terms of the changes in respiration rate during hyperthyroidism, but other ATPases are also involved and the total involvement is lower than originally proposed.

D. Chronic Renal Failure

As renal function diminishes during the course of progressive renal failure, increasing demands are placed on the residual nephrons to maintain solute balance. As the glomerular filtration rate (GFR) decreases, sodium chloride balance is achieved by a progressive decrease in reabsorption per nephron unit. This is reflected in the exponential rise in the fractional excretion of sodium. The factors involved in this adaptive process are complex and are thought to be related to the uremia-induced changes in the composition of the plasma and to hormonal changes which result from the increased extracellular fluid volume (71). The adaptation is so well regulated that sodium balance is fairly well maintained until the final stages of chronic renal failure, when dietary sodium chloride must be carefully restricted. The failure to do so results in clinically overt extracellular fluid volume overload, with edema, hypertension, and congestive heart failure. Too strict a reduction can lead to volume depletion as the urinary sodium concentration becomes fixed. Hence management of salt balance at this stage requires obsessional attention.

E. Liver Disease

Acute and chronic liver failure are both associated with hyponatremia. The classical theory attributes the renal sodium and water retention to a decrease in the effective circulatory volume which accompanies ascites formation. However, it is now known that renal sodium and water retention can be observed before ascites formation. It is thought that the decreased effective blood volume is secondary to splanchnic venous pooling, hypo-albuminemia, and a decrease in total peripheral resistance (72).

F. Interactions Between Potassium and Calcium Intakes and Sodium Balance in Disease States

It has been proposed that dietary intakes of potassium and calcium as well as that of sodium are involved in the pathogenesis of hypertension (73). As discussed above, epidemiologic studies have shown that sodium intake is directly related to blood pressure; such studies have also shown that potassium intake is inversely related to blood pressure (74–76). Furthermore it has been proposed that a low potassium intake is an important risk factor for the development of hypertension (77), and potassium depletion results in increases in blood pressure in both hypertensive (78) and normotensive individuals (79). Calcium intake has also been claimed to be important in the control of blood pressure, so that an increased intake mitigates the development of hypertension. Abnormalities in calcium homeostasis have been described in hypertensive individuals, and lower calcium intakes have been reported for hypertensives in comparison with controls (73).

The exact mechanisms through which these nutrients affect blood pressure are not understood. However, it has been suggested that in predisposed individuals the ability to excrete salt through the kidney is impaired and the sodium retention and the consequential volume expansion result in the release of a natriuretic substance which inhibits the renal tubular Na-K ATPase (80). This substance has been given various names, the most common of which are the digoxinlike immunoreactive substance, endogenous digitalis factor, and the digoxinlike circulating factor. It has also been shown that the inhibition of Na-K ATPase in vascular smooth muscle will increase blood pressure through a change in the intracellular concentration of calcium (81,82). It has been proposed that the mechanism for the effects of dietary potassium and calcium is similar (78). Studies in rats have shown that dietary calcium supplementation will decrease the plasma concentration of the digoxinlike immu-noreactive factor (83).

VI. DISORDERED SALT METABOLISM

The nutritionist's traditional concern with body composition has particular benefits in the management of disordered salt and water metabolism.

A. Sodium Chloride Retention and Edema

1. Pathophysiology

Edema, or any acute increase of weight not correlated with appropriate increase of energy intake, should be recognized as *prima facie* evidence of salt retention, no matter what is coincidentally happening to sodium or chloride concentration in extracellular fluid. One kilogram of weight gain is equivalent to the retention of approximately 140 mmol Na^+, depending on the concentration of sodium in the serum.

Edema is always evidence of an expanded extracellular volume. If edema can be detected at all, the expansion is of the order of 15% (84); i.e., unless serum sodium has fallen by >15%, edema cannot be explained by water retention alone. Similarly, albumin concentration will fall by greater than 15% with any acute development of edema, without any necessary alteration in protein metabolism or albumin mass. It appears that with protein deficiency this theoretical fall in albumin concentration is mitigated by a mechanism for the redistribution of total albumin from the extravascular to the vascular space so that a greater proportion is contained in the vascular space (85).

Before edema appears, weight gain in the absence of positive energy balance must mean positive sodium balance. Because weight can be measured to ±100 g, clinicians should detect positive sodium balance long before the 1–2 kg of extracellular fluid necessary to produce edema has been retained. Although the specific mechanism in any particular case may not be known, the general mechanism is always inappropriate retention of sodium by the kidney. It is therefore prudent to monitor renal excretion of sodium in all seriously ill subjects at risk for disordered sodium balance. If, as is often the case, very little sodium is being excreted, the appropriate therapy is to reduce intake to less than output, at which point sodium balance must begin to return to normal. Continuous monitoring of renal output of sodium, which is cheap and easy, will indicate when a natriuresis occurs and liberalization of sodium intake is therefore acceptable. The general principle is that even when it is difficult to modify renal function directly, it is usually possible to adjust intake to match the renal malfunction. It requires some persuasive powers to introduce a zero sodium intake in the management of an edematous subject with hyponatremia.

From the nutritionist's point of view, it is extremely interesting that the return of appropriate natriuretic responses in the kidney is often correlated with a return to energy balance. In primary malnutrition the impairment of renal blood flow and glomerular filtration rate is well documented, as is the inability of malnourished children to handle anything more than 2 mmol/kg of Na^+ per day without developing a pathologic positive balance. The relationship between energy balance and sodium balance is worthy of much more research. At present it appears that in the acutely sick, two errors must be avoided; giving supra-maintenance amounts of energy, which are associated with increased morbidity and mortality possibly dependent on redistribution of salt within the body (86), and allowing the development of acute weight loss, >10% of body weight, which carries similar consequences (87).

2. Etiological Theories

The question of the etiology of nutritional edema is still a debated issue, but some points now seem incontrovertible and they indicate that hypoalbuminemia is more likely to be an effect than a cause of edema. The pertinent facts are as follows:

1. Children born without any serum albumin do not suffer from edema. It follows that hypoalbuminemia is not an inevitable cause of edema. Increased lymphatic flow can compensate for the disordered Starling forces.
2. Marasmic children have lower lean body mass values than children with kwashiorkor and may have normal albumin values. Therefore it is not the extent of protein deficiency per se which causes edema.

3. The edema of children with kwashiorkor can be relieved without provision of any protein or amino acids. It follows that there was no specific protein or amino acid deficiency responsible for the edema in the first place (88).

4. The incidence of kwashiorkor varies with season, is never more than a few percent of the total number of malnourished children, and is clearly related to other factors such as epidemics of measles.

5. Only two types of biochemical measurement clearly distinguish marasmus and kwashiorkor: red cell and white cell sodium transport rates, and red cell glutathione levels. Golden has used these data to advance the hypothesis that kwashiorkor is a free-radical disease (89). He accepted the argument that edema must represent sodium retention (90) and proposed that free-radical damage to membranes impairs the capacity of the kidney to excrete sodium, possibly by increasing the permeability of the tubular cells.

6. There is evidence that in both renal and cirrhotic edema, the fall in albumin is secondary rather than primary (91).

B. Sodium Chloride Deficit

Sodium chloride deficit, a common cause of death, is eminently treatable with minimal facilities provided some very basic principles are remembered.

1. Body-weight changes are the best guide to deficit.
2. Except in the presence of imminent circulatory collapse, oral treatment is usually possible. It does not matter if losses continue as long as overall balance is improving.
3. Volume must be corrected before concentration.
4. Except in cholera, the colon usually responds to aldosterone, and quite low sodium concentrations are adequate for the rehydration solutions. In cholera, near-isotonic solutions are necessary.

VII. FUTURE RESEARCH

There are several areas where progress can be clearly expected. Further exploration of the interrelationships between energy balance and electrolyte physiology is needed. Identification of the critical factors inducing adaptation with be particularly informative. Some experiments involving studies of electrolyte physiology in wasting states associated with hypermetabolism would clearly be interesting. Moreover, it should now be possible to take the newly emerging insights about the genetic determinants of membrane transport of sodium and chloride and see whether they will allow further delineation of subsets of those diseases known to have associated transport defects.

VIII. CONCLUSION

Despite the availability of simple, precise, and accurate methods for the measurement of sodium and chloride, our understanding of their physiology and of their role in disease is still far from complete. Nutritionists and other clinicians still frequently contribute to the perpetuation of simplistic myths such as equating edema with protein deficiency or attributing too great a role to dietary sodium in hypertension. A greater understanding of the detailed physiology of sodium chloride within the body and within individual tissues will be necessary before we can claim to understand the role of salt in human health and disease.

REFERENCES

1. Maxwell MH, Kleeman CR, Nairns RG. Clinical Disorders of Fluid and Electrolyte Metabolism. New York: McGraw-Hill, 1987.
2. Albrink MJ, Hald PM, Man EB, Peters JP. Displacement of serum water by the lipids of hyperlipidemic serum: a new method for the rapid determination of serum water. J Clin Invest 1955; 34: 1483–1488.
3. Smith K. Fluids and Electrolytes: A Conceptual Approach. New York: Churchill Livingstone; 1980: 8–24.
4. Ganong WF. Review of Medical Physiology. Los Altos, CA: Lange, 1981: 23.
5. Koletzko S, Stringer DA, Cleghorn GJ, et al. Lavage treatment of distal intestinal obstruction syndrome in children with cystic fibrosis. Pediatrics 1989; 83: 727–733.
6. Navar LG, Rosivall L. Contribution of the renin-angiotension system to the control of intrarenal hemodynamics. Kidney Int 1984; 25: 857–868.
7. Hall JE. Control of sodium excretion by angiotension II: intrarenal mechanisms and blood pressure regulation. Am J Physiol 1986; 250: R960–R972.
8. Sealy JE, Laragh JH. The integrated regulation of electrolyte balance and blood pressure by the renin system. In: Seldin DW, Giebisch G, eds. The Regulation of Sodium and Chloride Balance. New York: Raven Press, 1990: 133–193.
9. Whittam R. Active cation transport as a pacemaker of respiration. Nature 1961; 191: 603–604.
10. Whittam R, Willis JS. Ion movements and oxygen consumption in kidney cortex slices. J Physiol 1963; 168: 158–177.
11. Whittam R, Blond DM. Respiratory control by an adenosine triphosphatase involved in active transport in brain cortex. Biochem J 1964; 92: 147–158. .
12. Yeagle PL. Lipid regulation of cell membrane structure and function. FASEB J 1989; 3: 1833–1842.
13. Stubbs CD, Smith AD. The modification of mammalian membrane polyunsaturated fatty acid composition in relation to membrane fluidity and function. Biochim Biophys Acta 1984; 779: 89–137.
14. Skou JC. The energy coupled exchange of Na^+ for K^+ across the cell membrane. The Na^+,K^+-pump. FEBS Lett 1990; 268: 314–324.
15. Patrick J, Michael J, Golden MH, Golden BE, Hilton PJ. The effect of zinc on leucocyte sodium transport in vitro. Clin Sci Molec Med 1978; 54: 585–587.
16. Sweadner K. Overview: subunit diversity in the Na,K-ATPase. In: Kaplan JH, De Weer P, eds. The Sodium Pump: Structure, Mechanism and Regulation. New York: Rockefeller University Press, 1991: 63–71.
17. Goto A, Yamada N, Yagi M, Yoshiola M, Sugimoto T. Physiology and pharmacology of endogenous digitalis-like factors. Pharmacol Rev 1992; 44: 377–399.
18. Blaustein MP. Physiological effects of endogenous ouabain: control of intracellular Ca^{2+} stores. Am J Physiol 1994; 264: C1367–1387.
19. Cournillon L, Pouyssegur J. Molecular biology and hormonal regulation of vertebrate Na^+/H^+ exchanger isoforms. In: Reuss L, Russel JM, Jennings ML, eds. Molecular Biology and Function of Carrier Proteins. New York: Rockefeller University Press, 1993: 169–186.
20. Haas M. The Na-K-Cl cotransporters. Am J Physiol 1994; 267: C869–885.
21. Lytle C, Forbush B. The Na-K-Cl cotransport protein of the shark rectal gland. 2. Regulation by direct phosphorylation. J Biol Chem 1992; 2267: 25438–25443.
22. Lauf P. Erythrocyte K-Cl cotransport: properties and regulation. Am J Physiol 1992; 263: C917–932.

23. Willis JS. On thermal stability of ion gradients in mammalian cells. In: Willis JS, ed. Advances in Cellular and Molecular Biology. Vol. 17. Greenwich, CT: JAI Press. In press.

24. Blaustein MP, Goldman WF, Fontana G, et al. Physiological roles of the sodium-calcium exchanger in nerve and muscle. Ann NY Acad Sci 1991; 639: 254–274.

25. Flatman PW. Mechanisms of magnesium transport. Ann Rev Physiol 1991; 53: 259–271.

26. Xu W, Willis JS. Sodium transport through the amiloride-sensitive Na-Mg pathway of hamster red cells. J Memb Biol 1994; 141: 277–287.

27. Strühmer W, Conti F, Suzuki H, et al. Structural parts involved in activation and inactivation of the sodium channel. Nature 1989; 339: 597–603.

28. Smith PR, Benos DJ. Epithelial Na$^+$ channels. Ann Rev Biochem 1991; 53: 509–530.

29. Duchatelle P, Ohara A, Ling BN, et al. Regulation of renal epithelia Na$^+$ channels. Mol Cell Biochem 1992; 114: 27–34.

30. Hoffmann EK, Simonsen LO. Membrane mechanisms in volume and pH regulation in vertebrate cells. Physiol Rev 1989; 69: 315–382.

31. Redon J, Battle D. Regulation of intracellular pH in the spontaneously hypertensive rat. Hypertension 1994; 23: 503–512.

32. Cliff WH, Frizzell RA. Separate Cl$^-$ conductance activated by cAMP and Ca^{2+} in Cl$^-$-secreting epithelial cells. Proc Natl Acad Sci (USA) 1990; 87: 4956–4960.

33. Welsh MJ, Denning GM, Ostedgaard LS, Anderson MP. Dysfunction of CFTR bearing the delta F508 mutation. J Cell Sci 1993; S17: 235–239.

34. Schwiebert EM, Flotte T, Cutting GR, Guggino WB. Both CFTR and outwardly rectifying chloride channels contribute to cAMP-stimulated whole cell chloride channels. Am J Physiol 1994; 266: C1464–1477.

35. Riordan JR. The cystic fibrosis transmembrane conductance regulator. Ann Rev Physiol 1993; 55: 609–630.

36. Marty A. The physiological role of calcium-dependent channels. Trends Neurolog Sci 1989; 12: 420–424.

37. Pusch M, Jentsch TJ. Molecular physiology of voltage-gated chloride channels. Physiol Rev 1994; 74: 813–827.

38. Nilius B, Oike M, Zahradnik I, Droogmans G. Activation of a Cl$^-$ current by hypotonic volume increase in human endothelial cells. J Gen Physiol 1994; 103: 787–805.

39. McCance RA. Experimental sodium chloride deficiency in man. Proc Roy Soc Lond Ser B 1936; 119: 245–268.

40. Strauss MB, Lamdin E, Smith WP, Bleifer BJ. Surfeit and deficit of sodium. Arch Intern Med 1958; 102: 527–536.

41. Goldberg M, McCurdy DK, Ramirez MA. Differences between saline and mannitol diuresis in hydropenic man. J Clin Invest 1965; 44: 182–192.

42. Gibson RS. Precision in dietary assessment. In: Principles of Nutritional Assessment. New York: Oxford University Press, 1990: 97–116.

43. Liu K, Cooper R, McKeever J, et al. Assessment of the association between habitual salt intake and high blood pressure: methodological problems. Am J Epidemiol 1979; 110: 219–226.

44. Luft FC, Aronoff GR, Sloan RS, Fineberg NS. Intra- and interindividual variability in sodium intake in normal subjects and in patients with renal insufficiency. Am J Kidney Dis 1986; 7: 375–380.

45. Sanchez-Castillo CP, Branch WJ, James WP. A test of the validity of the lithium-marker technique for monitoring dietary sources of salt in man. Clin Sci 1987; 72: 87–94.

46. Edelman IS, Liebman J, O'Meara MP, Birkenfield LW. Interrelations between serum sodium concentration, serum osmolality and total exchangeable sodium, total exchangeable potassium and total exchangeable water. J Clin Invest 1976; 37: 1236–1256.

47. Swales JD. Sodium Metabolism in Disease. London: Lloyd-Luke, 1975.

48. Overman RR, Feldman HA. The effect of fatal *P. knowlesi* malaria on simian circulatory and body fluid compartment physiology. J Clin Invest 1947; 26: 1049–1056.

49. Metcoff S, Frenk S, Yoshida T, Torres-Pinedo R, Kaiser E, Hansen JDL. Cell composition and metabolism in kwashiorkor. Medicine 1966; 45: 365–390.

50. Kaplay SS. Erythrocyte membrane Na^+ and K^+ activated adenosine triphosphatase in protein-calorie malnutrition. Am J Clin Nutr 1978; 31: 579–584.

51. Kaplay SS. Modified kinetics of erythrocyte membrane Na^+,K^+ adenosine triphosphatase in protein-energy malnutrition. Biochem Med 1979; 22: 282–287.

52. Patrick J, Golden MHN. Leukocyte electrolytes and sodium transport in protein energy malnutrition. Am J Clin Nutr 1977; 30: 1478–1481.

53. Willis JS, Golden MHN. Active and passive transport of sodium and potassium ions in erythrocytes of severely malnourished Jamaican children. Eur J Clin Nutr 1988; 42: 635–645.

54. Patrick J. Death during recovery from severe malnutrition and its possible relationship to sodium pump activity in the leucocyte. Br Med J 1977; 1: 1051–1054.

55. Patrick J, Golden BE, Golden MHN. Leukocyte sodium transport and dietary zinc in protein energy malnutrition. Am J Clin Nutr 1980; 33: 617–620.

56. Golden MHN, Golden BE, Harland PSEG, Jackson AA. Zinc and immunocompetence in protein-energy malnutrition. Lancet 1977; II: 1057–1059.

57. Patrick J, Michael J, Golden MHN, Golden BE, Hilton PJ. The effect of zinc on leucocyte sodium transport in vitro. Clin Sci Mol Med 1978; 54: 585–587.

58. Harper ME, Patrick J, Willis JS. The absence of adapted sodium and potassium transport in erythrocytes of cerebral palsied children with secondary malnutrition. Eur J Nutr 1990; 14: 549–558.

59. Oliver WJ, Cohen EL, Neel JV. Blood pressure, sodium intake, and sodium related hormones in the Yananamo Indians, a "no-salt" culture. Circulation 1975; 52: 146–151.

60. Intersalt Cooperative Research Group. Intersalt: an international study of electrolyte excretion and blood pressure. Results for 24 hour urinary sodium and potassium excretion. Br Med J 1988; 297: 319–328.

61. Donovan DS, Solomon CG, Seely EW, Williams GH, Simonson DC. Effect of sodium intake on insulin sensitivity. Am J Physiol 1993; 264: E730–734.

62. Koch C, Hoiby N. Pathogenesis of cystic fibrosis. Lancet 1993; 341: 1065–1069.

63. Folke M, Sestoft L. Thyroid calorigenesis in isolated perfused rat liver: minor role of active sodium-potassium transport. J Physiol 1977; 269: 407–419.

64. Ismail-Beigi F, Edelman IS. Mechanism of thyroid calorigenesis: role of active sodium transport. Proc Natl Acad Sci (USA) 1970; 67: 1071–1078.

65. Wardlaw GM. The effect of ouabain on basal and thyroid hormone stimulated muscle oxygen consumption. Int J Biochem 1986; 18: 279–281.

66. Whittam R, Willis JS. Ion movements and oxygen consumption in kidney cortex slices. J Physiol 1963; 168: 158–177.

67. Harper ME, Brand MD. The quantitative contributions of mitochondrial proton leak and ATP turnover reactions to the changes respiration rates of hepatocytes from rats of different thyroid status. J Biol Chem 1993; 268: 14850–14860.

68. Dauncey MJ. Thyroid hormones and thermogenesis. Proc Nutr Soc 1990; 49: 203–215.

69. Clausen T, van Hardeveld C, Everts ME. Significance of cation transport in control of energy metabolism and thermogenesis. Physiol Rev 1991; 71: 733–774.

70. Nobes CD, Lakin-Thomas PL, Brand MD. The contribution of ATP turnover by the Na^+,K^+ ATPase to the rate of respiration of hepatocytes. Effects of thyroid status and fatty acids. Biochim Biophys Acta 1989; 976: 241–245.

71. Eknoyan G. Diagnosis of disturbances. In: Seldin DW, Giebisch G, eds. The Regulation of Sodium and Chloride Balance. New York: Raven Press, 1990: 253–258.

72. Meyer-Lehnert H, Schrier RW. Hyponatemia: diagnosis and treatment. In: Seldin DW, Giebisch G, eds. The Regulation of Sodium and Chloride Balance. New York: Raven Press, 1990: 442–443.

73. Luft FC, McCarron DA. Heterogeneity of hypertension: the diverse role of electrolyte intake. Annu Rev Med 1991; 42: 347–355.

74. Krishna GG. Effect of potassium intake on blood pressure. J Am Soc Nephrol 1990; 1: 43–52.
75. Khaw KT, Barret-Connor E. Dietary potassium and blood pressure in a population. Am J Clin Nutr 1984; 39: 963–968.
76. Langford HG. Dietary potassium and hypertension. Ann Intern Med 1983; 98: 770–772.
77. Witteman JCM, Willett WC, Stampfer MJ, et al. Prospective study of nutritional factors and hypertension among United States women. Circulation 1989; 80:1320–1327.
78. Krishna GG, Kapoor SC. Potassium depletion exacerbates essential hypertension. Ann Intern Med 1991, 115: 77–83.
79. Krishna GG, Miller E, Kapoor SC. Increased blood pressure during K depletion in normotensive man. Engl J Med 1989; 320: 1177–1182.
80. DeWardener He, MacGregor CA. The natriuretic hormone and essential hypertension. Lancet 1983; i: 1450–1454.
81. Blaustein MP. Sodium ions, calcium ions, blood pressure regulation and hypertension. a reassessment and hypothesis. Am J Physiol 1977; 232: C165–C173.
82. Haddy FJ. Digitalis-like circulating factor in hypertension: potential messenger between salt balance and intracellular sodium. Cardiovasc Drug Ther 1990; 4: 343–349.
83. Doris PA. Digoxin-like immunoreactive factor in rat plasma: effect of sodium and calcium intake. Life Sci 1988; 42: 787–790.
84. Chobanian AV, Burrows BA, Hollander WN. Body fluid and electrolyte composition in cardiac patients were severe heart disease but without peripheral oedema. Circulation 1961; 24: 743–753.
85. James WPT, Hay AM. Albumin metabolism: effect of nutritional state and the dietary protein intake. J Clin Invest 1968; 47: 1558–1572.
86. Chang RW, Lee B, Jacobs S. Identifying ICU patients who would not benefit from total parenteral nutrition. JPEN 1989; 13: 535–538.
87. Buzby GP, Mullen JL, Matthews DC, Hobbs CL, Rosato EF. Prognostic nutritional index in gastrointestional surgery. Am J Surg 1980; 139: 160–167.
88. Hansen JDL, Jenkinson V. Electrolyte and nitrogen metabolism in kwashiorkor. S Afr J Lab Clin Med 1956; 2: 206–231.
89. Golden MHN, Ramdath D. Free radicals in the pathogenesis of kwashiorkor. Proc Nutr Soc 1987; 46 53–68.
90. Patrick J. Oedema in protein energy malnutrition: the role of the sodium pump. Proc Nutr Soc 1979; 38: 61–68.
91. Brenner BM, Stein JH. Sodium and Water Homeostasis. New York: Churchill Livingstone, 1978.

5

Magnesium

MAURICE EDWARD SHILS
Bowman Gray School of Medicine, Wake Forest University,
Winston-Salem, North Carolina

I. INTRODUCTION

Magnesium plays an essential role in a very wide variety of fundamental cellular reactions. Hence, it is not surprising that deficiency in the organism may lead to serious biochemical and symptomatic changes. McCollum and associates made the first systematic observations of magnesium deficiency in rats (1) and then in dogs in the early 1930s. The first description of clinical depletion in humans was published in 1934 for a small number of patients with various underlying diseases (2). Flink and associates, in the early 1950s, initiated long-term studies documenting depletion of this ion in alcoholics and in patients on magnesium-free intravenous solutions (3). Although the diets consumed by healthy Americans do not appear to lead to clinically significant hypomagnesemia, an increasing number of clinical disorders has been found to be associated with magnesium depletion. Experimental and clinical observations have revealed important interrelations of this essential ion with other electrolytes, second messengers, hormones and growth factors and their membrane receptors, signal pathways, ion channels, parathyroid hormone secretion and action, vitamin D metabolism, and bone functions.

II. ANALYTICAL METHODS

A. Total Magnesium

Early chemical analytical methods, which were replaced for the most part by the use of atomic absorption spectrophotometry (AAS), have been reviewed (4). While the latter procedure was widely employed in clinical chemistry laboratories, it has been replaced for the most part by one of four different automated colorimetric methods. These have varying degrees of coefficient of variation compared to AAS, which still remains the analytic standard (5). For the rapid determination following wet ashing of a number of minerals including magnesium in foods, inductively coupled argon plasma emission spectroscopy is a useful method (6).

B. Ionized Serum Magnesium

Ionized serum magnesium may be determined by ultrafiltration techniques (7), or less accurately by measuring total magnesium and calculating the concentration of ionized Mg^{2+}, which depends on serum protein concentration and pH, or by a new specific ion-selective electrode, e.g., using the ionophore ETH 5282 (7,8).

C. Cytosolic Free Magnesium

As methods have been developed that achieve reasonably accurate and reproductible data, there has been a major surge of interest in the roles of free intracellular magnesium $[Mg^{2+}]_i$.

1. Nuclear Magnetic Resonance Methods

A number of small endogenous compounds exist in equilibrium between uncomplexed and complexed Mg^{2+}. Since the resonances of such molecules may shift upon Mg^{2+} complexation, nuclear magnetic resonance (NMR) spectra can provide information on the level of free Mg^{2+} in the cell. ATP is the most useful NMR endogenous indicator because of the presence of ^{31}P nuclei and its high concentration and broad distribution in cells (9,10). The observed shift difference between alpha and beta phosphate resonances is the parameter of choice. Technical issues related to the ^{31}P shift of ATP for this measurement have been discussed (10).

Exogenous NMR indicators have been developed to measure cystolic Mg^{2+}; such indicators gain sensitivity and selectivity, for example, by utilizing fluoridated compounds which have essentially no fluoride background resonance. Since the dissociation constant for Ca^{2+} is several hundredfold greater than the basal cytosolic Ca^{2+} level of most cells, the Ca^{2+} binding is not generally a significant problem. (+)Fluorocitrate has been utilized as a magnesium indicator in the form of a membrane-permeable ester which is hydrolyzed by intracellular enzymes. Biological and technical issues with these indicators have been reviewed (10).

2. Fluorescent Indicators

The presence of Mg^{2+} causes a measurable shift in the excitation spectrum of suitable fluorescent magnesium chelators such as mag-fura-2 (Furaptra), which allows determination of the ion concentration in cell suspensions and in individual cells by the ratio method of excitation wavelength. A limitation for this probe is its relatively high affinity for Ca^{2+}. The use of fluorescent indicators, technical issues, and limitations have been reviewed (10,11).

3. Ion-Selective Microelectrodes

A recently available resin, ETH 5214, apparently overcomes a problem with earlier resins in which Mg^{2+} measurements were dependent on concentration of K^+ and Na^+ in the calibration solutions (12). These newer techniques are enlarging our understanding of the role(s) of free intracellular magnesium, the mechanisms controlling its changes in concentration, and the effect of deficiency.

D. Magnesium Isotopes

Magnesium isotopes have been used as biological tracers in to follow absorption, distribution in the body, and excretion of this ion. The radioisotope ^{28}Mg has been used in human studies (13); its value is limited by its radioactivity and its short half-life of 21.3 h. Three stable isotopes of magnesium occur in nature, 78.99% ^{24}Mg, 10.0% ^{25}Mg, and 11.01% ^{26}Mg; the latter has been used for tracer studies by labeling magnesium in vegetables (14), and ^{25}Mg has been utilized in absorption studies in humans (15).

III. BODY COMPOSITION

The distribution of magnesium in various compartments of apparently healthy adult individuals is summarized in Table 1. Somewhat more than half of the total is in bone, with almost all of the rest in soft tissue. Magnesium is second in quantity to that of potassium as an intracellular inorganic cation.

TABLE 1 Distribution and Concentrations of Magnesium in a Healthy Adult [Total Body: 833–1170 mmol[a] (20–28 g)]

Percent distribution	Concentration
Bone, 60–65%	0.5% of bone ash
Muscle, 27%	3.5–5 mmol/kg wet weight
Other cells, 6–7%	3.5–5 mmol/kg wet weight
Extracellular, <1%	1.65–2.73[b] mmol/L[b-c]
Erythrocytes	
Serum:	0.65–0.88[b] mmol/L[d]
55% free Mg^{2+} (13% complexed with citrate, phosphate, etc.)	0.48–0.66[b] mmol/L (ultrafilterable)
	or
	0.59 (range ± 0.07)[e] mmol/L (ion electrode)
32% bound, primarily to albumin	0.1–0.3 mmol/L
Mononuclear blood cells[f]	2.91 ± 0.6 fmol/cell[1]
	2.79 ± 0.6 fmol/cell[2]
	3.00 ± 0.04 fmol/cell[3]
Cerebrospinal fluid	1.25 mmol/L
55% free Mg^{2+}	
45% complexed	
Sweat	0.3 mmol/L (in hot environment)
Secretions (saliva, gastric, bile)	0.3 – 0.7 mmol/L

[a]1 mmol = 2 mEq = 24.3 mg.
[b]Hossseini E. Trace Elem Med 1988; 5: 47–51.
[c]Mg falls slowly with cell aging.
[d]Similar at various ages.
[e]Altura, Altura Magnes Trace Elem 1991–1992; 10: 90–98.
[f]Monocytes and lymphocytes in venous blood:
1. Elin, Hossini, Clin Chem 1985; 31: 377.
2. Reinhart et al. Clin. Clinica Acta 1987; 167: 187.
3. Yang et al. J Am Coll Nutr 1990; 9: 328.
From Shils ME. Magnesium. In: Shils ME, Olson JA, Shike M, eds. Modern Nutrition in Health and Disease. 8th ed. Philadelphia: Lea & Febiger, 1994: 166 (with slight modification).

The greater proportion of intracellular magnesium exists in bound form. For example, as measured by ^{31}P NMR, frog muscle cells contained 5.8 mM magnesium bound to ATP, 1.7 mM to phosphocreatine, and 0.3 mM to myosin; $[Mg^{2+}]_i$ was 0.6 mM (16). Magnesium as well as calcium forms complexes with phospholipids of various cell membranes as well as with nucleotides. The ratio of cystolic magnesium to total in guinea pig heart was 0.85. Other values for $[M^{2+}]_i$ are noted below.

With relatively limited data available, magnesium values in human bone cluster about 200 mmol (4.8 g)/kg of bone ash (17). Of total bone magnesium, 30% is in a surface-limited pool, either within the hydration shell or in the crystal surface. In adult men, the large fraction of bone magnesium does not appear to be associated with bone matrix, but is an integral part of the bone crystal (18).

IV. HOMEOSTATIC MECHANISMS

The homeostasis of the individual with respect to mineral balance is dependent on the amount ingested and the intestinal and renal absorption and excretion and all factors affecting them. A scheme for magnesium metabolism is given in Figure 1.

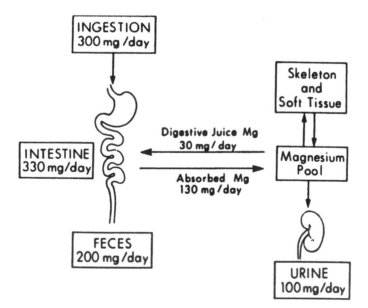

FIGURE 1 Magnesium homeostasis in the human. A schematic representation of its metabolic economy, indicating (a) its relatively poor absorption from the alimentary tract, (b) its distribution into a number of tissue pools with approximate distribution into bone and soft tissue, and (c) its dependence on the kidney for excretion. Homeostasis depends on the integrity of intestinal and renal absorptive processes. (From Slatapolsky E. In: Klahr S, ed. Pathophysiology of Calcium, Magnesium and Phosphorus Metabolism in the Kidney and Body Fluids. New York: Plenum Publishing Corp., 1984, with permission.)

A. Dietary Intake

The amount of magnesium ingested obviously plays a critical role in maintaining its homostasis. Magnesium is widely distributed in plant and animal sources but in widely differing concentrations (19). Data on the intakes of various population groups in the United States, the recommended dietary allowances (RDA) of the National Research Council, and issues concerning the adequacy of the American diet are discussed in the section on dietary needs for health.

B. Gastrointestinal Absorption

1. Laboratory Animals

Studies with rats utilizing segment perfusion or everted intestinal sacs—many using ^{28}Mg—have supported, for the most part, the concept that magnesium is often better absorbed in the ileum and colon than in the jejunum (reviewed in Ref. 20). As measured in stripped mucosa with the Ussing chamber, magnesium was found to be secreted across the duodenum (21) but absorbed in the ileum (22) and in the colon (23). Passive and nonpassive cellular transport processes of magnesium were noted in the ileum and colon (22,23).

2. Human Studies

The percentage absorption of ingested magnesium by healthy individuals is influenced by its dietary concentration and, to a variable extent, by the presence of inhibiting or promoting dietary components. Absorptive studies have been conducted in which the amounts of ingested magnesium [as ^{28}Mg (24) or magnesium acetate (25)] were varied progressively from very small to large amounts utilizing the same healthy subjects. Fractional absorption fell progressively from approximately 65–70% with intakes of 0.3 to 1.5 mmol (7–36 mg), to 11–14% with intakes of 40 mmol (960–1000 mg) (24,25). Absorption as a function of intake was curvilinear. The curved portion is compatible with a saturable process (facilitated diffusion or active absorption), and the linear function reflects passive diffusion as was suggested in children by Milla et al. (26). Estimates of the absorptive fraction related to passive diffusion were 10% (24) and 7% (25), respectively. Using intestinal perfusion techniques in human subjects, magnesium was absorbed in both the jejunum and ileum; it was fully saturable in the ileum but not in the jejunum (27). If it is analogous to that in the rat, human colonic absorption is significant.

With daily magnesium intake of 7.9–14.3 mmol (189–342 mg), healthy adult males in long-term balance studies excreted 35–68% in stool with a fixed daily calcium intake of 5 mmol (200 mg) (28). When free-living adults eating self-selected diets were evaluated periodically over the course of a year, absorption of men averaged 21% and of women 27%; their average daily intakes were 13.4 mmol (323 mg) and 9.75 mmol (234 mg), respectively (29).

A review of long-term balance studies in healthy individuals have, for the major part, indicated that increasing oral calcium intake did not significantly affect magnesium absorption or retention (30). Others have found that with increased calcium intake, the fractional absorption of magnesium was variably increased (depending on the calcium source); however, because of resulting increased urinary excretion, there was no change in net magnesium retention (31). With increased oral phosphate, some reports indicate a decrease in magnesium absorption at high levels of phosphate, while others found no consistent effect on absorption and/or retention (20). Increased amounts of magnesium in the diet have been associated with either decreased calcium absorption (20) or no effect (25). Increased amounts of absorbable oral magnesium have been noted to decrease phosphate absorption (20,25).

The influence of vitamin D and its metabolites on magnesium absorption has been studied extensively under eumagnesemic conditions, with conflicting results. However, the data appear increasingly to favor the concept that, unlike calcium and phosphate, magnesium absorption is not calcitriol-dependent under conditions in which relatively physiologic doses are administered (32). Absorption of magnesium has been noted in individuals with no detectable plasma calcitriol, nor is there a significant correlation between plasma calcitriol and absorption of magnesium (32,33). Furthermore, individuals with absorptive hypercalciuria resulting from increased calcium absorption have normal magnesium absorption (34).

C. Renal Excretion and Regulation: Filtration and Tubular Absorption

Magnesium is either retained for tissue growth (including bone) or used as turnover replacement; the remainder of absorbed magnesium is excreted in the urine. The kidney plays a critical role in magnesium homeostasis (35). Approximately 70% of serum magnesium is ultrafilterable in humans at the glomerulus. Approximately one-third of the filtered load is absorbed in the convoluted tubule. The thick ascending limb of the loop of Henle appears to be the major site of magnesium reabsorption and the major site of control of excretion, with 50–60% of filtered magnesium being reabsorbed between the thin descending limb and the early distal tubule (35). Changes in concentration of magnesium in the tubular lumen and in the plasma affect renal absorption in this segment. The distal convoluted tubule has limited reabsorption ability (< 5% of the filtered load), and the collecting tubules and ducts normally absorb very little. The healthy kidney with an average intake of magnesium reabsorbs about 95% of the filtered magnesium. Tubular secretion, if it occurs, must be a minor factor.

Even with a significant degree of renal disease, with its progressive loss of functioning nephrons, serum magnesium with usual daily intakes is well maintained as the result of increased excretion of a larger-than-normal filtered load per nephron. When creatinine or inulin clearance declines below approximately 10 ml/min, serum magnesium rises progressively unless dietary intake is progressively restricted (36).

When magnesium intake is severely restricted in human subjects with normal kidney function, magnesium output becomes very small within 5 to 7 days (Fig. 2) (37). Supplementary dietary intake increases urinary excretion without altering serum levels, provided that renal function is normal and the amounts given do not exceed maximum glomerular filtration. The intestinal and renal absorptive and excretory mechanisms in normal individuals permit homeostasis over a wide range of intakes. Magnesium reabsorption in the nephron is influenced by a number of physiologic and metabolic factors as well as by drugs and disease states. These have been discussed (35) and summarized elsewhere.

V. BIOCHEMICAL AND PHYSIOLOGIC FUNCTIONS

A. Mg²⁺ as an Enzyme Cofactor

Magnesium is involved as a cofactor in many enzymatic reactions (at least 300) by which food constituents are metabolized and new products formed (39–41). Even a listing of a

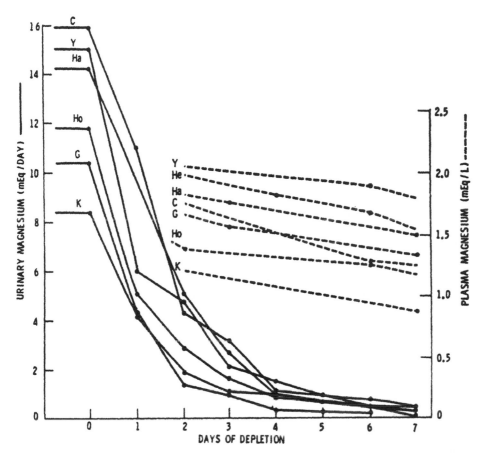

FIGURE 2 Plasma and urine concentrations of magnesium during the week following omission of magnesium from the control diet of human subjects developing experimental deficiency. The rapid decrease in urinary excretion is depicted for 6 subjects. By the tenth day, all plasma values except that of Y were more than 2 standard deviations below the normal mean for the method used. (From Ref. 37 with permission.)

relatively few of the magnesium associated enzymes is sufficient to emphasize the many points in intermediary metabolism at which this ion exerts an essential function. Mg^{2+} is involved in essentially all kinase reactions. The phosphate-donating substrate is not ATP but rather Mg^{2+}-ATP, whose structure is depicted in Figure 3. For example, in the classic hexokinase reaction,

$$\text{Glucose} + \text{ATP} \xrightarrow{Mg^{2+}} \text{glucose 6-phosphate} + \text{ADP}$$

magnesium does not interact directly with the enzyme but forms a "substrate-bridged" complex which can be represented as "enzyme–substrate–metal." However, muscle pyruvate kinase and phosphoenolpyruvate carboxykinase do not form such Mg^{2+} complexes. Protein kinases, the enzymes which catalyze the transfer of the gamma phosphate of Mg^{2+}-ATP to a protein substrate, constitute a large and diverse family, currently numbering more than 100 (42). Since most of the ATP in cells is associated with Mg^{2+}, it follows that most

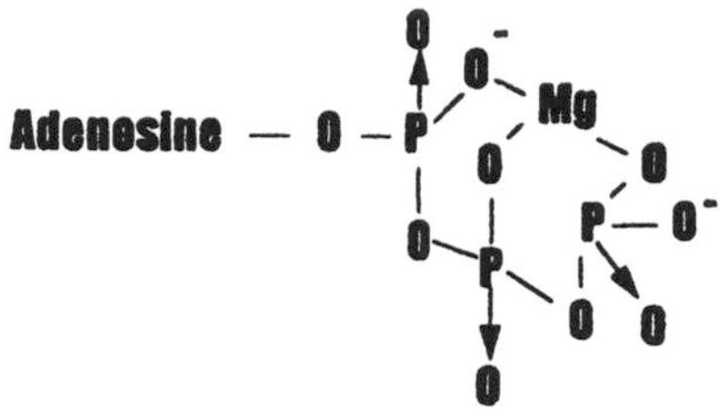

FIGURE 3 Magnesium-adenosine triphosphate complex. Mg^{2+} interacts with the negatively charged ATP^{4-} to form the substrate for most kinase-catalyzed reactions.

enzymatic reactions involving ATP and ADP (as well as GTP and GDP) are Mg^{2+}-dependent.

In the glycolytic cycle which converts glucose to pyruvate there are seven key enzymes that require Mg^{2+} alone or in association with ATP or AMP. These are hexokinase, phosphoglucoisomerase, phosphofructokinase, phosphoglycerate kinase, phosphoglycerate mutase, enolase, and pyruvate kinase. Other examples of Mg^{2+}-dependent reactions that are important in metabolism include those catalyzed by the following enzymes (with their products):

1. Thiamin pyrophosphotransferase (thiamin pyrophosphate), a key coenzyme involved in oxidative decarboxylation.
2. Succinyl-CoA synthetase (succinate and GTP formation in the citrate cycle).
3. Acyl CoA synthetase (fatty acyl CoA, the first product in the beta oxidation of fatty acids).
4. Adenylate cyclase [cyclic adenosine monophosphate (cAMP), the first "second messenger" identified]. The enzyme is activated by a hormone–receptor interaction, and the catalytic product, cAMP, in turn activates a protein kinase which leads to a cellular response (43,44).

B. Intracellular Free Magnesium Ion

The development of precise and sensitive methods for determining the concentration of intracellular free magnesium ion, $[Mg^{2+}]_i$ has significantly lowered earlier estimates and directed attention to the role(s) of this form of magnesium. The newer values are in the range at which certain enzymatic system have their K_m values. Most of the intracellular magnesium is associated with organic compounds and particularly with ATP, as noted above. Hence, relatively small percentage changes in the amount of bound magnesium will cause major changes in the amount of $[Mg^{2+}]_i$. Such variation within the range of 0.5–1.0 mM (or lower) is consistent with its possible function as a physiologic modulator.

On the basis of their own work and that of other investigators, White and Hartzell have proposed that $[Mg^{2+}]_i$ is carefully regulated and its alterations can have profound effects (45). In cardiac physiology, for example, "autonomic control of the heart is dependent upon Mg^{2+} in numerous ways: binding of neurotransmitters to their receptors, coupling of receptors to adenylate cyclase, activation of G proteins and adenylate cyclase, activation of proteins by Mg^{2+}-dependent phosphotransferases," and by modulating various types of ion channels and maintaining intracellular free Ca^{2+} at resting levels.

The known and postulated mechanisms by which $[Mg^{2+}]_i$ regulates ion movements have been reviewed (46–50). For example, the mechanism in cardiac muscle and other cells that allows K^+ to move readily into the cell but not out (inwardly rectifying K^+ channel) is related to its blocking by intracellular Mg^{2+}; the latter ion moves into the aqueous channel pore, thus blocking K^+ efflux. The Mg^{2+} cannot pass through the pore because of an outer energy barrier, and it stays until it is driven intracellularly again at a negative voltage by inward-moving K^+ (48). In this manner $[Mg^{2+}]_i$ modulates at least four such K^+ channels (47,48). Agus and Morad list additionally two Ca^{2+}, a Cl^-, and a Na^+ channel in cardiac cells of frogs and rodents (52). Many channels are markedly potentiated by phosphorylation involving cAMP and are modulated by cytosolic magnesium (47). Another example of the controlling role of Mg^{2+} relates to glutamate-activated receptor ion channels in the vertebrate central nervous system (Fig. 4). The N-methyl-D-aspartate receptor is part of a cation-selective channel with a high calcium permeability and sensitivity to magnesium blockage (49). Not only do the concentrations of $[Mg^{2+}]_i$ affect various cellular processes, but also the concentrations of Mg–nucleotide complexes play a role; the two forms often exert opposite effects, e.g., on ion channels (50).

Magnesium concentration in most cells at resting membrane potential is maintained below electrochemical equilibrium with the external ionized magnesium concentration. Under these circumstances, magnesium should slowly accumulate in cells by passive diffusion. Since this change has not been observed, the existence of one or more magnesium transport systems is suggested, some of which must be capable of active magnesium extrusion. Observations on squid axone, barnacle muscle, guinea pig papillary muscle, and skeletal muscle and red cells from several species indicate that a Na^+-dependent magnesium efflux may be the primary mechanism for keeping $[Mg^{2+}]_i$ below electrochemical equilibrium (12,51). Using ion-sensitive electrodes for measuring $[Mg^{2+}]_i$ in ferret papillary muscle, others have concluded that a simple system for Na^+–Mg^{2+} exchange is not the primary mode, nor does a Mg^{2+} extrusion mechanism involving steady-state ion exchange explain the data (52). There is some evidence for the existence of Na^+-independent

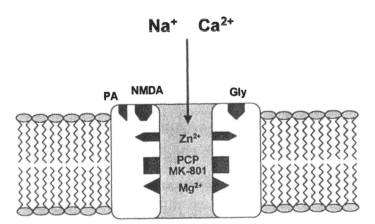

FIGURE 4   Schematic of the N-methyl-D-aspartate (NMDA) receptor-channel complex depicting the NMDA (glutamate) and glycine receptors and inhibitors, including Mg^{2+} and Zn^{2+}, of the Ca^{2+} channel. (Adapted with permission from Nakanishi, Science 1992; 258: 599.)

magnesium transport systems (51). The transport of magnesium across the rat placenta appeared to be sodium-dependent (53). A calcium channel blocker inhibited Mg^{2+} influx into magnesium-depleted embryonic chick myocytes (54); a Mg^{2+}-specific current elicited in voltage-clamped paramecium was inhibited when external Ca^{2+} was omitted or a Ca^{2+} chelator was injected (55). These observations suggest a role for Ca^{2+} in Mg^{2+} influx.

It has been suggested that $[Mg^{2+}]_i$ plays the role of a long-term regulatory ion which controls a set-point process in cell function (56); this contrasts to the very rapid, acute, and transient signaling induced by variations in Ca^{2+} movements.

VI. ASSESSMENT OF MAGNESIUM NUTRITURE

The desirability of having a reliable marker or markers for diagnosing magnesium depletion and its severity is obvious, both in terms of clinical usefulness and in providing more precise data on magnesium requirements in healthy individuals. Values for normal concentrations in both fluids, intact cells and cell partitions are given in Table 1.

A. Total Versus Ionized Magnesium in Serum Plasma

Protein-bound magnesium is subject to variations associated with changes in albumin and acid–base conditions (acidosis decreasing and alkalosis increasing the bonding); hence, the level of ionized or ultrafiltrable magnesium may be a more relevant determinant of deficiency than that of total serum magnesium (8,57).

Ultrafilterable magnesium obtained by Amicon micropartition systems, following human plasma or serum centrifugation with measurement by AAS, correlated closely ($r = 0.94$) with magnesium concentration determined by an ion-selective electrode (ISE) (8). In healthy individuals the difference in concentrations between least and most ionized magnesium as determined by ISE was 140 µM, which was appreciably less than that for total magnesium, which was 260 µM. Ionized plasma or serum magnesium averaged 71% of the total (8). There was virtually no difference in ionized magnesium by this technique when measured in whole blood, plasma, or serum.

2. Free Intracellular Mg^{2+}

The ability to measure change in $[Mg^{2+}]_i$ accurately in various blood cells and tissues together with ions such as K^+, Na^+, and Ca^{2+} will undoubtedly help to clarify, in various diseases, the concentrations of these ions in multiple tissues to those of serum, and cellular total magnesium. This may aid in the diagnosis of depletion. When ^{31}P NMR spectroscopy was applied to erythrocytes obtained from 24 normal subjects before and after 3 weeks' subsistence on a magnesium-restricted diet, the $[Mg^{2+}]_i$ fell from 209 ± 9.8 µM to 162 ± 9.3 µM ($p < 0.001$) (58).

C. Blood Mononuclear Cells

In experienced hands, the analyzed magnesium content of mononuclear blood cells is reproducible; however, variations in the proportion of isolated lymphocytes and monocytes in the analytic sample can influence the results (59). Its concentrations in human mononuclear cells have been claimed to be a better guide to magnesium nutriture than is the serum level (60,61). However, in patients with mild to severe congestive heart failure, magnesium concentrations in serum, circulating mononuclear cells, and skeletal muscle were of little predictive value in assessing the magnesium status of myocardial magnesium (62).

D. Urine Level of Magnesium

The urine level of magnesium can be helpful in determining the physiologic cause of hypomagnesemia: If the intake of magnesium is known to be reasonably good, then a low urinary magnesium level indicates intestinal malabsorption, while a urine output near or above intake levels suggests renal tubular dysfunction.

A fairly rapid entry of magnesium into one or more body pools is indicated by its increased retention when given as an intravenous infusion to patients depleted of magnesium as a result of prior diuretic therapy (63). This uptake may be assessed by a semiquantitative load test involving measurement of urinary magnesium following an infusion of a given amount of diluted magnesium salt (e.g., 63,64).

VII. DIETARY NEEDS FOR HEALTH

A number of factors affect the estimated requirements for healthy individuals. These include not only biological needs but also bioavailability of magnesium in the dietary source and accuracy in estimating intake and assessing need (65–67). Bioavailability factors are discussed in Section IX.

Growth rate of young animals is commonly used to assess nutrient requirement. The dietary requirements of several species, compiled primarily by the National Academy of Sciences, are presented in Table 2. In the adult human, metabolic balance studies are recognized as an important means of providing quantitative data on requirements. However, it is essential that measurements of intake and excretion be complete and accurate; that sufficient time be allotted for equilibrium between studies and prior to collection; that there be adequate numbers of individuals with stratification for age, sex, physiologic status to give statistical validity; that, in the case of magnesium, the amounts of other nutrients or nonnutrient dietary factors that may affect balance are understood and controlled, e.g., phosphate (20), calcium (30,31), acidosis (68), and perhaps vitamin B_6 (69); and finally, that systematic gradations of nutrient intake levels are utilized to cover the spectrum from negative to positive balances for the subjects. The latter point is critical; the normal intestinal and renal mechanisms can vary in their efficiency of absorption depending on the amounts presented, so that magnesium, like sodium, may be extremely well conserved at

TABLE 2 Dietary Magnesium Adequate for Growth of Laboratory Animals

Species	Percent of diet	Reference
Rat	0.04	(105)
Mouse	0.05–0.073	(105)
Gerbil	0.093–1.67	(105)
Guinea pig	0.10–0.30[a]	(105)
Golden hamster	0.06	(105)
Dog	0.018	(106)

[a]Depending on the concentrations of calcium, phosphorus, and potassium in the diet.

relatively low intakes. Balance studies which are not based on analysis of aliquots of the foods actually consumed are unacceptable because of the variability of magnesium data listed in various tables of food composition (70). Because of methodologic problems, including those of collection periods and analytic techniques, skepticism (71,72) is advised concerning older data (73). There is also considerable variance of data in more recent balance studies (71,72).

The specific 1989 RDA value for males and females 19 years and older is 350 mg and 280 mg, respectively; it is 320 mg for pregnant women, and 355 mg and 340 mg for the first 6 months and second 6 months of lactation, respectively. Females from 11 to 14 and from 15 to 18 years have RDAs of 280 and 300 mg; males in these age groups have 270 and 400 mg, respectively. The RDA for infants of 40–60 mg increases progressively to 170 mg for the age group 7–10 years (72).

Infants and children 1–5 years old in the United States consistently ingest magnesium at levels at or above the RDA (65,66); even those in the lowest fifth percentile, at ages 1–5 years, achieve intakes of about 90% of the RDA (65,66). It has been concluded that "magnesium deficiency is very unlikely to result from low dietary intake alone" (65).

Serum magnesium levels were determined by AAS on a U.S. population sample of 15,820 persons between 1971 and 1974 in NHANES 1 (74). Ninety-five percent of adults aged 18–74 had serum levels in the range 0.75–0.96 mmol/L (1.50–1.92 mEq), mean 0.85 mmol/L. The levels of the fifth percentile were at or above the lower levels of normal that are generally used in clinical laboratories (i.e., 0.70–0.73 mmol/L). In this author's opinion, the serum magnesium level in a healthy individual is a good index of magnesium nutriture; hence, these data indicate that magnesium deficiency in the U.S. population in 1970–1974 and presumably now is very uncommon in younger and older adults.

VIII. DEFICIENCY SIGNS

A. Laboratory and Domesticated Animals

Hypomagnesemia is the hallmark of experimental magnesium deficiency in all species that have been studied. However, there are other manifestations of deficiency which vary qualitatively and quantitatively within and among species, as mentioned below and summarized in Table 3.

The pathophysiologic changes occurring in the deficient rat are considered in some detail as a basis for comparison with other species. Acute deficiency in the young rat induces a spectacular series of events with the following typical sequence: usually after 3–5 days redness (hyperemia) and swelling of the ears, nose, and foot pads develop secondary to peripheral vasodilation; the hyperemia increases over the next several days and then diminishes; the animals then become progressively hyperkinetic when disturbed and exhibit frantic running about the cage, terminated by tonic-clonic convulsions and frequently by death (1). Hence magnesium deficiency has become associated with neuromuscular abnormalities.

The hyperemia has been associated with increased levels of histamine in certain tissues, blood, and urine, with mast cell activity and degranulation, and with eosinophilia (75,76). A transient leucocytosis also occurs. Skin ulceration and patchy alopecia appear after the hyperemia regresses. In more chronic depletion, there is growth retardation, edema, and overgrowth of the gums. Depending on the calcium and phosphorus contents of the diet and the presence of the parathyroid gland, soft tissue calcification often occurs (Table 3).

TABLE 3 Pathophysiologic Changes Induced by Magnesium Deficiency in Laboratory Animals

Sign	Affected species (reference)
Vasodilation	Rat (1)
Neuromuscular:	
Hyperkinetic activity	Rat (1); chick (91); duckling (92); rabbit (81); dog (87); pig (94); calf (95,100); lamb (95)
Convulsions	Rat (1); mouse (85); gerbil (105); chick (91); dog (87); duckling (92); rabbit (81); pig (94); lamb (95); calf (95,100); monkey (89)
Muscle weakness and/ or tremors/spasm	Chick (91); duckling (92); dog (87); pig (94); guinea pig (81); calf (100)
Growth retardation; anorexia	Rat (77,78); mouse (85,93); guinea pig (81); dog (87); calf (95); lamb (95); chick (91); duckling (92)
Skin lesions; alopecia	Rat (1,96); gerbil (105)
Gum hypertrophy	Rat (1)
Soft tissue calcification:	
Kidney	Rat (77,78); mouse (KK strain) (97); guinea pig (98); dog (87)
Skeletal/cardiac muscle	Rat (99); guinea pig (86); calf (100)
Aorta	Dog (106); pig (94)
Bone abnormalities	Rat (17,111); chick (17); pig (17); dog (17)
Thymic changes/ splenomegaly	Rat (83)
Anemia	Rat—fetal (80) and adult (103); guinea pig (104)

1. Calcification of Soft Tissues

In the rat kidney, calcification begins morphologically with the appearance of micro-crystalline bodies within the brush border and endocytotic vacuoles of the cortical proximal tubular cells and coincides with virtual disappearance of magnesium in the urine (77). Larger luminal renal calcium phosphate concretions occur primarily in the thin loop of Henle and in the ascending tubule (77,78). Tubular occlusion and functional renal impairment may result (78). Other organs and tissue undergo calcification in dogs and guinea pigs. Fig. 5 illustrates calcification in the dog aorta.

2. Electrolytes in Serum and Tissue

In the case of young rats on the high dietary calcium intakes usually used, serum or plasma calcium levels in the majority of reports were elevated above those of replete controls; in some reports, and especially when older rats were used, there were no differences between deficient and control animals (reviewed in Ref. 89). When dietary calcium was reduced to 0.14%, deficient rats developed hypercalcemia of a mild but statistically significant degree compared to pair-fed controls after 14 and 21 days; in some experiments, ad libitum-fed controls (which had gained considerably more weight) had serum calcium levels similar to deficient rats (85), while in other studies using this diet, the ad libitum-fed controls had lower calcium levels (111). With very severe dietary calcium restriction of magnesium deficient and control rats, hypocalcemia occurred with either no difference in degree between the groups (111) or with the magnesium-depleted becoming more hypocalcemic (90).

In marked contrast to the rat, the deficient mouse, guinea pig, chick, dog, pig, lamb, calf, monkey, and human either became hypocalcemic or remained eucalcemic with

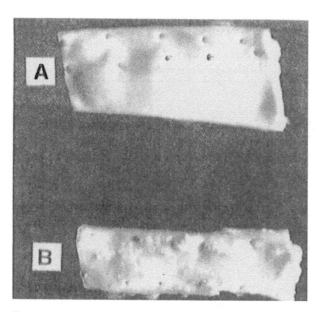

FIGURE 5   Aortic calcification in magnesium-deficient dog. A. Lumen of a normal aorta from a beagle pup fed 180 ppm. B. Lumen of a litter mate fed 80 ppm of magnesium. (From Ref. 106.)

controls (Table 4) (reviewed in Ref. 89). While differences in serum calcium in these species are attributable in part to factors such as age, the severity of hypomagnesemia, and dietary calcium levels, it is clear that there is a basic difference in physiologic control of serum calcium between the rat and the others. When the rat, mouse, dog, monkey, and human were maintained on similar magnesium-deficient diets containing 0.14% calcium, only the rat became hypercalcemic, the others became hypocalcemic (reviewed in Refs. 37, 85, and 89). Dunn performed thyroidectomy on magnesium-depleted hypocalcemic Rhesus monkeys and observed no increase in serum calcium as compared to thyroid-intact deficient animals; this experiment ruled out an effect of calcitonin on serum calcium levels (101). Bone cells in magnesium-depleted dogs become resistant to the effects of parathyroid hormone (102).

Hypophosphatemia in growing magnesium-deficient rats is commonly noted (Table 4) (37,85,114). In mice on a 0.14% calcium diet, hyperphosphatemia occurred during magnesium deficiency (85). Hyperphosphatemia was also present in dogs (89,106) and in guinea pigs (107) which were fed the more usual calcium and phosphate diets during deficiency. Phosphorus levels in deficient human subjects were variable; administration of magnesium caused a significant fall in one-half of the symptomatic individuals (37).

Hypokalemia and hyponatremia have not been observed generally in most species (37,107–109). Hypokalemia is often marked in deficient humans (37). Depressed serum albumin (84), immunoglobulin G (84), and alkaline phosphatase (110,111) occur in deficient rats.

Magnesium and potassium are usually reduced in the cardiac and skeletal muscles of deficient rats with little or no change in liver and kidney, whereas sodium and calcium are elevated on diets with usual amounts of calcium and phosphate (summarized in Ref. 112). Decreased cardiac magnesium and potassium have been noted in deficient mice (109). In deficient guinea pigs the concentration of these electrolytes changes in the same direction as noted in rats except for potassium, which is unchanged from control values (107). There

TABLE 4 Serum/Plasma Electrolyte Changes from Controls in Experimental Magnesium Deficiency[a]

	Mg	Ca	P	K		Mg	Ca	P	K
Rat	↓	↑	↓	→	Dog	↓	↓	↑	
Mouse	↓	↓→	↑	→	Calf	↓	↓→	→	
Guinea pig	↓	↓→	↑	→	Monkey	↓	↓	V	→
Chick	↓	↓	→		Human	↓	↓	V	↓

[a]See text for references and variability. V = variable.

were no changes in the calcium or phosphate content of the kidneys of deficient rats and mice on a diet with calcium restricted to 0.14% (85). In adult dogs, magnesium deficiency induced little or no change in skeletal muscle magnesium and potassium, but decreased the phosphorus and increased the sodium and calcium (113).

B. Humans

Signs of magnesium deficiency in the human have been observed experimentally and clinically. Symptomatic deficiency develops in a setting of predisposing and complicating disease states (Table 5). These are usually associated with impaired intake and intestinal or renal tubular malabsorptive conditions.

1. Experimental Deficiency

In a depletion study in which signs and symptoms occurred, the experimental diet provided about 6–10 mg (0.25–0.4 mmol) of magnesium per day; this followed a baseline period with a complete diet including adequate magnesium (37). Plasma magnesium fell progressively in six of the seven subjects with normal intestinal and renal functions to levels that were 10–30% those of control periods. Erythrocyte magnesium declined more slowly and to a lesser degree. Urine (Fig. 2) and fecal magnesium decreased to extremely low levels within 7 days. Hypomagnesemia, hypocalcemia, and hypokalemia were present in all of the five consistently symptomatic patients. The course of plasma ion concentrations in one patient is shown in Figure 6. In general, good intestinal absorption of calcium and low urinary output resulted in positive calcium balance. Serum phosphate values varied among the subjects. Negative potassium balance occurred as the result of increased urinary losses. Serum sodium remained normal, although the subjects were in positive sodium balance in association with a negative potassium balance.

Abnormal neuromuscular function occurred in five of the seven subjects after deficiency periods ranging from 25 to 110 days. All symptoms and signs (including personality changes and gastrointestinal symptoms) reverted to normal with reinstitution of magnesium. A characteristic finding during repletion was the delayed rise in serum calcium and potassium despite the rapid return to normal of serum magnesium (Fig. 6); a week or longer intervened before they returned to baseline levels. Potassium balances became strongly positive when sodium balances became negative as the result of appropriate changes in urinary excretion.

2. Clinical Deficiency

The signs and symptoms noted above in experimental deficiency have been described individually or in various combinations in clinical cases with hypomagnesemia (reviewed

TABLE 5   Clinical Conditions Contributing to Magnesium Depletion

Malabsorption syndromes
  Inflammatory bowel disease
  Gluten enteropathy; sprue
  Intestinal fistulas, bypass, or resection
  Bile insufficiency states, e.g., ileal dysfunction with steatorrhea
  Immune diseases with villous atrophy
  Radiation enteritis
  Lymphangiectasia; other fat absorbtive defects
  Primary idiopathic hypomagnesemia
  Gastrointestinal infections
Renal dysfunction with excessive losses
  Tubular diseases
  Metabolic disorders
  Hormonal effects
  Nephrotoxic drugs
Endocrine disorders
  Hyperaldosteronism
  Hyperparathyroidism with hypercalcemia
  Postparathyroidectomy ("hungry bone" syndrome)
  Hyperthyroidism
Pediatric genetic and familial disorders
  Primary idiopathic hypomagnesemia
  Renal wasting syndrome
  Bartter's syndrome
  Infants born of diabetic or hyperparathyroid mothers
  Transient neonatal hypomagnesemic hypocalcemia
Inadequate intake, provision, and/or retention of magnesium
  Alcoholism
  Protein-calorie malnutrition (usually with infection)
  Prolonged infusion or ingestion of magnesium-low nutrient solutions or diets
  Hypercatabolic states (burns, trauma), often associated with item immediately above
  Excessive lactation

From Shils ME. Magnesium, In: Shils ME, Olson JA, Shike M, eds. Modern Nutrition in Health and
Disease. 8th ed. Philadelphia: Lea & Febiger, 1994: 170.

in Ref. 37). They include Trousseau and Chvostek signs, normal or depressed deep tendon
reflexes, muscle fasciculations, tremor, muscle spasm, personality changes, anorexia,
nausea, and vomiting. Frank tetany, myoclonic jerks, athetoid movements, convulsions,
and coma also have been reported. Convulsions with or without coma occur more frequently in acutely deficient infants than in adults.

The closest disease-related condition to "pure" experimental human magnesium
deficiency is an uncommon congenital primary (idiopathic) hypomagnesemia related to a
specific defect in intestinal absorption of this ion (26,115). Hypomagnesemia, hypomag-
nesuria, hypocalcemia, and hypokalemia with tetany, often with convulsions, were corrected with magnesium supplements. Calcium and vitamin D supplements without magnesium were ineffective in maintaining normocalcemia.

The cellular loss of potassium during deficiency appears to be secondary to func-

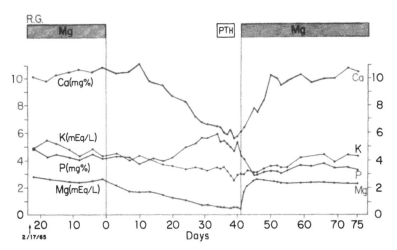

FIGURE 6 Blood cations in a subject during experimental magnesium depletion. Mg was omitted after the patient had been on the control diet for 1 month. The rise in serum inorganic phosphate (P) with Mg depletion in this patient was unique among the depleted subjects. On depletion day 25, Trousseau and Chvostek signs first occurred; the former became progressively stronger as plasma Ca, Mg, and K continued to decline. On depletion day 35, parathyroid hormone (PTH) was given intramuscularly at 50 units three times daily for 5 days; this had no effect on plasma Ca but appeared to decrease P. On day 41, anorexia, nausea, parathesias, and generalized muscle spasticity developed; 17 mEq of Mg I.V. was then given followed by similar amounts 12 and 15 hours later. Clinical improvement occurred. Dietary Mg (40 mEq daily) was resumed on the third repletion day. (From Ref 37, with permission.)

tional impairment of the magnesium-dependent Na,K-ATPase, the membrane sodium pump; potassium is lost and sodium ions accumulate intracellularly (116).

3. PTH Levels in Deficient Humans

The first reported depleted patient (one with idiopathic hypomagnesemia) assayed for circulating immunoparathyroid hormone (iPTH) had undetectable levels of iPTH which rose markedly when magnesium was given. A good calcemic response followed, indicating that depletion was associated with a failure of the parathyroid gland either to manufacture or to secrete the hormone (124). As more cases of deficiency were reported with iPTH measurements, it became apparent that the situation was more complex and that several types of responses were involved. In earlier stages of deficiency there was a fall in calcium caused in part by a decreased reactivity of bone to PTH, with increased circulating PTH resulting from the hypocalcemic stimulus to increased PTH production (89,102). With further progression of deficiency, impairment of PTH secretion occurred which responded rapidly to appropriate magnesium injection (118,119) (Fig. 7). The overall sequence may be summarized as follows.

1. *Initiation of hypocalcemia.* The initiating factor is probably the failure of the normal heterionic exchange of bone calcium for magnesium at the labile bone mineral surface (120). Impairment of receptor responsiveness to PTH of the osteoclasts follows, with reduction of active bone resorption (102). At this stage hypocalcemia persists despite increased levels of circulating PTH (89,119).

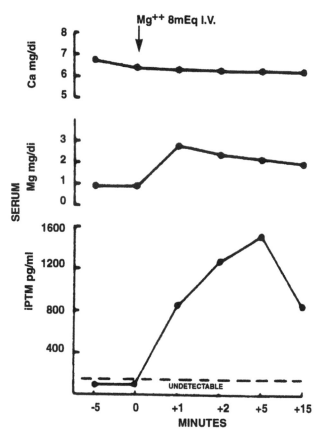

FIGURE 7 Effect of rapid intravenous magnesium administration on serum iPTH in a magnesium deficient hypocalcemic patient. Prior to the magnesium injection the iPTH had been undetectable, but within a minute after its injection, iPTH increased, along with serum magnesium, and continued to high levels while serum calcium remained low. (From Ref. 119, reprinted with permission of the Endocrine Society.)

   2. *Accentuation of electrolyte, PTH, and clinical abnormalities.* As depletion progresses, secretion of PTH diminishes to very low levels despite adequate intraparathyroid gland hormonal reserves (118,119). The signs of severe magnesium depletion are present at this stage, i.e., very low circulating PTH, unresponsive bone, hypocalcemia, hypocalciuria, hypokalemia, sodium retention, and neuromuscular and other clinical signs and symptoms (37).

   3. *Regression of magnesium depletion and associated changes.* Following administration of adequate magnesium, serum magnesium rises rapidly, presumably with restoration of heterionic calcium–magnesium exchange. Little or no detectable change in circulating calcium occurs in this early phase despite the increase in circulating PTH (Fig. 7), probably a result of the time required for bone cell receptors to regain responsiveness to PTH. As serum calcium increases, plasma

PTH levels decline appropriately. The delayed rise in serum potassium is presumably secondary to the time period required to restore the normal activity of the cellular membrane Na-K ATP-ase pump leading to renal tubular conservation. Clinical signs and symptoms disappear in a matter of hours to a few days.

C. Other Pathologies in Various Species

1. Resistance to Vitamin D in Magnesium Deficiency

The calcemic effect of vitamin D—even in high dose—is blunted in the presence of magnesium depletion in human rickets, in D-deficient laboratory animals, in human malabsorption, and in idiopathic or surgically induced hypoparathyroidism (reviewed in Ref. 38). PTH is necessary for the formation of calcitriol, while calcitriol is necessary for PTH to exert its effect on calcium mobilization from bone (121); nevertheless, despite low levels of calcitriol in the majority of reported cases with magnesium depletion, serum calcium has been found to rise following magnesium repletion (38). Magnesium depletion in rats did not prevent normal in-vivo conversion of calcidiol to calcitriol, nor did it modify the in-vitro activity of 1-alpha hydroxylase in renal mitochondria (122). Vitamin D resistance induced by magnesium depletion appears to be the consequence of impaired skeletal response to calcitriol.

2. Citrate Relationships

The influence on citrate excretion of vitamin D deficiency (decreased), parathyroid hormone (increased), magnesium concentration (decreased), and alkalosis (increased) has been known for many years (123,124). In magnesium-deficient rats with the usual calcium and phosphate intakes, the common serum electrolyte pattern persists (Table 4) with renal calcinosis. They were noted to have moderately elevated serum citrate and markedly decreased urinary citrate as compared to controls (123); the lower urine citrate was attributable to increased renal tubular reabsorption. With alkalosis induced by sodium bicarbonate, the deficient rats excreted somewhat more citrate; while this amount was only about one-fourth that of the stimulated controls, it was associated with a major reduction in kidney calcification. Patients who were acutely or chronically depleted of magnesium also markedly decreased their urinary excretion of citrate secondary to increased renal tubular citrate reabsorption (125). In the presence of malabsorption-associated hyperoxaluria, the reduced urine citrate concentration together with the reduced magnesium content pose a risk for oxalate kidney stone formation.

3. Lipids, Lipoproteins, and Prostanoids

Magnesium deficiency in rats has been associated with increased serum/plasma phospholipids, triglycerides, variable total cholesterol, low free cholesterol, increased levels of oleic and linoleic acids, decreased levels of stearic and arachidonic acids, and modifications of lipid and lipoprotein concentrations (126). Plasma prostanoids (PGE_2, $PGF_{2\alpha}$, 6-keto-$PGF_{1\alpha}$, and TBX_2) were significantly elevated in plasma and tissues of deficient rats as compared to controls (127), and in the outflow of the vessels of the mesenteric arterial bed (128). It has been hypothesized that magnesium depletion, by inhibiting adenylate cyclase activity and thereby lowering c-AMP levels, permits increased cyclooxygenase activity and stimulation of prostanoid synthesis (127). Comparison with other species is necessary before assuming that such effects in the deficient rat can be generalized.

D. Disease States That Induce Magnesium Deficiency

The list of causes of magnesium depletion (Table 5) emphasizes that deficiency may be a fairly common in acutely or chronically ill patients. A few examples make the point. Of 2300 patients surveyed in a Veterans Affairs hospital, 6.9% were hypomagnesemic (129); patients in medical and surgical intensive care units (ICUs) had a particularly high prevalence of hypomagnesemia; 65% of patients admitted with normal renal function had hypomagnesemia (130); of 193 adult postoperative ICU patients, 117 (63%) were hypomagnesemic and 10 (5%) were hypermagnesemic (131); in 32 pulmonary ICU patients, 9% had low serum magnesium and 47% had low muscle values (132).

1. Alcoholism

Magnesium depletion in acute and chronic alcoholism has been documented over many years. Causes include poor intake, increased urinary losses, vomiting, diarrhea, and ketosis (133).

2. Diabetes

Loss of magnesium in diabetic ketoacidosis has also been known for many years (134). There are a number of reports of hypomagnesemia in ambulatory diabetic patients without renal insufficiency; in insulin-dependent pregnant women; in infants born to diabetic mothers; and in diabetic children with insulin dependency (summarized in Ref. 38).

3. Malabsorption

Intestinal malabsorption is one of the more common causes of magnesium depletion. Syndromes vary from the more common gastrointestinal disorders associated with steatorrhea to the relatively rare and specific disorder, primary hypomagnesemia. Serious depletion may occur because of one or more of the following: (a) impaired transport across a diseased bowel, (b) reduced absorptive surface associated with surgical resection, bowel bypass, or radiation damage, (c) very rapid transit and loss secondary to choleralike disease, and (d) decreased intraluminal solubility of dietary or secreted magnesium in association with unabsorbed fatty acids and loss in stool; in the latter circumstance, restriction of dietary fat can reduce fecal magnesium losses (135,136).

4. Protein-Energy Malnutrition

Magnesium depletion occurs in children with inadequate food intakes in association with malabsorption, persistent vomiting and/or diarrhea, and infection. Serum or plasma magnesium was noted to be low in a significant proportion of such children in various studies in Africa (137) and Central America (138).

5. Kidney Disease and Nephrotoxic Drugs

A number of factors may modify adversely the critical role of the kidney in magnesium homeostasis. When glomerular filtration is seriously impaired, hypermagnesemia is usual. However, hypomagnesemia may occur in patients with renal failure because of poor food intake and concomitant losses associated with vomiting, diarrhea, malabsorption, diuretics, nephrotoxic drugs, chronic acidosis, and/or use of a magnesium-low dialysate. Increased excretion is also associated with postobstructive nephropathy, chronic glomerulonephritis, acute tubulo-intestinal nephritis, and post-renal transplantation. In congenital urinary magnesium wasting syndromes, the magnesium deficiency is often severe and symptomatic (139).

6. Postparathyroidectomy Hypomagnesemia

Symptomatic hypomagnesemia may follow parathyroidectomy for primary hyperparathyroidism in association with the expected hypocalcemia, presumably as part of the "hungry bone" syndrome, which occurs as the result of rapid uptake of calcium and magnesium by bone (140).

7. Hypertension

There are contradictory reports differentiating serum magnesium levels in hypertensives from those in nonhypertensives, so no conclusions can be drawn on this point. Of more relevance are the results of a series of intervention studies. Several have reported that hypertensive patients on thiazide diuretics who were also given magnesium supplements had a subsequent drop in blood pressure. Others reported no effect of magnesium in comparison with a placebo in patients with varying degrees of hypertension, all of whom had normal serum magnesium initially. An 8-month controlled study in subjects with mild hypertension and not on diuretics compared the effects of either placebo or potassium alone or in combination with magnesium; potassium alone or with magnesium caused a significant reduction in blood pressure, but magnesium did not have an additive effect to that of potassium. In another controlled study with hypertensive men given a placebo, hydrochlorothiazide alone or in association with potassium, or with potassium *and* magnesium, the only groups that did *not* have a significant fall in systolic blood pressure were those on a placebo and those given thiazide with potassium and magnesium. The data increasingly suggest that there is no antihypertensive effect of magnesium when given in physiologic amounts. This topic has been reviewed in more detail recently (38).

8. Coronary Artery Disease

In recent years the literature has been concerned with the possible preventive and therapeutic roles of magnesium in relation to coronary artery disease (CAD). The argument has been advanced that the American public has a significant amount of asymptomatic magnesium deficiency and that this is a contributing factor in the prevalence of CAD (141). Data presented above contradicts the concept of any significant magnesium deficiency in healthy Americans; this fact, together with the continuing decline in age-adjusted death rate from ischemic heart disease in the United States make this claim an unlikely one.

There is some epidemiologic data suggesting a decreased mortality from CAD in populations living in "hard" water areas (i.e., relatively high in calcium, magnesium, and fluoride) as compared to those in "soft" water areas (summarized in Ref. 141). Contrary data from various countries indicate no association between myocardial disease and mortality and the concentrations of magnesium or calcium in drinking water (142–144).

An older literature which noted low serum/plasma magnesium values in patients with suspected or proven myocardial infarction suggested that a primary state of magnesium depletion was involved. As noted above, such claims are contradicted by contrary evidence. Furthermore, more recent data indicate that a number of clinical factors affect serum and cardiac magnesium concentrations variably in such patients. These include (a) the time of drawing of blood following onset of chest pain, (b) the degree of pain, (c) the prior and often chronic use of diuretics (which may induce magnesium and potassium depletion), (d) postinfarction lipolysis (also induced by ethanol withdrawal, epinephrine, and surgery) causing increased serum fatty acids which lower serum magnesium, and (e) the extent of the infarction per se. This literature has been reviewed in Ref. 38.

In recent years there have been many reports suggesting that i.v. magnesium given early after suspected acute myocardial infarction reduces the frequency of serious arrythmias and mortality. These have been summarized in recent meta-analyses which suggest but do not prove benefit (145,146). We now have a recent report of a major randomized, double-blinded placebo-controlled study (LIMIT-2) which summarized the observations on 2316 patients with suspected acute myocardial infarction; patients were given either i.v. physiological saline or i.v. $MgSO_4$ over 24 h (147). The number of patients observed is many times the number in the largest study included in the two meta-analyses noted above. Mortality from all causes was 7.8% in the magnesium group and 10.3% in the placebo group ($p = 0.04$), a relative reduction of 24% [95% confidence interval (C.I.) 1–43%]. In coronary care unit (CCU) patients, left ventricular failure was reduced by 25% (C.I. 57–39%) in the magnesium group ($p = 0.009$). A number of hypotheses were tested because of claims made in prior studies; it was concluded that (a) there was no effect modification by magnesium related to diuretic therapy, (b) magnesium was acting pharmacologically rather than by correcting a deficit, (c) magnesium did not affect the progression to acute myocardial infarction among patients with unstable coronary artery disease, and (d) magnesium did not have antiarrhythmic actions.

While LIMIT 2 findings suggested a safe and worthwhile benefit of i.v. magnesium in patients with suspected myocardial infarction, the wide confidence interval reported was of some concern. This was responsible in part for continued recruitment in another major randomized trial of magnesium, the Fourth International Study of Infarct Survival (ISIS-4) the results of which have been published (148).

The Fourth International Study of Infarct Survival was a much larger randomized trial with 58,050 patients with suspected acute myocardial infarction; the study was designed to assess the benefits and risks and three treatments vs. placebo or open control. One treatment was intravenous magnesium sulfate given over 24 hours vs. open control; the magnesium infusion was 8 mmol (192 mg) in 15 minutes followed by 72 mmol infused over 24 hours. There was no significant reduction in 5-week mortality either overall (2216 magnesium allocated deaths [7.64%] vs. 2103 [7.24%] control deaths) or in any subgroup examined (i.e., treated early or late, in the presence or absence of fibrinolytic or antiplatelet therapies, or at high risk of death). There was a significant excess of mortality with magnesium in heart failure patients or those in cardiogenic shock. The conclusion was that intravenous magnesium was ineffective.

IX. FACTORS THAT AFFECT MAGNESIUM DEFICIENCY

Several intrinsic and environmental factors affect the signs of magnesium deficiency. Included among these factors are pregnancy, age, species, and dietary levels of calcium and phosphorus.

A. Pregnancy

The essentiality of magnesium in many critical enzymatic reactions suggests that its deficiency during pregnancy would be particularly harmful to the developing fetus. This is indeed the case; a severely magnesium-restricted diet fed to pregnant rats from the 6th to the 14th day of pregnancy produced fetal death and resorption or gross congenital malformations, anemia, and edema (79,80).

B. Age

The older the rat at onset of deficiency, the less marked are the signs. As the deficiency continues and the rate of growth diminishes, the degree of hypomagnesemia becomes less. Similarly, the degree of magnesium restriction in the diet and in the levels of accompanying nutrients such as calcium, phosphate, or potassium (e.g., Ref. 81) and protein (82) play a role in the expression of the severity of signs and biochemical changes.

C. Species

There are similarities and both qualitative and quantitative differences in the manifestation of deficiency between and among the rat and other species. The rat appears to be the only species that develops hyperemia (Table 3). On the other hand, the rat and almost all species studied develop neuromuscular signs including convulsions (Table 3); in the mouse, the convulsion is a single tonic and lethal one (85), but in the guinea pig, convulsions are rare (81).

D. Dietary Calcium and Phosphorus

The increased deposits of calcium in various species is of interest for several reasons. When renal calcification is advanced, tubular obstruction occurs, leading to filtration and absorption problems resulting in azotemia with serum acid–base changes, increased phosphate and potassium, and lowered calcium (78,86). The degree of calcification is affected not only by the extent of magnesium depletion but also by increased levels of calcium and phosphate in the diet; this is true for the rat (78), the guinea pig (81), and the dog (87,106).

Increased dietary levels of calcium and phosphate (especially the latter) exacerbate magnesium depletion signs in these species and raise the amount of magnesium required to maintain growth and avoid calcification. Furthermore, in the rat (88), guinea pig (81,88), and dog (87,106), an increase in phosphate is more deleterious than is an increase in calcium.

The amounts of calcium and phosphate incorporated into diets used for magnesium deficiency studies have varied among studies. In many instances, calcium has been incorporated in the basal diet for rats in the range of 0.4–0.9 grams percent with many at the 0.6% level and, on occasion, at higher levels for comparative purposes. In the guinea pig 0.9% has been a baseline value used by O'Dell and associates (81), but with test levels as high as 1.7% and 2.5%. The chick diet has usually contained calcium at about 1.2% (81), the pig at 0.7% (94), the calf at about 1.0 (81), and the dog with a basal diet of 0.6%, varying in test diets from 0.3% to 0.9% (87). In contrast, in experiments utilizing an experimental human diet (37) fed to rats and mice (83,85) and to dogs and monkeys (89), the calcium content was 0.14%. Diets providing still lower amounts (i.e., 0.070, 0.002, and 0.010%, respectively) have been used to observe the effects on serum calcium during magnesium deficiency (89,90,111).

Phosphorus as phosphate (plus that from casein when used) has been used in basal diets for mammalian species from 0.4 to 0.7% and for the chick from 0.4 to 0.8%. In the studies with various species on the diet containing 0.14% calcium (83,85,89), the P content was 0.375% including the phosphorus in the casein.

It is apparent that an accurate comparison of the manifestations of magnesium depletion in and among species requires knowledge of the many interacting factors operative in a particular experiment.

E. Magnesium Losses During Depletion

In young animals of various species, the source of tissue loss of magnesium is the skeleton, which can amount to 30% or more of that present; in older animals the loss is very much less (17,95), with the loss being proportionately greater from soft tissues. Chronic acidosis in starving adult humans leads to significant bone and muscle losses (68).

F. Magnesium–Parathyroid Interrelations

The electrolyte changes noted commonly in the magnesium-deficient rat (Table 4) are those seen in hyperparathyroidism whereas those occurring in other species suggested hypoparathyroid state. This initiated many studies on parathyroid function. Parathyroidectomy of the magnesium-deficient rat either eliminated the hypercalcemia or else induced a mild hypocalcemia (108,114) (reviewed in Ref. 89). Prior thyro-parathyroidectomy (T-PTX) of young dogs induced the expected hypocalcemia; subsequent magnesium deficiency further lowered the serum calcium. Injection of parathyroid extract (PTE) normalized the calcium in both deficient and control dogs. In T-PTX, magnesium-depleted rats, the response to PTE as compared to injected controls has been either similar or blunted (reviewed in Ref. 89).

The calcium responses of PTE of parathyroid-intact depleted rats, dogs, and monkeys have been similar to their controls; however, the deficient chick has been found to be resistant to PTE (reviewed in Ref. 89). Hence, these data do not explain the basis for the difference in serum calcium between the rat and other species.

The elevated serum calcium and decreased phosphate and the failure of the parathyroidectomized rat to develop hypercalcemia suggest that the intact deficient rat should have an elevated level of circulating PTH. Serial measurements of serum iPTH, calcium, and phosphorus were made in groups of young rats on the deficient and control diets (118,119). In both studies the hypomagnesemia and the rise in serum calcium were associated with a marked rise in plasma/serum iPTH; the latter peaked at day 14 in the report of Rayssiguier et al. (149) and at about the fourth or fifth day in the study of Anast et al. (150) (Fig. 8). The iPTH they proceeded to decrease to control levels by the 20th day (149) or below control levels by the 6th day (150), while the hypercalcemia continued without any apparent relation to the iPTH.

Hence, after the expected initial iPTH response to hypercalcemia, the PTH production fell. There was no difference between the deficient and control groups in the assays for intestinal calcium binding protein (149); this was an additional argument against the concept that hypercalcemia occurred because of increased calcium absorption (149). Circulating iPTH was greatly increased in both magnesium-deficient and magnesium-replete animals which were chronically hypocalcemic as the result of either calcium or vitamin D deficiencies (150). These data demonstrated (a) that magnesium depletion per se did not inhibit PTH production and (b) that the increasing hypercalcemia eventually inhibited PTH production. Because of other findings of *decreased* bone resorption in the magnesium deficient rat (17,111), it was concluded that the hypercalcemia in the deficient rat is secondary to unknown factors.

G. Mg^{2+}–Ca^{2+} Interactions

The complementary or antagonist effects of magnesium and calcium ions on rat renal cortical adenylate cyclase activity in vitro under parathyroid stimulation are demonstrated in Figure 9. $[Mg^{2+}]$ or $[Ca^{2+}]$ were varied while the level of one of these two ions were fixed (90). Addition of Mg^{2+} progressively activated the enzyme at any fixed $[Ca^{2+}]$ not exceeding 1.5 mM, its approximate physiologic concentration in extracellular fluid. With $[Mg^{2+}]$ up to 0.5 mM (its approximate normal physiologic extracellular concentration), addition of 0.5 mM Ca^{2+} stimulated enzyme activity, but higher $[Ca^{2+}]$ either was ineffective or reduced the cyclic AMP formed. At higher $[Mg^{2+}]$, addition of Ca^{2+} progressively inhibited the enzyme. Similar types of studies utilizing purified adenylate cyclase derived from rat or pig parathyroid membranes have confirmed the competitive actions of these two divalent ions on PTH secretion (151,152). The porcine enzyme has two Ca^{2+} inhibitory sites, with Mg^2 influencing the relative inhibitory contribution of Ca^{2+} at these sites (152). These data suggest that when magnesium is very depleted in vivo, the marked Ca^{2+} inhibitory effect on the enzyme reduces parathyroid secretion and its effects. There is increasing evidence that Mg^{2+} also influences PTH secretion by enhancing activation of the adenylate cyclase system by endogenous guanine nucleotides.

There are a number of studies with parathyroid tissue in vitro as well as infusion studies of rat and of goat, calf, and sheep parathyroid glands in vivo which demonstrate (a) the essentiality of magnesium at a basic minimum concentration for PTH formation and (b) the interplay between magnesium and calcium concentrations in the bath or perfusion fluids in which magnesium can replace calcium in inhibiting parathyroid function (reviewed in Ref. 89).

X. HYPERMAGNESEMIA AND MAGNESIUM TOXICITY

A. Hypermagnesemia with Normal Renal Function

High-dose parenteral magnesium sulfate is the drug of choice in North America for preventing eclamptic convulsions that may occur with severe hypertension in late pregnancy or during labor (153). It has been given also in an effort to prevent premature labor (154). A loading dose is given, followed by maintenance doses with the objective of maintaining high serum levels, e.g., 2.0 to 3 mmol. The high doses used clinically rarely cause a degree of hypermagnesemia likely to be associated with serious side effects (see next section), because the magnesium is excreted rapidly because of good renal function and because the patients are closely monitored.

The interdependent and often competitive relations of Mg^{2+} and Ca^{2+} are further demonstrated by the changes in serum Ca^{2+} and circulating PTH levels in patients with such therapeutic hypermagnesia. With the rise in serum magnesium, a fall in PTH may occur, with an associated hypocalcemia (155,156). Although some preeclamptic pregnant women developed hypocalcemia with little or no change in PTH levels (156,157), their fetuses at delivery had low calcium and very low PTH levels (157).

Infusion of magnesium into grown pigs increased plasma calcitonin in a linear fashion as plasma magnesium rose above 3 to 4 mEq/L (158). This was associated with the expected decline in total and ionized calcium and was prevented by thyro-parathyroidectomy.

In an animal model, magnesium sulfate infusions increased the circulating levels of vitamin K-dependent bone-specific protein osteocalcin, presumably as the result of its known inhibition of osteocalcin binding to hydroxyapatite, an effect that can be overcome by calcium (159). These and many other Mg^{2+}–Ca^{2+} interactions have led to the designation of magnesium as a "mimic-weak Ca^{2+} antagonist" and "the mimic/antagonist of calcium" (160,161).

Increased magnesium in vitro relaxes vascular smooth muscle and reduces pressor

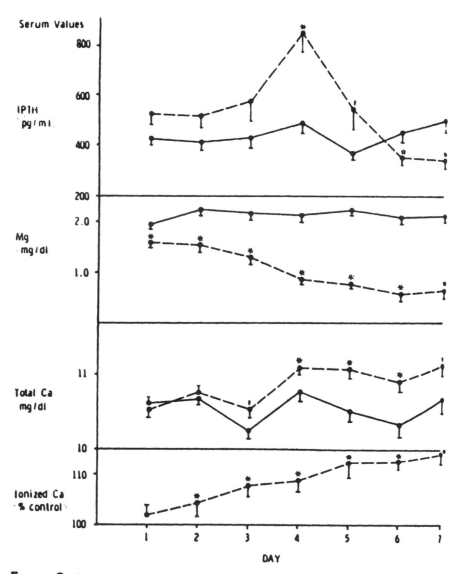

FIGURE 8 Serum iPTH, magnesium, total and ionized calcium (X ± SEM) in rats fed a control
(————) or a magnesium-deficient diet (— — —) for a 7-day period (left panel). The same parameters are shown for rats subsisting on the same diets for a 30-day period (right panel). ★ = significantly different from control, $p < 0.05$; † = significantly different from control, $p < 0.02$; * = significantly different from control, $p < 0.01$. (From Ref. 150, with permission.)

responses (160). Infusion of magnesium sulfate into normal human subjects over a 3-h period raised serum magnesium from an average of 0.83 mmol/L to 1.75 mmol/L; this was associated with declines in systolic and diastolic blood pressures and increased renal blood flow (162). Urinary excretion of 6-keto-$PGF_{1\alpha}$ (the stable metabolite of prostacyclin) increased markedly, whereas urinary PGE_2 did not change. Cyclooxygenase inhibitors (indomethacin, ibuprofen) completely blocked the magnesium-induced fall in blood pressure, and the rise in urinary 6-keto-$PGF_{1\alpha}$. These findings show that the effect of magne-

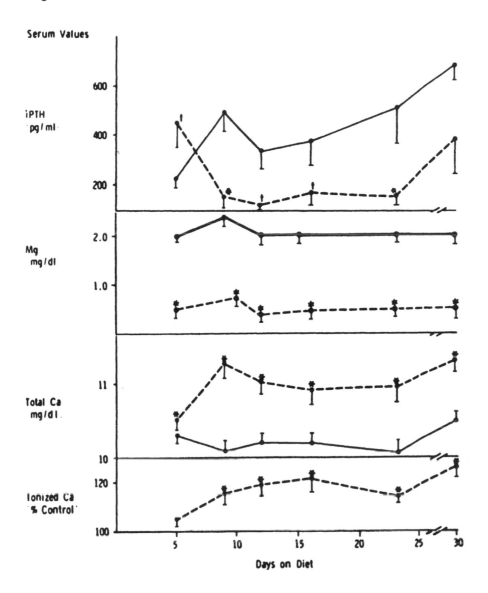

sium was mediated by prostacyclin release, which may be influenced by changes in Ca^{2+} flux. When intravenous magnesium was infused into pregnant women, either to delay premature delivery or to treat severe hypertension, only the former group demonstrated an increase in renal excretion of PGI_2 (prostacyclin) metabolites (163).

B. Magnesium Toxicity

In contrast to the planned therapeutic hypermagnesemia noted above, elevated serum levels can occur when magnesium-containing drugs, usually antacids or cathartics, are ingested chronically by individuals with serious renal insufficiency; this occurs because 20% or more of Mg^{2+} from various salts may be absorbed. In acute renal failure with oliguria, especially when accompanied by metabolic acidosis and trauma, tissue release in associa-

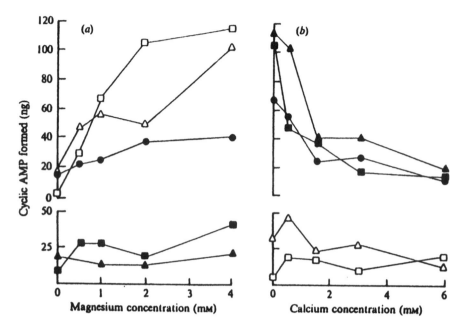

FIGURE 9   Influence of (*a*) magnesium and (*b*) calcium on parathyroid hormone-stimulated renal cortical adenylate cyclase activity in vitro, in the presence of various concentrations of the other ion. (*a*) Ca^{2+} concentrations (mM): ▲, 6.0; ■ 3.0; ●, 1.5; △, 0.5; □, 0.0. (*b*) Mg^{2+} concentrations (mM): ▲, 4.0; ■, 2.0; ●, 1.0; △, 0.5; □, 0.0. Each point represents the mean of duplicate determinations. (From Ref. 90, with permission.)

tion with magnesium ingestion or parenteral administration may result in hypermagnesemia.

The many and potentially toxic and even lethal effects of magnesium excess have been reviewed (164) and are summarized in Figure 10. Calcium infusion can counteract magnesium toxicity. Avoidance of magnesium-containing medications in patients with significant renal disease is recommended unless there is good reason and close monitoring. Hypermagnesemia should be suspected in instances of low anion gap in stable patients and a normal anion gap in severely ill, acidotic patients.

X.   PERSPECTIVES

More than 60 years have passed since the first detailed report was published concerning the manifestations of magnesium deficiency in the rat. This chapter has summarized briefly many, but certainly not all, of the many advances that have accrued in our knowledge of this essential ion. The advances concerning the roles of essential nutrients are increasingly those derived from molecular biology. A major lesson for the young investigator dedicated to nutrition research is the need to be versed in the newer aspects of molecular biology and its techniques, so as to direct his or her research efforts in that direction. It is also wise to be aware of the relevant clinical literature, since important leads may well arise from that area.

The technical ability to measure with reasonable accuracy the concentration of intracellular free Mg^{2+} will provide increasing information on its role in the control of cellular reactions. The role of this ion in various signal, receptors, channel, and enzymatic

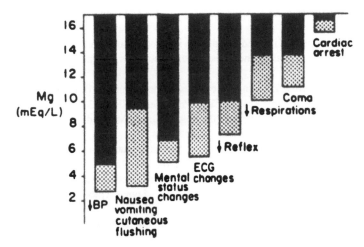

FIGURE 10 Summary of the toxic effects of increasing hypermagnesemia. The stippled sections of each bar graph depict the concentration range in which the signs and/or symptoms occur inconstantly and the solid area that in which they are constant. Nausea, vomiting, and hypotension may occur variability in the range 3–9 mEq/L and uniformly above that range; bradycardia and urinary retention also occur in that range. Electrocardiographic changes, hyporeflexia, and secondary central nervous system depression may appear in the range 5–10 mEq/L, followed at higher concentrations by life-threatening respiratory depression, coma, and asystolic cardiac arrest. (From Ref. 164, with permission of the American Society of Pharmacology and Experimental Therapeutics.)

reactions needs to be better known to understand their influences in health and in disease. It is this author's opinion that the role of magnesium in many areas of the complex field of immunology has not been given the attention it deserves.

The important molecular interplay between Mg^{2+} and Ca^{2+} as noted in adenylate cyclase undoubtedly has many other interacting sites with this mimic-antagonist relationship. Better understanding may help explain the still unresolved issue of why the rat, in contrast to all other species, develops hypercalcemia on the usual calcium intake.

REFERENCES

1. Kruse HD, Orent ER, McCollum EV. Studies on magnesium deficiency in animals. I. Symptomatology resulting from magnesium deprivation. J Biol Chem 1932; 96: 519–536.
2. Hirschfelder AD, Haury VG. Clinical manifestation of high and low plasma magnesium. JAMA 1934; 102: 1138–1141.
3. Flink EB, Stutzman FL, Anderson AR, Konig T, Fraser R. Magnesium deficiency after prolonged parenteral fluid administration and after chronic alcoholism complicated by delirium tremens. J Lab Clin Med 1954; 43: 169–183.
4. Alcock NW. Development of methods for the determination of magnesium. Ann NY Acad Sci 1969; 162: 707–716.
5. Elin RJ. Determination of serum magnesium concentrations by clinical laboratories. Magnes Trace Elem 1991–92; 10: 60–66.
6. Hunt CD, Shuler TR. Open-vessel, wet ash, low temperature digestion of biological materials for inductively coupled argon plasma spectroscopy (ICOP) analysis of boron and other elements. J Micronutrient Anal 1990; 6: 161–174.

7. Elin RJ. Laboratory tests for the assessment of magnesium status in humans. Magnes Trace Elem 1991; 10:172–181.

8. Altura BT, Altura BM. Measurement of ionized magnesium in whole blood, plasma and serum with a new ion-selective electrode in healthy and diseased human subjects. Magnes Trace Elem 1991–1992; 10: 90–98.

9. Gupta RK, Gupta P, Yushok WD, Rose ZB. On the noninvasive measurements of intracellular free magnesium by ^{31}P NMR spectroscopy. Physiol Chem Phys Med NMR 1983; 15:265–280.

10. London RE. Methods for measurement of intracellular magnesium: NMR and fluorescence. Annu Rev Physiol 1991; 53: 241–258.

11. Grubbs RD, Beltz PA, Koss KL. Practical consideration for using mag-fura-2 to measure cytosolic free magnesium. Magnes Trace Elem 1991–1992; 10: 142–150.

12. Blatter LA. Estimation of intracellular free magnesium using ion-selective microelectrodes: evidence for a Na/mg exchange mechanism in skeletal muscle. Magnes Trace Elem 1991–1992; 10: 67–79.

13. Aikawa JK, Gordon GS, Rhoades EL. Magnesium metabolism in human beings: studies with Mg^{28}. J Appl Physiol 1960; 15: 503–507.

14. Schwartz R. ^{26}Mg as a probe in research on the role of magnesium in nutriture and metabolism. Fed Proc 1982; 41:2709–2713.

15. Schuette SA, Ziegler EE, Nelson SE, Janghorbani M. Feasibility of using the stable isotope ^{25}Mg to study Mg metabolism in infants. Ped Res 1990; 27: 36–40.

16. Gupta RK, Moore RD. ^{31}P NMR studies of the interaction of intracellular free Mg^{2+} in intact frog skeletal muscle. J Biol Chem 1980; 255: 3987–3993.

17. Wallach S. Effects of magnesium on skeletal metabolism. Magnes Trace Elem 1990; 9: 1–14.

18. Alfrey AC, Miller NL. Bone magnesium pools in uremia. J Clin Invest 1973; 52: 3019–3027.

19. Bloch AS, Shils ME, Table A20. In: Shils ME, Olson JA, Shike M, eds. Appendix of Modern Nutrition in Health and Disease. 8th ed. Philadelphia: Lea & Febiger, 1994.

20. Hardwick LL, Jones MR, Brautbar N, Lee DBN. Magnesium absorption: mechanisms and the influence of vitamin D, calcium and phosphate. J Nutr 1991; 121: 13–23.

21. Karbach U, Schmitt A, Hakan Saner F. Different mechanisms of magnesium and calcium transport across rat duodenum. Dig Dis Sci 1991; 36: 1611–1618.

22. Karbach U, Rummel W. Cellular and paracellular magnesium transport across the terminal ileum of the rat and its interaction with calcium transport. Gastroenterology 1990; 98: 985–992.

23. Karbach U. Cellular mediated and diffusive magnesium transport across the colon descendems of the rat. Gastroenterology 1989; 96: 1282–1299.

24. Roth P, Werner E. Intestinal absorption of magnesium in man. Int J Appl Rad Isot 1979; 30: 523–526.

25. Fine KD, Santa Ana CA, Porter JL, Fordtran JS. Intestinal absorption of magnesium from food and supplements. J Clin Invest 1991; 88: 396–402.

26. Milla PJ, Aggett PJ, Wolff OH, Harries T. Studies in primary hypomagnesemia: evidence for defective carrier-mediated intestinal transport of magnesium. Gut 1979; 20: 1028–1033.

27. Brannan PG, Vergne-Marini P, Pak CYC, Hull AR, Fordtran JS. Magnesium absorption in the human small intestine. Results in normal subjects, patients with chronic renal disease, and in patients with absorptive hypercalcemia. J Clin Invest 1976; 57: 1412–1418.

28. Spencer H, Lesniak M, Gatza LA, Osis D, Lender M. Magnesium absorption and metabolism in patients with chronic renal failure and in patients with normal renal function. Gastroenterology 1980; 79: 26–34.

29. Lakshmann FL, Rao RB, Kim WW. Magnesium intakes, balances and blood levels of adults consuming self-selected diets. Am J Clin Nutr 1984; 40(suppl 6): 1380–1389

30. Spencer H, Osis D. Studies of magnesium metabolism in man. Original data and review. Magnesium 1988; 7: 271–280.

31. Lewis NM, Marcus MSK, Behling AR, Greger JL. Calcium supplements and milk: effects on

acid-base balances and on retention of calcium, magnesium and phosphorus. Am J Clin Nutr 1989; 49: 527–533.

32. Hodgkinson A, Marshall DH, Nordin BEE. Vitamin D and magnesium absorption in man. Clin Sci 1979; 57: 121–123.

33. Wilz DR, Gray RW, Dominguez JH, Lemann J Jr. Plasma 1,25 (OH)$_2$ vitamin D concentrations and net intestinal calcium, phosphate and magnesium absorption in humans. Am J Clin Nutr 1979; 32: 2052–2060.

34. Norman DA, Fordtran JS, Brinkley LJ, et al. Jejunal and ileal adaptation to alterations in dietary calcium: changes in calcium and magnesium absorption and pathogenic role of parathyroid hormones and 1,25 dihydroxy vitamin D. J Clin Invest 1981; 67: 1599–1603.

35. Quamme GA, Dirks JH. The physiology of renal magnesium handling. In: Wyndhagen EE, ed. Handbook of Physiology, Section 8, Renal Physiology. Vol. II. New York: American Physiology Society, Oxford University Press, 1992.

36. Steele TH, Wen S-F, Evenson MA, Rieselbach RE. The contribution of the chronically diseased kidney to magnesium homeostasis in man. J Lab Clin Med 1968; 71: 455–463.

37. Shils ME. Experimental human magnesium deficiency. Medicine (Balto) 1969; 48: 61–65.

38. Shils ME. Magnesium. Chap 8. In: Shils ME, Olson JA, Shike M, eds.), Modern Nutrition in Health and Disease. Philadelphia, Lea & Febiger, 1994.

39. Devlin TM, ed. Textbook of Biochemistry with Clinical Correlations. 3d ed. New York: Wiley-Liss, 1992.

40. Vernon WB. The role of magnesium in nucleic acid and protein metabolism. Magnesium 1988; 7: 234–248.

41. Garfinkel D, Garfinkel L. Magnesium and regulation of carbohydrate metabolism at the molecular level. Magnesium 1988; 7: 249–261.

42. Knighton DR, Zheng J, Ten Eyck LF, et al. Crystal structure of the catalytic subunit of cyclic adenosine monophosphate-dependent protein kinase. Science 1991; 253: 407–414.

43. Birnbaumer LA. Transduction of receptor into modulation of effector activity by G proteins. The first 20 years or so. FASEB J 1990; 4: 3178–3188.

44. Seuwen K, Pouyssegur J. G protein-controlled transduction pathways and the regulation of cell proliferation. Adv Cancer Res. 1992; 58: 75–94.

45. White RE, Hartzell HC. Magnesium ions in cardiac function. Regulator of ion channels and second messengers. Biochem Pharmacol 1989; 38: 859–867.

46. Stanfield PR. Intracellular Mg^{2+} may act as a cofactor in ion channel function. Trends Neurosci 1988; 11: 475–477.

47. Agus ZS, Morad M. Modulation of cardiac ion channels by magnesium. Annu Rev Physiol 1991; 53: 299–307.

48. Matsuda H. Magnesium gating of the inwardly rectifying K^+ channel. Annu Rev Physiol. 1991; 53: 289–298.

49. Bunashev N, Schoepfer R, Monyer H, et al. Control by asparagine residues of calcium permeability and magnesium blockade in the NDMA receptor. Science 1992; 257: 1415–1419.

50. O'Rourke B, Backx PH, Marban E. Phosphorylation-independent modulation of L-type calcium channels by magnesium-nucleotide complex. Science 1992; 257: 245–248.

51. Flatman PW. Mechanisms of magnesium transport. Annu Rev Physiol 1991; 53: 256–271.

52. Hall SK, Fry CH, Buri A, McGuigan JAS. Use of ion sensitive microelectrodes to study intracellular free magnesium concentration and its regulation in mammalian cardiac muscle. Magnes Trace Elem 1991–1992; 10: 80–89.

53. Shaw AJ, Mughal MZ, Maresh MJA, Sibley CP. Sodium dependent magnesium transport across in situ perfused rat placenta. Am J Physiol 1991; 261: R369–372.

54. Quamme GA, Rabkin SW. Cystosolic free magnesium in cardiac myocytes: identification of a Mg^{2+} influx pathway. Biochem Biophys Res Commun 1990; 167: 1406–1412.

55. Preston RR. A magnesium current in *Paramecium*. Science 1990; 250: 285–288.

56. Grubbs RD, Maguire ME. Magnesium as a regulatory cation: criteria and evaluation. Magnesium 1987; 6:113–127.

57. Zaloga GP, Wilkens R, Tourville J, Wood D, Klyme DM. A simple method for determining physiologically active calcium and magnesium concentrations in critically ill patients. Crit Care Med 1987; 15: 813–816.

58. Rude RK, Stephen A, Nadler J. Determination of red blood cell intracellular free magnesium by nuclear magnetic resonance as an assessment of magnesium depletion. Magnes Trace Elem 1991–1992; 10: 117–121.

59. Yang XY, Hosseini JM, Ruddel ME, Elin RJ. Comparison of magnesium in human lymphocytes and mononuclear blood cells. Magnesium 1989; 8: 100–105.

60. Reinhart RA. Magnesium metabolism: a review with special reference to the relationship between intracellular content and serum levels. Arch Intern Med 1988; 148: 2415–2420.

61. Ryzen E. Magnesium homeostasis in critically ill patients. Magnesium 1989; 8: 201–212.

62. Ralston MA, Murnane MR, Kelley RE, et al. Magnesium content of serum, circulating mononuclear cells, skeletal muscle, and myocardium in congestive heart failure. Circulation 1989; 80:573–580.

63. Rasmussen HS, McNair P, Goransson L, et al. Magnesium deficiency in patients with ischemic heart disease with and without acute myocardial infarction uncovered by an intravenous loading test. Arch Intern Med 1988; 148: 329–332.

64. Ryzen E, Elbaum N, Singer FR, Rude R. Parenteral magnesium tolerance testing in the evaluation of magnesium deficiency. Magnesium 1985; 4: 137–147.

65. Department of Health and Human Services, U.S. Department of Agriculture. Nutrition monitoring in the U.S. An update report on nutrition monitoring. DHHS Publ 89-1255. Hyattsville, Md, Washington, DC: U.S. Government Printing Office, Sept 1989.

66. Pennington JAT, Wilson DB. Daily intakes of nine nutritional elements: analyzed vs calculated values. J Am Diet Assoc 1990; 90: 375–381.

67. Pennington JAT, Young B. Total diet study nutritional elements, 1982–1989. J Am Diet Assoc 1991; 91: 179–183.

68. Drenick EG, Hunt JF, Swendseid ME. Magnesium depletion during prolonged fasting of obese males. J Clin Endocrinol 1969; 29: 1341–1348.

69. Turnlund JR, Betschart AA, Liebman M, et al. Vitamin B_6 depletion followed by repletion with animal or plant-source diets and calcium and magnesium metabolism in young women. Am J Clin Nutr 1992; 56: 905–910.

70. Nieman DC, Butterworth DE, Nieman CN, et al. Comparison of six microcomputer dietary analysis systems with the USDA Nutrient Data Base for Standard Reference. J Am Diet Assoc 1992; 92: 48–56.

71. Shils ME. Magnesium. In: Shils ME, Young VR, eds.), Modern Nutrition in Health and Disease. 7th ed. Philadelphia: Lea Febiger, 1988.

72. National Research Council. Recommended Dietary Allowances. 10th ed., Washington, DC: National Academy Press, 1989.

73. Seelig MS. The requirements of magnesium by the normal adult. Summary and analyses of published data. Am J Clin Nutr 1964; 14: 342–390.

74. Lowenstein FW, Stanton MF. Serum magnesium levels in the United States: 1971–74. J Am Coll Nutr 1986; 5: 399–414.

75. Belanger LF, Van Erkel GA, Jakerow A. Behavior of the dermal mast cells in magnesium-deficient rats. Science 1957; 126: 29–30.

76. Kraeuter SL, Schwartz R. Blood and mast cell histamine levels in magnesium-deficient rats. J Nutr 1980; 110: 851–858.

77. Bunce GC, Saacke RG, Mullins J. The morphology and pathogenesis of magnesium deficiency-induced nephrocalcinosis. Exp Mol Pathol 1980; 33: 203–210.

78. Whang R, Oliver J, Welt LG, MacDowell M. Renal lesions and disturbance of renal function in rats with magnesium deficiency. Ann NY Acad Sci 1969; 162: 766–774.

79. Hurley LS, Cosens G, Theriault LL. Teratogenic effects of magnesium deficiency in rats. J Nutr 1976; 106: 1254–1260.

80. Cosens G, Diamond I, Theriault LL, Hurley LS. Magnesium deficiency anemia in the rat fetus. Pediatr Res 1977; 11: 758–764.

81. O'Dell BL. Magnesium requirement and its relation to other dietary constituents. Fed Proc 1960; 19: 648–654.

82. Schwartz R, Wang FL, Woodcock NA. Effect of varying dietary protein-magnesium ratios on nitrogen utilization and magnesium retention in growing rats. J Nutr 1969; 97: 185–193.

83. Alcock NW, Shils ME, Lieberman PH, Erlandson RA. Thymic changes in the magnesium-depleted rat. Cancer Res 1973; 33: 2196–2204.

84. Alcock NW, Shils ME. Serum immunoglobulin G in the magnesium depleted rat. Proc Soc Exp Biol Med 1974; 145: 855–858.

85. Alcock NW, Shils ME. Comparison of Magnesium deficiency in the rat and mouse. Proc Soc Exp Biol Med 1974; 146: 137–141.

86. Morris ER, O'Dell BL. Effect of magnesium deficiency in guinea pigs on kidney function and plasma ultrafilterable ions. Proc Soc Exp Biol Med 1969; 132: 105–110.

87. Bunce GE, Chiemchaisri V, Phillips PH. The mineral requirement of the dog. IV. Effect of certain dietary and physiologic factors upon the magnesium deficiency syndrome. J Nutr 1962; 76: 23–29.

88. O'Dell BL, Morris ER, Regan WO. Magnesium requirement of guinea pigs and rats. J Nutr 1960; 70: 103–110.

89. Shils ME. Magnesium, calcium, and parathyroid hormone interactions. Ann NY Acad Sci 1980; 355: 165–180.

90. Ashby JP, Heaton FW. Effect of magnesium deficiency and parathyroid hormone on cyclic AMP metabolism in renal cortex. J Endocrinol 1975; 67: 105–112.

91. Almquist HJ. Magnesium requirement of the chick. Proc Soc Exp Biol Med 1942; 49: 544.

92. Van Reen R, Pearson PB. Magnesium deficiency in the duck. J Nutr 1953; 51: 191–203.

93. Leroy J. Necessite' du magnesium pour la croissance de la Souris. CR Soc Biol 1926; 94: 431–433.

94. Miller ER, Urlrey DE, Zutaut CL, et al. Magnesium requirements of the baby pig. J Nutr 1965; 85: 13–20.

95. Rook JAF, Storry JE. Magnesium in the nutrition of farm animals. Nutr Abstr Rev 1962; 32: 1055–1077.

96. Heroux O, Peter D, Heggtveit A. Long term effect of suboptimal dietary magnesium and calcium contents of organs, on cold tolerance and on lifespan, and its pathological consequences in rats. J Nutr 1977; 107: 1640–1652.

97. Hamuro Y, Shino A, Suzuoki Z. Acute induction of soft tissue calcification with transient hyperphophatemia in the KK mouse by modification in dietary contents of calcium, phosphorus and magnesium. J Nutr 1970; 100: 404–412.

98. O'Dell BL, Moroni RI, Regan WO. Interaction of dietary fluoride and magnesium in guinea pigs. J Nutr 1973; 103: 841–850.

99. Heggtveit HA. Myopathy in experimental magnesium deficiency. Ann NY Acad Sci 1969; 162: 758–765.

100. Blaxter KL, Rook JAF, MacDonald AM. Experimental magnesium deficiency in calves. I. Clinical and pathological observations. J Comp Pathol Therap 1954; 64: 157–175.

101. Dunn MJ. Magnesium depletion in the Rhesus monkey: induction of magnesium-dependent hypocalcemia. Clin Sci 1971; 41: 333–344.

102. Freitag JJ, Martin KJ, Conrades NB, et al. Evidence for skeletal resistance to parathyroid hormone in magnesium deficiency. Studies in isolated perfused bone. J Clin Invest 1979; 64: 1238–1244.

103. Elin RJ, Alling DW. Survival of normal and magnesium-deficient erythrocytes in rats: effect of magnesium deficient diet vs splenectomy. J Lab Clin Med 1978; 91: 666–672.

104. Morris ER, O'Dell BL. Relationship of excess calcium and phosphorus to magnesium requirement and toxicity in guinea pigs. J Nutr 1963; 81: 175–181.

105. Subcommittee on Laboratory Animal Nutrition, National Academy of Science. Nutrient requirements of laboratory animals. 3d rev ed. Washington, DC: National Academy of Science, 1978.

106. Bunce GE, Jenkins J, Phillips PH. The mineral requirement of the dog. III. The magnesium requirement. J Nutr 1962; 76: 17–22.

107. Grace ND, O'Dell BL. Interrelationship of dietary magnesium and potassium in the guinea pig. J Nutr 1970; 100: 37–44.

108. Gitelman HJ, Kukolj S, Welt G. The influence of the parathyroid glands on the hypercalcemia of experimental magnesium deficiency in the rat. J Clin Invest 1968; 47: 118–126.

109. Goldman RH, Kleiger RE, Schweizer E, Harrison DC. The effect on myocardial ^{3}H-digoxin of magnesium deficiency. Proc Soc Exp Biol Med 1971; 136: 747–749.

110. Loveless BN, Heaton FW. Changes in alkaline phosphatase and inorganic pyrophatase activities in rat tissues during magnesium deficiency. The importance of controlling feeding pattern. Br J Nutr 1976; 36: 487–495.

111. Mirra JM, Alcock NW, Shils ME, Tanenbaum P. Effects of calcium and magnesium deficiencies on rat skeletal development and parathyroid gland area. Magnesium 1982; 1: 16–33.

112. Guenther T. Biochemistry and pathobiochemistry of magnesium. Artery 1981; 9: 167–181.

113. Cronin RE, Ferguson ER, Shannon WA Jr, Knochel JP. Skeletal muscle injury after magnesium depletion in the dog. Am J Physiol 1982; 243: F113–F120.

114. Heaton FW. The parathyroid glands and magnesium metabolism in the rat. Z Clin Sci 1965 : 543–553.

115. Yamamoto T, Kabata H, Yagi R, et al. Primary hypomagnesemia with secondary hypocalcemia. Report of a case and review of the world literature. Magnesium 1985; 4: 153–164.

116. Whang R, Whang DD. Update: mechanism by which magnesium modulates intracellular potassium. J Am Coll Nutr 1990; 9: 84–85.

117. Anast CS, Mohs JM, Kaplan SL, Burns TW. Evidence for parathyroid failure in magnesium deficiency. Science 1972; 177: 606–608.

118. Anast CS, Winnacker JL, Forte LR, Burns TW. Impaired release of parathyroid hormone in magnesium deficiency. J Clin Endocrinol Metab 1976; 42: 707–717.

119. Rude RK, Oldham SB, Sharp CF Jr, Singer FR. Parathyroid hormone secretion in magnesium deficiency. J Clin Endocrinol Metab 1978; 47: 800–806.

120. Johannsesson AJ, Raisz LG. Effects of low medium magnesium concentration on bone resorption in response to parathyroid hormone and 1:25-dihydroxyvitamin D in organ culture. Endocrinology 1983; 113: 2294–2298.

121. Garabedian M, Tanaka Y, Holick MF, DeLuca HF. Response of intestinal calcium transport and bone calcium mobilization to 1α, 25-dihyroxyvitamin D_3 in thyroparathyroidectomized rats. Endocrinology 1974; 94: 1022–1027.

122. Carpenter TO, Carnes DL Jr, Anast CS. Effect of magnesium depletion on metabolism of 25-hydroxyvitamin D in rats. Am J Physiol 1987; 253: E106–E113.

123. Lifshitz F, Harrison HC, Bull EC, Harrison HE. Citrate metabolism and the mechanism of renal calcification induced by magnesium depletion. Metabolism 1967; 16: 345–357.

124. Simpson DP. Citrate excretion: a window on renal metabolism. Am J Physiol 1983; 244: F233–F234.

125. Rudman D, Dedonis JL, Fountain MT, et al. Hypocitraturia in patients with gastrointestinal malabsorption. N Engl J Med 1980; 303: 657–661.

126. Geuex E, Mazur A, Cardot P, Rayssiguier Y. Magnesium deficiency affects plasma lipoproteins in rats. J Nutr 1991; 121: 1222–1227.

127. Nigam S, Averdunk R, Gunther T. Alterations of prostanoid metabolism in rats with magnesium deficiency. Prostaglandins, Leukotrienes and Med 1986; 23:1–10.

128. Soma M, Cunnane SC, Horrobin DF, et al. Effects of low magnesium diet on the vascular prostaglandin and fatty acid metabolism in rats. Prostaglandins 1988; 36: 431–441.

129. Whang R, Oei T, Aikawa JK, et al. Predictors of clinical hypomagnesemia, hypokalemia, hypophosphatemia, hyponatremia, and hypocalcemia. Arch Intern Med 1984; 144: 1794–1796.

130. Ryzen E, Wagers PW, Singer FR, Rude RK. Magnesium deficiency in a medical ICU population. Crit Care Med 1985; 13: 19–21.

131. Chernow B, Bamberger S, Stoiko M, et al. Hypomagnesemia in patients in post operative intensive care. Chest 1987; 95: 391–397.

132. Fiaccadori E, del Canale S, Coffrini E, et al. Muscle and serum magnesium in pulmonary intensive care patients. Crit Care Med 1988; 16: 751–760.

133. Flink EB. Magnesium deficiency in alcoholism. Alcoholism 1986; 10: 590–594.

134. Butler AM. Diabetic coma. N Engl J Med 1950; 234: 648–656.

135. Booth CC, Barbouris N, Hanna S, McIntyre I. Incidence of hypomagnesaemia in intestinal malabsorption. Br Med J 1963; 2: 141–144.

136. Motil KJ, Altschuler SI, Grand RJ. Mineral balance during nutritional supplementation in adolescents with Crohn's disease and growth failure. J Pediatr 1985; 107: 473–479.

137. Rosen EU, Campbell G, Moosa GM. Hypomagnesemia and magnesium therapy in protein-calorie malnutrition. J Pediatr 1970; 77: 709–714.

138. Nichols BL, Alvarado J, Hazelwood CF, Viteri F. Magnesium supplementation in protein-calorie malnutrition. Am J Clin Nutr 1978; 31: 176–188.

139. Evans RA, Carter JN, George CRP, et al. The congenital "magnesium losing kidney." Q J Med N.S. 1981; 50: 39–52.

140. Jones CT, Sellwood RA, Evanson JM. Symptomatic hypomagnesaemia after parathyroidectomy. Br Med J 1973; 3: 391–392.

141. Marier JR. Quantitative factors regarding magnesium status in the modern-day world. Magnesium 1982; 1: 3–15.

142. Elwood PC, Sweetman PM, Beasley WH, et al. Magnesium and calcium in the myocardium: cause of death and area differences. Lancet 1980; 2: 720–722.

143. Hammer DI, Hayden S. Water hardness and cardiovascular mortality. An idea that has served its purpose. JAMA 1980; 243: 2399–2400.

144. Leoni V, Fabiani L, Tichiarelli L. Water hardness and cardiovascular mortality rate in Abruzzo. Arch Environ Health 1985; 40: 274–278.

145. Teo KK, Yusuf S, Collins R, et al. Effects of intravenous magnesium in suspected acute myocardial infarction: overview of randomized trial. Br Med J 1991; 303: 1499–1503.

146. Lau J, Antman EM, Jimenez-Silva J, Chalmers TC. Cumulative meta-analysis of therapeutic trials for myocardial infarction. N Engl J Med 1992; 327: 248–254.

147. Woods KL, Fletcher S, Roffe C, Haider Y. Intravenous magnesium sulphate in suspected acute myocardial infarction: results of the second Leicester Intravenous Magnesium Intervention Trial (LIMIT-2). Lancet 1992; 339: 1553–1558.

148. Collins R, Peto R, Flather M, et al. for ISIS-4 Collaborative Group. A randomized factorial trial assessing early oral captopril, oral mononitrate, and intravenous magnesium sulphate in 58,050 patients with suspected acute myocardial infarction. Lancet 1995; 345: 669–685.

149. Rayssiguier Y, Thomasset M, Garel J-M, Barlet J-P. Plasma parathyroid hormone levels and intestinal calcium binding protein in magnesium deficient rats. Horm Metab Res 1982; 14: 379–382.

150. Anast CS, Forte LF. Parathyroid function and magnesium depletion in the rat. Endocrinology 1983; 113: 184–189.

151. Mahaffey DD, Cooper CW, Ramp WK, Ontjes DA. Magnesium promotes both parathyroid hormone production and adenosine 3'5' monophosphate production in rat parathyroid tissues and reverses the inhibitory effects of calcium on adenylate cyclase. Endocrinology 1982; 110: 487–495.

152. Oldham SB, Rude RK, Molloy CT, Lipsor LG. The effects of magnesium on calcium inhibition of parathyroid adenylate cyclase. Endocrinology 1984; 115: 1183–1890.

153. Cunningham FG, Lindheimer MD. Hypertension in pregnancy. N Engl J Med 1992; 326: 927–932.

154. Cholst IN, Steinberg SF, Tropper PJ, et al. The influence of hypermagnesemia on serum calcium and parathyroid hormone levels in human subjects. N Engl J Med 1984; 310: 1221–1225.

155. Eisenbud E, LoBue CL. Hypocalcemia after therapeutic use of magnesium sulfate. Arch Intern Med 1976; 136: 688–691.

156. Cruikshank DP, Pitkin RM, Reynolds WA, et al. Effects of magnesium sulfate treatment on perinatal calcium metabolism I. Maternal and fetal responses. Am J Obstet Gynecol 1979; 134: 243–249.

157. Donovan EF, Tsang RC, Steichen JJ, et al. Neonatal hypermagnesemia: effect on parathyroid hormone and calcium homeostasis. J Pediatr 1980; 96: 305–310.

158. Littledike ET, Arnaud CD. The influence of plasma magnesium concentrations on calcitonin secretion in the pig. Proc Soc Exp Biol Med 1971; 136: 1000–1006.

159. Wians FH Jr, Strickland DM, Hankins GDV, Snyder RS. The effect of hypermagnesemia on serum levels of osteocalcin in an animal model. Magnes Trace Elem 1990; 9: 28–35.

160. Altura BM, Altura BT. Magnesium ions and contraction of vascular smooth muscles: relationship to some vascular diseases. Fed Proc 1981; 40: 2672–2679.

161. Levine BS, Coburn JW. Editorial. Magnesium, the mimic/antagonist of calcium. N Engl J Med 1984; 310: 1253–1254.

162. Rude R, Manoogian C, Ehrlich P, et al. Mechanisms of blood pressure regulation by magnesium in man. Magnesium 1989; 8: 266–273.

163. O'Brien WF, Williams MC, Benoit R, Sawai SK, Knuppel RA. Effect of magnesium sulfate infusion on systemic and renal prostacyclin production. Prostaglandins 1990; 40: 529–538.

164. Mordes JP, Wacker EC. Excess magnesium. Pharmacol Rev 1978; 29: 274–300.

6
Potassium in Nutrition

LINDA N. PETERSON
University of Ottawa, Ottawa, Ontario, Canada

I. INTRODUCTION

Potassium is classified as a macro essential element. It is normally plentiful in the diet, and mechanisms exist in the body to regulate its distribution and concentration in extracellular fluid. However, derangements in potassium metabolism may occur which have major physiologic consequences. Deficiency or excess of most essential minerals will gradually disrupt physiologic functions and may cause chronic illness. In contrast, small deviations in potassium concentration, specifically in the extracellular fluid compartment, can cause sudden death due to cardiac dysfunction. For this reason a thorough understanding of the factors affecting potassium balance, i.e., intake, distribution, and excretion, is warranted. This is particularly true for those interested in nutrition, in view of the lessons that have been learned about the dangers of bulimia, anorexia nervosa, and fad dieting, as well as the abuse of diuretics and laxatives (1). In the pages which follow, the reader will learn about the distribution of potassium in the body and the molecular mechanisms which determine and regulate this process. Later, the mechanism and regulation of potassium excretion by the kidney, one of the most important physiologic systems in potassium metabolism, will be analyzed. The physiologic importance of potassium, and the causes and effects of abnormal potassium balance, will be examined. Lastly, some insight into active areas of research will be described. Since it is not possible to address the above topics in detail, the reader will be referred to timely reviews and recent or classic research papers.

II. CHEMISTRY AND ANALYSIS

A. Chemistry

Potassium was discovered in 1807 by Sir Humphry Davy, who isolated the metal from "pot ash" (potash) (2,3). Potash was the term given to the residue remaining from burned plant material, such as wood ashes, hence the name *potassium*. However, the chemical symbol, K, is taken from the Latin name *kalium*, which means "alkali" (2). Potassium metal is not found free in nature and must be obtained from naturally occurring salts. These salts are found in plant and animal tissues, fertile soils, and rich deposits in certain locations in the world. Potassium constitutes about 2.4% of the earth's crust, making it the seventh most abundant element. It has an atomic weight of 39 and an atomic number of 19. Because elemental potassium has a low ionization potential, it readily loses one electron and reacts violently when placed in contact with water (potassium liberates hydrogen gas, which ignites). Obviously, the metal is not compatible with living systems, but the potassium cation is essential to plant and animal life. Traditionally, concentrations of such ions, which serve as electrolytes, were reported in units of charge, i.e., equivalents. In this chapter potassium concentrations will usually be reported in millimoles per liter, mmol/L or mM. However, milliequivalents per liter, mEq/L, is equally correct. When discussing dietary sources and requirements, the weight of potassium in various foods will be used, following the common practice in nutrition. The following conversion factors for potassium may prove useful: Each mmol weighs 39 mg; and the reciprocal conversion, each milligram of potassium contains 0.026 mmol.

The greatest commercial use of potassium is in the production of fertilizers (2). It is also used in fireworks (it emits a violet light when burned), and matches among other things (3). Readers may be interested to know that potassium superoxide is used in the self-contained breathing apparatus utilized by firefighters (4). This substance reacts with water from exhaled breath to release oxygen gas. Potassium hydroxide which is formed reacts with carbon dioxide and traps it as potassium bicarbonate. The term *potassium* used in subsequent portions of this chapter refers to the potassium ion.

B. Analysis

Potassium, like sodium, can be measured in body fluids by flame photometry, ion-selective electrodes, and atomic absorption spectrophotometry (2,3,5). Total body potassium content can be estimated by measuring the amount of naturally occurring isotopes (e.g., ^{40}K) by whole-body counting (6), or the distribution of administered radioactive isotope (i.e., ^{45}K) (7). Based on these measurements, total body potassium is estimated to be about 55 mmol/kg body weight. Total-body potassium content is of little use in the evaluation of patients with abnormal potassium metabolism, so the measurement is seldom, if ever, performed. Rather, accurate measurement of extracellular potassium concentration is of prime importance and is constantly monitored in high-risk situations. In research studies, radioactive rubidium (^{86}Rb) is frequently used as an analog to track the movement of potassium across cell membranes (8).

III. INTAKE AND REQUIREMENTS

North American diets supply about 60–150 mmol of potassium, primarily in the form of vegetables, meats, and fruits (6,9,10). Tables listing the content of macroelements in common foods are of value when making specific dietary recommendations for patients who must ingest or avoid potassium (11). The minimum daily requirement for adults is approximately 0.3–0.4 mmol/kg body weight (6,10). This is the amount an individual could consume without developing symptoms of potassium deficiency. The normal dietary potassium intake in adults is 1–2 mmol/kg/day, which is equivalent to 2–4 g of potassium (10). Since potassium is present in so many foods ingested in a normal diet, only inadequate food intake, e.g., in anorexia, bulimia, and alcoholism, will cause significant potassium depletion. The poor and the elderly tend to have low potassium intake due to less-than-ideal diets. Net potassium intake may also be decreased by the ingestion of clay soil, a behavior which impairs intestinal potassium absorption. This is more common in pediatric populations. Even in the face of reduced potassium intake, the possible contribution of increased loss should be evaluated.

Recommended daily intake for human infants is 8 mmol (320 mg)/day (12). This amount is supplied by breast milk ([K] = 13 mM) or cow's milk (35 mM), since infants consume about 1 L/day. In premature neonates, potassium is given in proportion to caloric intake, i.e., 2.4 mmol of potassium/100 kcal (13). The amount of potassium administered to patients receiving total parenteral nutrition (TPN) is 2–3 mmol/kg daily (10).

As long as potassium intake increases gradually over a period of days, balance can be maintained even at a potassium intake almost 10 times greater than normal. Prior to the Potato Famine of 1848, most of the caloric intake of the Irish population had been sustained by a diet consisting almost exclusively of potatoes, a high-potassium food (14). This type of diet contained between 20 and 40 g of potassium. In contrast, the single ingestion of 25 g of potassium (about 0.6 mol) by a person who has been consuming a normal diet (2–4 g of potassium daily), is associated with life-threatening acute toxicity (10). Adaptation to a high-potassium diet as seen in the Irish population was due to an enhanced capacity of the kidney to excrete potassium, thereby allowing them to tolerate otherwise lethal amounts of this ion. As might be expected, rapid intravenous administration of much smaller amounts of potassium can also be fatal. The oral route of potassium ingestion results in lower plasma concentrations because insulin release is stimulated by small increases in portal blood potassium concentration. Insulin increases the rate of cellular potassium uptake, thereby blunting the increase in plasma potassium concentration (see Sec. VI). Also, the rate of intestinal potassium absorption is slower, thereby gradually increasing plasma potassium concentration.

IV. METABOLISM

A. Distribution and Concentration in Body Fluids

The relation among intake, distribution, and excretion of potassium is illustrated in Figure 1. Potassium is the most abundant cation in the body, with total body potassium stores in adults amounting to 3000–4000 mmol. In contrast to sodium, more than 98% is found in intracellular fluid. It is clear that the small extracellular fluid (ECF) compartment is in intimate contact with cells containing potentially lethal amounts of potassium. Logically, cell death from any cause will lead to the introduction of potassium into the ECF. The concentration of potassium in ECF is about 4 mM (see Sec. VI). (Note: the terms *extracellular* and *plasma* will be used interchangeably when referring to potassium concentration.) The concentration of freely exchangeable potassium in all cell types is not known and probably varies. The approximate concentration of potassium in most cells is 150 mM. In

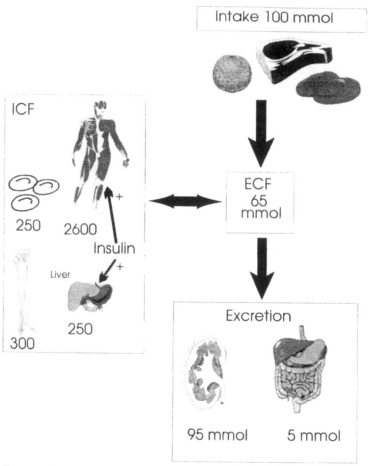

FIGURE 1 Quantitative relation among intake, distribution, and excretion of potassium in humans. Quantitative amounts (mmol) of potassium in red blood cells, bone, liver, and muscle. Uptake into liver and muscle is stimulated (+) by insulin. Total potassium in extracellular fluid (ECF) can be affected by intake, distribution between ECF and intracellular fluid (ICF), and excretion by the kidneys and large intestine.

later discussion of the effects of potassium on the electrical properties of cell membranes, it will be assumed that all potassium in intracellular fluid is freely diffusable.

Muscle represents the largest tissue storage site, containing about 75% of intracellular potassium. Potassium uptake into skeletal muscle is affected by hormones (see Sec. VI.B) and participates in the regulation of plasma potassium concentration. A small amount of potassium can be found in the liver. This fraction is readily exchangeable and is affected by hormones (see Sec. VI.B). A similar amount of potassium is located in red blood cells. Although potassium in red blood cells does not normally participate in the regulation of plasma potassium concentration, excessive hemolysis can create a life-threatening increase in ECF potassium concentration. The reporting of falsely elevated values of plasma potassium concentration can occur due to hemolysis either while the blood sample is taken, or after it has been removed from the patient (15). The amount of potassium in bones is similar to that in liver and red blood cells, but it is not readily exchangeable.

B. Absorption

Virtually all of the potassium ingested in a meal is absorbed (16). It is absorbed primarily in the small intestine as a consequence of bulk fluid absorption (17). The distal colon is also capable of active absorption of potassium by a process which appears to be mediated by an apical H,K-ATPase (16) (see Sec. V.B). Potassium efflux across the basolateral membrane occurs through conductance channels. Potassium absorption in the small intestine and colon is unregulated.

C. Excretion

1. Renal

Normal individuals ingesting 100 mmol of K each day remain in balance by excreting 95% of the ingested K in the urine, and the remaining 5% in the stool (18). Within a 24-h period, the kidneys will eliminate the daily dietary load of potassium; however, it should be mentioned that extrarenal mechanisms exist to buffer transient changes in plasma K (see Sec. VI.B). To the extent that the kidney fails to excrete the daily intake, demands will be placed on the intestinal tract and intracellular buffering to offset increases in plasma potassium concentration. Extrarenal tissues have a limited capacity to store potassium. On the other hand, the kidney can be the cause of accelerated losses of potassium if excretion is inappropriately stimulated. This is often the cause of potassium deficiency.

2. Gastrointestinal

The gastrointestinal tract eliminates only 5–10% of the daily intake of potassium (18). Most of the excreted potassium is derived from epithelial cell secretion in the large intestine. These colonic cells respond to many of the factors that stimulate potassium secreting cells of the kidney (6,19). In chronic renal failure, the colon may excrete more than 30% of the dietary burden (6). Because of the capacity of the colon to secrete potassium, it can be useful in the elimination of excess potassium in patients, yet it should not be forgotten that abnormal stimulation of colonic secretion can be a source of significant potassium loss. The concentration of potassium in lower GI secretions can exceed 80 mM (19). Diarrhea due to a multitude of etiologies, including cholera, and laxative and enema abuse (bulimia), can be associated with excessive stool potassium losses and potassium deficiency. Potassium losses associated with diarrhea are due to stimulation of potassium secretion in the proximal and distal portions of the colon (16,20). Potassium secretion occurs in parallel with chloride secretion. Potassium and chloride ions enter the cell across the basolateral membrane via a bumetanide-sensitive Na-2Cl-K cotransporter and exit across the apical membrane through potassium and chloride conductance channels. Usually potassium and chloride secretions occur at low rates unless specifically stimulated.

Potassium concentration in gastric fluid is usually less than 10 mM. This only partially explains the potassium deficiency in patients that results from vomiting. Rather, increased renal losses and increased cellular uptake largely account for potassium depletion and reduced plasma potassium concentration in this setting (6,15,19).

V. MOLECULAR MECHANISMS UNDERLYING POTASSIUM MOVEMENT THROUGH CELL MEMBRANES

The striking compartmentalization of potassium in intracellular fluid and of sodium in extracellular fluid is a condition established and maintained by active transport across cell plasma membranes. It should be emphasized that in the absence of active transport pumps, cotransporters, and conductance channels, directional, selective, rapid, and regulated movement of potassium or sodium through cell membranes would be impossible. The major molecular pathways of potassium permeation through plasma membranes are Na,K-ATPase, H,K-ATPase, Na-2Cl-K cotransporter, and K conductance channels. There is evidence for the existence of a K-Cl cotransporter in principal cells of the cortical collecting duct (CCD) (21), but this mechanism has not been the subject of intensive investigation.

A. Na,K-ATPase

The membrane-bound Na,K-ATPase pump, expressed in virtually every cell in the body, transports potassium ions into cells while simultaneously extruding sodium ions (Fig. 2)

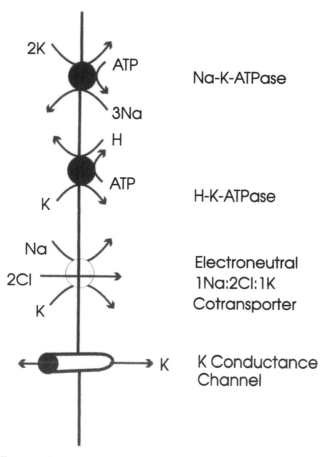

FIGURE 2 Molecular mechanisms of potassium permeability. The major molecular pathways of permeation through biological membranes are the two primary active transport pumps, i.e., sodium-potassium-ATPase (Na,K-ATPase) and hydrogen-potassium-ATPase (H,K-ATPase), and the electro-neutral sodium-potassium-chloride cotransporter (Na-2Cl-K) and potassium (K) conductance channels. The Na,K-ATPase transports 3 Na out of the cell and 2 K ions into the cell. The H,K-ATPase transports 1 H ion out of the cell and 1 K ion into the cell. The Na-2Cl-K cotransporter normally moves 1 Na, 2 Cl and 1 K ion into the cell.

driven by the simultaneous breakdown of ATP. Both ions are transported against their electrochemical concentration gradients. Since the protein complex has intrinsic ATPase activity, it is called a primary active transporter. It is well known that potassium rapidly exits from red cells after blood has been removed from the body and refrigerated. The plasma potassium concentration can rise to a lethal level in this stored blood. However, when the blood is rewarmed, potassium is quickly transported into the cells and a normal extracellular concentration is reestablished. The pump is electrogenic, since only two positive ions are pumped into the cell for every three that are extruded. Accelerated operation of the pump increases the net negative charge inside the cell (see Sec. VIII.A). The energy in ATP is transformed into ion gradients for sodium and potassium, which subsequently provides the energy for the operation of secondary active Na- and K-dependent cotransporters, and Na- and K-selective conductance channels. The molecular structure and kinetics of pump activity are described in the chapter on sodium and chloride. Recently attempts have been made to image the pump in order to understand better how the ions traverse the membrane within the molecular structure (22). It is possible that the active transport pumps have a structural domain very similar to the conductance channels, i.e., a pore. Investigators are attempting to understand the mechanism(s) by which factors (hormones) stimulate or inhibit the active transport pump (i.e., the signal transduction systems and the role of phosphorylation/dephosphorylation cycles) (23).

B. H,K-ATPase

The H,K-ATPase protein complex is also membrane bound and a primary active transporter. It moves hydrogen ions out of the cell and potassium ions into the cell against their electrochemical concentration gradients. The Na,K-ATPase pump is responsible for proton secretion by parietal cells in the gastric mucosa (stomach). Although there is no net transport of potassium across the parietal cell, potassium must participate in several transport steps across the apical and basolateral membranes in order for HCl secretion to occur (24). Potassium enters the cell via the H,K-ATPase in the apical membrane and the Na,K-ATPase in the basolateral membrane. It exits from the cell through potassium conductance channels in both apical and basolateral membranes. If the potassium conductance channels in the apical membrane are blocked, e.g., by barium, potassium will be reabsorbed by the parietal cell. On the other hand, if potassium conductance channels are blocked in the basolateral membrane, then potassium will be secreted into the stomach.

It does not appear that coupling of K to the desired movement of protons confers any advantage that is obvious to this author. For example, HCl secretion could be accomplished by a H-ATPase with chloride movement through a channel. The coupling of potassium to proton movement is probably the consequence of the common origin which the H,K-ATPase pump shares with the Na,K-ATPase.

In order for H and Cl secretion to occur, potassium conductance channels must be present and open. It is not clear how the potassium conductance channels interact with the H,K-ATPase pump, but the potassium conductance of the apical membrane is low until the pump inserts. Perhaps potassium and chloride channels interact with another channel protein similar to the cystic fibrosis transmembrane regulator (CFTR) (25) in order to activate and regulate ion movement. Recent work suggests that the chloride channel which operates during proton secretion may be an integral part of H,K-ATPase (26).

The gastric form of the H,K-ATPase is expressed in intercalated cells of the cortical collecting duct of the kidney (27). It mediates reabsorption of potassium and bicarbonate.

The activity of this pump increases in potassium-depleted animals, suggesting that it plays a role in potassium conservation rather than in acid–base homeostasis (27,28). In these kidney cells, the H,K-ATPase primarily transports potassium, whereas in the gastric parietal cell, the same pump transports hydrogen ions primarily.

C. Na-2Cl-K Cotransporters

This protein simultaneously binds and translocates 1Na:2Cl:1K to the cell interior, driven by the inwardly directed sodium concentration gradient established by the Na,K-ATPase pump. Since the cotransporter does not breakdown ATP, it is called a secondary active transporter. It was first fully characterized by Geck in Ehrlich ascites cells (29), and two forms have recently been cloned from mammalian cells (30,31). Both cloned proteins are composed of a single polypeptide chain with ion-binding regions and multiple phosphorylation sites (32,33). In the thick ascending limb of the loop of Henle, a sodium chloride-reabsorbing epithelium, the transporter is located in the apical membrane. In secretory epithelia, e.g., the small intestine, and many other sites, e.g., red blood cells, inner medullary collecting duct, and certain regions of the brain, a different gene product is present and is usually located in the basolateral membrane (31). Both forms of the cotransporter are inhibited by the loop diuretic, furosemide, and its more potent analogs, e.g., bumetanide. The diuretics appear to bind to the second chloride site on the molecule (33,34). The affinity of the cotransporter for Na and K is very high, the Michaelis-Menton constants (K_m values) being less than 2 mM, while the affinity for chloride is low, the K_m being about 50 mM (35). In the thick ascending limb, luminal chloride concentration determines the velocity of transport. If chloride delivery increases, the rate of transport increases. In the thick ascending limb, little or no potassium is reabsorbed directly by the cotransporter. However, coupling of potassium to the cotransporter doubles the efficiency of NaCl reabsorption. The thick ascending limb cotransporter has been shown to operate in a potassium-independent mode under certain conditions (8). This nephron segment also produces message for splice variants of the cotransporter (36). It is possible that one of these messenger RNAs codes for the K-independent form of the bumetanide-sensitive cotransporter.

There is over 70% homology between the bumetanide-sensitive cotransporters and another 1Na:1Cl cotransporter that is inhibited by another type of diuretic, thiazide. It is now recognized that the bumetanide-sensitive and the thiazide-sensitive cotransporters belong to a family of related proteins referred to as the electroneutral NaCl cotransporters (32).

D. K Conductance Channels

Ion conductance channels allow rapid, selective movement through the membrane driven by the electrochemical gradient (37). Presently, six types of potassium channels have been identified and are listed in Table 1 (38). These channels are highly selective for potassium over other cations and are inhibited by barium. Also, channel conductance is increased by

TABLE 1 Classes of Potassium Channels

1.	Voltage gated	4.	Nucleotide gated
2.	Calcium activated	5.	Stretch activated
3.	Ligand gated	6.	Chemoreceptive

elevating ECF potassium concentration and reduced by decreasing ECF potassium concentration (37). The channels differ in their gating properties and conductance to potassium (38). Structural variations underlie these functional differences. The voltage-regulated and calcium-activated channels have six transmembrane regions and are open when membrane potential is more positive than -30 mV (38). In contrast, the ATP-gated (K_{ATP}) and ligand-gated potassium channels have only two transmembrane regions and conduct potassium inwardly when the interior of the cell is hyperpolarized (inward rectification).

All potassium channels consist of, at least, an α-polypeptide chain which contains the ion pore region, and they may have several phosphorylation sites as well as ligand-binding sites. An inward rectifying potassium channel was recently isolated and cloned from rat outer medulla (ROMK1), and its putative structure is illustrated in Figure 3 (39). ROMK1 is the K_{ATP} channel which operates with the bumetanide-sensitive cotransporter in the thick ascending limb in the reabsorption of NaCl, and is the K channel responsible for potassium secretion across the apical membrane of principal cells in the cortical collecting duct (39); see Sec. VI.C.1.

Typically, α-subunits alone are able to conduct potassium when expressed in vitro, but the channels do not exhibit the gating properties characteristic of their native state.

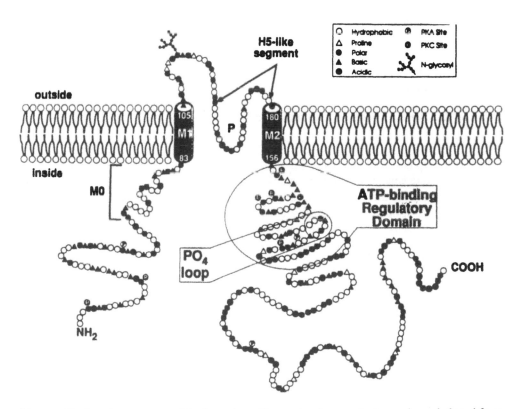

FIGURE 3 Putative structure of the inward-rectifyng potassium conductance channel cloned from the outer medulla of the kidney (ROMK1). This is a representative ATP-gated potassium conductance channel. The figure illustrates the typical two transmembrane spaning domains, the ATP-binding region, the glycosylation site, and phosphorylation sites for protein kinase A and C (PKA, PKC). (From Ref. 39, with permission.)

Current opinion favors the view that these channels have subunit structures similar to that of sodium channels (40). Recently, the voltage gating property of the potassium channel has been attributed to a β-subunit (41), and the sulfonylurea-binding site of the ligand-gated K channel regulating insulin release has been localized to a β-subunit (42).

VI. DEFENSE OF EXTRACELLULAR POTASSIUM CONCENTRATION

Following the ingestion of K, only half is excreted by the kidneys over the first 4–6 h. The remaining 50% is taken up by peripheral tissues. For example, if all the potassium contained in two 10-oz bags of potato chips (70 mmol) was ingested and distributed exclusively in the extracellular compartment, plasma potassium concentration would double. This increase in plasma potassium concentration would cause life-threatening electrical disturbances in the heart.

A. Definition of Terms

The range of normal plasma potassium concentration, i.e., normokalemia, is defined as 3.5–5.0 mM (6,15). Hypokalemia is defined as a reduction in plasma potassium below 3.5 mM. *Hypokalemia* applies only to a decrease in extracellular potassium concentration, while the term *potassium depletion* refers to a reduction in cellular potassium stores (6). Potassium depletion is not always accompanied by hypokalemia, if cellular uptake is impaired simultaneously. Hyperkalemia is defined as a plasma potassium concentration greater than 5.0 mM. Both hypo- and hyperkalemia are associated with potentially fatal cardiac arrhythmias.

B. Regulation of Tissue Distribution

1. Insulin

A feedback loop has been identified that establishes a role for insulin in the regulation of plasma potassium concentration. Increases in plasma potassium of only a few tenths of a millimole are sufficient to stimulate insulin release into the portal circulation (43,44). Insulin stimulates potassium uptake by liver and skeletal muscle. The activated insulin receptor increases its Na,K-ATPase activity, driving potassium uptake via the pump. Additional potassium may enter the cell through potassium conductance channels due to hyperpolarization.

2. Catecholamines

Muscular activity causes an increased potassium concentration in extracellular fluid due to potassium efflux during repolarization. The consequent increase in the conductance of potassium channels is beneficial in accelerating muscle repolarization, and in shortening the refractory period. The increase in extracellular potassium concentration also mediates vasodilatation, which increases muscle blood flow. Usually, exercise is associated with increased sympathetic nervous system activity and release of adrenal medullary catecholamines. Catecholamines blunt the rise in plasma potassium concentration associated with vigorous exercise (45). Activation of β_2 receptors increases cyclic AMP, which is associated with stimulation of Na,K-ATPase activity. Increased pump activity as well as membrane hyperpolarization accounts for accelerated potassium uptake. This is a normal homeostatic mechanism to maintain plasma potassium concentration (43,44).

C. Regulation of Renal Excretion

Since the kidney is the major route of potassium elimination from the body, a disturbance in renal potassium handling can be the cause of excess potassium loss or retention. Depending on the magnitude of the potassium imbalance and the status of nonrenal tissue to buffer the change, the ability to regulate plasma potassium concentration may be severely impaired.

1. Potassium Transport in the Nephron

The fate of potassium as it traverses the nephron is illustrated in Figure 4. Only the highlights of transport can be presented, and the reader is directed to more detailed sources for more in-depth coverage (21,46–48). The amount of nonfiltrable potassium bound to albumin can be ignored. If the glomerular filtration rate (GFR) is 180 L per day for a 70-kg man, and plasma potassium is 4 mM, the daily amount of potassium filtered by the nephron is 720 mmol (180 L × 4 mM). Potassium is extensively reabsorbed (580 mmol in this example) in the proximal tubule, driven passively by the electrical gradient which the tubule generates (21). Only 20% of the amount originally filtered is present at the end of the proximal tubule.

The thick ascending limb is the next site of significant potassium transport. This segment reabsorbs approximately 15% of the filtered potassium. Potassium participates in the active reabsorption of NaCl and as a consequence generates an electrical gradient which

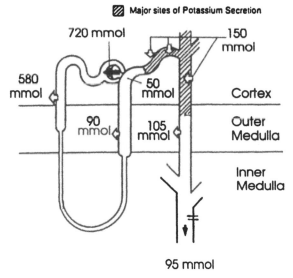

FIGURE 4 Quantitative amounts of potassium filtered, reabsorbed, and secreted along the mammalian nephron. In this example, the amount of potassium transported by 2 million nephrons of the human kidney are combined and illustrated as a single nephron. Potassium enters the glomerulus by filtration, indicated by the large arrow. About 80% is reabsorbed by the proximal tubule, and 15% is reabsorbed by the thick ascending limb, leaving 50 mmol of the filtered potassium in the lumen. Potassium is secreted by the principal cells in the cortical collecting duct, indicated by the hatched region. The amount secreted is equivalent to about 20% of the original filtered potassium. Subsequently, some potassium is reabsorbed by intercalated cells in the outer medullary collecting duct. Under normal conditions, there is no net movement of potassium in the terminal collecting duct. The amount excreted, 95 mmol, represents 95% of the daily intake.

is largely responsible for its own reabsorption. Net reabsorption of sodium chloride is driven by the primary active transport of sodium and potassium across the basolateral membrane via the Na,K-ATPase pump coupled to electrically silent uptake of sodium, chloride, and potassium ions by the Na-2Cl-K luminal cotransporter (33,35). Although the uptake step is electrically silent, a lumen-positive potential develops due to potassium reentry into the lumen through the K_{ATP} channel. The lumen-positive voltage is responsible for passive potassium reabsorption and drives approximately 50% of sodium chloride reabsorption between cells (paracellular pathway). If potassium reabsorption by the thick ascending limb is inhibited by a K_{ATP} channel antagonist, there is little change in potassium excretion since potassium is reabsorbed in the collecting duct (49).

Under normal circumstances, urinary excretion is determined primarily by potassium secretion along the cortical collecting duct (CCD) (21,46,47) (Fig. 4). Potassium secretion in the CCD can increase dramatically, to the point where the amount of potassium in luminal fluid exceeds the amount that was originally filtered. In the example illustrated in Figure 4, 150 mmol of K are secreted into tubular fluid by the principal cells which reside in the cortical collecting duct. This region of the nephron, and portions of the collecting duct in the medulla of the kidney, also contain potassium-reabsorbing cells i.e., intercalated cells, which become active when potassium retention is required. Previously, one cell type was thought to be capable of secreting and reabsorbing potassium. However, it is now known that there are distinct cells resident in the CCD that are responsible for the variability of potassium transport. This discussion will focus on the potassium-reabsorbing and -secreting cells of the CCD.

2.   Site and Mechanism of Potassium Secretion

The Na,K-ATPase pump and ion conductance channels in the principal cells that are involved in secretion are illustrated in Figure 5. Potassium secretion involves active uptake across the basolateral membrane by the Na,K-ATPase pump. Energy expended by the active transport pump is translated into the establishment of large concentration gradients for potassium and sodium across the luminal and peritubular membranes. Potassium preferentially exits across the luminal membrane through potassium conductance channels due to the favorable electrochemical concentration gradient. The electrical potential across the luminal membrane is depolarized due to inwardly directed Na movement through Na conductance channels. The luminal membrane of the principal cell permits the inwardly directed sodium gradient to provide the electrical driving force for potassium secretion. Net secretion of potassium stops if Na conductance channels in the luminal membrane are blocked. When sodium channels close, the luminal membrane voltage increases to approximately -70 mV. Under these conditions, the chemical concentration gradient which favors potassium secretion is opposed by an equivalent electrical gradient oriented in the opposite direction, which retards potassium exit from the cell. There is uncertainty regarding the mechanism of chloride reabsorption; however, recent evidence suggests that chloride is reabsorbed passively between cells driven by the lumen negative potential (47).

3.   Factors Affecting Potassium Secretion

Several factors affect potassium secretion by the CCD; some have direct effects on principal cells, while others exert indirect effects (48). Aldosterone, the principal mineralo-corticoid hormone in humans, and sodium reabsorption (delivery) in principal cells are two most important factors affecting potassium secretion.

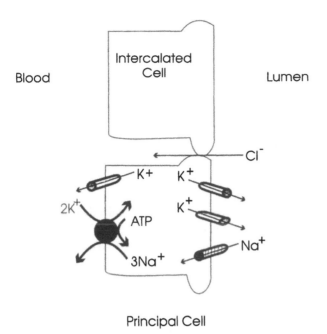

FIGURE 5 Molecular basis of potassium secretion in principal cells. Potassium is pumped into the principal cell by the Na,K-ATPase. Some K exits via conductance channels in the basolateral membrane. However, most potassium leaves the cell through conductance channels in the apical membrane. A favorable electrical gradient is created by the inward movement of Na through apical Na conductance channels. Chloride appears to be reabsorbed paracellularly, driven by the lumen negative transepithelial potential.

Aldosterone

Aldosterone excess or deficiency always disturbs potassium balance. Normal rates of potassium secretion do not occur in the absence of aldosterone. Adrenal insufficiency causes potassium retention and sodium-wasting, which can be reversed by aldosterone, but not by glucocorticoid hormone (50). On the other hand, excess mineralocorticoid hormone stimulates sodium reabsorption and potassium secretion. The role of plasma potassium concentration in the regulation of aldosterone has been established by identification of a feedback loop involving stimulation of aldosterone by increasing plasma potassium concentration. Aldosterone plays an important regulatory role in the excretion of potassium after each meal (51,52).

The principal cell is the major target of aldosterone in the kidney. Within an hour after introduction of the hormone via a genomic signal transduction mechanism, sodium conductance of the luminal membrane increases, thus enhancing the driving force for potassium secretion. This involves activation of previously existing sodium channels. After several hours, there is increased synthesis and insertion of luminal sodium and potassium conductance channels and Na,K-ATPase pumps on the basolateral membrane (50,53). Activity of the Na,K-ATPase pump can be so great that the voltage across the basolateral membrane hyperpolarizes, causing passive entry of potassium through basolateral potassium conductance channels (47). Aldosterone enhances the intrinsic capacity of the principal cell to secrete potassium. Higher aldosterone concentrations are associated with greater stimulation of principal cells, which will persist as long as the hormone concentration is above normal. The actual amount of potassium secreted, however, will depend on the status of the other factors which modulate potassium secretion.

Sodium Reabsorption (Sodium Delivery)

Potassium secretion will not occur if luminal sodium channels are closed. Continuous inward movement of sodium is required to depolarize the luminal cell membrane to permit potassium secretion (21). The major factor affecting the rate of inward Na movement is the chemical concentration gradient for sodium across the luminal membrane of the principal cell. Thus, provided the channel is open, maintenance of a high luminal sodium concentration will increase inward sodium movement and maximize depolarization of the luminal membrane. Normally, when fluid flow rate through the cortical collecting duct increases, a high luminal sodium concentration is maintained. At low flow rates in the CCD, sodium concentration declines as sodium is reabsorbed. At the end of the CCD, there is no gradient for sodium entry into principal cells. In contrast, when flow rate increases, despite high rates of Na reabsorption through Na conductance channels, sodium concentration barely declines by the end of the CCD. Therefore, a favorable gradient for sustained sodium reabsorption exists along the entire CCD and stimulates potassium secretion continuously. This is the mechanism underlying increased potassium secretion associated with loop, thiazide, and proximally acting diuretics, including osmotic diuresis (untreated diabetes mellitus, mannitol, and some antibiotics).

The dependence of potassium secretion on sodium reabsorption explains inhibition of secretion in the presence of the potassium-sparing diuretics which block sodium channels. These drugs, amiloride and triamterene, prevent potassium secretion in response to any stimulus (21), and are frequently combined with thiazide or loop diuretics to prevent potassium loss that normally occurs (54). Although useful in preventing diuretic-induced K deficiency, these drugs may cause hyperkalemia in patients at risk, or if abused. Recently, hyperkalemia in some patients with AIDS was shown to be associated with the use of trimethoprim to treat pneumonia. Later, this antibiotic was found to block sodium channels in the cortical collecting duct (55).

4. Potassium Reabsorption

The mammalian kidney is very efficient in excreting large amounts of potassium and rather inefficient in conserving potassium when intake decreases. An analysis of urinary excretion rates of potassium and sodium in geographically isolated people shows that potassium excretion varies from 100 to greater than 600 mmol/day with a sodium excretion rate of less than 10 mmol/day. The excretion rates reflect the abundance of potassium and scarcity of sodium in these inland terrestrial locations. These and other data suggest that the ability of the kidney to excrete large amounts of potassium and conserve sodium were traits selected in evolution (56). Since the kidney is so seldom called upon to conserve potassium, it may explain the existence of an inefficient reabsorptive system. In mammals, once intake falls below the minimum daily requirement, negative potassium balance ensues. Renal potassium conservation in humans requires about 1–2 weeks to activate fully, and during this time excretion will exceed intake by a significant degree (9,19).

Potassium reabsorption by the cortical collecting duct is mediated by type A (α) intercalated cells in this segment. Intercalated cells are distinguished by the absence of Na,K-ATPase activity, the expression of two luminal primary active acid-secreting pumps, and a basolateral HCO_3-Cl antiporter (21). One of the proton pumps is linked to the simultaneous reabsorption of potassium (H,K-ATPase) and is virtually identical to the form expressed by gastric epithelial cells (27). The other pump transports hydrogen ions (H-ATPase). The type A (α) cells work in unison with bicarbonate secreting, type B (β), intercalated cells. Under normal circumstances, it has been estimated that there is little or no movement of H^+ or HCO_3^- because the transport is antagonistic (47). On the other hand, during dietary potassium depletion the type A cells mediate active potassium reabsorption. In potassium-depleted animals there is increased expression and activity of the H,K-ATPase pump in type A cells in the CCD and in the outer medullary collecting duct (28). When the kidney must conserve potassium, the activity of principal cells declines due to decreased aldosterone, and the activity of type A intercalated cells increases (28,47).

VII. CAUSES OF POTASSIUM DEFICIENCY AND EXCESS

A. Potassium Deficiency and Hypokalemia

The principal causes of hypokalemia are listed in Table 2. They can be derived from the relation among intake, distribution, and excretion. If intake is reduced below the ability of the kidney to conserve potassium, then a deficit will develop. It has been noted in Section II that only rarely is insufficient intake the sole cause of potassium deficiency. Reduced intake in anorexia is probably responsible for potassium deficiency and reduced plasma potassium concentration in these individuals. Usually, however, increased loss via the kidney or GI tract is a contributory factor. Thus, in bulemic patients, in whom intake may be low, a component of increased intestinal (secondary to simultaneous laxative abuse) and renal (secondary to the existence of metabolic acidosis) losses, or renal losses due to metabolic alkalosis secondary to vomiting, largely account for potassium deficiency (21). Continuing this line of reasoning, if excretion exceeds the simultaneous intake (even when intake is

TABLE 2 Major Causes of Hypokalemia

1. Reduced potassium intake[a]
   (a) Deficient diet
   (b) Inadequate absorption
2. Increased renal losses
   (a) Diuretic use
   (b) Osmotic diuresis[b]
   (c) Excess mineralocorticoid
3. Increased intestinal losses
   (a) Diarrhea[c]
   (b) Laxative abuse
4. Redistribution of potassium
   (a) Excess catecholamines
   (b) Excess insulin
   (c) Abnormal skeletal muscle calcium channels

[a]Usually insufficient by itself to cause potassium depletion; see text.
[b]Hypokalemia does not occur in untreated diabetic patients due to insulin deficiency; see text.
[c]Depends on acid–base status; see text.

normal), a deficit will develop. This is the most common situation and explains the potassium deficit seen in patients treated vigorously with loop or thiazide diuretics, or patients abusing these drugs (e.g., for weight reduction). Patients with a potassium deficit will be hypokalemic as long as factors affecting cellular distribution of potassium are normal.

Increased sodium reabsorption in principal cells will occur when above-normal amounts of sodium are delivered to the cortical collecting duct for reasons other than diuretic use. One of the most common causes is the osmotic diuresis that is seen in patients with untreated diabetes mellitus ("sugar" diabetes). In this situation, NaCl reabsorption in the proximal tubule is disturbed by the presence of increased amounts of glucose. The increased delivery of Na to principal cells stimulates potassium secretion. Due to the diuretic action of glucose, the patient loses significant amounts of NaCl and water, leading to a reduction in effective circulating volume (48). This stimulates aldosterone release, which subsequently further stimulates potassium secretion. These patients develop large potassium deficits, but in their untreated state, do not have hypokalemia. This is due to the absence of insulin, which impairs normal uptake into muscle and liver. When insulin is administered, however, potassium quickly moves into cells and the patient rapidly becomes hypokalemic. This explains why current treatment includes simultaneous administration of insulin and potassium.

Large amounts of potassium can be lost due to diarrhea or inappropriate use of laxatives because of the ability of colonic epithelial cells to secrete potassium. Potassium deficiency should be expected in these patients. Hypokalemia may not be observed because the patient will have inorganic metabolic acidosis, which causes potassium to leave cells, thus masking the deficit (48).

Hypokalemia can occur as a result of increased uptake of potassium into cells. As expected, increased catecholamines (via activation of β_2 receptors) or insulin, either exogenous or endogenous, can cause hypokalemia. Both of these agents are used in the treatment of severe hyperkalemia to stimulate uptake of potassium from ECF.

Lastly, intrinsic defects in skeletal muscle ion channels which disturb potassium distribution have been identified (57). These are the periodic familial hypo- and hyper-kalemic paralyses. Patients suffer intermittent muscle paralysis associated with changes in plasma potassium concentration. Due to the profound effect of plasma potassium concentration on resting membrane potential, variations in plasma potassium concentration are usually the initiating stimulus provoking the attack, and plasma potassium concentration is consequently affected by the change in muscle function. Potassium channels are normal in these patients.

A defect in skeletal muscle calcium channels exists in the more common hypo-kalemic disorders (57). This abnormality is genetically linked to the voltage-sensitive calcium channel (dihydropyridine receptor) which participates in excitation–contraction coupling. Mutations in the affected gene causes calcium channels to become inactivated at lower membrane potentials (58). Attacks are precipitated by a reduction in plasma potassium concentration, e.g., after a carbohydrate-rich meal (insulin), or rest after vigorous exercise (catecholamines), factors which normally cause membrane hyperpolarization. In response to these stimuli, calcium current decreases the muscle hyperpolarizes, extracellular potassium moves into muscle, thereby decreasing potassium concentration, and paralysis ensues. The cause-and-effect relation between these changes is unknown. The following facts are known: (a) The defect resides only in skeletal muscle; (b) skeletal paralysis is not due to hypokalemia; and (c) cardiac disturbances are expected due to the hypokalemia.

B. Potassium Excess and Hyperkalemia

The body has a limited capacity to increase body stores of potassium. Usually, plasma potassium concentration increases, i.e., hyperkalemia develops, with relatively small increments of potassium, e.g., 100 mmol. The major causes of hyperkalemia are listed in Table 3. Increased intake by itself is seldom the sole cause of significant hyperkalemia. As long as potassium intake increases gradually, mechanisms exist to defend plasma potassium concentration. Adaptation to a high-potassium diet requires increased cellular buffering, elevated plasma potassium concentration, and marked stimulation of renal secretion by aldosterone (21,43). Accelerated intake from either exogenous or endogenous sources can cause a transient increase in plasma potassium concentration. However, sustained hyperkalemia usually indicates an underlying defect in renal K excretion or impaired K distribution. The most common exogenous source is KCl supplements or salt substitutes (lite salt). Simultaneous use of K-sparing diuretics, underlying renal disease, advanced age, or diabetes mellitus are present in over 50% of patients who develop hyperkalemia while taking KCl supplements or salt substitutes. Other common sources of excess potassium are large doses of potassium penicillin, or administration of old stored blood which has a high extracellular potassium concentration (15).

The factors listed under reduced renal losses cause hyperkalemia by reducing potassium secretion. This can be due to insufficient sodium delivery (acute renal failure), insufficient numbers of functioning cortical collecting ducts (end-stage renal disease), or reduced activity of potassium-secreting principal cells (mineralocorticoid deficiency and potassium-sparing diuretics via different mechanisms) (15,48).

Hyperkalemia can also occur by increased movement of potassium from ICF into ECF, i.e., redistribution. Destruction of cells by any means will result in potassium addition to extracellular fluid. Traumatic injury may be particularly difficult, since acute renal failure may also develop secondary to myoglobin exposure, or ischemia associated with blood loss (6,43).

As anticipated, catecholamine antagonists (used for hypertension) can cause hyperkalemia in settings when enhanced potassium uptake is required, e.g., strenuous exercise.

TABLE 3 Major Causes of Hyperkalemia

1. Excess potassium intake[a]
2. Reduced renal losses
    (a) Acute renal failure
    (b) End-stage renal disease
    (c) Mineralocorticoid deficiency
    (d) Potassium-sparing diuretics
3. Redistribution of potassium
    (a) Hemolysis
    (b) Necrosis
    (c) Muscle injury
    (d) Catecholamine antagonists
    (e) Insulin deficiency[b]
    (f) Abnormal skeletal muscle sodium channels

[a]Excess intake by itself rarely causes hyperkalemia; see text.
[b]Hyperkalemia does not occur in untreated diabetic patients due to accelerated renal potassium loss; see text.

Likewise, insulin deficiency would be expected to cause hyperkalemia. However, the primary disturbance in regulating plasma glucose concentration in diabetes mellitus causes a diuresis which increases renal potassium loss. Because cellular uptake of potassium is impaired in the absence of insulin, plasma potassium concentration does not decrease and may actually be slightly elevated in these potassium-deficient patients.

Lastly, there is a rare genetic disease, hyperkalemic periodic familial paralysis, which can cause skeletal muscle paralysis and hyperkalemia. A population of abnormal Na channels which fail to inactivate normally has been identified in patients with this disorder (57). Under resting conditions, inward sodium current is greater than normal. In these patients, if plasma potassium concentration increases, for example, after a meal, the resultant depolarization increases conductance of all sodium channels. Inward sodium current persists because the abnormal channels do not inactivate. This causes further depolarization of the muscle. Normal sodium channels become inactivated due to the sustained subthreshold depolarization, causing paralysis. Increased potassium efflux occurs secondary to cellular depolarization. It is important to note that (a) this defect is expressed only in skeletal muscle cells, (b) skeletal muscle paralysis is not due to hyperkalemia, and (c) hyperkalemia would be expected to affect cardiac function adversely. The disease is inherited as a single-gene autosomal dominant trait, hence only half of the sodium channels are abnormal. It has been suggested that a disease in which all the sodium channels were affected would be nonviable.

VIII. PHYSIOLOGIC FUNCTIONS OF POTASSIUM

The major function of potassium relates to its role in maintenance of the cell membrane potential. Thus, it is intimately associated with muscle and nerve physiology. The physiological function of these excitable tissues depends on the generation of action potentials. See Hypokalemia, Cardiac Muscle, in Section IX for discussion of the phenomenon. Potassium has minimal known catalytic or regulatory roles, so a separate section on biochemical function is not justified.

A. Potassium is the Major Determinant of Resting Membrane Potential

As a result of the activity of the Na,K-ATPase pump, intracellular potassium concentration is normally maintained at about 150 mM, while intracellular sodium concentration is about 15 mM. An intracellular negative voltage develops as a consequence of outward diffusion of potassium through a population of open potassium channels (Fig. 6). The negative potential inside the cell increases until the electrical force holding potassium in the cell is equal to the chemical force favoring potassium exit. This condition of electrochemical equilibrium for potassium is reached at about −90 mV. The steady-state resting membrane potential is about 15 mV less negative than this, due to the inward movement of sodium down its electrochemical gradient through sodium conductance channels. Activity of the Na,K-ATPase is required intermittently to maintain the chemical concentration gradients. If pump activity increases above baseline, the cell hyperpolarizes due to the extrusion of 3 sodium ions in exchange for only 2 potassium ions pumped into the cell. The electrochemical gradients for potassium and sodium drive or participate in a number of processes in the body. These include nerve conduction, synaptic transmission, muscle contraction, fluid transport, hormone release, and embryonic development.

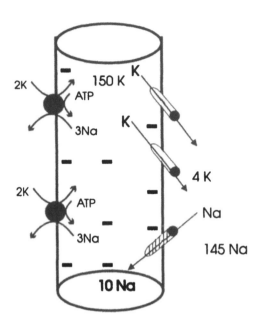

Resting membrane potential = -75 mV

FIGURE 6 Potassium permeability determines the resting membrane potential. The Na,K-ATPase pump creates the chemical concentration gradients for sodium and potassium across the cell membrane. Potassium is the most permeant ion due to the number of open conductance channels in most cell membranes. Potassium diffusion down its chemical concentration gradient without an accompanying anion contributes to the cell negative potential. The resting membrane potential is less than the potassium equilibrium potential (Nernst), due to the inward movement of some sodium ions through sodium conductance channels.

Because the majority of ion channels that are open in the resting muscle cell membrane are potassium channels, variations in the potassium concentration gradient will determine the magnitude of the resting membrane potential. The electrical potential equivalent to the potassium concentration gradient can be calculated using the Nernst equation: Membrane potential $= 61.5 \times \log([K]_{ICF}/[K]_{ECF}$ (37). In our example, given an intracellular [K] of 150 mM and ECF concentration of 4 mM, the concentration ratio is 38:1 and the predicted equilibrium potential is -90 mV. If the extracellular compartment sustained the loss of 20–30 mmol, plasma potassium concentration would be reduced by about 50%. The potassium concentration ratio changes from the normal of 38:1 (150/4) to 75:1 (150/2). Due to the reduction in extracellular potassium concentration, the driving force for outward potassium movement is increased and cells hyperpolarize (Fig. 7). The opposite change in membrane potential occurs if plasma potassium concentration increases from 4.0 to 6.0 mM, the ratio decreases to 25:1, and the membrane potential becomes less negative, i.e., the cell depolarizes (Fig. 7). There are pathophysiological consequences of sustained hyperpolarization or depolarization in electrically excitable tissue which will be discussed in Section IX.

A reduction in intracellular potassium stores in the absence of hypokalemia does not disturb excitable tissue. The following example is offered by way of explanation. Typical potassium deficits in adults amount to 200–300 mmol, which would reduce intracellular

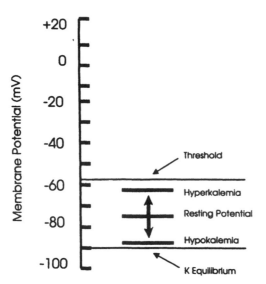

FIGURE 7 The effect of extracellular potassium concentration on resting membrane potential. Since potassium is the most permeant ion, small changes in ECF potassium concentration cause significant changes in resting membrane potential (see text for details). A decrease in ECF potassium below 3.5 mM (hypokalemia) hyperpolarizes cell membranes, while an increase in ECF potassium above 5.0 mM (hyperkalemia) depolarizes cell membranes. The direction of the change in membrane potential is indicated by an arrow. The threshold potential is the voltage at which sodium channels open and an action potential occurs in electrically excitable cells. Variations in ECF potassium affect the resting membrane potential, but not the threshold potential. See text for details about K equilibrium potential.

potassium concentration by about 5–8%. Since the ratio of potassium concentration across the cell membrane barely changes from 38:1 (intracellular/extracellular, 150/4) to 36:1 (144/4), there is a minimal effect on resting membrane potential.

Although potassium depletion unaccompanied by hypokalemia does not disturb cardiac and skeletal muscle, it is vital to realize that these patients are at risk for developing sudden hypokalemia during the course of treatment when underlying disturbances in potassium distribution are corrected, e.g., administration of insulin to patients with diabetes mellitus. If hypokalemia occurs, all of the disturbances in excitable tissue will be evident.

B. Growth

Normal intracellular potassium concentration is required in protein synthesis and cellular growth. Early experiments in intact cells and cell-free systems demonstrated a linear relation between intracellular potassium concentration and cell growth and incorporation of amino acids into protein (59). Impaired protein biosynthesis is manifested as growth retardation in young animals (60,61). This effect probably contributes to failure to obtain positive nitrogen balance during potassium-deficient hyperalimentation (62) as well as failure-to-thrive in children in children with Bartter's syndrome. Growth retardation may also be a consequence of impaired growth hormone release, or altered protein synthesis due to relative insulin deficiency (63). Although somatic growth is impaired in potassium-depleted subjects, renal growth is disproportionately increased (61). This may be due to the effects of elevated angiotensin II on the kidney.

C. Blood Pressure

Epidemiologic surveys suggest that populations ingesting diets that are low in potassium are more susceptible to the development of hypertension. Several clinical studies have demonstrated that potassium depletion is associated with an increase in blood pressure, while potassium supplementation exerts the opposite effect (64,65). The mechanism underlying the increase in blood pressure during potassium depletion is not well understood. Sodium retention, which accompanies potassium depletion, most likely plays an important role, as the hypertensive effect of potassium depletion fails to become manifest if sodium intake is curtailed.

IX. SYMPTOMS OF HYPO- AND HYPERKALEMIA

Since the resting membrane potential depends primarily on the potassium gradient across the cell membrane, variations in extracellular potassium concentration have a profound effect on the excitability of smooth, skeletal, and cardiac muscle. Effects on the heart are potentially fatal. Neurons are affected minimally by variations in ECF potassium, so one sees little or no change in nerve conduction, synaptic transmission, and central nervous system function. Nerve cell function may be spared due to the physical isolation of neurons by cerebral spinal fluid, glial cell attachment, or myelination.

A. Hypokalemia

Chronic hypokalemia is common and causes several types of disturbances, including muscular, renal, and endocrine, as well as impaired water homeostasis. The muscle and cardiac effects are potentially life-threatening. Severe potassium depletion can result in two major complications: paralysis and muscle cell death with release of contractile proteins (rhabdomyolysis) (45). Hypokalemia, whether produced by redistribution or potassium depletion, can alter the function of all muscles, i.e., skeletal, smooth, and cardiac. The specific effects on cardiac muscle will be discussed subsequently. An increase in the intracellular-to-extracellular potassium ratio hyperpolarizes the membrane, which increases the voltage required to reach threshold for initiating an action potential (Fig. 7). Even after an action potential has arisen at the neuromuscular junction, spread along the muscle fiber will be greatly impaired. As the degree of hypokalemia worsens, the decrease in the conductance of potassium channels allows the underlying sodium and calcium conductances to have a greater effect on the resting membrane potential. It is not uncommon for the resting muscle in patients with severe hypokalemia (1–2 mM) to depolarize. Sustained depolarization near or above the threshold potential inactivities sodium channels which renders the muscle completely inexcitable.

1. Skeletal Muscle

Plasma potassium levels below 3.0 mM are often associated with complaint of muscle weakness. Skeletal muscle dysfunction can also be attributed to other defects associated with potassium depletion: (a) impaired muscle blood flow and absence of exercise-induced vasodilatation, (b) a depletion of energy (glycogen) stores, (c) total loss of cellular integrity which can result in muscle necrosis (rhabdomyolysis). Paralysis affects lower limbs initially and subsequently moves up the trunk. If a patient does not experience cardiac dysfunction, death may occur due to respiratory muscle paralysis.

2. Smooth Muscle

Hypokalemia paralyzes small intestinal smooth muscle (by the same mechanism as described in skeletal muscle), causing abdominal distension, anorexia, nausea, vomiting, and constipation. Urinary bladder mobility is also decreased as a result of potassium depletion.

3. Cardiac Muscle

The cardiac effects are the most serious consequence of hypokalemia. Reductions in plasma potassium concentration are associated with marked changes in the action potential recorded in cardiac muscle cells. A single action potential recorded in a ventricular muscle cell in the presence of a normal ECF potassium concentration is illustrated in Figure 8, along with the changes caused by hypo- and hyperkalemia. The duration of the action potential at a normal heart rate (70 beats/min) is about 300 ms, which allows for a sustained contraction of the muscle fiber. Ventricular muscle cells are "paced" by the electrical currents flowing through the conduction system of the heart and subsequently from cell to

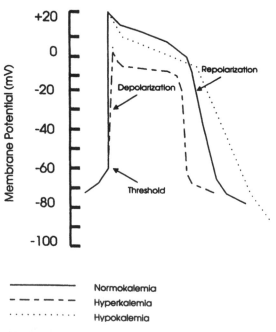

FIGURE 8   The effect of hypo- and hyperkalemia on the action potential in cardiac muscle. The solid line represents the spontaneous change in membrane voltage which occurs when cardiac muscle cells are depolarized to the voltage called threshold. Once threshold is reached, the cell rapidly depolarizes and gradually repolarizes, restoring membrane voltage to the resting value. Increased sodium and calcium channel activity are responsible for depolarization, while increased potassium channel activity is responsible for repolarization. Hypokalemia reduces the conductance of potassium channels, which causes a marked delay in repolarization (dotted line), whereas hyperkalemia delays depolarization, reduces the peak voltage that is reached, and increases the rate of repolarization (dashed line). See text for further details.

cell so that the muscle fibers contract in a coordinated manner. Once the depolarizing current arrives at the individual ventricular muscle cell, the membrane potential depolarizes until a certain membrane voltage is reached, at which time an "all or none" spontaneous change in potential occurs. This spontaneous change in voltage is called an *action potential*, and the voltage at which it occurs is called *threshold potential*. At the threshold potential, sodium and calcium conductance channels open, allowing sodium and calcium to rush into the cell. This causes the membrane voltage to depolarize rapidly, which generates the upstroke or rising phase of the action potential. The voltage increases until the sodium equilibrium potential is reached, at which time net sodium entry ceases. Inside the cell, calcium stores are released which activate the contractile process. Muscle contraction will persist as long as the cell is depolarized. As shown in Figure 8, following the peak of the action potential, the cell remains depolarized for a considerable period of time due to sustained calcium conductance. However, sodium channels rapidly close or inactivate in a time-dependent manner after they have been activated at threshold. Sometime during this stable period of depolarization (plateau phase), potassium channels become activated. Since the voltage inside the cell is positive at this time, there is a large driving force for potassium to exit from the cell. As potassium leaves the cell, the membrane voltage gradually returns to the resting potential, which is close to the potassium equilibrium potential. Therefore, opening of sodium channels is responsible for depolarization (i.e., the upstroke of the action potential), and opening of potassium channels is responsible for repolarization.

When plasma potassium concentration is reduced, the principal effect is a decrease in the conductance of potassium channels. This means that the rate at which potassium leaves the cell during repolarization is reduced, causing the falling phase of the action potential to be prolonged as seen in Figure 8. Hyperkalemia has the reverse effect on potassium conductance and causes the rate of repolarization to increase. In addition, hyperkalemia by causing sustained subthreshold depolarization (Fig. 7) adversely affects sodium channel activity (79). As resting membrane potential remains closer to threshold, a fraction of sodium channels open and then close, i.e., inactivate, and will not open again until the membrane hyperpolarizes. The number of sodium channels inactivated will be related to the magnitude of membrane depolarization (i.e., proximity to threshold), which is related directly to the increase in plasma potassium concentration. Depending on the severity of the increase in plasma potassium concentration, fewer sodium channels will be able to produce an action potential. The above phenomenon is called sodium inactivation. Note in Figure 8 that the rate of raise of the action potential is reduced in hyperkalemia. This means that it will take more time to depolarize ventricular muscle fully. Note also that the peak voltage is reduced in hyperkalemia. Since more sodium channels are closed, the membrane potential is affected by calcium channels, so the potential moves toward the calcium equilibrium potential. Severe hyperkalemia by inactivating sodium channels can render the heart inexcitable, causing death.

Cardiac muscle currents can be recorded on the surface of the body in an electrocardiogram (ECG) illustrated in Figure 9. The P wave, the first wave in the ECG, is the sum of all the depolarizing currents in the atria and represents atrial contraction. Atrial muscle repolarization occurs shortly after and is masked by the larger currents flowing in the ventricules. As the ventricules depolarize, the sum of all the upstrokes of the action potentials is recorded in the ECG as the QRS wave or complex. The plateau phase of the action potential occurs during the S-T segment. As the ventricules repolarize to return to the resting membrane potential, the sum of all these repolarizing currents is recorded as the T

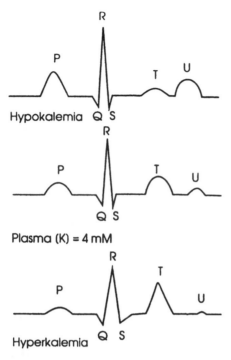

FIGURE 9 The effect of plasma potassium concentration on the electrocardiogram (ECG). A schematic of an ECG pattern for one cardiac cycle in an individual with a plasma potassium concentration of 4 mM is illustrated in the center panel. The upper panel shows the effect of lowering plasma potassium (hypokalemia) to diminish the size of the T wave, which represents ventricular repolarization, and increase the size of the U wave. P waves, which represent atrial depolarization, are actually increased in amplitude. In contrast, increasing plasma potassium concentration (hyperkalemia) causes the T wave to peak and the U wave to minimize. Notice the widening of the QRS complex and virtual disappearance of the P wave. See text for details.

wave. As expected, hypokalemia will cause characteristic changes in the electrocardiogram (ECG) (66). In hypokalemia, since the falling phase of the action potential becomes progressively less steep (Fig. 8), it is manifested in the ECG by the flattening of the T wave (Fig. 9). Delayed repolarization contributes in a major way to the increased duration of the action potential. Normally, the U wave represents repolarization of Purkinje fibers. In severe hypokalemia (1–2 mM), the T wave and U wave combine. ECG evidence of hypokalemia is based primarily on S-T segment depression and abnormalities in T and U waves (66,67).

The greatest cardiac risk in hypokalemia is the threat of reentry currents arising during the prolonged repolarization phase, leading to the development of arrhythmias (15,66). The increased incidence of arrhythmias in hypokalemia may also be related to the activation of sodium channels secondary to hyperpolarization of the resting membrane potential, causing increased automaticity. Hypokalemia appears to be related to serious ventricular ectopy such as ventricular tachycardia and fibrillation, particularly in the setting of coronary artery disease and acute myocardial infarction (15,68,69).

4. Endocrine

Carbohydrate intolerance is the most common metabolic disorder associated with potassium depletion (6). Impairment in glucose regulation during K depletion is due to diminished insulin secretion secondary to diminished β-cell response to glucose. Glucose intolerance in hyperaldosteronism or vigorous thiazide therapy is observed only in patients who are hypokalemic. This can now be understood in view of the role of potassium channels in mediating insulin release (38,42).

Potassium depletion stimulates renin production, with a consequent increase in Ang II; however, aldosterone secretion decreases (6,70–72). Potassium stimulates aldosterone synthesis directly and potentiates stimulation by Ang II and ACTH. The decline in aldosterone is beneficial in defending body stores of potassium during potassium depletion. The decrease in aldosterone augments stimulation of renin production, which is enhanced by potassium depletion itself.

5. Renal

Potassium depletion has both structural and functional effects on the kidney, which are reviewed thoroughly elsewhere (6,19,48). Briefly, potassium depletion decreases renal blood flow; impairs concentrating ability; increases ammonium production, bicarbonate reabsorption, and sodium reabsorption; and impairs phosphate reabsorption (6,19,73,74).

Impaired urinary concentrating ability is associated with increased urine output (polyuria) and increased water intake (polydipsia). There are two components to the polyuria: (a) diminished urinary concentrating ability (i.e., nephrogenic diabetes insipidus) due to inhibition of thick ascending limb NaCl reabsorption (71,75), and (b) a primary increase in thirst (see below).

Hypokalemia causes increased production of ammonium (NH_4^+) and bicarbonate by the proximal tubular cells. Bicarbonate is added to the blood, causing metabolic alkalosis which worsens the hypokalemia (6,15), and NH_4^+ is excreted in the urine (76).

6. Water Homeostasis

Hypokalemia stimulates increased water intake secondary to elevated Ang II. Ang II activates receptors in discrete regions of the wall of the third ventricle. Type 2 Ang II receptors (AT2) mediate the effect on water intake. Destruction of this area of the brain (77), or a reduction in Ang II by converting enzyme inhibition (72), prevent increased water intake in potassium-depleted rats. The osmotic threshold for antidiuretic hormone (ADH) release is reset to a lower osmolality in potassium-depleted animals (78). Increased water intake and reset of ADH release are adaptations which aid in the defense of ECF volume in the absence of aldosterone in these hypokalemic animals.

B. Hyperkalemia

The effects of chronic and acute hyperkalemia are usually restricted to skeletal and cardiac muscle. Due to the fatality associated with the cardiac disturbances associated with hyperkalemia, chronic severe hyperkalemia is not commonly observed.

1. Skeletal Muscle

Hyperkalemia causes skeletal muscle weakness and paralysis (45). Skeletal muscle cells elicit action potentials, which are similar to cardiac action potentials (Fig. 8) except being of shorter duration. An increase in plasma potassium concentration causes sustained subthreshold depolarization, which inactivates sodium channels as discussed previously (Sec. IX). The extent of sodium channel inactivation can be so great that the muscle fiber can be depolarized above threshold and remain completely inexcitable. In hyperkalemia, despite normal synaptic transmission, the motor end plate and the entire muscle cell membrane can be inexcitable. Severe muscle paralysis in hyperkalemia will usually not be seen, because of the fatality associated with cardiac arrhythmias which begin to develop as plasma potassium concentration increases.

2. Cardiac Effects

The cardiac effects are the most serious consequence of hyperkalemia (66,67). Increases in plasma potassium concentration are associated with characteristic changes in the ECG, which are shown in Figure 9. As plasma potassium concentration increases, resting membrane potential depolarizes from -75 mV to a value closer to threshold. Sustained subthreshold depolarization causes the abnormal delay in atrial and ventricular depolarization (due to sodium inactivation, Sec. IX.A, Cardiac Muscle) during an action potential manifested by the flattening and eventual loss of the P wave, and progressive widening of the QRS complex. However, ventricular repolarization is enhanced causing peaked T waves. This is due to an increase in the conductance of potassium channels as a consequence of the increase in plasma potassium concentration. Peaked T waves are diagnostic of the existence of hyperkalemia. With severe hyperkalemia, the classic sine-wave pattern is seen due to the merging of the widened QRS complex with the peaked T waves. Ventricular arrhythmias or cardiac arrest may occur at any point after changes in the ECG have occurred. Cardiac arrest is more common in hyperkalemia than hypokalemia.

X. ACTIVE AREAS OF RESEARCH

Recently, the molecular mechanism underlying Liddle's syndrome was discovered. These patients are hypokalemic and hypertensive, and were said to have pseudo-hyperaldosteronism since plasma aldosterone levels were actually suppressed (80). The defect resides in the β and γ subunits of the sodium channel expressed in principal cells of the cortical collecting duct (81). These sodium channels are virtually unregulated and have an open probability approaching 100%. Thus sodium reabsorption is increased and potassium secretion is increased as expected. The search is currently underway to find the molecular basis of other diseases which disrupt potassium homeostasis. Bartter's syndrome is a classic example. It generally presents early in life and is associated with hypokalemia, metabolic alkalosis, hyperaldosteronism, hyperreninemia, marked hypertrophy and hyperplasia of the juxtaglomerular apparatus, growth retardation, normal blood pressure, insensitivity to exogenous angiotensin II, polyuria, polydipsia, decreased concentrating ability, and elevated synthesis of vasodilator prostaglandins (prostaglandin E_2 and prostacyclin) (82). It is currently diagnosed by exclusion of other causes. Clustering of cases suggests a genetic component. The findings described above are compatible with a primary defect in sodium chloride reabsorption in the medullary thick ascending limb of the loop of Henle. Another disorder, Gitelman's syndrome, which appears to be a variant of Bartter's, causes hypokalemia and magnesium wasting (83). The underlying molecular basis of this disease is currently unknown.

Another area of intense investigation is in elucidation of the subunit structure of potassium channels and their molecular interactions. Much effort is currently focused on the structure, function, and regulation of voltage-gated and ATP-gated channels in view of their diverse roles in multiple physiological systems. Lastly, studies will continue to elucidate the regulation and structure of the primary active transport pumps and as well as the 1Na:2Cl:1K cotransporter. This work will lead to a better understanding of the sites that confer potassium specificity in the various transporters. Further information is required to understand the coupling between apical and basolateral transport events in all transporting epithelia. This will involve the understanding of cross-talk among active transport pumps, cotransporters, and ion channels.

XI. ABBREVIATIONS AND DEFINITIONS

ACTH   Adrenocorticotropic hormone: Anterior pituitary hormone which regulates cortisol secretion by the adrenal cortex. It can transiently stimulate aldosterone secretion.

ADH   Antidiuretic hormone: Posterior pituitary hormone which stimulates water reabsorption by the cortical collecting duct in the kidney.

AIDS   Acquired immunodeficiency syndrome: Failure of the immune system due to destruction of T lymphocytes by human immunodeficiency virus (HIV).

Ang II   Angiotensin II: Peptide hormone produced by the renin-angiotensin system with multiple actions in the kidney, adrenal cortex, and brain. Angiotensin II stimulates salt and water conservation.

AT2   Angiotensin II type 2 receptor: Type 2 receptors mediate most of the effects of angiotensin II on vasoconstriction, aldosterone release, kidney salt conservation, and thirst.

Ca-ATPase   Calcium adenosine triphosphatase: A protein complex which moves calcium through cell membranes at the expense of ATP breakdown (simultaneous hydrolysis of ATP).

CCD   Cortical collecting duct: Portion of the collection duct located in the cortex of the kidney (see Fig. 4). This segment reabsorbs sodium, secretes potassium, and reabsorbs water in the presence of ADH.

CFTR   Cystic fibrosis transmembrane regulator: Protein product of the gene which when defective causes cystic fibrosis. It functions as a chloride channel, but more important, it confers regulation on other ion channels. Chloride and sodium channels in the lungs and sweat glands are regulated by CFTR.

ECG   Electrocardiogram: Variations in voltage due to the contraction of cardiac muscle that can be recorded at the body surface. The electrocardiogram is the sequence of recorded voltages.

ECF   Extracellular fluid: Body fluid found outside cells. Ions found in high concentrations are sodium, chloride, and bicarbonate. Ions found in low concentrations are potassium, calcium, magnesium, phosphate, citrate, and sulfate.

GI   Gastrointestinal tract.

HCO_3-Cl   Bicarbonate-chloride antiporter. A protein complex that moves bicarbonate and chloride ions in opposite directions through cell membranes. It is driven by the difference in bicarbonate and chloride ions across the membrane and is not linked directly to the breakdown of ATP. It is a secondary active transporter.

H,K-ATPase   Hydrogen, potassium-ATPase. A protein complex that moves hydrogen ions out of the cell and potassium ions into the cell at the expense of simultaneous breakdown of ATP. It is a primary active transport pump.

ICF   Intracellular fluid: Body fluid found exclusively inside cells. Ions found in high concentrations are potassium, phosphate, and magnesium to some extent. Ions found in low concentrations are sodium, chloride, bicarbonate, and calcium.

K_{ATP} ATP-regulated potassium channels: A type of potassium selective ion channel in which ATP causes the channel to open.

K_m Michaelis-Menton constant: Characterizes rates of reaction by enzymes and rates of transport by cotransporters and pumps. The Michaelis-Menton constant for a transporter is the ion concentration at which the transport rate is 50% of maximal. The lower the K_m for an ion, the greater is the affinity of that transporter for the ion.

mM   Millimoles per liter (concentration term).

mmol   Millimoles (a quantity).

mV   Millivolts.

Na-2Cl-K   Sodium-2 Chloride-Potassium cotransporter: A membrane protein that simultaneously moves 1 sodium ion, 2 chloride ions, and 1 potassium ion in the same direction through the membrane. It is driven by the difference in sodium concentration across the membrane and does not depend directly on the breakdown of ATP for energy. It is called a secondary active transporter.

Na,K-ATPase   Sodium, Potassium-ATPase: A membrane protein complex that moves sodium ions out of the cell and potassium ions into the cell at the expense of ATP breakdown. This primary active pump is found in virtually every cell in the body.

P wave   Voltage deflection on an electrocardiogram caused by atrial depolarization.

QRS wave   Voltage deflection on an electrocardiogram caused by ventricular depolarization.

ROMK1   Rat outer medullary potassium channel (1 = first cloned). This is the ATP-gated channel which participates in NaCl reabsorption in the thick ascending limb, and potassium secretion in the cortical collecting duct.

T wave   Voltage deflection on an electrocardiogram caused by ventricular repolarization.

U wave   Voltage delection on an electrocardiogram caused by Purkinji fiber repolarization.

REFERENCES

1. Drossman DA. Eating disorders. In: Wyngaarden JB, Smith LH Jr, eds. Cecil Textbook of Medicine. 18th ed. Philadelphia: Saunders, 1988: 1215–1219.

2. Potassium. In: McGraw-Hill Encyclopedia of Science and Technology. 7th ed. New York: McGraw-Hill, 1992: 221–222.

3. Potassium. In: Encarta 95. Redmond, WA: Microsoft, 1994.

4. Masterson WL, Hurley CN. Chemistry: Principles and Reactions. 2d ed. Philadelphia: Saunders, 1993: 530.

5. Nash LA, Peterson LN, Nadler SP, et al. Determination of sodium and potassium in nanoliter volumes of biological fluids by furnace atomic absorption spectrometry. Anal Chem 1988; 60: 2413–2418.

6. Tannen RL. Potassium disorders. In: Kokko JP, Tannen RL, eds. Fluids and Electrolytes. Philadelphia: Saunders 1986: 150–228.

7. Corsa L Jr, Sidney JM, Steenburg RW, et al. The measurement of exchangeable potassium in man by isotope dilution. J Clin Invest 1950; 29: 1280–1294.

8. Sun A, Grossman EB, Lombardi M, et al. Vasopressin alters the mechanism of apical Cl entry from Na:Cl to Na:K:2Cl cotransport in mouse medullary thick ascending limb. J Membr Biol 1991; 120(1): 83–94.

9. Lemann J Jr. Internal and external solute balance. In: Seldin DW, Giebisch G, eds. The Kidney: Physiology and Pathophysiology. 2d ed. New York: Raven Press, 1992: 45–59.

10. Alfin-Slater RB, Mirenda R. Nutrient requirements: what they are and basis for recommendation. In: Alfin-slater RB, Kritchevsky D, eds. Nutrition and the Adult—Macronutrients. New York: Plenum Press, 1980: 1–48.

11. Appendix D: nutrient composition of common foods. In: Mitch WE, Klahr S, eds. Nutrition and the Kidney 2d ed. Boston: Little, Brown, 1993: 399–448.

12. Avery GB. The newborn. In: Jelliffe DB, Jelliffe EF, eds. Human Nutrition. Vol. 2. Nutrition and Growth. New York: Plenum Press, 1979: 129–152.

13. Nelson's Textbook of Pediatrics. 14th ed. Philadelphia: Saunders, 1992.

14. Potato, Irish. In: McGraw-Hill Encyclopedia of Science and Technology. 7th ed. New York: McGraw-Hill, 1992: 222–224.

15. Rose BD. Clinical Physiology of Acid–Base and Electrolyte Disorders. 4th ed. New York: McGraw-Hill, 1994.

16. Halm DR, Frizzell RA. Ion transport across the large intestine. In: Schultz S, ed. Handbook of Physiology, Sec. 6: The Gastrointestinal System, Intestinal Absorption and Secretion. Bethesda, MD: American Physiological Society, 1991; 287–301.

17. Gilman A, Koelle E, Ritchie JM. Transport of potassium ions in rat intestine. Nature 1963; 197: 1210–1211.

18. Smith JD, Bia M, DeFronzo RA. Clinical disorders of potassium metabolism. In: Arieff A, DeFronzo RA, eds. Fluid, Electrolyte, and Acid–Base Disorders. New York: Churchill Livingstone, 1985: 413–509.

19. Mujais SK, Katz AI. Potassium deficiency. In: Seldin DW, Giebisch G, eds. The Kidney: Physiology and Pathophysiology. 2d ed. New York: Raven Press, 1992: 2249–2278.

20. Field M, Rao MC, Chang EB. Intestinal electrolyte transport and diarrheal disease, part 1. N Engl J Med 1989; 321: 800–806.

21. Wright FS, Giebisch G. Regulation of potassium excretion. In: Seldin DW, Giebisch G, eds. The Kidney: Physiology and Pathophysiology. 2d ed. New York: Raven Press, 1992: 2209–2247.

22. Paul JK, Nettikadan SR, Ganjeizadeh M, et al. Molecular imaging of Na,K-ATPase in purified kidney membranes. FEBS Lett 1994; 346: 289–294.

23. Aperia A, Holtback U, Syren M-L, et al. Activation/deactivation of renal Na,K-ATPase: a final common pathway for regulation of natriuresis. FASEB J 1994: 8: 436–439.

24. Forte JG, Soll A. Cell biology of hydrochloric acid secretion. In: Schultz S, ed. Handbook of Physiology, Sec. 6: The Gastrointestinal System III. Bethesda, MD: American Physiological Society, 1992: 207–228.

25. Schwiebert EM, Egan ME, Hwang T-H, et al. CFTR regulates outwardly rectifying chloride channels through an autocrine mechanism involving ATP. Cell 1995; 81: 1063–1073.

26. Takeguchi N, Tomiyama Y, Ohshika M, et al. The apical chloride channel as part of the function of gastric H,K-ATPase. Jpn J Physiol 1994; 44(suppl 2): S157–S159.

27. Wingo CS, Smolka AJ. Function and structure of H,K-ATPase in the kidney. Am J Physiol 1995; 269: F1–F16.

28. Wingo CS, Armitage FE. Potassium transport in the kidney: regulation and physiological relevance of H,K-ATPase. Sem Nephrol 1993; 13: 213–224.

29. Geck P, Pietrzyk C, Burckhart B-C, et al. Electrically silent cotransport of Na, K, and Cl in Ehrlich cells. Biochem Biophys Acta 1980; 600: 432–447.

30. Gamba G, Miyanoshita A, Lombardi M, et al. Molecular cloning, primary structure, and characterization of two members of the mammalian electroneutral sodium-(potassium)-chloride cotransporter family expressed in the kidney. J Biol Chem 1994; 269: 17713–17722.

31. Delpire E, Rauchman MI, Beier DR, et al. Molecular cloning and chromosome localization of a putative basolateral Na-K-2Cl cotransporter from mouse inner medullary collecting duct (mIMCD-3) Cells. J Biol Chem 1994; 269: 25677–25683.

32. Hebert SC, Gullans SR. The electroneutral sodium-(potassium)-chloride co-transporter family: a journey from fish to the renal co-transporters. Curr Opin Nephrol Hyperten 1995; 4: 389–391.

33. Haas M. The Na-K-Cl cotransporters. Am J Physiol 1994; 267: C869–C885.

34. Forbush B III, Palfrey HC. ^{3}H bumetanide binding to membranes isolated from dog kidney outer medulla. J Biol Chem 1983; 258: 11787–11792.

35. Reeves WB, Andreoli TE. Sodium chloride transport in the loop of Henle. In: Seldin DW, Giebisch G, eds. The Kidney: Physiology and Pathophysiology. 2d ed. New York: Raven Press, 1992: 1975–2001.

36. Payne JA, Forbush B III. Alternatively spliced isoforms of the putative renal Na-K-Cl cotransporter are differentially distributed within the rabbit kidney. Proc Natl Acad Sci (USA) 1994; 91: 4544–4548.

37. Dawson DC. Principles of membrane transport. In: Schultz S, ed. Handbook of Physiology, Sec. 6: The Gastrointestinal System, Intestinal Absorption and Secretion. Bethesda, MD: American Physiological Society, 1991: 1–44.

38. Desir GV. The structure, regulation and pathophysiology of potassium channels. Curr Opin Nephrol Hyperten 1995; 4: 402–405.

39. Hebert SC, Ho K. Structure and functional properties of an inwardly rectifying ATP-regulated K channel from rat kidney. Renal Physiol Biochem 1994; 17: 143–147.

40. Canessa CM, Schild L, Buell G, et al. Amiloride-sensitive epithelial Na channel is made of three homologous subunits. Nature 1994; 367: 463–467.

41. Rettig J, Heinemann SH, Wunder F, et al. Inactivation properties of voltage-gated K channels altered by presence of β-subunit. Nature 1994; 369: 289–292.

42. Aguilar-Bryan L, Nichols CG, Wechsler SW, et al. Cloning of the b-cell high-affinity sulfonyl-urea receptor: A regulator of insulin secretion. Science 1995; 268: 423–425.

43. DeFronzo RA. Clinical disorders of hyperkalemia. In: Seldin DW, Giebisch G, eds. The Kidney: Physiology and Pathophysiology. 2d ed. New York: Raven Press, 1992: 2279–2337.

44. Rosa RM, Williams ME, Epstein FH. Extrarenal potassium metabolism. In: Seldin DW, Giebisch G, eds. The Kidney: Physiology and Pathophysiology. 2d ed. New York: Raven Press, 1992: 2165–2190.

45. Knochel JP. Potassium gradients and neuromuscular function. In: Seldin DW, Giebisch G, eds. The Kidney: Physiology and Pathophysiology. 2d ed. New York: Raven Press, 1992: 2191–2208.

46. Schlatter E. Potassium transport in the cortical collecting duct. Sem Renal Physiol 1993; 65: 169–179.

47. Stokes JB. Ion transport by the collecting duct. 1993; Sem Nephrol 13: 202–212.

48. Peterson LN, Levi M. Disorders of potassium metabolism. In Schrier RW, ed. Renal and Electrolyte Disorders. 5th ed. Boston: Little, Brown, 1996: chap 5.

49. Wang T, Wang W-H, Klein-Robbenhaar G, et al. Effects of glyburide on renal tubule transport and potassium channel activity. Renal Physiol Biochem 1995; 18: 169–182.

50. Stanton BA. Regulation of Na and K transport by mineralocorticoids. Sem Nephrol 1987; 7: 82–90.

51. Adam WR, Ellis AG, Adams BA. Aldosterone is a physiologically significant kaliuretic hormone. Am J Physiol 1987; 252: F1048–F1054.

52. Rabelink RJ, Koomans HA, Hene RJ, et al. Early and late adjustment to potassium loading in humans. Kidney Int 1990; 38: 942–947.

53. O'Niel RG. Aldosterone regulation of sodium and potassium transport in the cortical collecting duct. Sem Nephrol 1990; 10: 365–374.

54. Rose BD. Diuretics. Kidney Int. 1991; 39: 336–352.

55. Velazquez H, Perazella MA, Wright FS, et al. Renal mechanism of trimethoprim-induced hyperkalaemia. Ann Intern Med 1993; 119: 296–301.

56. Sebastian A, Hernandez RE, Schambelan M. Disorders of renal handling of potassium. In: Brenner BM, Rector FC, eds. The Kidney. 3d ed. Philadelphia: Saunders, 1986: 519–549.

57. Hoffman EP, Lehmann-Horn F, Rudel R. Overexcited or inactive: ion channels in muscle disease. Cell 1995; 80: 681–686.

58. Ptacek LJ, Rawil R, Griggs RC, et al. Dihydropyridine receptor mutations cause hypokalemic periodic paralysis. Cell 1994; 77: 863–868.

59. Lubin M, Ennis H. On the role of intracellular potassium in protein synthesis. Biochem. Biophys Acta 1964; 80: 614–631.

60. Brokaw A. Renal hypertrophy and polydipsia in potassium deficient rats. Am J Physiol 1953; 172: 333–346.

61. Peterson LN, Carpenter B, Guttierrez G, et al. Potassium depletion enhances renal compensatory hypertrophy in the nephrectomized rat. J Min Elect Met 1987; 13: 57–62.

62. Rudman D, Millikan WJ, Richardson TJ, et al. Elemental balances during intravenous hyperalimentation of underweight adult subjects. J Clin Invest 1975; 55: 94–104.

63. Podolsky S, Melby JC. Improvement of growth hormone response to stimulation in primary aldosteronism with correction of potassium deficiency. Metabolism 1976; 25: 1027–1032.
64. Krishna GG, Kapoor SC. Potassium depletion exacerbates essential hypertension. Ann Intern Med 1991; 115: 77–83.
65. Linas SL. The role of potassium in the pathogenesis and treatment of hypertension. Kidney Int 1991; 39: 771–786.
66. Surawicz B. Relationship between electrocardiogram and electrolytes. Am Heart J 1967; 73(6): 814–834.
67. Surawicz B. Contributions of cellular electrophysiology to the understanding of the electrocardiogram. Experientia 1987; 43: 1061–1068.
68. Podrid PH. Potassium and ventricular arrhythmias. Am J Cardiol 1990; 65: 33E–44E.
69. Schulman M, Narins RG. Hypokalemia and cardiovascular disease. Am J Cardiol 1990; 65: 4E–9E.
70. Linas SL, Peterson LN, Anderson RJ, et al. Mechanism of renal potassium conversion in the rat. Kidney Int. 1979; 15: 601–611.
71. McKay AJ, Peterson LN. K infusion corrects thick ascending limb Cl reabsorption in K-depleted rats by an aldosterone-independent mechanism. Am J Physiol 1993; 264: F792–F799.
72. McKay AJ, Poirier CD, Peterson LN. Converting-enzyme inhibition abolishes polydipsia induced by dietary NaCl and K depletion. Am J Physiol 1990; 258(Regulatory Integrative Comp Physiol 27): F1164–F1172.
73. Agnoli GC, Borgatti R, Cacciari M, et al. Effects of angiotensin-converting enzyme inhibition on renal dysfunction induced by moderate potassium depletion in healthy women. Clin Physiol 1994; 14: 205–222.
74. Tizianello A, Garibotto G, Robaudo C, et al. Renal ammoniagenesis in humans with chronic potassium depletion. Kidney Int. 1991; 40: 772–778.
75. Gutsche HU, Peterson LN, Levine DZ. In vivo evidence of impaired solute transport by the thick ascending limb in potassium depleted rats. J Clin Invest 1984; 73: 908–916.
76. Halperin ML. Biochemistry and physiology of ammonium excretion. In: Seldin DW, Giebisch G, eds. The Kidney: Physiology and Pathophysiology. 2d ed. New York: Raven Press, 1992: 1471–1489.
77. Saikaley A, Bichet D, Kucharczyk J, et al. Neuroendocrine factors mediating polydipsia induced by Na, Cl, and K depletion. Am J Physiol 251 (Regulatory Integrative Comp Physiol 1986; 20): R1071–R1077.
78. Peterson LN, Mathur S, Borzecki JS. Reset of the osmotic threshold for vasopressin in rats fed a low NaCl, K-free diet. Can J Physiol Pharmacol 1992; 70: 645–650.
79. Catterall WA. Molecular mechanisms of inactivation and modulation of sodium channels. Renal Physiol Biochem 1994; 17: 121–125.
80. Botero-Velez M, Curtis JJ, Warnock DG. Brief report: Liddle's syndrome revisited—a disorder of sodium reabsorption in the distal tubule. N Engl J Med 1994; 330: 178–181.
81. Shimkets RA, Warnock DG, Bositis CM, et al. Liddle's syndrome: heritable human hypertension caused by mutations in the b-subunit of the epithelial sodium channel. Cell 1994; 79: 407–414.
82. Stein JH. The pathogenetic spectrum of Bartter's syndrome. Kidney Int. 1985; 28: 85–93.
83. Sutton RAL, Mavichak V, Halabe A, et al. Bartter's syndrome: evidence suggested a distal tubular defect in a hypocalciuric variant of the syndrome. Miner Electrolyte Metab 1992; 18: 43–51.

7

Zinc

JOHN K. CHESTERS
Rowett Research Institute, Bucksburn, Aberdeen, Scotland

I. INTRODUCTION AND HISTORY

Although the presence of zinc in animal tissues had been known since the end of the nineteenth century, clear evidence of a biological function for zinc was not available until 1934, when the effects of an experimental zinc deficiency in rats were first described (1). Furthermore, it took another 20 years before naturally occurring zinc deficiency was recognized as the cause of parakeratotic lesions of the skin of pigs (2); then, shortly afterwards, lack of zinc was shown to result in poor growth, feathering, and skeletal development in poultry (3,4).

Clinical deficiency of zinc was first diagnosed in humans in the early 1960s (5), but the extent of naturally occurring zinc deficiency in the human is still controversial—largely because of a dearth of satisfactory indicators of zinc status (6). However, overt deficiencies of zinc have been found repeatedly in association with the use of highly purified solutions for intravenous nutrition (7), and in 1974, the rare inherited disease acrodermatitis enteropathica was related to an inability to absorb adequate zinc from normal diets (8).

In 1939, recognition of zinc as an integral component of the enzyme carbonic anhydrase established the first biochemical role for zinc (9). Subsequently, numerous other zinc enzymes have been discovered (10), and recently a second group of zinc proteins, probably more numerous than the zinc enzymes, have been shown to function as transcription factors (11).

The earliest clinical studies identified the common manifestations of dietary zinc deficiency as reduction in growth and the appearance of skin lesions. More recent biochemical studies have provided a plethora of potential candidates for the underlying causes of these clinical signs of the deficiency, and many of these have been studied extensively (12). However, none of the known functions of zinc has yet been linked directly to the clinical symptoms, and there is still plenty of scope for further research into the fundamental roles of zinc in animals.

II. CHEMICAL PROPERTIES OF ZINC

Zinc is a group IIb metal with a completed d subshell. As such, it possesses only one oxidation state in biological systems and is thus distinguished from the remaining cationic essential trace metals. The lack of unpaired electrons and a complete $3d$ shell make its detection by physicochemical techniques difficult, and this delayed recognition of its importance in biology. It is present in biological systems as the divalent cation but very little as the free ion, the vast majority being complexed to organic ligands. The latter are mainly proteins and amino acids, preferred ligands being cysteine and histidine, but in a number of enzymes glutamate and aspartate also contribute to zinc binding (12). Zinc is often present in tetrahedral coordination, but it can also adopt square pyramidal, trigonal bipyramidal, and octahedral geometries with five and six ligands. Frequently, one of the ligands is a water molecule, which is activated by its environment to take part in the catalytic activity of an enzyme.

III. ANALYTICAL METHODS

A. Contamination

In addition to the usual problems of sample contamination when dealing with analytes present in only trace amounts, there has been a long history of specific contamination of samples with zinc. The major source of this problem is the very high concentration of zinc found in rubber. Common sources of contamination are rubber stoppers for evacuated blood collection tubes (13), bladder catheters made from latex rubber (14), and sealing gaskets in ultrafiltration apparatus (15). Silicon rubber is often a useful alternative, since it is essentially devoid of exchangeable zinc.

B. Estimation of Total Zinc

Table 1 lists a number of analytical techniques of varying sensitivity for estimating the zinc content of biological samples. However, atomic absorption is the method against which others are normally assessed (16). It is highly specific, sensitive, and subject to few interferences, but it requires specialized equipment and has a relatively narrow response range of not more than two orders of magnitude. For some samples, preparation may be minimal. Simple dilution of plasma or serum samples approximately fourfold with a suitable aqueous solution permits estimation of zinc by direct flame atomic absorption (17,18). However, for solid samples and for various other liquid samples, prior treatment to reduce organic matter is often necessary. This may be achieved by dry ashing or by wet digestion using strong acids. With zinc, there is a risk of elemental loss if dry ashing is performed at temperatures in excess of 400–450°C (32–34). Generally, a mixture of acids is used for wet ashing (35). Great care must be exercised when ashing samples that are rich in lipid or that contain perchloric acid, as there is a risk of sudden violent oxidation. Flame atomic absorption has a lower limit of useful sensitivity of about 25 μg zinc/L, but much lower detection limits are readily obtainable with various electrothermal atomic absorption systems. These use very small samples which are atomized directly into the beam of the

TABLE 1 Analytical Methods

Method	Working limit[a] (μg/L)	Advantages	Disadvantages	Refs.
Flame atomic absorption	25	Specific	Requires specialist equipment	16–18
Electrothermal atomic absorption	0.5	Specific Very sensitive	Requires specialist equipment	19,20
Spectrophotometry	100	Simple apparatus	Low sensitivity and specificity	21,22
ICP emission spectroscopy	5	Multielement analysis	Expensive equipment	23
Neutron activation	Depends on neutron flux	Multielement analysis Can yield isotope ratios	Requires nuclear reactor	24–29
Mass spectroscopy	5	Can yield isotope ratios	Expensive equipment	30–32

[a]These are not detection limits, but rather attempts to indicate minimum concentrations which can be estimated with confidence under practical conditions.

atomic absorption instrument. Zinc concentrations below 1 μg/L can be determined, and problems are more likely to arise from sample contamination than from lack of sensitivity (19).

C. Ionic and Ultrafilterable Zinc

Estimation of ionic zinc is a highly desirable objective which has previously proved elusive but which may now be becoming feasible with the development of fluorescent probes such as MagFura II. Estimation of zinc present in low-molecular-weight complexes may prove a useful alternative to measuring free ionic zinc (15).

IV. METABOLISM

A. General

Figure 1 presents an overview of zinc kinetics in the human. The human body contains about 2–2.5 g of zinc, approximately 55% of this being located in muscle and 30% in bone, with the rest fairly evenly distributed among the other tissues (37). Kinetic measurements of zinc such as those in Figure 1 underestimate the total body content by 20–30%, the difference probably representing zinc with a very slow turnover (36). Thus, much of the zinc in bone is probably associated with the bone mineral being incorporated into bone during ossification (38). Physiologic stores of zinc are very limited, particularly in the rat, and growth failure associated with zinc deficiency occurs before any major reduction in zinc concentration other than in plasma. However, prolonged deficiency releases a significant quantity of zinc from bone (38), and stimulation of bone resorption by feeding of a low-calcium diet during early pregnancy has been shown to liberate sufficient zinc to prevent fetal abnormalities (39,40).

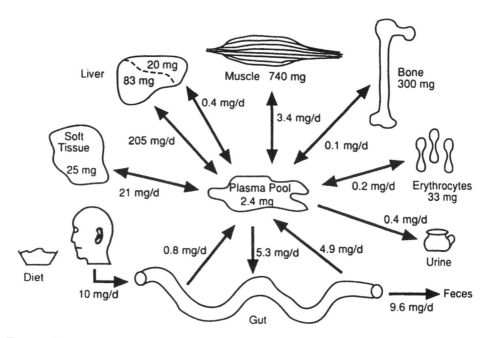

FIGURE 1 Exchangeable zinc in humans. The figure illustrates the daily fluxes of zinc between the gut and the pool in rapid equilibrium with plasma. It also presents both the size of those zinc pools within the body, which show appreciable exchange of zinc with plasma within a period of 9 months, and the fluxes of zinc from these pools to that in rapid equilibrium with plasma. The data are based on those in Ref. 35.

B.   Absorption

Despite widespread agreement that zinc homeostasis is achieved largely through metabolic controls acting on the gut, the nature of these controls and the mechanism by which homeostasis is achieved remain substantially unresolved (41,42).

1.   Sites of Absorption

The site(s) of absorption of zinc have been investigated by studying zinc uptake from portions of gut isolated by ligation (43,44), by intestinal perfusion at a range of sites (45,46), and by following the loss of [65]Zn injected at sites between the pylorus and caecum (47). Neither the stomach nor the caecum and colon appear to contribute significantly to zinc absorption (42). However, ligation of the gut restricts the flow of digesta and the subjects used with the other techniques were fasted, which has been shown to increase the efficiency of zinc absorption (31). Unambiguous evidence on the relative contributions of the different regions of the small intestine to zinc absorption in the normal-fed animal still needs to be obtained.

2.   Mucosal Entry

The intestinal mucosa is covered on its luminal surface by a layer of mucus, the glycocalyx. Fasting increased both its quantity and the proportion of an intragastric dose of zinc which bound to it in the duodenum (48), but whether it acts as a barrier to absorption or as a store for zinc awaiting absorption remains unknown.

At least two components of zinc uptake have been identified in isolated brush border membrane vesicles (49–51). One showed saturation kinetics with a K_m of 70–350 μM (40,49,52), comparable to normal intraluminal zinc concentrations which range from 50 to 150 μM following a meal (46,53). The second responded linearly to zinc concentrations up to 2 mM (50,54), and is probably a minor contributor under physiologic conditions. Studies with isolated, doubly perfused rat guts suggested that the saturable component of mucosal uptake has a K_m between 30 and 55 μM (55,56). Some of the variation in the above estimates of K_m probably arose from the difficulties of deconvoluting the absorption curves into saturable and nonsaturable components (Fig. 2). Dietary deficiency of zinc did not alter the affinity of the isolated membranes for zinc, but increased the maximum capacity of the saturable carrier twofold (49). Similarly, uptake of zinc from the lumen of Zn-deficient rats was substantially greater than that in controls, suggesting that mucosal uptake acts as a major site for homeostatic regulation of zinc (45,55,56).

3. Regulation Within the Mucosa

Zinc uptake into the circulation appears to involve two pools, one mediating rapid transfer to the blood and the other exchanging with the endogenous zinc of the mucosa and thereby resulting in a slower transfer to the circulation (45,46). Transfer of the mucosal [65]Zn to the circulation was increased by dietary zinc deficiency, but inability to determine its specific activity meant that the relative sizes of the zinc fluxes from the control and zinc-deficient guts could not be estimated (56,57). However, the fractional turnover rate of the Zn-deficient mucosal to vascular pool was substantially greater than that observed with control tissue (Table 2). Plasma zinc concentration per se does not seem to affect the transfer of zinc from the mucosa to the vasculature. Thus, Zn-deficient rats given an i.p. injection of zinc 6 h before absorption was measured had highly elevated zinc concentrations in both plasma and mucosa but still absorbed as much zinc as noninjected rats (46). Furthermore, injection of rats with interleukin-1 depressed plasma zinc by 70% but did not alter zinc absorption (58).

The nature and importance of the pools of zinc within the mucosa have been the

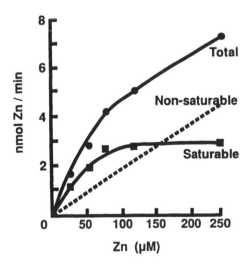

FIGURE 2 Zinc absorption by the doubly perfused Zn-deficient rat small intestine deconvoluted into the saturable and nonsaturable components. (Based on Ref. 55.)

TABLE 2   Mucosal Metallothionein: Rate of Zinc Uptake by Mucosa and Fractional Turnover Rate of Mucosal to Vascular Transfer Pool in Perfused Rat Guts

Rat	Metallothionein (μg/g)	Luminal to mucosal transfer (%/h)	Fractional turnover rate of mucosal to vascular pool (x/h)
Control	19.0	34	2.3
Zn-deficient	12.8	64	3.8
Fasted	28.8	46	0.8

Based on Ref. 57.

subject of extensive investigation and debate. High dietary zinc concentrations can induce gut metallothionein (see below), which has been postulated to sequester zinc and thereby prevent toxic levels of the metal entering the circulation (57,59). However, the initial evidence for this hypothesis related to absorption of ^{65}Zn and an alternative explanation has been proposed based on variations in ^{65}Zn specific activity rather than zinc flux (60,61). Recently, a cysteine-rich protein (CRIP) which binds zinc but is not metallothionein has been isolated from rat small intestine (62,63). At low doses of zinc, ^{65}Zn absorbed from the gut initially accumulated preferentially on CRIP, but at higher intakes or when intestinal metallothionein was induced by peritoneal injection of zinc, the fraction of label on metallothionein increased at the expense of that on CRIP (62). In Zn-deficient rats, the proportion of zinc absorbed into the circulation increased substantially, and this was associated with a high proportion of newly absorbed mucosal zinc on CRIP with little on metallothionein (Fig. 3) (64). CRIP therefore exhibits the properties expected of an intramucosal zinc carrier, facilitating transfer of zinc from the brush border to the basolateral membranes. It seems likely that metallothionein and CRIP compete for newly absorbed zinc and that the final balance depends both on the instantaneous flux of zinc through the cells and on the extent to which metallothionein has previously been induced.

4.   Biological Availability

Numerous factors influence the extent to which dietary zinc is absorbed into the circulation and the proportion of the absorbed zinc which is rapidly reexcreted into the gut. The latter can be estimated by determining the loss of labeled zinc given parenterally (47,65–67). Estimation of the fraction absorbed initially requires isotopic labeling of the dietary zinc. Only rarely has the label been incorporated naturally into the food items being investigated (intrinsic labeling). More commonly, labeled inorganic zinc has been added to the diet (extrinsic labeling), on the presumption that the fate of the added zinc will match that of the endogenous metal. With milk-based diets, extrinsic labeling has generally proved satisfactory (68–70). However, with other dietary ingredients, significant differences have been found between intrinsic and extrinsic labels (71–75).

Although reference is often made to the biological availability of zinc from particular diets, this is not an intrinsic property of the diet. Thus stimulation of anabolism by i.p. injection of a Zn-free nutrient solution into fasted rats increased net zinc absorption by more than 40% (67). Furthermore, the zinc status of the animal can alter the efficiency of zinc absorption from a diet. In human studies, onset of low zinc status was accompanied by a compensatory doubling in the efficiency of zinc absorption from a given diet (32,76), which was also shown to depend on the age of the subject (32). Biological availability is

LUMEN   MUCOSA   PLASMA

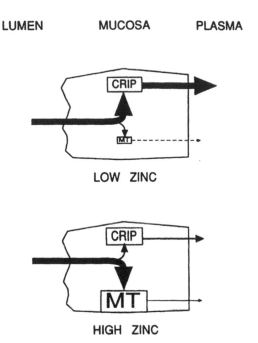

FIGURE 3   Diagrammatic representation of the roles of cysteine-rich intestinal protein (CRIP) and metallothionein (MT) in the transfer of labeled zinc from the gut lumen to plasma in animals offered either a low- or a high-zinc diet. The sizes of the boxes indicate the relative sizes of the zinc pools associated with these two proteins in the mucosa. The thicknesses of the arrows indicate the extent of the initial channeling of the labeled zinc into and through these pools. (Based on Ref. 64.)

therefore a composite of all the factors which influence absorption and is not independent of the test animal.

Milk provides a simple and important whole diet in which the factors influencing zinc availability may be assessed, yet these factors have engendered intense debate. Recognition that a failure to absorb adequate zinc underlies the rare inherited disease, acrodermatitis enteropathica, stimulated interest in the availability of zinc to humans from different milks (8). Symptoms of the disease are rarely manifest while babies are still receiving human milk, but appear abruptly when the infants are transferred to diets based on cows' milk. There seems little doubt that zinc is more available to people from human milk than from cows' milk, even in normal subjects (77,78). However, this difference has been variously attributed to picolinate (79), citrate (80), and the content and type of casein (81–83). Lactoferrin has also been both postulated and discounted as having a role in zinc uptake from human milk (84–86).

In solid diets, fiber has been proposed to influence zinc availability, but the experimental observations are inconsistent (87–92). Probably "fiber" is too broad a category to expect consistent effects, and studies of more precisely defined ingredients will be needed. Undoubtedly, the clearest evidence of a dietary ingredient influencing zinc availability relates to the polyphosphoinositols or phytic acids commonly found in plants. Recent studies have indicated that probably only the hexa- and pentaphosphate derivatives of inositol are relevant to zinc absorption (93), but these can produce profound effects in nonruminants (94–96). Insoluble and thus nonavailable calcium–zinc–phytate complexes are formed, and the availability of zinc from diets containing phytate depends not only on the concentration of the latter but also on that of calcium (94,96,97). Initially this relationship was expressed as a critical molar ratio of phytate/zinc, values exceeding about 15 being considered to indicate a risk of reduced zinc absorption (98,99). However, the importance of the dietary calcium concentration had been recognized in the early studies (94), and eventually this led to the derivation of a composite ratio including calcium, zinc, and phytate (97). Using data from at least 40 experiments in which effects of dietary calcium, zinc, and phytate on growth had been reported, effects on growth could be predicted from the ratio

$$\frac{(\text{Calcium}) \times (\text{phytate})}{(\text{Zinc})}$$

where the constituents are expressed as moles per kilogram diet. Ratios in excess of 3.5 were associated with a significant reduction in growth rate (Fig. 4).

In practical diets, phytate and fiber are often closely associated, but most evidence suggests that it is the phytate content which influences zinc availability (100,101). The actual content of phytate in a particular diet depends not only on the nature of the raw ingredients but also on their preparation. Thus, leavening of bread and exposure to wet heat lower phytate content and significantly increase zinc availability (102–104). However, although phytate is generally the main factor influencing zinc availability from plant sources, a recent study indicated that another agent is probably also contributing to the low availability of zinc from beans (105).

C. Transport

1. Carriers

Albumin is generally thought to be the major zinc transport protein in blood. During gel exclusion chromatography of plasma or serum, about 60–70% of plasma zinc cochromato-

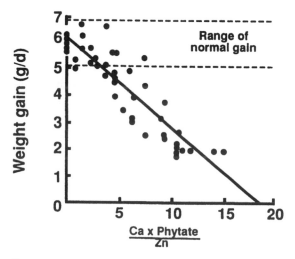

FIGURE 4   Relationship between the rate of weight gain of young rats and the dietary calcium-zinc-phytate molar ratio. The data presented are a compilation of published experiments and were initially presented in Ref. 97.

graphs with albumin and 30% with high-molecular-weight proteins (106,107). Zinc binds to albumin at a number of similar sites through tetrahedral ligation to sulfur atoms (108), and since albumin is generally present at 30- to 40-fold molar excess with respect to the zinc, competition for sites is minimal. The affinity constant for the albumin–zinc complex has been estimated to be about 10^7 M, which allows ready exchange of zinc with other components of plasma (109).

The majority of the zinc that is not bound to albumin is present in a high-molecular-weight fraction and was initially reported to be associated in human plasma with α-2-macroglobulin, to which it bound firmly (106). However, in both porcine (110) and rat (111) plasma, the high-molecular-weight zinc was found to exchange with other plasma proteins. It appears that in certain species there is either another high-molecular-weight component in plasma with a significant capacity to bind zinc, or the zinc on human α-2-macroglobulin is more firmly bound than that of other species.

Transferrin has been reported to transport zinc in plasma, especially in the portal circulation (112). However, in a vascularly perfused rat gut preparation, saturation of transferrin in the perfusate with iron failed to influence zinc absorption (113), and in experiments designed to mimic conditions in plasma, zinc was shown to bind preferentially to albumin rather than transferrin (110,114). The competition for zinc between transferrin and albumin has been subjected to computer modeling with conflicting results (30,110, 115), but on balance, it seems likely that the majority of exchangeable zinc in plasma is bound to albumin.

Ultrafilterable zinc probably accounts for between 0.5% and 2% of total plasma zinc, accurate estimates being difficult to obtain because the filtration apparatus often has an appreciable affinity for zinc. Computer simulation suggests that most of this zinc is present in various complexes with the amino acids cysteine and histidine (116). The free zinc concentration in plasma has been estimated by computer simulation (117,118) and by enzymatic methods (119) to be about 1 nM, while intracellular ionic zinc was reported as 3 nM (120).

2. Kinetics

Plasma contains only about 0.1% of the total zinc of the body, and substantial changes in plasma zinc concentration do not necessarily reflect significant alterations in the body's zinc economy. However, plasma provides the medium for zinc transport around the body, and the kinetics of zinc flux in an animal have been investigated by introduction into the blood of a dose of labeled zinc. Deconvolution of the disappearance curve of labeled zinc from blood yields a number of exponential functions considered to represent the loss and return of zinc from separate body pools (Fig. 1). The loss of labeled zinc in urine and feces can also be measured, and in certain pioneering studies of [69m]Zn in the human, the appearance and loss of activity in liver and thigh muscle were followed by external counting (121).

The kinetics of loss of zinc from plasma have generally been resolved into either two or four exponential components (111,121–124). Although they are interesting, the biological relevance of these equations and the theoretical pools which they characterize become increasingly difficult to assess as the number of pools detected increases. Several reports have concentrated on the early period after zinc injection, when the experimental data approximate to a two-term exponential equation. This has provided a useful insight into the relative effects of dietary deficiency and stress in reducing plasma zinc concentration (111,122,123), but assumptions have to be made even with this simplified system. Figure 5 illustrates two possible two-pool models. Loss of zinc from the second pool to other tissues

(a)

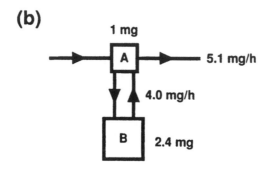

(b)

FIGURE 5 Alternative models for zinc flux through a two-pool system. In model (a), loss of zinc from the system occurs through pool B, whereas in (b) zinc is lost directly from pool A. The size of pool A and flux of zinc from it are the same in both models, but the equivalent values for B are totally dependent on the model. The data presented are based on an individual pig from the experiments reported in Ref. 122.

may be either direct or via return to the initial pool. Theoretical consideration of these models indicates that, even for the same disappearance curve from plasma, the calculated relative sizes of the first and second pools will differ significantly depending on the model chosen (125). Therefore, attempts to fit model data to biological entities may in practice be constrained by prior conceptions of their biological relevance. One group, however, has greatly extended these models for the human by taking into account data for plasma, erythrocytes, liver, muscle, and gut as well as urinary and fecal losses (Fig. 1) (121).

In pigs (122) and in rats (111), dietary zinc deficiency decreased the quantity of zinc in both the first and second pools but did not alter their fractional turnover rates. In the pigs, the effects of endotoxin stress on zinc kinetics assessed at the time of maximal depression of plasma zinc concentration were indistinguishable from those produced by dietary deficiency of zinc. In contrast, the sizes of both zinc pools were increased in the endotoxin-treated rats, but these were assessed 24 h after endotoxin injection—at a time when the maximum effect on plasma zinc concentration would have been past (126). The fraction of total body zinc equilibrating with the labile plasma pool during the first 90 min was less than 1% in pigs (122) and only about 10% in rats (124) and humans (121) 4 or 5 days after injection with labeled zinc. If readily exchangeable zinc is crucial for growth, the observations that it makes such a small contribution to total zinc and the substantial decrease in this component in the deficient animal help to explain how a remarkably slight reduction in whole-body zinc content in Zn-deficient rats can result in total growth failure.

D. Cellular Uptake and Storage

Zinc uptake by the liver contributes significantly to the regulation of overall zinc flux both by sequestering newly absorbed zinc (121,127) and by removing zinc from the circulation in response to stress (125). In cultured hepatocytes, zinc uptake is a two-stage process involving a rapid saturable phase followed by a slower linear accumulation (128–130). The initial uptake is temperature-dependent and stimulated by glucocorticoids but not by sex hormones, aldosterone, insulin, growth hormone, ACTH, T3, or prostaglandins (131). Furthermore, the concentrations of glucocorticoid required for maximal stimulation are within the normal physiologic range. Glucocorticoid-stimulated uptake corresponds with de-novo induction of the synthesis of metallothionein, to which most of the extra zinc is bound.

Metallothionein is a protein with a molecular weight of approximately 6200, contains about 30% cysteine residues, and can bind 7 g atoms of zinc/mol. Although it is present in most tissues, it is particularly concentrated in liver, kidney, pancreas, and intestine, with especially high concentrations in the fetus and neonate. Tissue concentrations of metallothionein vary with zinc supply, being virtually nondetectable in Zn-deficient animals and increasing when induced by oral or parenteral loading with zinc (59,132). Metallothionein appears to act as a temporary store for zinc, particularly when the element is present in excess over immediate requirements. The mechanisms of its induction by zinc and by hormonal stimulation are considered in Section VI.C.

Zinc uptake has also been investigated with fibroblasts (133,134), proximal tubule cells of the kidney (135), and lymphocytes (136,137). As with hepatocytes, each of these cell types exhibited a biphasic uptake, with initial saturable and subsequent linear accumulation. Fibroblast uptake was temperature-sensitive and inhibited by N-ethyl maleimide and dithioerythritol, suggesting an involvement of thiol groups, but was unaffected by metabolic inhibitors which reduced intracellular ATP (133,138).

The form of zinc involved in transmembrane uptake remains uncertain. Ionic zinc (134), a calcitonin-dependent form (137), and transferrin-bound zinc (136) have all been implicated. α-2-Macroglobulin does not seem to be involved (134). Although the data quoted above suggest that transferrin is unlikely to be a major carrier of zinc in plasma, it is interesting that uptake of zinc by erythrocytes appears to be an anionic process that depends on bicarbonate ions (120,139). These have also been shown to be critical for zinc binding to transferrin (115), and the possibility exists that an anionic complex of zinc with both bicarbonate and transferrin is involved in transmembrane transport. Such a role for transferrin would be compatible with the ability of inorganic iron to inhibit zinc uptake, since the affinity of transferrin for iron is several orders of magnitude greater than that of zinc (115,140).

E. Excretion

Zinc is lost from the body via a number of routes, including hair, sweat, desquamation of skin, bile and pancreatic juices, seminal fluid, and urine, but secretions into the gut and loss of mucosal cells provide the main components of endogenous loss (Table 3) (76,141–144). Interestingly, there appears to be a major enterohepatic circulation of endogenous zinc. The combined secretions from bile and pancreas introduce a significant quantity of Zn into the upper small intestine of the human (145). This underlies the difference in the estimates of total zinc per day returning from plasma to the gut (Fig. 1) and the estimates of daily endogenous loss in feces. The site of reabsorption of this endogenous zinc and whether

TABLE 3 Losses of Endogenous Zinc in Normal and Zn-Depleted Men

Route of loss	Endogenous loss (mg/day)	
	Normal	Depleted
Feces	1.4	0.7
Urine	0.3	0.2
Integument	0.7	ND[a]
Semen (per ejaculation)	0.6	0.3

[a]ND = not determined.
Based on Refs. 76, 141, and 144.

whether it is preferentially absorbed compared with dietary zinc remain unknown. In pigs, the relative contributions of bile and pancreatic secretions to luminal zinc were found to be roughly comparable (142).

F. Homeostasis

Homeostasis of zinc is achieved through a number of mechanisms, but undoubtedly the first level of regulation is at the gut during absorption as discussed in Section IV.B. Zinc deficiency also results in a significant reduction in urinary excretion and in endogenous secretion into the gut (75,123,141,142). With adequate zinc nutrition and relatively normal diets, zinc absorption probably ranges from 20% to 50%, and although it is reduced at high dietary intakes, this is normally insufficient to prevent an elevated total absorption. Thus, a man offered a diet that supplied 110 μmol/day absorbed approximately 50% of the zinc, but when the dietary content was increased fourfold the fractional absorption of zinc decreased by only half (146). However, the extra zinc absorbed was matched by a corresponding increase in endogenous zinc secretion, with essentially no change in the amount of zinc retained. Parenteral administration of zinc indicated that by far the most important route of

TABLE 4 Signs of Zinc Deficiency

Sign	Species	Time to onset
Depressed plasma zinc concentration	Humans, rodents, pigs, ruminants, birds	Very short
Slowed growth	Humans, rodents, pigs, ruminants, birds	Short
Decreased voluntary food intake	Humans, rodents, pigs, ruminants, birds	Short
Excessive salivation	Ruminants	Moderate
Parakeratotic skin lesions	Humans, rodents, pigs, ruminants	Prolonged
Abnormalatities of hoof and horn	Ruminants	Prolonged
Impaired feathering	Birds	Prolonged
Peripheral neuropathy	Rodents, birds	Prolonged
Impaired immune response	Humans, rodents	Prolonged
Testicular malfunction	Humans, rodents, pigs, ruminants	Prolonged
Erythrocyte osmotic fragility	Rodents, pigs	Prolonged

For details see the reviews in Refs. 147–150.

excretion was through endogenous losses to the gut. When diets ranging in zinc content from 5.6 to 141 mg/kg were investigated, true absorption increased steadily but less rapidly than endogenous excretion into the gut, until the latter accounted for almost half the absorbed zinc (143).

V. PHYSIOLOGICAL FUNCTIONS AND PATHOLOGY OF DEFICIENCY

A. Growth and Food Intake

Table 4 lists the signs of zinc deficiency in a range of species. Despite minor variations, the dominant early features in most species are slow growth and depressed food intake. In the young rat, growth virtually ceases within 5 days of introducing a severely deficient diet, mean food intake drops to approximately 60% of normal, and a cyclic pattern of daily intake begins (Fig. 6) (53,151–153). With hygienic housing, the appearance of skin lesions, which are the most characteristic clinical feature of the deficiency in most species, may be delayed in rats for as much as 3–5 weeks.

There has been disagreement regarding the precise relationship between the depressions of growth and food intake in zinc-deficient rats (152,154–156). However, there is little difference in growth rate between deficient rats and individually matched pair-fed controls, and at least part of any growth increment in the controls is likely to be due to more efficient utilization of nutrients associated with "meal eating" (157). Experiments in which the food intake of Zn-deficient rats was normalized by force-feeding indicated that the lack of growth was not solely the result of depressed food intake but arose from an inherent metabolic defect (152,158–160). Investigations of the factors influencing food intake in Zn-deficient rats have implicated energy demand (153), amino acid intake (153,155,161) (Table 5), and brain catecholamines (156,162–164). The cyclic pattern of intake is accompanied by inverse fluctuations in plasma zinc concentration, which appear to result from a fall in plasma zinc following the anabolic demands of a high food intake rather than from an increase in appetite consequent upon a systemic increase in availability of zinc (153). Furthermore, the sizes of meals eaten were not affected by the deficiency, suggesting that short-term control of ingestion was not altered and that cycles of intake result from extended satiety following a normal meal (153).

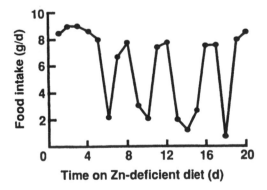

FIGURE 6 Daily food intakes of an individual rat of approximately 80 g transferred to a Zn-deficient diet on day 0.

TABLE 5 Factors Influencing Daily Food Intake by Young Male Rats Weighing 110 g

Dietary modifications	Zn content (mg/kg)	Environmental temperature (°C)	Food intake (g/d)	Food intake (kJ/d)	Cycling[a] (g/d)	Cycling[a] (kJ/d)
Standard						
None	40	22	12.2	229	1.1	21
High fat	40	22	7.5	232	0.8	26
Zn-deficient						
None	<1	22	6.8	128	3.4	64
High fat	<1	22	4.1	127	2.4	74
None	<1	10	13.0		3.7	
40% protein	<1	22	6.8		2.9	
5% protein	<1	22	8.9		1.3	
5% protein + NEAA	<1	22	9.5		1.7	
5% protein + EAA	<1	22	6.4		3.6	
5% protein + Met, Phe, Tyr, Try	<1	22	6.5		2.3	

[a]Cycling was assessed as the standard deviation of day-to-day intake.
The standard diet contained 20% protein, 65% sucrose, 10% lipid, and alterations were compensated by adjusting the sucrose content.
Based on Ref. 153.

In addition to effects on food intake, lack of adequate zinc has been shown to induce abnormalities of taste in both rats and humans (165–167). The combination of effects on intake and taste has led to considerable interest in a possible involvement of zinc in anorexia nervosa (168–171), but further double-blind supplementation trials are needed before any definite conclusions can be drawn.

B. Stress Response

A wide range of factors loosely grouped as stresses decrease the plasma zinc concentration of an animal to about the same extent as severe dietary deficiency of zinc and greatly complicate the diagnosis of inadequate zinc supply (see Sec. VII.A). They include infection (172), bacterial endotoxins (173), surgery (174,175), burns (176,177), and pregnancy (178). This response to stress is initially mediated by a factor originally called leukocyte endogenous mediator (179) and now thought to be interleukin-1 (IL-1). It is associated with increased uptake of zinc principally by liver but also by thymus and bone marrow (180). In the liver, the extra zinc is bound to metallothionein, which may be induced by glucocorticoids in response to stress (see Sec. IV.C). However, the response to IL-1 is more likely mediated through its induction of the synthesis of IL-6, which, unlike IL-1 stimulates zinc uptake by liver cells directly (181). The induction of metallothionein would then result from increased hepatic zinc concentration.

Measurements of zinc flux in endotoxin-treated pigs (122) indicated that stress decreased the passage of zinc through the plasma to an extent comparable to that induced by dietary deficiency of zinc, yet prior to the stress these animals were of normal zinc status (Table 6). However, when the plasma zinc concentration of stressed pigs was maintained in

TABLE 6 Effect of Dietary Zinc Deficiency and Endotoxin
Stress on Pool Sizes and Zinc Flux in Pigs[a]

Animal	Pool A (mg)	Flux A→B (mg/h)	Pool B (mg)	Flux out of B (mg/h)
Control	8.8	0.96	4.8	5.2
Control + endotoxin	4.7	0.44	3.0	3.3
Zn-deficient	4.1	0.23	2.4	2.4

[a]Results were calculated using model (a) in Figure 5.
Based on Ref. 122.

the normal range by i.v. infusion of zinc bound to porcine albumin, 3 of 7 pigs died, whereas comparable pigs infused with saline alone all survived (122). A similar phenomenon has recently been reported with rats (182). These observations suggest that zinc supplementation following stress would not be beneficial. In contrast, the survival of both rats (183) and mice (184) was improved when they were dosed with zinc either shortly before or at the time of administration of endotoxin. Severe trauma can result in significant zinc loss (185), but this is thought to be associated with muscle catabolism and is unlikely per se to induce a reduction in zinc availability (186). There is clearly a need to investigate further the relationship between zinc and stress.

C. Immunology

Virtually every aspect of the immune system may be impaired by dietary zinc deficiency (187–189). T-cell-mediated responses have consistently been found to be defective in Zn-deficient animals (190–193), and inadequate zinc invariably results in atrophy of the thymus (194–197). Many but not all reports suggest that B-cell function is also disrupted (190,191,197–199), and Zn-deficient rats appear to be particularly sensitive to challenge with parasites (200,201). Impaired immune responses in children suffering from kwashiorkor and marasmus have also been shown to respond to zinc supplementation (202,203). Sensitivity of the immune system to lack of zinc extends to its ontogeny. When mice were supplied with Zn-deficient diet from day 7 of pregnancy until parturition, their offspring had markedly lower IgM concentrations than control animals, even though both the dams and their pups were returned to control diets immediately after parturition (204). Furthermore, even in the absence of further exposure to zinc deficiency, this defect extended to the second generation offspring.

In view of the impairment of T-cell function, it is interesting that thymulin, a peptide hormone involved in maintaining thymus integrity, requires zinc for its physiological activity (205,206) and is present in lower quantity or functional activity in Zn-deficient rats (207–210). Recent evidence suggests that a similar effect occurs in humans (211). The impact of zinc deficiency on the individual components of the cellular immune response is less clear. The number of responsive cells undoubtedly decreases with zinc deficiency (197,212,213). However, the magnitude of the response by individual cells may be either unaffected (191,197,214) or decreased (213,215–217). The proportions of T-cell subtypes did not differ between control and Zn-deficient cells, and differences in response were attributable during early zinc deficiency to the altered macrophage function (Table 7) (218). Longer zinc deprivation was required to impair the responsiveness of lymphocytes, prob-

TABLE 7   Effects of the Origin of the Macrophages and T Lymphocytes on Thymidine Incorporation in Recombined Cultures of Cells from 6- or 12-week Zn-Deficient and Pair-Fed Rats

| | | Incorporation (% of 6-week control) T-lymphocyte source | |
		Pair fed	Zn-deficient
6 weeks' deficiency			
Macrophage source	Pair fed	100	98
	Zn-deficient	75	74
12 weeks' deficiency			
Macrophage source	Pair fed	33	22
	Zn-deficient	26	21

Based on Ref. 218.

ably because of their relatively long lifespan. In agreement with this, a previous study showed that at least 4 weeks' repletion was necessary to overcome loss of responsiveness after an extended period of zinc depletion (219).

D. Neurobiology

Although the zinc content of brain as a whole is rather low, certain areas and the hippocampus in particular have appreciably higher concentrations (220,221). In humans the zinc content of the brain has essentially stabilized by the time of parturition, but in the rat it increases significantly during the first 3 weeks of life (222). Postnatal zinc deficiency has relatively little effect on the brain zinc content of rats (223,224), but in pigs it resulted in about a 10–15% reduction in zinc in most regions of the brain (225).

Prenatally, the brain is very sensitive to zinc deprivation. Inadequate zinc in the first third of pregnancy led to fetal abnormalities in rats, many of which were associated with the developing brain and central nervous system (226,227). When the period of zinc deprivation was delayed until the last third of pregnancy or into the suckling period, visible abnormalities of the fetus were absent but brain development was still impaired (228). Brain size and cellularity were decreased (154) and subsequent behavior (227–234) and learning ability disturbed, even though the rats were fed Zn-adequate diets from weaning (230). Similar phenomena were observed in rats maintained on Zn-deficient diets from 30 days of age (231). Despite uncertainties as to the primary or secondary nature of the effects of zinc deprivation on brain function (232), behavioral changes associated with a generalized loss of "well-being" in humans are sufficiently characteristic to have been listed among the syndromes to be expected in cases of human zinc deficiency (149).

A recent study showed that drug binding of hippocampal zinc produced selective disruption of spatial-working memory (233). Hippocampal zinc is concentrated in vesicles within the boutons of the mossy fibers (234–236), where it can attain concentrations of the order of 300 μM. These are too high to be present as ionic zinc, and a cysteine-rich protein very similar in properties to metallothionein has been isolated from the hippocampus and probably acts a temporary store for zinc (237). The zinc in the vesicles is thought to be involved in synaptic function (236,238). Thus, repeated stimulation of the mossy fibers resulted in decreasing synaptic field potentials in Zn-deficient but not in control rats (234). Furthermore, stimulation resulted in release of zinc from hippocampal slices (239), and this zinc was derived at least in part from the mossy fibers (240). Zinc is also involved in the metabolism of the inhibitory neurotransmitter gamma aminobutyric acid (GABA) (237). These observations all point to a role for zinc in modulating nerve conduction in the brain, and recent reports have indicated that the peripheral neuropathy seen in Zn-deficient chickens and guinea pigs is associated with impaired nerve conduction velocities (241, 242). Studies of the effects of zinc deficiency on brain amino acids indicated that lack of zinc may also affect other neurotransmitters. In one set of experiments, zinc deficiency increased tyrosine concentrations in brain (163); but in another, these responded more to level of food intake than to the deficiency (161). Brain catecholamine levels were reported to be either unaffected by the deficiency (161,243) or increased (244). However, the concentrations of neither tryptophan nor serotonin appear to be influenced by lack of zinc (161,163).

Zinc may also have an impact on the brain through its effects on tubulin polymerization. Early studies indicated that zinc could facilitate tubulin polymerization, but the concentrations of zinc used (about 1 mM ionic zinc) were totally nonphysiologic (245). Zinc was shown to bind directly to tubulin but with a relatively high K_d of 110 μM, which is unlikely to be physiologically relevant (246,247). On the other hand, when brain homogenates were cooled to depolymerize the endogenous tubulin and its repolymerization upon rewarming followed, extracts from Zn-deficient brain were slower to polymerize than control extracts (248,249). Addition of zinc to extracts from Zn-deficient brain accelerated polymerization at concentrations around 1 μM (249). This concentration of free zinc is substantially higher than predicted intracellular concentrations (see Sec. IV.C), and a recent study of Zn-deficient chicks and guinea pigs failed to demonstrate any effect on the rate of tubulin polymerization (250). The rate was, however, depressed in extracts from Zn-deficient rat brains, but only to the extent induced by the restricted food intake in pair-fed controls.

E. Reproduction

Studies with rats have provided clear evidence for the importance of zinc in all stages of pregnancy. Rats which had been offered Zn-deficient diet prior to mating failed to conceive (226,251). When rats were transferred to a Zn-deficient diet immediately after mating, a high incidence of fetal abnormalities was observed (226). These included deformities of skull, limbs, brain, eyes, heart, and lungs, and even at the earliest stages of pregnancy abnormalities of blastocyst development were observed (252). The induction of fetal abnormalities is exquisitely sensitive to zinc availability, as even the small variations in zinc availability accompanying the cycles of food intake in deficient dams influenced the incidence of abnormalities induced during the period of tissue differentiation on days 8 and 9 of pregnancy (Table 8) (253). These effects have also been reproduced in 9.5- day embryos cultured for 2 days in vitro (254,255).

Imposition of a low zinc intake during the third trimester did not induce fetal abnormalities, presumably because the main stages of differentiation are already complete, but it did result in low-birth-weight pups (256). Furthermore, parturition was prolonged and difficult, but this could be prevented by providing Zn-supplemented diet from day 19 of pregnancy (257,258). This effect has been associated with irregular and poorly syn-

TABLE 8 Effect of Short-Term Food Intake on the
Induction of Fetal Abnormalities in Pregnant Zn-Deficient
Rats[a]

Pattern of food intake		Period of gestation	
	High	Days 8, 9	Days 6, 7, 10, 11
	Low	Days 6, 7, 10, 11	Days 8, 9
		Abnormalities (% of all fetuses)	
Incomplete flexion		51	1.3
Neural tube defects		32	1.3
Anophthalmia		21	1.3
Heart defects		10	1.3
No forelimbs		26	1.3

[a]Rats were offered Zn-deficient diet in a synchronized cyclical pattern mimicking the natural cycles of intake of Zn-deficient rats.
Based on Ref. 253.

chronized pressure surges in the oxytocin-stimulated uterus, possibly related to fewer myometrial gap junctions in the deficient rats (259,260). Plasma progesterone levels were if anything higher in the Zn-deficient rat near term (261), but there was a delayed increase in 20-α-hydroxysteroid dehydrogenase (259).

Many of the effects of zinc deprivation seen in rats have also been observed in monkeys fed a marginal zinc diet from 1 year before conception (262). When the marginal diet was introduced only following conception, plasma zinc concentrations remained normal during the period of tissue differentiation and no overt fetal abnormalities occurred (263). However, skeletal maturation was delayed, and this resulted in defective mineralization similar to a rachitic syndrome (264).

The relevance of the above effects to human pregnancy is still highly debatable (265). The normal decline in plasma zinc concentration during pregnancy and an absence of satisfactory indicators of zinc status complicate assessment, but in four double-blind zinc supplementation trials, three indicated no effect on birth weight and the fourth, with women at risk of delivering small-for-gestational-age babies, pointed toward a significant benefit (266–269). The latter study was, however, based on too few subjects for firm conclusions to be drawn.

One of the earliest recognized effects of zinc deficiency is an impairment of testicular development and a cessation of spermatogenesis (150,270,271). This is associated with shrinkage of the seminiferous tubules and an early reduction in size of Leydig cells (272–274). Serum testosterone concentrations in rats were reduced in comparison with ad-libitum and pair fed controls, but not with respect to weight-restricted animals (275). Response to pituitary gonadotrophin-releasing hormone was normal (275), but human chorionic gonadotrophin stimulated a much greater increase in testosterone in the weight-restricted than in the Zn-deficient animals. This has been suggested to result from a loss of 3-β-hydroxysteroid dehydrogenase (276) rather than inadequate androgen-binding protein (277). Sperm acquire additional zinc from the seminal fluids during ejaculation (278), and sperm quality as indicated by motility (279,280) and chromatin stability (281,282) depend on the availability of zinc. There appears to be growing evidence that some cases of infertility in human males can be improved by zinc supplementation (279,283).

F. Clinical Significance of Deficiency

In the past, zinc deficiency was relatively common in pigs and poultry fed corn-based rations that were rich in phytic acid, but routine supplementation of rations with zinc has now virtually eliminated the problem. Phytic acid appears to be fully hydrolyzed in the rumen and thus does not present a problem for ruminant nutrition, dietary zinc deficiency occurring only in relatively rare situations where the diet is naturally low in zinc (284).

Severe deficiency of zinc in humans is also uncommon. Acrodermatitis enteropathica [and its bovine equivalent, A46 or Adema disease (285)] is a rare inherited disease which proved fatal until the recognition that it is caused by an impaired ability to absorb zinc and can be totally overcome by zinc supplementation (8). Zinc deficiency has been encountered sporadically where patients have been maintained on total parenteral nutrition with highly purified solutions which lacked adequate zinc (7,286). There have also been at least seven reports of zinc deficiency in young, often premature, infants, who either received insufficient zinc in their mother's milk or had not yet developed the ability to absorb adequate amounts from milk (287–293). In mice there is a mutant strain, lethal milk (lm), in which low zinc in the milk of the homozygous dam proves fatal to the offspring (294,295).

A beneficial response to zinc has been obtained in a number of other clinical conditions, including protein energy malnutrition (202,296) and patients with Crohn's disease (297). Less severe manifestations of the deficiency are thought to retard growth in at least a subgroup of the general population, and in about a third of subjects suffering from loss of taste acuity, zinc supplementation proved beneficial (186).

The clinical importance of zinc as a stimulant to wound healing has a long and mixed pedigree dating back to the ancient Egyptians (298). Following a more recent report of improved wound healing after oral zinc supplementation (299), numerous other studies produced conflicting results (298,300). The general consensus seems to be that supplementation with zinc is beneficial only when the patient or tissue has below-normal physiologic levels of available zinc. However, it has been emphasized that such situations may be more common than was previously supposed (298).

VI. BIOCHEMICAL FUNCTIONS

A. Zinc Enzymes

There are known to be many enzymes that require zinc, precisely how many depending in part on whether similar enzymes from different species are counted individually or as a group. They have been shown to catalyze at least 50 separate reactions, and zinc is unique among the trace elements in that Zn-containing enzymes are present in all six Enzyme Commission classes (12). The functions of zinc in these enzymes have been subdivided into catalytic, coactive (cocatalytic), and structural (Fig. 7). Catalytic zinc atoms are typically coordinated with three protein amino acid side chains and a water molecule involved in the enzyme's catalytic function (Fig. 8). The most common amino acid to act as a ligand at a catalytic site is histidine, followed by glutamic and aspartic acids (Table 9) (301). Most zinc enzymes appear to have two of the ligand groups provided by amino acids separated from each other by only 1–3 residues in the polypeptide chain. The third protein-derived ligand

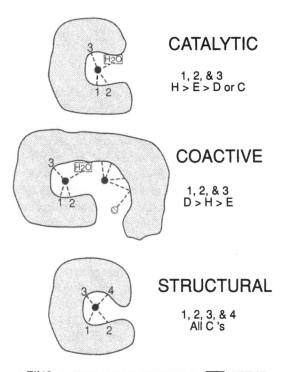

● ZINC   ◎ ZINC OR MAGNESIUM   H2O WATER

FIGURE 7 Diagrammatic representation of the different forms of ligation of zinc within zinc proteins. (Based on Ref. 12.)

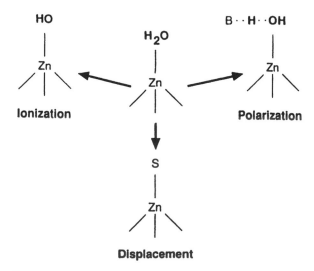

FIGURE 8 Schematic of the functions of the water molecule in the active zinc sites of zinc enzymes. S, substrate; B, amino acid base. Activation of the site involves ionization, polarization, or displacement of the water molecule. (Based on Ref. 301.)

is generally situated at a considerable distance from the other two in the linear amino acid sequence of the protein (11). It is suggested that the first two ligands provide an "anchor" for the zinc atom, while the flexibility of positioning of the third ligand allows adjustment of the active site to provide specificity for its substrate. Only rarely does cysteine participate in zinc ligation at a catalytic site, but it is the most common ligand where the zinc functions to provide structural stability to the protein (Table 9) (12). Coactive zinc atoms are relatively unusual and involve two zinc atoms at the active site, only one of which is essential for enzyme activity. Such a situation is present in phospholipase C (302) and alkaline phosphatase (303,304).

The zinc enzymes have been further subdivided on the basis of their affinity for the metal into zinc-activated enzymes which are readily dissociated from the metal (305,306), and zinc metalloenzymes which bind zinc firmly and probably constitute the majority of Zn-dependent enzymes (303). However, there are intermediate forms such as α-mannosidase, which retains zinc avidly at pH 7 and above but is inactive at this pH. Lowering the pH activates the enzyme but decreases its affinity for zinc, which is still, however, essential for its activity (307). With certain zinc metalloenzymes it has proved possible to replace the zinc atom with cobalt, the spectral and paramagnetic properties of which have allowed the geometry of the active sites to be investigated (10). These studies indicated that, unlike atoms occupying a structural role, the ligand geometries at active sites appear to be distorted (308). It has been suggested that this distortion introduces strains within the site which are conducive to its catalytic function, and the metal atoms subjected to these forces are said to be in an "entatic" state (309,310). This hypothesis is supported by the observations that binding of inhibitors and alterations in pH which inactivate these enzymes often result in loss of the distorted geometry of the binding site (303,310). However, as indicated above, the chemistry of zinc prevents this type of investigation being performed on the native enzyme, and the possibility remains that at least some of the strained configurations observed have been introduced along with the cobalt atoms.

TABLE 9 Amino Acids Acting as Zinc Ligands in Zinc Enzymes and Metalloproteins

Protein	Ligands
Catalytic Zn	
Alcohol dehydrogenase	Cys (2), His (1)
Carboxypeptidase A	Glu (1), His (2)
Thermolysin	Glu (1), His (2)
β-lactamase	His (3)
Phospholipase C	Glu (1), His (2)
Alkaline phosphatase	Asp (1), His (2)
Carbonic anhydrase	His (3)
Structural Zn	
Aspartate transcarbamylase	Cys (4)
TFIIIA	Cys (2), His (2)
Steroid receptor	Cys (4)
Protein kinase C	Cys (3), His (1)
Alcohol dehydrogenase	Cys (4)

Based on Ref. 12.

With so many known zinc enzymes, a plausible hypothesis for the failure of growth that is characteristic of Zn-deficient animals would be a functional inadequacy of one or more of them. Many zinc enzymes, including several dehydrogenases, show tissue-specific decreases in activity in Zn-deficient rats (311,312). Some, such as plasma alkaline phosphatase, rapidly decline in activity when rats are transferred to a Zn-deficient diet (313) and have been suggested to have diagnostic potential (314). However, despite numerous investigations, none of the Zn-dependent enzymes has yet been linked directly to the critical function of zinc which influences the growth of animals. Typical of the situation is the observation that while a Zn-deficient diet induced a marked fall in pancreatic carboxypeptidase A activity in rats, digestion and absorption of a radioactive protein by the rats was unaffected (315). Similarly, liver fructose 1,6 bisphosphatase activity decreased to less than half its control activity in Zn-deficient rats, but plasma glucose concentrations were unaffected (316).

B. Growth and Cell Replication

As discussed above, neither the reduction in food intake nor the loss of activity of a Zn-dependent enzyme can explain the lower growth rate of Zn-deficient animals. Early attempts to assess the underlying cause of the failure of growth indicated that DNA synthesis was more severely affected than was protein synthesis (317). Thymidine incorporation was used as a measure of DNA synthesis, and thymidine kinase has subsequently been shown to be influenced by zinc supply (318,319), raising the possibility that DNA synthesis was not affected to the same extent as thymidine incorporation. However, more recent studies have indicated that they were equally affected by lack of zinc (320) and that protein synthesis in vivo was not specifically inhibited by zinc deficiency (321,322), whereas DNA synthesis and cell replication were (160,322). These effects on cell replication were not overcome by supplementation with growth hormone (323), and although IGF1 concentrations were reduced by the deficiency (324), this seemed to relate to the reduction in food intake rather than lack of zinc per se (325).

A similar sensitivity of DNA synthesis to lack of zinc has been observed in cell culture (326–328), and investigations of the timing of the requirement within the cell cycle indicated that a critical period extends from mid-G1 until shortly before the onset of S phase (326,328,329). This is a period leading up to the induction of the enzymes required for DNA synthesis, and experiments have shown that the activities of thymidine kinase, thymidylate synthase, and DNA polymerase decrease to similar extents in the absence of adequate zinc (318,329,330). Furthermore, a lack of zinc in liver resulted in parallel falls in thymidine incorporation and in the number of cells labeled (331). These observations point toward an impaired commitment of individual cells to entry into S phase rather than the specific loss of an individual enzyme activity.

Extensive studies of *Euglena gracilis* have resulted in broadly similar conclusions being drawn (332). When the cells were allowed to grow until they exhausted the zinc in the medium, they arrested in G2 rather than G1; but when they were placed in Zn-deficient medium they also exhibited a requirement for zinc during passage through G1. Certain other features of zinc deficiency in these cells, such as the replacement of histones with an arginine-rich polypeptide and the presence of only a single RNA polymerase, have not been observed in mammalian systems. However, these studies again implicated zinc in alterations of gene expression (333).

C. Differentiation and Change in Gene Expression

The effects of zinc deficiency on DNA synthesis appear to be most easily explained by an inability of the deficient cells to induce the enzymes required for DNA synthesis. This suggests an impaired ability to alter gene expression which was supported by the finding that the reduction in thymidine kinase activity in Zn-deficient cells was associated with an equal fall in the concentration of its mRNA (Table 10) (334). If zinc is required for certain changes in gene expression, lack of zinc might be expected to hinder cell differentiation. This has indeed been observed in the fetal rat, where even transitory loss of adequate zinc resulted in the appearance of fetal abnormalities (336). The parakeratosis characteristic of Zn-deficient skin, buccal mucosa, and esophagus is consistent with slower differentiation of cells migrating from the basal layer (337). Despite a reduced zinc content, the esophagus exhibits an elevated mitotic index probably associated with impaired differentiation of the basal cells allowing continuing replication. Finally, lack of zinc prevented differentiation of cultured myoblasts into myotubes and inhibited to equal extents the associated increases in both creatine kinase activity and its mRNA (Table 10) (335). All these observations suggest that zinc is critically involved in modifying gene expression, which adds particular interest to the recent recognition that an extensive range of transcriptional regulators contain zinc.

D. Transcription Factors

The Zn-dependent transcription factors (Fig. 9) were originally called Zn finger proteins because of the structure of the first to be recognized. This protein, TFIIIA, was shown to

TABLE 10 Effects of Zinc Deprivation on the Activities and mRNA Concentrations of Thymidine Kinase in 3T3 Cells and Creatine Kinase in Chick Myoblasts

	Thymidine kinase	
	Activity (nmol/min/mg protein)	mRNA ratio[a] (TK/ribosomal S6)
Control	ND	0.50
Zn-deprived	0.2	0.03
Zn-repleted	3.3	0.49

	Creatine kinase	
	Activity (units/mg protein)	mRNA ratio[a] (CK/ribosomal S6)
Control	2.4	1.40
Zn-deprived	0.3	0.15
Zn-repleted	2.3	1.20

[a]Enzyme mRNA concentrations were standardized by comparing them to the concentration of the constitutive mRNA for S6 ribosomal protein.
ND = not determined.
Based on Refs. 334 and 335.

bind to an internal region of the 5S ribosomal RNA gene and activate its transcription by RNA polymerase III (338,339). The protein contains a series of polypeptide "loops," each held together at their base by a zinc ion ligated to two cysteine residues on one side of the loop and two histidines on the other (339). The series of "loops" give rise to the term "Zn finger," and the human genome has been estimated to contain around 300 such proteins (11), but it has become clear that they do not form a homogeneous group nor is the original concept of a finger correct (340). Because of the configuration of ligand groups around the zinc ion, the original Zn finger proteins are known as the C2H2 series, and they typically contain three or more similar "fingers." Structural investigations have shown that the "loops" actually contain a hairpinlike zone consisting of two antiparallel beta sheets containing the Zn-binding cysteines plus a C-terminal α-helical region incorporating the two histidines with the helix facing into the major groove of the DNA (Fig. 9) (341,342). Unlike TFIIIA, most of the C2H2 proteins bind to response elements in the upstream promoters of genes transcribed by RNA polymerase II. Transcriptional activation depends on regions outside the Zn-finger DNA-binding zones, but an understanding of the mechanism of activation is only just beginning to emerge. The most extensively studied of the C2H2 proteins, Sp1, often has multiple binding sites within the promoter, and transcriptional activation seems to depend on an interaction between one or more Sp1 molecules and the TATA-box binding protein (343–345).

A second series of transcriptional activators contain zinc, and these were originally classed as Zn finger proteins. They include the nuclear receptors for steroid and thyroid hormones, for retinoids, and for vitamin D (346). However, they always have just two zinc ions per molecule, each of which is coordinated to four cysteine residues (C4 proteins) with an additional cysteine residue located at the C-terminal side of the second "finger" (Fig. 9) (347). Unlike the C2H2 proteins, the two C4 fingers differ substantially in structure (348,349) and interact at right angles to each other to form a rigid structure. The latter is stabilized by the C-terminal finger, with the specificity for DNA binding residing in the N-terminal finger (350–352). This specificity is determined by the amino acids bridging its two C-terminal cysteine residues and those immediately C-terminal to the finger. The proteins generally contain an N-terminal zone involved in transcriptional activation, a central DNA-binding region containing the Zn fingers, and a C-terminal portion responsible for hormone recognition and receptor dimerization (350,352). The receptors interact with the DNA as dimers recognizing response elements which are generally palindromic. The recognition sequences for estrogen and glucocorticoid receptors have comparable spacing of the two halves of the palindrome but differ in sequence, whereas the estrogen and thyroid receptors have identical palindromic sequences but differ in the spacing between them (352).

There is also a third group of transcription factors known to contain zinc. They are all fungal in origin and are typified by the Gal4 transcription factor. Their structure is totally different from the Zn finger proteins, each containing a Zn2Cys6 cluster reminiscent of metallothionein (353).

Metallothioneins encompass a number of different isoforms which vary with species and tissue and have distinctive promoters (Fig. 10) (357,358). Within these promoters are response elements for SP1 and AP1 (thought to be involved in basal levels of synthesis), glucocorticoids, and a series of metal response elements (MRE) (Fig. 10) (359). The interrelationships among these elements can yield complex responses to environmental stimuli, and a recent study of cultured liver cells suggested that "metallothionein was

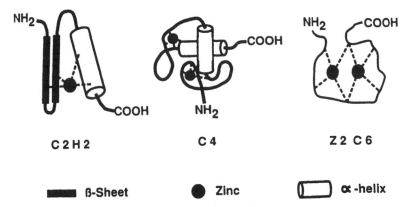

FIGURE 9 Zinc-containing transcription factors. The diagrams illustrate the structures of the zinc-binding sites of the three basic groups of Zn finger proteins. The C_2H_2 proteins contain a series of "fingers" of similar structure shown here diagrammatically. Each contains two antiparallel β sheets and an α helix with the Zn residue coordinated with two cysteine in the β sheets and two histidines in the helical region. The two "fingers" comprising the C4 transcription factors have individual structures which differ from each other, interact at approximately right angels, and each contain a Zn ion coordinated with four cysteine residues. The Gal4 type of transcription factor contains two Zn ions coordinated with six cysteines in a binuclear cluster. The diagrams are based on Refs. 341, 342, 347, and 353.

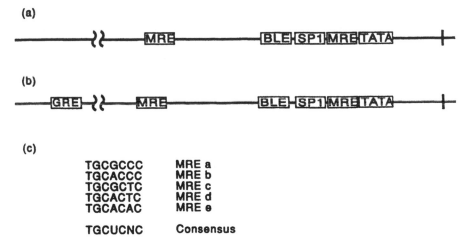

FIGURE 10 Distribution of transcription factor-binding sites within the promoters of (a) human metallothionein-If and (b) human metallothionein-IIa. The locations of response elements for gluco-corticoids (GRE) and metals (MRE) are indicated, together with binding sites for a basal level enhancer (BLE) and for the general transcription factor Sp1. Also marked are the positions of the TATA box and the transcription initiation site, represented by a vertical bar. Part (c) lists the sequences of the five MREs present in the rat metallothionein-I promoter, together with their consensus sequence. (Figure based on Refs. 357 and 358.)

synergistically induced by either a cytokine or a heavy metal with a glucocorticoid hormone and was additively induced by the combination of a cytokine and a heavy metal" (360).

The MREs have a consensus sequence

5'-TGCUCNC-3'

which is sufficient to confer metal responsiveness on heterologous promoters (361). Furthermore, the mouse metallothionein promoter has been used experimentally to provide metal inducible expression of an extensive range of proteins both in cell culture (362) and in transgenic animals (363). The MREs interact with protein(s) which act as transcriptional enhancers and require the presence of a metal, commonly zinc or cadmium, in order to bind to the MRE (364–367). At least one of these proteins appears to be specific for zinc (368).

E. Membrane Stability and Free Radicals

Studies of the interactions between zinc and biological membranes have been comprehensively reviewed (369,370). Membrane fractions from a range of sources contain quite high concentrations of zinc (370), and early studies suggested a role for zinc in the stabilization of membranes (371,372). However, many of these investigations related to ionic zinc added in vitro at concentrations far in excess of those likely to be encountered in vivo. On the other hand, there have been several observations which suggest that zinc deficiency increases the fragility of certain membranes both in vivo and in vitro (370). Some (373,374) but not all (375) reports have suggested that erythrocytes from Zn-deficient animals are osmotically more fragile than those from control animals. Others have observed increased sensitivity of erythrocytes to hemolysis by a range of nonspecific stressors (376).

Zinc has been postulated to protect membranes from oxidative damage by competing for binding sites with redox metals which catalyze oxidation (377). However, superoxide dismutase activities were not altered by zinc deficiency in either erythrocytes (373,375) or liver (378). Conversely, liver microsomes from Zn-deficient rats produced higher concentrations of lipid peroxides than those in control preparations when challenged with NADPH (379). Another report indicated only a trend toward higher free-radical generation by liver microsomes from Zn-deficient rats but significantly increased free-radical production by lung microsomes (380). However, the iron content of the lung microsomes was increased fivefold by zinc deficiency, whereas there was only a twofold increase in the liver. Since Fe^{2+} ions are well known to catalyze free-radical production, the differences in free-radical generation may have been secondary to the changes in iron content. Finally, when rats were exposed to lethal levels of ozone, the survival time of the rats was not decreased by previously deficient zinc intake (381). The physiologic relevance of zinc as a natural antioxidant still requires clarification. Similarly, there have been various reports of zinc involvement in transmembrane signaling events, but the location and identity of the proteins involved remain unknown (370).

VII. NUTRITIONAL ASSESSMENT AND REQUIREMENTS

A. Diagnosis of Deficiency

There have been at least four reviews of the assessment of zinc status since 1987 (314,382–384), but the present situation was summarized in one sentence: "In conclusion, a simple, reliable clinical measure of zinc deficiency is lacking" (384). Table 11 gives a simplified

TABLE 11 Criteria for the Diagnosis of Zinc Deficiency

Criterion	Response	Advantages	Complicating factors	References
Plasma zinc concentration	< 0.5 mg/L, indicative of deficiency	Simple methodology	Equally susceptible to lowering by stresses	122,383,385
Leukocyte zinc concentration	Decreased by deficiency	May better reflect tissue concentrations	Complex methodology Influenced by proportions of leukocyte subtypes	384,386,387
Hair zinc concentration	Decreased by deficiency	Easily sampled Integrative index of status	Very variable Response slight Contamination	314
Plasma thymulin concentration	Decreased by deficiency	Specific for zinc	Complexity of assay	211
Erythrocyte ^{65}Zn uptake	Increased by deficiency	Simple methodology	Requires radioisotope May be affected by stress	384,388,389
Zinc enzymes	Lowered plasma alkaline phosphatase (AP'ase) activity	Easy to assay	AP'ase affected by many other conditions Other enzymes less accessible	314,388
Blood metallothionein concentrations	Lowered by deficiency	Elevated by stress	Complex assay Complicated by Fe or protein deficiency	390–394

overview of techniques which have been considered, but readers should refer to the above reviews for a more detailed treatment of the subject than is attempted here.

Although it is still the main diagnostic parameter, the value of plasma zinc concentration as an indicator of zinc deficiency is very seriously impaired by its response to stress (see Sec. V.B). In uncomplicated deficiency, zinc concentrations below about 0.5 mg/L in serum or plasma are generally associated with a Zn-responsive condition (383). However, there are numerous reports of low plasma or serum values associated with a wide range of infectious diseases or other stressful conditions. Few of these are likely to indicate a situation meriting supplementation with zinc, but a real problem stems from the probability that some might benefit (298) while in other cases extra zinc could prove harmful. A better indicator is sorely needed.

Recently, the increase in ^{65}Zn uptake by Zn-deficient erythrocytes was found to be less susceptible to stress when assayed under standardized conditions (389). Zn-deficient plasma has been shown to contain an inactive form of thymulin that is capable of reactivation in vitro, and the difference in thymulin activity between unmodified and Zn-supplemented plasma may have diagnostic potential (211). In rats, plasma metallothionein concentrations appear to depend largely on those in liver, and thus they decrease in dietary deficiency and increase with stress (390). A low value for both plasma zinc and metallothionein would therefore indicate zinc deficiency, but a low zinc with a high metallothionein content would be characteristic of a stressed animal. A stressed zinc-deficient animal is unable to produce liver metallothionein and would thus be indistinguishable from one suffering from simple zinc deficiency, but the deficiency could still be recognized (393).

Each of these measures may in future provide the basis of an improved index of zinc status. In the meantime, it is clear that both in humans and other animals, growth can be affected without the deficiency being sufficient to induce overt clinical signs (151,395). In practice, confirmation of possible zinc deficiency still rests largely on a response to judicious zinc supplementation. Fortunately, the toxicity of zinc is generally very low, and responses to zinc are normally obtained with only modest supplementation.

B. Requirements

An animal's requirement for zinc tends to be expressed in terms of an adequate concentration in the diet. This may be appropriate where the dietary composition varies little from day to day, but the nature and composition of human diets are more varied and requirements are therefore normally listed as amounts of zinc required per day.

Zinc requirements may be estimated by either empirical or factorial methods. Empirical estimates obtained by investigating a response to increasing supplementation of a particular diet with zinc are truly applicable only to that diet. In contrast, the factorial approach involves summation of all the zinc accretion required for growth and all obligatory losses of zinc to provide a figure for the minimum quantity of zinc needed to be absorbed per day. Although fraught with problems, these calculations can now be achieved with reasonable precision; however, they then have to be converted to dietary requirements by providing an estimation of the biological availability of zinc from the diet.

Some of the numerous factors which influence availability have been considered in Section IV.B. Their significance, however, depends on both the object of the exercise and the extent to which allowance is made for increased efficiencies of absorption from diets that are low in zinc. The object may be to define minimum requirements for assessing when intervention is vital. Alternatively, the object may be to provide an estimate of the intakes desirable to ensure that all normal members of the population have a sufficient zinc intake. Although increased efficiency of uptake at low zinc dietary concentrations has been clearly demonstrated (31,76), there is at present no evidence to indicate whether, as with iodine intake, this is accompanied by undesirable side effects. Consideration must therefore be given to the provision of safety margins in assessing requirements.

In practice, a dietary concentration of zinc of 20 mg/kg dry matter is likely to prove adequate for most animals fed diets lacking specific antagonists of absorption. With nonruminants consuming diets high in phytate and calcium, supplementation to 50 or even 100 mg/kg may prove beneficial and is highly unlikely to prove toxic. The present WHO/FAO estimates of requirement for humans (Table 12) are based on factorial estimates and assume an availability of dietary zinc of 20% with supplementary values for 10% or 40% absorption.

VIII. PHARMACOLOGY AND TOXICITY

For most practical purposes, zinc appears to be nontoxic. Toxicities do occur where metal workers are exposed to zinc fumes or where wet feed or acid drinking water is in prolonged contact with galvanized vessels, but the tolerance of zinc is generally very high (147). Rats show few deleterious effects at dietary concentrations up to about 1000 mg/kg. Above this,

TABLE 12 WHO Recommendations for Zinc Intake by Humans: 1993 Proposals

Age (yr)	Sex	Zn requirement (mg/day) Dietary availability		
		High	Medium	Low
1–6	M & F	4	6	12
6–10	M & F	5	8	15
10–18	M	7	12	24
18–>60	M	6	9	19
10–18	F	6	10	20
18–>60	F	4	7	13
Pregnant, third trimester	F	8	13	27
Lactating 0–3 months	F	8	13	25

Based on Ref. 396.

signs of anemia may appear, mainly as a result of impaired copper availability. Similar considerations probably also apply to pigs and poultry. Certain reports seem to suggest that ruminants may be more at risk of zinc toxicity, particularly when young or pregnant, but others have reported no ill effects from diets containing 500–1000 mg/kg. It is possible that some of their increased sensitivity to zinc relates to direct effects on rumen organisms rather than on the animal itself.

In humans, sporadic cases of toxicity have been reported (397). Excessive supplements of zinc taken alone can cause nausea, vomiting, and diarrhea while chronic ingestion of high doses has been known to result in cooper deficiency, but problems associated with high zinc intake in humans are nevertheless rare.

A. Free Zinc Concentration

One of the prime limitations to understanding zinc metabolism is our inability to measure free zinc concentrations. While these are virtually certain to be no more than nanomolar, they may still be presumed to be the medium through which most Zn-dependent processes compete for available zinc. There are two approaches to their estimation. One involves a theoretical simulation of zinc binding in situations of interest such as plasma. For this the major needs are more biologically relevant estimations of stability constants and a method of incorporating multiligand macromolecules into the simulations. The other approach is through the use of experimental techniques. These must be both specific and sensitive, and because of this, methods based on enzyme activation seem worthy of further consideration.

B. Gene Expression

One of the most exciting areas of zinc metabolism is the apparent convergence of studies aimed at explaining problems with growth and differentiation in Zn-deficient animals with a growing awareness of a whole range of Zn-dependent transcription factors whose metabolic importance and sensitivity to zinc depletion remain largely unknown. The integration of these aspects should prove one of the major areas for research on zinc in the foreseeable future.

C. Cellular Zinc Transport

Another area demanding further study is the mechanism(s) by which passage of zinc across cell membranes is facilitated and regulated, since this in turn determines the balance of zinc within an organism.

D. Neurobiology

Finally, there appear to be a whole class of neurons in which zinc performs some important but as yet ill-defined function. The elucidation of the role of zinc in their physiology and function could be of profound importance to understanding the effects of its deficiency on learning and behavior.

REFERENCES

1. Todd WR, Elvehjem CA, Hart EB. Zinc in the nutrition of the rat. Am J Physiol 1934; 107: 146–156.
2. Tucker HF, Salmon WD. Parakeratosis or zinc deficiency disease in the pig. Proc Soc Exp Biol Med 1955; 88: 613–616.
3. O'Dell BL, Savage JE. Potassium, zinc and distillers dried solubles as supplements to a purified diet. Poultry Sci 1957; 36: 459–460.
4. O'Dell BL, Newberne FM, Savage JE. Significance of dietary zinc for the growing chick. J Nutr 1958; 65: 503–523.
5. Prasad AS, Halsted JA, Nadimi M. Syndrome of iron deficiency anaemia, hepatospleno-megaly, hypogonadism, dwarfism and geophagia. Am J Med 1961; 31: 532–546.
6. White CL. Zinc deficiency in man and animals: endemic or imaginary? Proc Nutr Soc Austr 1992; 17: 115–124.
7. Ortega SS, Cachaza JA, Tovar IV, Feijoo MF. Zinc deficiency dermatitis in parenteral nutrition: an EM study. Dermatologica 1985; 171: 163–169.
8. Moynahan EJ. Acrodermatitis enteropathica: a lethal inherited human zinc-deficiency disor-der. Lancet 1974; ii: 399–400.
9. Keilin D, Mann T. Carbonic anhydrase. Nature 1939; 144: 442–443.
10. Vallee BL, Galdes A. The metallobiochemistry of zinc enzymes. Adv Enzymol 1984; 56: 283–430.
11. Berg JM. Zinc finger domains—hypotheses and current knowledge. Annu Rev Biophys Biophys Chem 1990; 19: 405–421.
12. Vallee BL, Falchuk KH. The biochemical basis of zinc physiology. Physiol Rev 1993; 73: 79–118.
13. de Haan KE, de Groot C, Boxma H, van den Hamer CJ. Zinc contamination due to the collection tube. Clin Chim Acta 1987; 170: 111–112.
14. de Haan KE, Woroniecka UD. Bladder catheters and zinc contamination of urine. Clin Chem 1989; 35: 888.
15. Foote JW, Delves HT. Determination of non-protein-bound zinc in human serum using ultrafiltration and atomic absorption spectrometry with electrothermal atomisation. Analyst 1988; 113: 911–915.
16. Falchuk KH, Hilt KL, Vallee BL. Determination of zinc in biological samples by atomic absorption spectrometry. Meth Enzymol 1988; 158: 422–434.
17. Kelson JR. Criticism of the proposed selected method of direct measurement of zinc in plasma by atomic absorption spectroscopy. Clin Chem 1980; 26: 349–350.
18. Perry DF. Flame atomic absorption spectrometric determination of serum zinc: collaborative study. J Assoc Offic Anal Chem 1990; 73: 619–621.
19. Accominotti M, Pegon Y, Vallon JJ. Determination of zinc in blood serum by electrothermal atomic absorption spectrometry with matrix modification. Clin Chim Acta 1988; 173: 99–106.

20. Arnaud J, Favier A. Determination of ultrafilterable zinc in human milk by electrothermal atomic absorption spectroscopy. Analyst 1992; 117: 1593–1598.

21. Herrador MA, Jimenez AM, Asuero AG. Spectrophotometric determination of zinc in potable water and insulin with methylglyoxal bis(4-phenyl-3-thiosemicarbazone). Analyst 1987; 112: 1237–1246.

22. Makino T. A sensitive, direct colorimetric assay of serum zinc using nitro-PAPS and microwell plates. Clin Chim Acta 1991; 197: 209–220.

23. Chappuis P, Poupon J, Rousselet F. A sequential and simple determination of zinc, copper and aluminium in blood samples by inductively coupled plasma atomic emission spectrometry. Clin Chim Acta 1992; 206: 155–165.

24. Janghorbani M, Young VR. Accurate analysis of stable isotopes ^{68}Zn, ^{70}Zn and ^{58}Fe in human feces with neutron activation analysis. Clin Chim Acta 1980; 108: 9–24.

25. Lavi N, Alfassi ZB. Determination of trace amounts of cadmium, cobalt, chromium, iron, molybdenum, nickel, selenium, titanium, vanadium and zinc in blood and milk by neutron activation analysis. Analyst 1990; 115: 817–822.

26. Gokmen IG, Aras NK, Gordon GE, Wastney ME, Henkin RI. Radiochemical neutron activation analysis of zinc isotopes in human blood, urine, and feces for in vivo tracer experiments. Anal Chem 1989; 61: 2757–2763.

27. Dybczynski R, Aldabbagh SS. Selective separation of zinc from other elements on the amphoteric resin retardion 11A8 and its use for the determination of zinc in biological materials by neutron activation analysis. Analyst 1987; 112: 449–453.

28. Janghorbani M, Young VR. Use of stable isotopes to determine bioavailability of minerals in human diets using the method of fecal monitoring. Am J Clin Nutr 1980; 33: 2021–2031.

29. Lo GS, Steinke FH, Ting BTG, Janghorbani M, Young VR. Comparative measurement of zinc absorption in rats with stable isotope ^{70}Zn and radioisotope ^{65}Zn. J Nutr 1981; 111: 2236–2239.

30. Eagles J, Fairweather-Tait SJ, Portwood DE, Self R, Gotz A, Heumann KG. Comparison of fast atom bombardment mass spectrometry and thermal ionization quadrupole mass spectrometry for the measurement of zinc absorption in human nutrition studies. Anal Chem 1989; 61: 1023–1025.

31. Friel JK, Naake VL Jr, Miller LV, Fennessey PV, Hambidge KM. The analysis of stable isotopes in urine to determine the fractional absorption of zinc. Am J Clin Nutr 1992; 55: 473–477.

32. August D, Janghorbani M, Young VR. Determination of zinc and copper absorption at three dietary Zn-Cu ratios by using stable isotope methods in young adult and elderly subjects. Am J Clin Nutr 1989; 50: 1457–1463.

33. Gorsuch TT. Radiochemical investigation of the recovery for analysis of trace elements in organic and biological materials. Analyst 1959; 84: 135–173.

34. Edward JB, Benfer RA, Morris JS. The effects of dry ashing on the composition of human and animal bone. Biol Trace Elem Res 1990; 25: 219–231.

35. Clegg MS, Keen CL, Lonnerdal B, Hurley LS. Influence of ashing techniques on the analysis of trace elements in animal tissues. I. Wet ashing. Biol Trace Elem Res 1981; 3: 107–115.

36. Wastney ME, Aamodt RL, Rumble WF, Henkin RI. Kinetic analysis of zinc metabolism and its regulation in normal humans. Am J Physiol 1986: 251: R398–R408.

37. Haumont S. Distribution of zinc in bone tissue. J Histochem Cytochem 1961; 9:141–145.

38. Brown ED, Chan C, Smith JC. Bone mineralization during a developing zinc deficiency. Proc Soc Exp Biol Med 1978; 157: 211–214.

39. Hurley LS, Tao S-H Alleviation of teratogenic effects of zinc by simultaneous lack of calcium. Am J Physiol 1972; 222: 322–325.

40. Masters DG, Keen L, Lonnerdal B, Hurley LS. Release of zinc from maternal tissue during zinc deficiency or simultaneous zinc and calcium deficiency in the pregnant rat. J Nutr 1986; 116: 2148–2154.

41. Cousins RJ. Absorption, transport and hepatic metabolism of copper and zinc: special reference to metallothionein and ceruloplasmin. Physiol Rev 1985; 65: 238–309.

42. Lonnerdal B. Intestinal absorption of zinc. In: Mills CF, ed. Zinc in Human Biology. London: Springer-Verlag, 1988: 33.

43. Van Campen DR, Mitchell EA. Absorption of Cu^{64}, Zn^{65}, Mo^{99} and Fe^{59} from ligated segments of the rat gastrointestinal tract. J Nutr 1965; 86: 120–124.

44. Methfessel AH, Spencer H. Zinc metabolism in the rat. I. Intestinal absorption of zinc. J Appl Physiol 1973; 34: 59–62.

45. Antonson DL, Barak AJ, Vanderhoof JA. Determination of the site of zinc absorption in rat small intestine. J Nutr 1979; 109: 142–147.

46. Davies NT. Studies on the absorption of zinc by rat intestine. Br J Nutr 1980; 43: 189–203.

47. Jackson MJ, Jones DA, Edwards RHT. Zinc absorption in the rat. Br J Nutr 1981; 46: 15–27.

48. Quaterman J. A possible role for the glycocalyx in metal absorption. J Physiol 1981; 322: 23.

49. Menard MP, Cousins RJ. Zinc transport by brush border membrane vesicles from rat intestine. J Nutr 1983; 113: 1434–1442.

50. Tacnet F, Watkins DW, Ripoche P. Studies of zinc transport into brush-border membrane vesicles isolated from pig small intestine. Biochim Biophys Acta 1990; 1024: 323–330.

51. Turnbull AJ, Blakeborough P, Thompson RP. The effects of dietary ligands on zinc uptake at the porcine intestinal brush-border membrane. Br J Nutr 1990; 64: 733–741.

52. Blakeborough P, Salter DN. The intestinal transport of zinc studied using brush-border membrane vesicles from the piglet. Br J Nutr 1987; 57: 45–55.

53. Solomons NW, Jacob RA, Pineda O, Viteri F. Studies on the bioavailability of zinc in man. II. Absorption of zinc from organic and inorganic sources. J Lab Clin Med 1979; 94: 335–343.

54. Lee HH, Prasad AS, Brewer GJ, Owyang C. Zinc absorption in human small intestine. Am J Physiol 1989; 256: G87–G91.

55. Steel L, Cousins RJ. Kinetics of zinc absorption by luminally and vascularly perfused rat intestine. Am J Physiol 1985; 248: G46–G53.

56. Hoadley JE, Leinart AS, Cousins RJ. Kinetic analysis of zinc uptake and serosal transfer by vascularly perfused rat intestine. Am J Physiol 1987; 252: G825–G831.

57. Hoadley JE, Leinart AS, Cousins RJ. Relationship of ^{65}Zn absorption kinetics to intestinal metallothionein in rats: effects of zinc depletion and fasting. J Nutr 1988; 118: 497–502.

58. Hempe JM, Carlson JM, Cousins RJ. Intestinal metallothionein gene expression and zinc absorption in rats are zinc-responsive but refractory to dexamethasone and interleukin 1 alpha. J Nutr 1991; 121: 1389–1396.

59. Richards M, Cousins RJ. Mammalian zinc homeostasis: requirement for RNA and metallothionein synthesis. Biochem Biophys Res Commun 1975; 64: 1215–1223.

60. Sugawara N. Role of metallothionein in zinc uptake from rat jejunum. In: Foulkes EC, ed. Biological Roles of Metallothionein. Amsterdam: Elsevier/North Holland, 1982: 151.

61. Flanagan PR, Haist J, Valberg LS. Zinc absorption, intraluminal zinc and intestinal metallothionein levels in zinc-deficient and zinc-replete rodents. J Nutr 1983; 113: 962–972.

62. Hempe JM, Cousins RJ. Cysteine-rich intestinal protein binds zinc during transmucosal zinc transport. Proc Natl Acad Sci (USA) 1991; 88: 9671–9674.

63. Birkenmeier EH, Gordon JI. Developmental regulation of a gene that encodes a cysteine-rich intestinal protein and maps near the murine immunoglobulin heavy chain locus. Proc Natl Acad Sci (USA) 1986; 83: 2516–2520.

64. Hempe JM, Cousins RJ. Cysteine-rich intestinal protein and intestinal metallothionein: an inverse relationship as a conceptual model for zinc absorption in rats. J Nutr 1992; 122: 89–95.

65. Wastney ME, Henkin RI. Calculation of zinc absorption in humans using tracers by fecal monitoring and a compartmental approach. J Nutr 1989; 119: 1438–1443.

66. Heth DA, Hoekstra WG. Zinc-65 absorption and turnover in rats. J Nutr 1965; 85: 367–374.

67. Hallmans G, Nilsson U, Sjostrom R, Wetter L, Wing K. The importance of the body's need for

zinc in determining Zn availability in food: a principle demonstrated in the rat. Br J Nutr 1987; 58: 59–64.

68. Egan CB, Smith FG, Houk RS, Serfass RE. Zinc absorption in women: comparison of intrinsic and extrinsic stable-isotope labels. Am J Clin Nutr 1991; 53: 547–553.

69. Serfass RE, Ziegler EE, Edwards BB, Houk RS. Intrinsic and extrinsic stable isotopic zinc absorption by infants from formulas. J Nutr 1989; 119: 1661–1669.

70. Sandstrom B, Keen CL, Lonnerdal B. An experimental model for studies of zinc bio-availability from milk and infant formulas using extrinsic labeling. Am J Clin Nutr 1983; 38: 420–428.

71. Bedi SPS, Chesters JK. Assessment of the availability of dietary copper and zinc to sheep using radioisotopes. Nutr Rep Int 1982; 25: 277–283.

72. Neathery MW, Lassiter JW, Miller WJ, Gentry RP. Absorption, excretion and tissue distribution of natural organic and inorganic ^{65}Zn in the rat. Proc Soc Exp Biol Med 1975; 149: 1–4.

73. Meyer NR, Stuart MA, Weaver CM. Bioavailability of zinc from defatted soy flour, soy hulls and whole eggs as determined by intrinsic and extrinsic labeling techniques. J Nutr 1983; 113: 1255–1264.

74. Fairweather-Tait SJ, Fox TE, Wharf SG, Eagles J, Crews HM, Massey R. Apparent zinc absorption by rats from foods labeled intrinsically and extrinsically with ^{65}Zn. Br J Nutr 1991; 66: 65–71.

75. Janghorbani M, Istfan NW, Pagounes JO, Steinke FH, Young VR. Absorption of dietary zinc in man: comparison of intrinsic and extrinsic labels using a triple stable isotope method. Am J Clin Nutr 1982; 36: 537–545.

76. Taylor CM, Bacon JR, Aggett PJ, Bremner I. Homeostatic regulation of zinc absorption and endogenous losses in zinc-deprived men. Am J Clin Nutr 1991; 53: 755–763.

77. Casey CE, Walravens PA, Hambidge KM. Availability of zinc: loading tests with human milk, cow's milk and infant formulas. Pediatrics 1981; 68: 394–396.

78. Sandstrom B, Cederblad A, Lonnerdal B. Zinc absorption from human milk, cow's milk and infant formulas. Am J Dis Child 1983; 137: 726–729.

79. Evans GW, Johnson PE. Characterisation and quantification of a zinc-binding ligand in human milk. Pediatr Res 1980; 14: 876–880.

80. Hurley LS, Lonnerdal B. Picolinic acid as a zinc-binding ligand in human milk: an unconvincing case. Pediatr Res 1981; 15: 166–167.

81. Holt C. Zinc binding ligands in milk: both arguments err seriously. J Nutr 1981; 111: 2240–2241.

82. May PM, Smith GL, Williams DR. Computer calculation of Zn(II) complex distribution in milk. J Nutr 1982; 112: 1990–1993.

83. Cousins RJ, Smith KT. Zinc-binding properties of bovine and human milk in vitro: influence of changes in zinc content. Am J Clin Nutr 1980; 33: 1083–1087.

84. Ainscough EW, Brodie AW, Plowman JE. Zinc transport by lactoferrin in human milk. Am J Clin Nutr 1980; 33: 1314–1315.

85. Blakeborough P, Salter DN, Gurr MI. Zinc binding in cow's milk and human milk. Biochem J 1983; 209: 505–512.

86. Lonnerdal B, Hoffman B, Hurley LS. Zinc and copper binding proteins in human milk. Am J Clin Nutr 1982; 36: 1170–1176.

87. Jiang K. Zinc and copper absorption in rats fed dietary cellulose. Fed Proc 1985; 44: A6408.

88. Gruden N, Buben M, Ciganovic M. The effects of cellulose and zinc on ^{65}Zn absorption in infant rats. Nutr Rep Int 1979; 20: 757–762.

89. Urabe K, Hayakawa F. Relationship between zinc and cellulose intakes in growing rats. Int J Vit Horm Res 1990; 60: 159–167.

90. Lei KY, Davis MW, Fang MM, Young LC. Effect of pectin on zinc, copper and iron balances in humans. Nutr Rep Int. 1980; 22: 459–466.

91. Fairweather-Tait SJ, Wright AJ. The effects of sugar-beet fibre and wheat bran on iron and zinc absorption in rats. Br J Nutr 1990; 64: 547–552.

92. Cossack ZT, Rojhani A, Musaiger AO. The effects of sugar-beef fibre supplementation for five weeks on zinc, iron and copper status in human subjects. Eur J Clin Nutr 1992; 46: 221–225.

93. Lonnerdal B, Sandberg AS, Sandstrom B, Kunz C. Inhibitory effects of phytic acid and other inositol phosphates on zinc and calcium absorption in suckling rats. J Nutr 1989; 119: 211–214.

94. Oberleas D, Muhrer ME, O'Dell BL. Dietary metal-complexing agents and zinc availability in the rat. J Nutr 1966; 90: 56–62.

95. Davies NT, Nightingale R. The effects of phytate on intestinal absorption and secretion of zinc and whole body retention of zinc, copper, iron and manganese in rats. Br J Nutr 1975; 34: 243–258.

96. Morris ER, Ellis R. Effect of dietary phytate/zinc molar ratio on growth and bone zinc response of rats fed semipurified diets. J Nutr 1980; 110: 1037–1045.

97. Davies NT, Carswell AJP, Mills CF. The effect of variation in dietary calcium intake on the phytate-zinc interaction in rats. In: Mills CF, Bremner I, Chesters JK, eds. Trace Elements in Man and Animals—5. Slough: Commonwealth Agricultural Bureau 1985: 456.

98. Lo GS, Settle SL, Steinke FH, Hopkins DT. Effect of phytate:zinc molar ratio and isolated soyabean protein on zinc availability. J Nutr 1981; 111: 2223–2225.

99. Davies NT, Olpin SE. Studies on the phytate: zinc molar contents in diets as a determinant of zinc availability to young rats. Br J Nutr 1979; 41: 590–603.

100. Andersson H, Navert B, Bingham SA, Englyst HN, Cummings JH. The effects of breads containing similar amounts of phytate but different amounts of wheat bran on calcium, zinc and iron balance in man. Br J Nutr 1983; 50: 503–510.

101. Franz KB, Kennedy BM, Fellers DA. Relative bioavailability of zinc from selected ceraels and legumes using rat growth. J Nutr 1980; 110: 2272–2283.

102. Kratzer FH, Allred JB, Davis PN, Marshall BJ, Vohra P. The effect of autoclaving soyabean protein and the addition of ethylenediaminetetraacetic acid on the biological availability of dietary zinc for turkey poults. J Nutr 1959; 68: 313–322.

103. Navert B, Sandstrom B, Cederblad A. Reduction of the phytate content of bran by leavening in bread and its effect on zinc absorption. Br J Nutr 1985; 53: 47–53.

104. Lonnerdal B, Bell JG, Hendrickx AG, Burns RA, Keen CL. Effect of phytate removal on zinc absorption from soy formula. Am J Clin Nutr 1988; 48: 1301–1306.

105. Rubio LA, Grant G, Bardocz S, Dewey P, Pusztai A. Mineral excretion of rats fed on diets containing faba beans (*Vicia faba* L.) or faba bean fractions. Br J Nutr 1992; 67: 295–302.

106. Parisi AF, Vallee BL. Isolation of a zinc alpha 2-macroglobulin from human serum. Biochemistry 1970; 9: 2421–2426.

107. Giroux EL. Determination of zinc distribution between albumin and alpha 2-macroglobulin in human serum. Biochem. Med 1975; 12: 258–266.

108. Zhou Y, Hu X, Dou C, Liu H, Wang S, Shen P. Structural studies on metal-serum albumin IV. The interaction of Zn(II), Cd(II) and Hg(II) with HSA and BSA. Biophys Chem 1992; 42: 201–211.

109. Giroux EL, Henkin RI. Competition for zinc among serum albumin and amino acids. Biochim Biophys Acta 1972; 273: 64–72.

110. Chesters JK, Will M. Zinc transport proteins in plasma. Br J Nutr 1981; 46: 111–118.

111. Lowe NM, Bremner I. Jackson MJ. Plasma ^{65}Zn kinetics in the rat. Br J Nutr 1991; 65: 445–455.

112. Evans GW, Winter TW. Zinc transport by transferrin in rat portal blood plasma. Biochem Biophys Res Commun 1975; 66: 1218–1224.

113. Smith KT, Failla ML, Cousins RJ. Identification of albumen as the plasma carrier for zinc absorption by perfused rat intestine. Biochem J 1979; 184: 627–633.

114. Charlwood PA. The relative affinity of transferrin and albumin for zinc. Biochim Biophys Acta 1979; 581: 260–265.

115. Harris WR. Thermodynamic binding constants of the zinc-human serum transferrin complex. Biochemistry 1983; 22: 3920–3926.

116. Hallman PS, Perrin DD, Watt AE. The computed distribution of Cu(II) and Zn(II) ions among seventeen amino acids present in human blood plasma. Biochem J 1971; 121: 549–555.

117. Harris WR, Keen C. Calculations of the distribution of Zn in a computer model of human serum. J Nutr 1989; 119: 1677–1682.

118. May PM, Linder PW, Williams DR. Computer simulation of metal-ion equilibria in biofluids: models for the low molecular weight complex distribution of Ca (II) Mg (II) Mn (II) Fe (II) Cu (II) Zn (II) and Pb (II). J Chem Soc (Dalton) 1977: 588–595.

119. Magneson GR, Puvathingal JM, Ray WJ Jr. The concentrations of free Mg^{2+} and free Zn^{2+} in equine blood plasma. J Biol Chem 1987; 262: 11140–11148.

120. Kalfakakou V, Simons TJ. Anionic mechanisms of zinc uptake across the human red cell membrane. J Physiol (Lond) 1990; 421: 485–497.

121. Foster DM, Aamodt RL, Henkin RI, Berman M. Zinc metabolism in humans: a kinetic model. Am J Physiol 1979; 237: R340–R349.

122. Chesters JK, Will M. Measurement of zinc flux through plasma in normal and endotoxin-stressed pigs and the effects of zinc supplementation during stress. Br J Nutr 1981; 46: 119–130.

123. Love NM, Green A, Rhodes JM, Lombard M, Jalan R, Jackson MJ. Studies of human zinc kinetics using the stable isotope [70]Zn. Clin Sci 1993; 84: 113–117.

124. House WA, Welch RM, Van Campen DR. Effect of phytic acid on the absorption, distribution and endogenous excretion of zinc in rats. J Nutr 1982; 112: 941–953.

125. Shipley RA, Clark RE. Tracer Methods for in Vivo Kinetics. New York: Academic Press, 1972.

126. Pekarek RS, Beisel WR. Effect of endotoxin on serum zinc concentration in the rat. Appl Microbiol 1969; 18: 482–484.

127. Keeling PWN, Ruse W, Bull J, Hannigan B, Thompson RPH. Direct measurement of the hepatointestinal extraction of zinc in cirrhosis and hepatitis. Clin Sci 1981; 61: 441–444.

128. Failla ML, Cousins RJ. Zinc uptake by isolated rat liver parenchymal cells. Biochim Biophys Acta 1978; 538: 435–444.

129. Stacey MH, Klaassen CD. Zinc uptake by isolated rat hepatocytes. Biochim Biophys Acta 1981; 640: 693–697.

130. Patterson SE, Cousins RJ. Kinetics of zinc uptake and exchange by primary cultures of rat hepatocytes. Am J Physiol 1986; 250: E667–E685.

131. Failla ML, Cousins RJ. Zinc accumulation and metabolism in primary cultures of adult rat liver cells. Biochim Biophys Acta 1978; 549: 293–304.

132. Bremner I, Davies NT. The induction of metallothionein in rat liver by zinc injection and restricted food intake. Biochem J 1975; 149: 733–738.

133. Guiraud P, Lepee M, Monjo AM, Richard MJ, Favier A. Cultured human skin fibroblasts absorb [65]Zn—optimization of the method and study of the mechanisms involved. Biol Trace Elem Res 1992; 32: 213–225.

134. Ackland ML, McArdle HJ. Significance of extracellular zinc-binding ligands in the uptake of zinc by human fibroblasts. J Cell Physiol 1990; 145: 409–413.

135. Gachot B, Tauc M, Morat L, Poujeol P. Zinc uptake by proximal cells isolated from rabbit kidney: effects of cysteine and histidine. Pflugers-Arch 1991; 419: 583–587.

136. Phillips JL. Subcellular distribution of transferrin-bound zinc incorporated by PHA-stimulated and unstimulated human lymphocytes. Biol Trace Elem Res 1980; 2: 291–301.

137. Chausmer AB, Chausmer AL, Dajani N. Effect of mitogenic and hormonal stimulation on zinc transport in mixed lymphocyte cultures. J Am Coll Nutr 1991; 10: 205–208.

138. Ackland ML, Danks DM, McArdle HJ. Studies on the mechanism of uptake of zinc by human fibroblasts. J Cell Physiol 1988; 135: 521–526.

139. Torrubia JO, Garay R. Evidence for a major route for zinc uptake in human red blood cells: [Zn(HCO_3)_2Cl]^- influx through the [Cl^-/HCO_3^-] anion exchanger. J Cell Physiol 1989; 138: 316–322.

140. Solomons NW. Competitive interactions of iron and zinc in the diet: consequences for human nutrition. J Nutr 1986; 116: 927–935.

141. Baer MT, King JC. Tissue zinc levels and zinc excretion during experimental zinc depletion in young men. Am J Clin Nutr 1984; 39: 556–570.

142. Sullivan JF, Williams RV, Wisecarver J, Etzel K, Jetson MM, Magee DF. The zinc content of bile and pancreatic juice in zinc deficient swine. Proc Soc Exp Biol Med 1981; 166: 39–43.

143. Weigand E, Kirchgessner M. True total efficiency of zinc utilisation: determination and homeostatic dependence upon the zinc supply status in young rats. J Nutr 1980; 110: 469–480.

144. Jacob RA, Sandstead HH, Munoz JM, Klevay LM, Milne DB. Whole body surface loss of trace metals in normal males. Am J Clin Nutr 1981; 34: 1379–1383.

145. Anonymous. On the enteropancreatic circulation of endogenous Zn. Nutr Rev 1981; 39: 162–163.

146. Jackson MJ, Jones DA, Edwards RHT, Swainbank IG, Coleman ML. Zinc homeostasis in man: studies using a new stable isotope-dilution technique. Br J Nutr 1984; 51: 199–208.

147. Jackson MJ. Physiology of zinc: general aspects. In: Mills CF, ed. Zinc in Human Biology. London: Springer-Verlag, 1988: 1.

148. Hambidge KM. Zinc. In: Mertz W, ed. Trace Elements in Human and Animal Nutrition. Vol. 2. 5th ed. New York: Academic Press, 1986: 1.

149. Aggett P. Severe zinc deficiency. In: Mills CF, ed. Zinc in Human Biology. London: Springer-Verlag 1988: 259.

150. Prasad AS. Clinical and biochemical spectrum of zinc deficiency in human subjects: In: Prasad AS, ed. Clinical, Biochemical and Nutritional Aspects of Trace Elements. New York: Liss, 1982: 3.

151. Williams RB, Mills CF. The experimental production of zinc deficiency in the rat. Br J Nutr 1970; 24: 989–1003.

152. Chesters JK, Quarterman J. Effects of zinc deficiency on food intake and feeding patterns of rats. Br J Nutr 1970; 24: 1061–1069.

153. Chesters JK, Will M. Some factors controlling food intake by zinc-deficient rats. Br J Nutr 1973; 30: 555–566.

154. Duerre JA, Ford KM, Sandstead HH. Effect of zinc deficiency on brain and liver of suckling rats. J Nutr 1977; 107: 1082–1093.

155. Wallwork JC, Fosmire GJ, Sandstead HH. Effect of zinc deficiency on appetite and plasma amino acid concentrations in the rat. Br J Nutr 1981; 45: 127–136.

156. Kasarskis EJ, Sparks DL, Slevin JT. Changes in hypothalamic noradrenergic systems during the anorexia of zinc deficiency. Biol Trace Elem Res 1986; 9: 25–35.

157. Fabry P, Braun T. Adaptation to the pattern of food intake: some mechanisms and consequences. Proc Nutr Soc 1967; 26: 144–152.

158. Masters DGH, Keen CL, Lonnerdal B, Hurley LS. Zinc deficiency teratogenicity: the protective role of maternal tissue catabolism. J Nutr 1983; 113: 905–912.

159. Faraji B, Swendseid ME. Growth rates, tissue zinc levels and activity of selected enzymes in rats fed a zinc-deficient diet by gastric tube. J Nutr 1983; 113: 447–455.

160. Park JHY, Grandjean CJ, Antonson DL, Vanderhoop JA. Effect of short-term isolated zinc deficiency on intestinal growth and activity of several brush border enzymes in weanling rats. Pediatr Res 1985; 19: 1333–1336.

161. Reeves PG, O'Dell BL. Short-term zinc deficiency in the rat and self-selection of dietary protein level. J Nutr 1981; 111: 375–383.

162. Reeves PG, O'Dell BL. The effect of dietary tyrosine levels on food intake in zinc-deficient rats. J Nutr 1984; 114: 761–767.

163. Wallwork JC, Sandstead HH. Effect of zinc deficiency on appetite and free amino acid concentrations in rat brain. J Nutr 1983; 113: 47–54.

164. Essatara MB, McClain LJ, Levine AS, Morley JE. Zinc deficiency and anorexia in rats: the effect of central administration of norepinephrine, muscinol and bromerogocryptine. Physiol Rev 1984; 32: 479–482.

165. Wright AL, King JC, Baer MT, Citron LJ. Experimental zinc depletion and altered taste perception for sodium chloride in young adult rats. Am J Clin Nutr 1981; 34: 848–852.

166. Henkin RI. Zinc in taste function—a review. Biol Trace Elem Res 1984; 6: 263–280.

167. Shatzman AR, Henkin RI. Gustin concentration changes relative to salivary zinc and taste in humans. Proc Natl Acad Sci (USA) 1981; 78: 3867–3871.

168. Bryce Smith D, Simpson RID. Case of anorexia nervosa responding to zinc sulphate. Lancet 1984; ii: 350.

169. Varela P, Marcos A, Navarro MP. Zinc status in anorexia nervosa. Ann Nutr Metabol 1992; 36: 197–202.

170. Katz RL, Keen CL, Litt IF, Hurley LS, Kellams-Harrison KM, Glader LJ. Zinc deficiency in anorexia nervosa. J Adolesc Health Care 1987; 8: 400–406.

171. Mira M, Stewart PM, Abraham SF. Vitamin and trace element status of women with disordered eating. Am J Clin Nutr 1989; 50: 940–944.

172. Pekarek RS, Burghen GA, Bartelloni PJ, Calia FM, Bostian KA, Beisel WR. The effect of live attenuated Venezuelian equine encelphomyelitis virus vaccine on serum iron, zinc and copper concentrations in man. J Lab Clin Med 1970; 76: 293–303.

173. Kincaid RL, Miller WJ, Gentry RP, Neathery MW, Hampton DL, Lassiter JW. The effect of endotoxin upon zinc retention and intracellular liver distribution in rats. Nutr Rep Int 1976; 13: 65–70.

174. Hallbook T, Hedelin H. Zinc metabolism and surgical trauma. Br J Surg 1977; 64: 271–273.

175. Lindeman RD, Bottomley RG, Cornelison RL, Jacobs LA. Influence of acute tissue injury on zinc metabolism in man. J Lab Clin Med 1972; 79: 452–460.

176. Powanda MC, Villarreal Y, Rodriguez E, Braxton G, Kennedy CR. Redistribution of zinc within burned and burned infected rats. Proc Soc Exp Biol Med 1980; 163: 296–301.

177. Cunningham JJ, Lydon MK, Briggs SE, DeCheke M. Zinc and copper status of severely burned children during TPN. J Am Coll Nutr 1991; 10: 57–62.

178. Hambidge KM, Droegemueller W. Changes in plasma and hair concentrations of zinc, copper, chromium and manganese during pregnancy. Obstet Gynec NY 1974; 44: 666–672.

179. Pekarek RS, Beisel WR. Characterisation of the endogenous mediator(s) of serum zinc and iron depression during infection and other stresses. Proc Soc Exp Biol Med 1971; 138: 728–732.

180. Cousins RJ, Leinhart AS. Tissue-specific regulation of zinc metabolism and metallothioncin genes by interleukin-1. FASEB J 1988; 2: 2884–2890.

181. Schroeder JJ, Cousins RJ. Interleukin 6 regulates metallothionein gene expression and zinc metabolism in hepatocyte monolayer cultures. Proc Natl Acad Sci (USA) 1990; 87: 3137–3141.

182. Cossack ZT. The role of zinc in endotoxin fever. Int J Vitam Nutr Res 1991; 61:57–60.

183. Sobocinski PZ, Powanda MC, Canterbury WJ, Machotka SV, Walker RL, Snyder SL. Role of zinc in the abatement of hepatocellular damage and mortality incidence in endotoxemic rats. Infect Immun 1977; 15: 950–957.

184. Snyder SL, Walker RI. Inhibition of lethality in endotoxin-challenged mice treated with zinc chloride. Infect Immun 1976; 13: 998–1000.

185. Cuthbertson DP, Fell GS, Smith CM, Tilstone WJ. Metabolism after injury. I. Effects of severity, nutrition and environmental temperature on protein, potassium, zinc and creatine. Br J Surg 1972; 59: 925–931.

186. Jackson MJ, Jones DJ, Edwards RHT. Tissue zinc levels as an index of body zinc status. Clin Physiol 1982; 2: 333–343.

187. Fraker PJ, Jardieu P, Cook J. Zinc deficiency and immune function. Arch Dermatol 1987; 123: 1699–1701.

188. Cunningham-Rundles S, Bockman RS, Lin A, et al: Physiological and pharmacological effects of zinc on immune response. Ann NY Acad Sci 1990; 587: 113–122.

189. Keen CL, Gershwin ME. Zinc deficiency and immune function. Annu Rev Nutr 1990; 10: 415–431.

190. Fraker PJ, Gershwin ME, Good RA, Prasad AS. Interrelations between Zn and immune function. Fed Proc 1986; 45: 1474–1479.

191. Carlomagno MA, McMurray DN. Chronic zinc deficiency in rats: its influence on some parameters of humoral and cell-mediated immunity. Nutr Res 1983; 3: 69–78.

192. Fernandes G, Nair M, Onoe K, Tanaka T, Floyd R, Good RA. Impairment of cell-mediated immunity functions by dietary Zn deficiency in mice. Proc Natl Acad Sci (USA) 1979; 76: 457–461.

193. Nash L, Iwata T, Fernandes G, Good RA, Incefy GS. Effect of Zn deficiency on autologuos rosette-forming cells. Cell Immunol 1979; 48: 238–243.

194. Fraker PJ, Haas SM, Luecke RW. Effect of Zn deficiency on the immune response of the young adult A/J mouse. J Nutr 1977; 107: 1889–1895.

195. Fraker PJ, DePasquale-Jardieu P, Zwicki CM, Luecke RW. Regeneration of T cell helper function in Zn-deficient adult mice. Proc Natl Acad Sci (USA) 1978; 75: 5660–5664.

196. Fernandes G, Nair M, Onoe K, Tanaka T, Floyd R, Good RA. Impairment of cell-mediated immunity functions by dietary Zn deficiency in mice. Proc Natl Acad Sci (USA) 1979; 76: 457–461.

197. Fraker PJ, Hildebrandt K, Luecke RW. Alteration of antibody-mediated responses of suckling mice to T-cell dependent and independent antigens by maternal marginal Zn deficiency: restoration of responsivity by nutritional repletion. J Nutr 1984; 114: 170–179.

198. Pekarek RS, Powanda MC, Hoagland AM. Effect of Zn deficiency on the immune response of the rat. Fed Proc 1976; 35: 360.

199. Anonymous. Zinc and immunocompetence. Nutr Rev 1980; 38: 288–289.

200. Fraker PJ, Caruso R, Kierszenbaum F. Alteration of the immune and nutritional status of mice by synergy between zinc deficiency and infection with *Trypanosoma cruzi*. J Nutr 1982; 112: 1224–1229.

201. Wirth JJ, Fraker PJ, Kierszenbaum F. Zinc requirement for macrophage function: effect of zinc deficiency on uptake and killing of a protozoan parasite. Immunology 1989; 68: 114–119.

202. Golden MHN, Golden BE, Harland PSEG, Jackson AA. Zinc and immunocompetance in protein-energy malnutrition. Lancet 1978; i: 1226–1228.

203. Castillo-Duran C, Heresi G, Fisberg M, Uauy R. Controlled trial of zinc supplementation during recovery from malnutrition: effects on growth and immune function. Am J Clin Nutr 1987; 45: 602–608.

204. Beach RS, Gershwin ME, Hurley LS. Gestational zinc deprivation in mice: persistence of immunodeficiency for three generations. Science 1982; 218: 469–471.

205. Kaiserlian D, Savino W, Dardenne M. Studies of the thymus in mice bearing the Lewis lung carcinoma. II. Modulation of thymic natural killer activity by thymulin (FTS-Zn) and the antimetastatic effect of zinc. Clin Immunol Immunopathol 1983; 28: 192–204.

206. Dardenne M, Wade S, Savino W, Nabarra B, Prasad AS, Bach J-F. Thymulin and zinc deficiency. In: Prasad AS, ed. Essential and Toxic Trace Elements in Human Health and Disease. New York: Liss, 1988: 329.

207. Iwata T, Incefy GS, Tanaka T, et al. Circulating thymic hormone levels in Zn deficiency. Cell Immunol 1979; 47: 100–105.

208. Chandra RK, Au B. Single nutrient deficiency and cell-mediated immune responses. 1. Zinc. Am J Clin Nutr 1980; 33: 736–738.

209. Bach J-F, Pleau J-M, Savino W, Laussac J-P, Dardenne M. The role of zinc in the biological activity of thymulin, a thymic metallopeptide hormone. In: Prasad AS, ed. Essential and Toxic Trace Elements in Human Health and Disease. New York: Liss, 1988: 319.

210. Dardenne M, Savino W, Wade S, Kaiserlian D, Lemonnier D, Bach J-F. In vivo and in vitro studies of thymulin in marginally Zn-deficient mice. Eur J Immunol 1984; 14: 454–458.

211. Prasad AS, Meftah S, Abdallah J, et al. Serum thymulin in human zinc deficiency. J Clin Invest 1988; 82: 1202–1210.

212. DePasquale-Jardieu P, Fraker PJ. The role of corticosterone in the loss of immune function in the Zn-deficient A/J mouse. J Nutr 1979; 109: 1847–1855.

213. Beach RS, Gershwin ME, Makishima RK, Hurley LS. Impaired immunological ontogeny in postanatal Zn deprivation. J Nutr 1980; 110: 805–815.

214. Dowd PS, Kelleher J, Guillou PJT. Lymphocyte subsets and interleukin-2 production in Zn-deficient rats. Br J Nutr 1986; 55: 59–69.

215. Gross RL, Osdin N, Fong L, Newberne PM. Depressed immune function in zinc-deprived rats as measured by mitogen response of spleen, thymus and periferal blood. Am J Clin Nutr 1979; 32: 1260–1265.

216. Flynn A. Control of in vitro lymphocyte proliferation by Cu, Mg and Zn deficiency. J Nutr 1984; 114: 2034–2042.

217. Haynes DC, Golub MS, Gershwin ME, Hurley LS, Hendrickx AG. Long-term marginal zinc deprivation in Rhesus monkeys. II. Effects on maternal health and fetal growth at midgestation. Am J Clin Nutr 1987; 45: 1503–1513.

218. James SJ, Swendseid M, Makinodan T. Macrophage-mediated depression of T cell proliferation in zinc-deficient mice. J Nutr 1987; 117: 1982–1988.

219. De Pasquale-Jardieu P, Fraker PJ. Interference in the development of a secondary immune response in mice by zinc deprivation: persistence of effects. J Nutr 1984; 114: 1762–1769.

220. Barbeau A, Zinc, taurine and epilepsy. Arch Neurol 1974; 30: 52–58.

221. Donaldson J, Pierre TSt, Minnich JL, Barbeau A. Determination of Na^+, K^+, Mg^{2+}, Cu^{2+}, Zn^{2+} and Mn^{2+} in rat brain regions. Can J Biochem 1973; 51: 87–92.

222. Prohaska JR. Functions of trace elements in brain metabolism. Physiol Rev 1987; 67: 858–901.

223. Dreosti IE, Manuel SM, Buckley RA, Fraser FJ, Record IR. The effect of late prenatal and/or early postnatal zinc deficiency on the development and some biochemical aspects of the cerebellum and hippocampus in rats. Life Sci 1981; 28: 2133–2141.

224. Wensink J, Lenglet WJ, Vis RD, Van den Hamer CJ. The effect of dietary zinc deficiency on the mossy fiber zinc content of the rat hippocampus. A microbeam PIXE study. Histochemistry 1987; 87: 65–69.

225. Hesketh JE, Aggett P, Crofton RW, Humphries WR, Mills CF. Effect of zinc deficiency on zinc concentrations in various regions of pig brain: particular sensitivity of the cerebellum. Nutr Res 1985; 5: 1223–1226.

226. Hurley LS, Swenerton H. Congenital malformations resulting from zinc deficiency in rats. Proc Soc Exp Biol Med 1966; 123: 692–696.

227. Sandstead HH, Fosmire GJ, McKenzie JM, Halas ES. Zinc deficiency and brain development in the rat. Fed Proc 1975; 34: 86–88.

228. Oberleas D, Caldwell DF, Prasad AS. Trace elements and behaviour. Int Rev Neurobiol Suppl 1972; 1: 83–103.

229. Golub MS, Gershwin ME, Vijayan VK. Passive avoidance performance of mice fed marginally or severely zinc deficient diets during post-embryonic brain development. Physiol Behav 1983; 30: 409–413.

230. Golub MS, Gershwin ME, Hurley LS, Hendrickx AG. Studies of marginal zinc deprivation in Rhesus monkeys. VIII. Effects in early adolescence. Am J Clin Nutr 1988; 47: 1046–1051.

231. Caldwell DF, Oberleas D, Clancy JJ, Prasad AS. Behavioural impairment in adult rats following acute zinc deficiency. Proc Soc Exp Biol Med 1970; 133: 1417–1421.

232. File SE. Zinc and behaviour. In: Mills CF, ed. Zinc in Human Biology. London: Springer-Verlag 1988: 225.

233. Frederickson RE, Frederickson CJ, Danscher G. In situ binding of bouton zinc reversibly disrupts performance on a spatial memory task. Behav Brain Res 1990; 38: 25–33.

234. Hesse GW. Chronic zinc deficiency alters neuronal function of hippocampal mossy fibers. Science 1979; 205: 1005–1007.

235. Haug F-MS. Electron microscopical localization of zinc in hippocampal fibre synapses by a modified sulphide silver procedure. Histochimie 1967; 8: 355–368.

236. Frederickson CJ, Danscher G. Zinc-containing neurons in hippocampus and related CNS structures. Prog Brain Res 1990; 83: 71–84.

237. Ebadi M, Murrin LC, Pfeiffer RF. Hippocampal zinc thionein and pyridoxal phosphate modulate synaptic functions. Ann NY Acad Sci 1990; 585: 189–201.

238. Xie XM, Smart TG. A physiological role for endogenous zinc in rat hippocampal synaptic neurotransmission. Nature 1991; 349: 521–524.

239. Asaf SY, Chung S-H. Release of endogenous Zn^{2+} from brain tissue during activity. Nature 1984; 308: 734–736.

240. Aniksztejn L, Charton G, Ben-Ari Y. Selective release of endogenous zinc from the hippocampal mossy fibers in situ. Brain Res 1987; 404: 58–64.

241. O'Dell BL, Conley-Harrison J, Browning JD, Besch-Williford C, Hempe JM, Savage JE. Zinc deficiency and peripheral neuropathy in chicks. Proc Soc Exp Biol Med 1990; 194: 1–4.

242. O'Dell BL, Conley-Harrison J, Besch-Williford C, Browning J, O'Brien D. Zinc status and peripheral nerve function in guinea pigs. FASEB J 1990; 4: 2919–2922.

243. Halas ES, Wallwork JC, Sandstead HH. Mild zinc deficiency and undernutrition during the pre- and post-natal periods in rats: effects on weight, food consumption and brain catecholamine. J Nutr 1982; 112: 542–551.

244. Wallwork JC, Botnen JH, Sandstead HH. Influence of dietary zinc on rat brain catecholamines. J Nutr 1982; 112: 514–519.

245. Nickolson VJ, Veldstra H. The influence of various cations on the binding of colchicene by rat brain homogenates. Stabilization of intact neurotubules by zinc and cadmium ions. FEBS Lett 1972; 23: 309–319.

246. Hesketh JE. Zinc binding to tubulin. Int J Biochem 1983; 15: 743–746.

247. Zombola RR, Himes RH. Tubulin-zinc interactions: binding and polymerization studies. Biochemistry 1983; 22: 221–228.

248. Oteiza PI, Hurley LS, Lonnerdal B, Keen CL. Effects of marginal zinc deficiency on microtubule polymerization in the developing rat brain. Biol Trace Elem Res 1990; 24: 13–23.

249. Hesketh JE. Zinc stimulated microtubule assembly and evidence for zinc binding to tubulin. Int J Biochem 1982; 14: 983–990.

250. Spurlock ME, Browning JD, O'Dell BL. Low zinc status in guinea pigs does not decrease reassembly rate of brain microtubules. J Nutr Biochem 1992; 3: 594–598.

251. Apgar J. Effect of zinc deficiency on maintenance of pregnancy in the rat. J Nutr 1977; 100: 470–476.

252. Hurley LS, Schraeder RE. Abnormal development of preimplantation rat eggs after 3d of maternal zinc deficiency. Nature 1975; 254: 427–429.

253. Record IR, Dreosti IE, Tulsi RS, Manuel SJ. Maternal metabolism and teratogenesis in zinc-deficient rats. Teratology 1986; 33: 311–317.

254. Mieden GD, Keen CL, Hurley LS, Klein NW. Effects on whole rat embryos cultured on serum from zinc and copper deficient rats. J Nutr 1986; 116: 2424–2431.

255. Record IR, Dreosti IE, Tulsi RS. In vitro development of zinc-deficient and replete rat embryos. Austr J Exp Biol Med Sci 1985; 1: 65–71.

256. McKenzie JM, Fosmire GJ, Sandstead HH. Zinc deficiency during the latter third of pregnancy: effects on fetal rat brain, liver and placenta. J Nutr 1975; 105: 1466–1475.

257. Apgar J. Effect of zinc repletion late in gestation on parturition in the zinc-deficient rat. J Nutr 1973; 103: 973–981.

258. Caldwell DF, Oberleas D, Prasad AS. Reproductive performance of chronically mildly zinc deficient rats and the effect on behaviour of their offspring. Nutr Rep Int 1973; 7: 309–319.

259. Lytton FDC, Bunce GE. Dietary zinc and parturition in the rat. 1. Uterine pressure cycles. Biol Trace Elem Res 1986; 9: 151–163.

260. Haynes DC, Golub MS, Gershwin ME, Hurley LS, Hendrickx AG. Long-term marginal zinc deprivation in Rhesus monkeys. II. Effects on maternal health and fetal growth at midgestation. Am J Clin Nutr 1987; 45: 1503–1513.

261. Dylewski DP, Lytton FDC, Bunce GE. Dietary zinc and parturition in the rat. 2. Myometrial gap junctions. Biol Trace Elem Res 1986; 9: 165–175.

262. Swenerton H, Hurley LS. Zinc deficiency in Rhesus and Bonnet monkeys including effects on reproduction. J Nutr 1980; 110: 575–583.

263. Golub MS, Gershwin ME, Hurley LS, Baly DL, Hendrickx AG. Studies of marginal zinc deprivation in Rhesus monkeys. II. Pregnancy outcome. Am J Clin Nutr 1984; 39: 879–887.

264. Leek JC, Vogler JB, Gershwin ME, Golub MS, Hurley LS, Hendrickx AG. Studies of marginal zinc deficiency in Rhesus monkeys. V. Fetal and infant skeletal effects. Am J Clin Nutr 1984; 40: 1203–1212.

265. Apgar J. Zinc and reproduction—an update. J Nutr Biochem 1992; 3: 266–278.

266. Swanson CA, King JC. Zinc and pregnancy outcome. Am J Clin Nutr 1987; 46: 763–771.

267. Cherry FF, Sandstead HH, Rojas P, Johnson LK, Batson HK, Wang XB. Adolescent pregnancy: associations among body weight, zinc nutriture, and pregnancy outcome. Am J Clin Nutr 1989; 50: 945–954.

268. Mahomed K, James DK, Golding J, McCabe R. Zinc supplementation during pregnancy: a double blind randomised controlled trial. Br Med J 1989; 299: 826–830.

269. Simmer K, Lort-Phillips L, James C, Thompson RP. A double-blind trial of zinc supplementation in pregnancy. Eur J Clin Nutr 1991; 45: 139–144.

270. Barney GH, Orgebin-Crist MC, Macapinlac MP. Genesis of esophageal parakeratosis and histologic changes in the testis of the zinc-deficient rat and their reversal by zinc repletion. J Nutr 1969; 95: 526–534.

271. Underwood EJ, Somers M. Studies of zinc nutrition in sheep. I. The relation of zinc to growth, testicular development and spermatogenesis in young rams. Austr J Agr Res 1969, 20: 889–897.

272. Taneja SK, Nirmal. Histopathology of testis of mice on zinc-deficient diets. Int J Exp Biol 1980; 18: 1411–1414.

273. Hafiez AA, el-Kirdassy ZH, el-Malkh NM, el-Zayat EM. Role of zinc in regulating the testicular function. Part 3. Histopathological changes induced by dietary zinc deficiency in testes of male albino rats. Nahrung 1990; 34: 65–73.

274. Hesketh JE. Effect of dietary zinc deficiency on Leydig cell ultrastructure in the boar. J Comp Pathol 1982; 92: 239–247.

275. McClain CJ, Gavaler JS, Van Thiel DH. Hypogonadism in the zinc-deficient rat: localization of the functional abnormality. J Lab Clin Med 1984; 104: 1007–1015.

276. Mansour MM, Hafiez AA, el-Kirdassy ZH, el-Malkh MN, Halawa FA, el-Zayat EM. Role of zinc in regulating the testicular function. Part 2. Effect of dietary zinc deficiency on gonadotropins, prolactin and testosterone levels as well as 3-β-hydroxysteroid dehydrogenase in testes of male albino rats. Nahrung 1989; 33: 941–947.

277. Meftah SP, Prasad AS, DuMouchelle E, Cossack ZT, Rabbaani P, Testicular androgen binding protein in Zn-deficient rats. Nutr Res 1984; 4: 437–446.

278. Sansone G, Martino M, Abrescia P. Binding of free and protein-associated zinc to rat spermatozoa. Comp Biochem Physiol [C] 1991; 99: 113–117.

279. Kynaston HG, Lewis-Jones DI, Lynch RV, Desmond AD. Changes in seminal quality following oral zinc therapy. Andrologia 1988; 20: 21–22.

280. Oka N, Matsumoto O, Kamidono S. Experimental studies of male infertility and zinc. Hinyokika-Kiyo 1988; 34: 1–10.

281. Kvist U, Bjorndahl L, Kjellberg S. Sperm nuclear zinc, chromatin stability, and male fertility. Scanning Microsc 1987; 1: 1241–1247.

282. Kvist U, Kjellberg S, Bjorndahl L, Hammar M, Roomans GM. Zinc in sperm chromatin and chromatin stability in fertile men and men in barren unions. Scand J Urol Nephrol 1988; 22: 1–6.

283. Tikkiwal M, Ajmera RL, Mathur NK. Effect of zinc administration on seminal zinc and fertility of oligospermic males. Indian J Physiol Pharmacol 1987; 31: 30–34.

284. Legg SP, Sears L. Zinc sulphate treatment of parakeratosis in cattle. Nature 1960; 186: 1061–1062.

285. Kroneman J, v.d. Mey GJW, Helder A. Hereditary zinc deficiency in Dutch Friesian cattle. Zbl Vet Med A 1975; 22: 201–208.

286. Weismann K, Kvist N, Kobayasi T. Bullous acrodermatitis due to zinc deficiency during total parenteral nutrition: an ultrastructural study of the epidermal changes. Acta Derm Venerol 1983; 63: 143–146.

287. Zimmerman AW, Hambidge KM, Lepow ML, Greenberg RD, Stover ML, Casey CE. Acrodermatitis in breast-fed premature infants: evidence for a defect of mammary zinc secretion. Pediatrics 1982; 69: 176–183.

288. Kuramoto Y, Igarashi Y, Kato S, Tagami H. Acquired zinc deficiency in two breast-fed mature infants. Acta Dermatol Venerol 1986; 66: 359–361.

289. Bonifazi E, Rigillo N, De Simone B, Meneghini C. Acquired dermatitis due to zinc deficiency in a premature infant. Acta Dermatol Venerol 1980; 60: 449–450.

290. Aggett PJ, Atherton DJ, More J, Davey J, Delves HT, Harries JT. Symptomatic zinc deficiency in a breast-fed pre-term infant. Arch Dis Child 1980; 55: 547–550.

291. Roberts LJ, Shadwick CF, Bergstresser PR. Zinc deficiency in two full-term breast-fed infants. J Am Acad Dermatol 1987; 16: 301–304.

292. Weismann K, Arroe M. Zinc deficiency in a premature infant. Ugeskr Laeger 1990; 152: 2571–2572.

293. Khoshoo V, Kjarsgaard J, Krafchick B, Zlotkin SH. Zinc deficiency in a full-term breast-fed infant—unusual presentation. Pediatrics 1992; 89: 1094–1095.

294. Piletz JE, Ganschow RE. Lethal milk mutation results in dietary zinc deficiency in nursing mice. Am J Clin Nutr 1978; 31: 560–562.

295. Piletz JE, Lonnerdal B, Hurley LS, Berry W, Ganschow RE, Herschman HR. Zinc and copper in milk of nursing lethal milk mutant mice. J Nutr 1987; 117: 83–90.

296. Golden MHN, Golden BE, Jackson AA. Skin breakdown in kwashiorkor responds to zinc. Lancet 1980; i: 1256.

297. Heimburger DC, Tamura T, Marks RD. Rapid improvement in dermatitis after zinc supplementation in a patient with Crohns disease. Am J Med 1990; 88: 71–73.

298. Van Rij AM. Zinc supplements in surgery. In: Prasad AS, ed. Clinical, Biochemical and Nutritional Aspects of Trace Elements. New York: Liss, 1982: 259.

299. Pories WJ, Henzel JH, Rob CG, Strain WH. Acceleration of wound healing in man with zinc sulphate given by mouth. Lancet 1967; i: 121–127.

300. Carruthers R. Oral zinc in cutaneous healing. Drugs 1973; 6: 161–164.

301. Vallee BL, Auld DS. Active-site zinc ligands and activated H_2O of zinc enzymes. Proc Natl Acad Sci (USA) 1990; 87: 220–224.

302. Hough E, Hansen LK, Birknes B, et al. High-resolution crystal structure of phospholipase C from *Bacillus cereus*. Nature 1989; 338: 357–360.

303. Wacker WEC. Metalloenzymes. Fed Proc 1970; 29: 1462–1468.

304. Coleman JE. Zinc proteins—enzymes, storage proteins, transcription factors, and replication proteins. Annu Rev Biochem 1992; 61: 897–946.

305. Chang LMS, Bollum FJ. Multiple roles of divalent cations in the terminal deoxynucleotidyl-transferase reaction. J Biol Chem 1990; 265: 17436–17440.

306. Churchich JE, Scholz G, Kwok F. Activation of pyridoxal kinase by metallothionein. Biochim Biophys Acta 1989; 996: 181–186.

307. Snaith SM. Characterization of jack-bean meal alpha-D-mannosidase as a zinc metalloenzyme. Biochem J 1975; 147: 83–90.

308. Argos P, Garavito RM, Ewentoff W, Rossman MG. Similarities in the active centre geometries of zinc-containing enzymes, proteases and dehydrogenases. J Mol Biol 1978; 126: 141–158.

309. Prince RH. Some aspects of the bioinorganic chemistry of zinc. Adv Inorg Chem Radiochem 1979; 22: 249–440.

310. Vallee BL, Williams RJP. Metalloenzymes: the entatic nature of their active sites. Proc Natl Acad Sci (USA) 1968; 59: 498–505.

311. Prasad AS, Oberleas D. Biochemical effects of zinc deficiency: changes in activities of zinc-dependent enzymes and ribonucleic and desoxyribonucleic acid content of tissues. J Lab Clin Med 1971; 77: 144–152.

312. Huber AM, Gershoff SN. Effects of dietary zinc on zinc enzymes in the rat. J Nutr 1973; 103: 1175–1181.

313. Kirchgessner M, Roth HP. Estimation of metabolic availability of zinc and assessment of zinc requirements from changes in Zn-metalloenzymes. Arch Tierernahr 1975; 25: 83–92.

314. Hambidge KM. Assessing the trace element status of man. Proc Nutr Soc 1988; 47: 37–44.

315. Mills CF, Quarterman J, Williams RB, Dalgarno AC. The effects of zinc deficiency on pancreatic carboxypeptidase activity and protein digestion and absorption in the rat. Biochem J 1967; 102: 712–718.

316. Cowen LA, Bell DE, Hoadley JE. Influence of dietary zinc deficiency and parenteral zinc on rat liver fructose 1,6 bisphosphatase activity. Biochem Biophys Res Commun 1986; 134: 944–950.

317. Williams RB, Chesters JK. The effects of early zinc deficiency on DNA synthesis and protein synthesis in the rat. Br J Nutr 1970; 24: 1053–1059.

318. Duncan JR, Hurley LS. Thymidine kinase and DNA polymerase activity in normal and zinc deficient developing rat embryos. Proc Soc Exp Biol Med 1978; 159: 39–43.

319. Record IR, Dreosti IE. Effects of zinc deficiency on liver and brain thymidine kinase activities in the fetal rat. Nutr Rep Int 1979; 20: 749–755.

320. Baker GW, Duncan JR. Possible site of zinc control of hepatoma cell division in Wistar rats. J Natl Cancer Inst 1983; 70: 333–336.

321. Giugliano R, Millward DJ. The effects of severe zinc deficiency on protein turnover in muscle and thymus. Br J Nutr 1987; 57: 139–155.

322. Southon S, Livesey G, Gee JM, Johnson IT. Intestinal cell proliferation and protein synthesis in zinc-deficient rats. Br J Nutr 1985; 53: 595–603.

323. Prasad AS, Oberleas D, Wolf P, Horwitz JP. Effect of growth hormone on nonhypophysec-tomized zinc-deficient rats and zinc on hypophysectomzied rats. J Lab Clin Med 1969; 73: 486–494.

324. Cossack ZT. Somatomedin-C and zinc status in rats as affected by zinc protein and food intake. Br J Nutr 1986; 56: 163–169.

325. Bolze MS, Reeves RD, Lindbeck FE, Elders MJ. Influence of zinc on growth somatomedin and glycosaminoglycan metabolism in rats. Am J Physiol 1987; 252: E21–E26.

326. Chesters JK. The role of zinc ions in the transformation of lymphocytes by phytohaemag-glutinin. Biochem J 1972; 130: 133–139.

327. Rubin H. Inhibition of DNA synthesis in animal cells by EDTA and its reversal by zinc. Proc Natl Acad Sci (USA) 1972; 69: 712–716.

328. Chesters JK, Petrie L, Vint H. Specificity and timing of the $zinc^{2+}$ requirement for DNA synthesis by 3T3 cells. Exp Cell Res 1989; 184: 499–508.

329. Watanabe K, Hasegawa K, Ohtake H, Tohyama C, Koga M. Inhibition of DNA synthesis by EDTA and its cancellation by zinc in primary cultures of adult rat hepatocytes. Biomed Res 1993; 14: 99–110.

330. Lieberman I, Abrams R, Hunt N, Ove P. Levels of enzyme activity and deoxyribonucleic acid synthesis in mammalian cells cultured from the animal. J Biol Chem 1963; 238: 3955–3962.

331. Fujioka M, Lieberman I. A Zn^{2+} requirement for synthesis of deoxyribonucleic acid by rat liver. J Biol Chem 1964; 239: 1164–1167.

332. Vallee BL, Falchuk KH. Zinc and gene expression. Phil Trans Roy Soc B 1981; 294: 185–197.

333. Crossley LG, Falchuk KH, Vallee BL. Messenger ribonucleic acid function and protein synthesis in zinc-deficient *E. gracilis*. Biochemistry 1982; 21: 5359–5363.

334. Chesters JK, Petrie L, Travis AJ. A requirement for Zn^{2+} for the induction of thymidine kinase but not ornithine decarboxylase in 3T3 cells stimulated from quiescence. Biochem J 1990; 272: 525–527.

335. Petrie L, Chesters JK, Franklin M. Inhibition of myoblast differentiation by lack of zinc. Biochem J 1991; 276: 109–111.

336. Dreosti IE, Record I, Manuel SJ. Zinc deficiency and the developing embryo. Biol Trace Elem Res 1985; 7: 103–122.

337. Chen S-Y. Autoradiographic study of cell proliferation in acanthotic buccal epithelium of zinc-deficient rabbits. Arch Oral Biol 1986; 31: 535–539.

338. Hanas JS, Hazuda DJ, Bogenhagen DF, Wu FY-H, Wu C-W. Xenopus transcription factor A requires zinc for binding to the 5S RNA gene. J Biol Chem 1983; 258: 14120–14125.

339. Klug A, Rhodes D. Zinc fingers: a novel protein motif for nucleic acid recognition. Trends Biochem Sci 1987; 12: 464–469.

340. Berg JM. Zinc fingers and other metal-binding domains—elements for interactions between macromolecules. J Biol Chem 1990; 265: 6513–6516.

341. Berg JM. Proposed structure for the zinc-binding domains from transcription factor IIIA and related proteins. Proc Natl Acad Sci (USA) 1988; 85: 99–102.

342. Elbaradi T, Pieler T. Zinc finger proteins—what we know and what we would like to know. Mech Devel 1991; 35: 155–169.

343. Pugh BF, Tjian R. Mechanism of transcriptional activation by Sp1—evidence for coactivators. Cell 1990; 61: 1187–1197.

344. Mastrangelo IA, Courey AJ, Wall JS, Jackson SP, Hough PVC. DNA looping and Sp1 multimer links—a mechanism for transcriptional synergism and enhancement. Proc Natl Acad Sci (USA) 1991; 88: 5670–5674.

345. Smale ST, Schmidt MC, Berk AJ, Baltimore D. Transcriptional activation by Sp1 as directed through Tata or initiator—specific requirement for mammalian transcription factor IID. Proc Natl Acad Sci (USA) 1990; 87: 4509–4513.

346. Sunderman FW, Barber AM. Finger-loops, oncogenes and metals. Ann Clin Lab Sci 1988; 18: 267–288.

347. Zilliacus J, Dahlmanwright K, Carlstedtduke J, Gustafsson JA. Zinc coordination scheme for the C-terminal zinc binding site of nuclear hormone receptors. J Steroid Biochem Mol Biol 1992; 42: 131–139.

348. Gronemeyer H. Transcription activation by estrogen and progesterone receptors. Annu Rev Genet 1991; 25: 89–123.

349. Freedman LP. Anatomy of the steroid receptor zinc finger region. Endocrinol Rev 1992; 13: 129–145.

350. Danielsen M, Hinck L, Ringold GM. Two amino acids within the knuckle of the first zinc finger specify DNA response element activation by the glucocorticoid receptor. Cell 1989; 57: 1131–1138.

351. Green S, Kumar V, Theulaz I, Wahli W, Chambon P. The N-terminal DNA-binding "zinc finger" of the estrogen and glucocorticoid receptors determines target gene specificity. EMBO J 1988; 7: 3037–3044.

352. Schwabe JWR, Rhodes D. Beyond zinc fingers—steroid hormone receptors have a novel structural motif for DNA recognition. Trends Biochem Sci 1991; 16: 291–297.

353. Tao P, Coleman JE. Gal4 transcription factor is not a zinc finger but forms a zinc(II)2Cys6 binuclear cluster. Proc Natl Acad Sci (USA) 1990; 87: 2077–2081.

354. Varshney U, Jahroudi N, Foster R, Gedamu L. Structure, organization, and regulation of human metallothionein IF gene: differential and cell-type-specific expression in response to heavy metals and glucocorticoids. Mol Cell Biol 1986; 6: 26–37.

355. Labbe S, Prevost J, Remondelli P, Leone A, Seguin C. A nuclear factor binds to the metal regulatory elements of the mouse gene encoding metallothionein-I. Nucleic Acids Res 1991; 19: 4225–4231.

356. Hamer DH. Metallothionein. Annu Rev Biochem 1986; 55: 913–951.

357. Peterson MG, Mercer JF. Differential expression of four linked sheep metallothionein genes. Eur J Biochem 1988; 174: 425–429.

358. Paynter JA, Camakaris J, Mercer JF. Analysis of hepatic copper, zinc, metallothionein and metallothionein-Ia mRNA in developing sheep. Eur J Biochem 1990; 190: 149–154.

359. Stuart GW, Searle PF, Chen HY, Brinster RL, Palmiter RD. A twelve base pair motif that is repeated several times in metallothionein gene promoter confers metal regulation to a heterologous gene. Proc Natl Acad Sci (USA) 1984; 81: 7318–7322.

360. Iijima Y, Fukushima T, Bhuiyan LA, Yamada T, Kosaka F, Sato JD. Synergistic and additive induction of metallothionein in Chang liver cells. A possible mechanism of marked induction of metallothionein by stress. FEBS Lett 1990; 269: 218–220.

361. Imbert J, Culotta V, Furst P, Gedamu L, Hamer D. Regulation of metallothionein transcription by metals. Adv Inorg Biochem 1990; 8: 139–164.

362. Dai Z, Takahasi SI, van Wyk JJ, D'Ercole AJ. Creation of an autocrine model of insulin-like growth factor-I action in transfected FRTL-5 cells. Endocrinology 1992; 30: 3175–3183.

363. Behringer RR, Lewin TM, Quaife CJ, Palmiter RD, Brinster RL, Dercole AJ. Expression of insulin-like growth factor stimulates normal somatic growth in growth hormone-deficient transgenic mice. Endocrinology 1990; 127: 1033–1040.

364. Andersen RD, Taplitz SJ, Oberbauer AM, Calame KL, Herschman HR. Metal-dependent binding of a nuclear factor to the rat metallothionein-I promoter. Nucleic Acids Res 1990; 18: 6049–6055.

365. Garg LC, Dixit A, Webb ML, Jacob ST. Interaction of a positive regulatory factor(s) with a 106 bp upstream region controlling transcription of metallothionein-1 gene in the liver. J Biol Chem 1989; 264: 2134–2138.

366. Imbert J, Zafarullah M, Culotta VC, Gedamu L, Hamer D. Transcription factor MBF-I interacts with metal regulatory elements of higher eukaryotic metallothionein genes. Mol Cell Biol 1989; 9: 5315–5323.

367. Seguin C, Felber BK, Carter AD, Hamer DH. Competition for cellular factors that activate metallothionein gene transcription. Nature 1984; 312: 781–785.

368. Koizumi S, Yamada H, Suzuki K, Otsuka F. Zinc-specific activation of a HeLa cell nuclear protein which interacts with a metal responsive element of the human metallothionein-IIa gene. Eur J Biochem 1992; 210: 555–560.

369. Bettger WJ, O'Dell BL. A critical physiological role of zinc in the structure and function of biomembranes. Life Sci 1981; 28: 1425–1438.

370. Bettger WJ, O'Dell BL. Physiological roles of zinc in the plasma membrane of mammalian cells. J Nutr Biochem 1993; 4: 194–207.

371. Warren L, Glick MC, Nass MK. Membranes of animal cells. I. Method of isolation of the surface membrane. J Cell Physiol 1966; 68: 269–288.

372. Chvapil M. New aspects in the biological role of zinc: a stabilizer of macromolecules and biological membranes. Life Sci 1973; 13: 1041–1049.

373. Bettger WJ, Fish TJ, O'Dell BL. Effects of copper and zinc status of rats on erythrocyte stability and superoxide dismutase activity. Proc Soc Exp Biol Med 1978; 158: 279–282.

374. Johanning GL, Browning JD, Bobilya DJ, Veum TL, O'Dell BL. Effect of zinc deficiency and food restriction in the pig on erythrocyte fragility and plasma membrane composition. Nutr Res 1990; 10: 1463–1471.

375. Record IR, Macqueen SE, Dreosti IE. Zinc, iron, vitamin-E, and erythrocyte stability in the rat. Biol Trace Elem Res 1990; 23: 89–96.

376. Paterson PG, Bettger WJ. Effect of dietary zinc intake on the stability of the rat erythrocyte membrane. In: Mills CF, Bremner I, Chesters JK, eds. Trace Elements in Man and Animals—5. Slough, UK: Commonwealth Agricultural Bureau, 1985: 79.

377. O'Dell BL. Metabolic functions of zinc—a new look. In: Howell JMc, Gawthorne JM, White CL, eds. Trace Elements in Man and Animals—4. Canberra: Australian Academy of Science 1981: 319.

378. Dreosti IE, Record IR. Superoxide dismutase (EC 1.15.1.1), zinc status and ethanol consumption in maternal and foetal livers. Br J Nutr 1979; 44: 399–402.

379. Sullivan JF, Jetton MM, Hahn HKJ, Burch RE. Enhanced lipid peroxidation in liver microsomes of Zn-deficient rats. Am J Clin Nutr 1980; 33: 51–56.

380. Hammermueller JD, Bray TM, Bettger WJ. Effects of zinc and copper deficiencies on microsomal NADPH-dependent active oxygen generation in rat lung and liver. J Nutr 1987; 117: 894–901.

381. Kang HK, Harnish RA. Zinc nutritional status and response to lethal level of ozone exposure in rats. Bull Environ Contam Toxicol 1979; 21: 206–212.

382. King JC. Assessment of zinc status. J Nutr 1990; 120(suppl 11); 1474–1479.

383. Mills CF. Biochemical and physiological indicators of mineral status in animals: copper, cobalt and zinc. J Animal Sci 1987; 65: 1702–1711.

384. Thompson RP. Assessment of zinc status. Proc Nutr Soc 1991; 50: 19–28.

385. Pekarek RS, Burghen GS, Bartelloni PJ, Calia FM, Bostian KA, Beisel WR. The effect of live attenuated Venezuelan equine encephalomyelitis virus vaccine on serum iron, zinc and copper concentrations in man. J Lab Clin Med 1970, 76: 293–303.

386. Prasad AS, Rabbani P, Abbasii A, Bowersox E, Fox MRS. Experimental zinc deficiency in humans. Ann Intern Med 1978; 89: 483–445.

387. van den Broek AH, Stafford WL. Diagnostic value of zinc concentrations in serum, leucocytes and hair of dogs with Zn-responsive dermatosis. Res Vet Sci 1988; 44: 41–44.

388. Chesters JK, Will M. The assessment of zinc status of an animal from the uptake of [65]zinc by the cells of whole blood *in vitro*. Br J Nutr 1978; 38: 297–306.

389. Van Wouwe JP, Veldhuizen M, De Goeij JJ, Van den Hamer CJ. Laboratory assessment of early dietary, subclinical zinc deficiency: a model study on weaning rats. Pediatr Res 1991; 29: 391–395.

390. Sato M, Mehra RK, Bremner I. Measurement of plasma metallothionein in the assessment of the zinc status of zinc-deficient and stressed rats. J Nutr 1984; 114: 1683–1689.

391. Bremner I, Morrison JN, Wood AM, Arthur JR. Effects of changes in dietary zinc, copper and selenium supply and of endotoxin administration on metallothionein. I. Concentrations in blood cells and urine in the rat. J Nutr 1987; 117: 1595–1602.

392. Grider A, Bailey LB, Cousins RJ. Erythrocyte metallothionein as an index of zinc status in humans. Proc Natl Acad Sci (USA) 1990; 87: 1259–1262.

393. Bremner I, Morrison JN. Assessment of zinc, copper and cadmium status in animals by assay of extracellular metallothionein. Acta Pharmacol Toxicol 1986; 59(suppl 7): 502–509.

394. Walravens PA, Hambidge KM, Koepfer DM. Zinc supplementation in infants with a nutritional pattern of failure to thrive: a double-blind, controlled study. Pediatrics 1989; 83: 532–538.

395. Bremner I, Wood A, Noble NA, Robertson A. Assessment of nutritional status by immunoassay of metallothionein. In: Klassen CD, Suzuki KT, eds. Metallothionein in Biology and Medicine. Boston: CRC Press, 1991: 323.

396. World Health Organization. Zinc. In: Trace Elements in Human Nutrition and Health. Geneva: World Health Organization 1996: 72.

397. Fox MRS. Zinc Excess. In: Mills CF, ed. Zinc in Human Biology. London: Springer-Verlag 1989: 365.

8

Copper

EDWARD D. HARRIS
Texas A&M University, College Station, Texas

I. INTRODUCTION

Befitting its definition as a trace metal, copper is present in tissues and fluids at parts per million (ppm or μg/g) or parts per billion (ppb, ng/g) concentration. With few exceptions—namely, electron-carrying blue copper proteins and cytochrome c oxidase found in some cyanobacteria and aerobic bacteria—copper enzymes and proteins belong almost exclusively to the domain of eukarotic organisms (1). Its use as a cofactor for enzymes (cuproenzymes) is well established. A first estimate of significance, therefore, is to consider that copper is linked intimately to the reactions served by these enzymes. Such reactions embrace systems that generate oxidative energy, oxidize ferrous iron, synthesize neurotransmitters, bestow pigment to hair and skin, give strength to bones and arteries, assure competence of the immune system, and stabilize the matrices of connective tissues. Biochemically, most cuproenzymes belong to the class of *oxidases*, which are enzymes that catalyze the transfer of electrons from a substrate to molecular oxygen. Nonenzyme functions, however, such as angiogenesis, neurohormone release, oxygen transport, and the regulation of genetic expression, are also a part of copper's overall necessity. Copper deficiency, predictably, has devastating consequences on physiologic systems. Its propensity to bind sulfhydryl and amine groups and to catalyze one-electron "radical-forming" transfer reactions is the basis of copper toxicity. In response to this threat, organisms from bacteria to mammals have developed mechanisms to cope with abnormally high amounts or dangerous chemical forms of copper. An interesting observation is that toxicity prevention and the more commonplace mechanisms for transporting and storing copper tend to overlap. Toxicity, therefore, is never a question of presence, only amount of copper. Even more imposing are exquisitely sensitive systems that recognize infinitesimally small amounts of copper and can execute functions at such low levels. The discovery of pathways and intermediates for copper continues to be a focus of significant new information about the nutrition of this metal. Studies of copper deficiency through dietary omission or inborn errors have further elevated insights into the metal's specific functions. Although there is much still to be learned, it seems clear that animals, plants, and microorganisms have all adapted special needs for copper, and no metal can replace copper in the functions performed. Numerous books and reviews have addressed diverse aspects of copper function, nutrition, and biochemistry (2–9).

II. CHEMICAL PROPERTIES

Copper, element 29, is a member of the first transition series, which, along with vanadium, chromium, manganese iron, cobalt, nickel, and zinc, constitute eight of the nutritionally essential metals. First transition metals with partially filled $3d$ orbitals tend to give rise to highly colorful complexes. Copper is no exception. Two examples are the proteins ceruloplasmin, whose prefix "cerulo" denotes a "heavenly blue," and azurin, a small blue protein in bacteria. Configured as $3d^{10}4s^1$ in the ground state, copper forms Cu(I) or cuprous ion upon losing its single $4s$ electron. The resulting Cu^+ is unstable in solution and is readily oxidized by O_2 to Cu^{2+}. The $3d^{10}$ configuration of Cu^+ is analogous to Zn(II), which perhaps explains why zinc competes with copper in transport and absorption. Cu(II) ($3d^9$), the common biological form, is referred to as cupric. Its single unpaired electron gives paramagnetic properties, permitting Cu(II) to be analyzed by electron paramagnetic resonance (EPR, also referred to as ESR or electron spin resonance). Water molecules, amino- and sulfhydryl groups bind to cupric copper, creating charge-transfer complexes that give a visible blue color. A third valence, Cu(III), is highly unstable and is of questionable biological significance.

A. Analysis of Copper

Colorimetric tests for copper ions exploit chelators that give colorful chromogens. Some chelators, e.g., bathocuproine sulfonate and 2,2′-biquinoline, react only with Cu(I) (10,11). Others, such as cuprizone, are specific for Cu(II) (12). Copper chelators tend to be nonspecific, and interference by other divalent metal ions (Zn^{2+}, Fe^{2+} in particular) presents problems. Although it is a convenient laboratory procedure, colorimetry has lower sensitivity than other methods, and interference by reducing agents, detergents, and acids limits its application.

Atomic absorption spectrophotometric analysis is the preferred method for quantitating copper ions in biological samples. The procedure is rapid, precise, and has good sensitivity at copper levels found in most biological fluids and tissues. The instrumentation is of modest cost and can be adapted to most laboratories. Before the analysis, it is common to remove all organic matter from the copper by digesting the sample with boiling $HClO_4$-HNO_3, a technique referred to as "wet-ashing." The clear hydrolysate is then injected directly into an air-acetylene flame or graphite furnace atomizer connected to an atomic absorption spectrophotometer (AAS). A hollow-cathode lamp radiating at 324.8 nm (maximum for the copper) provides the radiation. Limits of detection are 0.01–0.1 µg/mL for flame AAS and 0.01–1.0 ng/mL for graphite furnace AAS.

A procedure called inductively coupled plasma (ICP) applies radiofrequency energy to argon gas in a sealed chamber to atomize the sample. ICP has the advantage of uniform heating down to the core. Used with *atomic emission spectrophotometry* (AES), ICP extends linearity over a wider concentration range and at least four orders of magnitude. The sensitivity of AES, however, is on a par with the graphite furnace technique (AAS). One drawback to AES is that spectral lines can overlap if there are multiple metals present in the sample. Consequently, AES is more effective with purified samples. Another method, *Neutron Activation Analysis* (NAA), uses neutron bombardment of copper samples to generate ^{64}Cu/^{66}Cu, two radioactive nuclides which are identified and quantitated by their gamma emissions. This process, referred to as thermoneutron capture, has a very good sensitivity due to the large capture capability of the copper atom but, because of the special equipment and shielded environment needed, the procedure has limited application in most laboratories.

Electron paramagnetic resonance (EPR) exploits the unpaired electron property of the Cu^{2+} ($3d^9$). A signal is generated because of the magnetic moment created when the spinning electron is aligned with or against an applied magnetic field. EPR was formerly used only to distinguish Cu(II) from Cu(I), because the latter gives no EPR signal. Advancements in the technology, however, have now made EPR the most common tool for probing the fine details of Cu(II) sites in proteins and low-molecular-mass complexes. The hyperfine splitting identifies ligands, geometric distortions, and specific numbers of susceptible copper atoms. EPR is the basis for designating "types" of copper in specific binding sites (see below).

X-ray structure analysis is used to probe the finer atomic details of copper sites in proteins, contributing valuable information as to number of ligands, bond distances, and site geometry around each copper atom. By comparing such spectrum with known "model" compounds, one is able to distinguish specific structural features in the unknown.

B. Copper Proteins

1. Copper Centers in Proteins

Most of the copper in fluids and cells is bound to proteins. In binding to a protein, copper ions form chemical bonds with amino acid side chains (ligands) on the surface or within. These sites must be available to the copper ions, which means that the protein must have a special sequence of amino acids and must fold in the correct manner to accommodate the tetrahedral [Cu(I)] or square planar [Cu(II)] geometry of the copper atom. Such stereo constraints restrict the number of possible copper-binding sites in proteins. Characteristic spectrophotometric and magnetic parameters permit copper sites to be classified as types. Their properties, along with a recently described "trinuclear" site, are discussed briefly below.

Blue Copper

The blue copper proteins possess a "type 1 Cu," a blue Cu center that absorbs light around 600 nm with $\epsilon = 3000$–5000 M^{-1} cm^{-1}, and a relatively low reduction potential ($+300$ to $+500$ mV). The intense blue color results from a cysteine thiolate metal ligand charge-transfer transition (13).

Normal Copper

Normal copper has a center that exhibits electronic spectra (EPR, optical extinction) typical of small-molecular-weight copper complexes. Normal copper is practically colorless and has been designated "type 2 Cu" or EPR-detectable Cu in multicopper oxidases.

Binuclear Copper

The binuclear copper center, designated "type 3 Cu," exists as a Cu(I)–Cu(I) couple. O_2 binds as a stable peroxide species bridging and oxidizing the Cu(I) pairs to Cu(II) (14). The close proximity of the Cu(II) atoms, approximately 3.5 Å (15), cancels the unpaired spin effects that would normally give a Cu(II) EPR spectrum. When oxygenated, the center gives a characteristic strong absorption band at 330 nm.

Trinuclear Copper Center

The trinuclear copper center, sometimes referred to as a "copper cluster," is defined by the close proximity of the single type 2 and binuclear type 3 coppers in the protein (16,17). X-ray crystallography has determined that the center in laccase, cucumber ascorbate oxidase, and ceruloplasmin exhibits the same basic geometry—namely, an isoceles triangular arrangement with the binuclear Cu at the base and the type 2 Cu at the apex, as shown in Figure 1 (18).

2. Mono(site) Copper Proteins

Small, blue copper proteins with a single type 1 copper atom are quite common in chloroplasts, bacteria, and fungi, where they function primarily in electron transfer reactions (19). Some of the more familiar are *Stellacyanin*, from the latex of *Rhus vernicifera*, a Japanese lacquer tree, which has the lowest redox potential (+184 mV) of all blue Cu proteins (20); *azurins*, which transfer electrons in a wide variety of bacteria; and *pseudo-azurin*, which also transfers electrons and in one species, *Achromobacter cycloclastes*, is linked with the enzyme nitrite reductase (21). *Plastocyanin* is a prominent component of chloroplasts, functioning as a mobile electron-transfer protein between photosystem II and photosystem I. Although it is smaller than azurin, plastocyanin has a similar β-sheet structure and active-site geometry. *Amicyanin* belongs to a newly discovered subclass of blue bacterial Cu proteins, 100–106 amino acids, that has three of four copper ligands in a tight loop and one pH-sensitive ligand to histidine (22). Amicyanin mediates electron transfer between methylamine dehydrogenase and cytochrome c (23). Amicyanin is inducible in *Paracoccus denitrificans*. *Plantacyanin* is a basic glycoprotein purified from spinach leaves and cucumber peelings, the two sources giving rise to antigenically distinct proteins (24).

By genetic analysis it has been learned that almost all small, blue copper proteins display a signal peptide designed to permit the protein to pass across a biological membrane. Plastocyanin, for example, is synthesized as a preprotein, molecular weight 17 kDa, which is processed to 10.5 kDa in the plastid (25). Genetic analysis has also established that the small blue proteins of bacteria and fungi bear strong structural features to the multicopper oxidases of higher organisms (see below). A cDNA for cucumber ascorbate oxidase, for example, has four histidine-rich regions that show amazing sequence homology to ceruloplasmin, laccase, and plastocyanin (26).

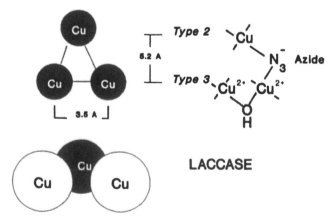

FIGURE 1 The trinuclear center in multicopper oxidases. The center is created by the close proximity of type 2 and type 3 coppers as shown for laccase, a nonmammalian protein. The overall geometry resembles an isosceles triangle with the two type 3 coppers at the base. The center was discovered when it was observed that a molecule of azide could straddle both centers simultaneously. The distance is such as to permit an interaction among all three copper atoms. Only the type 3 center binds O_2.

Only two proteins, hemocyanin and tyrosinase, have the binuclear center as the only copper in the protein. Designed to bind dioxygen, the center is used for two entirely different purposes. Hemocyanin, a protein prominent in members of the phyla arthropoda (lobsters, crab) and mollusks (snails, octopus), binds dioxygen reversibly for the purpose of transport (27).

$$Cu(I)Cu(I) + O_2 = Cu(II)_2 \cdot O_2^{2-}$$

On the other hand, tyrosinase, a monooxygenase, splits the dioxygen molecule and adds one of the oxygen atoms to a substrate. When O_2 binds to the center, the two Cu(I) are oxidized to Cu(II) and the O_2 is reduced to the oxidation state of a peroxide. Although the Cu is Cu(II), there is no EPR signal because the two unpaired electrons couple their spins and cancel the effect. The propinquity of the two coppers is designed specifically to accommodate the dimensions of a dioxygen molecule.

3. Multi(site) Copper Proteins

All known members of the family of multicopper oxidases are enzymes and include laccase, ceruloplasmin, and ascorbate oxidase. Each catalyzes a four-electron addition to dioxygen, splitting the molecule and forming two molecules of water. Electrons pass rapidly through the centers and over great distances, 2 nm or more (28). Additional information about each is discussed under "Copper Enzymes."

III. METABOLISM

Metabolism is a broad term that encompasses all events and components that take part in the postdigestive transfer of copper from a food source to its ultimate location in a tissue or cell. A single copper atom may encounter numerous biochemical agents in the blood, capillaries, cell membrane, and cytosol before arriving at its final destination, viz., an enzyme, binding, or storage protein. Together, these components form a metabolic pathway for copper, a pathway that is both progressive and integrated with important body organs. Figure 2 shows the distribution of copper throughout a normal human. Of the 1–2 mg taken in daily, only about half is absorbed through the intestines and passes to the liver, a principal storage site. The nonabsorbed fraction continues into the large intestine, where it is excreted in the feces. Copper that is trapped in desquamated epithelial cells is part of this fraction. Also contributing to fecal excretion is copper released into the bile. This can be about 0.4 mg/day, or close to half of the fecal copper. Thus, copper not absorbed and copper released into the bile account for nearly all of the daily intake for adults in balance. Liver cells synthesize ceruloplasmin and albumin, the major copper-binding proteins in plasma. Liver receives copper from both the intestine (via the portal circulation) and the general circulation. Copper is mobilized from the liver bound to ceruloplasmin (29). The liver is thus the major organ for distributing copper to tissues and excreting copper from the system. Transport, the extracellular phase of metabolism, occurs as part of the distribution of copper from the liver to the peripheral cells. Copper that is destined for biliary excretion must be metabolized, i.e., converted to a different chemical form, to prohibit its reabsorption into the system. These changes are all part of a system designed to move copper progressively through the system depending on need, thereby maintaining the proper homeostasis of the metal.

Whereas liver, brain, and kidney have the highest concentrations, muscle and bone, because of their overall greater mass, account for 50–70% of the total body load (Table 1). Liver contains about 10% of the body copper. In Table 1, "Other" includes body fluids such as plasma, cerebrospinal fluid, salivary secretions, bile, and intestinal secretions, each known to contain copper, but at different concentrations.

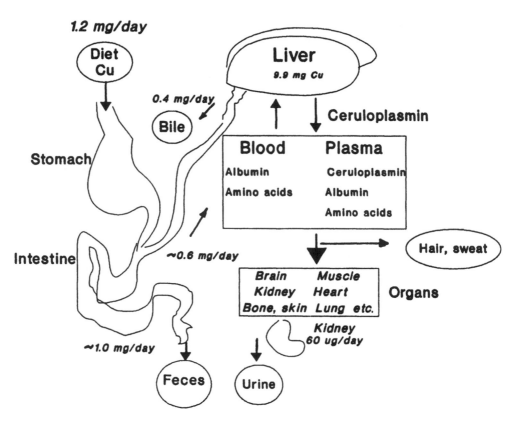

FIGURE 2 Overview of copper absorption, transport, and excretion. The liver receives copper from the intestine via the portal circulation and redistributes the copper to the tissue via ceruloplasmin, albumin, and amino acids. Nearly half of the copper consumed is not absorbed and passes into the feces. Another two-thirds of the daily intake is returned to the liver and released into the bile. Fecal excretion, therefore accounts quantitatively for nearly all of the copper consumed as the system endeavors to stay in balance. A small amount is excreted by the kidney via the urine, and still lesser amounts appear in hair and sweat. This interplay among the various systems maintains homeostasis and balance throughout the organism. The values in the figure are based on a dietary input of 1.2 mg/day. (Adapted from Ref. 239 with modifications to fit values for humans.)

A.   Body Burden and Tissue Distribution

Based on balance studies, an adult human male requires about 1.3 mg of copper per day to replace copper lost through fecal and urinary excretion, hair, and skin (30). An expert committee of the World Health Organization recommends 30 μg/kg, which is equivalent to about 2.1 mg/day for a 70-kg male (31). Thus 1–2 mg is the daily intake required to keep an average human male healthy and in balance. In rats, the value is about 300 μg/day (32). As a reference figure, one can estimate that an average adult vertebrate has about 1.5–2.5 μg copper per gram of fat-free tissue. Young children in stages of rapid growth have a proportionately higher need for copper than the recommended amount (33,34).

It is worth noting that food sources with more than 1 mg of copper per 1000 kcal (oysters, green vegetables, and many varieties of fish) are considered high in copper (35). Organ meats, nuts, dried fruit, and chocolate also meet the criterion (36). Those with less

TABLE 1 Copper Content of Major Body Organs and Blood: Percent Total

Tissue/organ	Copper concentration (μg/g)	Total for 70-kg person (mg)	Percent total
Skeleton	4.1	45.5	40.4
Muscle	0.9	26.2	23.3
Liver	6.2	9.9	8.8
Brain	5.2	8.8	7.8
Blood	1.1	6.2	5.5
Skin	0.8	3.8	3.4
Kidney	12.7	3.2	2.8
Adipose	0.2	3.0	2.7
GI tract	1.9	2.8	2.5
Other	—	3.1	2.8

After Ref. 9.

than 0.5 mg of copper per 1000 kcal (dairy products, breads, mutton, and beef) are deemed poor in copper (35). Cow's milk is particularly low (less than 0.2 mg per 1000 kcal).

Upon entering cells, copper relocates to enzymes, binding to proteins and organelles including (not necessarily in order of priority) nuclei, lysosomes, mitochondria, and peroxisomes (Fig. 3). The cytosol or "soluble fraction" features three major protein fractions that comprise the bulk of the cytosolic copper sites, although intracellular distribution to each varies with the particular organ (37). Metallothionein, superoxide dismutase, and an unidentified high-molecular-weight fraction appear consistently in chromatograms of newly incorporated cytosolic copper. By adding ^{64}Cu directly to extracts, Ettinger and colleagues recently detected an additional copper-binding protein in the cytosol of liver (38). Glutathione complexes of copper have been postulated to be a cytosolic transport form (39) and immediate precursors of enzyme-bound copper (40). Figure 3 suggests that glutathione might also be involved in the transport of copper into organelles and its release from membrane binding sites.

Since most of the information on Cu distribution in liver and other tissues has come from studies of copper-loaded animals, there has been biased and perhaps unjustified emphasis on metallothionein in copper metabolism. When trace doses of ^{67}Cu are administered, the ^{67}Cu distribution is quite different, the most salient feature being a considerably diminished presence of copper in metallothionein. Marceau and Aspin showed that Cu,Zn-superoxide dismutase (CuZnSOD; formerly cytocuprein) is a principal recipient of ^{67}Cu from ceruloplasmin (41). Work with aortas in culture (42) and K562 cells (43) shows that CuZnSOD is also a major recipient of the newly incorporated ^{67}Cu. More recent studies (44) suggest that liver may contain a constitutive pool of apoCuZnSOD poised to bind newly absorbed copper (44). Prins and van den Hamer observed that 86% of the copper given as a small dose of ^{67}Cu was bound to CuZnSOD; only 9% was bound to metallothionein, and 5% was in an unidentified macromolecule (45).

B. Absorption

Net absorption is the difference between dietary intake and fecal excretion, and *retention* is the difference between dietary intake and the sum of fecal and urinary excretion (36). As

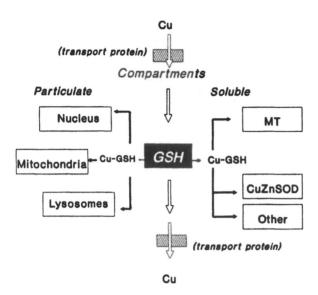

FIGURE 3 Status of copper within the cell. Upon entering via a membrane-transport protein, copper ions are distributed to the various organelles including nuclei, mitochondria, and lysosomes. The initial contact appears to be with glutathione (GSH), a cysteine-containing tripeptide. Some of the copper is distributed to soluble components in the cytosol, which include enzymes and storage proteins. Other copper ions are excreted to the exterior. The data suggest that copper as a Cu-GSH complex can engage with components in the various intracellular compartments.

pointed out earlier, only about half of the dietary copper is absorbed into the system. The remaining copper ingested either escapes uptake or, if absorbed, is trapped in mucosal epithelial cells that are shed periodically. Absorption begins within the acidic environment of the stomach. Most of the copper in the diet is bound to organic foodstuffs. The stomach secretions dissociate this bound copper, permitting small amounts to diffuse through the stomach lining. The largest portion, however, passes into the duodenum and ileum, where the major absorption occurs. Because the alkalinity of the intestine works against solubility, copper must complex with amino acids, organic acids, or other chelators to remain soluble in this region of the intestinal tract. pH is thus a critical determinant of absorption efficiency. Studies with isolated gut segments suggest that copper enters mucosal cells by simple diffusion and that the transfer across to the serosal side of the intestine is a different mode of transport (46). Chemical form, valence state, and relative concentrations of competing metals all determine the quantity absorbed. Sodium ions also may play a role in the overall transmembrane movement (47). Fibers in fruits and vegetables as well as phytate in grains have been noted to impair intestinal absorption of copper (48), but whether these substances are natural deterrents to absorption is still controversial. Amino acids also influence absorption, but again, the data are not firm. For example, supplementing a diet with free histidine, one of the most important ligands for copper in serum, appears to offer no advantage in improving the rate of absorption of copper (as ^{64}Cu) over the free metal (49). One of the biggest deterrents to absorption are copper-binding proteins (metallothioneins) that are synthesized in mucosal cells. By binding copper, metallothionein prevents its serosal transfer. Zinc can obstruct copper absorption indirectly by enriching the level of metallothionein through induced synthesis (50,51) and antagonizing copper exiting from mucosal cells (52). While induction of metallothionein may explain in part the antagonistic effects of zinc on copper metabolism, recent evidence (52a) suggests that another mechanism may be involved. Mucosal metallothionein concentration decreases after long-term consumption of high levels of zinc, but copper absorption does not increase. High concentrations of metallothioneins in the intestine offer protection against accidental copper overload and thus protect the organism against copper toxicity (53). In summary, studies of the mechanism suggest that copper absorption is a pH-dependent, two-stage transfer process that requires ligands, is competitive with zinc, is blocked by metallothionein, and may be facilitated by select amino acids and sodium ions.

C. Transport

Transport implies the movement of copper toward a defined target from a remote location. In plasma, two proteins, albumin and transcuprein (54), have been identified with transporting copper to the liver from the intestine. In time, extrahepatic organs take up copper from ceruloplasmin (55). Albumin, ceruloplasmin, and transcuprein, working asynchronously, transport copper from the intestine to body cells.

1. Transport in Plasma

Blood copper concentration provides a first approximation of nutritional adequacy. The copper levels in blood (plasma) differ between species and within individual members of a species. For example, human values for copper in plasma range between 0.5 and 1.5 μg/mL (8–24 μM), whereas domestic fowl is only one-third this level [0.2–0.35 μg/mL (3–5 μM)] (56). Plasma copper values fluctuate with age, exercise, and health status. Copper in plasma does not increase after a meal nor decrease during short-term fasting (57). In pregnancy, plasma copper almost doubles just before parturition. Besides plasma proteins and small-molecular-weight complexes, copper in the blood is also found in the cells of the blood. Copper in erythrocytes, for example, is partitioned between two major fractions, superoxide dismutase and a labile pool of amino acids. Erythrocyte copper tends to remain fixed and stable and serves only the needs of erythrocytes; i.e., it is not a source of tissue copper. When given orally or intravenously, ^{64}Cu binds quickly to albumin in the blood (55,58).

Albumin is the most prominent protein in blood plasma. This protein transports amino acids, bilirubin, vitamins, and, with its one high-affinity site for copper on a histidine three residues from the N terminus (59), is particularly suited for copper transport (60). The half-life of copper on albumin is about 10 min (61). In effect, albumin discharges copper very soon after it binds it. Furthermore, there is evidence for a ternary histidine–albumin–Cu complex that may exist in equilibrium with albumin to facilitate the discharge of copper from the protein (62). This conclusion is questioned, however, because the brief half-life may not allow histidine to equilibrate with the copper–albumin complex (63). Thus, the ternary complex, if it exists, may not keep pace with the on/off movement of the copper ions. An important property of albumin is the ability to bind copper ions in situ, i.e., at chance encounters with the metal outside the liver. This property is not shared by ceruloplasmin, which binds copper only at the assembly site in the liver (64–66). Consequently, some of the copper ions in albumin may represent ions that have disengaged from ceruloplasmin molecules or else released as free copper ions by cells. A role for albumin in extrahepatic transport, however, cannot be disregarded (42).

Ceruloplasmin is the major repository of copper in plasma, representing 60–95% of the total copper in serum of vertebrates (67). Soon after delivery to the liver, ^{64}Cu is incorporated into ceruloplasmin and released from the liver. Purified ceruloplasmin from normal human serum gives the appearance of a heterogeneous mixture of four proteins, one major and three minor bands, distinguishable by electrophoretic mobility and copper content. Ceruloplasmin is present in human plasma at around 0.2–0.5 g/L (68). Ceruloplasmin concentration in pig serum is higher than in human serum, while domestic fowl, on the other end of the scale, contains barely detectable amounts (69). Its presence in plasma and its ability to engage cells (see below) has made ceruloplasmin a strong candidate for a copper transport protein. Moreover, ceruloplasmin's role in transport has been considered analogous to that of transferrin, the iron transport protein. Copper ions aside from those at the oxidase site are believed to exchange with tissues and become incorporated into cellular enzymes that require copper for function. Which copper atoms in the protein are released has not been determined. These concepts are not without criticism, since the tight binding of copper to ceruloplasmin is grounds for considering ceruloplasmin's copper metabolically unusable (70).

Recent insights into the transport mechanism, however, have tended to give a clearer understanding of ceruloplasmin's role as a transport factor. In transporting copper, ceruloplasmin recognizes receptors on plasma membranes of cells and in tissues and organs (8). Copper is believed to be released at the membrane site, and the protein itself does not penetrate, a mechanism that differs from the endocytotic mechanism used by transferrin. The disengagement of copper from the protein requires an exogenous reducing agent and possibly a conformational change in the three-dimensional structure of ceruloplasmin (71). Ascorbic acid (vitamin C) has been suggested as the factor in vivo that reduces and facilitates the release of copper from the protein (72), thus allowing copper as the free ion to enter (most likely complexed to the membrane or an internal copper-binding agent). Ceruloplasmin shows a time-dependent release of one of its bound copper atoms to albumin. This reaction can be monitored by the appearance of an EPR signal below $g = 2.0$, which in effect signifies formation of an axial Cu–albumin bond. The signal is not seen when ceruloplasmin is removed from the plasma, nor is it stimulated by raising the temperature, adding ascorbate, or treating the ceruloplasmin with trypsin (73). The identity of the plasma factor(s) catalyzing the exchange is unknown, as is the significance of the reaction to copper transport.

2. Membrane Transport

Early experiments performed with liver slices supported a role for amino acids, histidine in particular, in tissue copper uptake (74). When these experiments were extended to liver cells and fibroblasts in culture, however, the need for histidine was not as obvious (75,76). Moreover, uptake studies, generally of short duration, have shown that hepatocytes take up copper very rapidly and against a concentration gradient, yet do not require a carrier or ATP (75). Expanding these studies to other cells has shown that the membrane transport mechanism is not the same for all cell types (77). For example, fibroblasts and liver carcinoma (Hep-G2) cells do not recognize a dihistidine–copper complex, whereas transport is more effective in normal hepatocytes when copper is present in this form (78). Copper atoms appear to disengage from the complex, however, before penetrating the membrane (78).

Recently, human cells have been shown to contain a gene that encodes a membrane-bound, copper-transporting protein similar to copper-transporting proteins in bacteria. The protein is the product of the *Mc1* gene. The gene's transcript is expressed in muscles, heart,

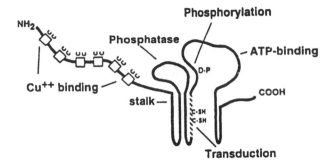

FIGURE 4 Membrane copper-transporting ATPase. The putative structure as deduced from a cDNA from human fibroblasts shows the key features of a metal-transport protein which includes a copper-binding site, a highly conserved ATP and phosphorylation site, a phosphatase domain, and six membrane-spanning domains which allow the protein to be inserted into a cell membrane and a transduction region to allow copper ions to pass through the membrane. (After Ref. 79, with permission.)

placenta, and kidney cells (79). As deduced from a cDNA, the *Mc1* gene product is a single polypeptide chain, 1500 amino acids, with a molecular mass estimated at 163 kDa (Fig. 4). At least six heavy metal-binding sites, identified by the sequence Gly-Met-X-Cys-X-X-Cys, appear in the N-terminal third of the molecule. There is also a strongly conserved phosphate-binding aspartate residue in the sequence Asp-Lys-Thr-Gly-Thr-Ile-Thr, which fits the structural motif of proteins classified as P-type ATPases. Amino acid sequences in the protein are analogous to ion-motive ATPases. More important, the gene contains regions of homology with bacterial genes known to manifest copper resistance (80,81). Cells from patients afflicted with Menkes' disease, a disorder characterized by abnormal cellular copper retention, express very low levels of the *Mc1* transcript (79,82), implying that the gene product participates in intracellular copper homeostasis. The data, although very inchoate at this stage, suggest that the gene codes for a membrane protein that actively removes copper ions from cells, forcing their movement through membrane barriers.

D. Excretion

The major excretory route for copper is through the bile, a further testament to the liver's role in maintaining balance and homeostasis. Less than 60 µg are excreted via the kidney into the urine, and smaller amounts move through skin and hair. The origin of biliary copper continues to be elusive. Strong evidence suggests that this copper fraction arises from secretions via lysosomes. In liver cells, the biliary canaliculi are literally surrounded by lysosomes, thus making direct passage into the bile a short trip. Moreover, a metallothionein–copper complex isolated from canine liver lysosomes (83) and the presence of fragments of ceruloplasmin (84) suggest that liver copper proteins that are catabolized in the lysosomes may provide the biliary copper (83). Biliary excretion is a saturable process that proceeds against a concentration gradient. Further metabolism is evident, however, because copper appears in multiple components that form at different rates and with different stabilities (85), with a high copper intake favoring a fast-forming, unstable component. The scheme is more complex, however, since the binding factors themselves show differences depending on rat strain, suggesting that genetic factors, yet to be identified, regulate biliary copper composition (86). Glutathione may play a role in excretion, but only at the intracellular copper transport stage (85). The function of such complexes is subject to speculation, although an obvious implication is that a bound copper fraction cannot be reabsorbed into the system. A shutdown of biliary excretion leads to a build up of liver copper and emulates the major symptoms seen in Wilson's disease (see below).

IV. PHYSIOLOGIC FUNCTIONS OF COPPER: SIGNS OF DEFICIENCY

Decisive insights into the necessity of copper has been gained by studying the impairments produced when animals (and sometimes humans) are fed low-copper diets. The temporary imbalances can be corrected by enriching the copper content of the diet, a fact which not only establishes copper as the causative agent, but also provides a means for tracing copper from its source to the functional components. Essentiality is shown by the fall of specific enzyme activities as well as the emergence of gross pathologic lesions. Suffice it to say that organs respond in select ways to copper depletion (87), and the underlying cuproenzymes show a decline in activity that varies with both organ and species (88). Although numerous symptoms of copper deficiency have been described in humans (89), the underlying biochemical factors for some of these is still unknown (Table 2). The major signs are discussed below by organ systems.

A. Cardiovascular System

Of all the symptoms of copper deficiency, none more dramatically illustrates the essential nature of copper than sudden death by aortic rupture (90). Aortic rupture was first described in chicks and pigs as a pathology reflecting defects in the connective tissue proteins of the major blood vessels (56). In cattle, a copper deficiency led to "falling disease," and, as the

TABLE 2 Correlation of Physiologic and Biochemical Function with Specific Cuproenzymes in Vertebrates

Function	Impaired activity	References
Cardiovascular system integrity	Lysyl oxidase	56,90,153
Heart size	Lysyl oxidase	93,95,231
Lung elasticity	Lysyl oxidase	97–99
Bone and cartilage stability	Lysyl oxidase	101,102,104
Egg shell shape	Lysyl oxidase	105,106
Hematopoiesis	Ferroxidase, ferrireductase	108,110,111
Immune system competence	IL-2	115,168
Catecholamine metabolism	Dopamine-monooxygenase	90,121
Nerve transmission	Dopamine-monooxygenase	90,125
Pigmentation	Tyrosinase	129,172,173
CNS hormones	α-Amidating enzyme	174,176,232
Electron transport system	Cytochrome c oxidase	89,179
Keratinization	Sulfhydryl oxidase?	131,132
Antioxidant activity	CuZnSOD, ceruloplasmin	184–186
Lipid metabolism	Fatty acyl monodesaturase	136,137,142
Neovascularization	Unknown	143–145

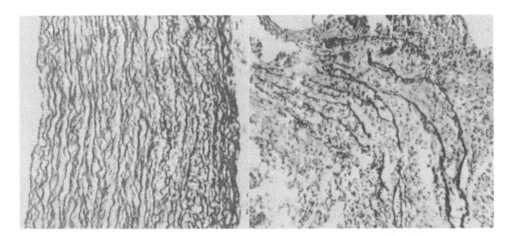

FIGURE 5 Histological sections of chick aortas. The left panel shows a cross section of an aorta from a normal control; the right panel is from a copper-deficient chick. In the deficient, note that the elastic laminae (shown as dark squiggly bands) appear less abundant and are more highly fragmented than controls. This is typical of the pathology created when elastin molecules fail to polymerize due to insufficient crosslinks of the type shown in Figure 7. (After Ref. 90, with permission.)

name implies, was characterized by the sudden collapse of an apparently healthy animal. The pathology behind the rupture is known to involve collagen and elastin in the connective tissues and results when these proteins are not properly crosslinked. The histology has been most revealing in that major arteries from deficient animals show extensive fragmentation in the fibrous elastic lamina, betraying a weakening of the superstructure internally (Fig. 5). Such sparse and fragmented fibers cannot support the demands of a vigorously swelling and contracting aorta. Biochemically, the defect is due in large part to a failure of the elastin precursor (proelastin) to polymerize into a fibrous elastic sheath (90). As a consequence, focal lesions develop where the stresses were greatest (generally at branch points) or where the underlying tissue layer is richest in elastin. These lesions lead first to balloonlike aneurysm and then to a full rupture. In a copper deficiency, the synthesis de novo of proelastin and procollagen is normal; only the posttranslational processing—specifically, the oxidation of peptidyl lysine residues that form lysine-derive aldehydes (allysines)—is altered (see below).

In intact animals, dietary copper restriction enhances the risk of myocardial infarction. The heart muscle and valves are targets, but each responds at different copper levels (91). A mild depletion raises the coronary perfusion pressure and contractive force of rat heart muscle, whereas a severe deficiency causes ventricular aneurysms. EKG parameters are abnormal (92). Heart muscle depends on an extensive extracellular matrix surrounding and connecting muscle fibers and cells. Collagen, primarily type I and type III, is the major protein in heart fibers. In rats, a copper deficiency decreases the pyridinium crosslinks in both right and left ventricles (93), which ultimately lowers the total collagen content of the heart muscle (94). A deficiency not only impairs collagen crosslinking but alters the tissue-specific type of collagen in the heart ventricle (95). One of the most salient features is an enlargement of the heart muscle itself, which exhibits eccentric or concentric hypertrophy caused by larger ventricles and thinner walls and intraventricular septa (Fig. 6). In seeking a

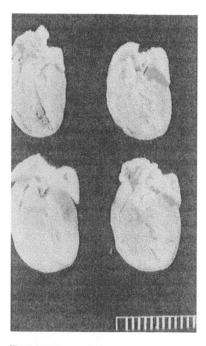

FIGURE 6 Longitudinal view of hearts from rats fed copper-adequate and copper-deficient diets. Hearts from rats fed adequate copper are shown in the top row. The rats (Long-Evans) were fed the respective diets for 5 weeks. Deficient diets contained about 0.4 µg Cu/g diet. Hypertrophy in deficient is predominantly concentric, whereby the left and right ventricular free walls and the intraventricular septum are thickened and the ventricular lumens smaller as compared to hearts from copper-adequate rats. Scale = 1 cm. (Photo courtesy of Dr. Denis Medeiros.)

cause, one should realize that the heart and major arteries are rich in connective tissue proteins, principally collagen and elastin (see below).

B. Lung

Since elastin comprises 8% of the dry weight of lung (96), one would anticipate lung tissue to be especially sensitive to copper deficiency. This prediction has been confirmed in experimental animals. Symptoms of copper deficiency closely resemble pulmonary emphysema in humans, a basic defect characterized by the lack of elasticity in aveoli and an enlargement of the distal air spaces. Rats (97) and chicks (98) consuming diets that are deficient in copper have less elastin and show ultrastructural modifications to bronchi, arterioles, and aveolar ducts (99). These defects are permanent and cannot be reversed by refeeding copper-rich diets. Some studies have suggested that a copper deficiency may lower CuZnSOD activity in rat lung (100), which raises the susceptibility of lung to edema and other factors associated with oxygen toxicity. The issue, however, is not fully resolved.

C. Bone and Cartilage

The so-called "hard" connective tissues, which include bone and cartilage, also appear to depend on copper for tissue integrity. Low-copper diets have been related to incidences of osteoporosis, fractures, and epiphyseal separations in young domestic animals and pups. Baxter, Van Wyck, and colleagues were the first to link copper deficiency to bone defects and showed further that copper prevented or even reversed the symptoms (101). An important observation by Rucker et al. showed that collagen in the organic matrix was the more likely biochemical site of the defect (102). Failure to form the proper pattern of crosslinks in the collagen led to an abnormal collagen matrix on which to deposit the mineralized bone material (102). In other instances, copper deficiency in human infants nourished by total parenteral nutrition gives rise to ephiphyseal separation, demineralization of bone surface areas, and scurvylike metaphyseal spurs (103). The articular surface of bone from young horses fed high zinc to suppress dietary copper absorption is characterized by extensive lesions of the articular surface cartilage, causing the animals to suffer crippling joint swelling and lameness (104). These studies have shown a priority role for copper in bone formation, mineralization, and growth-plate integrity.

Somewhat related to bone structure is the role of copper in egg shell formation. Mature hens fed deficient diets before or during egg production lay eggs that are abnormal in size, shape, and shell thickness (105). The calcification of the egg occurs in the shell gland and results when calcium as calcium carbonate ($CaCO_3$) is deposited around the thin filamentous structure supporting and enclosing the yolk and albumen. This membrane is composed of elastinlike material, suggesting a requirement for the cuproenzyme lysyl oxidase (see below) in its formation, and indeed the enzyme has been located in the membrane-forming (isthmus) region of the oviduct (106). Copper deficiency lowers the content of desmosine and isodesmosine in the egg shell membrane, thus weakening the force that opposes the osmotic pressure-induced increase in the volume of the egg's filling. Since the amount of $CaCO_3$ deposited is the same, eggs from deficient hens with a greater volume and outer circumference have thinner shells and, in some cases, no shell at all (105).

D. Hematopoietic System

The roles for copper in iron metabolism are many and varied. Interestingly, the first investigation that led to the recognition of copper as an essential nutrient (107) was, in fact, to identify the cause of iron-resistant anemia in laboratory animals. The missing nutrient turned out to be copper. Later studies showed that reticulocytes from copper-deficient swine assimilate iron poorly and are handicapped in heme synthesis (108). Cordano and Graham reported that an anemic condition that was prevalent in Peruvian children was due to a restricted amount of copper in their diet (109). These data show clearly that animals and humans need copper to utilize iron. This nutritional interdependence between the two essential metals, however, has yet to be fully clarified. In a copper deficiency, mucosal and liver tissues accumulate the iron that under normal circumstances would be transported to hematopoietic tissue for hemoglobin synthesis (110). A suggested site in vivo is the protein ceruloplasmin, whose ferroxidase activity is believed to be required to oxidize Fe(II) to Fe(III) preparatory to and necessary for iron to bind to transferrin (111).

More recently, copper–iron interaction have been clarified at the cellular level. K562 cells, an undifferentiated human erythroleukemic cell line, are primed for hemoglobin biosynthesis in response to iron from hemin. Percival has recently shown that concomitant with a greater influx of iron, 8 μM copper in the growth medium significantly enhances the pool of ferritin iron in K562 cells (112). Ferritin is a major source of iron for hemoglobin synthesis in these cells. *Saccharomyces cerevisiae* (baker's yeast cells) accumulate iron by multiple mechanisms, but the major transport system with the highest affinity uses a plasma membrane ferrireductase and a ferrous transporter (113). The *FRE1* locus appears to be responsible for the membrane-bound iron reductase activity, and a second gene encodes the high-affinity ferrous transporter. Ferrous iron transport requires a third gene product (FET3 for ferrous transport), a multicopper oxidase that catalyzes oxidation of Fe^{2+} to Fe^{3+} and is necessary for iron transport by the high-affinity transporter (113). Copper transport in these yeast appears to be a function of the *CTR1* gene product, a membrane-spanning protein that displays 11 Met-X_2-Met metal-binding sequences (114). Two items of importance attest to the significance of these observations. First, the *FET3* gene product (FET3 protein) has structural similarity to the blue copper-containing oxidases (114); second, *CTR1* mutants are profoundly deficient in ferrous iron uptake, suggesting that copper plays a critical role in that mechanism. Likewise, a deficiency in copper in the growth medium of wild-type cells also decreases ferrous ion transport (113). These data suggest that the copper domain of the FET3 is responsible for iron accumulation by these cells and that iron deficiency results from copper deficiency. Such interactions could have a bearing on the apparent anemia witnessed in copper-deficient animals.

E.   Immune System Functions

Copper-deficient rats have a lowered ability to withstand infection from *Salmonella typhimurium*. Copper-deficient mice have depressed T- and B-lymphocyte numbers, and the cells produced are functionally impaired (115). The respiratory burst activity of macrophages, an index of phagocytotic "killing" activity, is also compromised (116). Moreover, the production of interleukin-2, which mediates the cell-responsive defense of T cells, is also much less, and thus T cells cannot mount a coordinate defense against invading microbes. Refeeding a diet supplemented with copper reverses these defects (117).

F.   Central Nervous System

The brain and central nervous system (CNS) are particularly vulnerable to copper deprivation. Classically, neuropathologies resulting from copper deficiency were first seen in newborn lambs. The symptoms were incoordination of the hindquarters, with ataxia, tremors, and a swaying gait. Known as "swayback" (enzootic ataxia), the condition could be suppressed strongly by giving pregnant ewes supplements of copper (56). Guinea pigs, rats and mice show similar signs of copper deficiency (117a). In humans, a dementia, dysarthria with soft staccato speech, accompanied by involuntary movements and gait disturbances, has been observed in adult twin males that display abnormally low levels of serum copper and ceruloplasmin (118). The ataxia, tremors, clonic seizure, hypomyelination, or demyelination seem to be associated with reduced levels of sphingolipids and a reduction in the steady-state concentrations of norepinephrine in the CNS (117a). The low norepinephrine probably relates to depressed levels of dopamine-β-monooxygenase, a copper-dependent enzyme (see below). In the swayback lamb (119) and the deficient rat (119a), necrosis occurs in selected areas of the brain, notably the corpus striatum. In these species, copper deficiency results in decreased dopamine as well as norepinephrine levels. As in Parkinson's disease, the low striatal dopamine level associated with the symptoms is the result of neuron loss (120). This literature has been reviewed (121).

  Further research, however, has shown that the scope, severity, and location of central nervous system lesions in copper deficiency depends on species. For example, sheep suffer from extensive hypomyelination of brain cells and demyelination of nerve fibers in the spinal chord. Rodents, however, experience myelin loss in the cerebellum and brain stem.

Guinea pigs display extensive brain necrosis, and the cerebellar folia may be missing or deformed (122). Practically all species show a Parkinson-like tremor and involuntary movements. Sun and O'Dell recently found that brain dopamine, a neurotransmitter, was actually lowered in brain of second-generation copper-deficient female rats. The deficiency was accompanied by a severe degeneration of the striatal neurones and was accompanied by an increase in glial fibrillary acidic proteins (GFAP) (120). Linoleic acid [18:2(n-6)] in brain myelin was quite elevated, but no correlation with the hypomyelination was apparent (123).

Interestingly, the biochemical alterations induced by copper deficiency in experimental animals have parallels in some of the abnormalities found in brain tissue from Menkes' patients, and brindled and macular mice (124). In all three, brain development is arrested due to a genetic impairment in the mechanism transporting copper to brain neurones. The lethal effect, therefore, is a copper deficiency in the brain (125,126). GFAP levels in Menkes' patients are likewise elevated, and *synaptophysin*, a marker for presynaptic vesicle membranes, is decreased (127). Elevated GFAP suggests that glial cells may proliferate or expand to compensate for the neuronal loss. Neurodegeneration in select regions of the brain is common in brindled mice (125). Moreover, the protein *spectrin*, a membrane microfilament-anchoring protein, is more prone to degradation in brindled mouse brain than normal (128). Astrocytes from macular mice accumulate excessive amounts of copper over controls, thus prohibiting its transfer to the surrounding neurones (124). This sets the stage for neurodegeneration, as dietary studies have so clearly illustrated (120).

G. Hair, Wool, and Integument

A deficiency in copper causes skin and hair to lose color and affects the pigmentation of the eye. Fur, feathers, and wool are also affected. In one of the more vivid examples, black rats and black sheep made copper deficient through the diet take on a light gray appearance in their fur and wool, respectively. The copper-sensitive factor at the root of all these symptoms appears to be the enzyme *tyrosinase* (monophenol monooxygenase), an essential enzyme in melanin biosynthesis (129). Complete loss of pigmentation produces *albinism* a clinical manifestation of an inheritable metabolic defect in melanocytes. Albinism in humans is rare and is not related to copper, however. In one study, for example, it was noted that the serum ceruloplasmin in 20 albino negros between the ages of 9 and 54 was higher (not lower) (508 mg/L versus 340 mg/L) than in a control group of the same age range, but plasma copper levels for the two groups were similar (130).

Patients with Menkes' syndrome have hair fibers with twisted shafts, giving the hair a texture that is kinky or steely. The term "steely" describes the straight-line growth of the fibers and a diminished amount of curl or crimp (131). Lack of crimp is a prominent feature in wool sheared from copper-deficient sheep. The crimp is restored, however, when the deficient sheep are given copper supplements. These data support an unmistakable need for copper for normal keratinization of wool and hair. Biochemically, steely hair has been shown to have more sulfhydryl groups along the hair protein's surface. Hair keratin from a Menkes' patient, for example, may have a ninefold increase in sulfhydryl groups over normal hair keratin (132). Although these data are consistent with a copper-dependent oxidase designed specifically for hair or wool proteins, no such enzyme has been found in hair follicles or isolated from tissues. The putative enzyme is believed to catalyze formation of disulfide bonds, which in keratin are needed to align the protein molecules in the fiber in the proper order (133). Suffice to say that both hair color and texture are abnormal in a copper deficiency.

H. Lipid Synthesis

First reported in rats (134), hypercholesterolemia occurs in all species (humans included) that have inadequate amounts of copper in the diet (135). Typically, the deficiency stimulates cholesterol synthesis de novo (136) and results in a more rapid clearance of the newly made cholesterol from the liver into the plasma (137). The rate-controlling enzyme, 3-hydroxy-3-methylglutaryl coenzyme A (HMG-CoA) reductase, is also stimulated, but a direct regulation by copper is not likely (138). Hypercholesterolemia is reflected by nonuniform changes in pool sizes and composition of plasma VLDL, LDL, and HDL (139). Recently, Kim et al. (140) found that copper-deficient rats given buthionine sulfoxamine, a drug that lowers cellular levels of glutathione, fail to show hypercholesterolemia and elevated cholesterol HMG-CoA reductase activity. These data suggest that the copper status may influence glutathione levels, which in turn could impact positively on the HMG-CoA reductase activity. Although it seems clear that copper has a physiologic role in cholesterol production, the details and site of interaction have yet to be worked out.

Copper deficiency also alters the lipid composition of organs and tissues. The catalytic properties and stability of the microsomal desaturase enzyme, one of the enzymes responsible for desaturation of stearic acid, is known to be influenced (141). Liver stearoyl desaturase activity is lowered by two-thirds but quickly restored upon copper repletion (142). As a general principle, copper deficiency tends to shift fatty acid synthesis to products with higher degrees of unsaturation. Arachidonic acid, a prostaglandin precursor, is one of the preferred products.

I. Angiogenesis

Angiogenesis (neovascularization) plays a profound role in diseases such as cancer, diabetes, and arthritis. $CuSO_4$ and copper complexes induce growth of new blood vessels, as demonstrated in the rabbit cornea (143). Elvax pellets containing 10–75 μg of $CuSO_4$ or other copper sources implanted beneath the corneal sheath induce the formation of endothelial cells which create the capillaries and a well-defined canal system with tributaries for conducting blood flow. The effect can persists for more than 2 months. The role of copper in inducing angiogenesis is not understood, although collagenase from leukocytes is believed to be a fundamental factor in the induction mechanism. Recently, it was shown that low to moderate amounts of copper ions (0.01–0.2 mM) in a suspension of rabbit peritoneal leukocytes stimulated collagenase production in a dose-dependent manner and promoted the release of the enzyme from the cells (144). The copper did not appear to act directly on collagenase. Moreover, the collagenase in fibroblasts or endothelial cells was not affected. Other metal ions, such as Zn(II), Fe(III), or Mg(II) had less than 10% of the activity of Cu(II). Since the invasive effects of certain tumors requires angiogenesis, a deficiency in copper paradoxically can benefit tumor-bearing animals by depriving the copper needed for tumor blood vessels to form. While still in its early stages, some studies have actually shown that low dietary copper combined with penicillamine (a copper chelator) treatment inhibits the infiltrative spread of invasive brain tumors in rats (145). The same treatment fails to inhibit tumor growth in thigh muscle (146). The studies clearly show a need for copper in angiogenesis, and suggest a dietary approach to dealing with inoperable tumors.

V. BIOCHEMICAL FUNCTIONS OF COPPER (CUPROENZYMES, CYTOKINES, AND THEIR RELATIONSHIP TO PATHOLOGY)

Connective tissue weakness, anemia, loss of pigmentation, and other symptoms of copper deprivation have a primary defect in cuproenzymes which for lack of copper have lost their catalytic effectiveness. The symptoms one observes many times fit the function(s) of the failing enzyme in question. An example is the enzyme lysyl oxidase, whose function in crosslinking of collagen and elastin was suspected long before lysyl oxidase was isolated and shown to have a copper cofactor. A clear one-to-one relationship with enzymes, however, does not exist for all symptoms. Indeed, some symptoms have not been linked to a specific biochemical factor. Following are important enzymes recognized for their need for copper.

A. Lysyl Oxidase

Lysyl oxidase (EC 1.4.3.13) (LO) is a factor in the posttranslational processing of both collagen and elastin. In the reaction, uni- and multichain condensations form first as aldocondensates and Schiff bases. More extensive condensations give rise to desmosines and isodesmosines, crosslinks that unite the coiled springlike chains of elastin into a uniform protein sheet (Fig. 7). In mammalian systems the mature form of LO is a 32-kDa monomer with one Cu(II) firmly bound (147). LO catalyzes posttranslational deamination of lysine and hydroxylysine residues in specific environments of collagen and elastin precursor molecules to form allysine residues, the aldehyde derivative (148):

$$\text{Peptidyl-L-lysyl-peptide} + H_2O + O_2 = \text{Peptidyl-allysyl-peptide} + NH_3 + H_2O_2$$

Human LO maps to chromosome 5, specifically, 5q23.3-31.2 (149). Structural information obtained by analyzing cDNAs from the human placenta and rat aorta reveal a single polypeptide chain of 417 amino acids with a 21-residue presequence signal peptide. Copper is both a cofactor and a regulator of LO expression in tissues. The singe copper atom is projected to be present in a histidine-rich pocket referred to as "talon" (150). Dietary Cu deficiency rapidly depresses the LO oxidase activity in chick aorta (151) and lung (98), causing the percentage of salt-extractable (noncrosslinked) collagen and elastin to increase (Fig. 8). Micromolar amounts of $CuSO_4$ administered i.p. to a copper-deficient animal raises the enzyme to near normal levels in hours (152). The activity also can be restored in vitro by adding copper salts to the aorta in culture medium (153). No other metal can substitute for Cu in either in-vivo or in-vitro activation. As much as 6–8% of the [67]Cu incorporated into rat skin binds to LO, with an estimated 2.7–7.5 nmol of the enzyme in 1 g of skin (154). Lysyl oxidase is highly associated within connective tissues (148). Immuno-fluorescence analysis has detected the enzyme in aorta, dermal connective tissue, and fibroblasts, as well as the cytoskeleton of endothelial cells, basal cells, biliary epithelial, and glomular epithelium (155).

B. Ferroxidase

Ferroxidase is a name given originally to ceruloplasmin to signify an ability to catalyze the oxidation of ferrous ions at neutral pH:

$$4Fe^{2+} + O_2 + 4H^+ \rightarrow 4Fe^{3+} + 2H_2O$$

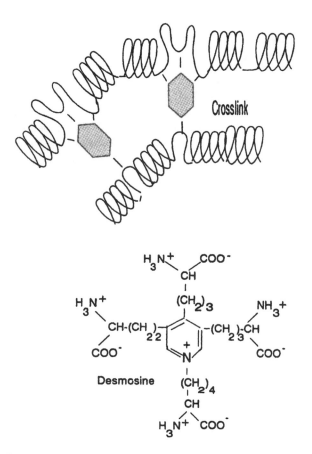

FIGURE 7   Role of desmosine in crosslinking elastin. Elastin monomers depend on intermolecular crosslinks to form a polymerized three-dimensional network of fibers. The desmosines and other crosslinks are formed by oxidation of the ε-carbon of lysine residues in the precursor proteins to form allysine. Condensations of allysines from neighboring chains eventually give rise to the desmosine structure shown in the figure or an isomer. The role of the desmosine in uniting the chains is also shown. Elastic fibers are bands of criss-crossing strands that are embedded in the tissue and surrounding a tubelike structure of the blood vessel. In copper deficiency, these fibers are much sparser, fragmented or incomplete, and are incapable of providing the elastic support for the vessel (see Fig. 5).

The function was considered unique until a second plasma factor with ferroxidase activity was discovered (156). That discovery prompted a change in nomenclature, and ceruloplasmin was called ferroxidase I and this second component ferroxidase II. Ferroxidase II is a cuproprotein with lipophilic properties, comprised of two subunits, whose combined atomic mass is about 800 kDa. Unlike ceruloplasmin, ferroxidase II is yellow, with only one Cu(II) essential for catalytic activity (157). Ferroxidase II activity is not inhibited by sodium azide (156), which would be expected since type 2 and type 3 copper centers are not in the molecule. Ceruloplasmin (ferroxidase I) has been shown to have three binding sites for ferrous ion (158).

It is still argued, however, as to whether the ferroxidase activity of ceruloplasmin or

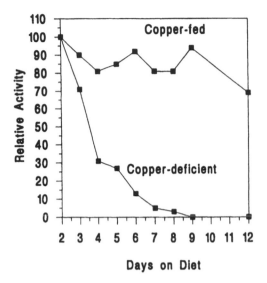

FIGURE 8 Lysyl oxidase activity in copper deficiency. The data are for newly hatched chicks. Half were fed a diet containing less than 1 μg/g copper. The other half consumed a normal, control diet with adequate copper. Lysyl oxidase activity in the aorta falls sharply in copper deficiency. By 9 days, no activity was detectable in the aortic tissue. Controls receiving adequate copper maintained a steady amount of enzyme activity in the tissue.

ferroxidase II has a physiologic function (159). In support of the hypothesis, it has been noted that the mobilization of iron from its storage sites in mucosal and hepatic parenchymal cells does not take place at normal rates in copper deficiency (110). Importantly, injections of ceruloplasmin into deficient swine result in an immediate rise in the plasma iron (160,161). In a perfused dog liver, as little as 4 nM ceruloplasmin in the perfusing medium stimulates the release of Fe as an Fe(III)–transferrin complex (162). The quantity of complex formed is proportional to the amount of ceruloplasmin used. Ceruloplasmin is more effective than $CuSO_4$ in stimulating release, and the rapidity of the response suggests that the effect is direct. Rat ceruloplasmin, which has less ferroxidase activity than human ceruloplasmin, is also less effective in mobilizing iron (160). Moreover, as an oxidant of ferrous iron, ceruloplasmin is superior to HCO_3^-, orthophosphate, citrate, apo-transferrin, or albumin, either alone or in combination (163). In opposing the feroxidase hypothesis, some studies have suggested that the ferroxidase activity in plasma is attributable to citrate (164), and what has been called azide-resistant ferroxidase activity is merely copper released from ceruloplasmin by storage or some other protein modification (165). Part of the lingering uncertainty regarding the physiologic significance of ferroxidase stems from a failure to pursue vigorously the properties and function of ferroxidase II, and the recognition that in patients suffering from Wilson's disease, with characteristic diminished levels of ceruloplasmin, iron metabolism appears to be normal.

C. Interleukin-2

Both humoral and cellular factors of the immune system are suppressed by copper deficiency. Copper deficiency decreases the relative percentages of splenic T lymphocytes and T-helper cells in rodents and impairs the ability of these and phagocytic cells to respond to proliferation signals (166). In contrast, B cells and monocytes in blood from deficient animals are increased. Normally, mitogenic signals induce T cells to move into the S phase of the cell cycle and initiate DNA synthesis. In the fully coordinated response, the synthesis of interleukin-2 (IL-2), a helper T-cell hormone, activates unstimulated cells and macrophages (167). Cells from deficient animals synthesize less IL-2 and release less hormone upon stimulation (168). The cells, however, continue to express normal levels of receptors for the stimuli. IL-2 added back to mitogen-treated deficient cells, however, allows DNA synthesis to follow its normal course, suggesting that the apparent weak response was a function of IL-2 availability. In less than 1 week of copper repletion, cells are able to respond at nearly full levels (168). With this has come a realization that inadequate copper in the diet reversibly suppresses IL-2 and the maturation and function of splenic T-helper cells.

D.   Dopamine β-Monooxygenase

Dopamine β-monooxygenase (EC 1.14.17.1)(DMO), also referred to as dopamine β-hydroxylase, is a member of a class of enzymes that require copper as a cofactor and use ascorbate as an electron donor (169). The enzyme catalyzes the conversion of dopamine to the neurotransmitter norepinephrine. There are both soluble and membrane-bound forms of the enzyme, the latter in association with chromaffin granules of the adrenal medulla (170). Catalytically active DMO is a tetramer with two copper atoms per monomer, making this enzyme one of the most complicated of all copper enzymes. The reaction uses two electrons donated from ascorbic acid.

3,4-Dihydroxyphenylethylamine (dopamine) + ascorbate + O_2 = norepinephrine + dehydroascorbate + H_2O

The adrenal medulla is known to be a rich source of ascorbate. An electron-transport mechanism with a membrane-bound cytochrome b_{561} is used to recycle the oxidized ascorbate. Recent data have revealed a remarkable structural similarity between DMO and α-amidating enzyme (see below) (171).

E.   Tyrosinase

Tyrosinase (E.C. 1.14.18.1) is present in melanocytes, where melanin is formed. The synthesis of melanin occurs in multiple steps with tyrosinase catalyzing three of the reactions (172):

(1)   (2)
Tyrosine → L-DOPA → dopaquinone → dopachrome → 5,6-dihydroxyindole +
              (3)
5,6-dihydroxyindole-2-carboxylate →→→ pheomelanin and eumelanin

The first step in the pathway is the conversion of tyrosine to the intermediate L-3,4-dihydroxyphenylalanine (L-DOPA). L-DOPA is then oxidized to dopaquinone, which cyclizes spontaneously to form dopachrome, which in turn rearranges and forms 5,6-dihydroxy indole and 5,6-dihydroxyindole-2-carboxylic acid. Further condensations and oxidations give rise to pheomelanin (reddish brown) and eumelanin (dark brown to black), the typical biopigments. An interesting anomaly regarding the enzyme is that depleting glutathione levels in melanocytes with buthionine sulfoxamine (BSO) strongly elevates tyrosinase activity and melanin formation (173).

F. α-Amidating Monooxygenase

α-Amidating monooxygenase (E.C. 1.14.17.3)(α-AE) is also an ascorbate-dependent monooxygenase, α-AE catalyzes the posttranslational conversion of peptides with a carboxy-terminal glycine to the amide (174). The overall reaction is

Peptidylglycine + ascorbate + O_2 = peptidyl(2-hydroxyglycine) + dehydroascorbate + H_2O + desglycine peptide amide + glyoxylate

The reaction occurs in two steps. α-AE is bifunctional, and the first step is catalyzed by a peptide component that requires two copper atoms for activity (174a). Hydrolysis of the first product, peptidyl(2-hydroxyglycine), is catalyzed by a specific lyase component of the peptide, forming glyoxylate and a peptide amide, i.e., the original peptide less the two glycine carbons (referred to as desglycine peptide amide). In the reaction, two electron equivalents from ascorbate are transferred to the peptide substrate. Vasopressin, calcitonin, gastrin, and oxytocin are a few of the peptides whose C-terminal residues have been amidated by the enzyme. Its distribution is widespread. Adrenal medulla, pituitary, pancreas, and cardiac atria have been shown to be sources of α-AE (175), and cDNAs prepared from bovine pituitary, atrial tissue, and thyroid carcinoma cells give evidence for multiple mRNAs coding for α-AE. All α-AEs isolated thus far require exogenous copper (2 μM) and ascorbate (3 mM) in the assay medium to obtain maximal enzyme activity (176). Zinc, calcium, iron, magnesium, nickel, cobalt, and manganese ions have no effect on the activity (177).

G. Cytochrome *c* Oxidase

Cytochrome *c* oxidase (EC 1.9.3.1) in aerobic oxidation catalyzes a four-electron reduction of O_2 in mitochondria and is directly responsible for establishing the high-energy proton gradient across the inner mitochondrial membrane (178):

4 cytochrome *c* (Fe^{2+}) + O_2 + 4 H^+ → 4 cytochrome *c* (Fe^{3+}) + 2 H_2O

This gradient retains the energy of electron transport for the synthesis of ATP. Cytochrome oxidase is a multisubunit complex consisting of at least nine and possibly more subunits. The larger subunits (I–III) are synthesized on mitochondria genes and engage four spectrographically distinct metals, two irons and two copper, bound to two dissimilar heme groups (heme a and a_3), and in close proximity to permit fascile electron transfer. The binding site for dioxygen is located on heme a_3 and consists of a copper–iron pair that interacts magnetically and physically. Cytochrome *c* oxidase receives electrons directly from cytochrome c and mediates their passage to dioxygen. Restricting copper in the diet severely suppresses the cytochrome *c* oxidase activity in a number of rat organs, thus potentiating a possible fall in ATP production (179). These observations link copper with the major energy-generating system of the cell.

H. Superoxide Dismutase

Mammalian cells contain two forms of superoxide dismutase (EC 1.15.1.1), a mangano and a cupro/zinc form. These enzymes are major defenses against oxygen toxicity, and a deficiency of copper weakens that defense. The dismutation reaction for superoxide anion is

$O_2^-\cdot$ + $O_2^-\cdot$ + 2H^+ = H_2O_2 + O_2

The Cu_2,Zn_2 form of this enzyme has relevance to the present discussion. It is present in all mammalian tissues. The enzyme is a 32-kDa homodimer located in a cytosolic compartment identified recently with the peroxisomes (180,181). The type 2 Cu-binding site in the enzyme has four histidines, one of which binds both copper and zinc on opposite sides of an imidazole ring. The bovine erythrocyte enzyme, one of the better-characterized forms, is known to be a dimer with identical 151 residue subunits and with active sites that face away from one another. Copper sits in a deep cleft and zinc is completely buried within the protein (182). Studies performed at different ranges of pH and temperature suggest that copper is the more mobile factor (183). In catalysis, copper is reduced by the first O_2^- and then reoxidized by the second O_2^- to yield O_2 and H_2O_2 (see above). Cu deficiency depresses CuZnSOD activity in numerous animal tissues (88,179). Erythrocyte CuZnSOD activity is restored by copper but not by zinc (184). Yeast cells (*Saccharomyces cerevisiae*) require at least 150 nM Cu^{2+} in the growth medium to sustain steady-state levels of the enzyme (185). Cu is thus a key to the CuZnSOD activity in tissues (186). Substitution of one of the histidines with cysteine (His 46 to Cys 46) leads to a stable copper site mutant with a new binding site closely resembling a type 1 copper site (187).

Experimentally, lowered intakes of copper suppress SOD activity in numerous tissues (186). SOD activity is restored by dietary copper supplementation or by injecting small doses of copper salts intraperitoneally (42,188). Reactivation is rapid and depends on the dose of copper given; 0.5 μmol injected i.p., for example, will suffice to activate the enzyme in the aorta of a 50-g chick. The extreme sensitivity to copper perhaps portrays a transport system that functions at nanomolar levels of copper. Zinc deficiency, surprisingly, does not lower CuZnSOD activity in erythrocytes of rats and chicks (184,189), while a copper deficiency strongly suppresses the enzyme. These data suggest that cells must incorporate copper continuously to sustain a steady-state level of functional CuZnSOD activity. Although zinc can be replaced by cadmium, mercury, or cobalt ions (190), no metal can substitute for copper to restore or retain activity. As measured by an enzyme-linked immunosorbent assay (ELISA), the enzyme protein stays relatively constant during short-term copper omission (44,188). Thus, apo-enzyme synthesis is likely to go on unabated despite a short supply of a critical metal cofactor.

I. Other Enzymes

1. Amine Oxidases

Copper-containing amine oxidases (EC 1.4.3.6) are quite versatile enzymes. Functioning primarily in the oxidative deamination of biogenic primary amines, these enzymes produce an oxidized organic product (generally an aldehyde) and form NH_3 and H_2O_2 as side products. Two of the better characterized are the bovine serum amine oxidase and porcine benzylamine oxidase. Copper-dependent amine oxidases, surprisingly, are not found in bacteria. Amine oxidases in general are composed of two identical subunits with two nonequivalent copper ions per subunit and an organic (carbonyl) cofactor which, in the resting oxidized enzyme, was recently identified as the quinone of 3-(2,4,5-trihydroxy-phenyl)-L-alanine (topa), a cofactor derived from one of the tyrosine residues in the protein (191). Whether topa is the cofactor for all amine oxidases seems unlikely, but is still under investigation.

2. Galactose Oxidase

Galactose oxidase (EC 1.6.6.4) is an extracellular enzyme that catalyzes the oxidation of most primary alcohols to the corresponding aldehyde; molecular oxygen is the substrate and peroxide is a product. The enzyme is of interest because it catalyzes a two-electron redox reaction using a single Cu(II) site:

$$RCH_2OH + O_2 = RCHO + H_2O_2$$

This single Cu(II) is ligated to a tyrosine. During catalysis, the protein, not the metal, is activated by a one-electron transfer (192). This happens when the tyrosine–copper complex becomes a free radical. Thus, the copper in the enzyme is associated with a stable free radical within the structure, a unique copper–enzyme interaction. The extreme sensitivity of the enzyme for copper is exemplified in *Gibberella*, where nanomolar amounts of Cu(II) are all that are needed to activate the enzyme (193).

3. Nitrite Reductase and Nitrous Oxide Reductase

Nitrite reductase (21) and nitrous oxide reductase (194) are two of the better-known copper enzymes in plants. Each functions in the denitrification pathway leading to the formation of N_2. In *Acromobacter cycloclastes*, nitrite reductase is a dimer with subunits of 69 kDa and three Cu atoms per dimer. Cupredoxin, a small type-1 blue copper protein, donates electrons to nitrite reductase. Nitrous oxide reductase contains two identical subunits with eight copper atoms and a molecular weight of 71 kDa.

4. Multicopper Oxidases

Laccase

Laccase (EC 1.10.3.2) (urishiol oxidase) is the simplest of the multicopper oxidases. As with all multioxidases, laccase contains three copper centers: one blue, one normal, and a coupled binuclear. Laccase thus supports the concept that only four copper atoms are needed to perform full oxidase function, i.e., the complete reduction of dioxygen to H_2O by a four-electron transfer. The enzyme is found in fungi and plants, and the substrates for this enzyme span a wide variety of phenols and diamines.

Ascorbate Oxidase

Ascorbate oxidase (EC 1.10.3.3)(AO) is found strictly in the cell walls of higher plants (195). The name is a misnomer, since organic acids other than ascorbic acid can serve as substrates. Green zucchini AO, one of the better characterized, is a homodimer of $M_r = 140,000$, with eight copper atoms per protein.

Ceruloplasmin

Ceruloplasmin (EC 1.16.3.1) (ferroxidase) (Cp) is the only multicopper oxidase present in humans and vertebrates. Isolated from plasma, ceruloplasmin has been studied extensively for its role in biological oxidations (organic and inorganic), antioxidant functions, and copper distribution to tissues. The human protein is a single polypeptide chain, 1046 amino acid residues, with four asparagine-linked oligosaccharide chains and 6–7 g-atoms of copper per 132,000 g of protein. One of the coppers could be a Cu(I), and in recognition of this unusual feature, has been designated type 4 copper by Rydén (196). The two blue type 1 coppers differ in redox potential (197), and one or both may be partially reduced (198); only one type 1 copper is involved in the transfer of electrons to O_2.

Ceruloplasmin is highly versatile—one of the few enzymes in nature capable of oxidizing both organic and inorganic substrates. Its oxidase activity toward aromatic amines, diamines, and ferrous ions is brought about by four Cu(II) ions at the C-terminal region of the protein (see Fig. 9). *p*-Phenylenediamine, N,N'-dimethyl-*p*-phenylene-

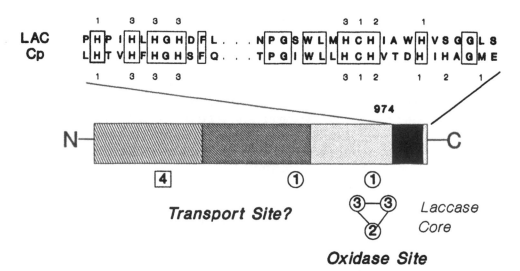

FIGURE 9 Comparison of copper centers in ceruloplasmin and laccase. Ceruloplasmin's structure gives evidence for a triple repeat in the overall sequence. The C-terminal end of the 1046-residue molecule bears a striking sequence homology to the oxidase site of laccase (200). Residues showing sequence identity are in boxes. The different types are indicated by number, with the trinuclear site shown in a triangular arrangement. The three homologous regions in Cp (approximately 340 residues) are shown by different stippling. The dark region on the C-terminal gives rise to the Cp sequences shown; not all are included. Four of the six copper atoms in Cp are present in the C-terminal region; the Cu are present as types 1–3. Because of sequence similarity and functional overlap, the region can be referred to as the "laccase core" in the molecule, suggesting that all copper so named function in the oxidase activity of the protein. Two additional coppers, one type 1 and one type 4 (square), are located in other regions of the protein. These two coppers have no functional assignment and could be involved in copper transport.

diamine, and *o*-dianisidine are substrates commonly employed to assay ceruloplasmin oxidase activity. The copper atoms are bound with different affinities, and the peptide chain of Cp is highly susceptible to proteases. Two trypsin-sensitive bonds are believed to be present, and their ease of cleavage led earlier investigators to conclude erroneously that Cp was oligomeric. The lability of some copper atoms leads to variable copper content of the isolated protein. A labile trinuclear center, similar to laccase, is also found in ceruloplasmin (199). One type 1 copper is coupled to the trinuclear center, comprising what may be called the "laccase core."

The transport function of Cp is poorly understood. Of the 114 residues in the C-terminal domain of Cp, 27 align in register with laccase (200). Figure 9 shows the extensive sequence homology in this short segment. If the C-terminal is the oxidase site, then the unassigned Cu atoms, viz., the second blue type 1 and the Cu(I), could be used for transport. Which Cu atoms in Cp actually exchange with cells during transport has not been determined.

5. Intracellular and Extracellular Copper-Binding Proteins

Storage of copper is a function of *metallothionein*, a cysteine-rich protein that binds many metals including copper. Next to ferritin, metallothionein (MT) is the most metal-rich protein known. Metallothioneins, however, do not bind iron (201). Human liver contains about 200 mg of MT, but this amount can be increased as much as 40 times when the cells are exposed to heavy metals (202). The complete amino acid sequences for human and equine liver MT are known (202). Metallothionein in all species are composed of about 60 amino acids, one-third of which are cysteine. There are no aromatic amino acids or disulfides. These low-molecular-weight proteins are present in most eukaryotic cells, but the better characterized are in the liver and kidney of various animal species. Similar proteins have been described in lower vertebrates, invertebrates, and microorganisms (203). The two major isoforms, metallothionein I and II, differ slightly in composition. Each contains 61 amino acids and has a calculated molecular weight of 6800. For native metallothionein, it is not unusual to find two or more different metals bound to the same molecule. The metals most commonly found in active metallothionein, Zn^{2+}, Cd^{2+}, and Cu^+, are bound to two separate metal clusters, one containing four metals and the other three. Designated A and B, respectively, each cluster coordinates a metal ion via four cysteinyl sulfurs. Copper is known to bind selectively to the three-metal cluster B sites (204). Cadmium ions bind almost exclusively to cluster A and can displace zinc. Cadmium is not a strong displacer of copper, however, suggesting that zinc and copper do not share the same cluster (205). The copper in metallothionein has been shown to restore enzymatic activity to metal-free dopamine β-monooxygenase (206) and tyrosinase (207), intimating that a copper–MT complex could be involved in the intracellular transport of copper to enzymes.

When cDNAs for blood-clotting Factors V and VIII were sequenced, it was noted that they bore close sequence homology to ceruloplasmin, giving rise to the speculation that these blood-clotting factors could bind copper and were likely to be cuproteins (208). Atomic absorption analysis has subsequently confirmed the validity of the concept for both factors (209,210). One gram-atom of copper per mole of protein is known to be present, presumably to help stabilize the interaction between the light and heavy chains of each factor.

VI. GENETIC DISEASES

Insights into the mechanism of copper-based diseases has contributed immensely to our understanding of normal metabolic pathways for copper in a living system. Two diseases stand out over the years: Menkes' syndrome and Wilson's disease. Both remain enigmas, but both have had major advancements in understanding of cause. Suffice it to say that both have their roots in genetic factors that maintain copper homeostasis and distribution in cells.

Menkes' disease, first described by John Menkes, an American pediatrician, is a fatal progressive neurologic disorder characterized by a "kinky-type" hair texture. The disease is X-linked and recessive, affecting mostly infant males (211). The kinky-hair descriptive derives from the presence of microscopic twists in the hair shafts (referred to as *pili torti*). Depending on severity, a Menkes' sufferer seldom lives beyond 2 years of age. Menkes' disease has its counterpart in animals in what has been described as a spontaneous mutation in inbred C57BL mice, referred to as brindled mottled (*Mo^{br}*) mutant. A second mouse mutant referred to as "macular" also expresses the disease (212). These mice have provided animal models of the clinical disorder (213). In both humans and animals, the disease has been traced to a mismanagement of copper at levels of absorption and tissue distribution. David Danks in Australia was the first to point out that Menkes' disease

Metal-Binding Site

32   *61*

Wilson   I L <u>G M T C</u> O <u>S C V</u> K S I E D R I S N L K G I I S M <u>K V S L</u>

Menkes   V E <u>G M T C</u> N <u>S C V</u> W TI E Q Q I G K V N G V H H I <u>K V S L</u>

14   *43*

Transduction Domain

806   *834* ·

Wilson   <u>G G K F P V D G</u> K V L E G N T M A <u>D E S L I T G E A M P V</u>

Menkes   <u>G G K F P V D G</u> R V I E G H S M V <u>D E S L I T G E A M P V</u>

853   *881*

Channel Phosphorylation

985   *1004*

Wilson   <u>E M A H K</u> I K T V M F <u>D K T G T I</u> I H G

Menkes   <u>E M A H K</u> V K V V V F <u>D K T G T I</u> T H G

1034   *1053*

ATP Binding

1227   *1255*

Wilson   G K K V <u>A M V G D G</u> V <u>N D S P A L A</u> O A D M G V <u>A I G T G</u>

Menkes   G K R V <u>A M V G D G</u> I <u>N D S P A L A</u> M A N V G I <u>A I G T G</u>

1293   *1321*

FIGURE 10   Alignment similarities of amino acid sequences in the Wilson's and Menkes' disease proteins. The data are derived from an analysis of the two genes. Four different domains are shown: metal-binding, transduction, channel phosphorylation, and ATP-binding. Letters are codes for the individual amino acids. Underline shows sequences that are common to both proteins. Numbers indicate the residue position in the protein.

closely resembled a pattern seen in animals with severe copper deficiency (132). Particularly noticeable was a strange twisting of abdominal, visceral, and femoral blood vessels. Subsequently, it was shown that Menkes' patients had serum copper values one-third normal, and less copper was present in brain and liver. Although they were able to clear copper from the plasma at normal rates, Menkes' patients were blocked in transferring copper from the mucosa to the blood.

Wilson's disease is a progressive hepatolenticular degeneration first thought to be a familial cirrhosis by its discoverer, Sir S. A. Kinnier Wilson (214). The incidences of the disease are 1/4000 in certain Middle Eastern populations to 1/40,000 in the Untied States (215). The disorder is inherited as an autosomal recessive pattern associated with chromosome 13 (216). Wilson's disease affects most organs, but pathologies are evident mostly in liver and brain. Its most outstanding pathology is an excess accumulation of copper in liver and brain (217). Biliary copper excretion is practically nonexistent (218). Low ceruloplasmin levels, once considered a hallmark of the disease, are seen in about 85% of afflicted individuals. A significant advance has been the isolation of a gene from human liver that is believed to encode the defective factor (219). The data have shown that the Wilson gene protein is a P-type ATPase that bears a striking similarity in certain features to the Menkes' gene protein (220,221). Figure 10 illustrates this point. Sequences of amino acids derived from the two genes reveal long strings of almost identical sequence throughout the different protein domains. For example, like the Menkes', the Wilson protein contains six copper-binding sites, denoted by the presence of GMTCxSC, in the N-terminus region of the protein, the sequence DKTGTI in the channel phosphorylation site (recall D, aspartic acid, forms a chemical bond with phosphate from ATP), and the sequence GxNDSPALA in the ATP-binding site. The overall sequence identity between the two proteins is 57%, but as high as 79% in certain regions (220).

VII. TOXICOLOGY

Copper finds its way into the environment in metal utensils, copper coins, plumbing fixtures, valves on dispensing machines, bacteriocides, and numerous industrial applications. This has increased the probability of humans and animals becoming exposed to copper at toxic levels. For example, a 1–2% copper solution (referred to as Bordeaux mixture) is used as a fungicidal spray on grape vines (222). Copper sprays are toxic to bacteria and are commonly used to control the growth of phytopathogenic species. Health problems, however, occur in vineyard workers who spray vines with copper sulfate. Health problems also arise by accidental ingestion, causing gastrointestinal disturbances and nausea (53). Cu_2O is a toxic pigment used to prevent barnacle growth on ship bottoms. Of interest to nutritionists is that some microorganisms develop resistance to copper exposure. Such resistance, although poorly characterized, has a genetic basis associated with conjugative plasmids harbored in the organism. For the latter, the precise regulator sites and functions of gene products have yet to be fully elucidated. These finding have affected how we view the mechanism for handling copper in mammalian cells (see below).

VIII. GENETIC REGULATION

Pioneering studies by a number of laboratories have shown that metal ions can regulate genes for heavy metal-binding and storage proteins. As discussed below, cells have adapted a variety of strategies to exploit these interaction. This has made a metal such as copper a major determinant of genetic expression. The subject has been reviewed (223).

Studies of the genetic apparatus of bacteria, yeast, and algae have uncovered a remarkable capacity for copper ions to regulate the genetic expression of proteins that sequester copper ions for storage, electron transport, or catalytic activity. Through such intervention, copper literally is able to control its own metabolic destiny in cells. In one interesting example, chloroplasts and cyanobacteria use a c-type cytochrome, cytochrome c-552 (containing iron), to conduct electron transfer in photosynthesis. These organisms also use plastocyanin (PC), a cuproprotein, for the same biological reaction. Thus, PC and cytochrome c-552 are functionally interconvertible. Which transport factor is selected depends on the amount of copper in the cell or accessible to the cell from the culture medium. That amount, in turn, is a determinant of the level of PC mRNA levels in the cells and the turnover time of the apo (copper-free) PC. Mature PC is synthesized only when the medium copper concentration exceeds 8 μM (224). Less than this amount will decrease the steady-state levels of PC mRNA and hastens the destruction of apoPC (half-life 16–18 min) (25). The synthesis of PC is accompanied by the presence of a repressor that blocks the synthesis of cytochrome c-552 mRNA. Only when PC has reached its functional biological concentration is the repressing factor at sufficient amounts to stop cytochrome c_{552} synthesis (225). These remarkable observations show how exacting and specific copper can be in regulating the expression of cell proteins. Although the mechanism may not be universal, its interesting to note that a similar phenomenon has been shown in green alga, *Pediastrum boryanum*. In these cells, 2 μM $CuSO_4$ leads to the accumulation of (apo)plastocyanin, whereas no added copper favors accumulation of (apo)cytochrome c-553 (226). Thus, copper ions appear to regulate synthesis of two photosynthetic electron carriers proteins at a pretranslational (transcriptional or posttranstranscriptional) level. Copper is the switch that determines if an iron or copper protein takes part in the photosynthetic reaction.

Perhaps analogous to the above is the capacity of copper ions to regulate genetic expression in cultures of common Baker's yeast, *Sacchromyces cerevisae*. Yeasts are able to tolerate copper because of an ability to synthesize metallothionein, a small, cysteine-rich protein which in this yeast is encoded by the *CUP1* gene. Regulation of the expression of *CUP1* is a function of ACE1, an 11-kDa cysteine-rich protein that activates transcription (227). ACE1 (which means Activation of *CUP1* Expression) contains 225 amino acids and a C terminus that is rich in acidic amino acids and an N-terminal portion rich in cysteine residues that bind Cu^+ in a manner analogous to metallothionein. ACE1 binds to DNA in the promoter region only when Cu^+ (or Ag^+) ions are bound to the protein. The presence of the metal allows recognition of two consensus sequences at -180 and -240 base pairs upstream from the start site. Recent evidence has shown that ACE1 also regulates the enzyme CuZnSOD in yeast (228). Figure 11 shows that this is brought about by having nearly identical ACE1 recognition sequences in the promoter region upstream from the start site of both *CUP1* and *SOD1*. The necessity for having both genes turn on simultaneously is still not clear, but could be related to the way these cells cope with high copper exposure. A second regulatory factor, AMT1, is a copper-dependent DNA-binding factor that has recently been identified in the yeast strain *Candida glabrata* (229). In this yeast, copper detoxification is more closely linked with higher organisms in that a family of three metallothionein (MT) genes take an active part: a *MT-I* gene that is unique for this yeast, a tandemly amplified *MTIIa* gene, and a single unlinked *MT-IIb* gene. AMT1 shows a striking sequence similarity to ACE1 at the N-terminus region. Kinetic data have shown that AMT1 mRNA accumulates very rapidly in the presence of copper. This AMT1-

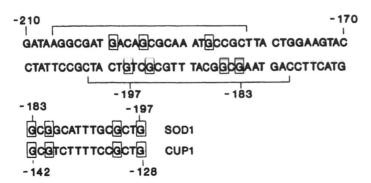

FIGURE 11 Comparative sequences of ACE1-binding site in the *SOD1* promoter. Upper figure shows the ACE1 site of the *SOD1* promoter. Brackets indicate the approximate location where ACE1 binds as determined by a DNAse I cleavage protection assay. Boxes show the location of guanines residues whose methylation will interrupt ACE1 binding in vitro. The lower figure compares the ACE1-binding site sequence of *SOD1* with an analogous sequence on the coding strand of promoter region for *CUP1*, the gene that codes for metallothionine in the yeast. (After Ref 228.)

positive autoregulation rapidly establishes a strong defense against high environmental copper.

Further evidence that copper ions control the expression of genes coding copper-binding proteins and enzymes has been derived from studies of heavy metal tolerance in bacteria. Table 3 summarizes those most important for copper. Copper is used as a bacteriocide for microorganisms that attack plants and animals. Invariably, such organisms acquire a tolerance to the toxic effects. *Pseudomonas syringae* carry an operon, *CopABCD*, that determines the extent to which copper ions accumulate in the periplasm and outer membrane. *CopABCD* is a copper-inducible operon borne on a plasmid that is harbored

TABLE 3 Genes Associated with Copper Resistance and Transport in Bacteria

Gene	Function or gene product	References
CopA	Periplasmic binding protein	230,233–235
CopB	Outer membrane-binding protein	230,233–235
CopC	Periplasmic binding protein	230,234,235
CopD	Inner membrane-binding protein	230,234,235
pcoA	Copper efflux	230,236
pcoB	Metal efflux	230,236
pcoC	Copper-binding protein, 26 kDa	230,236
pcoR	Transacting repressor	230,236
cutA	Nonspecific copper uptake	236,237
cutB	Copper-specific uptake	236,237
cutC	Copper efflux (low-level copper)	236,237
cutD	Copper efflux (low-level copper)	236,237
cutE	Intracellular copper transport/storage (regulation)	230,237,238
cutF	Intracellular copper transport/storage (regulation)	236,237
cutR	Intracellular copper transport/storage (regulation)	236,237

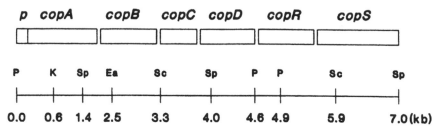

FIGURE 12 Physical map of *cop* operon genes in *P. Syringae*. Shown are the order of *cop* genes and the approximate size of each relative to the overall operon. Letters above the line refer to restriction nuclease sites, which are denoted as P, *PstI*; K, *KpnI*; Sp, *SphI*; Ea, *EagI*; p, promoter. (After Ref. 234.)

inside plant pathogenic and saprophytic bacteria (Fig. 12). *CopRS* appear to perform regulatory functions. Full copper resistance requires expression of all operon genes.

Another bacterium, *Escherichia coli*, uses a bank of linked genes encoded in a plasmid (pRJ1004), the *pco* cluster (*pcoA*, *pcoB*, *pcoC*, and *pcoR*), to control copper accumulation in the cell (230). The plasmid also contains determinants for low-level copper resistance: *cdr*. The latter are associated with the repair of DNA caused by exposure to low copper. Besides plasmid genes, there is a series of chromosomal genes referred to as *cut* (copper uptake), *cut*ACDEFR, to transport and store copper. Resistance to high copper exposure (up to 22 mM) is mainly a function of the *pco* cluster, which, when stimulated, produces a series of proteins that either sequesters or removes copper from the cell. For example, PcoC is a cytoplasmic transport and storage protein for copper whereas PcoA and PcoB function in copper efflux. The latter are P-type ATPase-driven mechanisms that actively extrude copper from the cell. A similar mechanism also operates in *Enterococcus hirae* (80). As discussed above, the active extrusion of copper by an energy-dependent (ATP) mechanism is believed to be the function of the *Mc1* gene product in human cells and is believed to be a major factor regulating cellular copper homeostasis in cells other than liver. Such a factor could be missing or defective in Menkes' and Wilson's disease. It is interesting to consider that mammals may have retained and in some cases expounded upon the basic bacterial mechanisms for dealing with copper.

IX. PERSPECTIVES FOR FUTURE RESEARCH

In looking ahead, one sees that the nutritional role for copper can be understood only when systems and components that depend on this metal are known. Studies of absorption, transport, and metabolism of copper are making important strides. More revealing, perhaps, are the studies that have defined the molecular basis of copper-deficiency symptoms. By learning the pathway components, we come closer to identifying the specific genes that regulate the transport and storage of copper. Human and animal diseases based on defective or missing genes in the copper pathway are providing the direction. We may now ask what other genes encode factors that regulate copper functions. Copper homeostasis in higher animals is only beginning to be understood. Bacteria learned how to handle copper long before any animal or plant first made its appearance on the earth. Those ancient, remarkable, and effective mechanisms should not be ignored, especially since the carry over to copper–cell interactions in higher animals shows remarkable parallels.

As pointed out in this chapter, the importance of copper in the nutrition of humans and animals extends beyond enzymes. It is thus a challenge to learn how copper exerts a biological effect when it is not part of an enzyme. Nonvertebrates use copper to transport oxygen, perhaps predating iron (hemoglobin) as an oxygen transporter. Its role in angiogenesis, immunocompetence, and blood clotting seems established, but a link with specific copper factors has not been discovered. In yeast, copper activates the expression of genes for its binding and storage proteins, and in plants and algae copper determines which metal–protein complex conducts electron transport in photosynthesis. These observations show the power of copper to alter the metabolic machinery of cells. Copper ions have a capability for regulating transport and storage proteins, and for engaging in cofactor control of enzyme activity. These phenomena are established, but insights into the mechanism are still far from being realized.

Finally, the role of copper in the aging process should not go unnoticed. This single area of copper research is of profound importance, yet is virtually unexplored. If we consider that many of the symptoms of aging, including wrinkling of skin, brain memory loss, graying of hair, and blood vessel and heart pathologies, are all seen in the young, copper-deficient animal, we have reason to suspect that copper is an underlying factor in the aged individual who displays similar symptoms. To date, copper's ability to intercede in early developmental stages has been a major focus of the research on this metal. Its potential to predispose the mature animal to tissue and organ failure could be a major factor in aging phenomena. Copper has unprecedented importance in nutrition regardless of the stage of the life cycle.

REFERENCES

1. Ochiai E-I. Copper and the biological evolution. Biosystems 1983; 16: 81–86.
2. Mason KE. A conspectus of research on copper metabolism and requirements of man. J Nutr 1979; 109: 1979–2066.
3. Biological Roles of Copper. Ciba Foundation Symp. Ser 79. Amsterdam: Excerpta Medica, 1980.
4. Harris ED. Copper in human and animal health. In: Rose J, ed. Trace Elements in Health. A Review of Current Issues. London: Butterworths, 1983: 44–73.
5. Rydén L. Evolution of blue copper proteins. In: King TE, Mason HS, Morrison M, eds. Oxidases and Related Redox Systems. New York: Liss, 1988: 349–366.
6. Kies, C. Copper Bioavailability and Metabolism. Adv in Exp Med. and Biology. Vol. 258. New York: Plenum Press, 1989.
7. Adman ET. Copper protein structures. Adv Protein Chem 1991; 42: 145–198.
8. Harris ED. Copper transport: an overview. Proc Soc Exp Biol Med 1991; 196: 130–140.
9. Linder, MC. Biochemistry of Copper. New York: Plenum Press, 1991.
10. Blair D, Diehl H. Bathophenanthrolinedisulphonic acid and bathocuproinedisulphonic acid, water soluble reagents for iron and copper. Talanta 1961; 7: 163–174.
11. Hanna PM, Tamilarasan R, McMillin DR. Cu(I) analysis of blue copper proteins. Biochem J 1988; 256: 1001–1004.
12. Peterson RE, Bollier ME. Spectrophotometric determination of serum copper with biscyclohexanoneoxalyldihydrazone. Anal Chem 1955: 27: 1195–1197.
13. McMillin DR, Holwerda RA, Gray HB. Preparation and spectroscopic studies of cobalt(II)-stellacyanin. Proc Natl Acad Sci (USA) 1984; 71: 1339–1341.
14. Solomon EI. Coupled binuclear copper proteins: catalytic mechanisms and structure-reactivity correlations. In: King TE, Mason HS, Morrison M, eds. Oxidases and Related Redox Systems. New York: Liss, 1988: 309–329.

15. Volbeda A, Hol WGJ. Structure of arthropodan hemocyanin. In: King TE, Mason HS, Morrison M, eds. Oxidases and Related Redox Systems. New York: Liss, 1988: 291–307.

16. Allendorf MD, Spira DJ, Solomon EI. Low-temperature magnetic circular dichroism studies of native laccase: spectroscopic evidence for exogenous ligand bridging at a trinuclear copper active site. Proc Natl Acad Sci (USA) 1985; 82: 3063–3067.

17. Spira-Solomon DJ, Allendorf MD, Solomon EI. Low-temperature magnetic circular dichroism studies of native laccase: confirmation of a trinuclear copper active site. J Am Chem Soc 1986; 108: 5318–5328.

18. Messerschmidt A, Huber R. The blue oxidases, ascorbate oxidase, laccase and ceruloplasmin. Modelling and structural relationships. Eur J Biochem 1990; 187: 341–352.

19. Gray HB, Solomon EI. Electronic structures of blue copper centers in proteins. In: Spiro TG, ed. Metal Ions in Biology. Vol. 3. New York: Wiley-Interscience 1981; 3–39.

20. Thomann H, Bernardo M, Baldwin MJ, Lowery MD, Solomon EI. Pulsed ENDOR study of the native and high pH perturbed forms of the blue copper site in stellacyanin. J Am Chem Soc 1991; 113: 5911–5913.

21. Denariaz G, Payne WJ, LeGall J. The denitrifying nitrite reductase of *Bacillus halodenitrificans*. Biochim Biophys Acta 1991; 1056: 225–232.

22. Lommen A, Pandya KI, Koningsberger DC, Canters GW. EXAFS analysis of the pH dependence of the blue-copper site in amicyanin from thiobacillus versutus. Biochim Biophys Acta 1991; 1076: 439–447.

23. Husain M, Davidson VL. An inducible periplasmic blue copper protein from *Paracoccus denitrificans*. Purification, properties, and physiological role. J Biol Chem 1985; 260: 14626–14629.

24. Nersissian AM, Nalbandyan RM. Studies of plantacyanin. III. Structural data obtained by CD and MCD methods and antigenic properties of the protein. Biochim Biophys Acta 1988; 957: 446–453.

25. Merchant S, Bogorad L. Rapid degradation of apoplastocyanin in Cu(II)-deficient cells of *Chylamydomonas reinhardtii*. J Biol Chem 1986; 261: 15850–15853.

26. Ohkawa J, Okada N, Shinmyo A, Takano M. Primary structure of cucumber (*Cucumis sativus*) ascorbate oxidase deduced from cDNA sequence: homology with blue copper proteins and tissue-specific expression. Proc Natl Acad Sci (USA) 1989; 86: 1239–1243.

27. Solomon EI. Binuclear copper active site. Hemocyanin, tyrosinase, and type 3 copper oxidases. In: Spiro TG, ed. Metal Ions in Biology. Vol. 3. New York: Wiley-Intersciences, 1981: 41–108.

28. Farver O, Pecht I. Electron transfer in proteins: in search of preferential pathways. FASEB J 1991; 5: 2554–2559.

29. Sternlieb I. Copper and the liver. Gastroenterology 1980; 78: 1615–1628.

30. Klevay LM, Reck SJ, Jacob RA, Logan GH, Munoz JM, Sandstead H. Human requirement for copper. I. Healthy men fed conventional, American diet. Am J Clin Nutr 1980; 33: 45.

31. World Health Organization. Trace elements in human nutrition. Copper. WHO Tech Rep 532 15, 1973.

32. Owen CAJ. Distribution of copper in the rat. Am J Physiol 1964; 207: 446–448.

33. Cordano A, Baerti JM, Graham GG. Copper deficiency in infancy. Pediatrics 1964; 34: 324–336.

34. Cordano A. Copper requirements and actual copper recommendation per 100 kilocalories of infant formula. Pediatrics 1974; 54: 524.

35. Solomons N. Zinc and copper in human nutrition. In: Karcioglu ZA, Sarper RM, eds. Zinc and Copper in Medicine. Springfield, IL: Charles C Thomas 1980: 224–275.

36. Delves HT. Dietary sources of copper. In: Biological Roles of Copper. Ciba Foundation Symposium 79 (new series). Amsterdam: Excerpta Medica 1980: 5–22.

37. Terao T, Owen CA Jr. Copper in supernatant fractions of various rat organs. Studies with [67]Cu. Mayo Clin Proc 1974; 49: 376–381.

38. Palida FA, Ettinger MJ. Identification of proteins involved in intracellular copper metabolism. Low levels of A ≈ 48-kDa copper-binding protein in the brindled mouse model of Menkes disease. J Biol Chem 1991; 266: 4586–4592.

39. Freedman JH, Peisach J. Intracellular copper transport in cultured hepatoma cells. Biochem Biophys Res Commun 1989; 164: 134–140.

40. Ciriolo MR, Desideri A, Paci M, Rotilio G. Reconstitution of Cu,Zn-superoxide dismutase by the Cu(I)·glutathione complex. J Biol Chem 1990; 265: 11030–11034.

41. Marceau N, Aspin N. The association of the copper derived from ceruloplasmin with cyto-cuprein. Biochim Biophys Acta 1973; 328: 351–358.

42. Dameron CT, Harris ED. Regulation of aortic Cu,Zn-superoxide dismutase with copper. Ceruloplasmin and albumin transfer copper and reactivate the enzyme in culture. Biochem J 1987; 248: 669–675.

43. Harris ED, Percival SS. Copper transport: insights into a ceruloplasmin-based delivery system. In: Kies C, ed. Copper Bioavailability and Metabolism. New York: Plenum Press, 1989: 95–102.

44. Chung K, Romero N, Tinker D, Keen CL, Amemiya K, Rucker RB. Role of copper in the regulation and accumulation of superoxide dismutase and metallothionein in rat liver. J Nutr 1988; 11(8): 859–864.

45. Prins HW, van den Hamer CJA. Comparative studies of copper metabolism in liver and kidney of normal and mutated brindled mice—with special emphasis on metallothionein. Comp Biochem Physiol 1981; 70C: 255–260.

46. Bremner I. Absorption, transport and distribution of copper. In: Biological Roles of Copper. Ciba Foundation Symposium 79 (new series). Amsterdam: Excerpta Medica, 1980: 23–48.

47. Wapnir RA, Stiel L. Intestinal absorption of copper: effect of sodium. Proc Soc Exp Biol Med 1987; 185: 277–282.

48. Kelsay JL, Jacob RA, Prather S. Effect of fiber from fruits and vegetables on metabolic responses of human subjects. III. Zinc, copper and phosphorus balances. Am J Clin Nutr 1979; 32: 2307–2311.

49. Marceau N, Aspin N, Sass-Kortsak A. Absorption of copper 64 from gastrointestinal tract of the rat. Am J Physiol 1970; 218: 377–383.

50. Hall AC, Young BW, Bremner I. Intestinal metallothionein and the mutual antagonism between copper and zinc in the rat. J Inorgan Biochem 1979; 11: 57–66.

51. Scarino ML, Poverini R, Di Lullo G, Bises G. Metallothionein gene expression in the intestinal cell: modulation of mRNA and protein synthesis by copper and zinc. Biochem Soc Trans 1991; 19: 283S.

52. Oestreicher P, Cousins RJ. Copper and zinc absorption in the rat: mechanism of mutual antagonism. J Nutr 1985; 115: 159–166.

52a. Reeves PG, Rossow KL, Bobilya DJ. Zinc-induced metallothionein and copper metabolism in intestinal mucosa, liver and kidney of rats. Nutr Res 1993; 13: 1419–1431.

53. Harris ED. Biological monitoring of iron, zinc, and copper. In: Dillon HK, Ho MH, eds. Biological Monitoring of Exposure to Chemicals: Metals. New York: John Wiley, 1991: 175–196.

54. Weiss KC, Linder MC. Copper transport in rats involving a new plasma protein. Am J Physiol 1985; 249: E77–E88.

55. Owen CA Jr. Metabolism of radiocopper (Cu64) in the rat. Am J Physiol 1965; 209: 900–904.

56. Underwood EJ. Copper. In: Underwood EJ, ed. Trace Elements in Human Nutrition. New York: Academic Press, 1977: 56–108.

57. Gubler CJ, Lahey ME, Cartwright GE, Wintrobe MM. Studies on copper metabolism. X. Factors influencing the plasma copper level of the albino rat. Am J Physiol 1952; 171: 652–658.

58. Bearn AG, Kunkel HG. Localization of 64Cu in serum fractions following oral administration: an alteration in Wilson's disease. Proc Soc Exp Biol Med 1954; 85: 44–48.

59. Masuoka J, Hegenauer J, Van Dyke BR, Saltman P. Intrinsic stoichiometric equilibrium constants for the binding of zinc(II) and copper(II) to the high affinity site of serum albumin. J Biol Chem 1993; 268: 21533–21537.

60. Breslow E. Comparison of cupric ion-binding sites in myoglobin derivatives and serum albumin. J Biol Chem 1964; 239: 3252–3259.

61. Marceau N, Aspin N. Distribution of ceruloplasmin-bound 67Cu in the rat. Am J Physiol 1972; 222: 106–110.

62. Lau S-J, Sarkar B. Ternary co-ordination complex between human serum albumin, copper (II), and L-histidine. J Biol Chem 1971; 246: 5938–5943.

63. Laurie SH, Pratt DE. Copper-albumin: what is its functional role. Biochem Biophys Res Commun 1986; 135: 1064–1068.

64. Sternlieb I, Morell AG, Tucker WD, Green MW, Scheinberg IH. The incorporation of copper into ceruloplasmin in vivo: studies with copper-64 and copper-67. J Clin Invest 1961; 40: 1834–1840.

65. Holtzman NA, Gaumnitz BM. Studies on the rate of release and turnover of ceruloplasmin and apoceruloplasmin in rat plasma. J Biol Chem 1970; 245: 2354–2358.

66. Sato M, Gitlin JD. Mechanisms of copper incorporation during the biosynthesis of human ceruloplasmin. J Biol Chem 1991; 266: 5128–5134.

67. Wirth PL, Linder MC. Distribution of copper amount components of human serum. J Natl Cancer Inst 1985; 75: 277–284.

68. Morell AG, Scheinberg IH. Heterogeneity of human ceruloplasmin. Science 1960; 131: 930–932.

69. Evans GW, Wiederanders RE. Blood copper variations among species. Am J Physiol 1967; 213: 1183–1185.

70. Sarkar B. Recent trends in the application of coordination chemistry in biology and medicine. In: Banerjea D, ed. (IUPAC) Coordination Chemistry–20. Oxford/New York: Pergamon Press, 1980: 191–200.

71. Goode CA, Dinh CT, Linder MC. Mechanism of copper transport and delivery in mammals: review and recent findings. In: Kies C, ed. Copper Bioavailability and Metabolism. New York: Plenum Press, 1989: 131–144.

72. Percival SS, Harris ED. Ascorbate enhances copper transport from ceruloplasmin into human K562 cells. J Nutr 1989; 119: 779–784.

73. Musci G, Bonaccorsi di Patti MC, Carlini P, Calabrese L. Ceruloplasmin in human plasma and its relationships with the copper-albumin complex. Eur J Biochem 1992; 210: 635–640.

74. Harris DIM, Sass-Kortsak A. The influence of amino acids on copper uptake by rat liver slices. J Clin Invest 1967; 46: 659–677.

75. Schmitt RC, Darwish HM, Cheney JC, Ettinger MJ. Copper transport kinetics by isolated rat hepatocytes. Am J Physiol 1983; 244: G183–G191.

76. Stockert RJ, Grushoff PS, Morell AG, et al. Transport and intracellular distribution of copper in a human hepatoblastoma cell line, HepG2. Hepatology 1986; 6: 60–64.

77. McArdle HJ, Guthrie J, Ackland ML, Danks DM. Albumin has no role in copper uptake by fibroblasts. J Inorg Biochem 1987; 31: 123–131.

78. McArdle HJ, Gross SM, Danks DM. Uptake of copper by mouse hepatocytes. J Cell Physiol 1988; 136: 373–378.

79. Vulpe C, Levinson B, Whitney S, Packman S, Gitschier J. Isolation of a candidate gene for Menkes disease and evidence that it encodes a copper-transporting ATPase. Nature Genet 1993; 3: 7–13.

80. Odermatt A, Suter H, Krapf R, Solioz M. An ATPase operon involved in copper resistance by *Enterococcus hirae*. Ann NY Acad Sci 1992; 671: 484–486.

81. Solioz M, Mathews S, Fürst P. Cloning of the K^+-ATPase of *Streptococcus faecalis*. Structural and evolutionary implications of its homology to the KdpB-protein of *Escherichia coli*. J Biol Chem 1987; 262: 7358–7362.

82. Mercer JFB, Livingston J, Hall B, et al. Isolation of a partial candidate gene for Menkes disease by positional cloning. Nature Genet 1993; 3: 20–25.

83. Stockert RJ, Morell AG, Sternlieb I. Purification of canine hepatic lysosomal copper-metallothionein. Meth Enzymol 1991; 205: 286–291.

84. Iyengar V, Brewer GJ, Dick RD, Owyang C. Studies of cholescystokinin-stimulated biliary secretions reveal a high molecular weight copper-binding substance in normal subjects that is absent in patients with Wilson's disease. J Lab Clin Med 1988; 111: 267–274.

85. Nederbragt H. Effect of the glutathione-depleting agents diethylmaleate, phorone and buthionine sulfoximine on biliary copper excretion in rats. Biochem Pharmacol 1989; 38: 3399–3406.

86. Nederbragt H, Lagerwerf AJ. Strain-related patterns of biliary excretion and hepatic distribution of copper in the rat. Hepatology 1986; 6: 601–607.

87. Prohaska JR. Biochemical changes in copper deficiency. J Nutr Biochem 1990; 1: 452–461.

88. Paynter DI, Moir RJ, Underwood EJ. Changes in activity of the Cu-Zn superoxide dismutase enzyme in tissues of the rat with changes in dietary copper. J Nutr 1979; 109: 1570–1576.

89. Danks DM. Copper deficiency in humans. Annu Rev Nutr 1988; 8: 235–257.

90. O'Dell BL. Roles for iron and copper in connective tissue biosynthesis. Phil Trans R Soc Lond B 1981; 294: 91–104.

91. Medeiros DM, Davidson J, Jenkins JE. A unified perspective on copper deficiency and cardiomyopathy. Proc Soc Exp Biol Med 1993; 203: 262–273.

92. Viestenz KE, Klevay LM. A randomized trial of copper therapy in rats with electrocardiographic abnormalities due to copper deficiency. Am J Clin Nutr 1982; 35: 258–266.

93. Farquharson C, Duncan A, Robins SP. The effects of copper deficiency on the pyridinium crosslinks of mature collagen in the rat skeleton and cardiovascular system. Proc Soc Exp Biol Med 1989; 192: 166–171.

94. Dawson R, Milne G, Williams RB. Changes in the collagen of rat heart in copper-deficiency-induced cardiac hypertrophy. Cardiovascular Res 1982; 16: 559–565.

95. Vadlamudi RK, McCormick RJ, Medeiros DM, Vossoughi J, Failla ML. Copper deficiency alters collagen types and covalent cross-linking in swine myocardium and cardiac valves. Am J Physiol Heart Circ Physiol 1993; 264: H2154–H2161.

96. Briscoe AM, Loring WE. Elastin content of the human lung. Proc Soc Exp Biol Med 1958; 99: 162–164.

97. O'Dell BL, Kilburn KH, McKenzie MS, Thurston RJ. The lung of the copper-deficient rat. Am J Pathol 1978; 91: 413–432.

98. Harris ED. Biochemical defect in chick lung resulting from copper deficiency. J Nutr 1986; 116: 252–258.

99. Buckingham K, Heng-Khoo CS, Dubick M, Cross C, Julian L, Rucker R. Copper deficiency and elastin metabolism in avian lung. Proc Soc Exp Biol Med 1981; 166: 310–319.

100. Jenkinson SG, Lawrence RA, Grafton WD, Gregory PE, McKinney MA. Enhanced pulmonary toxicity in copper-deficient rats exposed to hyperoxia. Fund Appl Toxicol 1984; 4: 170–177.

101. Baxter JH, Van Wyk JJ. A bone disorder associated with copper deficiency. I. Gross morphological roentgenological and chemical observations. Bull Johns Hopkins Hosp 1953; 93: 1.

102. Rucker RB, Parker HE, Rogler JC. Effect of copper deficiency on chick bone collagen and selected bone enzymes. J Nutr 1969; 98: 57–63.

103. Levy J, Berdon WE, Abramson SJ. Epiphyseal separation simulating pyarthrosis, secondary to copper deficiency in an infant receiving total parenteral nutrition. Br J Radiol 1984; 57: 636–638.

104. Bridges CH, Harris ED. Experimentally induced cartilaginous fractures (osteochondritis dissecans) in foals fed low-copper diets. J Am Vet Med Assoc 1990; 193: 215–221.

105. Baumgartner S, Brown DJ, Salevsky EJ, Leach RMJ. Copper deficiency in the laying hen. J Nutr 1978; 108: 804–811.

106. Harris ED, Blount JE, Leach RMJ. Localization of lysyl oxidase in hen oviduct. Implications in egg shell membrane formation and composition. Science 1980; 208: 55–56.

107. Hart EB, Steenbock H, Waddell J, Elvehjem CA. Iron in nutrition. VII. Copper as a supplement to iron for hemoglobin building in the rat. J Biol Chem 1928; 77: 797–812.

108. Williams DM, Loukopoulos D, Lee GR, Cartwright GE. Role of copper in mitochondrial iron metabolism. Blood 1976; 48: 77–85.

109. Cordano A, Graham GG. Copper deficiency complicating severe chronic intestinal malabsorption. Pediatrics 1966; 38: 596–604.

110. Chan W-Y, Rennert OM. The role of copper in iron metabolism. Ann Clin Lab Sci 1980; 10: 338–344.

111. Osaki S, Johnson DA. Mobilization of liver iron by ferroxidase (ceruloplasmin). J Biol Chem 1969; 244: 5757–5758.

112. Percival SS. Iron metabolism is modified by the copper status of a human erythroleukemic (K562) cell line Proc Soc Exp Biol Med 1992; 200: 522–527.

113. Askwith C, Eide D, Van Ho A, et al. The *FET3* gene of *S. cerevisiae* encodes a multicopper oxidase required for ferrous iron uptake. Cell 1994; 76: 403–410.

114. Dancis A, Yuan DS, Haile D, et al. Molecular characterization of a copper transport protein in *S. cerevisiae*: an unexpected role for copper in iron transport. Cell 1994; 76: 393–402.

115. Prohaska JR, Lukasewycz OA. Copper deficiency suppresses the immune response of mice. Science 1981; 213: 559–561.

116. Babu U, Failla ML. Respiratory burst and candidacidal activity of peritoneal macrophages are impaired in copper-deficient rats. J Nutr 1990; 120: 1692–1699.

117. Babu U, Failla ML. Copper status and function of neutrophils are reversibly depressed in marginally and severely copper-deficient rats. J Nutr 1990; 120: 1700–1709.

117a. O'Dell BL, Prohaska JR. Biochemical aspects of copper deficiency in the nervous system. In: Dreosti IE, Smith RM, eds. Neurobiology of the Trace Elements. Vol. 1. Clifton, NJ: Humana Press, 1983: 41–81.

118. Ono S, Kurisaki H. An unusual neurological disorder with abnormal copper metabolism. J Neurol 1988; 235: 397–399.

119. O'Dell BL, Smith RM, King RA. Effect of copper status on brain neurotransmitter metabolism in the lamb. J Neurochem 1976; 26: 451–455.

119a. Morgan RF, O'Dell BL. Effect of copper deficiency on the concentration of catecholamines and related enzyme activities in the rat brain. J Neurochem 1977; 28: 207–213.

120. Sun SH-H, O'Dell BL. Elevated striatal levels of glial fibrillary acidic protein associated with neuropathology in copper-deficient rats. J Nutr Biochem 1992; 3: 503–509.

121. Prohaska JR. Functions of trace elements in brain metabolism. Physiol Rev. 1987; 67: 858–901.

122. Everson GJ, Shrader RE, Wang T. Chemical and morphological changes in the brains of copper-deficient guinea pigs. J Nutr 1968; 96: 115–125.

123. Sun SH-H, O'Dell BL. Low copper status of rats affects polyunsaturated fatty acid composition of brain phospholipids, unrelated to neuropathology. J Nutr 1992; 122: 65–73.

124. Kodama H, Meguro Y, Abe T, et al. Genetic expression of Menkes disease in cultured astrocytes of the muscular mouse. J Inherited Metab Dis 1991; 14: 896–901.

125. Hunt DM, Johnson DR. An inherited defect in noradrenaline biosynthesis in the brindled mouse. J Neurochem 1972; 19: 2811–2819.

126. Williams RS. Marshall PC, Lott IT, Caviness VS. The cellular pathology of Menkes' steely hair syndrome. Neurology 1978; 28: 575–583.

127. Goto S, Hirano A, Rojas-Corona RR. A comparative immunocytochemical study of human cerebellar cortex in X-chromosome-linked copper malabsorption (Menkes' kinky hair disease) and granule cell type cerebellar degeneration. Neuropathol Appl Neurobiol 1989; 15: 419–431.

128. Seubert P, Peterson C, Vanderklish P, Cotman C, Lynch G. Increased spectrin proteolysis in the brindled mouse brain. Neurosci Lett 1990; 108: 303–308.

129. Hearing VJ, Tsukamoto K. Enzymatic control of pigmentation in mammals. FASEB J 1991; 5: 2902–2909.

130. Silverstone B, Mendelsohn D. Copper metabolism in oculocutaneous albinism. Metabol Ped Syst Ophthal 1983; 7: 95–99.

131. Davis GK, Mertz W. Copper. In: Mertz W, ed. Trace Elements in Human and Animal Nutrition. Vol. 1. San Diego, CA: Academic Press 1987: 301–364.

132. Danks DM, Campbell PE, Walker-Smith J, et al. Menkes' kinky-hair syndrome. Lancet 1972; 1: 1100–1103.

133. Steinert PM, Parry DA. The conserved H1 domain of the type II keratin 1 chain plays an essential role in the alignment of nearest neighbor molecules in mouse and human keratin 1/keratin 10 intermediate filaments at the two- to four-molecule level of structure. J Biol Chem 1993; 268: 2878–2887.

134. Klevay L. Hypercholesterolemia in rats produced by an increase in the ratio of zinc to copper ingested. Am J Clin Nutr 1973; 26: 1060–1068.

135. Lei KY. Plasma cholesterol response in copper deficiency. In: Lei KY, Carr TP, eds. Role of Copper in Lipid Metabolism. Boca Raton, FL: CRC Press, 1990: 1–23.

136. Allen KGD, Klevay LM. Copper deficiency and cholesterol metabolism in the rat. Atherosclerosis 1978; 31: 259–271.

137. Sho MSJ, Lei KY. Conversion of [2-^{14}C]mevalonate into cholesterol, lanosterol and squalene in copper-deficient rats. J Nutr 1980; 110: 859–867.

138. Yount NY, McNamara J, Al-Othman AA, Lei KY. The effect of copper deficiency on rat hepatic 3-hydroxy-3-methylglutaryl coenzyme A reductasee activity. J Nutr Biochem 1990; 1: 21–27.

139. Al-Othman AA, Rosenstein F, Lei KY. Copper deficiency alters plasma pool size, percent composition and concentration of lipoprotein components in rats. J Nutr 1992; 122: 1199–1204.

140. Kim S, Chao PY, Allen KGD. Inhibition of elevated hepatic glutathione abolishes copper deficiency cholesterolemia. FASEB J 1992; 6: 2467–2471.

141. Thompson EH, Allen CE, Meade RJ. Influence of copper on stearic acid desaturation and fatty acid composition in the pig. J Animal Sci 1973; 36: 868–873.

142. Wahle KWJ, Davies NT. Effects of dietary copper deficiency in the rat on fatty acid composition of microsomes. Br J Nutr 1975; 34: 105–112.

143. Parke A, Bhattacherjee P, Palmer RMJ, Lazarus NR. Characterization and quantification of copper sulfate-induced vascularization of the rabbit cornea. Am J Pathol 1988; 130: 173–178.

144. Lin MT, Chen YL. Effect of copper ion on collagenase release. Invest Opthorhol Vls Sci 1992; 33: 558–563.

145. Brem S, Tsanaclis AMC, Zagzag D. Anticopper treatment inhibits pseudopodial protrusion and the invasive spread of 9L gliosarcoma cells in the rat brain. Neurosurgery 1990; 26: 391–396.

146. Brem SS, Zagzag D, Tsanaclis AMC, Gately S, Elkouby M-P, Brien SE. Inhibition of angiogenesis and tumor growth in the brain. Suppression of endothelial cell turnover by penicillamine and the depletion of copper, an angiogenic cofactor. Am J Pathol 1990; 137: 1121–1142.

147. Gacheru SN, Trackman PC, Shah MA, et al. Structural and catalytic properties of copper in lysyl oxidase. J Biol Chem 1990; 265: 19022–19027.

148. Kagan HM. Characterization and regulation of lysyl oxidase. In: Mecham RP, ed. Biology of Extracellular Matrix: A Series. Regulation of Matrix Accumulation. Vol. 1. Orlando, FL: Academic Press, 1986; 321–398.

149. Hämäläinen E-R, Jones TA, Sheer D, Taskinen K, Pihlajaniemi T, Kivirikko KI. Molecular cloning of human lysyl oxidase and assignment of the gene to chromosome 5q23.3-31.2. Genomics 1991; 11: 508–516.

150. Krebs CJ, Krawetz SA, Lysyl oxidase copper-talon complex: a model. Biochim Biophys Acta Protein Struct Mol Enzymol 1993; 1202: 7–12.

151. Harris ED, Gonnerman WA, Savage JE, O'Dell BL. Connective tissue amine oxidase. II. Purification and partial characterization of lysyl oxidase from chick aorta. Biochim Biophys Acta 1974; 341: 332–344.

152. Harris ED. Copper-induced activation of aortic lysyl oxidase in vivo. Proc Natl Acad Sci (USA) 1976; 73: 371–374.

153. Rayton JK, Harris ED. Reaction of lysyl oxidase with copper. Properties of an in vitro system. J Biol Chem 1979; 254: 621–626.

154. Romero-Chapman N, Lee J, Tinker D, Uriu-Hare JY, Keen CL, Rucker RR. Purification, properties and influence of dietary copper on accumulation and functional activity of lysyl oxidase in rat skin. Biochem J 1991; 275: 657–662.

155. Wakasaki H, Ooshima A. Immunohistochemical localization of lysyl oxidase with monoclonal antibodies. Lab Invest 1990; 63: 377–384.

156. Topham RW, Frieden E. Identification and purification of a non-ceruloplasmin ferroxidase of human serum. J Biol Chem 1970; 245: 6698–6705.

157. Garnier A, Tosi L, Steinbuch M. Ferroxidase II. The essential role of copper in enzymatic activity. Biochem Biophys Res Commun 1981; 98: 66–71.

158. Mcdermott JA, Huber CT, Osaki S, Frieden E. Role of iron in the oxidase activity of ceruloplasmin. Biochim Biophys Acta 1968; 151: 541–557.

159. Mareschal JC, Rama R, Crichton RR. The role of ceruloplasmin in Fe(III)-transferrin formation in vitro. FEBS Lett 1980; 110: 268–270.

160. Roeser HP, Lee GR, Nacht S, Cartwright GE. The role of ceruloplasmin in iron metabolism. J Clin Invest 1970; 49: 2408–2417.

161. Ragan HA, Nacht S, Lee GR, Bishop CR, Cartwright GE. Effect of ceruloplasmin on plasma iron in copper-deficient swine. Am J Physiol 1969; 217: 1320–1323.

162. Osaki S, Johnson DA, Frieden E. The mobilization of iron from the perfused mammalian liver by a serum copper enzyme, ferroxidase I. J Biol Chem 1971; 246: 3018–3023.

163. Carver FJ, Farb DL, Frieden E. The effect of albumin, ceruloplasmin, and other serum constituents on Fe(II) oxidation. Biol Trace Element Res 1982; 4: 1–19.

164. Williams DM, Christensen DD, Lee GR, Cartwright GE. Serum azide-resistant ferroxidase activity. Biochim Biophys Acta 1974; 350: 129–134.

165. Evans PJ, Bomford A, Halliwell B. Non-ceruloplasmin copper and ferroxidase activity in mammalian serum. Ferroxidase activity and phenanthroline-detectable copper in human serum in Wilson's disease. Free Rad Res Commun 1989; 7: 55–62.

166. Bala S, Failla ML, Lunney J. T-cell numbers and mitogenic responsiveness of peripheral blood mononuclear cells are decreased in copper deficient rats. Nutr Res 1990; 10: 749–760.

167. Failla ML, Bala S. Cellular and biochemical functions of copper in immunity. In: Chandra RK, ed. Nutrition and Immunity. St. John's, NF, Canada: ARTS Publishers, 1992: 129–141.

168. Bala S, Failla ML. Copper repletion restores the number and function of CD4 cells in copper-deficient rats. J Nutr 1993; 123: 991–996.

169. Stewart LC, Klinman JP. Cooperativity in the dopamin β-monooxygenase reaction. Evidence for ascorbate regulation of enzyme activity. J Biol Chem 1991; 266: 11537–11543.

170. Huyghe BG, Klinman JP. Activity of membranous dopamine β-monooxygenase within chromaffin granule ghosts. Interaction with ascorbate. J Biol Chem 1991; 266: 11544–11550.

171. Southan C, Kruse LI. Sequence similarity between dopamine β-hydroxylase and peptide α-amidating enzyme: evidence for a conserved catalytic reaction. FEBS Lett 1989; 255: 116–120.

172. Körner A, Pawelek J. Mammalian tyrosinase catalyzes three reactions in the biosynthesis of melanin. Science 1982; 217: 1163–1165.

173. Del Marmol V, Solano F, Sels A, et al. Glutathione depletion increases tyrosinase activity in human melanoma cells. J Invest Dermatol 1993; 101: 871–874.

174. Eipper BA, Mains RE. Peptide α-amidation. Ann Rev Physiol 1988; 50: 333–344.

174a. Kulathila R, Consalvo AP, Fitzpatrick PF, et al. Bifunctional peptidylglycine alpha-amidating enzyme requires two copper atoms for maximum activity. Arch Biochem Biophys 1994; 311: 191–195.

175. Glembotski CC, Eipper BA, Mains RE. Characterization of a peptide α-amidation activity from rat anterior pituitary. J Biol Chem 1984; 259: 6385–6392.

176. Beaudry GA, Mehta NM, Ray ML, Bertelsen AH. Purification and characterization of functional recombinant α-amidating enzyme secreted from mammalian cells. J Biol Chem 1990; 265: 17694–17699.

177. Graham L, Gallop PM. Peptidylglycine α-amidating monooxygenase activity in spinal cord, dorsal roots, and dorsal root ganglia of *Macaca fascicularis*. Brain Res 1989; 491: 371–373.

178. Frausto da Silva JJR, Williams RJP. The Biological Chemistry of the Elements. The Inorganic Chemistry of Life, Oxford: Clarendon Press, 1991.

179. Prohaska JR. Changes in Cu,Zn-superoxide dismutase, cytochrome *c* oxidase, glutathione peroxidase and glutathione transferase activities in copper-deficient mice and rats. J Nutr 1991; 121: 355–363.

180. Keller G-A, Warner TG, Steimer KS, Hallewell RA. Cu,Zn superoxide dismutase is a peroxisomal enzyme in human fibroblasts and hepatoma cells. Proc Natl Acad Sci (USA) 1991; 88: 7381–7385.

181. Dhaunsi GS, Gulati S, Singh AK, Orak JK, Asayama K, Singh I. Demonstration of Cu-Zn superoxide dismutase in rat liver peroxisomes. Biochemical and immunochemical evidence. J Biol Chem 1992; 267: 6870–6873.

182. Tainer JA, Getzoff ED, Richardson JS, Richardson DC. Structure and mechanism of copper, zinc superoxide dismutase. Nature 1983; 306: 284–287.

183. Valentine JS, Pantoliano MW, McDonnell PJ, Burger AR, Lippard SJ, pH-dependent migration of copper(II) to the vacant zinc-binding site of zinc-free bovine erythrocyte superoxide dismutase. Proc Natl Acad Sci (USA) 1979; 76: 4245–4249.

184. Bettger WJ, Fish TJ, O'Dell BL. Effects of copper and zinc status of rats on erythrocyte stability and superoxide dismutase activity. Proc Soc Exp Biol Med 1978; 158: 279–282.

185. Greco MA, Hrab DI, Magner W, Kosman DJ. Cu,Zn superoxide dismutase and copper deprivation and toxicity in *Saccharomyces cerevisiae*. J Bacteriol 1990; 172: 317–325.

186. Harris ED. Regulation of antioxidant enzymes. FASEB J 1992; 6: 2675–2683.

187. Lu Y, Gralla EB, Roe JA, Valentine JS. Redesign of a type 2 into a type 1 copper protein: construction and characterization of yeast copper-zinc superoxide dismutase mutants. J Am Chem Soc 1992; 114: 3560–3562.

188. Dameron CT, Harris ED. Regulation of aortic CuZn-superoxide dismutase with copper. Effects in vivo. Biochem J 1987; 248: 663–668.

189. Bettger WJ, Savage JE, O'Dell BL. Effects of dietary copper and zinc on erythrocyte superoxide dismutase activity in the chick. Nutr Rep Int 1979; 19: 893–900.

190. Beem KM, Rich WE, Rajagopalan KV. Total reconstitution of copper-zinc superoxide dismutase. J Biol Chem 1974; 249: 7298–7305.

191. Brown DE, McGuirl MA, Dooley DM, Janes SM, Mu D, Klinman JP. The organic functional group in copper-containing amine oxidases. Resonance Raman spectra are consistent with the presence of topa quinone (6-hydroxydopa quinone) in the active site. J Biol Chem 1991; 266: 4049–4051.

192. Whittaker MM, Whittaker JW. The active site of galactose oxidase. J Biol Chem 1988; 263: 6074–6080.

193. Aisaka K, Uwajima T, Terada O. Reactivation of gibberella apoglactose-oxidase by copper. Agric Biol Chem 1984; 48: 2157–2158.

194. Scott RA, Zumft WG, Coyle CL, Dooley DM. *Pseudomonas stutzeri* N_2O reductase contains CuA-type sites. Proc Natl Acad Sci (USA) 1989; 86: 4082–4086.

195. Ohakwa J, Okada N, Shinmyo A, Takano M. Primary structure of cucumber (*Cucumis sativus*) ascorbate oxidase deduced from cDNA sequence: homology with blue copper proteins and tissue-specific expression. Proc Natl Acad Sci (USA) 1989; 86: 1239–1243.

196. Rydén L. Model of the active site in the blue oxidases based on the ceruloplasmin-plastocyanin homology. Proc Natl Acad Sci (USA) 1982; 79: 6767–6771.

197. Deinum J, Vanngard T. The stoichiometry of the paramagnetic copper and the oxidation-reduction potential of type 1 copper in human ceruloplasmin. Biochim Biophys Acta 1973; 310: 321–330.

198. Calabrese L, Leuzzi U. Presence of reduced type I copper in ceruloplasmin as revealed by reaction with hydrogen peroxide. Biochem Int 1984; 8: 35–39.

199. Calabrese L, Carbonaro M, Musci G. Presence of coupled trinuclear copper cluster in mammalian ceruloplasmin is essential for efficient electron transfer to oxygen. J Biol Chem 1989; 264: 6183–6187.

200. Lerch K, German UA. Evolutionary relationships among copper proteins containing coupled binuclear copper sites. In: King TE, Mason HS, Morrison M, eds. Oxidases and Related Redox Systems. New York: Liss, 1988: 331–348.

201. Kägi JHR, Schäfer A. Biochemistry of metallothionein. Biochemistry 1988; 27: 8509–8515.

202. Kojima Y, Kägi JHR. Metallothionein. Trends Biochem Sci 1978; 3: 90–93.

203. Kojima Y, Nordberg M. Metallothionein and other low molecular weight metal-binding proteins. In: Kägi JHR, Nordberg M, eds. Metallothionein. Basel: Birkhäuser, 1979: 41–124.

204. Byrd J, Berger RM, McMillin DR, Wright CF, Hamer D, Winge DR. Characterization of the copper-thiolate cluster in yeast metallothionein and two truncated mutants. J Biol Chem 1988; 263: 6688–6694.

205. Briggs RW, Armitage IM. Evidence for site-selective metal binding in calf liver metallothionein. J Biol Chem 1982; 257: 1259–1262.

206. Markossian KA, Melkonyan VZ, Paitian NA, Nalbandy RM. On the copper transfer between dopamine B-monooxygenase and Cu-thionein. Biochem Biophys Res Commun 1988; 153: 558–563.

207. Beltramini M, Lerch K. Copper transfer between neurospora copper metallothionein and type 3 copper apoproteins. FEBS Lett 1982; 142: 219–222.

208. Vehar GA, Keyt B, Eaton D, et al. Structure of human factor VIII. Nature 1984; 312: 337–342.

209. Mann KG, Lawler CM, Vehar GA, Church WR. Coagulation Factor V contains copper ion. J Biol Chem 1984; 259: 12949–12951.

210. Bihoreau N, Pin S, de Kersabiec A-M, Vidot F, Fontaine-Aupart MP. Metal identification in human antihemophilia A factor (factor VIII). C R Acad Sci Paris 1993; 316: 536–539.

211. Menkes JH, Alter M, Steigleder GK, Weakley DR, Sung JH. A sex-linked recessive disorder with retardation of growth, peculiar hair, and focal cerebral and cerebellar degeneration. Pediatrics 1962; 29: 764–779.

212. Shiraishi N, Aono K, Taguchi T. Copper metabolism in the macular mutant mouse: an animal model of Menkes' kinky-hair disease. Biol Neonate 1988; 54: 173–180.

213. Hunt DM. Primary defect in copper transport underlies mottled mutants in the mouse. Nature 1974; 249: 852–854.

214. Wilson SAK. Progressive lenticular degeneration: a familial nervous disease associated with cirrhosis of the liver. Brain 1912; 34: 295–307.

215. Yarze JC, Martin P, Muñoz SJ, Friedman LS. Wilson's disease: Current status. Am J Med 1992; 92: 643–654.

216. Farrer LA, Bowcock AM, Hebert JM, et al: Predictive testing for Wilson's disease using tightly linked and flanking DNA markers. Neurology 1991; 41: 992–999.

217. Owen CA Jr. Wilson's Disease. The Etiology, Clinical Aspects, and Treatment of Inherited Copper Toxicosis, Park Ridge, NJ: Noyes, 1981.

218. Sternlieb I, van den Hamer CJA, Morrell AG, Alport S, Gregariadis G, Scheinberg IH. Lysosomal defect of hepatic copper excretion in Wilson's disease (hepatolenticular degeneration). Gastroenterology 1973; 64: 99–103.

219. Yamaguchi Y, Heiny ME, Gitlin JD. Isolation and characterization of a human liver cDNA as a candidate gene for Wilson's disease. Biochem Biophys Res Commun 1993; 197: 271–277.

220. Bull PC, Thomas GR, Rommens JM, Forbes JR, Cox DW. The Wilson disease gene is a putative copper transporting P-type ATPase similar to the Menkes gene. Nature Genet 1993; 5: 327–336.

221. Tanzi RE, Petrukhin K, Chernov I, et al. The Wilson disease gene is a copper transporting ATPase with homology to the Menkes disease gene. Nature Genet 1993; 5: 344–350.

222. Aaseth J, Norseth T. Copper. In: Friberg L, Nordberg GF, Vouk V, eds. Handbook on the Toxicology of Metals. Amsterdam: Elsevier, 1986: 233–254.

223. Hamer DH, Winge DR. Metal Ion Homeostasis: Molecular Biology and Chemistry, New York: Liss, 1989.

224. Merchant S, Bogorad L. Regulation by copper of the expression of plastocyanin and cytochrome c552 in *Chlamydomonas reinhardi*. Mol Cell Biol 1986; 6: 462–469.

225. Merchant S, Hill K, Howe G. Dynamic interplay between two copper-titrating components in the transcriptional regulation of cyt *c6*. EMBO J 1991; 10: 1383–1389.

226. Nakamura M, Yamagishi M, Yoshizaki F, Sugimura Y. The syntheses of plastocyanin and cytochrome c-553 are regulated by copper at the pre-translational level in green alga, *Pediastrum boryanum*. J Biochem 1992; 111: 219–224.

227. Szczypka MS, Thiele DJ. A cysteine-rich nuclear protein activates yeast metallothionein gene transcription. Mol Cell Biol 1989; 9: 421–429.

228. Gralla EB, Thiele DJ, Silar P, Valentine JS. ACE1, a copper-dependent transcription factor, activates expression of the yeast copper, zinc superoxide dismutase gene. Proc Natl Acad Sci (USA) 1991; 88: 8558–8562.

229. Zhou P, Thiele DJ. Rapid transcriptional autoregulation of a yeast metalloregulatory transcription factor is essential for high-level copper detoxification. Genes Dev 1993; 7: 1824–1835.

230. Mergeay M. Towards an understanding of the genetics of bacterial metal resistance. TIBTECH 1991; 9: 17–24.

231. Derkachev EF, Shaposhnikov AM. The role of cytochrome c in redox reactions of ceruloplasmin. Biokhimiya 1971; 37: 174–177.

232. Beaudry GA, Mehta NM, Ray ML, Bertelsen AH. Purification and characterization of functional recombinant α-amidating enzyme secreted from mammalian cells. J Biol Chem 1990; 265: 17694–17699.

233. Odermatt A, Suter H, Krapf R, Solioz M. Primary structure of two P-type ATPases involved in copper homeostasis in *Enterococcus hirae*. J Biol Chem 1993; 268: 12775–12779.

234. Lim C-K, Cooksey DA. Characterization of chromosomal homologs of the plasmid-borne copper resistance operon of *Pseudomonas syringae*. J Bacteriol 1993; 175: 4492–4498.

235. Voloudakis AE, Bender CL, Cooksey DA. Similarity between copper resistance genes from *Xanthomonas campestris* and *Pseudomonas syringae*. Appl Environ Microbiol 1993; 59: 1627–1634.

236. Rouch D, Lee BTO, Camakaris J. Genetic and molecular basis of copper resistance in *Escherichia coli*. In: Hamer DH, Winge DR, eds. Metal Ion Homeostasis: Molecular Biology and Chemistry. New York: Liss, 1989: 439–446.

237. Rouch D, Camakaris J, Lee BTO. Copper transport in *Escherichia coli*. In: Hamer DH, Winge DR, eds. Metal Ion Homeostasis: Molecular Biology and Chemistry. New York: Liss, 1989: 469–477.

238. Rogers SD, Bhave MR, Mercer JFB, Camakaris J, Lee BTO. Cloning and characterization of *cutE*, a gene involved in copper transport in *Escherichia coli*. J Bacteriol 1991; 173: 6742–6748.

239. van den Berg GJ. Copper Metabolism in Rats Fed Ascorbic Acid or Restricted Amounts of Copper. Ph.D. thesis, Delft University of Technology, 1993.

9
Iron

John L. Beard and Harry D. Dawson
Pennsylvania State University, University Park, Pennsylvania

I. HISTORICAL PERSPECTIVE

Among all of the micronutrients, iron possesses the longest and best described history. Iron is the fourth most abundant terrestrial element, comprising approximately 4.7% of the earth's crust in the form of the minerals hematite, magnetite, and siderite. Primordial iron compounds were probably responsible for the catalytic generation of some of the atmospheric oxygen on which most modern life forms depend (1). Iron is an essential nutrient for all living organisms with the exception of certain members of the bacterial genera *Lactobacillus* and *Bacillus*. In these organisms, the functions of iron are replaced by other transition metals, especially manganese and cobalt, which appear next to iron in the periodic table. In all other life forms, iron is an essential component of, or cofactor for, hundreds of proteins and enzymes.

Based on extrapolations made from modern aboriginal societies, prehistoric humans had an adequate intake of iron (2). The ancient Arabs, Chinese, Egyptians, Greeks, and Romans, although ignorant of the nutritional importance of iron, attributed therapeutic properties to iron (3). For example, the ancient Greeks administered iron to their injured soldiers to improve muscle weakness, which probably derived from hemorrhagic anemia (4). Alchemists and physicians of the sixteenth century prescribed iron for medicinal use (5,6). Iron salts were given to young women to treat what was then described as chlorosis, an arcane term for anemia usually due to iron or protein deficiency (4). Various physicians during this time also prescribed iron pills for anemia and were unceremoniously ridiculed by their successors in the medical profession (7,8).

Iron was identified as a constituent of animal liver and blood in the early eighteenth century (3,9,10). In 1825, hemoglobin iron content was determined to be 0.35% (4), a value extremely close to the hemoglobin iron content of 0.347% (11) calculated by modern methods. Between 1832 and 1843 chlorosis was defined by low levels of iron in the blood and reduced number of red cells (3,9,10). Boussingault first described the nutritional essentiality of iron in 1872 (12). In 1895, Bunge accurately described the anemia of chlorosis in terms of nutritional iron deficiency (13). Key observations about iron nutrition were made during the first half of this century (4,9,10,14). For example, Moore discovered the enhancing effect of ascorbic acid on iron absorption (15). Later, Granick proposed the "mucosal block" theory for control of body iron (16). Although these fundamental observations on the metabolism of iron and its nutritional significance were made some time ago, the molecular mechanisms involved in iron metabolism are just now being described. We shall make these mechanisms the focus of this review.

II. WHOLE ANIMAL METABOLISM

A. Food Sources

Despite its abundance in the earth's crust, iron deficiency is a serious health issue in many parts of the world. The iron nutritional status of an individual and of populations is largely a function of the amount of dietary iron, the bioavailability of that iron, and the extent of iron losses. Many foods that are potentially good sources of iron are limited by the bioavailability of iron in those food (Table 1) (17). The bioavailability of iron is a function of its chemical form and the presence of food items that promote or inhibit absorption. We have summarized these factors in Table 2 (15,18–24). Basal obligatory iron losses in humans are approximately 1 mg/day and must be replaced by an equivalent amount of iron derived from the diet. The typical Western diet provides an average of 6 mg of heme and nonheme iron per 1000 kcal of energy intake (25,26). Heme iron is an important dietary source of iron because it is more effectively absorbed than nonheme iron. From 5% to 35%

TABLE 1 Good Sources of Dietary Iron

Representative food	Predominant type of iron	Typical serving size	Method of preparation	Total iron content (mg)	Estimated bioavailable iron[a] (mg)
Chicken liver	Heme	3 oz	Simmered	7.2	0.81
Oysters	Heme	6 medium	Raw	5.63	0.63
Beef liver	Heme	3 oz	Pan Fried	5.34	0.60
Beef chuck roast	Heme	3 oz	Braised	3.22	0.48
Lamb loin	Heme	3 oz	Roasted	2.07	0.31
Tuna, light meat	Heme	3 oz	Canned	2.72	0.31
Shrimp	Heme	3 oz	Moist heat	2.63	0.30
Black-strap molasses	Nonheme	1 tbs.	—	5.05	0.25
Raisin bran, enriched	Nonheme	1/2 cup	Dry	4.5	0.23
Potato, with skin	Nonheme	1 medium	Baked	2.75	0.14
Kidney beans	Nonheme	1/2 cup	Boiled	2.58	0.13
Tofu	Nonheme	2.5 × 2.75 × 1 in.	Raw	2.3	0.12

[a]Available iron for individuals with 500 mg of iron stores = [heme iron content (mg) × 23%] + [nonheme iron content (mg) × 5%]

An average heme iron content (mg) of 55% was used for beef and lamb, while 35% was used for liver and seafood. Adapted from Ref. 17.

TABLE 2 Dietary Intraluminal Factors Affecting Nonheme Iron Absorption (15,18–24)

Promotors	Inhibitors
Amino acids	Carbonates
Animal proteins	Calcium
Ascorbic acid	Egg yolk phosvitin
Hydrochloric acid	Fiber
Organic acids	Oxalates
Sugars	Phosphates
	Phytates
	Plant polyphenols
	Soy proteins

of heme iron is absorbed from a single meal, whereas nonheme iron absorption from a single meal can range from 2% to 20%, depending on the iron status of the individual and the ratio of enhancers and promoters in the diet. Thus, although it constitutes about 10% of the iron found in the diet, heme iron may provide up to one-third of total absorbed dietary iron (27).

Nonheme iron, which constitutes 90% of the remaining dietary iron, accounts for 60% of the iron from animal sources and about 100% of the iron found in vegetable material. Intentional iron fortification or iron contamination of food during preparation may account for as much as 10–15% of dietary nonheme iron (28). The primary overall effect of foodstuffs on nonheme iron absorption is inhibitory. The rat, which has been the standard model of iron absorption for humans, appears to be less sensitive to these factors when compared to humans. Therefore, the actual influence of these factors in humans may be underestimated (29). Conversely, the long-term contributions of these enhancers and promoters to body iron stores may be more limited than was first thought (30). The majority of human absorption studies have used single-meal designs which test for specific effects of particular food items on the absorption of iron (31). For example, ascorbic acid, a potent enhancer of iron absorption from single meals, had no effect on the iron status of a group of individuals in prolonged studies (32).

Attempts to alleviate iron deficiency through food fortification and diet supplementation have been largely successful in the United States. Many different forms of iron have been employed for this purpose. In the United States, fortification of food with iron started in the 1940s. The U.S. Food and Drug Administration has since upwardly revised standards for iron enrichment of cereal products and has issued guidelines for fortification of infant formulas. These actions have prompted much debate about potential iron overloading in people with adequate iron status (33,34). The issue of food fortification is likely to become more contentious in the future, since public health recommendations now focus on reducing red meat consumption, which contains the most assimilable form of iron, and increasing consumption of whole-grain products and cereals, which contain factors that inhibit iron absorption. Furthermore, concerns over the proposed relationship between body iron stores and the risk of cancer and heart disease have led some scientists and health professionals to recommend severe restrictions on iron intake (35–37). The effect of these recommendations may increase the prevalence of iron deficiency.

Supplementation, although more able to target specific populations at risk for iron deficiency, is limited by dosage requirements and potential side effects, all of which lead to noncompliance. Some side effects of iron supplementation, at high doses (> 200 mg Fe) are gastrointestinal distress and constipation. The addition of bovine hemoglobin to foods (38) and bovine lactoferrin to infant formulas (39) appears to be an effective method of iron supplementation that has minimal side effects. Other methods of long-lasting iron supplementation, such as slow-release intramuscular or intravenous iron dextran or iron chondroitin sulfate, may be effective in treating iron deficiency in populations in which dietary supplementation with iron or fortification of the food supply with iron is not practical or effective.

B. Iron Absorption

1. General

The vast amount of work that has contributed to our knowledge of iron absorption will not be extensively rereviewed in this chapter. We refer the readers to other recent and more comprehensive documents (40,41). We would like, however, to direct attention to some of the mechanistic aspects of iron absorption that have been suggested in recent years.

The process of iron absorption can be divided into three stages: (a) iron uptake, (b) intraenterocyte transport, and (c) storage and extraenterocyte transfer (Fig. 1). During the intestinal phase of digestion, iron binds to specific mucosal membrane sites, is internalized, and then is either retained by the mucosal cell or is transported to the basolateral membrane, where it is bound to transferrin in the plasma pool. The process of iron absorption is controlled by intraluminal, mucosal, and somatic factors. A multitude of intraluminal factors affects the amount of iron available for absorption as either inhibitors or promoters. Mucosal factors include the amount of mucosal surface and intestinal motility. Somatic factors which influence iron absorption include erythropoiesis and hypoxia.

2. Luminal Phase

No absorption of iron occurs in the mouth, esophagus, or stomach. However, the stomach contributes hydrochloric acid, which not only helps to remove protein-bound iron by protein denaturation but also helps in the solubilization of iron and the reduction of ferric iron to the ferrous state. Reduction of ferric iron is necessary because the majority of iron in the diet is found in the relatively insoluble ferric form (K_{sp} = 10^{-17} M) and is poorly absorbed (42,43). Decreased stomach acidity, due to overconsumption of antacids, ingestion of alkaline clay, or pathologic conditions such as achlorhydria or partial gastrectomy, may lead to impaired iron absorption (44,45). In addition to the actions of gastric acid, gastric pepsin liberates some nonheme iron from digestiva through its protease activity. The combined actions of gastric acid and pepsin account for slightly less than one-half of the release of conjugated dietary iron and the reduction of one-third of total dietary ferric iron.

Other gastrointestinal components have roles in iron absorption. Pancreatic ductal cells secrete bicarbonate, which, by raising the pH of the lumen, potentially decreases iron absorption. This effect is counterbalanced by pancreatic proteases which liberate nonheme iron from digestiva. Alterations in this balance may have potential consequences to patients with pancreatic insufficiency or cystic fibrosis (46). It has been suggested that consumption of pancreatic enzymes by these patients may predispose them to iron overload (47).

The majority of iron absorption takes place in the duodenum and upper jejunum (48,49). Factors which increase transit time through these areas decrease iron absorption

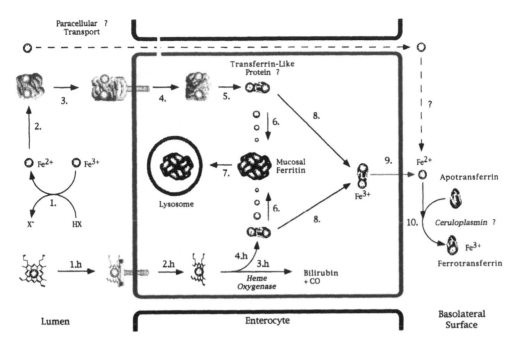

FIGURE 1 Enterocyte uptake and transfer of iron. *Nonheme iron.* A reductant such as ascorbate reduces nonheme ferric iron to ferrous iron (1). Chelators sequester and solubilize nonheme iron. Nonheme iron is then transferred to a binding protein(s) within the lumen (2). The iron-binding protein binds to a specific transporter on the luminal surface of the enterocyte (3). Nonheme iron is transported to the enterocyte interior (4). This iron is transferred either to low-molecular-weight chelates or to a transferrinlike protein (5). The transferrinlike protein delivers iron to either mucosal cell ferritin (6) or to the basolateral surface of the enterocyte (8). Absorbed iron that is not sequestered by ferritin is delivered to the basolateral surface of enterocytes (9) and oxidized for binding to transferrin (10). *Heme iron.* Heme binds to it receptor (1h) and is internalized (2h). After entering the cell, heme is degraded to iron, carbon monoxide, and bilirubin IXa by the enzyme heme oxygenase (3h). This iron enters the common intracellular (enterocyte) pool of iron (4h) (5) and is processed like nonheme iron (6–10).

(50). A multitude of dietary factors affect iron absorption during this phase. Heme iron appears to be affected only by animal proteins, which facilitate its absorption (51,52), and by calcium, which inhibits its absorption (53). In contrast to heme iron, a large number of factors affect nonheme iron absorption (Table 2). Ascorbic acid is qualitatively the most important enhancer of nonheme iron absorption in humans (54). For example, a dose of 75 mg of ascorbic acid can increase iron absorption from a meal by three to four times. Ascorbic acid maintains iron in a reduced form and forms a soluble chelate with iron. These actions are shared by other organic acids found in fruits and vegetables, including citric, lactic, malic, and tartaric acids (41). Sugars such as fructose and sorbitol enhance absorption, possibly by forming iron chelates (41). Singly administered free amino acids such as cysteine, glycine, histidine, lysine, and methionine also increase absorption of iron, as does cysteine-containing animal proteins (20,24,55,56).

A large number of extrinsic intraluminal factors decrease iron absorption. Dietary fiber (18) in the form of bran (57), hemicellulose, cellulose, pectin (58), and guar gum all inhibited the absorption of iron in feeding studies. The general mechanism of inhibition may be a reduction in intestinal transit time. Phytic acid (inositol hexaphosphate), found in wheat and soy products, inhibits iron absorption in rats (59) and humans (60). Polyphenolic compounds in tea, coffee, sorghum, legumes, spinach, and red wine (21) also inhibit iron absorption. Similarly, oxalates in foods such as spinach, rhubarb, and chocolate form insoluble iron oxalate, which is poorly absorbed. Finally, phosvitin, an iron-binding protein found in egg yolk, reduces intestinal absorption of iron (23).

3. Mineral–Metal Interactions

The absorption of iron is affected by interactions with other metal ions or minerals. Generally, very high amounts of divalent cations in the diet inhibit iron absorption. Conversely, the absorption of metal ions or minerals is affected in the same way by iron. Some of the nutritionally significant known metals–minerals interactions are summarized in Table 3 (61–63). The reader is referred to other chapters in this volume for a more complete description of these interactions. Early studies involving adult humans indicated that nonheme iron reduced absorption of inorganic zinc (64). Additional evidence to support this relationship came from infants receiving iron-fortified cow's milk and who had lower plasma zinc (65). However, in more recent studies, no evidence of zinc deficiency in infants was evident after iron supplementation (66–68). Although infants receiving iron-fortified formula absorbed less copper compared to those receiving unfortified formula (67), infants receiving iron-fortified formula have normal levels of plasma copper (65). Studies with humans indicate that nonheme iron intake affects manganese balance negatively (69). However, manganese intake does not affect iron balance (69). Humans studies have suggested that both heme and nonheme iron absorption are inhibited by calcium (53). However, in a recent study, 1000 mg of calcium administered for 12 weeks to premenopausal women did not influence iron status (70). The mechanism of the inhibitory effect of calcium on iron absorption appears to be located within the intestinal mucosal cell (53,71).

4. Mechanisms of Intestinal Cell Uptake

The complete pathway of iron absorption is largely unknown and is currently a matter of controversy. What is known is summarized in Figure 1. Heme iron metabolism will be discussed in the next section. At physiologic levels, iron uptake is mediated by a series of receptors and binding proteins. At higher levels, iron is apparently absorbed passively, via a paracellular pathway. During the intestinal phase of digestion, iron is present in the lumen as either heme iron or nonheme iron chelates. Heme iron is taken up directly by the enterocyte and, after enzymatic action, is processed in a manner analogous to nonheme iron. Nonheme iron is transferred to binding proteins within the lumen. Specific transporters exist for nonheme iron-binding proteins on the luminal surface of enterocytes (72).

TABLE 3 Nutritionally Significant Interactions of Iron with Other Minerals (61–63)

Absorption	Transport	Cellular uptake	Storage
Calcium	Chromium	Copper	Chromium
Copper	Manganese	Zinc	Copper
Manganese			Zinc
Zinc			

Nonheme iron is transported to the enterocyte interior, where it is bound to an iron-binding protein(s). This iron is transferred either to ferritin or to the basolateral side of the enterocyte. Given the observation of increased iron absorption with low iron stores and decreased absorption with high iron stores, it is tempting to speculate that there is genetic regulation of both receptors and binding proteins. This regulation appears to be exerted across the basolateral membrane in a manner which is correlated to whole-body iron stores. Iron is then either lost when the cell is sloughed or bound to transferrin in the circulation. The tools of molecular biology are now being used to determine what receptors, binding proteins, and cells contribute to iron absorption. Unfortunately, at this time the description of the process of iron absorption is incomplete.

Heme Iron

Heme is soluble in an alkaline environment; hence, no binding proteins are necessary for its luminal absorption. Specific transporters exist for heme on the surface of rat enterocytes (73,74); however, rats do not absorb heme iron as efficiently as humans (75). To date, a specific receptor/transporter for heme has not been described in humans. After binding to its receptor, the heme molecule is then internalized. After entering the cell, heme is degraded to iron, carbon monoxide, and bilirubin IXa by the enzyme heme oxygenase (27,76). This enzyme is not induced by oral administration of hemoglobin (a source of heme), but is induced by iron deficiency (76). Its distribution in the intestine is identical to the areas of maximal heme iron absorption (77). It is thought that the iron that is liberated from heme by heme oxygenase enters the common intracellular (enterocyte) pool of iron.

Luminal Nonheme Iron-Binding Proteins

Ferrous iron that has been liberated by gastric and pancreatic proteases is readily oxidized to the ferric form in an alkaline environment and would be rendered insoluble and biologically unavailable except for the presence of intraluminal iron-binding molecules. Various attempts have been made to identify these molecules. The interpretation of these and other studies seeking to identify physiologic iron-binding molecules are difficult because of the large amount of nonspecific binding by iron. Originally it was proposed that the enterocyte, or some other gastrointestinal entity such as the stomach or liver, synthesized transferrin (Tf) and that Tf was extruded into the lumen to sequester iron (78). This Tf, replete with dietary iron, was then absorbed by the enterocyte. Tf protein has been detected within duodenal mucosal cells (79,80), but most investigators have failed to detect Tf mRNA in these cells (81,82). Although one study has claimed to detect transferrin receptors (TfR) on the luminal surface of enterocytes (83), most others have failed to do so (84,85). Furthermore, even though Tf-bound iron is effectively absorbed by the rat (78), it is not effectively absorbed when it is administered to patients with achlorhydria (86). In addition, humans and mice with hypotransferrinemia become iron overloaded rather than iron deficient (87). Although the intestinal absorption of Tf-bound iron is an attractive hypothesis, most of the available evidence argues against this scenario and suggests a very limited role for Tf in the direct absorption of iron.

Several investigators have reported the presence of luminal iron-binding proteins which are distinct from Tf. One of these proteins is mucin, which binds ($K_d = 1.1 \times 10^{-4}$ M) and solubilizes ferric iron in an acidic milieu (88). Mucin also binds zinc, but with lower affinity (88). Iron chelates of histidine, ascorbate, and fructose, which enhance iron absorption in vivo, donate iron to mucin at neutral pH and may represent true in-vivo complexes. More stable chelates of anions which inhibit iron absorption in vivo, such as carbonate and oxalate, do not seem to donate iron to mucin in vitro.

Enterocyte Nonheme Iron-Binding Receptors

Numerous investigators have described putative enterocyte nonheme iron-binding receptors. A mouse enterocyte nonheme iron-binding site which exhibits increased binding after chronic hypoxia has been described (89). A 160-kDa glycoprotein from human microvillous membrane vesicles which may participate in facilitated transport of iron has also been described (72,90). This protein is composed of three identical 54-kDa monomers (90). Other iron-binding proteins of 35, 95, and 120 kDa have been isolated from cultured rat intestinal epithelial cells (91). The α (150-kDa) and β (90-kDa) subunits of integrin are insoluble membrane-bound iron-binding proteins isolated from intestinal homogenates (92). It is not clear at this time which of these enterocyte membrane iron-binding proteins are responsible for the transport of iron into the mucosal cell.

5. Intraenterocyte Transport and Storage

Transport of absorbed iron through the enterocyte may involve a Tf-like protein (93). A candidate for this Tf-like protein may be mobilferrin, a 56-kDa cytosolic protein isolated from rat and human duodenal mucosa which can bind iron ($K_d = 9 \times 10^{-5}$ M) (92). It is a homologue of calreticulin, which can also bind calcium, copper, and zinc (94). The multiple metal ion-binding properties of mobilferrin have been suggested as explanations of the interactions between the absorption of these elements. Mobilferrin coprecipitates with the α and β subunits of integrin during its purification, prompting Conrad to suggest that mobilferrin is involved in cytosolic acceptance of iron from membrane-bound integrin (92).

In the conceptual model of feedback regulation of iron absorption, iron status increases the amount of iron retained by the enterocyte. In this regard, ferritin has been proposed to act as an "iron sink" for intestinal mucosal cells. Iron that is not transferred to the plasma is stored in mucosal cell ferritin and is lost when the enterocyte dies and is subsequently shed (95,96). It is unlikely that any mucosal cell ferritin reaches the circulation before the enterocyte is shed.

The lower duodenal levels of ferritin mRNA found in iron-deficient subjects and higher duodenal levels of ferritin mRNA found in secondary iron overload support the role of mucosal ferritin as a major regulator of iron absorption (82). If ferritin is the mucosal "iron sink," dysregulation of mucosal ferritin mRNA expression could lead to iron deficiency or iron overload. Consistent with this hypothesis is the fact that the concentrations of mucosal cell ferritin mRNA and ferritin protein in patients with familial hemochromatosis are lower than those of patients with secondary iron overload (80,82,97).

6. Extraenterocyte Transfer

Absorbed iron is delivered and bound to Tf at the basolateral surface of enterocytes. It has been proposed that ceruloplasmin is the protein responsible for oxidation of iron, a process that is necessary for its binding to Tf at the basolateral membrane (98,99). The evidence for the involvement of ceruloplasmin in this process is largely circumstantial. Copper deficiency results in accumulation of iron in the mucosa and liver, reduced iron transport to peripheral tissues, and anemia (100). The classic explanation for this type of anemia is lack of basolateral mucosal cell ferroxidase I (ceruloplasmin) action. This explanation is not fully adequate, as brindled mice and patients with Menkes' or Wilson's disease all have low serum ceruloplasmin levels but do not exhibit iron-deficiency anemia (100).

7. Regulation of Iron Absorption

Mucosal Factors

As mentioned previously, the majority of iron absorption takes place in the duodenum and upper jejunum. These areas also adapt during iron deficiency to promote iron absorption (49). In these areas the amount of functional absorptive mucosal surface is important for iron absorption. Consequently, surgical removal of any part of the duodenum or upper jejunum or factors that increase enterocyte turnover decrease iron absorption (50). Clinical disorders that affect iron absorption at this level include malabsorption syndromes such as steatorrhea and tropical sprue (50).

Somatic Factors

The regulation of iron absorption involves somatic factors which signal the enterocyte about the need for iron absorption. It is clear that the iron status of an individual correlates inversely with the amount of iron absorbed (101). More recent investigations have shown that iron deficiency is the most potent somatic inducer of both heme and nonheme iron absorption. The mechanism(s) for this induction is largely unknown. One possible contributing factor is intestinal heme oxygenase, which is activated by somatic iron deficiency (76).

Hemoglobin and serum ferritin apparently have limited roles in signaling the enterocyte about the need for iron absorption (82,102,103). It has been suggested that internalized plasma ferro-Tf may allow the enterocyte to monitor body iron status and regulate iron absorption. Exposure to low intracellular amounts of plasma ferro-Tf would signal the enterocyte to upregulate iron entry into the body. Tf receptors are found only at the basolateral surface of enterocytes (104,105). The amount of enterocyte TfR mRNA and protein increase during iron deficiency and decrease during secondary iron loading (82,104,106). Acute hemolysis, which stimulates iron absorption, does not influence enterocyte basolateral TfR number (106). Interestingly, the levels of TfR and TfR mRNA in hemochromatosis patient mucosal cells are higher than suitably matched controls (82,105).

Abnormally low levels of plasma Tf or decreased expression of duodenal cell TfR would falsely induce the enterocyte to upregulate its absorption of iron. This could explain why both hypotransferrinemia (107) and hemochromatosis are associated with iron overloading. However, the fact that transfusing red cells to "normalize" hematocrit values can reduce iron absorption levels in hypotransferrinemic mice (87) argues against this hypothesis.

Since active erythropoiesis, induced by either bleeding (101) or acute hemolysis (108), increases the absorption of iron, it has been proposed that erythropoietin is an endogenous signal for iron absorption. There is limited evidence for this hypothesis. In fact, recombinant human erythropoietin does not increase intestinal iron absorption when given to iron-overloaded rats (109). Moreover, exchange transfusion of reticulocytes with a large number of TfRs into rats stimulates iron absorption in iron-replete animals, independently of erythropoietin production or active erythropoiesis (110).

Hypoxia increases iron absorption (111) independently of erythropoiesis (89,112). Increase plasma iron turnover, which occurs not only in erythropoiesis but also in disorders of ineffective erythropoiesis such as thalassemia, hemolytic anemias, and sideroblastic anemias, is associated with increased iron absorption (113).

Other clinical disorders such as hemochromatosis, congenital ferrochelatase deficiency, and porphyria cutanea tarda (50) results in an increase in iron absorption by as yet unexplained mechanisms. Finally, inflammatory processes may decreased iron absorption (114), probably by eliciting the production of cytokines which have a direct effect on the mucosal cell.

The application of some newer methods involving regulation of the expression of iron-regulatory binding protein(s) and its influence on the translation of TfR and ferritin mRNAs will help resolve questions of regulation of enterocyte iron movement.

C. Transport of Iron

Free iron, in addition to being oxidized to the insoluble ferric state in an oxygen-rich environment such as is found under physiologic conditions, is an extremely toxic substance capable of catalyzing many deleterious reactions. Natural selection has resulted in the survival of organisms with effective strategies to sequester and solubilize iron for transport to the tissues. Quantitatively, the most significant iron transport molecule in vertebrates is Tf. Not only is it responsible for delivery of iron from the basolateral surface of enterocytes to peripheral tissues, it also is responsible for redistribution of iron to various body compartments and protection of iron from glomerular filtration. A number of other systems may make small but important contributions to iron transport to the tissues, including heme-hemopexin, ferritin, lactoferrin, and the as yet uncharacterized low-molecular-weight pool of iron.

1. Transferrin

Tf is a single-chain, 80-kDa protein composed of two iron-binding half-site motifs. Each site binds ($K_d = 10^{-22}$ M) ferric iron in a ternary complex of protein ligands, bicarbonate, and water. Tf can also bind manganese and aluminum under physiologic conditions (115). Some investigators have suggested that because the two half-sites of Tf release iron at different pHs, they may be functionally distinct (116). However, recent evidence suggests that they are physiologically indistinct (117). In vivo, Tf is normally 25–50% saturated with iron (118). Thus, under normal physiologic circumstances, the iron-binding capacity of plasma is always in excess of iron concentration.

Tf belongs to a family of proteins which includes ovotransferrin, lactoferrin, melanotransferrin (p97 antigen), and a newly described protein, hemiferrin (119). In rats and humans, the primary site of synthesis is the liver; however, other sites, including brain, kidney, testes, and fetal muscle, also synthesize Tf. The human Tf gene has been localized to the 3q21-25 region of chromosome 3. The gene contains 17 exons and 16 introns. The coding region is 2.3 kb, which is lengthened to 3.5 kb by elongation of the intron regions. The 5' sequence of the human Tf gene contains elements which allow transcriptional regulation by heavy metals, glucocorticoids, and the acute-phase reaction signal (120). The Tf gene is also transcriptionally regulated by insulinlike growth factor, epidermal growth factor, platelet-derived growth factor (121), and retinoic acid (122). Iron regulates Tf gene expression in liver (123) but not in other tissues (81). Using the chloramphenicol acetyl transferase (CAT) reporter gene, it has been determined that Tf synthesis is regulated by iron posttranscriptionally (124).

2. Heme-Hemopexin

Free heme is detected in serum only in hemolytic conditions. Normally, serum heme is bound to either albumin ($K_d = 1 \times 10^{-8}$ M) or hemopexin (HPX) ($K_d < 1 \times 10^{-13}$ M) (125).

HPX is a 60-kDa glycoprotein (125). The gene for human HPX has been localized to chromosome 11 (125). HPX is synthesized by the liver and circulates in the plasma. Its synthesis has recently been detected in neurons (126). HPX transports heme to cells by binding (K_d = 6.8 × 10^{-7} M) to HPX receptors (M_r = 115 kDa) and is processed by endocytosis (127–129). Ultimately, heme released from HPX is degraded by heme oxygenase and its iron enters the common intracellular iron pool.

3. Lactoferrin

Lactoferrin is an 80-kDa iron-binding protein found in milk, plasma, and mucus secretions such as tears. It is secreted from some glandular epithelial tissues as well as from activated neutrophils. Human lactoferrin is composed of 703 amino acids and exhibits 59% sequence homology with Tf (130). Unlike Tf, however, iron does not appear to affect the transcription of the lactoferrin gene. Specific uptake of lactoferrin by hepatocyte has been described (131). Although its role in iron transport remains unclear, lactoferrin is considered to be part of the acute-phase response and to be bacterio- and fungistatic by virtue of its iron-sequestering ability (132).

4. Ferritin

In addition to its role as an iron-storage protein, ferritin can act as a cellular iron delivery agent. Kupffer cells release some of the iron that has been salvaged from senescent erythrocytes in the form of H-ferritin. This ferritin is ultimately scavenged by hepatocytes. Halliday et al. have described ferritin receptors of rat (K_d = 1.0 × 10^{-8} M) (133), pig (K_d = 2.9 × 10^{-9} M) (134), and human (K_d = 6.0 × 10^{-8} M) (135) hepatocytes. Separate, specific binding sites on Molt-4 cells have also been described for H-ferritin (K_d = 6.5 × 10^{-7} M) (136).

5. Extracellular Low-Molecular-Weight Species

When the iron-binding capacity of Tf is exceeded in hemochromatosis patients, iron is present in the serum as a low-molecular-weight species (137). In addition, non-Tf bound iron has also been detected in the serum of hypotransferrinemic mice (138). This iron has been localized to three molecular-weight fractions of >150 kDa, 40–80 kDa, and 1-kDa (138). In some cultured cells, the uptake of iron from sources such as iron citrate (139) and iron trinitriloacetate (14) is more rapid than that of Tf-bound iron. These observations have led several investigators to suggest that iron transport and cellular uptake of extracellular low-molecular-weight species of iron occurs independently of transferrin.

D. Storage and Mobilization of Iron

The molecular distribution of iron in the human body is summarized in Table 4 (141). The concentration of iron in the body is approximately 30–40 mg/kg body weight. However, that concentration varies as a function of the age and gender of the individual, and the specific tissues and organs within the individual that are being examined. About 85–90% of nonstorage iron is found in the erythroid mass. The storage iron concentration in the body varies from 0 to 15 mg/kg body weight, depending on the sex or the iron status of the individual. The distribution of this stored iron is not uniform, as the liver contains about 60% of the ferritin in the body. The remaining 40% is found in muscle tissues and cells of the reticuloendothelial system (118). Normally, 95% of the stored iron in liver tissue is found in hepatocytes as ferritin. Hemosiderin constitutes the remaining 5% and is found

TABLE 4 Molecular Distribution of Iron in Adult Male and Female

		Male (mg/kg)	Female (mg/kg)
Functional Compounds	Hemoglobin	31	28
	Myoglobin	4	3
	Heme enzymes	1	1
	Nonheme enzymes	1	1
	Transferrin iron	0.05	0.05
	Total functional	37	33
Storage compounds	Ferritin	9	4
	Hemosiderin	4	1
	Total storage	13	5
Total		50	38

Adapted from Ref. 141.

predominately in Kupffer cell lysosomal remnants. However, during iron overload, the mass of hemosiderin in the liver accumulates at 10 times the rate of ferritin (142).

1. Ferritin

The overall structure of ferritin is conserved among higher eukaryotes and in humans is composed of 24 polypeptide subunits. At least two distinct isoforms of the polypeptide subunits exist, and combinations of these subunits allow for considerable heterogeneity in the structure of the full protein. The isoform designated H ferritin is a 22-kDa protein composed of 182 amino acids. The L isoform is a 20-kDa protein containing 174 amino acids. The subunit composition of ferritin seems to be tissue specific. For example, the H form predominates in heart, whereas the L form predominates in liver (143). Numerous pseudo-genes exist for ferritin on multiple chromosomes; however, the actively transcribed gene for the H subunit is found on chromosome 11 (144) and that for the L form on chromosome 19 (145,146). The genes are 3 kb each, with 4 exons which are processed into 1-kb transcripts. The synthesis of both subunits of ferritin is stimulated by iron (147,148). The H subunit appears to be regulated only at the level of translation (149). The L subunit is apparently regulated at the level of transcription (149,150) and translation (147). By coupling these two mechanisms, a 25- to 50-fold change in the level of ferritin mRNA can be achieved (151). Theil has proposed that differential ferritin gene expression plays a role in the "housekeeping" of cellular iron, and the proportion of H- to L-chain ferritin is related to the developmental demands of the cells (152).

Theoretically, up to 4500 ferric iron atoms can be stored in a ferritin molecule (153). Even though ferritin with 1200 to 1400 molecules of iron appear to be the most efficient in the acquisition or release of iron, in vivo, ferritin is normally 20% saturated (800 of 4500 iron sites occupied) (154). The structure and composition of the mineralized core is analogous to a polymer of ferrihydrite ($5Fe_2O_3 \cdot 9H_2O$) with a variable amount of phosphate (155). The description of ferritin iron core formation has been reviewed recently by Chrichton and Ward (155) and will be discussed here only in limited detail. First, ferrous iron enters the protein through specific channels. Then iron is oxidized either at various sites within the protein or on the core surface. H-chain ferritin possesses a distinct ferroxidase site (s), and the homogeneous polymer of H-chain ferritin is capable of self-loading (156). The L-chain of ferritin lacks this site, but the homogeneous polymer of L-chain ferritin is evidently also capable of some self iron loading at physiologic pH (157). The L chain is also more efficient than the H chain in forming mineralization nuclei. Therefore it has been suggested that there is cooperativity between the H and L subunits in the process of iron loading (158). Alternatively, some investigators have proposed a model of ferritin iron loading in which ceruloplasmin is responsible for iron oxidation and subsequent incorporation into ferritin (159).

Iron is rapidly released from ferritin by reduction of the iron core. It has been suggested that ascorbic acid or reduced flavin mononucleotide are the endogenous reductant in this process in vivo. At the present time, however, the identity of the reductant is unknown. Ascorbic acid is sometimes used in in-vitro studies of iron oxidation to mobilize iron from iron-loaded ferritin. Some authors have suggested that excessive ascorbic acid intakes could lead to increased mobilization of storage iron, which could promote oxidative damage to tissues (160). There is little in-vivo evidence to suggest that this occurs in individuals with normal iron status or normal iron-handling capabilities. However, in iron-loaded thalassemics who are treated with desferoxamine, supplemental ascorbic acid may be toxic (161).

The rate of iron release from ferritin is influenced by several factors. For example, the last iron atoms entering the mineralized core of ferritin are more easily liberated than those loaded first (162). H-chain ferritin also release iron more rapidly than the L chain (158). In addition, heme binds to ferritin (163), which increases the rate of iron release (164). It has been proposed that ceruloplasmin is necessary for the oxidation of ferritin-derived iron and for its subsequent attachment to Tf. Copper-deficient rats accumulate liver iron in the form of ferritin (165). Liver perfusion of these animals with blood containing ceruloplasmin causes immediate transfer of ferritin-bound iron to Tf (166).

2. Hemosiderin

When the average tissue iron-storing content of ferritin approaches about 4000 atoms of iron per ferritin molecule, ferritin is degraded by lysosomal proteases to form hemosiderin, an insoluble iron-storage protein (167). By this process the protein shell of ferritin is partially degraded so that up to 40% of the mass of hemosiderin consists of iron. The description of the type of iron that is stored in hemosiderin depends on the sources and conditions under which it was obtained. These forms of iron include amorphous ferric oxide, ferrihydrite, and goethite (155). These forms of iron are less chemically reactive compared to those found in ferritin and may be less available for mobilization.

E. Iron Turnover and Redistribution

The absorption and loss of iron are balanced in individuals with normal iron status. However, disruptions of this balance are commonly seen during menstruation, pregnancy, and gastrointestinal bleeding. In order to meet tissue needs, iron must either be mobilized from storage or recycled in order to meet the iron requirements of the body. Iron turnover is a significant means of recycling iron in the body. For example, in a 70-kg individual with a normal iron status, about 35 mg/day of iron is turned over in the plasma (168) (Fig. 2).

Iron turnover is mediated primarily by destruction of senescent erythrocytes by the reticuloendothelial system (168). Erythrocytes, which contains about 80% of the body's functional iron, have a mean functional lifetime of 120 days in humans. At the end of their functional lifetime, they are recognized as senescent by changes in the structure of their

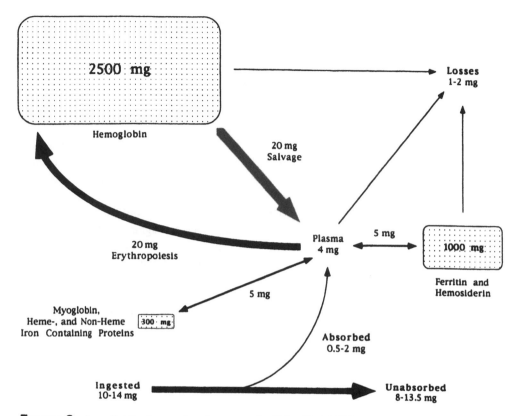

FIGURE 2 Iron distribution and exchange pools. (After Ref. 168.)

membranes and are catabolized at extravascular sites by Kupffer cells and spleen macrophages. After phagocytosis, the globin chains of hemoglobin are denatured, which releases bound heme. Intracellular unbound heme is ultimately degraded by heme oxygenase, which liberates iron. About 85% of the iron derived from hemoglobin degradation is re-released to the body in the form of iron bound to Tf or ferritin. Each day, 0.66% of the body's total iron content is recycled in this manner (168). Smaller contribution are made to plasma iron turnover by the degradation of myoglobin and iron-containing enzymes.

F. Iron Losses

The low solubility of iron precludes excretion as a major mechanism of maintaining iron hemostasis. Thus, in contrast to most other trace minerals whose homeostasis is maintained by excretion, the primary mechanism of maintaining whole-body iron homeostasis is to regulate the amount of iron absorbed so that it approximates iron losses. Iron losses can vary considerably with the gender of the individual. In male humans, total iron losses from the body have been calculated to be 1 mg/day. For premenopausal female humans, this loss is slightly higher. The predominant route of loss is from the gastrointestinal tract and amounts to 0.6 mg/day in adult males (169). Fecal iron losses derives from shed enterocytes, extravasated red blood cells, and biliary heme breakdown products which are poorly absorbed. Urogenital and integumental iron losses have been estimated to be >0.1 mg/day and 0.3 mg/day, respectively, in adult males (169). Menstrual iron loss, estimated from an average blood loss of 33 mL/month, equals 1.5 mg/day, but may range as high as 2.1 mg/day (170). Oral contraceptives reduce this loss (170,171), and intrauterine devices increase it (170,172,173). Pregnancy is associated with losses approximating 1 g, which consists of basal losses of 230 mg iron, increased maternal red cell mass of 450 mg iron, fetal needs of 270–300 mg iron, and placenta, decidua, and amniotic fluid iron content of 50–90 mg.

A number of clinical and pathologic conditions are attended by variable amounts of blood loss. These include hemorrhage, hookworm infestation, peptic gastric or anastomotic ulceration, ulcerative colitis, colonic neoplasia, cow's milk feeding to infants, aspirin, nonsteroidal antiinflammatory drugs, or corticosteroid administration and hereditary hemorrhagic telangiectasia (174–179). In addition to these conditions, a significant amount of iron (210–240 mg/unit) can be lost with regular blood donation (180).

III. INTRACELLULAR METABOLISM OF IRON

A. Acquisition of Iron via the Transferrin Receptor

Because most cellular iron acquisition occurs via Tf uptake, we will focus on the role of the TfR in maintaining intracellular iron homeostasis. The TfR (Fig. 3) is a 180-kDa glycoprotein composed of two identical 95-kDa subunits which are linked by two disulfide bridges (Cys-89 and Cys-98) (181). The human TfR gene has been localized to chromosome 3, region q26.2–∅ter (182,183). The promoter region of this gene contains several metal-response elements and appears to be transcriptionally (two- to threefold decrease) (184) and translationally (185) regulated by iron. The transcription of the gene is also negatively regulated by retinoic acid (186) and variably by 1,25-dihydroxyvitamin D_3. The mechanisms underlying the translational regulation of the TfR by iron will be discussed later, in the section on iron-response elements.

Each subunit of the TfR is composed of 760 amino acids (Fig. 3) (187). Specific sequences in the intracellular domain composed of Tyr-Thr-Arg-Phe (YTRF) appears necessary for aggregation in clathrin-coated pits (188). Serine 24 on the cytoplasmic domain of the TfR is phosphorylated by protein kinase C (189). The functional consequences of this phosphorylation are unknown but it is not required for internalization (190). The transmembrane region of the TfR consists of a single hydrophobic domain (24-28 AA) above positive 65. The transmembrane segment of the human TfR functions as a signal peptide and is necessary for translocation to the cell surface (191). This hydrophobic domain is also acylated in positions Cys-62 and possibly Cys-67 (181). This acylation is apparently not required for transport to the cell surface. The receptor is (N-linked) glycosylated on Asn-251, Asn-317, and Asn-727 (187). Glycosylation facilitates Tf-TfR binding through its effects on the tertiary and quaternary structure of the TfR.

Each TfR subunit binds one transferrin molecule with high affinity (192). The affinity of the TfR for Tf increases with Tf iron-binding site occupancy. The affinity is highest for diferric Tf ($K_d = 1.1 \times 10^{-8}$ M) and lowest for apoTf (4.6×10^{-6} M) (193). Since the concentration of Tf in plasma is $30–40 \times 10^{-6}$ M, cell surface TfRs are usually saturated with transferrin. Therefore, the regulation of cellular iron uptake is mediated by altering the number of TfRs present on the cell surface. At any one time about one-third of the cellular mass of TfRs is found on the cell surface. This number can be increased either by immediate translocation of cytoplasmic receptors to the surface or de-novo synthesis. The number of receptors present on the cell surface is a function of intracellular iron status, cell

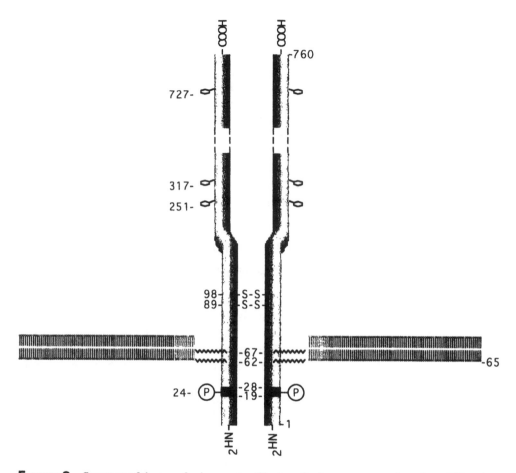

FIGURE 3 Structure of the transferrin receptor. The transferrin receptor consists of two 760 amino acid chains linked by two disulfide bonds at Cys-89 and Cys-98. The transferrin receptor is classified as a type II receptor, indicating that the amino terminus in lies in the cytoplasm. The amino terminus is phosphorylated on Ser-24. A sequence necessary (YTRF) for aggregation in clathrin-coated pits is found between residues 19 and 28. The transmembrane region of the TfR consists of a single hydrophobic domain (24–28 AA) above position 65. This segment of the TfR functions as a signal peptide and is necessary for translocation to the cell surface. This hydrophobic domain is also acylated in positions Cys-62 and possibly Cys-67. This helps anchor the TfR to membranes. The remaining 671 AA are extracellular. The receptor is (N-linked) glycosylated on Asn-251, Asn-317, and Asn-727. Glycosylation is apparently necessary not only for dimerization of the receptor but also for proper folding of the protein.

proliferative status, and metabolic need such as production of hemoglobin and myoglobin. Consequently erythroblasts (1×10^5) and reticulocytes (8×10^5) have the highest number of TfRs per cell, as their needs for iron are very high. As these cells mature into erythrocytes, they lose functioning TfR on their cell surfaces (194).

Ferro-Tf is taken up by TfR-mediated endocytosis (Fig. 4). Some researchers have demonstrated that internalization of the TfR can occur with apoTf attached (195), although others have shown that only ferro-Tf is internalized (196). After internalization, the

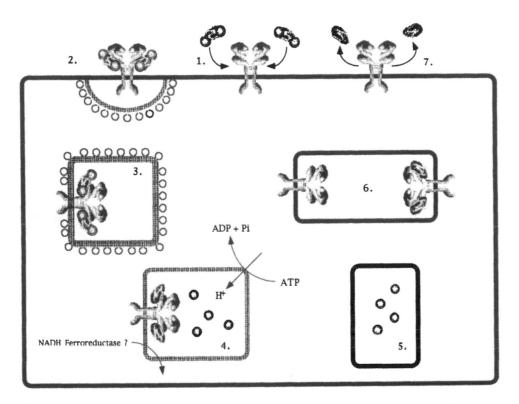

FIGURE 4 Cellular uptake of iron via the transferrin-transferrin receptor. (1) Each TfR subunit binds one transferrin molecule with high affinity. (2) Ferrotransferrin is then taken up by TfR-mediated endocytosis. (3) After internalization, the endosomal compartment sheds its clathrin coat. (4) An endosomal proton pump lowers the pH in the endosome to around pH 5–6. This acidic milieu releases iron by lowering the affinity of transferrin for iron. The endosome contains a molecule with NADH-ferric iron reductase activity, which reduces ferric iron to the ferrous state. (5) At this time the iron-containing portion of the endosome separates from the compartment containing the Tf-TfR complex. (6) The endosomal portion containing the apoTf-TfR complex travels to the Golgi apparatus, where it is packaged, along with newly synthesized receptors, for translocation to the cell surface. (7) ApoTf is released from the TfR when the TfR returns to the cell surface.

endosomal compartment containing the Tf-TfR complex sheds it clathrin coat. An endosomal proton pump (H^+-ATPase) then lowers the pH in the endosome to around pH 5–6. This acidic milieu lowers the affinity of Tf for iron. Binding of chloride to an anion-binding site of TfR-bound Tf facilitates the removal of iron from Tf (197). Additionally, part of the TfR also participates in this process (198). Some investigators have described an endosomal enzyme which uses nicotinamide adenine dinucleotide (NADH) to reduce Tf-derived ferric iron to the ferrous state (199,200). Other investigators have suggested that ascorbate may assist in this action nonenzymatically (201).

After iron is removed from Tf, the iron-containing portion of the endosome separates from the compartment containing the Tf-TfR complex. Iron in the endosomal compartment is transported across the membrane to the cytosol, where it appears either to enter a pool of low-molecular-weight iron chelates (202) or to be attached to an intracellular iron-binding protein. Recent evidence suggests that the endosomal proton pump (H^+-ATPase) may

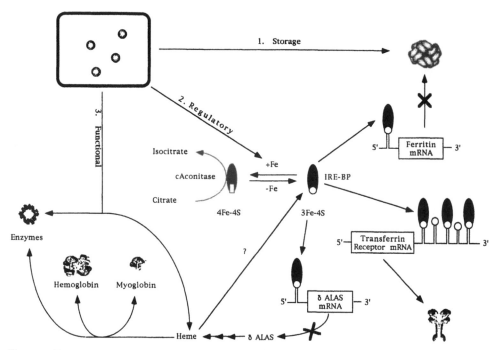

FIGURE 5 Intracellular iron metabolism. Iron in the endosomal vesicle or compartment is transported across the membrane to the cytosol, where it appears to enter a pool of low- molecular-weight iron chelates (upper left box). This iron can go to storage (path 1), be incorporated into functional protein (path 3), or can regulate the translation of the mRNAs of proteins involved in iron metabolism, including TfR, ferritin, and δ-aminolevulinic acid synthetase (ALAS). Putatively, the latter is accomplished by iron interacting with cytosolic (c) aconitase, which serves as the iron-response element-binding protein (IRE-BP). IRE-BP, the iron-deficient form of aconitase whose concentration is increased when iron is limiting, decreases ferritin synthesis, increases TfR mRNA, and decreases delta-ALAS.

participate in the transport of iron from the endosome to the cytosol (203). This iron is then channeled into one of three pathways: iron-regulatory protein(s), iron-utilizing proteins, or storage iron (Fig. 5).

The endosomal portion containing the TfR-apoTf complex travels to the Golgi apparatus, where it is packaged along with newly synthesized receptors and translocated to the cell surface. The affinity of the TfR for apoTf at pH 7.4 is much lower than that at pH 5.5. Consequently, apoTf is released when the TfR-apoTf complex returns to the cell surface. The complete cycling of TfR-Tf occurs in about 10 min and can occur repeatedly about 100 times before either TfR or Tf is degraded. In sheep and rat reticulocytes the TfR receptor can be actively shed from the cell surface (204,205). A truncated form of the TfR lacking cytoplasmic and transmembrane regions is found in human plasma bound to transferrin (206,207). It is not known whether the human TfR fragment arises from alternate splicing of the TfR gene or posttranslational cleavage. The fragment of TfR that circulates in plasma can be detected by ELISA and is the basis of a new method of determining the iron status of an individual.

B. Intracellular Low-Molecular-Weight Species

Several investigators have reported the presence of an intracellular pool of low-molecular-weight iron-containing species. The nature of this pool is largely speculative, and suggestions of its composition range from citrate, nucleotide, pyrophosphate, amino acid, and/or protein chelates or complexes of iron (208–210). The intracellular concentration of this pool is constant throughout conditions ranging from iron deficiency to iron overload (209).

C. Intracellular Iron Homeostasis

1. Iron Response Elements

Intracellular iron homeostasis requires the coordinated regulation of the synthesis and action of proteins involved in iron acquisition, utilization, and storage. When intracellular iron is scarce, the cell needs to increase its acquisition of iron either by mobilization of storage iron or acquisition of plasma iron. The cell also needs to prioritize its utilization of iron so that life-sustaining iron-containing proteins receive iron preferentially. Much of this process in animals is regulated at the genetic level by iron (Table 5) (124,184,211–214) (Fig. 5). In addition to the ill-defined transcriptional regulation by iron of Tf, TfRs, and ferritin, iron participates directly in its own homeostasis through binding to a cis-acting element(s) known as the iron-responsive element-binding protein(s) [IRE-BP(s)]. During intracellular iron deficiency, an IRE-BP binds to trans-acting iron-regulatory or -responsive elements (IREs) located in either the 3′ or 5′ untranslated region of some messenger RNAs. These IREs are a family of stem loop structures (Fig. 6) (215), which are highly conserved

TABLE 5 Eukaryotic Iron-Controlled Gene Expression (124,184,211–214)

Form of iron	Regulator	Level	Action	Gene product(s)
Fe	?	Transcription	↑ (5 to 6 ×)	Ferritin
			↓ (2 to 3 ×)	Transferrin receptor
Fe	IRE-BP	Translation	↓	Transferrin receptor
			↑ (5 to 6 ×)	Ferritin
			↑	e δ-ALAS
			↑	m-Aconitase
			↑	Transferrin ?
			?	β-Amyloid precursor protein
			?	m*Toll* (Drosophila)
Heme	?	Transcription	↓	e δ-ALAS,
			↑	Cytochrome P450 b/c
Heme	HPX	Transcription	↑	Heme oxygenase
			↑	Metallothionein
Heme	HAP-1	Transcription	↑	Catalase T (yeast)
			↑	iso-1-cytochrome c (yeast)
			↑	iso-2-cytochrome c (yeast)
			↑	cytochrome c1 (yeast)
Heme	HCI	Translation	↑	β-Globin
Heme	HRM	Translocation	↓	e δ-ALAS,
			↓	h δ-ALAS

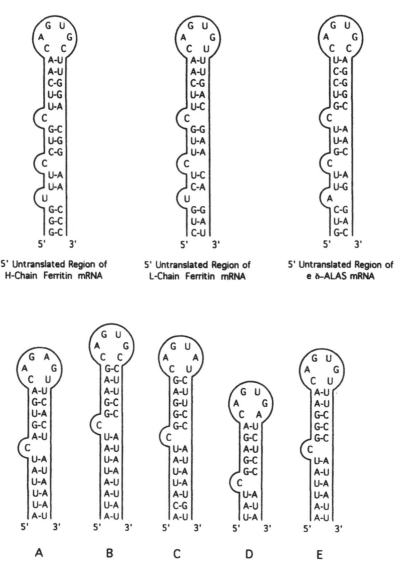

5' Untranslated Region of   5' Untranslated Region of   5' Untranslated Region of
H-Chain Ferritin mRNA   L-Chain Ferritin mRNA   e δ–ALAS mRNA

A   B   C   D   E

3' Untranslated Region of Transferrin Receptor mRNA

FIGURE 6 Structures of human iron response elements. Iron response elements of IREs are secondary structures located within the 5' and 3' untranslated regions of some mRNAs of proteins that contain iron or are involved in iron metabolism. Shown here are the three sets of stem loop structures for the transferrin receptor, ferritin, and δ-ALAS. Note the similarity both within and between structures where the 5' stems of the TfR mRNA are indicated as A–E and the other stems are labeled.

among species (216). Their secondary and tertiary structures are important for high-affinity binding of the IRE-BP.

The synthesis of the major proteins involved in the regulation of iron uptake and storage as well as the quantitatively most significant functional form of iron (heme) are regulated via the IRE-IRE-BP system (Fig. 5). Five IREs have been identified in the 3'

untranslated region of TfR mRNA (185,217–219). A single IRE has been located in the 5'
untranslated region of the mRNAs of ferritin, erythroid δ-aminolevulinate synthase (e-δ-
ALAS) (211), and mitochondrial isoform of aconitase (m-aconitase) (220), which repress
translation of these genes when an IRE-BP is bound (221–223). Other mRNAs in which an
IRE element have been located include the Drosophila *toll* maternal effect gene (211) and
the amyloid precursor protein (224,225). In contrast to e-δ-ALAS, which contains a
functional IRE, examination of the mRNA for housekeeping δ-aminolevulinate synthase
(h-δ-ALAS) did not reveal an IRE (211). Finally, although transferrin synthesis may be
regulated at the level of translation by iron (124), to date no IRE has been identified in the
mRNA for transferrin. Thus translational control of iron-containing proteins by the IRE-
IRE-BP system is widespread in animals but may not be universal.

The stabilization of TfR mRNA by the IRE-BP probably involves interactions with
3' untranslated region destabilizing sequence(s) (219). The position of the IRE in the
untranslated regions of the mRNA is also important for its ability to stabilize or block
translation of the mRNA (226,227). Furthermore, the IRE and base-paired flanking regions
of the ferritin mRNA exhibit positive translational control in the absence of IRE-BP (227).

2. Iron-Response Element-Binding Protein(s)

The iron-response element-binding protein(s) (IRE-BPs), also known as the ferritin repressor protein (228), the iron regulatory factor (229), or P-90 (230), shows broad tissue
distribution (231). The gene for one IRE-BP has been localized to chromosome 9 (232) and
has been cloned from a number of species (233). This IRE-BP has a molecular mass of 98
kDa, shows 95% homology among four different species, and shows considerable homology to m-aconitase (30%) and isopropylmalate isomerase (234). This IRE-BP has been
putatively identified as the cytosolic form of aconitase (c-aconitase) (235). Iron-replete
c-aconitase is an enzyme that converts citrate to isocitrate. The regulation of translation of
mRNA by this IRE-BP does not involve changes in the level of IRE-BP (236). Disassembly
of its iron-sulfur cluster (4Fe-4S) to (3Fe-4S) results in loss of aconitase activity and
promotes high-affinity binding to mRNA (237–239). However, simple reduction and
removal of the iron bound in the fourth coordination site of c-aconitase is insufficient to
produce the high-affinity RNA-binding properties found in the native IRE-BP. It appears
that endogenously produced nitric oxide serves to promote disassembly of the iron-sulfur
cluster of IRE-BP and enhances the high-affinity binding of IRE-BP to mRNA (240,241).
The IRE-BP is also phosphorylated by protein kinase C, which also enhances the high-
affinity binding of IRE-BP to mRNA (242). As attractive as this hypothesis of 3Fe/4Fe
switching is with regard to signaling IRE-BP binding to mRNA, other mechanisms also
seem likely, and further study of the binding region of IRE with IRE-BP is needed.

A second IRE-BP has recently been identified which differs from the above IRE-BP
in size (105 kDa) and tissue distribution (primarily brain and intestine) (243). The location
of the IREs and its binding proteins in tissues and cellular organelles will help clarify the
regulatory system within and between organ systems.

3. Heme

Heme synthesis accounts quantitatively for the largest utilization of functional iron (20 mg/
day). Heme, in addition to participating in oxygen transport and storage or functioning as a
cofactor in enzymes, regulates a number of different biochemical pathways. The metabolism of heme will not be discussed at length here, and we refer the reader to a more
comprehensive document for further reading (244). We will focus on heme's role in gene

expression as it relates to the process of heme/hemoglobin synthesis and degradation. This process is regulated by iron or heme at many levels (Fig. 7 and Table 5) and may be a model for other iron-containing proteins.

The formation of δ-ALAS is the rate-limiting step in the heme biosynthetic pathway. Two distinct forms of this enzyme occur in humans, an erythroid-specific (e-δ-ALAS) and a housekeeping-specific form (h-δ-ALAS). The regulation of each of these by iron or heme is different. As mentioned previously, an iron-regulatory element has been located in the 5′ untranslated region of e-δ-ALAS mRNA which inhibits ribosomal binding when the negative regulator protein, IRE-BP, is bound (211,223). Thus, in intracellular iron deficiency, the energetically expensive production of heme will be decreased because the synthesis of the first enzyme in its biosynthetic pathway is blocked by transitional control of the IRE-BP. At very high levels of heme, heme binds to IRE-BP (245), which inhibits IRE-BP binding to the IRE in vitro (246) and enhances IRE-BP degradation in vivo (247). This may be physiologically unimportant. Although e-δ-ALAS gene transcription is not changed by heme (248), heme inhibits its own production by inhibiting the transport of e-δ-ALAS preprotein from the cytoplasm to the mitochondria [via a heme regulatory motif (HRM)] (249).

The transcription of ferrochelatase, the enzyme responsible for insertion of ferrous iron into protoporphyrin IX, is positively regulated by iron in mouse erythroleukemia cells (250). Heme increases the transcription of ferrochelatase mRNA by inducing differentiation in these cells (250). This may be counterbalanced, however, by its inhibitory effect on ferrochelatase enzyme activity.

Transcription of erythroid-specific genes including β-globin is regulated by the erythroid transcription factor GATA-1. GATA-1 is a zinc-finger DNA-binding protein which also can bind to DNA as an iron complex (251). The physiologic significance of this DNA binding is unknown. Synthesis of β-globin is positively controlled at the level of mRNA translation by heme as follows. Translation of β-globin mRNA involves utilization and recycling of two proteins involved in initiation, eukaryotic initiation factor-2α (eIF-2α) and eukaryotic initiation factor-2β (eIF-2β). Reticulocytes contain an eIF-2α kinase called heme-controlled inhibitor (HCI). In the absence of heme, HCI is activated and phosphorylates eIF-2α, which promotes association of eIF-2α and eIF-2β, reducing the free concentration of each, and thereby inhibiting β-globin synthesis. Heme inactivates HCI and appears to promote the association of HCI with other related peptides (252). In summary, heme repletion assures translation of β-globin mRNA by preventing the inactivation of eIF-2α. It is not known whether this mechanism is limited solely to β-globin synthesis, but all protein synthesis that is dependent on eIF-2α will be affected by the heme concentration in erythroid cells (253).

In addition to its role in hemoglobin synthesis, heme regulates a number of other gene products which are either involved in its own metabolism or to which it is bound as a prosthetic group. In addition to feedback inhibiting the enzymatic activity of h-δ-ALAS, heme inhibits the transcription of pre h-δ-ALAS (254,255). In nonerythroid cells, heme also limits its own synthesis by binding to the mRNA for h-δ-ALAS. This action enhances h-δ-ALAS mRNA degradation (256). By binding to h-δ-ALAS preprotein, heme inhibits the transport of h-δ-ALAS from the cytoplasm to the mitochondria (257,258). Heme also induces the transcription of cytochrome P-450b/e (for which heme is a prosthetic group) and induces the synthesis of heme oxygenase (which degrades heme) (212,259). This latter induction involves specific heme or heme-HPX recognition sequences in the 5′ untranslated region of the mRNA for heme oxygenase (260).

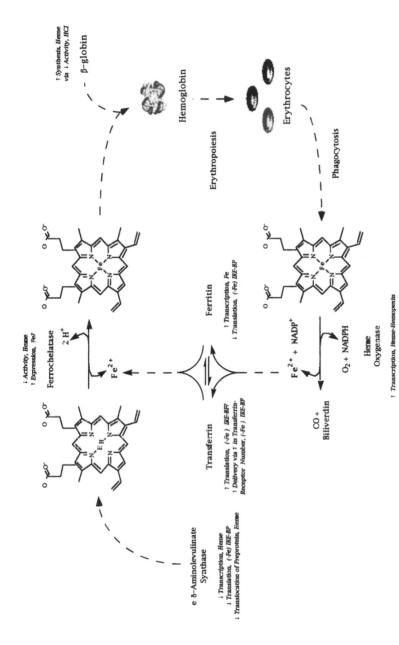

FIGURE 7 Regulation of the biosynthesis of heme by heme and iron. Heme biosynthesis accounts for the major functional usage of iron. Heme consists of a tetrapyrrole ring, protoporphyrin IX, conjugated to Fe²⁺. The biosynthesis and degradation of heme is regulated at many levels by iron and heme (see text for details) and may provide a model for other iron-containing molecules.

IV. CHEMICAL PROPERTIES AND BIOCHEMICAL FUNCTIONS OF IRON

A. Introduction

Iron is a d-block transition element, which can exist in oxidation states ranging from -2 to $+6$. In biological systems, these oxidation states are limited primarily to the ferrous $(+2)$, ferric $(+3)$, and ferryl $(+4)$ states. The interconversion of iron oxidation states is not only a mechanism whereby iron participates in electron transfer but also a mechanism whereby iron can reversibly bind ligands. Iron can bind to many ligands by virtue of its unoccupied d orbitals. The preferred biological ligands for iron are oxygen, nitrogen, or sulfur atoms. The electronic spin state and biological redox potential (from $+1000$ mV for some heme proteins to -550 mV for some bacterial ferredoxins) of iron can change according to the ligand to which it is bound. By exploiting the oxidation state, redox potential, and electron spin state of iron, nature can precisely adjust the chemical reactivity of iron. Thus iron is particularly suited to participate in a large number of useful biochemical reactions (Table 6) (261; see also Figs. 10 and 11, below). The general classification of these reactions are oxygen transport and storage, electron transfer, and substrate oxidation–reduction. We will discuss some of the iron-dependent reactions in only limited detail here, and we refer the reader to a more comprehensive review (262). It is important to recall that the activity of many of these enzymes decreases during tissue iron deficiency. Only rarely, however, have direct connections between biochemical events and clinical manifestations been firmly established.

Four major classes of iron-containing proteins (Fig. 8) carry out these reactions in the mammalian system: iron-containing proteins (hemoglobin and myoglobin), iron-sulfur enzymes, heme proteins, and iron-containing enzymes (noniron sulfur, nonheme enzymes). In iron-sulfer enzymes, iron can be bound to sulfur in four possible arrangements (FeS, 2Fe-2S, 4Fe-4S, 3Fe-4S). However, only three of these occur in humans (Fig. 9). In heme proteins, iron is bound to various forms of heme which differ not only in the composition of their side chains but also in the methods whereby they are attached to proteins. In humans the predominant form of heme is protoporphyrin-IX (PP-IX) (Fig. 7).

B. Oxygen Transport and Storage

The movement of oxygen from the environment to terminal oxidases is one of the key functions of iron, in which dioxygen is bound to porphyrin-ring iron-containing molecules, either as part of the prosthetic group of hemoglobin within red blood cells or as the facilitator of oxygen diffusion in tissue, myoglobin.

Hemoglobin is a tetrameric protein with two pairs of identical subunits ($\alpha 2$, $\beta 2$, $M_r = 64$ kDa) with either 141 or 142 amino acids in the α chain and 146 in the β chain. Each subunit has one prosthetic group, Fe-PP-IX, whose ferrous iron reversibly binds dioxygen (Fig. 10). The four subunits are not covalently attached to each other but do react cooperatively with dioxygen with specific modulation by pH, pCO_2, organic phosphates, and temperature. These modulators of the affinity of hemoglobin for iron determine the efficiency of transport of oxygen from the alveoli capillary interface in the lung to the red cell–capillary tissue interface in peripheral tissues. The allosteric effect of decreasing pH, the well-known Bohr effect, decreases binding affinity of heme-Fe for dioxygen via protonation of His-146 on beta chains and Val-1 on alpha chains in the presence of Cl^- and CO_2. CO_2 forms a Schiff base with the terminal amino acids of each chain and decreases dioxygen affinity. This favors the unloading of oxygen in tissues where the pH is lower and pCO_2 is higher than in arterial blood. 2,3-Diphosphoglycerate is a product of a side pathway within erythrocytes and binds to a specific region of the β chain to decrease $Hb-O_2$ binding affinity. This right shift of the dissociation curve is evident in times of greater need for oxygen delivery, such as in anemia, where the blood content of hemoglobin is significantly reduced and increased cardiac output is only partially compensatory.

Myoglobin is a single-chain hemoprotein of 17 kDa in cytoplasm and increases the rate of diffusion of dioxygen from capillary RBCs to cytoplasm and mitochondria. The concentration of myoglobin in muscle is drastically reduced in tissue iron deficiency, thus limiting the rate of diffusion of dioxygen from erythrocytes to mitochondria (263).

C. Electron Transport

The overall scheme of the electron transport chain and the forms of iron that participate in electron transport are summarized in Figure 11. The cytochromes contain heme as the active site, with the Fe-porphyrin ring functioning to reduce ferrous iron to ferric iron with the acceptance of electrons. The iron–sulfur proteins also act as electron carriers via the action of iron bound to either two or four sulfur atoms and cysteine side chains. The 40 different proteins that constitute the respiratory chain contain six different heme proteins, six iron-sulfur centers, two copper centers, as well as ubiquinone to connect NADH to oxygen.

D. Substrate Oxidation and Reduction (Table 6)

1. Oxidoreductases

The oxidoreductases are a diverse family of enzymes whose catalytic functions include oxidation of aldehydes, oxidation of inorganic sulfite, and the catabolism of purines. However, the most important member of this family is ribonucleotide reductase, the rate-limiting element in DNA synthesis.

2. Monooxygenases

Amino Acid Monooxygenases

The amino acid monooxygenases catalyze the formation of L-tyrosine, 5-OH L-tryptophan (a precursor to serotonin), and L-dopa (the precursor to dopamine).

Cytochrome P450

Several hundred enzyme activities have also been ascribed to the cytochrome P450 family of enzymes. Some demonstrate limited substrate specificity, but most exhibit broad substrate specificity, hence they have been termed the mixed-function oxidases. At least 39 rat and 28 human cytochrome P450 genes have been identified so far, and more are likely to be discovered (264). Because of the number and broad range of enzymes/enzymatic activity, our list cannot be exhaustive. Therefore we have chosen those enzymes which we feel are most related to nutrition and metabolism.

The microsomal P450 enzyme system participates in the biosynthesis of steroid hormones such as pregnenolone, corticosterone, aldosterone, and 1α25-OH-vitamin D_3. The microsomal P450 enzyme system participates in the metabolism of xenobiotics such as drugs and aromatic hydrocarbons. This system also participates in the biosynthesis of some steroid hormones such as 25-OH-vitamin D_3 and dihydroxyepiandrosterone (DHEA). This

Table 6 Mammalian Iron-Dependent Enzymes (261)

D. Substate Oxidation-Reduction

1. Oxido-reductases

Enzyme	E C Number	Type of Iron	Reaction
Aldehyde oxidase	[1.2.3.1]	2 (2Fe-2S)	R-CHO + O_2 → R-COOH + H_2O_2
Sulfite Oxidase	[1.8.3.1]	Heme b_5	Inorganic SO_3^{-3}+ O_2 → inorganic SO_4^{-3}+ H_2O_2
Xanthine dehydrogenase /(oxidase)	[1.1.1.204]	2 (2Fe-2S)	Xanthine + O_2 + NADH → uric Acid + NAD^+
Xanthine oxidase / (dehydrogenase)	[1.1.3.22]	2 (2Fe-2S)	Xanthine + O_2 → uric Acid + H_2O_2

Typical Mechanism:

Xanthine Uric Acid

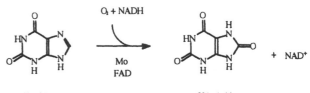

Xanthine dehydrogenase/(oxidase)

Enzyme	E C Number	Type of Iron	Reaction
Ribonucleotide reductase	[1.17.4.1]	2 Fe^{3+}	Ribonucleotide diphosphate + oxi-thioreoxin → 2' deoxyribonucleotide diphosphate

2. Monooxygenases

a. Amino Acid Monooxygenases

Enzyme	E C Number	Type of Iron	Reaction
Tryptophan 5-monooxygenase	[1.14.16.4]	Fe^{2+}	L-Tryptophan + BH_4 + O_2 → 5-OH L-tryptophan + BH_2 + H_2O
Phenylalanine 4-monooxygenase	[1.14.15.6]	Fe^{2+}	L-Phenylalanine + BH_4 + O_2 → L-tyrosine + BH_2 + H_2O
Tyrosine 3-monoxygenase	[1.14.16.2]	Fe^{2+}	L-Tyrosine + BH_4 + O_2 → 3,4-dihydroxyphenylalanine + BH_2 + H_2O

Typical Mechanism:

Phenylalanine Tyrosine

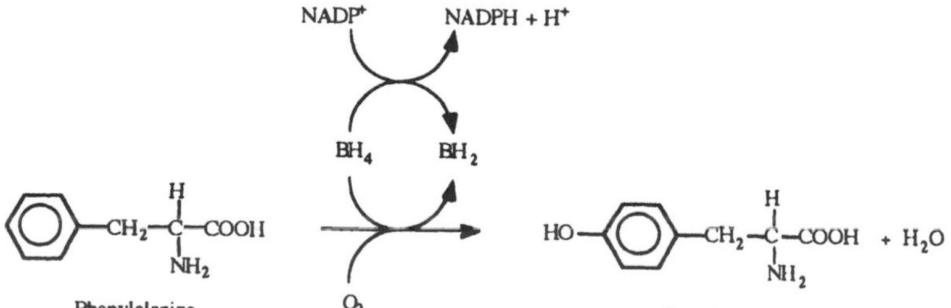

Phenylalanine 4-monooxygenase

TABLE 6 Continued

c. Fatty Acid Desaturases

Enzyme	E C Number	Type of Iron	Reaction
Linoleoyl-CoA (Δ6) desaturase	[1.14.99.25]	$2Fe^{2+}$, 2Cyt b_5	Linoleoyl-CoA + NADH + H^+ + O_2 → γ-linolenoyl-CoA + NAD$^+$ + 2 H_2O
Stearyl CoA (Δ9) desaturase	[1.14.99.5]	$2Fe^{2+}$, 2Cyt b_5	Stearoyl-CoA + NADH + H^+ + O_2 → oleoyl-CoA + NAD$^+$ + 2 H_2O
			Palmitoyl-CoA + NADH + H^+ + O_2 → palmitoleoyl-CoA + NAD$^+$ + 2 H_2O

<u>Typical Mechanism:</u>

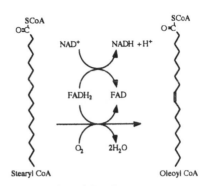

Stearyl CoA desaturase

3. Dioxygenases

a. Amino Acid or Amine Dioxygenases

Enzyme	E C Number	Type of Iron	Reaction
γ-Butyrobetaine dioxygenase	[1.14.11.1]	Fe^{2+}	γ-Butyrobetaine + O_2 + α-KG → L-carnitine + succinate + CO_2
Peptide-aspartate ß-dioxygenase	[1.14.11.16]	Fe^{2+}	Peptide L-aspartate + O_2 + α-KG → peptide 3-OH-L-aspartate + succinate + CO_2
Procollagen lysine 5-dioxygenase	[1.14.11.4]	4 Fe^{2+}	L-Lysine + O_2 + α-KG → 5-OH-L-lysine + succinate + CO_2
Procollagen proline 3-dioxygenase	[1.14.11.2]	4 Fe^{2+}	L-Proline + O_2 + α-KG → 3-OH-L-proline + succinate + CO_2
Procollagen proline4-dioxygenase	[1.14.11.7]	4 Fe^{2+}	L-Proline + O_2 + α-KG → 4-OH-L-proline + succinate + CO_2
Trimethyllysine dioxygenase	[1.14.11.8]	Fe^{2+}	N^6, N^6, N^6-Trimethylysine + O_2 + α-KG → 3-OH-N^6, N^6, N^6-trimethylysine + succinate + CO_2

<u>Typical Mechanism:</u>

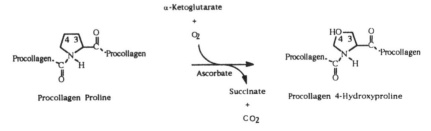

Procollagen-proline 4-dioxygenase

Enzyme	E C Number	Type of Iron	Reaction
Cysteamine dioxygenase	[1.13.11.19]	Fe^{2+}	Cysteamine + O_2 → hypotaurine
Cysteine dioxygenase	[1.13.11.20]	Fe^{2+}	Cysteine + O_2 → 3-sulfoalanine
Homogentisate 1,2-dioxygenase	[1.13.11.5]	Fe^{2+}	Homogentisate + O_2 → 4-maleylacetoacetate
3-OH anthranilate 3,4-dioxygenase	[1.13.11.6]	Fe^{2+}	3-Hydroxyanthranilate + O_2 → 2-amino-3-carboxymuconate semialdehyde

TABLE 6   Continued

Tryptophan 2, 3-dioxygenase   [1.13.11.11] Fe^{3+}-PP IX   Tryptophan + O_2 → L-N-formylkynurenine

b. Lipoxygenases

Enzyme	E C Number	Type of Iron	Reaction
Arachidonate 5-Lipoxygenase	[1.13.11.34]	Fe^{2+}	Arachidonic Acid + O_2 → 5-hydroperoxycosatetraenoic acid
Arachidonate 12-Lipoxygenase	[1.13.11.31]	Fe^{2+}	Arachidonic Acid + O_2 → 12-hydroperoxycosatetraenoic acid
Arachidonate 15-Lipoxygenase	[1.13.11.33]	Fe^{2+}	Arachidonic Acid + O_2 → 12-hydroperoxycosatetraenoic acid

Typical Mechanism:

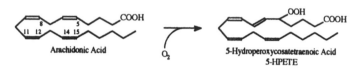

Arachidonate 5-Lipoxygenase

c. Peroxidases

Enzyme	E C Number	Type of Iron	Reaction
Catalase	[1.11.1.6]	Fe^{3+}-PP-IX	$2H_2O_2$ → $2H_2O + O_2$
Lactoperoxidase	[1.11.1.7]	Fe^{3+}-PP-IX	$AH_2 + H_2O_2$ → $2H_2O + A$
Myeloperoxidase	[1.11.1.7]	Fe^{3+}- chlorin	Cl^- → ClO^-
Prostaglandin-endoperoxide synthase	[1.14.99.1]	Fe^{3+}-PP-IX	Arachidonic Acid + $AH_2 + 2O_2$ → prostaglandin $H_2 + A + H_2O$
Thyroperoxidase	[1.11.1.7]	Fe^{3+}-PP-IX	Thyroglobulin-Tyr + $2I^- + H_2O_2$ → thyroglobulin-I-Tyr +2 H_2O + OH^-
			2 Thyroglobulin-I-Tyr → thyroglobulin-T_3 or T_4 + Thyroglobulin + serine + H_2O

c. Fatty Acid Desaturases

Enzyme	E C Number	Type of Iron	Reaction
Linoleoyl-CoA (Δ6) desaturase	[1.14.99.25]	$2Fe^{2+}$, 2Cyt b_5	Linoleoyl-CoA + NADH + H^+ + O_2 → γ-linolenoyl-CoA + NAD $^+$ + 2 H_2O
Stearyl CoA (Δ9) desaturase	[1.14.99.5]	$2Fe^{2+}$, 2Cyt b_5	Stearoyl-CoA + NADH + H^+ + O_2 → oleoyl-CoA + NAD $^+$ + 2 H_2O
			Palmitoyl-CoA + NADH + H^+ + O_2 → palmitoleoyl-CoA + NAD$^+$ + 2 H_2O

Typical Mechanism:

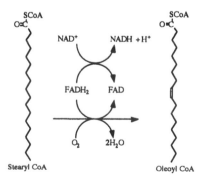

Stearyl CoA desaturase

TABLE 6 Continued

d. NO Synthases

Enzyme	E C Number	Type of Iron	Reaction
Nitric Oxide Synthase I and II	[1.14.13.39]	Fe^{3+}-PP-IX	L-Arginine + BH_4 + 1.5 NADPH + $2O_2$ → NO· + citrulline + BH_2 + 1.5 $NADP^+$ + H_2O

e. Others

Enzyme	E C Number	Type of Iron	Reaction
ß-Carotene 15, 15' dioxygenase	[1.13.11.21]	Fe^{2+}	ß-Carotene + O_2 → 2 retinal

E. Miscellaneous Iron-containing Enzymes

Enzyme	E C Number	Type of Iron	Reaction
Aconitase	[4.2.1.3]	(4Fe-4S)	Citrate → *cis*-aconitate → isocitrate

Mechanism:

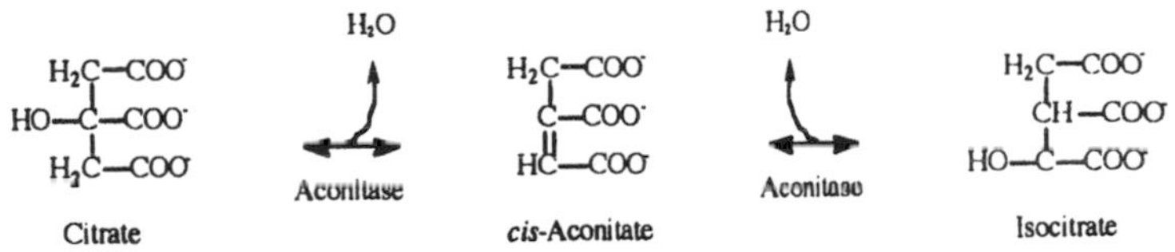

Aconitase

Enzyme	E C Number	Type of Iron	Reaction
Guanylate Cyclase		Fe^{2+}-PP-IX	GTP → cGMP + PP_i
Amidophosphoribosyltransferase	[2.4.2.14]	(4Fe-4S)	5-Phospho-a-D-ribose-1-diphosphate + Gln + H_2O → 5-phospho-β-D-ribosylamine + PP_i + Glu
Purple Acid Phosphatase /Uteroferrin	[3.1.3.2]	$2Fe^{2+}$	R-PO_4 + H_2O → PO_4^{-3} + ROH + H^+

enzyme system includes cholesterol 7α-monooxygenase, the rate-limiting reactant in bile acid synthesis. This enzyme system is also responsible for the formation of prostacyclin (PGI), thromboxane (TBX$_2$), and leukotrienes (LTs).

Fatty Acid Desaturases

The fatty acid desaturases catalyze the formation of the unsaturated fatty acids palmitoleic acid (16:1,9), oleic acid (18:1,9), and γ-linolenic acid (18:2;6,9,12).

3. Dioxygenases

Amino Acid or Amine Dioxygenases

The amino acid or amine dioxygenases catalyze the posttransalational hydroxylation of proline and lysine residues of proteins. These enzymes also synthesize L-carnitine, an important mediator of fatty acid metabolism. Finally, this family of enzymes participates in the degradation of cysteine, cysteamine, and tryptophan.

Lipoxygenases

The lipoxygenases generate 5-, 12-, and 15-hydroperoxyeicosatetraenoic (HPETE) acids, the parent compounds in leukotriene synthesis.

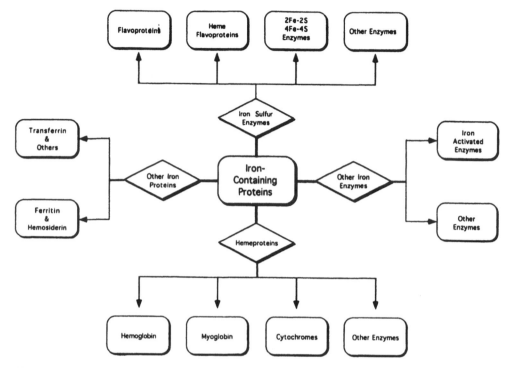

FIGURE 8   Classification of major mammalian iron-containing proteins.

Peroxidases

With the exception of the glutathione peroxidases, all mammalian peroxidases contain iron. Catalase degrades hydrogen peroxide formed as a by-product of some oxidase reactions. Myeloperoxidase forms hypochlorite anion, which is an important cytotoxic molecule produced by neutrophils. Thyroperoxidase is responsible not only for the organification of iodide but also for the conjugation of iodinated tyrosine residues on thyroglobulin. Finally, prostaglandin-endoperoxide synthase generates PGH$_2$, the parent compound in the synthesis of all prostaglandins.

NO Synthases

Nitric oxide (NO·) is a recently identified biological effector molecule. The growing list of physiologic functions in which NO· participates includes vasodilation, enzyme regulation, neurotransmission, and the immune response. NO synthase is a cytochrome P450-like protein which occurs in at least four isoforms. At least two of these forms, NO synthase I and II, contain iron in the form of PP-IX (265,266). They may also contain a catalytically active nonheme iron (267).

Others

The formation of retinal from β-carotene requires a dioxygenase, β-carotene 15,15'-dioxygenase.

4.   Miscellaneous Iron-Containing Enzymes

Other iron-containing enzymes include those in which iron does not participate in oxidation–reduction. Among these are aconitase, which is part of the citric acid cycle in

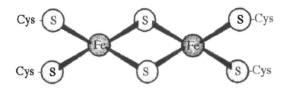

2 Fe-2 S

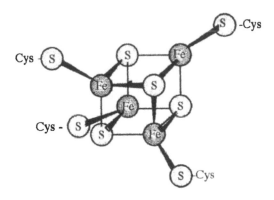

4 Fe-4 S

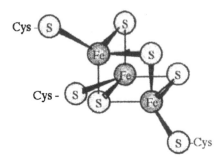

3 Fe-4 S

FIGURE 9 Structure of iron–sulfur clusters. Iron–sulfur clusters consist of nonheme iron bound to sulfur in iron in four possible arrangements (FeS, 2Fe-2S, 4Fe-4S, 3Fe-4S). In FeS (not shown), one Fe is tetrahedrally bound to four Cys residues. In 2Fe-2S, two Fe are bound to four Cys and two inorganic S residues. In 4Fe-4S clusters, four Fe are bound to four Cys and four inorganic S residues. Finally, in 3Fe-4S clusters, three Fe are bound to three Cys and four inorganic S residues. Processes which involve iron–sulfur proteins, such as electron transport and substrate oxidation–reduction, require the transfer of electrons from one molecule to another. Iron–sulfur proteins accomplish this by oxidation–reduction of their iron centers. Thus, a fully reduced ($4Fe^{3+}$) 4Fe-4S cluster is theoretically capable of accepting and transfering four electrons.

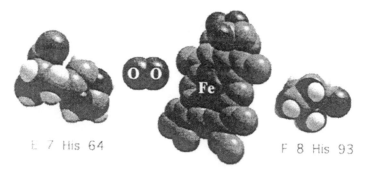

E 7 His 64   F 8 His 93

FIGURE 10 Oxygen binding to hemoglobin heme. In this magnified representation of the O_2-binding site of hemoglobuin, heme is noncovalently bound to a proximal His-93 and distal His-64 side chains of hemoglobin. O_2 binds to heme by occupying the 6th coordination position of the iron atom. This results in a conformational change in the porphyrin ring which is transmitted into a conformational change in the protein. The conformational change ultimately facilitates O_2 binding to the other three heme ring found in hemoglobin. This facilitation is known as cooperativity and is influenced by a number of other factors, including CO_2, pH, and 2,3-diphosphoglycerate.

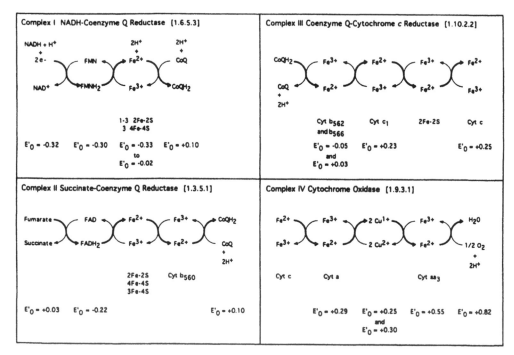

FIGURE 11 Role of iron in the electron-transport chain. The function of the electron-transport chain is to transfer electrons from NADH (or other intermediate electron donors) to molecular oxygen with the penultimate formation of H_2O. The electron-transport chain consists of at least five complexes of proteins containing 40 different proteins, including six distinct heme proteins, six iron sulfur centers, two copper centers, as well as ubiquinone. The cytochromes contain heme as the active site, with the Fe-porphyrin ring functioning to reduce ferrous iron to ferric iron with the acceptance of electrons. The iron–sulfur proteins also act as electron carriers via the action of iron bound to either two or four sulfur atoms and cysteine side chains.

mitochondria, guanylate cyclase, which forms the important intracellular second messenger cyclic GMP, and amino phosphoribosyltransferase, which is the rate-limiting reactant in the synthesis of purines such as adenine and guanine.

V. PHYSIOLOGIC FUNCTIONS OF IRON AND SIGNS OF IRON DEFICIENCY

A. General

The overt physical manifestations of iron deficiency are glossitis, angular stomatitis, koilonychia (spoon nails), blue sclera, esophageal webbing (Plummer-Vinson syndrome), and anemia (Table 7). Behavioral disturbances such as pica [which is characterized by abnormal consumption of nonfood items such as clay (geophagia) and ice (pagophagia)] are often present in iron deficiency. Physiologic manifestations of iron deficiency have also been noted in immune function, cognitive performance and behavior, thermoregulatory performance, energy metabolism, and exercise or work performance (263,268). Many of these manifestations of iron deficiency are not mutually exclusive events and do not occur independently from one another. Furthermore, many of these manifestations occur only during certain stages of iron deficiency.

The progression of iron deficiency occurs in two steps related to depletion of iron stores prior to depletion of functional iron: (1) bone marrow, spleen, and liver stores depletion; and (2) diminished erythropoiesis due to a negative iron balance leading to anemia and decreased activity of iron-dependent enzymes. Clinically, iron deficiency is frequently diagnosed by virtue of anemia secondary to long-term diminished erythropoiesis.

Depletion of the storage iron pool is generally without influence on physiologic function, with a few exceptions (269,270). In those studies, correlations were noted

TABLE 7 Symptomatology of Iron Deficiency[a]

A.	Anemia
B.	Impaired thermoregulation
C.	Impaired immune function
D.	Impaired mental function
E.	Impaired physical performance
F.	Glossitis
G.	Angular stomatitis
H.	Koilonychia
I.	Pica
J.	Complications of pregnancy
K.	Increased absorption of lead and cadmium
L.	Altered drug metabolism
M.	Increased insulin sensitivity
N.	Blue sclera
O.	Fatigue

[a]See text for details.

between electroencephalogram asymmetry (a CNS abnormality) and plasma ferritin within the iron adequate range. Nonetheless, nearly all functional consequences are more strongly related to human "anemia" rather than tissue iron deficits. The challenge of separating O_2 transport events from tissue iron deficits still looms large. Good examples are the decreases in muscle myoglobin content, cytochrome oxidase activity, and electron transport.

Several of the well-known consequences of iron deficiency that occurs after the depletion of iron stores is the decline in hemoglobin concentration, the decrease in mean corpuscular Hb concentration, a decrease in the size and volume of the new red cells, reduced myoglobin, and reduced amounts of both Fe–S and heme iron-containing cytochromes within cells. Diffusion of dioxygen from Hb into tissue becomes limited in this situation due to fewer erythrocytes packed close together in capillaries, increased membrane diffusivity, and a decreased tissue myoglobin concentration. The heterogeneity of distribution of mitochondria around and adjacent to capillary walls is well known but is not well studied in the iron-deficient individual or animal model. The delivery of red cells to tissue is under a complex regulation by both systemic and local regulatory features. While it is not a part of this review, the reader is urged to consider that the matching of oxygen delivery to tissue needs for oxygen are the ultimate goals of these regulators. In severe anemia, oxygen transport is clearly limiting to tissue oxidative function at anything but the resting condition (263), despite a significant right shifting of the Hb–O_2 dissociation curve (decreased affinity) and an increase in cardiac output in an attempt to increase TaO$_2$. Tissue extraction of oxygen is increased by this compensation, and mixed venous PO$_2$ is significantly lower in anemic individuals. While Hb–O_2 affinity compensation is reasonable at sea level, just the opposite direction of compensation occurs in anemic individuals at high altitudes (4000 m). The Hb–O_2 dissociation curve is "left shifted" in these hypobaric hypoxic conditions to increase O_2 loading in the lung at the expense of tissue delivery (271). The very significant decrease in myoglobin and other iron-containing proteins in skeletal muscle in iron-deficiency anemia contributes significantly to the decline in muscle aerobic capacity (263).

A recent study used ^{31}P NMR spectroscopy to examine the functional state of bioenergetics in iron-deficient and -replete rat gastrocnemius muscle (272) at rest and during 10 seconds of contraction at 2 Hz. Iron-deficient animals had a clear increase in phosphocreatine breakdown and a decrease in pH compared to controls, and a slower recovery of Pcr and Pi concentrations after exercise. During repletion for 2–7 days with iron dextran there was no substantial improvement in these indicators of muscle mitochondrial energetics. These authors concluded that "tissue factors" such as decreased mitochondrial enzyme activity, decreased number of mitochondria, and altered morphology of the mitochondria might be responsible for these observations. It is not uncommon for P:O ratios to be normal in iron deficiency, despite very significant alterations in activity of iron-containing respiratory-chain enzymes.

A more typical repair curve for muscle iron-containing and oxidative enzymes during iron-repletion experiments has been described (273). Pyruvate and malate oxidase were decreased to 35% of normal in iron-deficient muscle and improved to 85% of normal in 10 days of treatment. 2-Oxoglutarate oxidase was decreased to 47% of normal and improved to 90%; succinate oxidase, in contrast, was only 10% of normal in iron deficiency and improved to only 42% of normal after 10 days. Cytoplasmic enzymes hexokinase and lactate dehydrogenase were unaffected by iron status. The 50–90% decrease in both the Fe–S enzymes and in the heme-containing mitochondrial cytochromes are consistent with many other observations over the last two decades (263). What seems to determine the amount of decline in activity with iron deprivation is the rate of turnover of that particular iron-containing protein in the time of cellular deprivation of iron.

The last stage of iron deficiency is when stores are depleted and there is no longer sufficient iron to meet daily requirements. This stage of iron-deficient erythropoiesis leads to a significant compromise in cellular function in many organs (263). The rate at which individual tissues and cellular organelles within those tissues develop a true "deficit" in iron is dependent on the rate of turnover of iron-containing proteins, the rate of cell growth, and intracellular mechanisms for recycling iron (263).

B. Impaired Thermoregulation

Iron-deficiency anemia alters the ability of humans and rats to maintain body core temperature during acute cold exposure. Investigations have documented clear alterations in thermoregulation (274,275), the thyroid system (276,277), and the sympathetic nervous system (278,279).

Iron-deficient anemic (IDA) humans have significantly greater losses of core body temperature when cold stressed than controls (280), even when body fatness is accounted for in experimental settings (277,281). Nutritional iron-deficiency anemia also limits body temperature maintenance during acute cold (4°C) stress in rats (274,275). Anemia plays a key role in this defect, as nonanemic rats and nonanemic humans thermoregulate adequately despite tissue iron depletion. There is still the perception in humans, however, that iron-deficient people "feel cold." Consistent observations in humans and animal models have been a decrease in thyroid function and some increase in sympathetic activity.

Anemic humans and rats had low plasma hormone concentrations (T_3), and rats had a blunted thyroid-stimulating hormone response (TSH) to thyroid-releasing hormone or cold challenge if anemic (275,276). This does not occur if they are nonanemic. In addition, there is a decrease in activity of the peripheral production of T_3 from thyroxine and utilization of this hormone. While the deiodinase is selenium, not iron containing; there is a likely iron dependency (282).

Peripheral catecholamine metabolism appears to be altered dramatically in iron deficiency. Elevated levels of norepinephrine in urine of iron-deficient children (283), adults (280), and rats (278,279) are well documented. However, in these studies the level of epinephrine appeared to be unaffected. Early studies suggested that decreased monoamine oxidase activity was causal to these observations, though it is more likely that increased "spillover" into plasma is a significant contribution. Rat studies show dramatic large increases in norepinephrine turnover in many tissue (278). Thermoregulatory capacity in IDA can be improved dramatically by injection of large amounts of T_3 or infusion of TSH (284). These pharmacologic interventions seemingly override a defect in the generation of sufficient T_3 at local levels.

C. Impaired Immune Function

Although it is true that most pathogens require iron and have evolved sophisticated strategies for acquiring it, iron is also required by the host in order to mount an effective immune response. In the conceptual model of nutritional immunity, the host must effectively sequester iron away from pathogens and at the same time provide a supply of iron that is not limiting to its immune system (285). Extreme experimental manipulation of dietary iron may perturb the delicate balance between these two processes and may give results unrelated to those likely found in free-living humans. Additionally, the reduction in energy intake accompanying iron deficiency may contribute to immune dysfunction. Furthermore, the confounding presence of multiple nutritional deficiencies and unsanitary conditions limit what can be said about iron and immune function in the large number of clinical or intervention studies. These issues have been effectively reviewed by Dallman (286).

Experimental and clinical data suggest that there is an increased risk of infection during iron deficiency, although a small number of reports indicates otherwise. The molecular and cellular defects responsible for immune deficiency are complex, since almost every effector of the immune response is limited in number or action by experimental iron deficiency. Development of the immune system is retarded, sometimes irreversibly, by iron deficiency (287–289). In adult animals or humans with intact immune systems, nonspecific, cell-mediated, and humoral immunity are affected (to varying degrees) by iron deficiency.

Nonspecific immunity is affected by iron deficiency. Macrophage phagocytosis is generally unaffected by iron deficiency, although the bactericidal activity of macrophages is limited (290). Neutrophil function is also altered in iron deficiency, and may be due to reduced activity of the iron-containing enzyme, myeloperoxidase, which produces reactive oxygen intermediates responsible for intracellular killing of pathogens (291).

Delayed-type hypersensitivity, a measure of cell-mediated immune function, is depressed in iron-deficient children (290,291). Some studies have found decreases in both T-lymphocyte number and T-lymphocyte blastogenesis/mitogenesis in iron deficiency which are largely correctable with iron repletion (292,293). On the other hand, others have found a normal T-lymphocyte proliferative response to mitogens (294,295). In-vitro and in-vivo natural killer cell activity is also diminished in iron-deficient rats (296,297).

Humoral immunity appears to be less affected by iron deficiency than is cellular immunity. In iron-deficient animals there is often a profound decrease in B-lymphocyte blastogenesis as well as alterations in antibody production in response to antigen. However, antibody production in iron-deficient humans in response to immunization with most antigens is preserved (291,293,298).

Several possible mechanisms could explain the effects of iron deficiency on the immune system. DNA synthesis, initiated by the iron-containing enzyme ribonucleotide reductase, is a rate-limiting factor in cellular replication and may be limited by iron deficiency. In addition, Galen et al. have recently reported that in iron-deficient children there is a reduction in interleukin-2 (IL-2) production by activated lymphocytes (299). IL-2 is a key regulatory molecule in the immune system.

D. Impaired Mental Development and Function

Several recent reviews have covered the growing research area relating iron status to cognition and behavior (300–302). The studies reviewed in these articles demonstrate that iron-deficient children have alterations in attention span, lower intelligence scores, and some degree of perceptual disturbance. Interestingly, no such database exists in the literature on adult humans, though there is no clear reason to suggest that this relationship is developmentally linked except in certain studies where the nutritional insult could have interfered with the structural organization of the brain (303,304). The perception exists that the brain is resistant to changes in brain iron content and distribution within normal variations in iron status of individuals. There have been few systematic investigations, however, to test this assumption. Added stimulus for understanding iron entry into the brain is provided by current studies of the role of iron in neurologic pathology. Two reports (269,270) with adult subjects with serum ferritin concentration in the normal ranges suggested a greater amount of cortical asymmetry in electroencephalograph patterns as the plasma ferritin concentration was lowered. The biochemical alterations that occur in the brain with iron deficiency could in theory occur in adults in the same fashion as in children if the severity of the iron deficit is similar.

The mechanisms of causality of decreased cognition by iron deficiency remain unknown though much discussed. The key unresolved questions are: (a) how to differentiate the effects of acute iron deficiency from the effects of chronic iron deficiency; (b) what role the severity of iron deficiency has in these relationships; (c) whether there is a proven biologic and/or psychosocial causal model that will explain these relationships; (d) what are the appropriate theory-driven cognitive variables that test functionality in specific domains and contribute to models of causality.

Some of the background that led to those questions is now summarized. Oski et al. (305) observed increases in urinary norepinephrine in iron-deficient infants 9–26 months of age. These children also had significantly lower Bayley Mental Index (BMI) scores than controls. Both the BMI scores and urine catecholamine excretions were normalized within a short period of iron treatment. In a follow-up study, these psychomotor alterations were independent of anemia (305).

Subsequent studies observed a significant impact of iron-deficiency anemia on abnormal affective behavior in children. Several studies show poor affect in iron-deficient children related to poor performance on the BMI. The diminished interest of anemic children in this environment likely alters their performance on cognitive and psychomotor tasks (306). Costa Rican studies and those from Chile (307,308) both noted a failure to improve performance in many of the anemic children with active iron therapy despite prompt hematological response and normalization of iron status. In addition, children with storage-iron depletion, but no anemia, showed no measurable neurologic abnormalities.

Older children, average age 9.5 years, had a decreased efficiency in the Matching Familiar Figure Test that was significantly improved with 3 months of oral iron therapy (309). In a separate study, there was a significant improvement in Raven Progressive Matrices test performance with the only intervention being iron supplementation or anthelmintic drug treatment (310). An important point is that the cognitive domains tested by these achievement-oriented tests are far different from the developmental constructs applied to infants. That is, they test primary through tertiary memory as well as processing time and efficiency. These are not easily understood relative to the psychomotor tests used on infants. A possible explanation is that iron status affects a state variable such as attention or arousal, which in turn alters cognitive performance (311).

There is little doubt that iron deficiency has direct effects on central neurotransmitter metabolism in both animals (268,302) and humans (306,311). We recently reviewed the biological effects of iron deficiency on the brain; there is substantial support for concluding that the primary effect of iron-deficiency anemia in brain is on dopamine metabolism and related brain function (302).

The fundamental observations over a large number of studies (312) has been that caudate nucleus dopamine metabolism is perturbed in iron deficiency due to a downregulation in the number of D_2 receptors with subsequent changes in dopaminergic systems. There are no repeatable changes on dopamine receptor affinity, norepinephrine metabolism, or serotonin metabolism. However, alterations in the endogenous opiate system are indicated in iron deficiency. Administration of naloxone has significantly greater analgesic effects in anemic animals than in controls in their latency to respond to a noxious stimuli. This has been attributed to significant elevations in Met and Leu-enkephalin (313), which in turn are subject to dopaminergic influences. In addition, there was a significant effect of the diurnal cycle on this sensitivity. That is, iron-deficient animals exhibited a much greater sensitivity in the dark than during the light cycle and exhibited a reversal of the normal activity patterns. Iron repletion resulted in a normalization of these diurnal activity patterns within 2 weeks. This reversal in the normal activity pattern with the light–dark cycle is of great interest because it implies a perturbance of a central neural process. Not all investigators have been able to replicate this reversal of the diurnal cycle with iron deficiency (268,314).

The brain adapts to tissue iron deficiency by increasing TfR density, increasing uptake of iron across brain capillary endothelial cells, and altering ferritin concentration (302). The cellular distribution of iron in brain and the effects of iron nutriture are currently under investigation.

E. Impaired Physical Performance

Observations of lethargy, apathy, and listlessness are frequent symptoms of severe iron-deficiency anemia. These may well be associated with aforementioned alterations in cognition and behavior. However, it has been known for some time that iron deficiency is associated with decreased physical capacity (315–321). The mechanisms of this effect have been associated primarily with diminished oxygen transport, delivery of oxygen to exercising tissue, and oxidative capacity of muscle (322). Efficiency of oxygen extraction is improved but VO_2 max is decreased 30–50% in both animals and humans. Endurance is also decreased to the extent that earned income from physical labor (i.e., the harvesting of sugar cane) is significantly lower in iron-deficient people. The manifestations of depletion of essential body iron also have profound effects on skeletal muscle, with a significant decrease in mitochondrial iron–sulfur content (323), mitochondrial cytochrome content (316,319,324), and total mitochondrial oxidative capacity (317,319,324,325). The mitochondrial density and morphology changes as well. The activity of tricarboxylic acid cycle enzymes and oxidative capacity of mitochondria in other organs (263) is less strongly affected (319). These changes appear to be readily reversible with iron repletion. There is also a clear and apparently independent effect of tissue iron deficiency that leads to a pronounced lactic acidosis (325,327). Studies show that a complex set of changes in iron-containing enzymes in skeletal muscle are causally related to an increased rate of lactate production in muscle and utilization by liver in iron deficiency (319,328).

Increased insulin sensitivity in iron-deficient rats is a related observation (329,330). These studies using euglycemic clamps as well as radioisotope clearance methods demonstrate a clear preference for glucose oxidation to lactate in iron-deficient and anemic animals. Iron-deficient rats also have an increased glucose concentration and turnover (319,326) and an increased rate of glucose oxidation. These studies have not been replicated in humans to our knowledge, and the role of altering insulin sensitivity in humans in unclear.

A considerable number of lay publications argue that heavy exercise decreases iron status through a combination of decreased absorption and increased losses through feces, urine, and sweat. This analysis is more complicated than many appreciate, though it is likely that exercise does in some fashion change iron status.

F. Complications of Pregnancy

Maternal iron deficiency has been associated with retardation of fetal development in experimental animals. In humans, increased risk of premature delivery, low birth weight, and infant morbidity have been found in studies of iron-deficient mothers (331–333). The etiology of these complications is unknown, although it has been noted that the absorption of known fetotoxins such as cadmium (and probably lead) is increased in pregnant women (334).

VI. ASSESSMENT OF IRON STATUS

The nutritional iron status of humans can range from iron overload to iron-deficiency anemia. Historically, many different methods have been used for assessing the iron status of an individual, including dietary intake, hematocrit, hemoglobin, mean cellular hemoglobin, mean cell volume, erythrocyte mean index, free erythrocyte protoporphyrin, bone marrow iron stain, serum iron, total iron-binding capacity, serum transferrin, transferrin saturation, serum ferritin, and serum TfR. These methods vary considerably in their sensitivity and selectivity. The more commonly accepted diagnostic tests and their associated values are summarized in Table 8 (335,336).

TABLE 8 Diagnostic Criteria for Iron Deficiency

Parameters	Iron overload	Normal	Iron depletion	Iron-deficient erythropoiesis	Iron-deficiency anemia
Erythrocyte morphology	Normal	Normal	Normal	Normal	Microcytic/ hypochromic
Hemoglobin (g/dl)		>12.0	>12.0	>12.0	<12.0
Hematocrit (% PCV)		>36	>36	>36	<36
Plasma Iron (μg/dl)	>175	115 ± 50	115	<60	<40
RBC protoporphyrin (μg/dl)	30	30	30	100	200
RE marrow Fe	4+	2–3+	0–1+	0	0
Sideroblasts (%)	40–60	40–60	40–60	<10	<10
TIBC (μg/dl)	<300	330 ± 30	360	390	410
Tf saturation (%)	>60	35 ± 15	30	<15	<15
Plasma ferritin (μg/L)	>300	100 ± 60	20	10	<10
TfR relative amount		1	1.5	3	3–4
TfR (mg/L)		5.36 ± 0.82			13.9 ± 4.6

Adapted from Refs. 335 and 336.

A.   Hemoglobin/Hematocrit

Several reviews of iron metabolism in the last decade (263,337,338) have noted that the term *iron deficiency* means different things to different people. Since clinical sequelae are most frequently recognized only near the end stages of iron-depletion process, when body iron stores have been depleted, for clinicians the prevalence of iron deficiency is equated with the prevalence of iron-deficiency anemia. Perhaps the ease of assessment through the measurement of hemoglobin concentration is a factor (337), or perhaps the assumption that iron deficiency exerts its deleterious effects only if anemia is present (338), can explain the high use of this indicator. The use of hemoglobin and hematocrit as indices of iron status must be used carefully, as significant false positive indications occur (339). Although a single replicate has been determined to predict iron status accurately, significant variations due to age, sex, and race must be adjusted for in clinical assessment of iron status of individuals or populations. Hemoglobin concentrations are also altered in/by polycythemia, dehydration, cigarette smoking, chronic inflammation, chronic infection, hemorrhage, protein-energy malnutrition, vitamin B_{12} deficiency, folic acid deficiency, hemoglobinopathies, and pregnancy (340). Thus, considerable information about nutritional and health status is needed apart from hemoglobin determination if one is to use hemoglobin to assess iron status.

B.   Ferritin

A long-term negative iron balance leads eventually to the depletion of the storage iron pool, and plasma ferritin concentrations drop dramatically. To date, the most realistic tool in a nonclinical setting for assessment of the size of the storage pool is the measurement of serum or plasma ferritin concentrations. The concentration of serum ferritin reflects the size of the storage iron compartment if the subject is not also in an inflammatory state (341). In the range of 20 to 300 $\mu g/L$, each 1 $\mu g/L$ represents 10 mg of storage iron (154). Plasma ferritin concentration can increase dramatically with both acute and chronic inflammations, vitamin B_{12} deficiency, folic acid deficiency, liver disease, leukemia, Hodgkin's disease, alcohol intake, and hyperthyroidism (118,342–344). In addition, it is now known that there is a large within-subject day-to-day coefficient of variation (25–40%) in plasma ferritin concentrations (339).

C.   Transferrin Saturation

Once the storage iron pool is depleted due to a prolonged or acute negative iron balance, there is a decline in the transferrin saturation, and less than adequate iron is available for essential body iron proteins (345,346). Individuals in this stage of iron depletion have a transferrin saturation below 15–16% and an inadequate supply of iron for bone marrow to support normal erythropoiesis (346–348). The amount of erythropoiesis is clearly an important aspect in this iron delivery scheme, as decreased erythropoiesis can lower iron transport requirements by 50–80%.

D.   Transferrin Receptor

The measurement of the concentration of TfR in the plasma has diagnostic value for the assessment of iron-deficiency anemia and ineffective erythropoiesis (349–351). The amount of TfR in circulation has been shown to vary with the iron status of the subject. Plasma TfR concentrations increase even in mild iron deficiency of recent onset (352,353).

The plasma concentration of TfR is increased in β-thalassemia, autoimmune hemolytic anemia, sickle cell anemia, hereditary spherosis, hemoglobin H disease, polycythemia vera, secondary polycythemia, myelofibrosis, and chronic lymphocytic leukemia (349–351). The plasma TfR concentration is decreased in hemochromatosis, aplastic anemia-bone marrow ablation, posttransplantation anemia, and chronic renal failure (336,349–351). Unlike ferritin, levels of plasma TfR are not significantly affected by inflammation (353,354) or liver disease (336). Hence, the TfR is particularly useful in assessing iron status, because unlike most other methods of assessment, TfR concentration can be used to distinguish between ID anemia and other anemias, including the anemia of chronic disease (336).

VII. POPULATIONS AT RISK FOR IRON DEFICIENCY

Despite the effectiveness of interventional therapies, iron deficiency is the primary nutritional deficiency in the United States (355,356). Approximately 6–11% of reproductive-age females, 14% of 15- to 19-year-old females, and approximately 25% of pregnant women were iron deficient in the United States and Canada in the 1980s (356,357). Fortification of the food supply in combination with additional intakes of iron from supplements, and some changes in dietary patterns, has effectively eradicated iron deficiency from nearly all segments of the U.S. population except for pregnant women and a small proportion of young children, adolescents, and reproductive-age women. On a worldwide basis, the numbers are even more demonstrable of the immensity of the problem (358,359), with 15% of the world's population having iron-deficiency anemia. The WHO estimates that 1.3 billion people are anemic, with nearly half of them (500 to 600 million) having iron deficiency as the causal agent.

As noted in the various sections of this chapter, iron requirements are determined by growth and maintenance requirements. The range of requirements for humans is summarized in Table 9 (360). There are additional requirements associated with clinical and pathologic conditions leading to increased blood loss. Iron requirements in infancy, childhood, adolescence, and during pregnancy are covered in detail elsewhere (361–364). Menstrual blood losses during the reproductive years elevate iron requirements in females on average 5 mg/day above that of males. The requirements for adult male and postmenopausal women is 10 mg/day. A number of clinical and pathologic conditions that have blood loss associated with them can cause iron deficiency. In addition, treatments that actively increase iron requirements, such as erythropoietin therapy, can lead to iron deficiency (365,366).

VIII. TOXICOLOGY OF IRON EXCESS

Iron can be extremely toxic if acutely ingested in large amounts. Iron toxicity can also arise because of the chronic absorption or accumulation of iron in amounts that exceed normal iron transport and storage mechanisms. This situation occurs during primary hemochromatosis, a relatively common genetic disorder. Other genetic disorders associated with an increased iron burden include neonatal hemochromatosis, congenital atransferrinemia, β-thalassemia major, and Y-linked hypochromic anemia (50). Iron toxicity is also manifested during secondary hemochromatosis, which can arise from increased parenteral or enteral intake of iron or as a result of certain disease processes.

TABLE 9 NAS-NRC RDAs, Revised 1989, RDIs Revised 1987 (360)

Category	Age (years) or condition	Weight (kg)	(lb)	Height (cm)	(in)	Iron RDA (mg)	Iron RDI (mg)
Infants	0.0–0.25	6	13	60	24	6	—
	0.25–0.5	—	—	—	—	6	6.6
	0.5–1.0	9	20	71	28	10	8.8
Children	1–3	13	29	90	35	10	10
	4–6	20	44	112	44	10	10
	7–10	28	62	132	52	10	10[a]
Males	11–14	45	99	157	62	12	12
	15–18	66	145	176	69	12	12[b]
	19–24	72	160	177	70	10	10
	25–50	79	174	176	70	10	10
	51+	77	170	173	68	10	10
Females	11–14	46	101	157	62	15	15
	15–18	55	120	163	64	15	15
	19–24	58	128	164	65	15	15
	25–50	63	138	163	64	15	15
	51+	65	143	160	63	10	10
Pregnant						30	45
Lactating	1st 6 months					15	15
	2nd 6 months					15	15

[a]To 9 years of age.
[b]To 17 years of age.

A. Acute

Acute ingestion of iron in the amounts of 200–250 mg/kg are usually fatal. Unintentional ingestion of iron-containing supplements are the single largest cause of pediatric poisoning fatalities in the United States (367). The symptomatology (368,369) of iron poisoning is well known. The treatment of acute iron poisoning is primarily emesis, fluid and electrolyte replacement, and, in certain patients, systemic administration of chelating agents such as desferrioxamine.

B. Genetic

Primary hemochromatosis is an autosomal recessive trait characterized by increased dysregulated heme (370) and nonheme (371) iron absorption, leading to iron overload. Kinetic studies suggest that the defect lies in the transfer of iron to the plasma pool (372). The total excess iron burden due to this increased absorption is typically 20–40 g, compared to 3–5 g for a normal individual. The molecular defect leading to dysregulated iron absorption has not been characterized, but it has been localized to chromosome 6 around the region for the human leukocyte antigen (HLA) haplotype (373–375). Most of the obvious candidate genes have been ruled out, as they do not lie on this chromosome: transferrin (chromosome 3), TfR [chromosome 3 (182)], ferritin [chromosomes 11 (144) and 19 (145)], and the iron-response element-binding protein [chromosome 9 (232)]. Nevertheless, several interesting relationships exist between some of these gene products and hemochromatosis. The levels for the TfR mRNA in the mucosal cells from hemochromatosis patients are lower compared to iron-loaded controls (82). Additionally, mucosal cell ferritin mRNA and ferritin protein levels in patients with hemochromatosis are lower than one would expect when compared to secondary iron overload (80,82).

The gene prevalence is still speculative and the subject of much public clamor over excessive iron in the diet. The HLA-A3 alloantigen is present in 70% of patients with hemochromatosis. A positive test for the HLA-3 antigen does not always indicate hemochromatosis and must be followed by a liver biopsy in order to confirm the presence of the disease. The incidence of the disease in Caucasians of northern European ancestry, as calculated by HLA typing, ranges from 0.3% to 1.0%. In the largest study to date, the incidence among blood donors in Utah was 0.45% (376). Other methods of screening, including postmortem examination or liver biopsy, predict an incidence of 0.5–3.7%. Genetic homozygosity is required for expression of the disease, but not all genotypic homozygotes develop the full phenotypic profile. Heterozygous females, although displaying alterations in markers of iron status, develop the disease one-fifth to one-tenth as frequently as heterozygous males. Furthermore, the age of onset is delayed in females. These disparities are presumably due to menstrual iron losses. A recent population survey did not find an increase in the incidence of hemochromatosis due to food fortification with iron (377).

The pathophysiology of the disease and the rate of iron accumulation in heterozygotes is unclear due to insensitive early diagnostic measures. The pathophysiology is associated with parenchymal deposition of iron (378) which occurs in muscle, liver, pancreatic, and adrenal tissue. The sequelae of this deposition is a broad range of conditions which include congestive heart failure, diabetes mellitus, hypogonadism, idiopathic cardiomyopathy, hyperpigmentation, and primary liver cancer. Many of these conditions can be slowed or reversed by frequent phlebotomy and chelation therapy. This disease is not to be confused with secondary hemosiderosis or hemochromatosis that arises from increased parenteral intake of iron (379).

C. Iron and Free-Radical Pathology

Recent debate has focused on the chronic toxicity of iron particularly in regard to its relationship with cancer (380–382), atherosclerosis (383–385), and neurodegenerative disorders (386). Frequently the implied or stated causality is that a certain intake of iron, or elevated indices of iron status, lead to the aforementioned conditions. These hypotheses rely mostly on iron's ability to generate reactive oxygen species and/or to stimulate lipid peroxidation, modify proteins, or cause damage to nucleic acids. These reactions have been collectively categorized as "oxidant stress," and a recent census lists over 60 human diseases in which they are thought to play a role (387). In vitro experiments are the frequent paradigms, but these can provide only circumstantial evidence for iron's toxicity, for although it is true that free iron can catalyze a number of biologically undesirable reactions in vitro, under normal circumstances iron is always chelated to low-molecular-weight compounds or associated with macromolecules such as proteins, lipids, carbohydrates, and nucleic acids. The situation can change under pathologic or extreme conditions in vivo, when the capacity of the liver to produce transferrin is sufficiently impaired or the release of iron into the plasma pool is so high that iron-binding capacity is overwhelmed and free iron can be detected with a bleomycin assay.

IX. CONCLUSIONS AND FUTURE RESEARCH PERSPECTIVES

This chapter is not a comprehensive examination of all aspects of iron nutrition in health and disease. Rather, our intent is to review the current knowledge in key aspects of the field of iron nutrition and biology and, we hope, stimulate new intellectual efforts by scholars to understand better the role of iron in human biology. Scientific investigations spanning several decades have increased our understanding of the role of this mineral in many aspects of metabolism, but it is clear that many questions remain. For example, what are all of the components of the iron absorption pathway? What is the somatic regulator of iron absorption? What is the nature of the low-molecular-weight intra- and extracellular pools of iron? What are the full consequences of iron deficiency, particularly as it relates to cognitive function, and are they reversible? How does hemochromatosis arise? Finally, what role does iron, as found in the body under normal nutritional states, play in oxidative stress? We hope that scientists in the next decade will unravel some of these mysteries.

ACKNOWLEDGMENTS

The authors would like to thank Mr. Dale Brigham, Dr. Roland Leach, and Dr. Elizabeth Theil for their helpful commentaries regarding this manuscript.

REFERENCES

1. De Duve C. Prelude to a cell. The Sciences 1990; 30: 22–28.
2. Eaton SB, Konner M. Paleolithic nutrition. A consideration of its nature and current implications. N Engl J Med 1985; 312: 283–289.
3. Vannotti A, Delachaux A. Iron metabolism and its clinical significance. New York: Grune & Stratton, 1949.
4. Hughes ER. Human iron metabolism. In: Sigel H, ed. Metal Ions in Biological Systems. Iron in Model and Natural Compounds. New York: Marcel Dekker, 1977.
5. MacKay C. Memoirs of Extraordinary Popular Delusions. London: Richard Bently, 1841.
6. Marks G, Beatty WK. The Precious Metals of Medicine. New York: Charles Scribner, 1975.
7. Cule J. The iron mixture of Dr. Griffith. Pharm J 1967; CXCVIII: 399–400.
8. Fairbanks VF, Fahey JL, Bentler E. Clinical Disorders of Iron Metabolism. New York: Grune & Stratton, 1971.
9. McCollum EV. A History of Nutrition. Boston: Houghton Mifflin, 1957.
10. McCay CM. Notes on the History of Nutrition Research. Bern: Huber, 1973.
11. Blood–inorganic substances. In: Lentner C, ed. Geigy Scientific Tables. Physical Chemistry, Composition of Blood, Hematology, Somatometric Data. 8th ed. West Cadwell: Medical Education Division, Ciba-Geigy Corporation, 1984.
12. Boussingault JB. Du fer contenu dans le sang et dans les aliments. CR Acad Sci Paris 1872; 74: 1353–1359.
13. Schmidt JE, ed. Medical Discoveries. Springfield, IL: Charles C Thomas, 1959.
14. McCance RA, Widdowson EM. Absorption and excretion of iron. Lancet 1937; 2: 680–684.
15. Moore CV, Arrowsmith WR, Welch J, Minnich V. Studies in iron transportation and metabolism. IV. Observations on the absorption of iron from the gastrointestinal tract. J Clin Invest 1939; 18: 553–580.
16. Granick S. Protein apoferritin in iron feeding and absorption. Science 1946; 103: 107–113.
17. Iron in Human Nutrition. National Live Stock and Meat Board. 1990.

18. McCance RA, Widdowson EM. Mineral metabolism of healthy adults on white and brown bread dietaries. J Physiol 1942; 101: 44–85.
19. McCance RA, Edgecomb CN, Widdowson EM. Phytic acid and iron absorption. Lancet 1943; 2: 126–128.
20. Van Campen D, Gross C. Effect of histidine and certain other amino acids on the absorption of iron-59 by rats. J Nutr 1969; 99: 68–74.
21. Disler PB, Lynch SR, Charlton RW, Torrance JD, Bothwell TH. The effect of tea on iron absorption. Gut 1975; 16: 193–200.
22. Monsen ER, Cook JD. Food iron absorption in human subjects. IV. The effects of calcium and phosphate salts on the absorption of nonheme iron. Am J Clin Nutr 1976; 29: 1142–1148.
23. Breddy M, Chidambaram MV, Fonseca J, Bates GW. Potential role of in vitro iron bioavailability studies in combatting iron deficiency: a study of the effects of phosvitin on iron mobilization from pinto beans. USAid Cooperative Agreement 1976; 1: 1–45.
24. Layrisse M, Martinez-Torres C, Leets I, Taylor P, Ramirez J. Effect of histidine, cysteine, glutathione or beef on iron absorption in humans. Br J Nutr 1984; 52: 37–46.
25. Wretland A. In: Hallberg L, ed. Iron Deficiency. London: Academic Press, 1970.
26. Takkunen H, Seppänen R. Iron deficiency and dietary factors in Finland. Am J Clin Nutr 1975; 28: 1141–1147.
27. Bjorn-Rasmussen E, Hallberg L, Isaksson B, Arvidsson B. Food iron absorption in man. Application of the two-pool extrinsic tag method to measure heme and non-heme iron absorption. J Clin Invest 1974; 53: 247–256.
28. Cook JD, Reusser ME. Iron fortification: an update. J Food Sci 1983; 48: 1340–1349.
29. Reddy MB, Cook JD. Assessment of dietary determinants of nonheme-iron absorption in humans and rats. Am J Clin Nutr 1991; 54: 723–728.
30. Forbes RM, Erdman JW. The bioavailability of trace mineral elements. Annu Rev Nutr 1983; 3: 213–231.
31. Cook JD, Dassenko SA, Lynch SR. Assessment of the role of non-heme-iron availability in iron balance. Am J Clin Nutr 1991; 54: 717–722.
32. Cook JD, Watson SS, Simpson KM, Lipschitz DA, Skikne BS. The effect of high ascorbic acid supplementation on body iron stores. Blood 1984; 64: 721–726.
33. Beard J. Iron fortification—rationale and effects. Nutr Today 1986; 17–20.
34. Crosby WH. Yin, yang and iron. Nutr Today 1986; 14–16.
35. Sullivan JL. Stored iron and ischemic heart disease—empirical support for a new paradigm. Circulation 1992; 86: 1036–1037.
36. Lauffer R. Preventive measures for the maintenance of low but adequate iron stores. In: Lauffer R, ed. Iron and Human Disease. Boca Raton, FL: CRC Press, 1992.
37. Natow AB, Heslin J-A. The Iron Counter. New York: Pocket Books, 1993.
38. Walter T, Hertrampf E, Pizarro F, et al. Effect of bovine-hemoglobin fortified cookies on iron status of schoolchildren—a nationwide program in Chile. Am J Clin Nutr 1993; 57: 190–194.
39. Chierici R, Sawatzki G, Tamisari L, Volpato S, Vigi V. Supplementation of an adapted formula with bovine lactoferrin. 2. Effects on serum iron, ferritin and zinc levels. Acta Paediatr 1992; 81: 475–479.
40. Finch CA, Huebers HA. Iron absorption. Am J Clin Nutr 1988; 47: 102–107.
41. Carpenter CE, Mahoney AW. Contributions of heme and nonheme iron to human nutrition. Crit Rev Food Sci Nutr 1992; 31: 333–367.
42. Wollenberg P, Rummel W. Dependence of intestinal iron absorption on the valency state of iron. Naunyn Schmiedebergs Arch Pharmacol 1987; 336: 578–582.
43. Raja KB, Simpson RJ, Peters TJ. Comparison of $^{59}Fe^{3+}$ uptake in vitro and in vivo by mouse duodenum. Biochim Biophys Acta 1987; 901: 52–60.
44. Kelly KA, Turnbull EE, Cammock CT, Bombeck LM, Nyhus LM, Finch CA. Iron absorption after gastrectomy: an experimental study in the dog. Surgery, 1967; 62: 356–360.

45. Conrad ME. Iron absorption. In: Johnson LR, ed. Physiology of the Gastrointestinal Tract. 2d ed. New York: Raven Press, 1987.

46. Murry MJ, Stein N. Does the pancreas influence iron absorption? Gastroenterology 1966; 51: 694–700.

47. Zempsky WT, Rosenstein BJ, Carroll JA, Oski FA. Effect of pancreatic enzyme supplements on iron absorption. 1990; 67–93.

48. Hastings-Wilson T. Intestinal Absorption. Philadelphia: Saunders, 1962.

49. Schümann K, Elsenhans B, Ehtechami C, Forth W. Rat intestinal iron transfer capacity and the longitudinal distribution of its adaptation to iron deficiency. Digestion 1990; 46: 35–45.

50. Conrad ME. Regulation of iron absorption. In: Prasad AS, ed. Essential and Toxic Trace Elements in Human Disease: An Update. 2d ed. New York: Wiley-Liss, 1993.

51. Layrisse M, Martinez-Torres C. Model for measuring dietary absorption of heme iron: test with a complete meal. Am J Clin Nutr 1972; 25: 401–411.

52. Lynch SR, Dassenko SA, Morck RA, Beard JL, Cook JD. Soy protein products and heme iron absorption in humans. Am J Clin Nutr 1985; 41: 13–20.

53. Hallberg L, Rossanderhulthen L, Brune M, Gleerup A. Inhibition of haem-iron absorption in man by calcium. Br J Nutr 1993; 69: 533–540.

54. Sayers MH, Lynch SR, Jacobs P, et al. The effects of ascorbic acid supplementation on the absorption of iron in maize, wheat and soy. Br J Haematol 1973; 24: 209–218.

55. Cook JD, Monsen ER. Food iron absorption in human subjects. III. Comparison of the effect of animal proteins on non heme iron absorption. Am J Clin Nutr 1976; 29: 859–867.

56. Taylor PG, Martinez-Torres C, Romano EL, Latrisse M. The effect of cysteine-containing peptides released during meat digestion on iron absorption in human. Am J Clin Nutr 1986; 43: 68–71.

57. Simpson KM, Morris ER, Cook JD. The inhibitory effect of bran on iron absorption in humans. Am J Clin Nutr 1981; 34: 1469–1478.

58. Baig MM, Burgin CW, Cerda JJ. Effect of dietary pectin on iron absorption and turnover in the rat. J Nutr 1983; 113: 2615–2622.

59. Thompson DB, Erdman JEW. The effect of soy protein isolate in the diet on retention by the rat of iron from radio-labeled test meals. Am J Physiol 1984.

60. Cook JD, Morck TA, Lynch SR. The inhibitory effect of soy products on nonheme iron absorption in man. Am J Clin Nutr 1981; 34: 2630–2634.

61. Crichton R. Ferritin—the structure and function of an iron storage protein. In: Dunford HB, Dolphin D, Raymond KN, Sieker L, eds. The Biological Chemistry of Iron. Dordrecht, Holland: Reidel, 1982.

62. Schäfer SG, Förth W. The influence of tin, nickel, and cadmium on the intestinal absorption of iron. Ecotoxicol Environ Safety 1982; 7: 87–95.

63. Lönnerdal B, Keen CL, Hurley LS. Manganese binding proteins in human and cow's milk. Am J Clin Nutr 1985; 41: 550–559.

64. Solomons NW, Jacob RA. Studies on the bioavailability of zinc in humans IV: effects of heme and nonheme iron on the absorption of zinc. Am J Clin Nutr 1981; 34: 475–482.

65. Craig WJ, Balbach L, Harris S, Vyhmeister N. Plasma zinc and copper levels of infants fed different formulas. J Am Coll Nutr 1984; 3: 183–186.

66. Yip R, Reeves JD, Lönnerdal B, Keen CL, Dallman PR. Does iron supplementation compromise zinc nutrition in healthy infants. J Nutr 1983; 113: 2159–2170.

67. Haschke F, Zeigler EE, Edwards BB, Fomon SJ. Effect of iron fortification of infant formula on trace mineral absorption. J Ped Gastroenterol Nutr 1986; 5: 768–773.

68. Hambidge KM, Krebs NF, Sibley L, English J. Acute effects of iron therapy on zinc status during pregnancy. Obstet Gynecol 1987; 70: 593–596.

69. David CD, Malecki EA, Greger JL. Interactions among dietary manganese, heme iron, and nonheme iron in women. Am J Clin Nutr 1992; 56: 926–932.

70. Sokoll LJ, Dawson-Hughes B. Calcium supplementation and plasma ferritin concentrations in premenopausal women. Am J Clin Nutr 1992; 56: 1045–1048.

71. Hallberg L, Rossander-Hulten L, Brune M, Gleerup A. Calcium and iron absorption: mechanism of action and nutritional importance. Eur J Clin Nutr 1992; 46: 317–327.

72. Stremmel W, Lotz G, Niederau C, Teschke R, Strohmeyer G. Iron uptake by rat duodenal microvillous membrane vesicles: evidence for a carrier mediated transport system. Eur J Clin Invest 1987; 17: 136–145.

73. Conrad M, Burton B, Williams H, Foy A. Human absorption of hemoglobin-iron. Gastroenterology 1967; 53: 5–10.

74. Grasbeck R, Majuri I, Kouvonen I, Tenhun R. Spectral and other studies on the intestinal haem receptor of the pig. Biochim Biophys Acta 1982; 700: 137–147.

75. Weintraub LR, Conrad ME, Crosby WH. Absorption of hemoglobin iron by the rat. Proc Soc Exp Biol Med 1965; 120: 840–843.

76. Raffin SB, Woo CH, Roost KT, Price DC, Schmid R. Intestinal absorption of hemoglobin heme iron cleavage by mucosal heme oxygenase. J Clin Invest 1974; 54: 1344.

77. Rosenberg DW, Kappas A. Arch Biochim Biophys 1989; 274: 471–480.

78. Huebers HA, Huebers E, Csiba E, Rummel W, Finch CA. The significance of transferrin for intestinal iron absorption. Blood 1983; 61: 283–290.

79. Isobe K, Sakurami T, Ysobe Y. Studies on iron transport in human intestine by immunoperoxidase technique. I. The localization of ferritin, lactoferritin and transferrin in human duodenal mucosa. Acta Haematol Jpn 1978; 41: 294–299.

80. Fracanzani AL, Fargion S, Romano R, et al. Immunohistochemical evidence for a lack of ferritin in duodenal absorptive epithelial cells in idiopathic hemochromatosis. Gastroenterology 1989; 96: 1071–1078.

81. Idzerda KL, Huebers H, Finch CA, McKnight GS. Rat transferrin gene expression: tissue-specificity regulation by iron deficiency. Proc Natl Acad Sci (USA) 1986; 83: 3723–3727.

82. Pietrangelo A, Rocchi E, Casalgrandi G, et al. Regulation of transferrin, transferrin receptor, and ferritin genes in human duodenum. Gastroenterology 1992; 102: 802–809.

83. Diponkar B, Flanagan P, Cluett J, Valberg L. Transferrin receptors in the human gastrointestinal tract. Gastroenterology 1986; 91: 861–869.

84. Levine JS, Seligman PA. The ultrastructural immunocytochemical localization of transferrin receptor (TFR) and transferrin (TF) in the gastrointestinal tract (abstr). Gastroenterology 1984; 86: 1161.

85. Parmley RT, Barton JC, Conrad ME. Ultrastructural localization of transferrin, transferrin receptor, and iron-binding sites on human placental and duodenal microvilli. Br J Haematol 1985; 60: 81–89.

86. Bezwoda WR, MacPhail AP, Bothwell TH, Baynes RD, Derman DP, Torrance JD. Failure of transferrin to enhance iron absorption in achlorohydric human subjects. Br J Haematol 1986; 63: 749–758.

87. Buys SS, Martin CB, Eldridge M, Kushner JP, Kaplan J. Iron absorption in hypotransferrinemic mice. Blood 1991; 78: 3288–3290.

88. Conrad ME, Umbreit JN, Moore EG. A role for mucin in the absorption of inorganic iron and other metal cations. A study in rats. Gastroenterology 1991; 100: 129–136.

89. Raja KB, Simpson RJ, Pippard MJ, Peters TJ. In vivo studies on the relationship between intestinal iron (Fe^{3+}) absorption, hypoxia, and erythropoiesis in the mouse. Br J Haematol 1988; 68: 373–384.

90. Teichmann R, Stremmel W. Iron uptake by human upper small intestine microvillous membrane vesicles: indication for a facilitated transport mechanism mediated by a membrane iron-binding protein. J Clin Invest 1990; 86: 2145.

91. Nichols GM, Pearce AR, Alverez X, et al. The mechanisms of nonheme iron uptake determined in IEC-6 rat intestinal cells. J Nutr 1992; 122: 945–952.

92. Conrad ME, Umbreit JN, Peterson RDA, Moore EG, Harper KP. Function of integrin in duodenal mucosal uptake of iron. Blood 1993; 81: 517–521.

93. Pollack S, Lasky FD. A new iron-binding protein isolated from intestinal mucosa. J Lab Clin Med 1976; 87: 670–679.

94. Conrad ME, Umbreit JN, Moore EG. Rat duodenal iron-binding protein mobilferrin is a homologue of calreticulin. Gastroenterology 1993; 104: 1700–1704.

95. Hahn PF, Bale WF, Ross JF, Balfour WM, Whipple GH. Radioactive iron absorption by gastrointestinal tract: influence of anemia, anoxia and antecedent feeding distribution in growing dogs. J Exp Med 1943; 78: 169–188.

96. Granick S. Ferritin. IX. Increase of the protein apoferritin in the gastrointestinal mucosa as a direct response to iron feeding. The function of ferritin in the regulation of iron absorption. J Biol Chem 1946; 164: 737–746.

97. Whittaker P, Skikne BS, Covell AM, Flowers C, Cooke A, Lynch SL. Duodenal iron proteins in idiopathic hemochromatosis. J Clin Invest 1989; 83: 261–267.

98. Osaki S, Johnson DA, Freiden E. The possible significance of the ferrous oxidase activity of ceruloplasmin in normal human serum. J Biol Chem 1966; 241: 2746.

99. Wollenberg P, Malberg R, Rummel W. The valency state of absorbed iron appearing in the portal blood and ceruloplasmin substitution. Biometals 1990; 336: 1.

100. O'Dell BL. Copper. In: Brown ML, ed. Present Knowledge in Nutrition. 6th ed. Washington DC: International Life Sciences Institute Nutrition Foundation, 1990.

101. Bothwell TH, Pirzio-Biroli G, Finch CA. Iron absorption. I. Factors influencing absorption. J Lab Clin Med 1958; 51: 24–36.

102. Scade SG, Bernier GM, Conrad ME. Normal iron absorption in hypertransferremic mice. Br J Haematol 1969; 17: 187–190.

103. Cook JD, Dassenko S, Skikne BS. Serum transferrin receptor as an index of iron absorption. Br J Haematology 1990; 75: 603–609.

104. Banerjee D, Flanagan PR, Cluett J, Valberg LS. Transferrin receptors in the human gastrointestinal tract. Relationship to body iron stores. Gastroenterology 1986; 91: 861–869.

105. Lombard M, Bomford AB, Polson RJ, Bellingham AJ, Williams R. Differential expression of transferrin receptor in duodenal mucosa in iron overload. Evidence for a site-specific defect in genetic hemochromatosis. Gastroenterology 1990; 98: 976–984.

106. Anderson GJ, Powell LW, Halliday JW. Transferrin receptor distribution and regulation in the small intestine. Effect of iron stores and erythropoiesis. Gastroenterology 1990; 98: 576–584.

107. Buys SS, Martin CB, Eldridge M, Kushner JP, Kaplan J. Iron absorption in hypotransferrinemic mice. Blood 1991; 78: 3288–3290.

108. Erlandson ME, Walden B, Stern G, Hilgartner MW, Wehman J, Smith CH. Studies on congenital hemolytic syndromes. IV. Gastrointestinal absorption of iron. Blood 1962; 19: 359.

109. Adams PC, Chau LA, Lin E, Muirhead N. The effect of human recombinant erythropoietin on iron absorption and hepatic iron in a rat model. Clin Invest Med 1991; 14: 432–436.

110. Finch CA, Heuber H, Eng M, Miller L. Effect of transfused reticulocytes on iron exchange. Blood 1982; 59: 364–369.

111. Vassar PS, Taylor DM. Effect of hypoxia on iron absorption in rats. Proc Soc Exp Biol Med 1956; 93: 504–506.

112. Mendel GA. Studies on iron absorption. I. The relationship between the rate of erythropoiesis, hypoxia and iron absorption. Blood 1961; 18: 727.

113. Weintraub LR, Conrad ME, Crosby WH. The significance of iron turnover in the control of iron absorption. Blood 1964; 24: 19–24.

114. Hershko C. Storage iron kinetics. VI. The effects of inflammation on iron exchange in the rat. Br J Haematol 1977; 26: 67–75.

115. Aschner M, Aschner JL. Manganese transport across the blood brain barrier: relationship to iron homeostasis. Brain Res Bull 1990; 24: 857–860.

116. Princiotto JV, Zapolski FJ. Functional heterogeneity and pH dependent dissociation properties of human transferrin. Biochem Biophys Acta 1976; 428: 766–771.

117. van Der Heul C, Roos MJK, van Noort WL, van Eijk HG. No functional difference of the two iron-binding sites of human transferrin in vitro. Br J Haematol 1980; 46: 417–426.

118. Bothwell TH, Charlton RW, Cook JD, Finch CA. Iron metabolism in man. Oxford: Blackwell, 1979.

119. Stallard BJ, Collard MW, Griswold MD. A transferrin (hemiferrin) mRNA is expressed in the germ cells of rat testis. Mol Cell Biol 1991; 11: 1448–1453.

120. Adrian GS, Korinek BW, Bowman BH, Yang F. The human transferrin gene: 5' region contains conserved sequences which match the control elements regulated by heavy metals, glucocorticoids and acute phase reaction. Gene 1986; 49: 167–175.

121. Davis RJ, Czech MP. Regulation of transferrin receptor expression at the cell surface by insulin-like growth factors, epidermal growth factor and platelet-derived growth factor. EMBO J 1986; 5: 653–658.

122. Hsu SL, Lin YF, Chou CK. Transcriptional regulation of transferrin and albumin genes by retinoic acid in human hepatoma cell line Hep3B. Biochem J 1992; 283: 611–615.

123. McKnight GS, Lee DC, Hemmaplardh D, Finch CA, Palmiter RD. Transferrin gene expression. Effects of nutritional iron deficiency. J Biol Chem 1980; 255: 144–147.

124. Cox LA, Adrian GS. Posttranscriptional regulation of chimeric human transferrin genes by iron. Biochemistry 1993; 32: 4738–4745.

125. Muller-Eberhard U, Nikkilä H. Transport of tetrapyrroles by proteins. Semin Hematol 1989; 26: 86–104.

126. Morris CM, Candy JM, Edwardson JA, Bloxham CA, Smith A. Evidence for the localization of haemopexin immunoreactivity in neurones in the human brain. Neurosci Lett 1993; 149: 141–144.

127. Smith A, Morgan WT. Hemopexin-mediated heme transport to the liver. Evidence for a heme-binding protein in liver plasma membranes. J Biol Chem 1985; 260: 8325–8329.

128. Smith A, Hunt RC. Hemopexin joins transferrin as representative members of a distinct class of receptor-mediated endocytotic transport systems. Eur J Cell Biol 1990; 53: 234–245.

129. Potter D. In vivo fate of hemopexin and heme-hemopexin complexes in the rat. Arch Biochem Biophys 1993; 300: 98–104.

130. Metz-Boutique M-H, Jollés J, Marzurier J, et al. Human lactoferrin: amino acid sequence and structural comparison with other transferrins. Eur J Biochem 1984; 145: 659–676.

131. Ziere GJ, Van Dijk MC, Bijsterbosch MK, Van Berkel TJ. Lactoferrin uptake by the rat liver. Characterization of the recognition site and effect of selective modification of arginine residues. J Biol Chem 1992; 267: 11229–11235.

132. Baynes R, Bezwoda W, Bothwell T, Khan Q, Mansoor N. The non-immune inflammatory response: serial changes in plasma iron, TIBC, lactoferrin, ferritin, and C-reactive protein. Scand J Clin Lab Invest 1986; 46: 695–704.

133. Mack U, Powell LW, Halliday JW. Detection and isolation of a hepatic membrane receptor for ferritin. J Biol Chem 1983; 258: 4672–4675.

134. Adams PC, Mack U, Powell LW, Halliday JW. Isolation of a porcine hepatic ferritin receptor. Comp Biochem Physiol 1988; 90: 837–841.

135. Adams PC, Powell LW, Halliday JW. Isolation of a human hepatic ferritin receptor. Hepatology 1988; 8: 719–721.

136. Moss D, Fargion S, Fracanzani AL, Levi S, Cappellini MD, Arosio P, Powell LW, Halliday JW. Functional roles of the ferritin receptors of human liver, hepatoma, lymphoid and erythroid cells. J Inorg Biochem 1992; 47: 219–227.

137. Aruoma OI, Bomford A, Polson RJ, Halliwell B. Nontransferrin-bound iron in plasma from hemochromatosis patients: effect of phlebotomy therapy. Blood 1988; 72: 1416–1421.

138. Simpson RJ, Cooper CE, Raja KB, et al. Nontransferrin-bound iron species in the serum of hypotransferrinaemic mice. Biochim Biophys Acta 1992; 1156: 19–26.

139. Page MA, Baker E, Morgan EH. Transferrin and iron uptake by rat hepatocytes in culture. Am J Physiol 1984; 246: G28–G33.
140. Brock JH. The effect of iron and transferrin on the response of serum-free culture of mouse lymphocytes to Concanavalin A and lipopolysaccharides. Immunology 1981; 43: 387–392.
141. Hunt SM, Groff JL. Advanced Nutrition and Human Metabolism. St. Paul, MN: West, 1990.
142. Selden C, Owen JMP, Hopkins JMP, Peters TJ. Studies on the concentration and intracellular localization of iron proteins in liver biopsy specimens from patients with iron overload with special reference to their role in lysosomal disruption. Br J Haematol 1980; 44: 593.
143. Thiel EC. Ferritin: structure, gene regulation, and cellular function in animals, plants and microorganisms. Annu Rev Biochem 1987; 56: 289–315.
144. Cragg SJ, Drysdale J, Worwood M. Genes for the "H" subunit of human ferritin are present on a number of human chromosomes. Hum Genet 1985; 71: 108–112.
145. Lebo RV, Kan YW, Cheung MC, Jain SK, Drysdale J. Human ferritin light chain gene sequences mapped to several assorted chromosomes. Hum Genet 1985; 71: 325–328.
146. McGill JR, Naylor SL, Sakaguchi AY, et al. Human ferritin H and L sequences lie on ten different chromosomes. Hum Genet 1987; 76: 66–70.
147. Zahringer J, Baliga BS, Munro HN. Novel mechanism for translational control in regulation of ferritin synthesis by iron. Proc Natl Acad Sci (USA) 1976; 73: 857–861.
148. Aziz N, Munro HN. Both subunits of rat liver ferritin are regulated at translational level by iron induction. Nucleic Acids Res 1986; 14: 915–927.
149. White K, Munro HN. Induction of ferritin subunit synthesis by iron is regulated at both the transcriptional and translational level. J Biol Chem 1988; 263: 8938–8942.
150. Cairo G, Bardella L, Schiaffonati L, Arosio P, Levi S, Berneli-Zazzera A. Multiple mechanisms of iron-induced ferritin synthesis of HeLa cells. Biochem Biophys Res Commun 1985; 133: 314–321.
151. Coulson RMR, Cleveland DW. Ferritin synthesis is controlled by iron-dependent translational derepression and by changes in synthesis/transport of nuclear ferritin RNAs. Proc Natl Acad Sci (USA) 1993; 90: 7613–7617.
152. Thiel EC. Ferritin mRNA translation, structure, and gene transcription during development of animals and plants. Enzyme 1990; 44: 68–82.
153. Fishbach FA, Andreregg JW. An X-ray scattering study of ferritin and apoferritin. J Mol Biol 1965; 14: 458–473.
154. Cook JD, Skikne BS. Serum ferritin: a possible model for the assessment of nutrient stores. Am J Clin Nutr 1982; 35: 1180–1185.
155. Crichton R, Ward RJ. Iron metabolism—new perspectives in view. Biochemistry 1992; 31: 11255–11264.
156. Levi S, Luzzago A, Cesareni G, et al. Mechanism of ferritin iron uptake: activity of the H-chain and deletion mapping of the ferro-oxidase site. J Biol Chem 1988; 263: 18086–18092.
157. Levi S, Franceschinelli F, Cozzi A, Doerner MH, Arosio P. Expression and structure and functional properties of human ferritin L-chain from *Escherichia coli*. Biochemistry 1989; 28: 5179–5185.
158. Levi S, Yewdall SJ, Harrison PM, et al. Evidence that H- and L-chains have cooperative roles in the iron-uptake mechanism of human ferritin. Biochem J 1992; 288: 591–596.
159. De Silva D, Aust SD. Stoichiometry of Fe(II) oxidation during ceruloplasmin-catalyzed loading of ferritin. Arch Biochem Biophys 1992; 298: 259–264.
160. Herbert V. Viewpoint does mega-C do more good than harm, or more harm than good? Nutr Today 1993:28–32.
161. Roeser HP. The role of ascorbic acid in the turnover of storage iron. Semin Hematol 1983; 20: 91–100.
162. Treffry A, Harrison PM. Non-random distribution of iron entering rat liver ferritin in vivo. Biochem J 1984; 220: 857–859.
163. Kuhn LC, Hentze MW. Haem binding to ferritin and possible mechanisms of physiological iron uptake and release by ferritin. J Inorg Biochem 1992; 47: 175–181.

164. Kadir FH, al Massad F, Moore GR. Haem binding to horse spleen ferritin and its effect on the rate of iron release. Biochem J 1992; 282: 867–870.
165. Osaki S, Johnson DA, Freiden E. Mobilization of liver iron by ferroxidase (ceruloplasmin). J Biol Chem 1969; 244: 5757–5765.
166. Roeser HP, Lee GR, Nacht S, Cartwright GE. The role of ceruloplasmin in iron metabolism. J Clin Invest 1970; 49: 2408–2417.
167. Weir MP, Gibson JF, Peters TJ. Biochemical studies on the isolation and characterisation of human spleen haemosiderin. Biochem J 1984; 223: 31–38.
168. Finch CA, Deubelbliss K, Cook JD, et al. Ferrokinetics in man. Medicine 1970; 49: 17–53.
169. Green R, Charlton R, Seftel H, Bothwell TH, Mayet F. Body iron excretion in man. A collaborative study. Am J Med 1968; 45: 336–353.
170. Cole SK, Billewicz WZ, Thomson AM. Sources of variation in menstrual blood loss. J Obstet Gynaecol Br Commun 1971; 78: 933–939.
171. Frassinelli-Gunderson EP, Margen S, Brown JR. Iron stores in users of oral contraceptive agents. Am J Clin Nutr 1985; 41: 703–712.
172. Guillebaud J, Barnett MD, Gordon YB. Plasma ferritin levels as an index of iron deficiency in women using intrauterine devices. Br J Obstet Gynaecol 1979; 86: 51–55.
173. Kivijarvi A, Timonen H, Rajamaki A, Gronroos M. Iron deficiency in women using modern copper intrauterine devices. Obstet Gynecol 1986; 67: 95–98.
174. Pierson RNJ, Holt PR, Watson RM, Keating RP. Aspirin and gastrointestinal bleeding chromate blood loss studies. Am J Med 1961; 31: 259–265.
175. Layrisse M, Roche M. The relationship between anemia and hookworm infection. Results of a survey of a rural Venezuelan population. Am J Hyg 1964; 79: 279–301.
176. Fomon SJ, Ziegler EE, Nelson SE, Edwards BB. Cow milk feeding in infancy: gastrointestinal blood loss and iron nutritional status. J Pediatr 1981; 98: 540–545.
177. Flower RJ, Moncada S, Vane JR. Analgesic-antipyretics and anti-inflammatory agents; drugs employed in the treatment of gout. In: Gilman AG, Goodman LS, Rall RW, Murad F, eds. The Pharmacological Basis of Therapeutics. 7th ed. New York: Macmillan, 1985:682–728.
178. Haynes RC Jr, Murad F. Adrenocorticotropic hormone; adrenocortical steroids and their synthetic analogs; inhibitors of adrenocortical steroid biosynthesis. In: Gilman AG, Goodman LS, Rall TW, Murad F., eds. The Pharmacological Basis of Therapeutics. 7th ed. New York: Macmillan, 1985:1466–1496.
179. Peery WH. Clinical spectrum of hereditary hemorrhagic telangiectasia (Osler-Weber-Rendu disease). Am J Med 1987; 82: 989–997.
180. Finch CA, Cook JD, Labbe RF, Culala M. Effect of blood donation of iron stores as evaluated by serum ferritin. 1977; 50: 441–447.
181. Jing S, Trowbridge IS. Identification of the intermolecular disulfide bonds of the human transferrin receptor and its lipid attachment site. EMBO J 1987; 6: 327–331.
182. Enns CA, Suomalainen H, Gebhardt J, Schroder J, Sussman HH. Human transferrin receptor: expression of the receptor is assigned to chromosome 3. Proc Natl Acad Sci (USA) 1982; 79: 3241–3245.
183. Rabin M, McClelland A, Kuhn L, Ruddle FH. Regional localization of human transferrin receptor gene to 3q26.2 φter. Am J Hum Genet 1985; 37: 1112–1116.
184. Rao K, Harford JB, Rouault T, McClelland A, Ruddle FH, Klausner RD. Transcriptional regulation by iron of the gene for the transferrin receptor. Mol Cell Biol 1986; 6: 236–240.
185. Casey JL, Hentze MW, Koeller DM, et al. Iron-responsive elements: regulatory RNA sequences that control mRNA levels and translation. Science 1988; 240: 924–928.
186. Iturralde M, Vass JK, Oria R, Brock JH. Effect of iron and retinoic acid on the control of transferrin receptor and ferritin in the human promonocytic cell line U937. Biochim Biophys Acta 1992; 1133: 241–246.
187. McClelland A, Kuhn LC, Ruddle FH. The human transferrin receptor gene: genomic organisation and the complete primary structure of the receptor deduced from a cDNA sequence. Cell 1984; 39: 267–274.

188. Collawa JF, Stangel M, Kuhn LA, et al. Transferrin internalization sequence YXRF implicates a tight turn as the structural recognition motif for internalization. Cell 1990; 63: 1061–1072.

189. David RJ, Johnson GL, Kelleher DJ, Anderson JK, Mole JE, Czech MP. Identification of serine 24 as the unique site on the transferrin receptor phosphorylated by protein kinase C. J Biol Chem 1986; 261: 9034–9041.

190. Zerial M, Suomalainen M, Zanetti-Schneider M, Schneider C, Garoff H. Phosphorylation of the human transferrin receptor by protein kinase C is not required for endocytosis and recycling in mouse 3T3 cells. EMBO J 1987; 6: 2661–2667.

191. Zerial M, Melancon P, Schneider C, Garoff H. The transmembrane segment of the human transferrin receptor functions as a signal peptide. EMBO J 1986; 5: 1543–1550.

192. Wada HD, Hass PE, Sussman HH. Transferrin in human placental brush border membranes. J Biol Chem 1979; 254: 12629–12635.

193. Young SP, Bomford A, Williams R. The effect of iron saturation of transferrin on its binding and uptake by rabbit reticulocytes. Biochem J 1984; 219: 505–510.

194. Iacopetta BJ, Morgan EH, Yeoh GCT. Transferrin receptors and iron uptake during erythroid cell development. Biochim Biophys Acta 1982; 687: 204–210.

195. Watts CA. Rapid endocytosis of the transferrin receptor in the absence of bound transferrin. J Cell Biol 1985; 100: 633–637.

196. Klausner RD, Hartford J, van Renswoude J. Rapid internalization of the transferrin receptor in K562 cells is triggered by ligand binding or treatment with a phorbol ester. Proc Natl Acad Sci (USA) 1984; 81: 3005–3009.

197. Egan TJ, Zak O, Aisen P. The anion requirement for iron release from transferrin is preserved in the receptor transferrin complex. Biochemistry 1993; 32: 8162–8167.

198. Bali PK, Zak O, Aisen P. A new role for the transferrin receptor in the release of iron from transferrin. Biochemistry 1991; 30: 324–329.

199. Núñez MT, Gaete V, Watkins JA, Glass J. Mobilization of iron from endocytotic vesicles. J Biol Chem 1990; 265: 6688–6692.

200. Scheiber B, Goldenberg H. NAD(P)H:ferric iron reductase in endosomal membranes from rat liver. Arch Biochem Biophys 1993; 305: 225–230.

201. Escobar A, Gaete V, Núñez MT. Effect of ascorbate in the reduction of transferrin-associated iron in endocytic vesicles. J Bioenerg Biomembrane 1992; 24: 227–233.

202. Richardson DR, Baker E. Intermediate steps in cellular iron uptake from transferrin. Detection of a cytoplasmic pool of iron, free of transferrin. J Biol Chem 1992; 267: 21384–21389.

203. Li CY, Watkins JA, Glass J. The H^+-ATPase from reticulocyte endosomes reconstituted into liposomes acts as an iron transporter. J Biol Chem 1994; 269: 10242–19246.

204. Pan BT, Johnstone R. Selective externalization of the transferrin receptor by sheep reticulocytes in vitro. Response to ligands and inhibitors of endocytosis. J Biol Chem 1984; 259: 9776–9782.

205. Chitambar CR, Loebel AL, Noble NA. Shedding of transferring receptor from rat reticulocytes during maturation *in vitro*: soluble transferrin receptor is derived from receptor shed in vesicles. Blood 1991; 78: 2444–2450.

206. Kohgo Y, Nishisato T, Kondo H, et al. Circulating transferrin receptor in human serum. Br J Haematol 1986; 64: 277–281.

207. Shih YJ, Baynes RD, Hudson BG, Flowers CH, Skikne BS, Cook JD. Serum transferrin receptor is a truncated form of tissue receptor. J Biol Chem 1990; 265: 19077–19081.

208. Mulligan M, Linder M. The size of small molecular weight iron pools in rat tissues. In: Saltman P, Hagenaue J, eds. The Biochemistry and Physiology of Iron. New York: Elsevier, 1982.

209. Mulligan M, Althaus B, Linder MC. Non-ferritin, non-heme iron pools in rat tissues. Int J Biochem 1986; 18: 791–801.

210. Weaver J, Pollack S. Low molecular weight isolated from guinea pig reticulocytes as AMP-iron and ATP-iron complexes. Biochem J 1989; 261: 787–793.

211. Dandekar T, Stripecke R, Gray NK, et al. Identification of a novel iron-responsive element in

murine and human erythroid d-aminolevulinic acid synthase mRNA. EMBO J 1991; 10: 1903–1909.

212. Rangarajan PN, Padmanaban G. Regulation of cytochrome P-450 b/e gene expression by a heme- and phenobarbitone-modulated transcription factor. Proc Natl Acad Sci (USA) 1989; 86: 3963–3967.

213. Alam J, Smith A. Receptor-mediated transport of heme by hemopexin regulates gene expression in mammalian cells. J Biol Chem 1989; 264: 17637–17640.

214. Alam J, Smith A. Heme-hemopexin-mediated induction of metallothionein gene expression. J Biol Chem 1992; 267: 16379–16384.

215. Bettany A, Eisenstein RS, Munro HN. Mutagenesis of the iron-regulatory element further defines a role for rna secondary structure in the regulation of ferritin and transferrin receptor expression. J Biol Chem 1992; 267: 16531–16537.

216. Munro HN, Kikinis Z, Eisenstein RS. Iron-dependent regulation of ferritin synthesis. In: Berdanier C, Hargrove JL, eds. Nutrition and Gene Expression. Boca Raton, FL: CRC Press, 1993:525–545.

217. Müllner EW, Kühn LC. A stem-loop in the 3′ untranslated region mediates iron-dependent regulation of transferrin receptor mRNA stability in the cytoplasm. Cell 1988; 53: 815–825.

218. Owen D, Kuhn LC. Noncoding 3′ sequences of the transferrin receptor gene are required for mRNA regulation by iron. EMBO J 1987; 6: 1287–1295.

219. Casey JL, Koeller DM, Ramin VC, Klausner RD, Harford JB. Iron regulation of transferrin receptor mRNA requires iron-responsive elements and a rapid turnover determinant in the 4′ untranslated region of the mRNA. EMBO J 1989; 8: 3693–3699.

220. Zheng L, Kennedy MC, Blondin GA, Beinert H, Zalkin H. Binding of cytosolic aconitase to the iron responsive element of porcine mitochondrial aconitase mRNA. Arch Biochem Biophys 1992; 299: 356–360.

221. Aziz N, Munro HN. Iron regulates ferritin mRNA translation through a segment of its 5′ untranslated region. Proc Natl Acad Sci (USA) 1987; 84: 8478 8482.

222. Leibold EA, Munro HN. Cytoplasmic protein binds in vitro to a highly conserved sequence in the 5′ untranslated region of ferritin heavy- and light-subunit mRNAs. Proc Natl Acad Sci (USA) 1988; 85: 2171–2175.

223. Melefors Ö, Goossen B, Johansson HE, Stripecke R, Gray NK, Hentze MW. Translational control of 5-aminolevulinate synthase mRNA by iron-responsive elements in erythroid cells. J Biol Chem 1993; 268: 5974–5978.

224. Panter SS, Braughler JM, Hall ED. Clinically-silent mutation in the putative iron-responsive element in exon-17 of the beta-amyloid precursor protein gene. J Neuropathol Exp Neurol 1992; 51: 459–463.

225. Zubenko GS, Farr J, Stiffer JS, Hughes HB, Kaplan BB. Clinically silent mutation in the putative iron-response element in exon 17 of the β-amyloid precursor protein gene. J Neuropathol Exp Neurol 1992; 51: 459–466.

226. Goossen B, Hentze MW. Position is the critical determinant for function of iron-responsive elements as translational regulators. Mol Cell Biol 1992; 12: 1959–1966.

227. Dix DJ, Lin PN, Kimata Y, Theil EC. The iron regulatory region of ferritin mRNA is also a positive control element for iron-independent translation. Biochemistry 1992; 31: 2818–2822.

228. Walden WE, Daniels-McQueen S, Brown PH, et al. Translational repression in eukaryotes: partial purification and characterization of a repressor of ferritin mRNA translation. Proc Natl Acad Sci (USA) 1988; 85: 9503–9507.

229. Müllner EW, Neupert B, Kühn LC. A specific mRNA binding factor regulates the iron-dependent stability of cytoplasmic transferrin receptor mRNA. Cell 1989; 58: 373–382.

230. Harrell CM, McKenzie AR, Patino MM, Walden WE, Thiel EC. Ferritin mRNA: interactions of iron regulatory elements with translational regulator protein P-90 and the effect on base-paired flanking regions. Proc Natl Acad Sci (USA) 1991; 88: 4166–4170.

231. Müllner EW, Rothenberger S, Müller AM, Kühn LC. In vivo and in vitro modulation of the

mRNA-binding activity of iron-regulatory factor. Tissue distribution and effects of cell prolif-eration, iron levels and redox state. Eur J Biochem 1992; 208: 597–605.

232. Hentz MW, Senanez HN, O'Brien SJ, Hartford JB, Klausner RD. Chromosomal localization of nucleic acid-binding proteins by affinity mapping: assignment of the IRE-binding protein gene to human chromosome 9. Nucleic Acids Res 1989; 17: 6103–6108.

233. Yu Y, Radisky E, Leibold EA. The iron-responsive element binding protein—purification, cloning, and regulation in rat liver. J Biol Chem 1992; 267: 19005–19010.

234. Hentz MW, Argos P. Homology between IRE-BP, a regulatory RNA-binding protein, aconi-tase, and isopropylmalate isomerase. Nucleic Acids Res 1991; 19: 1739–1740.

235. Kennedy MC, Mende-Mueller L, Blondin GA, Beinert H. Purification and characterization of cytosolic aconitase from beef liver and its relationship to the iron-responsive element binding protein. Proc Natl Acad Sci (USA) 1992; 89: 11730–11734.

236. Tang CK, Chin J, Harford JB, Klausner RD, Rouault TA. Iron regulates the activity of the iron-responsive element binding protein without changing its rate of synthesis or degradation. J Biol Chem 1992; 267: 24466–24470.

237. Haile DJ, Rouault TA, Tang CK, Chin J, Hartford JB, Klausner RD. Reciprocal control of RNA-binding and aconitase activity in the regulation of the iron-responsive element binding protein—role of the iron-sulfur cluster. Proc Natl Acad Sci (USA) 1992; 89: 7536–7540.

238. Haile DJ, Rouault TA, Hartford JB, et al. Cellular regulation of the iron-responsive element binding protein: disassembly of the cubane iron-sulfur cluster results in high affinity RNA binding. Proc Natl Acad Sci (USA) 1992; 89: 11735–11739.

239. Emery-Goodman A, Hirling H, Scarpellino L, Henderson B, Kühn LC. Iron regulatory factor expressed from recombinant baculovirus—conversion between the RNA-binding apoprotein and Fe-S cluster containing aconitase. Nucleic Acids Res 1993; 21: 1457–1461.

240. Drapier JC, Hirling H, Wietzerbin J, Kaldy P, Kühn LC. Biosynthesis of nitric oxide activates iron regulatory factor in macrophages. EMBO J 1993; 12: 3643–3649.

241. Weiss G, Goossen B, Doppler W, et al. Translational regulation via iron-responsive elements by the nitric oxide/NO-synthase pathway. EMBO J 1993; 12: 3651–3657.

242. Eisenstein RS, Tuazon PT, Schalinske KL, Anderson SA, Traugh JA. Iron-responsive element binding protein. Phosphorylation by protein kinase C. J Biol Chem 1993; 268: 27363–27370.

243. Henderson BR, Seiser C, Kühn LC. Characterization of a second RNA-binding protein in rodents with specificity for iron-responsive elements. J Biol Chem 1993; 268: 27327–27334.

244. Beri R, Chandra R. The chemistry and biology of heme. Drug Metabol Rev 1993; 25: 49–152.

245. Lin J-J, Patino MM, Gaffield L, Walden WE, Smith A, Thach RE. Crosslinking of hemin to a specific site on the 90kDa ferritin repressor protein. Proc Natl Acad Sci (USA) 1991; 88: 6068–6071.

246. Lin J-J, Daniels-McQueen S, Patino MM, Gaffield L, Walden WE, Thach RE. Derepression of ferritin messenger RNA translation by hemin *in vitro*. Science 1990; 247: 74–77.

247. Goessling LS, Daniels MS, Bhattacharyya PM, Lin JJ, Thach RE. Enhanced degradation of the ferritin repressor protein during induction of ferritin messenger RNA translation. Science 1992; 256: 670–673.

248. Gardner LC, Smith SJ, Cox TM. Biosynthesis of δ-aminolevulinic acid and the regulation of heme formation by immature erythroid cells in man. J Biol Chem 1991; 266: 22010–22018.

249. Lathrop JT, Timko MP. Regulation by heme of mitochondrial protein transport through a conserved amino acid motif. Science 1993; 259: 522–525.

250. Chan RY, Schulman HM, Ponka P. Expression of ferrochelatase mRNA in erythroid and non-erythroid cells. Biochem J 1993; 292: 343–349.

251. Omichinski JG, Trainor C, Evans T, Gronenborn AM, Clore GM, Felsenfeld G. A small single-"finger" peptide from the erythroid transcription factor GATA-1 binds specifically to DNA as a zinc or iron complex. Proc Natl Acad Sci (USA) 1993; 90: 1676–1680.

252. Mendez R, Moreno A, de Haro C. Regulation of heme-controlled eukaryotic polypeptide chain initiation factor 2 alpha-subunit kinase of reticulocyte lysates. J Biol Chem 1992; 267: 11500–11507.

253. Samuel CE. The eIF-2α protein kinases, regulators of translation in eukaryotes from yeasts to humans. J Biol Chem 1993; 268: 7603–7606.

254. Srivastava G, Borthwick IA, Brooker JD, Wallace JC, May BK, Elliot WH. Hemin inhibits transfer of pre-δ-aminolevulinate synthase into chick embryo liver mitochondria. Biochem Biophys Res Commun 1983; 117: 344–349.

255. Srivastava G, Borthwick IA, Maguire DJ, et al. Regulation of 5-aminolevulinate synthase mRNA in different rat tissue. J Biol Chem 1988; 236: 5202–5209.

256. Drew PD, Ades IZ. Regulation of the stability of chicken embryo liver d-aminolevulinate synthase mRNA by hemin. Biochem Biophys Res Commun 1989; 162: 102–107.

257. Yamauchi K, Hayashi N, Kikucchi G. Translocation of d-aminolevulinate synthase from the cytosol to the mitochondria and its regulation by hemin in the rat liver. J Biol Chem 1980; 255: 1746–1751.

258. Srivastava G, Brooker JD, May BK, Elliot WH. Haem control in experimental porphyria. The effect of haemin on the induction of δ-aminolevulinate synthase in isolated chick-embryo liver cells. Biochem J 1983; 188: 781–788.

259. Eisenstein RS, Garcia-Mayol D, Pettingiell W, Munro HN. Regulation of ferritin and heme oxygenase synthesis in rats fibroblasts by different forms of iron. Proc Natl Acad Sci (USA) 1991; 88: 688–692.

260. Tyrrell RM, Applegate LA, Tromvoukis Y. The proximal promoter region of the human heme oxygenase gene contains elements involved in stimulation of transcription activity by a variety of agents including oxidants. Carcinogenesis 1993; 14: 761–765.

261. Webb EC. Enzyme Nomenclature. San Diego, CA: Academic Press, 1992.

262. Cammack R, Wriggleworth JM, Baum H. Iron-dependent enzymes in mammalian systems. In: Ponka P, ed. Iron Transport and Storage. Boca Raton, FL: CRC Press, 1990:17–39.

263. Dallman PR. Biochemical basis for the manifestations of iron deficiency. Annu Rev Nutr 1986; 6: 13–40.

264. Nebert DW, Nelson DR, Coon MJ, et al. The P450 superfamily: update on new sequences, gene mapping, and recommended nomenclature. DNA Cell Biol 1991; 10: 1–33.

265. Stuehr DJ, Ikeda SM. Spectral characterization of brain and macrophage nitric oxide synthases. Cytochrome P-450-like hemoproteins that contain a flavin semiquinone radical. J Biol Chem 1992; 267: 20547–20550.

266. White KA, Marletta MA. Nitric oxide synthase is a cytochrome P450 type hemoprotein. Biochemistry 1992; 31: 6627–6631.

267. Mayer B, John M, Heinzel B, et al. Brain nitric oxide synthase is a biopterin- and flavin-containing multi-functional oxidoreductase. FEBS Lett 1991; 288: 187–191.

268. Beard JL. Neuroendocrine alterations in iron deficiency. Prog Food Nutr Sci 1990; 14: 45–82.

269. Tucker DM, Sandstead HH. Spectral electroencephalographic correlates of iron status: tired blood revisited. Physiol Behav 1981; 26: 439–449.

270. Tucker DM, Sandstead HH, Swenson RA, Sawler BG, Penland JG. Longitudinal study of brain function and depletion of iron stores in individual subjects. Physiol Behav 1982; 29: 737–740.

271. Beard JL, Haas JD, Tufts H, Spielvogel E, Vargas E, Rodriguez C. Iron deficiency anemia and steady-state work performance at high altitude. J Appl Physiol 1988; 64: 1878–1884.

272. Thompson CH, Green YS, Ledingham JG, Radda GK, Rajagopalan B. The effect of iron deficiency on skeletal muscle metabolism of the rat. Acta Physiol Scand 1993; 147: 85–90.

273. Azevedo JL, Willis WT, Turcotte LP, Rovner AS, Dalman PR, Brooks GA. Reciprocal changes of muscle oxidases and liver enzymes with recovery from iron deficiency. Am J Physiol 1989; 256: E401–E405.

274. Dillman E, Gale C, Green W, Johnson DG, Mackler B, Finch CA. Hypothermia in iron deficiency due to altered triiodothyronine metabolism. Am J Physiol 1980; 239: R377–R381.

275. Beard JL, Green W, Finch CA. Effects of anemia and iron deficiency on thyroid hormone levels and thermoregulation during cold exposure. Am J Physiol 1984; 247: R114–R119.

276. Beard J, Tobin B, Green W. Evidence for thyroid hormone deficiency in iron-deficient anemic rats. J Nutr 1989; 119: 772–778.

277. Beard JL, Borel MJ, Derr J. Impaired thermoregulation and thyroid function in iron deficiency anemia. Am J Clin Nutr 1990; 52: 813–819.

278. Groeneveld D, Smeets HGW, Kabra PM, Dallman PR. Urinary catecholamines in iron deficient rats at rest and following surgical stress. Am J Clin Nutr 1985; 42: 263–269.

279. Beard J, Tobin B, Smith S. Norepinephrine turnover in iron deficiency at three environmental temperatures. Am J Physiol 1988: R90–R96.

280. Martinez-Torres C, Cubeddu L, Dillman E, et al. Effect of exposure to low temperature on normal and iron-deficient subjects. Am J Physiol 1984; 246: R380–R383.

281. Lukaski HC, Hall CB, Nielsen FH. Thermogenesis and thermoregulatory function of iron-deficient women without anemia. Aviat Space Environ Med 1990; 61: 913–920.

282. Moriarty PM, Hildenbrandt GR, Beard JL, Reddy CC. Decreased classical selenium-dependent glutathione peroxidase expression secondary to iron deficiency. J Nutr 1994; in press.

283. Voorhees ML, Stuart MJ, Stockman JA, Oski FA. Iron deficiency anemia and increased urinary NE excretion. J Pediatr 1975; 86: 542–547.

284. Beard JL, Green W, Finch CA. Interactions of iron deficiency anemia and thyroid hormone levels. Life Sci 30: 691.

285. Weinberg ED. Iron withholding: a defense against infection and neoplasia. Physiol Rev 1984; 64: 65–93.

286. Dallman PR. Iron deficiency and the immune response. Am J Clin Nutr 1987; 46: 329–334.

287. Rothenbacher H, Sherman AR. Target organ pathology in iron-deficient suckling rats. J Nutr 1980; 110: 1648–1654.

288. Kochanowski BA, Sherman AR. Cellular growth in iron-deficient rat pups. Growth 1982; 46: 126–134.

289. Kochanowski BA, Sherman AR. Cellular growth in iron-deficient rats: effect of pre- and postweanling iron repletion. J Nutr 1985; 115: 279–287.

290. Macdougall LG, Anderson R, McNab GM, Katz J. The immune response in iron-deficient children: impaired cellular defence mechanism with altered humoral components. J Pediatr 1975; 86: 833–843.

291. Chandra RK, Saraya AK. Impaired immunocompetence associated with iron deficiency. J Pediatr 1975; 86: 899–901.

292. Skikantia SG, Bhaskharam C, Prasad JS, Krishnamarachari KAVR. Anemia and immune response. Lancet 1976; II: 1307–1309.

293. Baliga BS, Kuvibidila S, Suskind RM. Effect of iron deficiency on the cell mediated immune response. Indian J Pediatr 1982; 49: 431–445.

294. Bhaskaram C, Reddy V. Cell-mediated immunity in iron and vitamin-deficient children. Br Med J 1975: 522–525.

295. Krantman HJ, Young SR, Jank BL, O'Donnell CM, Rachelefsky GS, Stiehm ER. Immune function in pure iron deficiency. Nutr Rep Int 1982; 26: 862–870.

296. Hallquist NA, McNeil LK, Lockwood JF, Sherman AR. Maternal-iron-deficiency effects on peritoneal macrophage and peritoneal natural-killer-cell cytotoxicity in rat pups. Am J Clin Nutr 1992; 55: 741–746.

297. Spear AT, Sherman AR. Iron deficiency alters DMBA-induced tumor burden and natural killer cell cytotoxicity in rats. J Nutr 1992; 122: 46–55.

298. Bagchi K, Mohanram M, Reddy V. Humoral immune response in children with iron-deficiency anaemia. Br Med J 1980; 280: 249–251.

299. Galan P, Thibault H, Preziosi P, Hercberg S. Interleukin 2 production in iron-deficient children. Biol Trace Element Res 1992; 32: 421–426.

300. Lozoff B. Behavioral alterations in iron deficiency. Adv Pediatr 1988; 35: 331–359.

301. Pollitt E. Iron deficiency and cognitive function. Annu Rev Nutr 1993; 13: 521–537.

302. Beard JL, Connor JR, Jones BC. Iron in the brain. Nutr Rev 1993; 51: 157–169.

303. Dallman PR, Siimes MN, Manies EC. Brain iron: persistent deficiency following short term iron deprivation in the young rat. Br J Haematol 1975; 31: 209–215.

304. Dallman PR, Spirito RA. Brain iron in the rat: extremely slow turnover in normal rat may explain the long-lasting effects of early iron-deficiency. J Nutr 1977; 107: 1075–1081.

305. Oski FA, Honig AS, Helu BPH. Effect of iron therapy on behavior performance in nonanemic, iron-deficient infants. Pediatrics 1983; 71: 877–880.

306. Lozoff B. Behavioural aspects of iron deficiency in infancy. Am J Clin Nutr 1989; 50(suppl): 641–655.

307. Walter T, Kovalskys J, Stekel A. Effect of mild iron deficiency on infant mental development scores. J Pediatr 1983; 102: 519–522.

308. Walter T. Iron deficiency and behaviour in infancy: a critical review. In: Dobbing J, ed. Brain, Behaviour and Iron in the Infant Diet. London: Springer-Verlag, 1990.

309. Soemantri AG, Pollitt E, Kim I. Iron deficiency anemia and educational achievement. Am J Clin Nutr 1985; 42: 1221–1228.

310. Pollitt E, Soemantri AG, Yunis F, Scrimshaw NS. Cognitive effects of iron deficiency anemia. Lancet 1985; 1: 158–162.

311. Pollitt E. Iron deficiency. In: The Impact of Poor Nutrition and Disease on Educational Outcomes. University of California, Davis, 1989.

312. Youdim MBH, Ben-Schachar D, Yehuda S. Putative biological mechanisms on the effects of iron deficiency on brain biochemistry. Am J Clin Nutr 1989; 50: 607–617.

313. Yehuda S, Youdim MBH, Zamir N. Iron deficiency induces increased brain met-enkephalin and dynorphin B and pain threshold in response to opiate peptides. Br J Pharmacol 1986; 87: 44.

314. Glover J, Jacobs A. Activity pattern of iron deficient rats. Br Med J 1972; ii: 627–628.

315. Edgerton VR, Gardner GW, Ohira Y, Gunawardena KA, Senewiratne B. Iron-deficiency anemia and its effect on worker productivity and activity patterns. Br Med J 1979; 2: 1546–1549.

316. McLane JA, Fell RD, McKay RH, Winder WW, Brown EB, Holloszy JO. Physiological and biochemical effects of iron deficiency on rat skeletal muscle function. Am J Physiol 1981; 241: C47–C54.

317. Davies KJA, Donovan CM, Refino CA, Brooks GA, Packer L, Dallman PR. Distinguishing effects of anemia and muscle iron deficiency on exercise bioenergetics in the rats. Am J Physiol 1984; 246: E535–E542.

318. Beard J, Green W, Miller L, Finch CA. Effect of iron deficiency anemia on hormone levels and thermoregulation during cold exposure. Am J Physiol 1984; 247: R114–R119.

319. Willis WT, Brooks GA, Henderson SA, Dallman PR. Effects of iron deficiency and training on mitochondrial enzymes in skeletal muscle. J Appl Physiol 1987; 62: 2442–2446.

320. Willis WT, Gohil K, Brooks GA, Dallman PR. Iron deficiency: improved exercise performance within 15 hours of iron treatment in rats. J Nutr 1990; 120: 909–916.

321. Willis WT, Jones PH, Chengson R, Dallman PR. Hepatic adaptations to iron deficiency and exercise training. J Appl Physiol 1992; 73: 510–515.

322. Finch CA, Miller LR, Inamdar R, Person R, Seiler K, Mackler B. Iron deficiency in the rat: physiological and biochemical studies of muscle dysfunction. J Clin Invest 1976; 58: 447–453.

323. Maguire JJ, Davies JKA, Dallman PR, Packer L. Effects of dietary iron deficiency on iron-sulfur proteins and bioenergetic functions of skeletal muscle mitochondria. Biochim Biophys Acta 1982; 679: 210–220.

324. McKay RH, Higuchi DA, Winder WW, Fell RD, Brown EB. Tissue effects of iron deficiency in the rat. Biochim Biophys Acta 1983; 757: 352–358.

325. Davies JKA, Maguire JJ, Brooks GA, Dallman PR, Packe L. Muscle mitochondrial bioenergetics, oxygen supply, and work capacity during dietary iron deficiency and repletion. Am J Physiol 1982; 242: E418–E427.

326. Henderson SA, Dallman PR, Brooks GA. Glucose turnover and oxidation are increased in the iron-deficient anemic rat. Am J Physiol 1986; 250: E414–E421.

327. Finch C, Gollnick PD, Hlastala MP, Miller LR, Dillman E, Mackler B. Lactic acidosis as a result of iron deficiency. J Clin Invest 1979; 64: 129–137.

328. Ohira Y, Chen CS, Hegenauer J, Saltman P. Adaptations of lactate metabolism in iron-deficient rats. Proc Soc Exp Biol Med 1986; 173: 213–216.

329. Farrell PA, Beard JL, Druckenmiller M. Increased insulin sensitivity in iron-deficient rats. H Nutr 1988; 118: 1104–1109.

330. Borel MJ, Beard JL, Farrell PA. Hepatic glucose production and insulin sensitivity and responsiveness in iron-deficient anemic rats. Am J Physiol 1993; 264: E662–E667.

331. Lieberman E, Ryan KJ, Monson RR, Schoenbaum SC. Association of maternal hematocrit with premature labor. Am J Obstet Gynceol 1988; 159: 107–114.

332. Murphy JF, O'Riordan J, Newcombe RG, Coles EC, F PJ. Relation of haemoglobin levels in first and second trimesters to outcome of pregnancy. Lancet 1986; 1: 992–994.

333. Scholl TO, Hediger ML, Fischer RL, Shearer JW. Anemia vs iron deficiency: increased risk of preterm delivery in a prospective study. Am J Clin Nutr 1992; 55: 985–988.

334. Wing-Moberg A, Wing K, Tholin K, Sjostrom R, Sandstrom B, Hallmans G. The relation of the accumulation of cadmium in human placenta to the intake of high-fibre grains and maternal iron status. Eur J Clin Nutr 1992; 46: 585–595.

335. Herbert V. Recommended dietary intakes (RDI) of iron in humans. Am J Clin Nutr 1987; 45: 679–686.

336. Ferguson BJ, Skikne BS, Simpson KM, Baynes RD, Cook JD. Serum transferrin receptor distinguishes the anemia of chronic disease from iron deficiency anemia. J Lab Clin Med 1992; 119: 385–390.

337. Beard JL, Finch CA. Iron deficiency. In: Clydesdale F, Weimer KL, eds. Iron Fortification of Foods. New York: Academic Press, 1985.

338. Finch CA, Heubers H. Perspectives in iron metabolism. N Engl J Med 1982; 306: 1520–1528.

339. Borel MJ, Smith SM, Derr J, Beard JL. Day-to-day variation in iron-status indices in healthy men and women. Am J Clin Nutr 1991; 54: 729–735.

340. Gibson RS. Principles of Nutritional Assessment. New York: Oxford University Press, 1990.

341. Measurement of Iron Status. Washington, DC: International Life Science Institute, 1984.

342. Lipschitz DA, Cook JD, Finch CA. A clinical evaluation of serum ferritin as an index of iron stores. Proc Soc Exp Biol Med 1975; 148: 358–364.

343. Macaron CI, Macaron ZG. Increased serum ferritin levels in hyperthyroidism. J Clin Endoc Metab 1985; 61: 672–676.

344. Leggett BA, Brown NN, Bryant SJ, Duplock L, Powell LW, Halliday JW. Factors affecting the concentration of ferritin in serum in a healthy Australian population. Clin Chem 1990; 36: 1350–1355.

345. Dallman PR. Tissue effects of iron deficiency. In: Jacobs A, Worwood M, eds. Iron in Biochemistry and Medicine. London: Academic Press, 1974.

346. Huebers HA, Finch CA. Transferrin: physiologic behavior and clinical implications. Blood 1984; 64: 763–767.

347. Dallman PR. Manifestations of iron deficiency. Semin Hematol 1982; 19: 19–30.

348. Siimes MA, Refino C, Dallman PR. Manifestations of iron deficiency at various levels of dietary iron intake. Am J Clin Nutr 1980; 33: 570–574.

349. Beguin Y. The soluble transferrin receptor: biological aspects and clinical usefulness as quantitative measures of erythropoiesis [editorial]. Haematologica 1992; 77: 1–10.

350. Cook JD, Skikne BS, Baynes RD. Serum transferrin receptor. Annu Rev Med 1993; 44: 63–74.

351. Thorstensen K, Romslo I. The transferrin receptor: its diagnostic value and its potential as therapeutic target. Scan J Clin Lab Invest 1993; 53(suppl 215): 113–120.

352. Carriaga MT, Skikne BS, Finley B, Cutler B, Cook JD. Serum transferrin receptor for the detection of iron deficiency in pregnancy. Am J Clin Nutr 1991; 54: 1077–1081.

353. Skikne BS, Flowers CH, Cook JD. Serum transferrin receptor: a quantitative measure of tissue iron deficiency. Blood 1990; 75: 1870–1876.

354. Beguin Y, Huebers HA, Josephson B, Finch CA. Transferrin receptors in rat plasma. Proc Natl Acad Sci (USA) 1988; 85: 637–640.

355. Nutrition monitoring in the United States. Washington, DC: U.S. Government Printing Office, 1986.

356. Group ESW. Summary of a report on assessment of the iron nutritional status of the United States population. Am J Clin Nutr 1985; 42: 1318–1330.

357. Seoane NA, Roberge AG, Page M, Allard C, Bouchard C. Selected indices of iron status in adolescents. J Can Diet 1985: 298–303.

358. DeMaeyer E, Adiels-Tegman M. The prevalence of anaemia in the world. Wld Hlth Statist Quart 1985; 38: 302–316.

359. Hillman RS, Finch CA, Red cell manual. 5th ed. Philadelphia: Davis, 1985.

360. National Research Council, Food and Nutrition Board. Recommended Dietary Allowances. 10th ed. Washington, DC: National Academy of Sciences, 1989.

361. Dallman PR. Changing iron needs from birth to adolescence. In: Fomon SJ, Zlotkin S, eds. Nutritional Anemias. New York: Vervey/Raven Press, 1992.

362. Hallberg L. Iron balance in pregnancy and lactation. In: Fomon SJ, Zlotkin S, eds. Nutritional Anemias. New York: Vervey/Raven Press, 1992.

363. Romslo I, Haram K, Sagen N, Augensen K. Iron requirements in normal pregnancy as assessed by serum ferritin, serum transferrin saturation and erythrocyte protoporphyrin determinations. Br J Obstet Gynaecol 1983; 90: 101–107.

364. Filer LJ. Dietary Iron: Birth to Two Years. New York: Raven Press, 1989.

365. Macdougall IC, Cavill I, Hulme B, et al. Detection of functional iron deficiency during erythropoietin treatment—a new approach. Br Med J 1992; 304: 225–226.

366. Humphries JE. Anemia of renal failure. Use of erythropoietin. Med Clin N Am 1992; 76: 711–725.

367. Litovitz T, Manoguerra A. Comparison of pediatric poisoning hazards: an analysis of 3.8 million exposure incidents. A report from the American Association of Poison Control Centers. Pediatrics 1992; 89: 999–1006.

368. Banner WJ, Tong TG. Iron poisoning. Pediatr Clin N Am 1986; 33: 393–409.

369. Injuries, poisonings, and resuscitation. In: Berkow R, Fletcher AJ, eds. The Merck Manual. Rahway, NJ: Merck, 1992.

370. Lynch SR, Skikne BS, Cook JD. Food iron absorption in idiopathic hemochromatosis. Blood 1987; 74: 2187–2193.

371. Chodos RB, Ross JF, Apt L, Pollycove M, Halkett JAE. The absorption of radioiron labeled foods and iron salts in normal and iron-deficient subjects and in idiopathic hemochromatosis. J Clin Invest 1957; 36: 314–321.

372. McLaren GD, Nathanson MH, Jacobs A, Trevett D, Thomson W. Regulation of intestinal iron absorption and mucosal iron kinetics in hereditary hemochromatosis. J Lab Clin Med 1991; 117: 390–401.

373. Simon M, Bourel M, Genetet B, Fauchet R. Idiopathic hemochromatosis. Demonstration of recessive transmission and early detection by family HLA typing. N Engl J Med 1977; 297: 1017–1021.

374. Dadone MM, Kushner JP, Edwards CQ, Bishop DT, Skolnick MH. Hereditary hemochromatosis. Analysis of laboratory expression of the disease by genotype in 18 pedigrees. Am J Clin Pathol 1982; 78: 196–207.

375. Edwards CQ, Griffen LM, Dadone MM, Skolnick MH, Kushner JP. Mapping the locus for hereditary hemochromatosis: localization between HLA-B and HLA-A. Am J Hum Genet 1986; 38: 805–811.

376. Edwards CQ, Griffen LM, Goldgar D, Drummond C, Skolnick MH, Kushner JP. The prevalence of hemochromatosis among 11,065 presumably healthy blood donors. N Engl J Med 1988; 318: 1355–1362.

377. Gable CB. Hemochromatosis and dietary iron supplementation: implications from US mortality, morbidity, and health survey data. J Am Diet Assoc 1992; 92: 208–212.

378. Charlton R, Hawkins DM, Mavor WO, Bothwell TH. Hepatic storage iron concentrations in different population groups. Am J Clin Nutr 1970; 23: 358–371.

379. Schafer AI, Ceron RG, Dluhy R, et al. Clinical consequences of acquired transfusional iron overload in adults. N Engl J Med 1981; 304: 319–324.

380. Stevens RG, Beasley RP, Blumberg BS. Iron-binding proteins and risk of cancer in Taiwan. Natl Cancer Inst 1986; 76: 605–610.

381. Selby JV, Friedman GD. Epidemiologic evidence of an association between body iron stores and risk of cancer. Int J Cancer 1988; 41: 677–682.

382. Stevens RG, Jones DY, Micozzi MS, Taylor PR. Body iron stores and the risk of cancer. N Engl J Med 1988; 316: 1047–1052.

383. Salonen JT, Nyyssonen K, Korpela H, Tuomilehto J, Seppanen R, Salonen R. High stored iron levels are associated with excess risk of myocardial infarction in eastern Finnish men. Circulation 1992; 86: 803–811.

384. Cooper R, Liao Y. Iron stores and coronary heart disease: negative findings in NHANES I epidemiologic follow-up study. Circulation 1993; 87: 686(abstr 33).

385. Rimm E, Ascherio A, Stampfer MJ, Colditz G, Giovannucci E, Willett W. Dietary iron intake and risk of coronary disease among men. Circulation 1993; 87: 692 (abstr P22).

386. Youdim M, Benshachar D, Riederer P. The possible role of iron in the etiopathology of Parkinson's disease—review. Movement Disord 1993; 8: 1–12.

387. Halliwell B. Oxidants and human disease: some new concepts. FASEB J 1987; 1: 358–364.

10
Manganese

ROLAND M. LEACH, JR.
Pennsylvania State University, University Park, Pennsylvania

EDWARD D. HARRIS
Texas A&M University, College Station, Texas

I. INTRODUCTION

Because he found copper, manganese, and zinc to be widely distributed in tissues of plants and animals, McHargue (1) attempted to assess the role played by these elements in the nutrition of animals. Rats were maintained in glass cages and fed a semipurified diet containing ingredients selected for low mineral content. It was concluded that "manganese definitely and possibly copper and zinc have important biological functions in animal metabolism." Subsequent research at Wisconsin by Kemmerer et al. (2) and by Orent and McCollum (3) at Johns Hopkins confirmed these observations. The recognition of the need for vitamin supplementation by these latter investigators provided stronger evidence than that provided by McHargue.

At about this same time in history, the raising of chickens moved from the barnyard to the chicken house. With this change in management, chickens became afflicted with a debilitating skeletal deformity called "perosis." Instead of alleviating the condition, additional supplements of calcium and phosphorus exacerbated it. However, one source of calcium and phosphorus supplement alleviated rather than exacerbated the condition, leading Wilgus et al. (4) to analyze for contaminating minerals. Testing the other elements present in the supplement showed that manganese was effective in preventing this debilitating skeletal deformity. Subsequent research at a number of Agricultural Experiment Stations showed that manganese was essential for all phases of the life cycle of avian species. Although manganese deficiency has been described in a wide variety of animal species, there is limited evidence of its essentiality for humans.

II. CHEMICAL PROPERTIES

Manganese ($3d^5$, $4s^2$), a first transition series metal, sits adjacent to iron ($3d^6$, $4s^2$) in the periodic table. Of its 11 oxidation states ($+7$ to -3), only Mn^{2+} is stable in dilute solutions at neutral pH. While Mn^{2+} has the potential to be a redox ion, its stability in neutral solution allows Mn^{2+} to behave as a simple divalent cation. The ionic radius of Mn^{2+} is 0.09 nm, which is midway between Mg^{2+} and Ca^{2+}, both of which Mn^{2+} readily replaces in vitro. Of greater interest is that the close juxtaposition to iron allows manganese to assume some of the properties of this metal as well, and hence iron–manganese interactions in biological systems are well known.

Manganous and ferric ions display a $3d^5$ configuration. Both tend to favor the formation of octahedral oxyanions (e.g., MnO_4^-, MnO_2) that have stability constants close to the oxyanion complexes of Mg^{2+} which also prefers octahedral complexes. Because of their similar properties, Mn^{2+} and Mg^{2+} have the potential to interchange cofactor roles in enzyme reactions, particularly when ATP is a substrate. Most of the biochemistry of manganese is dominated by the Mn^{2+} and Mn^{3+} forms, the former with five electrons in the partially filled $3d$ orbitals, leading to some interesting chemical properties. For one, movements of d electrons to form spin multiplicity are formally forbidden. As a consequence, manganese complexes are not boldly colorful like chromium or iron complexes, but are generally pale pink in color and exhibit a number of narrow spectral bands with small extinction coefficients. Cyanide ion (CN^-) is one of the few ligands capable of producing spin paring in Mn^{2+}, whereas all other complexes of the divalent ion are usually high spin, leading to the properties mentioned above. Mn^{3+} is more adept (compared to Mn^{2+}) at forming stable complexes with proteins. This fact is also important in biological properties of manganese. The free ion [$-MN(III)$] is unstable in solution and rapidly disproportionates to Mn(II) and Mn(IV), a reaction that may be responsible for some of the toxicity associated with manganese ions.

III. ANALYTICAL METHODOLOGY

Although manganese is about as common in the environment as iron and copper, its concentration in tissues and fluids is much smaller. Contaminants introduced during sample handling, therefore, are a special concern for this metal. For example, manganese is a component of steel (ferromanganese). Therefore, preparation of samples to be analyzed for manganese must avoid contact with stainless steel knives, homogenizer blades, spatulas, or mortar pestle handles. When it is practical, plastic is the preferred material for utensils and containers (5).

A. Neutron Activation Analysis

Given the concentration in samples, neutron activation analysis (NAA) is the most reliable and sensitive method for quantitating manganese in tissue samples. The technique was used in the 1960s by Cozias and co-workers (5). The protocol requires an atomic reactor capable of generating a neutron flux of 10^{12} to 10^{14} neutrons/cm^2/s. During the bombardment, the stable and more common ^{55}Mn is converted into radioactive ^{56}Mn in direct proportion to its quantity in the sample. ^{56}Mn decays by emitting gamma rays, which are readily detectable and distinguishable from other radioactive elements (6).

B. Atomic Absorption Spectrometry

While NAA is the method of choice for sensitivity and specificity, atomic absorption spectroscopy (AAS) is perhaps the most popular method. The standard protocol is to destroy organic matter via wet ashing with HNO_3 and measure manganese ions in the solution. A graphite furnace is generally used because it provides greater detection sensitivity than flame AAS.

C. Electron Paramagnetic Resonance

Mn^{2+}, with a spin of 5/2, generates five hyperfine splitting lines in an electron paramagnetic resonance (EPR) spectrum. On the other hand, Mn^{3+}, a $3d^4$ ion, has no unpaired electron and is EPR silent. Hence, EPR can be applied for the determination of the valence state of manganese ions in fluids such as blood or complexes.

IV. METABOLISM

A. Absorption

An overall scheme depicting our present knowledge of manganese metabolism is illustrated in Fig. 1. As with other mineral elements, the availability of manganese for absorption from the intestinal lumen is influenced by many factors, such as chemical form, presence of chelating or complexing agents, and the amount of calcium and phosphorus. The latter

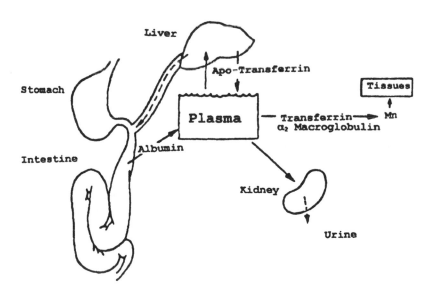

FIGURE 1 Manganese metabolism. While manganese is readily absorbed, it is excreted primarily by way of the intestine to establish homeostasis. Albumin plays a transport role from intestine to liver, and transferrin is involved in transport from liver to other tissues.

played a key role in the discovery of the importance of manganese in diets composed of natural ingredients for the avian species.

Little is known about the transport of manganese across the intestinal mucosa. Several lines of evidence indicate that manganese might share some features with the iron transport system (7). Manganese uptake is enhanced under conditions of iron deficiency and depressed by the presence of large amounts of nonheme iron. Also, mucosal tissue has been proposed to play a role in manganese homeostasis by sequestering manganese which is subsequently lost with sloughing of the intestinal mucosa.

B. Transport

Once absorbed, manganese is complexed with albumin in the portal blood for transport to the liver, the key organ in manganese metabolism (8,9). In the liver, manganese is found in both rapid- and slow-exchanging pools (9,10). The rapidly exchanging pool is hypothesized to be the precursor of biliary manganese, which represents a major route of manganese excretion from the body (10). The slow-exchanging pool likely serves as a source of manganese for liver as well as transferrin-bound manganese. Transferrin (11) and α_2-macroglobulin (12) have been proposed as the proteins responsible for transporting manganese to peripheral tissues (see below).

C. Cellular Uptake

Little is known at the present time about the uptake of manganese by cells at the tissue level. One obvious possibility involves movement into the cell by the same mechanism as that of iron, bound to transferrin (13). Transferrin binds numerous heavy metal cations, including Mn^{2+}. To be taken up by cells, manganese must form a tight complex with transferrin. Analogous to iron, transferrin can bind two trivalent ions (Mn^{3+}) in sites normally occupied by ferric (Fe^{3+}) iron (14). This means that the Mn^{2+} ions must be oxidized to Mn^{3+} in order to form a firm complex. Evidence suggests that ceruloplasmin, the copper protein in serum, catalyzes this oxidation reaction (15). Other than albumin and transferrin, manganese is also known to form a stable complex with α_2-macroglobulin (12). What role, if any, this complex plays in the cellular uptake of manganese is unknown.

D. Tissue Concentration and Storage

Manganese is fairly uniformly distributed in the soft tissues, with the liver containing the highest concentration (16). There are no storage forms for manganese such as exist for iron. Bone contains substantial quantities of manganese, a phenomenon that several investigators have used as an indicator of available manganese intake (17,18). However, this is a situation analogous to zinc, where there is no "recall" mechanism for releasing the mineral from bone. This should be considered passive storage, since these minerals are released only as a result of normal bone turnover or a situation accelerating bone resorption, such as a suboptimal calcium intake (19).

E. Excretion

Biliary excretion represents the major route of excretion of manganese from the body (8). Most researchers have concluded that this is a key mechanisms for maintaining manganese homeostasis. Little is known about the chemical form of manganese in bile except that the binding agent appears to be distinct from the compounds which bind copper (20). Recently, results of a detailed study of manganese metabolism led to the conclusion that gut absorption also influences homeostasis (10). As mentioned earlier, manganese present in the enterocyte would be lost to the feces in the normal process of enterocyte turnover. Similar to iron, this represents a mechanism of preventing entry of manganese into the body when dietary manganese exceeds physiologic needs.

F. Genetic Defects in Manganese Metabolism

Congenital ataxia has been found to be associated with genes affecting coat color in mice and mink (21–23). This ataxia is similar to that observed when normal mice are fed a manganese-deficient diet during pregnancy. When mutants are fed diets containing high levels of manganese during pregnancy, the occurrence of congenital ataxia is reduced. The levels of manganese needed to prevent the condition in mutant mice greatly exceed those required to prevent congenital ataxia in normal mice. Studies with radiomanganese demonstrated differences in metabolism between the two strains of mice (24).

V. PHYSIOLOGIC FUNCTIONS AND PATHOLOGY OF DEFICIENCY

A. Signs of Deficiency: Animals

1. Reproductive Failure

Reproductive failure was one of the earliest reported symptoms of manganese deficiency. Furthermore, the history of research on this topic serves to illustrate an important point, namely, that type and severity of symptoms depends on a number of factors. For example, Shils and McCollum (25) demonstrated several degrees of manganese deficiency in female rodents: (a) birth of viable young with ataxia, (b) nonviable young which die shortly after birth, and (c) disturbances in estrus cycle with no reproduction. The latter symptom has also been reported for cattle and swine (26–28). When manganese-deficient diets are fed to laying hens, decreases in egg production, egg shell quality, and hatchibility are observed (29,30). Embryonic development is also impaired, chondrodystrophy and congenital ataxia being the primary signs (31,32). Male reproductive capacity is also impaired by manganese deficiency, testicular degeneration being reported for a number of species (3,25,33,34).

2. Skeletal Development

When imposed in utero or in young growing animals, manganese deficiency has devastating effects on skeletal development. Symptoms include shortening of the limbs, enlargement of joints, twisting of legs, stiffness, and lameness (4,26,35–40). An example of manganese deficiency is shown in Fig. 2. Since manganese is a mineral element and bone contains 50% mineral, early research focused on the role of manganese in bone mineralization. These endeavors were not fruitful, since the actual effects of manganese on bone mineralization were minor compared to the effect of vitamin D (41). The seminal report of Wolbach and Hegsted (42) showed that endochondral bone rather than cortical bone was the site of the pathologic lesions associated with manganese deficiency. Subsequent research focused on the effect of manganese on the biochemical composition of the epiphyseal growth plate, the tissue responsible for endochondral bone growth. It was found

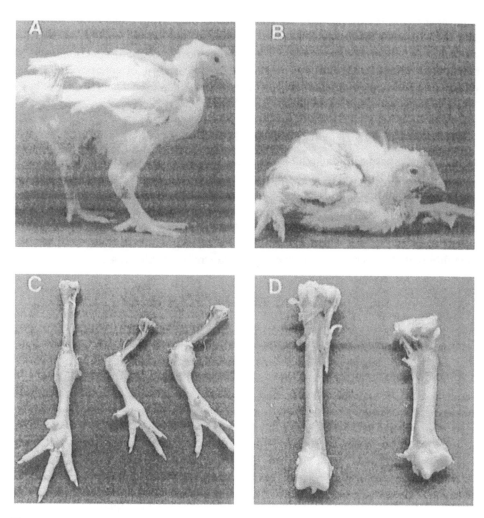

FIGURE 2 Manganese deficiency affects skeletal development. A. Normal 24-day-old chick. B. Same-age chick fed a manganese-deficient diet. C. Tibial and metatarsal bones from normal chick on left and from manganese-deficient chicks in center and on right. D. Tibia from control chick on left and from deficient chicks on right. Note swollen joints, shortened and twisted tibias.

that there is a substantial reduction in proteoglycans, a major extracellular matrix component of cartilage (43,44). This original observation with chicken cartilage was confirmed in a number of mammalian species, leading to the current concept that manganese plays an important role in proteoglycan biosynthesis (35,39).

Proteoglycans are huge macromolecules that play a key role in the integrity of cartilage, such as its ability to resist deformation from compressive loads. Aggregan, the major proteoglycan found in cartilage, is comprised of a core protein to which are attached glycosaminoglycan side chains and oligosaccharides (Fig. 3). Manganese deficiency results in a 40% reduction in cartilage polysaccharide content (45). In addition to the quantitative reduction in proteoglycan content, there were qualitative changes in the size and distribution of the polysaccharides isolated from manganese-deficient cartilage.

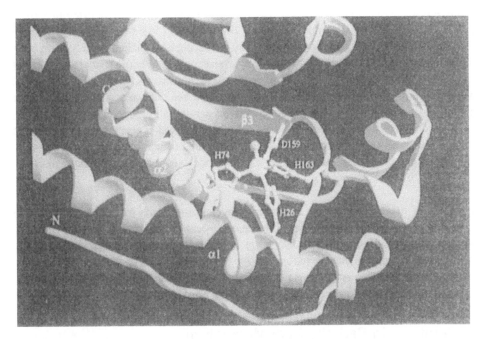

FIGURE 3 Location of the manganese ion in a subunit of human Mn-superoxide dismutase. The Mn^{2+} ion is complexed with histidines 26, 74, and 163 to aspartate 159. This three-dimensional model, determined by 2.2 Å resolution X-ray crystallography, was supplied courtesy of Dr. John Tainer.

3. Bone Mineralization

As discussed earlier, the influence of manganese on skeletal development was originally thought to be manifested via an effect on bone mineralization. The effects of manganese on chick bone mineralization are small compared to those of vitamin D (41). This concept is supported by the results with manganese-deficient rats (46). In these kinetic studies, manganese deficiency did not perturb any of the parameters of calcium metabolism, including pool size, endogenous fecal calcium, urinary calcium, or rates of calcium entering or leaving the bone. More recent studies (47) have implicated manganese as essential for maintenance of bone mineralization. In long-term studies, manganese deficiency resulted in lowered bone calcium concentrations and radiographic differences in bone mineralization. It should be noted that there are several peculiarities with regard to the performance of the rats in these experiments. For example, although manganese did not influence growth rate, there was a hypercalcemia associated with the manganese-deficient diet. These observations differ considerably from those described previously (46).

This research has been extended to a clinical trial with postmenopausal women (48). Participants received supplements of trace minerals (Cu, Zn, Mn), calcium (1000 mg) or a combination of calcium and trace minerals. Only the latter treatment reversed the loss in bone mineral density observed in individuals receiving the other treatments or the placebo. However, it is not known which trace element(s) was (were) acting in concert with the supplemental calcium to produce this effect.

The laying hen has been used as a model to study the potential role of manganese in the development of osteoporosis (49). The laying hen metabolizes 2 g of calcium daily, a quantity approximating that metabolized by a 70-kg human (50). Medullary bone, which plays a key role in the metabolism of calcium by the laying hen, differs from cortical bone in chemical composition, with larger amounts of proteoglycans being a characteristics of this tissue (51). This would theoretically provide a tissue sensitive to manganese deficiency. However, prolonged manganese deficiency in the laying hen did not perturb the amount or composition of medullary or cortical bone (49). In parallel studies with young chickens, manganese deficiency had a large impact on the amount and characteristics of cartilage proteoglycans. It was concluded that medullary bone and cortical bone are not sensitive to manganese deficiency in the laying hen, an animal model with a high rate of bone turnover.

4. Ataxia

Deprivation of manganese during embryonic development leads to congenital ataxia in mammals and newly hatched chicks. Subsequent research has shown that the ataxia is associated with defective otolith development in the utricular and saccular maculae (52). Data obtained by sulfate incorporation and by histochemical stain implicated defective proteoglycan metabolism as the cause of impaired otolith calcification. Thus, the skeletal lesions and postural defects appear to arise due to the need for manganese for proteoglycan biosynthesis (53,54).

5. Alterations in Carbohydrate Metabolism

Two reports were responsible for sustained interested in the possible relationship between manganese deficiency and carbohydrate metabolism. One was an anecdotal report that manganese improved glucose tolerance in a patient who did not respond to insulin (55). This concept was reinforced by the observation that manganese-deficient guinea pigs had impaired glucose tolerance (56). Subsequent laboratory research has focused on glucose and insulin metabolism in young rat pups derived from Mn-sufficient and Mn-deficient female rats (57,58). The deficient rats exhibited an abnormal glucose tolerance curve, decreased pancreatic release of insulin, depressed pancreatic insulin synthesis, and enhanced rate of insulin degradation. Subsequent research indicated that decreased preproinsulin mRNA levels may be a major factor contributing to the decreased insulinogenesis in the manganese-deficient rats (59). However, the mechanism whereby manganese affects insulin mRNA remains to be elucidated.

Manganese deficiency has also been found to influence the response to insulin in peripheral tissues (60). Adipocytes isolated from the offspring of manganese-deficient rats had decreased insulin-stimulated glucose transport. These cells also had a reduced level of insulin-stimulated glucose oxidation and glucose conversation to fatty acids. It was concluded that the defect in response to insulin was distal to the insulin receptor, since there were no differences observed in insulin receptor affinity.

The issue of the relationship of manganese to glucose tolerance has been addressed also with nondiabetic and type II diabetic human subjects (61). Oral administration of manganese with glucose did not alter glycemic or hormonal responses in either group of subjects. The authors concluded that these results did not support the concept that acute manganese supplementation alters glucose metabolism in the average diabetic subject.

The other approach to pancreatic function has been research on the relationship between manganese nutrition and exocrine function (62). Manganese-deficient rats had increased pancreatic amylase activity, while lipase and proteolytic enzyme activities remained normal. Manganese repletion did not reverse the elevated amylase activity, leading to the conclusion that manganese plays a complex role in the development of the exocrine pancreas.

6. Alterations in Lipid Metabolism

The earliest report linking aberrations in lipid metabolism with manganese deficiency showed that manganese had a lipotropic effect (63). This was confirmed in later research with mice, indicating that there were ultrastructural lesions associated with the accumulation of lipid in the liver (64).

Cholesterol metabolism in manganese-deficient animals has been subjected to close scrutiny. The major impetus for this research was the report that manganese enhanced cholesterol biosynthesis in liver homogenates (65). There has not been agreement in the results obtained with in-vivo experiments. Research with young chickens and laying hens led to the conclusion that manganese does not play a major role in cholesterol biosynthesis (66). Similar conclusions were reached by the same investigators when rats were used as the experimental animals (67). Later, it was reported that there are modest changes in HDL cholesterol metabolism associated with manganese deficiency in Sprague-Dawley, but not Wistar, rats (68). Davis and associates (69), also using Sprague-Dawley strain, observed that manganese deficiency decreased plasma and HDL cholesterol concentrations but had no effect on liver cholesterol content. The basal diet used in the latter investigations differed considerably from that used in the other laboratories. It contained higher levels of supplemental fat and used sucrose as the primary source of carbohydrate. Thus, in addition to strain of rat, dietary composition could have influenced the outcome of the research. Collectively, there is not overwhelming evidence that manganese plays a dominating role in cholesterol biosynthesis. Deficiency of the element results in modest changes in various measures of cholesterol metabolism which are not consistent across species or strains within a species.

B. Signs of Deficiency: Humans

Although manganese deficiency has been observed in many species of animals, there is little evidence of deficiency symptoms in humans (70). Since manganese does perform essential biochemical functions in animals, it is difficult to conceive that similar reactions in humans do not also require manganese. One can only conclude that the requirements are very low and the body has the ability to conserve manganese. It should be noted that for several animal species, manganese deficiency has to be imposed during pregnancy in order to produce severe deficiency signs. Thus, marginal intakes during pregnancy might suffice to prevent the development of deficiency symptoms during the prenatal and early postnatal period.

VI. BIOCHEMICAL FUNCTION

Enzymes that require manganese as a cofactor will not function optimally when there is a deficiency of manganese in the diet, but low enzyme activity suggests only that manganese is a component of a metalloenzyme. Definitive proof depends on the isolation of the purified enzyme and proof that manganese is part of its structure. Table 1 lists enzymes that have been shown to have a manganese cofactor or are activated by the addition of manganese to the assay medium. Mn^{2+} ions are nonspecific activators of a number of enzymes that have a nonstringent requirement for metal ions. These enzymes cover a broad range of

TABLE 1 Examples of Manganese-Metalloenzymes and Manganese-Activated Enzymes

Enzymes	Function	References
Manganese metalloenzymes		
Oxygen-evolving center in photosystem II	Photosynthesis	72
Mn-dependent superoxide dismutase	Antioxidant in bacteria, mitochondria	73, 75
Pyruvate carboxylase	Gluconeogenesis	83
Arginase	Urea cycle	85
Mn-dependent catalase	Antioxidant in bacteria	87
Manganese-activated enzymes		
Phosphoenolpyruvate carboxykinase	Gluconeogenesis	84
Glycosyl transferases	Glycoprotein biosynthesis	122
Glutamine synthetase	Ammonia metabolism	88
Farnesyl pyrophosphate synthetase	Cholesterol biosynthesis	123
Mn-dependent peroxidases	Antioxidant in bacteria	124

functions and include but are not limited to phosphatases, peptidases, kinases, decarboxylases, and transferases (71). Properties of known manganese-dependent enzymes are described below.

A. Dioxygen Synthesis

The enzyme system that generates dioxygen in chloroplasts of plants is the most actively studied manganese-requiring enzyme in biology. This most unique enzyme system shows that manganese, in contrast to iron or copper, has a role in oxygen formation. Iron and copper, it appears, are more suited for systems that transport dioxygen or split dioxygen during the course of a metabolic reaction. Splitting water to form dioxygen is the reverse of the more common catabolic reactions in animals. The reaction of the so-called water-splitting enzyme of photosystem II is

$$2H_2O \Leftrightarrow 4H^+ + O_2 + 4e^-$$

Energy for splitting H_2O molecules is obtained from photons of light channeled into the reaction center. The reaction furnishes electrons to activated chlorophyll centers whose electrons have been displaced from the molecule by the electron transport mechanism. The four manganese ions in the enzyme combine to form a cluster that accepts one electron at a time from the H_2O molecule while the latter is bound to the manganese ions (72). One key to the success of this reaction is that manganese readily assumes all the multivalence states that are required in the transition.

B. Mn-Dependent Superoxide Dismutase

One of the most intensely studied manganese enzyme in humans, Mn-dependent superoxide dismutase (MnSOD) is primarily of mitochondrial origin. The enzyme has received considerable attention for its role as a member of the family of antioxidant enzymes. MnSOD, therefore, is a factor in the prevention of oxygen toxicity, and autoimmune and degenerative diseases. Because mitochondria consume over 90% of the O_2 used by cells, mitochondrial are particularly vulnerable to oxygen toxicity. Indeed, the mitochondrial electron transport chain is a source of a large number of oxygen free radicals (73). Specifically, MnSOD catalyzes the dismutation of superoxide anion as shown below:

$$O_2^- + O_2^- + 2H^+ \Leftrightarrow H_2O_2 + O_2$$

SODs in general defend against oxygen toxicity and of late have been used in therapy for treatment of oxidative stress associated with postischemic reperfusion of organs (74). The half-life of MnSOD in serum is about 5–6 h, compared to only 6–10 min for Cu,ZnSOD (74). Eykaryotic MnSODs are usually tetrameric proteins, whereas prokaryotic MnSODs are generally dimeric (75), with each subunit of the dimer containing one atom of manganese. Tetrameric SODs appear to be more stable to heat and other denaturants than dimeric forms of the enzyme (76). The human enzyme uses amino acid residues in both the N-terminal helical hairpin and the C-terminal domains to bind Mn ion to the protein (Fig. 3) (77). MnSOD activity is decreased in numerous tissues of Mn-deficient rats and mice (78,79) and its loss could produce mitochondrial abnormalities (80). Regulation of the enzyme by manganese ions is not well established, however. For example, although dietary manganese deficiency lowers the enzyme activity, that of the liver and kidney enzyme is increased if the deficient animals has been exposed chronically to ethanol in the drinking water (81). Also, MnSOD mRNA can be induced by various cytokines such as tumor necrosis factor and interleukin-1 (82).

C. Pyruvate Carboxylase

Two manganese enzymes are believed to be required to catalyze the formation of phosphoenol pyruvate (PEP) from pyruvate, a key reaction in the synthesis of glucose in liver. One of these, pyruvate carboxylase, has a manganese ion firmly to its structure (83). The other enzyme, PEP carboxykinase, is activated by adding manganese ions (and other divalent ions) to the assay medium but may not be a mangano-metalloenzyme (84). Pyruvate carboxylase requires biotin and catalyzes the carboxylation of pyruvate in the mitochondria to form oxaloacetate as shown below:

$$\text{Pyruvate} + HCO_3^- + \text{ATP} \Leftrightarrow \text{oxaloacetate} + \text{ADP} + P_i + H^+$$

The oxaloacetate can then react with a second enzyme, PEP carboxykinase, which catalyzes the removal of the −COOH group concomitant with the phosphorylation of the carbonyl oxygen atom giving rise to phosphoenolpyruvate (PEP):

$$\text{Oxaloacetate} + \text{GTP} \Leftrightarrow \text{PEP} + \text{GDP} + HCO_3^-$$

D. Arginase

Arginase is the terminal enzyme in the urea cycle. It catalyzes the hydrolysis of L-arginine, giving rise to urea and ornithine according to the following reaction:

$$\text{L-arginine} + H_2O \Leftrightarrow \text{L-ornithine} + \text{urea}$$

Arginase is most highly concentrated in the liver, although the enzyme is also present in abundance in the mammary gland, which has no urea cycle and thus may be performing other functions, possibly to provide ornithine for proline synthesis. There is evidence that arginases in different organs are different proteins (85). Arginases from the livers of several mammalian sources appear to be tetrameric proteins with molecular weights between 115 and 120 kDa (86), although recent evidence suggests that liver arginase is a trimer of identical subunits (35 kDa). Each subunit contains a firmly bound manganese ion, but a total of six manganese ions are required for maximal activity (personal communication, David Ash).

E. Manganese-Dependent Catalase

Manganese-dependent catalase occurs in a number of bacterial species, functioning to destroy the potentially damaging peroxides that accumulate in the cytosol. The typical reaction is shown below. The enzyme in *Thermus thermophilus* obeys Michaelis-Menten kinetics and is not inhibited by its substrate (H_2O_2) at concentrations as high as 0.45 M (87). Two active-site manganese ions in close juxtaposition are required to prohibit one-electron chemistry, which could result in mixed-valence forms of the enzyme that are kinetically inactive.

$$2H_2O_2 \Leftrightarrow O_2 + 2H_2O$$

It is important to note that catalases from mammalian sources, as a rule, are iron-dependent enzymes, using heme iron as a cofactor. In the bacterial enzyme, however, manganese ions are bound firmly to the protein structure directly and are apparently able to catalyze decomposition of hydrogen peroxide with equal facility. The discovery of a manganese-dependent catalase points out the versatility of manganese as an enzyme cofactor and its close relationship with iron in biological molecules.

F. Glutamine Synthetase

Glutamine synthetases from a number of sources have been shown to be activated by manganese and magnesium ions, but there is little or no evidence that it is a metalloenzyme (88). The mammalian enzymes consist of a family of large octameric proteins with molecular weights of about 350–400 kDa. A subunit from the rat brain enzyme, for example, has a molecular weight of 49 kDa. The reaction catalyzed is

$$\text{L-glutamate} + \text{ATP} + NH_4^+ \Leftrightarrow \text{L-glutamine} + \text{ADP} + P_i + H^+$$

By contrast, glutamine synthetase in *Escherichia coli* has a molecular weight of 600 kDa and consists of 12 subunits each with a molecular weight of 50 kDa. Manganese in glutamine synthetase is believed to perform mainly a structural role and is not linked directly to the catalytic events.

G. Glycosyl Transferases

The devastating effects of manganese deficiency on skeletal development during the fetal and early postnatal period can be accounted for by severe reduction in proteoglycan content of the cartilage tissue. A defect in proteoglycan formation has led to one of the many biochemical functions of manganese. The ultimate cause of the skeletal defects may not be the proteoglycans per se, but the enzymes that synthesize these complex carbohydrates.

Glycosyl transferases are a family of enzymes responsible for the sequential addition of carbohydrate molecules to core proteins to form proteoglycans (Fig. 4). Defects in proteoglycan formation are responsible for ataxia (51) and abnormal egg shell formation (89,90). Aggregan, the major proteoglycan found in cartilage, is comprised of a core protein to which are attached numerous glycosaminoglycan side chains (91). Following the synthesis of the core protein, a trisaccharide linkage sequence and the glycosaminoglycan

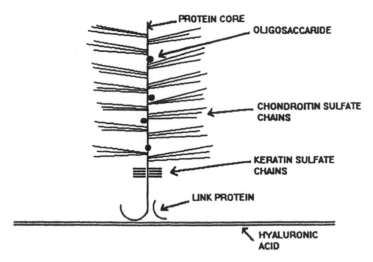

FIGURE 4 Structure of cartilage proteoglycan aggregan. The aggregate is complexed with hyaluronic acid via a link protein. Modified from Hascall (63) and Heinegard and Oldberg (64).

side chains are synthesized. The general reaction which occurs in the rough endoplasmic reticulum and Golgi apparatus can be described in the following manner:

$$UDP - sugar + acceptor \Leftrightarrow UDP + acceptor - sugar \text{ (product)}$$

There are specific glycosyltransferases for each UDP-sugar. When studied in vitro, a number of different divalent cations can participate in enzyme activity. In vivo, however, there appears to be a specific requirement for manganese for the activity of these enzymes. This conclusion is supported by in vitro studies on radioactive UDP-sugar incorporation by normal and manganese-deficient cartilage (92,93). Second, the products of these reactions are greatly reduced in cartilage tissue. In addition to a severe reduction in aggregan content, there is a reduction in the size of the glycoaminoglycan chains associated with the aggregan isolated from deficient cartilage (45). The mechanism of action of manganese in cartilage glycosyl transferases has been difficult to determine, since both the enzyme and acceptor are membrane bound. However, data are available for the soluble galactosyltransferase found in milk (94,95). This enzyme has two metal-binding sites which must be occupied for lactose synthesis to occur (96,97). A high-affinity binding site must be occupied for activation of the enzyme and binding of the substrate or binding of metals to the second binding site to occur. The second (low-affinity) binding site requires larger quantities of metal, with calcium readily replacing manganese at this site. It is likely that the active form of the enzyme in vivo contains Mn(II) at site 1 and Ca(II) at site 2 (98). Similar results have been obtained with glycosyl transferases involved in the glycosylation of hydroxylysine residues on collagen (99).

VII. NUTRITIONAL ASSESSMENT AND REQUIREMENTS

The avian species are the only ones likely to experience manganese deficiency when fed unsupplemented diets composed of natural feed ingredients. The National Research Council lists dietary requirements for manganese that range from 20 mg/kg for mature animals to

60 mg/kg for young, rapidly growing animals (100). Because of the poor absorption of manganese from the diet, these levels greatly exceed the actual available requirements (10 mg/kg). For many other animal species the requirements may be as low as 1–2 mg/kg (16).

Since manganese deficiency has not been observed in humans, little information is available on the human requirement. Most of the data for requirements were obtained from balance studies which have provided estimates in the range of 0.05–3.5 mg/day (101–104). Estimates of dietary intakes have been reported to range from 2 to 5 mg/day (105–107).

A wide variety of parameters has been used to evaluate manganese status. Use of the dietary balance technique can be misleading because of variable excretion in the feces. This method is useful only when endogenous losses are carefully estimated. Variable bone deposition could also render misleading values, because the amount deposited in bone increases as intake increases. The most sensitive noninvasive methods for evaluation of status include serum manganese, urinary manganese, lymphocyte manganese, and superoxide dismutase activity (108,109).

VIII. ROLE IN GENE EXPRESSION

More than half of the manganese in liver tissue is found in the nucleus (110). A nuclear location predicts a potential role for Mn in genetic-related events, possibly in connection with the regulation of genetic expression. Although no definitive information is at hand, there is support for the existence of specific Mn-dependent factors that regulate expression and non-enzyme-related cell functions such as cell signaling and response to hormones. For example, manganese is an important cofactor for RNA polymerase and could modulate the transcription of specific genes, although no manganese-dependent transcription factors have been found. Manganese is ubiquitous in cells, and the ability of manganese ions to modulate calcium and other ions connected with cells signaling and other regulatory pathways cannot be dismissed. It is difficult to draw conclusions as to the mechanism of action, since manganese could be acting through modulating insulin levels or the glucocorticoids. One study reported that manganese effects on pancreatic amylase mRNA levels as seen in Mn-deficient rats appear without perceivable changes in insulin and corticosterone levels (111).

IX. PHARMACOLOGY AND TOXICOLOGY

There are numerous citations in the literature that manganese is a pharmacologic agent capable of stimulating biochemical processes. For example, small doses of manganese salts given to normal rats stimulate insulin secretion and promote the release of pancreatic amylase (112). Manganese given intraperitoneally also raises blood sugar levels by stimulating glyconeogenesis and potentiating the action of glucagon and epinephrine on glycogen breakdown (113). Levels as low as 0.03 mM manganese in the culture medium of pancreatic acinar cells have the capacity to stimulate protein biosynthesis (114).

Like other heavy metals, however, manganese in excess is very toxic to living systems. Animals can tolerate 1 ppm manganese in the diet without disturbing iron metabolism. Slightly higher amounts, for example, 2 ppm, have been shown to inhibit hemoglobin regeneration in baby pigs, rabbits, and lambs (115) as measured by a drop in the rate of iron incorporation into hemoglobin (116). As noted previously, manganese in the diet is detrimental to iron absorption. In larger amounts, however, manganese affects the central nervous system, impairing cognitive functions and motor activity (see below). One of the concerns of environmentalists is the use of methylcyclopentadienyl tricarbonyl manganese as an antiknock agent in gasoline. Automobile emissions, therefore, can raise the manganese compounds in the air, especially in large metropolitan areas. An increase in air inhalation from 1 μg/day to 2 μg/day has been estimated since its introduction as an additive (117). One encouraging note, however, is that adult rats purposely exposed to exhaust fumes reportedly do not show any signs of manganese toxicity (118).

A. Manganese Toxicity in Humans

Toxicity to humans has been seen most often in countries that mine manganese ores. A shocking statistic is that from 1% to 4% of the exposed population in Chile to as high as 25% in India suffer from some form of manganese intoxication (119). Daily exposure by contact through the skin or by inhaling the dust from manganese-rich ores produces a Parkinson-like tremor in some subjects and causes hallucinations in others. A condition known as "manganic madness," which has all the signs of serious mental disturbances, has been seen in mine workers in Chile. Interestingly, the conditions is treatable by administration of large doses of L-DOPA. It is thought that manganese acts as a neurotoxin, affecting specific areas of the central nervous system, probably the striatal area.

B. Mechanism of Toxicity

The root causes for the symptoms of manganese poisoning are slowly coming to light. Controlled studies using animals as models have been able to reproduce many of the toxicity signs seen in humans and have given direct support to CNS involvement in the toxicity (120). Table 2 shows behavioral symptoms observed when different animal species are administered large doses of manganese oxide. Note the similarity of symptoms among species. Mena has pointed out that the extrapyramidal system of the CNS tissue bears the brunt of the toxicity (121).

In its capacity as a toxin, manganese is believed to target the biochemical synthesis of the catecholamine neurotransmitters, although the mechanism could involve cell death. In the catecholamine pathway, tyrosine is converted to norepinephrine by way of L-DOPA and dopamine:

$$\text{Tyrosine} \rightarrow \text{L-DOPA} \rightarrow \text{dopamine} \rightarrow \text{norepinephrine}$$

Both dopamine and norepinephrine are major neurotransmitters in the CNS. Although there is clear evidence that norepinephrine synthesis is lowered in manganese toxicity, most studies have focused on dopamine as the critical factor affected. One intriguing idea is that dopamine is oxidized to a trihydroxy compound, which in turn is a highly toxic agent that damages neurons producing neurotransmitters such as dopamine.

TABLE 2 Comparative Signs of Manganese Toxicity in Animals and Humans

Species	Signs	Reference
Dogs	Highly nervous activity, poor condition reflexes	119
Rhesus monkeys	Hyperexcitability, clumsy movements, rigidity, tremors	120
Humans	Hypokinesia, bradykinesia, rigidity, tremors	121

Manganese toxicity also impairs the normal functioning of the liver, pancreas, and respiratory tract. The signs and symptoms in these organs are less pronounced and often go unnoticed. Nonetheless, hepatitis, pancreatitis, and pneumonitis are known to occur in humans suffering from excess exposure to manganese.

X. SUMMARY AND FUTURE DIRECTIONS

Although it was one of the earliest trace elements to be recognized as nutritionally essential, manganese is perhaps the least understood of all the essential metals. The levels of manganese in tissues and body fluids are far below the concentrations of other trace elements; thus manganese borders on the ultratrace classification. Despite the small amount, it is clear that there are specific biochemical and nutritional systems that rely strictly on manganese, no other metal being capable of fulfilling these physiologic functions. The functions of manganese in photosynthesis, proteoglycan synthesis, and antioxidant enzyme function are well established. Manganese, however, appears to interact with humoral systems and may interface with mechanisms of genetic regulation. A surprising facet of manganese nutrition is the very low levels of manganese in tissues, yet its profound effects on metabolic processes in cells. The toxicity of manganese is also of interest. Manganese in excess seems to target the nervous system and affect the biosynthesis of neurotransmitters, dopamine in particular. Deficiencies of manganese, on the other hand, are most keenly seen in gross alterations to connective tissue (bone and cartilage), where the biochemical target appear to be the proteoglycans that make up a large proportion of connective tissue ground substance. One must bear in mind that the deficiencies seen in animal experiments may not extrapolate to humans. Nonetheless, the newer information on manganese and calcium interactions suggest that irregularities in bone attributed to calcium may have their basis in manganese deficiency or mismanagement. Calcium–manganese interactions require more detailed monitoring. Since manganese is a component of at least three metalloenzymes in mammals, it must be an essential element for humans. Nevertheless, this needs to be demonstrated through evidence of deficiency signs. The unique role that manganese plays in catalysis deserves further study.

REFERENCES

1. McHargue JS. Further evidence that small quantities of copper, manganese and zinc are factors in the metabolism of animals. Am J Physiol 1926; 77: 245–255.
2. Kemmerer AR, Elvehjem CA, Hart EB. Studies on the relation of manganese to the nutrition of the mouse. J Biol Chem 1931; 92: 623–630.
3. Orent ER, McCollum EV. Effects of deprivation of manganese in the rat. J Biol Chem 1931; 92: 651–678.
4. Wilgus HS Jr, Norris LC, Heuser GF. The role of certain inorganic elements in the cause and prevention of perosis. Science 1936; 84: 252–253.
5. Cotzias GC, Miller ST, Edwards J. Neutron activation analysis: the stability of the manganese concentration in human blood and plasma. J Lab Clin Med 1966; 67: 936–949.
6. Bird ED, Collins GH, Dodson MH, Grant LC. The effect of phenothiazine on the manganese concentration in the basal ganglia of sub-human primates by activation analysis. *Proc. Int. Congr. Neuro-Genet. Neuro-Ophthalmol. World Fed. Neurol 2nd, Vol. 1,* 1967:600–605.
7. Thomson ABR, Volberg LS. Intestinal uptake of iron, cobalt, and manganese in the iron deficient rat. Am J Physiol 1972; 223: 1327–1329.
8. Papavasiliou PS, Miller ST, Cotzias GC. Role of liver in regulating distribution and excretion of manganese. Am J Physiol 1966; 211: 211–216.

9. Schramm VL, Brandt M. The manganese (II) economy of rat hepatocytes. Fed Proc 1986; 45: 2817–2820.

10. Davis CD, Zech L, Greger JL. Manganese metabolism in rats: an improved methodology for assessing gut endogenous losses. PSEBM 1993; 202: 103–108.

11. Davidsson L, Lönnerdal B, Sandström B, Kunz C, Keen CL. Identification of transferrin as the major plasma carrier protein for manganese introduced orally or intravenously or after in vitro addition in the rat. J Nutr 1989; 119: 1461–1464.

12. Scheuhammer AM, Cherian MG. Binding of manganese in human and rat plasma. Biochim Biophys Acta 1985; 840: 163–169.

13. Klausner RD. From receptors to genes—insights from molecular iron metabolism. Clinical Res 1988; 36: 494–500.

14. Harris WR, Chen Y. Electron paramagnetic resonance and difference ultraviolet studies of Mn^{2+} binding to serum transferrin. J Inorg Biochem 1994; 54: 1–19.

15. Aschner M, Aschner JL. Manganese transport across the blood–brain barrier: relationship to iron homeostasis. Brain Res Bull 1990; 24: 857–860.

16. Hurley LS, Keen CL. Manganese. In: Mertz W, ed. Trace Elements in Human and Animal Nutrition. Vol. 1. New York: Academic Press, 1987:185–223.

17. Baker DH, Halpin KM. Research note: efficacy of a manganese-protein chelate compared with that of manganese sulfate for chicks. Poultry Sci 1987; 66: 1561–1563.

18. Henry PR, Ammerman CB, Miles RD. Relative bioavailability of manganese in a manganese-methionine complex for broiler chicks. Poultry Sci 1989; 68: 107–112.

19. Masters DG, Keen CL, Lönnerdal B, Hurley LS. Release of zinc from maternal tissues during zinc deficiency or simultaneous zinc and calcium deficiency in the pregnant rat. J Nutr 1986; 116: 2148–2154.

20. Rosenblum CI, Leach RM Jr. Biliary copper excretion in the chicken. Biol Trace Elem Res 1985; 8: 47–63.

21. Erway LC, Hurley LS, Fraser AS. Neurologic defect: manganese in phenocopy and prevention of a genetic abnormality of inner ear. Science 1966; 152: 1766–1768.

22. Rolfsen RM, Erway LC. Trace metals and otolith defects in mocha mice. J Hered 1984; 75: 158–162.

23. Erway LC, Mitchell SE. Prevention of otolith defect in pastel mink by manganese supplementation. J Hered 1973; 64: 111–119.

24. Cotzias GC, Tang LC, Miller ST, Sladic-Simic D, Hurley LS. A mutation influencing the transportation of manganese, L-Dopa, L-Tryptophan. Science 1972; 176: 410–412.

25. Shils ME, McCollum EV. Further studies on the symptoms of manganese deficiency in the rat and mouse. J Nutr 1943; 26: 1–19.

26. Bentley OG, Phillips PH. The effect of low manganese rations upon dairy cattle. J Dairy Sci 1951; 34: 396–403.

27. Dyer IA, Rojas MA. Manganese requirements and function in cattle. J Am Vet Med Assoc 1965; 147: 1393–1396.

28. Plumlee MP, Thrasher DM, Beeson WM, Andrews FN, Parker HE. The effects of a manganese deficiency upon the growth, development, and reproduction of swine. J Animal Sci 1956; 15: 352–367.

29. Lyons M, Insko WM Jr. Chondrodystrophy in the chick embryo produced by manganese deficiency in the diet of the hen. K Agric Exp Sta Bull 1937; 371: 61–75.

30. Lyons M. Some effects of manganese on eggshell quality. Arkansas Agric Exp Sta Bull 1939; 374: 1–18.

31. Gallup WD, Norris LC. The effect of a deficiency of manganese in the diet of the hen. Poultry Sci 1939; 18: 83–88.

32. Caskey CD, Norris LC. Micromelia in adult fowl caused by manganese deficiency during embryonic development. Proc Soc Exp Biol Med 1940; 44: 332–225.

33. Boyer PD, Shaw JH, Phillips PH. Studies on manganese deficiency in the rat. J Biol Chem 1942; 143: 417–423.

34. Smith SE, Medlicot M, Ellis GH. Manganese deficiency in the rabbit. Arch Biochem Biophys 1944; 4: 281–289.
35. Rojas MS, Dyer IA, Cassett WA. Manganese deficiency in the bovine. J Animal Sci 1965; 24: 664–667.
36. Hurley LS, Everson GJ, Wooten E, Asling CW. Disproportionate growth in offspring of manganese-deficient rats. 1. The long bones. J Nutr 1961; 74: 274–281.
37. Miller RC, Keith TB, McCarty MA, Thorp WTS. Manganese as a possible factor influencing the occurrence of lameness in pigs. Proc Soc Exp Biol Med 1940; 45: 50–51.
38. Ellis GH, Smith SE, Gates EM. Further effects of manganese deficiency in the rabbit. J Nutr 1947; 34: 21–31.
39. Tsai H-C, Everson GJ. Effect of manganese deficiency on the acid mucopolysaccharides in cartilage of guinea pigs. J Nutr 1967; 91: 447–452.
40. VanReen R, Pearson PB. Manganese deficiency in the duck. J Nutr 1955; 55: 225–234.
41. Combs GF, Norris LC, Neuser GF. The interrelationship of manganese, phosphatase and vitamin D in bone development. J Nutr 1967; 23: 131–140.
42. Wolbach SB, Hegsted DM. Perosis: epiphyseal cartilage in choline and manganese deficiencies in the chick. Arch Pathol 1953; 56: 437–453.
43. Leach RM Jr. Effect of manganese upon the epiphyseal growth plate in the young chick. Poultry Sci 1968; 47: 828–830.
44. Leach RM Jr, Muenster AM. Studies on the role on manganese in bone formation. I. Effect upon the mucopolysaccharide content of chick bone. J Nutr 1962; 78: 51–56.
45. Liu AC-H, Heinrichs BS, Leach RM Jr. Influence of manganese deficiency on the characteristics of proteoglycans of avian epiphyseal growth plate cartilage. Poultry Sci 1994; 73:663–669.
46. Hurley LS, Gowan J, Milhaud G. Calcium metabolism in manganese-deficient and zinc-deficient rats. Proc Soc Exp Biol Med 1969; 130: 856–860.
47. Strause LG, Hegenauer J, Saltman P, Cone R, Resnick D. Effects of long-term dietary manganese and copper deficiency on rat skeleton. J Nutr 1986; 116: 135–141.
48. Strause L, Saltman P, Smith KT, Bracker M, Andon MB. Spinal bone loss in postmenopausal women supplemented with calcium and trace minerals. J Nutr 1994; 124: 1060–1064.
49. Liu AC-H. The effect of manganese on the quantity and characteristics of proteoglycans found in cartilage and bone. M.Sc. thesis in Nutrition. The Pennsylvania State University, University Park, PA, 1990.
50. Mueller WJ, Schraer R, Schraer H. Calcium metabolism and skeletal dynamics of laying pullets. J Nutr 1964; 84: 20–26.
51. Candlish JK, Folt FJ. The proteoglycans of fowl cortical and medullary bone. Comp Biochem Physiol 1971; 40B: 283–293.
52. Hurley LS, Wooten E, Everson GJ, Asling CW. Anomalous development of ossification in the inner ear of offspring of manganese-deficient rats. J Nutr 1960; 71: 15–19.
53. Shrader RE, Everson GJ. Anomalous development of otoliths associated with postural defects in manganese-deficient guinea pigs. J Nutr 1967; 91: 453–460.
54. Shrader RE, Erway LC, Hurley LS. Mucopolysaccharide synthesis in the developing inner ear of manganese-deficient and pallied mutant mice. Teratology 1973; 8: 257–266.
55. Rubenstein AH, Leven NW, Elliott GA. Manganese-induced hypoglycemia. Lancet 1962; ii: 1348–1351.
56. Everson GH, Shrader RE. Abnormal glucose tolerance in manganese-deficient guinea pigs. J Nutr 1968; 94: 89–94.
57. Baly DL, Curry DL, Keen CL, Hurley LS. Effect of manganese deficiency on insulin secretion and carbohydrate homeostasis in rats. J Nutr 1984; 114: 1438–1446.
58. Baly DL, Curry DL, Keen CL, Hurley LS. Dynamics of insulin and glucagon release in rats: influence of dietary manganese. Endocrinology 1985; 116: 1734–1740.
59. Baly DL, Lee I, Doshi R. Mechanism of decreased insulinogenesis in manganese-deficient rats: decreased insulin mRNA levels. Fed Eur Biochem Soc 1988; 239: 55–58.

60. Baly DL, Schneiderman JS, Garcia-Welsh AL. Effect of manganese deficiency on insulin binding, glucose transport and metabolism in rat adipocytes. J Nutr 1990; 120: 1075–1079.

61. Walter RM Jr, Aoki TT, Keen CL. Acute oral manganese administration does not consistently affect glucose tolerance in non-diabetic and type II diabetic humans. J Trace Elem Exp Med 1991; 4: 73–79.

62. Brannon PM, Collins VP, Korc M. Alterations of pancreatic digestive enzyme content in the manganese-deficient rat. J Nutr 1987; 117: 305–311.

63. Amdur MO, Norris LC, Heuser GF. The lipotropic action of manganese. J Biol Chem 1946; 164: 783–784.

64. Bell LT, Hurley LS. Ultrastructural effects of manganese deficiency in liver, heart, kidney, and pancreas of mice. Lab Invest 1973; 29: 723–736.

65. Curran G. Effect of certain transition group elements on hepatic synthesis of cholesterol in the rat. J Biol Chem 210: 765–770.

66. Klimis-Tavantzis DJ, Kris-Etherton PM, Leach RM Jr. The effect of dietary manganese deficiency on cholesterol and lipid metabolism in the estrogen-treated chicken and the laying hen. J Nutr 1983; 113: 320–327.

67. Klimis-Tavantzis DJ, Leach RM Jr, Kris-Etherton PM. The effect of dietary manganese deficiency on cholesterol and lipid metabolism in the Wistar rat and in the genetically hypercholesterolemic RICO rat. J Nutr 1983; 113: 328–336.

68. Kawano J, Ney DM, Keen CL, Schneeman BO. Altered high density lipoprotein composition in manganese-deficient Sprague-Dawley and Wistar rats. J Nutr 1987; 117: 902–906.

69. Davis CD, Ney DM, Greger JL. Manganese, iron and lipid interactions in rats. J Nutr 1990; 120: 507–513.

70. Anonymous. Manganese deficiency in humans: Fact or fiction? Nutr Rev 1988; 46: 348–352.

71. O'Dell BL, Campbell BJ. Trace elements: metabolism and metabolic function. Comp Biochem 1971; 21: 179–226.

72. Dismukes CG, Siderer Y. Intermediates of a polynuclear manganese center involved in photosynthetic oxidation of water. Proc Natl Acad Sci (USA) 1981; 78: 274–278.

73. Weisiger RA, Fridovich I. Superoxide dismutase. J Biol Chem 1973; 248: 3582–3592.

74. Gorecki M, Beck Y, Hartman JR, et al. Recombinant human superoxide dismutases: production and potential therapeutical uses. Free Radical Res Commun 1991; 1: 401–410.

75. Hassan HM. Biosynthesis and regulation of superoxide dismutases. Free Radical Biol Med 1988; 5: 377–385.

76. Beyer W, Imlay J, Fridovich I. Superoxide dismutases. Prog Nucleic Acid Res Mol Biol 1991; 40: 221–253.

77. Borgstahl GEO, Parge HE, Hickey MJ, Beyers WF Jr, Hallewell RA, Tainer JA. The structure of human mitochondrial manganese superoxide dismutase reveals a novel tetrameric interface of two 4-helix bundles. Cell 1992; 71: 107–118.

78. Paynter DI. Changes in activity of manganese superoxide dismutase enzyme in tissues of the rat with changes in dietary manganese. J Nutr 1980; 110: 437–447.

79. De Rosa G, Keen CL, Leach RM, Hurley LS. Regulation of superoxide dismutase activity by dietary manganese. J Nutr 1980; 110: 795–804.

80. Zidenberg-Cherr S, Keen CL, Lonnerdahl B, Hurley LS. Superoxide dismutase activity and lipid peroxidation in the rat: developmental correlations affect by manganese deficiency. J Nutr 1983; 113: 2498–2504.

81. Dreosti IE, Manuel SJ, Buckley RA. Superoxide dismutase (EC 1.15.1.1), manganese and the effect of ethanol in adult and foetal rats. Br J Nutr 1982; 48: 205–210.

82. Wong GHW, Goeddel DV. Induction of manganous superoxide dismutase by tumor necrosis factor: possible protective mechanism. Science 1988; 242: 941–944.

83. Scrutton MC. Manganese and pyruvate carboxylase. In Schramm Vl, Wedler FC, eds. Manganese in Metabolism and Enzyme Function. New York: Academic Press, 1986:147–163.

84. Bentle LA, Lardy HA. Interactions of anions and divalent metal ions with phosphoenol pyruvate carboxykinase. J Biol Chem 1976; 251: 2916–2921.

85. Farron F. Arginase isozymes and their detection by catalytic staining in starch gel. Anal Biochem 1973; 53: 264–268.

86. Harell D, Sokolovsky M. Beef-liver arginase isolation and molecular properties. Eur J Biochem 1972; 25: 102–106.

87. Shank M, Barynin V, Dismukes GC. Protein coordination to manganese determines the high catalytic rate of dimanganese catalases. Comparison to functional catalase mimics. Biochemistry 1994; 33: 15433–15436.

88. Wedler FC, Toms R. Interactions of Mn(II) with mammalian glutamine synthetase. In: Schramm VL, Wedler FC, eds. Manganese in Metabolism and Enzyme Function. New York: Academic Press, 1986:221–238.

89. Leach RM Jr, Gross JR. The effect of manganese deficiency upon the ultrastructure of the eggshell. Poultry Sci 1983; 62: 499–504.

90. Longstaff M, Hill R. The hexosamine and uronic acid contents of the matrix of shells of eggs from pullets fed on diets of different manganese content. Br Poultry Sci 1972; 13: 377–385.

91. Hascall VC. Proteoglycans: the chondroitin sulfate/keratan sulfate proteoglycan of cartilage. Biochemistry 1988; 1: 189–198.

92. Leach RM Jr, Muenster A-M, Wien EM. Studies on the role of manganese in bone formation. II. Effect upon chondroitin sulfate synthesis in chick epiphyseal cartilage. Arch Biochem Biophys 1969; 133: 22–28.

93. McNatt ML, Fisher FM, Elders MJ, Kilgore BS, Smith WG, Hughes ER. Uridine diphosphate xylosyltransferase activity in cartilage from manganese-deficient chicks. Biochem J 1976; 160: 211–216.

94. Morrison JF, Ebner KE. Studies on galactosyltransferase. Kinetic investigations with glucose as the galactosyl group acceptor. J Biol Chem 1971; 246: 3985–3991.

95. Morrison JF, Ebner KE. Studies on galactosyltransferase. Kinetic effects of β-lactalbumin with N-acetylclucosamine and glucose as galactosyl group acceptors. J Biol Chem 1971; 246: 3992–3998.

96. Powell JT, Brew K. Metal ion activation of galactosyltransferase. J Biol Chem 1976; 251: 3645–3652.

97. Powell JT, Brew K. A comparison of the interactions of galactosyltransferase with a glycoprotein substrate (ovalbumin) and with β-lactalbumin. J Biol Chem 1976; 251: 3653–3663.

98. O'Keeffe ET, Hill RL, Bell JE. Active site of bovine galactosyltransferase: Kinetic and fluorescence studies. Biochemistry 1980; 19: 4954–4962.

99. Myllylä R, Anttinen H, Kivirikko KI. Metal activation of galactosylhydroxylysyl glucosyltransferase, an intracellular enzyme of collagen biosynthesis. Eur J Biochem 1979; 101: 261–269.

100. National Research Council. Nutrient Requirements of Poultry, 9th rev. ed. Washington, DC: National Academy Press, 1994.

101. McLeod BE, Robinson MF. Metabolic balance of manganese in young women. Br J Nutr 1972; 27: 221–227.

102. Friedman BJ, Freeland-Graves JH, Bales CW, et al. Manganese balance and clinical observations in young men fed a manganese-deficient diet. J Nutr 1987; 117: 133–143.

103. Freeland-Graves JH, Behmardi F, Bales CW, et al. Metabolic balance of manganese in young men consuming diets containing five levels of dietary manganese. J Nutr 1988; 118: 764–773.

104. Johnson PE, Lykken GI. Manganese and calcium absorption and balance in young women fed diets with varying amounts of manganese and calcium. J Trace Elem Exp Med 1991; 4: 19–35.

105. Schroeder HA, Balassa JJ, Tipton IH. Essential trace metals in man: manganese, a study in homeostasis. J Chron Dis 1966; 19: 545–571.

106. Wenlock RW, Buss DH, Dixon EJ. Trace nutrients 2. Manganese in British food. Br J Nutr 1979; 41: 253–261.

107. Guthrie BE, Robinson MF. Daily intakes of manganese, copper, zinc and cadmium by New Zealand women. Br J Nutr 1977; 38: 55–63.

108. Matsuda A, Kimura M, Kataoka M, Ohkuma S-I, Sato M, Itokawa Y. Quantifying manganese in lymphocytes to assess manganese nutritional status. Clin Chem 1989; 35: 1939–1941.

109. Davis CD, Malecki EA, Greger JL. Interactions among dietary manganese, heme iron, and nonheme iron in women. Am J Clin Nutr 1992; 56: 926–932.

110. Smeyers-Verbeke J, May C, Crochmans P, Massart DL. The determination of Cu, Zn, and Mn in subcellular rat liver fractions. Anal Biochem 1977; 83: 746–753.

111. Chang SC, Brannon PM, Korc M. Effects of dietary manganese deficiency on rat pancreatic amylase mRNA levels. J Nutr 1990; 120: 1228–1234.

112. Brannon PM, Collins VP, Korc M. Alterations of pancreatic digestive enzyme content in the manganese-deficient rat. J Nutr 1987; 117: 305–311.

113. Keen CL, Lonnerdal B, Hurley LS. Metabolism and biochemistry of manganese. In: Frieden E, ed. Biochemistry of the Essential Ultratrace Elements. New York: Plenum, 1984: 89–132.

114. Korc M. Manganese as a modulator of signal transduction pathways. In: Prasad AS, ed. Essential and Toxic Elements in Human Health and Disease: An Update. New York: Wiley-Liss, 1993:235–255.

115. Matrone G, Hartman RH, Clawson A. Studies of a manganese iron antagonism in the nutrition of rabbits and baby pigs. J Nutr 1959; 67: 309–317.

116. Hartman RH, Matrone G, Wise GH. Effect of high dietary manganese on hemoglobin formation. J Nutr 1955; 57: 429–439.

117. Mena I. Manganese. In: Bonner F, Coburn JW, eds. Disorders of Mineral Metabolism. Vol. 1. New York: Academic Press, 1981:233–270.

118. Exon JH, Koller LD. Effects of feeding manganese antiknock gasoline additive exhaust residues (Mn_3O_4) in rats. Bull Environ Contam Toxicol 1975; 14: 370–373.

119. Rjazanov VA. Criteria and methods for establishing maximum permissible concentrations of air pollution. Bull WHO 1965; 32: 389.

120. Neff NH, Barret RE, Costa E. Selective depletion of caudate nucleus dopamine and serotonin during chronic manganese dioxide administration to squirrel monkeys. Experientia 1969; 25: 1140–1141.

121. Mena I. In: Vinken PJ, Bruyn GW, eds. Handbook of Clinical Neurology. Amsterdam: North-Holland, 1979: 217–237.

122. McNatt ML, Fiser FM, Elders MJ, Kilgore BS, Smith WG, Hughes ER. Uridine diphosphate xylosyltransferase activity in cartilage from manganese-deficient chicks. Biochem J 1976; 160: 211–216.

123. Benedict CR, Kett J, Porter J. Properties of farnesyl pyrophosphate synthetase of pig liver. Arch Biochem Biophys 1965; 110: 611–621.

124. Pease EA, Andrawis A, Tien M. Manganese-dependent peroxidase from phanerochaete chrysosporium: primary structure deduced from cDNA. J Biol Chem 1989; 264: 13531–13535.

11
Cobalt

RICHARD M. SMITH
CSIRO, Adelaide, Australia

I. INTRODUCTION

Cobalt is not an abundant element in the earth's crust. Clarke (1) calculated that the igneous rocks of the earth's surface contain about 10 ppm cobalt, as compared with 200 ppm nickel, and later estimates are also of this order. Gold-quartz veins are the ultimate residual product of high-silica magmas, and these contain only traces of cobalt (2).

Although it is not abundant, cobalt is widely diffused in nature and occurs at relatively low concentrations in rocks, seawater, soils, plants, and animals. In its ionic form, cobalt is an essential nutrient only for certain bacteria and algae, in which its use is confined to the synthesis of a range of cobamides (cobalt-containing corrinoids) which include vitamin B_{12}. Preformed vitamin B_{12} is required by all forms of animal life, and vitamin B_{12} or other cobamides are required by certain bacteria, but cobamides appear not to be required or used by plants (see, however, Ref. 3). The essential requirement for vitamin B_{12} by animals thus reflects an ancient symbiotic relationship between animals and microorganisms in which no form of animal life evolved with the capacity to synthesize the corrin ring or to find a substitute for the remarkable catalytic properties of the bound cobalt atom. The symbiosis is direct in the case of ruminants. In these animals, vitamin B_{12} is produced during fermentation of food in the forestomach (rumen) and absorbed in the ileum for use by the animal's tissues.

The taxonomic classifications of organisms that produce cobamides and so require cobalt and those that require cobamides but do not produce them are shown in Figure 1. The symbiotic relationships to serve the latter must arise either directly or indirectly from the limited sources shown. Seawater, for example, contains enough algal or bacterial cobamides (0.1–50 ng/L) to meet the needs of most organisms that live there.

The vitamin B_{12} molecule has been said to be the most complex nonpolymeric

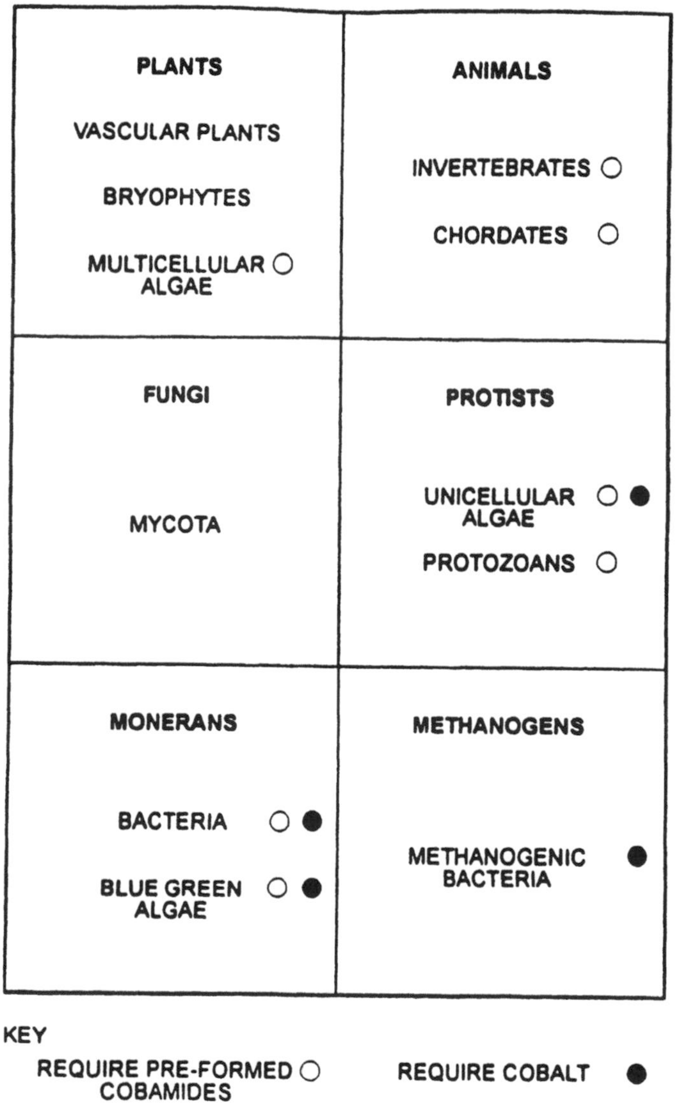

PLANTS	ANIMALS
VASCULAR PLANTS BRYOPHYTES MULTICELLULAR ○ ALGAE	INVERTEBRATES ○ CHORDATES ○
FUNGI	PROTISTS
MYCOTA	UNICELLULAR ○ ● ALGAE PROTOZOANS ○
MONERANS	METHANOGENS
BACTERIA ○ ● BLUE GREEN ○ ● ALGAE	METHANOGENIC ● BACTERIA

KEY

REQUIRE PRE-FORMED ○   REQUIRE COBALT ●
COBAMIDES

FIGURE 1 Cobalt and cobamide requirements of living organisms. Organisms that produce co-bamides and therefore require cobalt (●) or that require preformed cobamides (○) and so must live in symbiotic relationship with those that produce cobamides are shown in relationship to six kingdoms of living organisms. Except for the animal kingdom in which all members require preformed cobalamin, only a few members of each of the marked classifications may manufacture or require cobamides.

compound yet identified, and it appears to have arisen at a very early stage in the evolution of life on the planet. It was pointed out by Dickman (4) that some strains of the strictly anaerobic *Clostridia* produce corrinoids but do not produce porphyrins, and it was sug-gested that the requirement for cobalt-containing corrinoids may have emerged before the requirement for iron porphyrins. The primitive anaerobe *Clostridium thermoaceticum* brings about the synthesis of acetate solely from carbon monoxide or from hydrogen and carbon dioxide by a corrinoid-dependent pathway that presumably arose in a primordial atmosphere prior to the appearance of significant amount of oxygen (5). Somewhat similar reasoning applies to the production of B_{12} factor III, a related cobamide, by *Methanosarcina barkeri*. The methanogens have now been recognized on molecular biological grounds as a separate kingdom from the monerans and are thought to be very ancient indeed (6). If this reasoning is valid, then the unique catalytic possibilities of a cobalt atom constrained in a porphyrinlike ring were taken advantage of very early in evolutionary history by primitive life forms, and the detailed structural solution to the biochemical problems encountered then has remained unimproved.

The recognition of cobalt as a trace element essential for grazing sheep came in 1934 (7), fourteen years before the discovery of the anti-pernicious anemia factor from liver. This factor contained 4% cobalt and was named vitamin B_{12} (8). Sheep grazing on pastures grown on consolidated dunes of wind-blown calcareous sands in coastal regions of South Australia suffered a wasting condition known locally as coast disease. This disease could be prevented or reversed by moving the sheep periodically to sound pastures inland. A dual deficiency of copper and cobalt proved to prevail, but the effect of cobalt on the wasting disease was immediate and striking (7). The reported response to cobalt was followed almost at once by a report of a concurrent outcome in Western Australia (9). Accounts of the widespread occurrence of cobalt deficiency in ruminants have appeared worldwide over the intervening period, and the condition has been the subject of detailed biochemical study (10). All significant outcomes of cobalt deficiency in ruminant herbivores are attributable to a systemic deficiency of vitamin B_{12}. Two of the three demonstrated enzymic functions of vitamin B_{12} in animal tissues become critically depleted. The first of these is the action of methylmalonyl coenzyme A mutase, one of the sequence of reactions by which propionate produced in the rumen is introduced into the pool of common metabolites of the tricarboxylic acid cycle. Methylmalonyl coenzyme A mutase employs 5′-deoxyadenosylcobalamin as coenzyme. Failure of this sequence is linked closely to failure of appetite in ruminants (11). The second critical enzyme depletion is that of methionine synthetase, responsible for the remethylation of homocysteine. The latter is produced when S-adenosyl methionine donates its labile methyl group in any of a variety of biological methylation reactions. The reduced ability of the vitamin B_{12}-deficient animal to restore and sustain its S-adenosyl methionine and methionine status leads to such outcomes as severe depletion of tissue folates and the loss of lipotropic capacity (10).

With very few exceptions, the roles of cobalt in biology are played by cobamides, and a description of the biology of cobalt becomes a discussion of the modes of action of cobamides. The very few exceptions are of great interest, in that the cobalt fulfils the same function as a cobamide. The biological reactions served by cobalt are closely defined and highly conserved. The coordination chemistry of cobalt is fundamental to the unique biochemistry of the cobamides.

II. CHEMICAL PROPERTIES OF COBALT

A. Oxidation States

Cobalt is a Mendeleeff Group 8 element with atomic number 27 and atomic weight 58.94. It is a member of the iron triad of iron, cobalt, nickel. Orbital electron arrangement is written $1s^2$, $2s^2$, $3s^2$, $3p^6$, $3d^7$, $4s^2$. The stable valency of ionic compounds of cobalt is 2; the trivalent ionic cobalt compounds are unstable. Thus cobalt occupies an intermediate position between iron (trivalent stable) and nickel, for which trivalent ions probably do not exist.

B. Chelating and Binding Properties

Cobalt provides the classical example of the coordination chemistry of metallic atoms. The biochemical properties of the cobamides are a reflection of and an evolutionary biochemical exploitation of this feature of the chemistry of cobalt and of its capacity to exist in three oxidation states. Only complexes of Co(III) are considered here.

The cobaltammines [parent $Co(NH_3)_6]^{3+}$ are the exemplars of metal coordination in which coordination occurs through the two unshared electrons of the nitrogen atoms of ammonia molecules. By replacement of the ammonia molecules with various anions, a large series of pentammines, tetrammines, triammines, diammines, monammines, and finally, of compounds that contain no ammonia but retain the coordinated structure of cobaltammines, can be prepared. The structure is that of a Co(III) ion surrounded by six coordinately linked groups in the form of an octahedron. The structural integrity of the compound is attributable to the coordinate links, which here exhibit the stability usually associated with covalent bonds. For conceptual clarity, Pauling's valence bond (12) notation will be used in the following discussion, although matching and satisfactory renderings can be made for these substances by either the ligand field theory (13) or molecular orbital theory (14). According to valence bond theory, two of the five $3d$ orbitals of the Co(III) ion must be reserved for hybridization to form the six d^2sp^3 orbitals used for bonding by paired electrons from the six donor atoms. Thus the six remaining $3d$ electrons of Co(III) must be assigned to the three remaining $3d$ orbitals. The configuration of the octahedrally oriented d^2sp^3 orbitals is shown in Figure 2.

A spatial rendering of the 6-coordinate octahedral structure of CO(III) is given in Figure 3; such compounds may be isolated in the form of salts $[Co(NH_3)_6]X_3$, where X may be a monovalent anion, half of a bivalent anion, or one-third of a trivalent anion. Anion-substituted triammines are electrically neutral $[Co(NH_3)_3X_3]$ and do not form salts. Unlike the hexaaquated cobalt III complex, which is unstable and converts readily to ionic cobalt II, cobalt III hexammine is very stable (15). All of the hexacoordinated cobalt III cobamides are of the octahedral conformation.

C. Cobalt in the Cobamides

The general form of cobamides is shown in Figure 4. In crystalline form and often in solution, the cobalt atom is hexacoordinated in octahedral conformation, as in the hexammines with the square planar bonding electron pairs donated by the nitrogen atoms of the porphyrinlike corrin ring. The convention adopted here for structural representation and nomenclature of cobamides is that of Ref. 16. In vitamin B_{12}, or cobalamin, the α ligand is 5,6-dimethylbenzimidazole, and the β ligand is the cyano group linked in a carbon–cobalt bond to the central cobalt atom. The two metabolically active forms of cobalamin in animal tissues are 5-deoxyadenosyl cobalamin (Fig. 5) and methyl cobalamin, in which a methyl group substitutes for deoxyadenosine. Both substituents are linked to cobalt through carbon–cobalt bonds.

Bacterial cobamides exist in a variety of forms in which the α ligand may differ from that in the cobalamins. Forms in which the α (aglycon) ligand is other than 5,6-dimethyl-

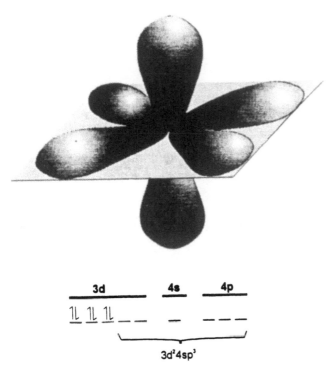

FIGURE 2 Valence bond treatment of octahedral d^2sp^3 hybrid bonds in coordination compounds of cobalt. Note that six orbitals, one s orbital, three p orbitals, and two of the five d orbitals, are involved in hybridization.

benzimidazole are not active in animal cells and are generally not well absorbed from the alimentary tract.

X-ray studies have shown that in the crystalline form of 5-deoxyadenosylcobalamin the adenine ring is approximately parallel to the corrin plane and that it is sterically hindered from free rotation about the cobalt carbon bond. It is also found that the corrin ring of 5-deoxyadenosyl cobalamin is buckled. Both distortions may be relevant to the mode of action of the coenzyme form of vitamin B_{12} (17).

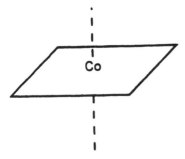

FIGURE 3 A spatial rendering of the 6-coordinate, octahedral structure of Co(III). Four of the coordinates are in a plane and two extend on either side of the plane.

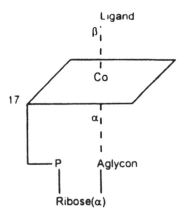

FIGURE 4 General structure of the cobamides with the α ligand below the plane and the β ligand above.

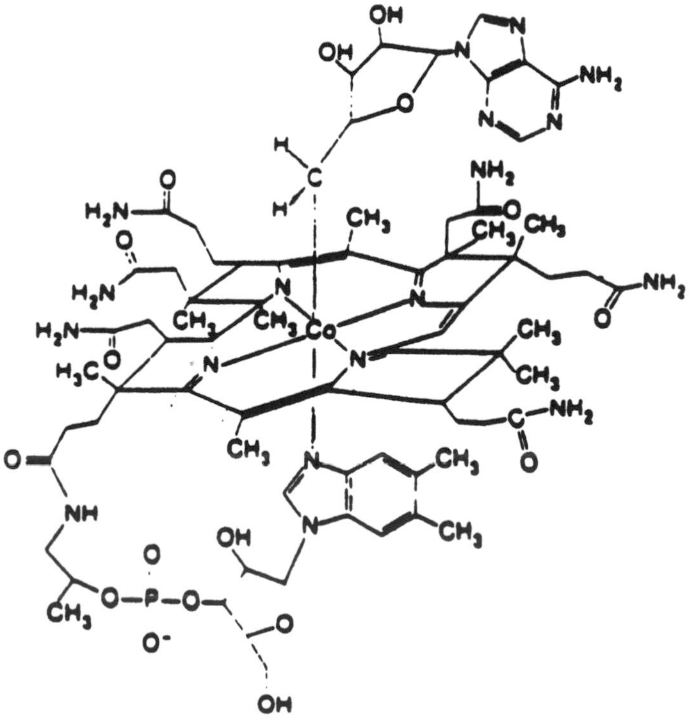

FIGURE 5 Structure of the 5′-deoxyadenosylcobalamin form of vitamin B_{12}. Deoxyadenosyl occupies the β position which may be occupied by methyl or by cyanide ion, the isolated form of vitamin B_{12} (cyanocobalamin).

In a review of the coordination chemistry of the vitamin B_{12}-dependent mutase reactions (of which 10 are known, with two of them occurring in animal tissues), Pratt (18) has advanced reasons for the inevitability of evolutionary selection of cobalt as the biochemical catalyst for the kind of intramolecular rearrangement in which vitamin B_{12} is involved. As will be described, the mutase actions of vitamin B_{12} involve the homopolar making and breaking of cobalt–carbon bond, with the formation of a 5'-deoxyadenosyl radical and a cobalt II atom. Both elements of these enzymes, the vitamin B_{12} molecule and the particular enzyme protein are involved in sequential components of these unique reactions. According to Pratt (18), only cobalt could have fulfilled all of the requirements for them and the reactions involving methyl cobalamin to occur.

III. ANALYTICAL METHODOLOGY

With recognition that the symptoms of cobalt deficiency in ruminants are entirely explicable in terms of a systemic deficiency of vitamin B_{12}, it became logically more appropriate as well as technically simpler to determine the vitamin B_{12} status of the animal than to determine its cobalt status. Recognition that the earliest indications of vitamin B_{12} deficiency are often to be found in the appearance in the bloodstream of increased concentrations of those intermediates whose further metabolism is hindered by the lack of vitamin B_{12} has led to the use of circulating levels of methylmalonic acid and of homocysteine as indices of vitamin B_{12} status. Plant and soil analysis for cobalt remains important, however, and modern cobalt methodology addresses these outcomes. Monitoring of industrial exposure to cobalt is also an important need. Preferred methodology for the estimation of cobalt, vitamin B_{12}, methylmalonic acid, and homocysteine will be discussed briefly.

A. Estimation of Cobalt

Concentrations of cobalt in biological materials of plant or animal origin are very low (seldom above 0.5 ppm dry matter and often below 0.1 ppm dry), and the determination of cobalt requires considerable skill and care. Preliminary wet digestion in nitric, perchloric, and sulfuric acids may be necessary. The analytical method of choice is graphite-furnace atomic absorption spectrophotometry (AAS) (19,20) although neutron activation analysis is also feasible (21). Flame atomic absorption spectrophotometry is insufficiently sensitive.

In the method described by Baruthio and Pierre (20), a detection limit of 1.9 nmol/L and a sensitivity (absorbance 0.044) of 3.4 nmol/L were obtained. The method is suitable for serum (normal concentration around 2.7 nmol/L) or urine (normal concentration around 6.7 nmol/L). Wet digestion is followed by extraction of cobalt from the neutralized digest with ammonium pyrrolidine dithiocarbamate into isobutylmethylketone prior to AAS of the organic phase. Interference from the iron in hemoglobin occurs and represents a limitation to the method as described.

B. Estimation of Vitamin B_{12}

Vitamin B_{12} as cyanocobalamin was first isolated and characterized in 1948. For many years, the standard form of assay was microbiological, employing *Lactobacillus leichmanii* (ATCC 7830 and ATCC 4797), an organism that requires either vitamin B_{12} or any deoxyribonucleotide. Other microbiological assays used *Escherichia coli* mutants requiring vitamin B_{12} or methionine or the protists *Euglena gracilis* or *Ochromonas malha-*

mensis. Whereas the latter two show a specific requirement for vitamin B_{12}, *E. coli* responds also to a number of the vitamin B_{12} analogs.

Vitamin B_{12} is chemically defined as cyanocobalamin, but the vitamin B_{12} in blood and tissues is present mainly in the coenzyme form, adenosyl cobalamin, with smaller amounts of a second coenzyme, methyl cobalamin, and some hydroxocobalamin. The distribution of cobalamins in human tissues is shown in Table 1, derived from the work of Linnell (22) with percentages of blood components derived by Beck (23). Material for microbiological assay was generally preextracted in the presence of hot buffered cyanide, which not only released protein-bound cobalamin but also converted all of the cobalamins into cyanocobalamin. The latter effect, however, was unrecognized at the time.

Later assays for cobalamins have used the newer isotope dilution techniques that employ binding proteins more or less specific for vitamin B_{12}. A satisfactory protein for this purpose is Castle's "intrinsic factor," the binding protein specific for cobalamins that is secreted by gastric parietal cells and that is essential to the absorption of vitamin B_{12} in the terminal ileum. Use of other binding proteins, for example, the R proteins, is less specific and has led to estimates of circulating vitamin B_{12} that exceed those obtained with *L. leichmanii* (24). The presence in plasma and tissues of such noncobalamin B_{12} analogs, although adequately confirmed (25), has not been resolved satisfactorily. Neither the nature nor the source of this material is known, although there is some evidence that absorption of them from the gastrointestinal tract is independent of intrinsic factor (26).

Specific methods must therefore be employed for estimation of vitamin B_{12} from any source. Recent developments include radioimmunoassay using antisera raised by immunizing rabbits with the monocarboxylic acid derivative of cyanocobalamin coupled to human serum albumin (27) or with 5'-0-succinyl cyanocobalamin coupled to chicken serum albumin (28). Automated enzyme-linked binding assays based on porcine intrinsic factor have also been developed (29), and a simplified microtiter-plate microbiological assay of vitamin B_{12} using *L. leichmanii* has been published (30). Until the nature of the analogs that interfere with binding assays is better known, microbiological assay of vitamin B_{12} using *L. leichmanii* or binding assays involving intrinsic factor are likely to remain as standards.

C. Assays for Accumulating Substrates of Vitamin B_{12}-Dependent Enzymes

The two substrate-derived substances concerned are circulating levels of methylmalonic acid (from unmetabolized methylmalonyl coenzyme A) and homocysteine awaiting re-

TABLE 1 Distribution of Cobalamins in Human Tissues (22)

Tissue	(Units)	Total	Ado-Cbl (%)	Me-Cbl (%)	OH-Cbl (%)	CN-Cbl (%)
Liver	(μg/g)	555	69.8	4.0	26.2	0
Kidney	(μg/g)	134	52.2	25.3	22.5	0
Spleen	(μg/g)	63	43.0	37.3	19.7	0
Brain	(μg/g)	81	61.1	11.4	27.5	0
Blood						
Plasma [a]	(μg/l)	385	29	70	1	1
Erythrocyte [a]	(μg/l)	202	54	12	24	10

[a]Proportions in blood plasma and erthyrocytes were derived by Beck (23) from Linnell's graphical data.

methylation to form methionine. Both are elevated in the blood of most patients with vitamin B_{12} deficiency (31,32). Circulating methylmalonic acid is also elevated in the blood of cobalt-deficient sheep (33,34).

Serum methylmalonic acid may be measured by solvent extraction followed by capillary gas chromatography (35,36). Homocysteine may be estimated following capillary gas chromatography by mass spectrometry (37). An improved method involves preliminary reduction of homocysteine with dithiothreitol followed by treatment with iodoacetamide and purification by cation exchange (32).

It is generally agreed for both human and ovine vitamin B_{12} deficiency that plasma (or serum) methylmalonic acid provides the most sensitive and reliable single indication of incipient deficiency, but that measurement of both intermediates and of circulating cobalamin as well is more satisfactory (36,38).

IV. METABOLISM OF COBALT AND COBALAMIN

A. Metabolism of Cobalt

Gastrointestinal absorption of cobalt by both humans and small laboratory animals is quite efficient. Thus normal mice absorbed 26.2% of an oral dose of labeled cobalt (39), and balance studies in humans show gastrointestinal absorption of from 20% to 97% of dietary cobalt (40,41). Absorption of cobalt by ruminants is much less complete. Oral or intra-ruminal administration of cobalt to sheep or cattle is followed by fecal excretion of 84–98% of the dose within 14 days (42–44). The poor absorption may be a result of the rapid binding of cobalt by rumen microorganisms (44).

In nonruminants (and perhaps in ruminants), absorption of cobalt appears to share a common intestinal mucosal transport system with iron (45,46). Cobalt and iron mutually inhibit one another's absorption, and cobalt absorption is enhanced in iron deficiency (W. Forth and R. Rummel in Ref. 46, pp. 173–191).

Tissue distribution of injected radiocobalt is similar in most experimental animals, with initial rapid uptake by liver and kidney, and to a lesser extent by spleen, pancreas, and parts of the gastrointestinal tract (43,47,48). Loss of this label is relatively rapid, and with elapsed time the differences in distribution between tissues become less marked (48).

Concentrations of cobalt in the human body have been assessed in the Report of the Task Group on Reference Man (49). The report lists: whole blood, 0.31 ng Co/g; blood plasma, 0.45 ng/Co/g; erythrocytes, 0.14 ng Co/g; liver, 0.22 ng/Co/g; spleen, < 0.16 ng Co/g; kidney, 0.06 ng Co/g; heart, 0.11 ng Co/g; and pancreas, < 0.08 ng Co/g.

Excretion of cobalt from the human body occurs mainly via the urine (50,51, and this is also true of animals (48,52).

B. Metabolism of Vitamin B_{12}

A mixed diet in Western countries supplies 5–30 μg of vitamin B_{12} daily, of which 1–5 μg is absorbed. Urinary excretion of the absorbed vitamin B_{12} is relatively small (< 250 ng), and the unabsorbed vitamin B_{12} is excreted in the feces together with the overflow from an active enterohepatic circulation via the bile (53). The total body content of vitamin B_{12} is 2–5 mg in an adult male (54), and the turnover is 0.02–0.03% of this content per day (55). Although imprecise, these estimates suggest that the daily requirements for vitamin B_{12} lie in the range 1–2 μg and will be adequately met by currently recommend adult allowances of 1–3 μg/day (56,57).

The observation that the daily turnover of vitamin B_{12} in the human body is a small proportion of the body load (53–55) rather than a fixed daily amount provides an explanation of the body's ability to sustain reasonably adequate vitamin B_{12} function during long periods of relative deprivation (58). Thus progressively lower body stores are accompanied by progressively smaller daily losses and, in addition, at low oral intakes of vitamin B_{12}, the efficiency of absorption is high (59).

On a body-weight basis, the requirement for parenterally administered vitamin B_{12} by humans is less than that of other mammals, including that of ruminants (60). Minimum requirement for parenteral or absorbed vitamin B_{12} in the sheep (40–50 kg body weight) is estimated at around 11 μg/day (61,62). Injections of 150 μg every 14 days were adequate for lambs fed a cobalt-deficient diet (63). On the other hand, oral requirements for vitamin B_{12} by sheep are higher than those of other species, and oral doses of 100 μg of vitamin B_{12} per day were not adequate for young sheep fed a diet deficient in cobalt (64). By extrapolation, an oral requirement of around 200 μg of vitamin B_{12} per day would be needed to meet the needs of such animals, suggesting an absorptive efficiency of around 5%. The absorptive efficiency of vitamin B_{12} from the human diet may be as high as 80% (59).

1. Absorption and Transport of Vitamin B_{12}

Dietary intakes of vitamin B_{12} by mammals tend to be only marginally greater than their minimum needs. Perhaps in consequence of this, a series of absorption and transport proteins has evolved which show very high affinity as well as high to very high specificity for the cobalamins. The three proteins are (a) gastric intrinsic factor (IF), a glycoprotein secreted by gastric parietal cells; (b) haptocorrin (HC), a family of closely related glycoproteins also known as the R proteins which is produced by various secretory and accessory digestive organs; and (c) transcobalamin II (TCII), an unglycated protein produced by many cells and responsible for the transport of cobalamin in blood plasma from the site of absorption in the ileum to somatic cells in the body. Both IF and TCII are essential components of the vitamin B_{12} economy, but the function of haptocorrins is less clear. Haptocorrin found in blood plasma was formerly referred to as transcobalamin I (TCI).

The sequence of events during absorption, plasma transport, and tissue-cell uptake is reviewed by Seetharam et al. (56) and may be summarized as follows.

Gastric Phase

Low gastric pH and pepsin release protein-bound cobalamin (Cbl) in food (mostly adenosyl Cbl and Me-Cbl). At low pH, Cbl is bound mostly to HC. The IF present in acidic gastric juice is not bound to Cbl.

Luminal Phase

In the intestinal lumen, the pancreatic proteins partially hydrolyze the HC part of the complex and Cbl is released to complex with IF. The IF-Cbl complex traverses the small intestine and in the terminal part of the ileum becomes attached to the IF-Cbl receptor situated in the microvillus pits of the apical brush border membrane of the ileal enterocytes. The carbohydrate on the IF molecule has no role in binding either to Cbl or to the receptor but may protect the protein from proteolytic degradation.

Mucosal Phase

The binding site of the receptor is on the luminal side of the apical brush border. Binding requires neutral pH and calcium ions and is facilitated by bile salts. Evidence suggests that IF-Cbl is internalized by receptor-mediated endocytosis. The process by which Cbl is released from IF and bound to TCII within the enterocyte is not well understood but may involve lysosomes. The Cbl, now complexed to TCII, is released after a delay of 2–4 h from the basolateral domain of the cell and into the bloodstream. Neither the mechanism by which TCII-Cbl traverses the basal membrane, nor the regulatory process which appears to control the amount of TCII-Cbl released into the bloodstream is known (see 56). The specificity of IF for cobalamin is very high, but there is evidence that human blood contains considerable amounts of noncobalamin compounds that bind to haptocorrins. These substances have not been identified but appear to be absorbed from the ileum by a mechanism that does not involve IF (26). Both vitamin B_{12} and the analogs are secreted in bile, where they are bound to haptocorrin (66).

The specificity of the binding proteins from human sources for cobalamin and for some known and synthetic analogs was examined by Stupperich and Nexø (67), and some of their findings are shown in Table 2. It is clear that both IF and TCII are highly specific for vitamin B_{12} and that HC is much less specific. The table also reveals the features of the vitamin B_{12} molecule that convey this specificity. Thus effective binding of corrinoids to either IF or TCII did not occur unless the α ligand was coordinated with the cobalt atom. This restriction did not apply to haptocorrin, which was also relatively insensitive to substitution or deletion of the α ligand.

The authors concluded that intrinsic factor acts as a filter for the intestinal absorption of cobamides which contain a cobalt-coordinated N-heterocyclic nucleotide base and that transcobalamin II fulfils an analogous function for cobalamin-requiring cells (67).

All three vitamin B_{12}-binding proteins show structural homology with one another, although these are not close enough to bring about immunological cross-reactivity (56). Thus both IF (69) and HC (70) are encoded by genes on human chromosome 11 and both are secreted by the same tissues in a range of species. The genomic structures of IF and HC from human sources show strikingly similar intron-exon structure and several positionally conserved splice sites, suggesting that both arose in the distant past from a single ancestral gene, presumably by duplication. Amino acid similarities in corresponding exons range from 32% to 65% (70). The human TCII gene, which resides on chromosome 22 (71),

TABLE 2 Binding of Corrinoids by Intrinsic Factor (IF) Transcobalamin (TC11) and Haptocorrin (HC)

Corrinoid	Structure of the α-ligand nucleotide base	Base-on $(+)^b$ or base-off $(-)$	IF	TC11	HC
Vitamin B_{12} [a]	5,6-Dimethylbenzimidazole	+	1	1	1
Factor III	5-Hydroxybenzimidazole	+	8×10^{-1}	1	8×10^{-1}
Imidazolyl cobamide (guided biosynthesis)	Imidazole	+	1×10^{-1}	3×10^{-1}	8×10^{-1}
Pseudo-vitamin B_{12}	Adenine	±	2×10^{-3}	8×10^{-1}	1
Amino vitamin B_{12} (chemical synthesis)	2-Amino-5,6-dimethylbenzimidazole	−	1×10^{-5}	5×10^{-4}	5×10^{-1}
Cobinamide (chemical synthesis)	No α ligand	−	1×10^{-5}	5×10^{-4}	5×10^{-1}

[a]Apparent affinity constants of vitamin B_{12} for IF = 20, for TCII = 50, and for HC = 10 nmol/L (68).
[b]Whether or not the N atom of the α ligand is coordinated with the Co atom.
Source: Abridged from Ref. 67.

shows > 50% nucleotide homology with both IF and HC (72). The regions of amino acid homology common to all three proteins are located in seven domains of the amino acid sequence. The authors speculate that one or more of these domains is likely to be involved in cobalamin binding and that all three proteins probably resulted from divergences of a common ancestral gene (72).

2. Tissue Concentrations and Storage of Vitamin B_{12}

The distribution of the various cobalamins in human tissues have been given in Table 1. In Table 3 is set out the distribution of vitamin B_{12} in subcellular fractions of the livers of normal rats and of rats made deficient of vitamin B_{12} by total gastrectomy (73). The mitochondria, in which is to be found the enzyme methylmalonyl coenzyme A mutase, contain the largest fraction of the vitamin B_{12}, mainly in the form of adenosyl cobalamin. The same is true of kidney. Methyl cobalamin is associated with folate metabolism and is found in the supernatant cytosolic fraction. From Table 3 it is clear that a deficiency of vitamin B_{12} arising from gastrectomy reduces all fractions to about the same extent.

These observations are consistent with the view that the distribution of vitamin B_{12}, at least in liver, is functional and does not represent passive storage of an accumulated excess. There is still much to learn about the mechanisms that regulate the retention of vitamin B_{12} in the body, but it is possible that the kidney may retain and then redistribute Cbl on a short-term basis.

3. Excretion of Vitamin B_{12}

There is little excretion of vitamin B_{12} in urine. This is attributable in part to the presence in the bloodstream of an excess of haptocorrin which, although binding most (75%) of the circulating vitamin B_{12}, still has substantial unoccupied binding capacity There is virtually no vitamin B_{12} in blood plasma that is not bound to a high-affinity binder. A second renal mechanism exists that may ensure retention in the body of Cbl taken up by the kidney proximal tubule cell as well as regulate secretion into urine. Uptake of Cbl by renal tubule cells normally takes place during periods of cellular loading via Cbl-TCII from plasma (74). Resecretion of the retained Cbl may take place either as Cbl-HC or as Cbl-TCII. It was found that opossum kidney epithelial tubular cells synthesize both of these Cbl binders but secrete them in directionally differentiated ways. Thus HC is secreted only through the

TABLE 3 Subcellular Distribution of Vitamin B_{12} in the Livers of Normal and Gastrectomized Rats

Centrifugal fraction of homogenate of liver in 0.25 M sucrose	Normal rats, ng B_{12}/g liver	Gastrectomized rats, ng B_{12}/g liver
Nuclear	17.7 ± 10.7	4.7 ± 0.3
Mitochondria	56.1 ± 22.7	10.5 ± 10.8
Microsomes	1.7 ± 1.2	0.4 ± 0.3
Supernatant	16.9 ± 11.1	3.4 ± 3.4
Whole homogenate	103.9 ± 35.2	23.7 ± 16.8

Wistar albino rats were gastrectomized 12 weeks prior to preparation and differential centrifugation of homogenates of liver in 0.25 M sucrose.
Source: Abridged from Ref. 73.

basolateral membrane of the cell (for tissue retention), whereas TCII was secreted both basolaterally and apically (for excretion) (75).

It is clear that most systemic vitamin B_{12} excretion takes place in the feces, presumably via biliary secretion in excess of what will then be reabsorbed in the ileum. Much further work needs to be done in understanding both the renal tubular mechanisms that allow for sorting of vitamin B_{12} between retention and excretion and the ileal mucosal cell mechanisms that regulate the uptake of Cbl as Cbl-IF and its release as Cbl-TCII.

V. PHYSIOLOGIC FUNCTIONS OF VITAMIN B_{12}

The wide spectrum of effects of vitamin B_{12} deficiency in the mammalian body must be attributed to lowered activity of only two vitamin B_{12}-dependent enzymes. These are methylmalonyl coenzyme A mutase, which converts methylmalonyl CoA arising during the metabolism of propionate to succinyl CoA (a mainline intermediate in the energy yielding tricarboxylic acid cycle), and N5 methyl tetrahydrofolate-homocysteine methyl transferase (methionine synthetase), responsible for the remethylation of homocysteine to re-form the methyl donor molecule methionine. Consequences arising from the partial failure of one or both of these reactions are presumably responsible for all of the very wide spectrum of physiologic effects seen in vitamin B_{12} deficiency of various mammalian species. While the biochemical changes underlying many of these effects are clear, there are others that are not. This section outlines both kinds.

In the case of vitamin B_{12} deficiency in ruminants, the cause of the deficiency is a dietary lack of cobalt. In the case of human vitamin B_{12} deficiency, the predominant cause is malabsorption of vitamin B_{12}, although direct dietary deficiency does occur either in very young infants because of a low vitamin B_{12} status of the mother, or in the elderly, although the latter, again, may be due mainly to malabsorption of vitamin B_{12}.

A. Human Vitamin B_{12} Deficiency

The most common form of human vitamin B_{12} deficiency due to malabsorption is pernicious anemia. It occurs in about 1% of the population and generally appears after the age of 60 years (76). The disease is attributable directly to lack of intrinsic factor and arises from atrophy of the gastric parietal cells, also the cause of achlorhydria. Progression of the disease is thought to be an autoimmune process in which antibodies arise both to intrinsic factor itself and to the gastric parietal cells that produce it. Rigorous identification of pernicious anemia depends on the detection of antibodies to intrinsic factor, but a positive outcome of the Schilling test for malabsorption of free vitamin B_{12} that can be corrected by intrinsic factor is generally accepted (77). In the Schilling test the absorption of radio-labeled vitamin B_{12} given orally is assessed by urinary excretion of label elicited by a swamping dose of vitamin B_{12} given intramuscularly. If low excretion of label ($< 6\%$ of the dose in 24 h) is found, the test is repeated with the addition of oral intrinsic factor. In cases of pernicious anemia, the latter step restores normal excretion of label (to $> 10\%$ in 24 h). With the recognition that many cases of malabsorption are due not to a lack of intrinsic factor but to a failure to release food-bound vitamin B_{12}, a modified Schilling test has been devised involving the administration of protein-bound vitamin B_{12} with and without manipulation of gastric secretion (78).

The essential features of advanced pernicious anemia are as follows:

1. A macrocytic anemia with mean cell volume > 110 fL, further characterized by the presence of megaloblasts. Such an anemia may also be produced by folate deficiency and is, in fact, attributable to the functional deficiency of folate brought about by the deficiency of vitamin B_{12}. In the early stages of vitamin B_{12} deficiency a lesser degree of macrocytosis without the presence of megaloblasts is seen (76).

2. Hypersegmentation of neutrophils, said to be the most sensitive early hematological indicator of vitamin B_{12} deficiency (79,80).

3. Impaired vitamin B_{12} absorption consequent upon a lack of gastric intrinsic factor.

4. A range of neurologic and neuropsychiatric consequences, the most characteristic of which are associated with the so-called subacute combined degeneration of the spinal cord or cortico-spinal tract disease.

The hematologic and neurologic consequences of pernicious anemia may also be produced by any of a number of conditions that induce severe vitamin B_{12} deficiency by interfering with absorption. Such conditions include partial or total gastrectomy (81), gastric bypass for morbid obesity (82), ileal resection for necrotizing enterocolitis in premature infants (83), atrophic gastritis associated with bacterial overgrowth (84), and Crohn's disease (85).

True dietary deficiency of vitamin B_{12} in humans is rare, and almost all cases prove to be associated with a very strict vegetarian diet in which no animal products whatever are consumed. But even at the very low vitamin B_{12} intakes provided by such "vegan" or "macrobiotic" diets, frank vitamin B_{12} deficiency rarely occurs. Long-term adherence to ovo-lactovegetarian or lacto-vegetarian diets in 44 elderly subjects produced levels of circulating vitamin B_{12} of only marginally deficient status as compared with omnivorous controls (235 pg B_{12}/L compared with 288 pg B_{12}/L for men, and 183 pg B_{12}/L compared with 268 pg B_{12}/L for women) (58). It is now suspected that many cases of low circulating vitamin B_{12} with or without vegetarianism are due to subtle vitamin B_{12} malabsorption (86,87) rather than to dietary intake.

Most reported cases of severe vitamin B_{12} deficiency on "vegan" diets have arisen in infants or young children who had been borne and nursed by vegan mothers. The outcomes described include megaloblastic anemia (88) and neurologic disorders (89). A macrobiotic diet (vegan-like but with some fish) gave rise to low plasma vitamin B_{12} levels and macrocytosis with stunting, the latter thought to arise from low energy intakes (90).

B. Possible Biochemical Basis of Vitamin B_{12} Deficiency Symptoms in Humans

As indicated, the main effects of vitamin B_{12} deficiency in humans are a macrocytic anemia and a progression of serious neurologic effects. Neither of these can be convincingly reproduced in nonprimate animal models, and so understanding of them is incomplete. There is, however, ample demonstration that in severe human vitamin B_{12} deficiency, the activity of both the vitamin B_{12}-dependent enzymes mentioned earlier are seriously depleted at the cellular level. Thus Stabler and co-workers (86) found that of those of their patients with low serum cobalamin (< 200 pg/mL) who responded hematologically or neurologically to cobalamin therapy, 94% showed levels of both methylmalonic acid and homocysteine in serum that were elevated by more than 3 SD above the mean for normal subjects.

Biochemical interpretations of the hematologic effects are less equivocal than those for the neurologic outcomes, in part because the effects can be reversed by administering folate or mimicked by a deficiency of folate. The megaloblastic condition of blood cells and bone marrow cells in human cobalamin deficiency is associated with impaired DNA synthesis, which is in turn attributed to diminished methylation of dUMP to form dTMP. This reaction is dependant on folate and one of the critical consequences of cobalamin deficiency is to create a secondary deficiency of folate. This manifests itself in a number of ways, including excessive urinary excretion of formiminoglutamate, a consequence of depletion of another folate-dependent enzyme. The mechanism by which vitamin B_{12} deficiency leads to a deficiency of folate is not completely clear, but there is reasonably good evidence to support the "methyl trap" hypothesis. The reactions involved are shown in Figure 6.

Depletion of the vitamin B_{12}-dependent methyl transferase activity leads to accumulation not only of homocysteine as observed, but also to accumulation of N^5-methyl tetrahydrofolate. The latter accumulation is not so readily observed except in some cases of blood plasma. Because there is no other way to discharge the methyl group on methylfolate, the body's folate reserves are converted progressively to the methyl form and there is less and less tetrahydrofolate available for other functions. The methyl trap hypothesis has received experimental support from work with vitamin B_{12}-deficient L1210 leukemia cells. Addition of 5-methyl tetrahydrofolate to the medium was followed by cessation of cell growth which could be restored by the addition of vitamin B_{12} or free folic acid (91). Reservations about the adequacy of the methyl trap hypothesis arise from observations of the effects of vitamin B_{12} deficiency on liver folate reserves in sheep. In this species the

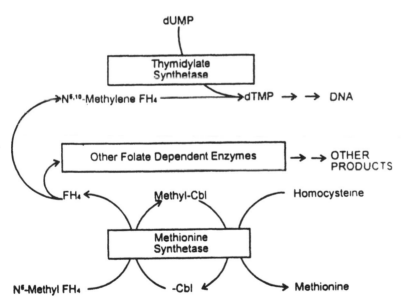

FIGURE 6 Interrelations of vitamin B_{12} and folate in the catalysis of reactions essential for the biosynthesis of DNA. According to the methyl trap hypothesis, when there is a deficiency of cobalamin, metabolically formed N^5-methyl FH_4 cannot be cleared and accumulates, leading to a diminishing tissue supply of FH_4 and hence to inhibition of all folate-dependent reactions, including the synthesis of DNA. There is an observed accumulation of homocysteine and a decreased level of methionine and especially of the methyl donor molecule S-adenosyl methionine.

effect of the deficiency is a massive depletion of all forms of folate in the liver, especially of the polyglutamate forms and including a depletion of methylfolates. It can be argued that the deficiency of metabolically available folate is more a reflection of this general deficit than of a trapping of folate in the methyl form (92). A further unexplained feature is the ability of injected methionine under these circumstances to restore folate function (93). It might have been anticipated that a heavy influx of further methyl groups would exacerbate rather than alleviate a functional folate deficiency induced by the extent of its own methylation. Whatever the mechanism, however, it is undoubtedly the deficit of free folate in vitamin B_{12} deficiency that underlies the macrocytosis and impaired cell division that characterizes the development of anemia.

The neurologic and neuropathologic effects of human vitamin B_{12} deficiency do not respond to folate and may become irreversible if not identified and treated at a relatively early stage. Early neurologic effects include symmetric parasthesias in the extremities (stocking and glove), with disturbances of proprioception and vibratory sensation. With later degenerative changes in the dorsal and lateral columns of the spinal cord, spastic ataxia becomes apparent. In the advanced condition there is weakness or paralysis of voluntary movement, with impaired motor function. The underlying pathology is a myelinopathy, and it is the etiology of this effect that is now examined.

Improved understanding of the pathology of demyelination in vitamin B_{12} deficiencies has followed the development of models in a primate (94,95), a fruit bat (96,97) and in the totally gastrectomized rat (98). All show a spongy demyelination process with vacuolation that may be prevented by administration of vitamin B_{12}. The biochemical basis of this process, however, remains unresolved. Beck (99) reviewed three currently tenable hypotheses to explain a defect in myelin synthesis:

1. Incorporation of abnormal fatty acids into the lipids in myelin. The accumulation of methylmalonic acid in blood reflects the hydrolysis of metabolically derived methylmalonyl CoA in the tissues. Since the normal substrate for elongation of fatty acids synthesized in tissues is malonyl CoA, substitution by endogenous methylmalonyl CoA can be envisaged with the consequent production of abnormal fatty acids either with branched chains or with an odd instead of an even number of carbon atoms (99). Production of unusual fatty acids with 15 and 17 carbon atoms has been observed in rat glial cells cultured in vitamin B_{12}-deficient medium in the presence of propionate. These cease to be produced when vitamin B_{12} is added to the medium (100). Similar acids were found to be synthesized from labeled proponate in nerves excised from patients with pernicious anemia (101). There is, however, no evidence that such events will cause derangement in myelogenesis, and there has been no correlation evident between circulating or urinary methylmalonic acid and neurologic disease. No such demyelinating disease is observed in infants exhibiting severe methylmalonic aciduria (102).

2. Impaired DNA synthesis. The encephalopathy that results from nitrous oxide exposure combined with dietary vitamin B_{12} deficiency in the fruit bat was reported to be accompanied by impairment of the cobalamin-dependent methyl transferase (103). Since myelin synthesis depends on replication of glial cells (oligodendrocytes), DNA synthesis must be involved and may be impaired by vitamin B_{12} deficiency. The hypothesis is essentially that of a lack of available folate as for the hematologic outcome, but unlike that outcome, the myelinopathy does not respond to administered folate.

3. A possible effect of cyanide. Endogenous or environmental cyanide may inactivate the coenzyme forms of cobalamin, and cobalamin-deficient tobacco smokers
show a high incidence of tobacco amblyopia and optic atrophy (for review, see
Ref. 104). Tobacco smoke contains cyanide, and ingestion of either cyanide or
certain cyanogenic compounds may have neuropathologic consequences (104).
However, while it is possible that in some cases cyanogenic compounds may
precipitate or exacerbate a vitamin B_{12} deficiency, it is difficult to believe that
they represent a common primary cause of the myelinopathies of vitamin B_{12}
deficiency.

A fourth hypothesis that may also be tenable is that the myelinopathy results not from
a lack of free folate inhibiting the synthesis of DNA, but from a lack of methylating
capacity within the central nervous system in some way impairing the production of
myelin. Both a lack of available folate and a lowered capacity for methylation will result
from lowered activity of the vitamin B_{12}-dependent methionine synthetase. Administered
folate does not prevent or reverse the myelinopathy of vitamin B_{12} deficiency, but there
have been some reports of a similar myelinopathy from long-term folate deficiency that
have not involved a deficiency of vitamin B_{12} (105,106). Severe neurologic effects and
spinal cord degeneration have also been observed in certain inborn errors of methyl folate
and methyl cobalamin metabolism (107,108). In a more recent report, three cases of inborn
errors involving folate-vitamin B_{12} metabolism have been reported in which a deficiency of
S-adenosyl methionine in cerebrospinal fluid was a common factor. In all cases, oral
therapy with appropriate methyl donors (respectively betaine, methionine, and S-adenosyl
methionine-toluene-sulfonate) led to clinical improvement with evidence of remyelination
(109). In the absence of convincing evidence in favor of any other proposed mechanisms,
the possibility that the effects of vitamin B_{12} (or folate) deficiency on the central nervous
system may lie in a reduced capacity for methylation has to be taken seriously.

C. Inborn Errors of Vitamin B_{12} Metabolism in the Human

A detailed description of the range of recognized inborn errors is beyond the scope of this
chapter, but because of their clinical importance and the light they throw on normal vitamin
B_{12}-related metabolism, a brief tabulation of the ones that affect excretion of methylmalonate or of homocysteine is assembled in Table 4.

Several points emerge from this information. First is the intracellular distinction
between an exclusively mitochondrial location for adenosyl cobalamin action and the
cytosolic production of homocysteine, so that a particular mutation may target one without
affecting the other. Second is the clear association of megaloblastic anemia only with those
mutations that give rise to homocysteinuria. Third is the wide range of responsiveness
between inborn errors to administered vitamin B_{12}, although it should also be noted that
there is often wide heterogeneity within the individual mutations in this respect. A final
point to note is that prognosis for several of these inherited disorders is unfavorable, they
generally become apparent early in life and they are frequently lethal. An extended review
was published by Cooper and Rosenblatt in 1987 (110).

D. Cobalt Deficiency in Ruminants

The physiologic changes that take place in cobalt-deficient ruminants are markedly different from those seen in vitamin B_{12}-deficient humans, but they stem from the same
immediate cause, a systemic deficiency of vitamin B_{12}. The requirement of sheep for cobalt

TABLE 4 Inherited Disorders of Vitamin B$_{12}$ Metabolism Presenting with Methylmalonic Aciduria or Homocysteinuria[a]

Identity	Defect	Clinical indicator	Prognosis	Treatment	Refs
mut^0	No activity of MM CoA mutase under saturating cofactor conditions.	Methymalonic aciduria	Very poor	Unresponsive to OH Cbl	111,112
mut$^-$	Partial activity of MM CoA mutase under saturating cofactor conditions. Reduced affinity for AdoCbl.	Methylmalonic aciduria	Variable	Unresponsive to OH Cbl	111,112
cbl A	Deficiency of mitochondrial reductase responsible for reduction of cobamide cobalt.	Methylmalonic aciduria	Favorable	90% of patients respond to OH Cbl	113
cbl B	Deficiency of deoxyadenosyl transferase in mitochondria.	Methylmalonic aciduria	Poor	< 40% of patients respond to OH Cbl	113
cbl C	Deficiency of cytosolic reductase responsible for reduction of cobamide cobalt.	Methylmalonic aciduria, homocysteinuria, megaloblastic anemia	Poor to very poor	Some patients respond to large doses of OH Cbl	114,115
cbl D	Deficiency of cytosolic reductase responsible for reduction of cobamide cobalt.	Methylmalonic aciduria, homocysteinuria, megaloblastic anemia	Poor	Some response to OH Cbl	115
cbl E	Decreased methyl cobalamin in cells.	Homocysteinuria, megaloblastic anemia	Good	All patients respond to OH Cbl	115,116
cbl F	Defective lysosomal release of cobalamin into cells after endocytosis of TCII-Cbl.	Methylmalonic aciduria, homocysteinuria	Poor	Partial response to OH Cbl	117
cbl G	Decreased methionine synthase activity; decreased methyl cobalamin in cell.	Megaloblastic anemia, homocysteinuria, possible demyelination	Good	All patients respond to OH Cbl	109,115,116

[a]MMCoA mutase; methylmalonyl coenzyme A mutase; cbl, cobalamin mutant prefix; AdoCbl, 5' deoxyadenosyl cobalamin; OHCbl, hydroxocobalamin; TCIICbl, transcobalamin II-cobalamin complex.

has been shown to be due entirely to the need for vitamin B_{12} by the animal's tissues (10). In ruminants the microbial population of the forestomach or rumen is responsible for digestion of dietary cellulose and other carbohydrates to produce the mixture of short-chain fatty acids which constitutes the energy source of the animal. Certain of these microorganisms extend the symbiotic relationship with the host by their ability to synthesize the vitamin B_{12} needed by its tissues. Because the body content of vitamin B_{12} in the normal cobalt-sufficient animal is considerable (the liver contains about 1 mg of vitamin B_{12}), the animal may consume a severely cobalt-deficient diet (< 0.05 μg Co/g dry) for 3–6 months before deficiency symptoms emerge (64,119).

The major physiologic effect of vitamin B_{12} deficiency in sheep is a progressive loss of appetite. The consequent progressive loss of body weight produces an emaciated animal in which several further consequences may become apparent. These include a fatty liver, a reduced immune status, heavily depleted folate reserves, and sometimes anemia (10), but the immediate and dramatic response of appetite and body weight to parenteral administration of vitamin B_{12}, even in the most advanced state of deficiency, makes clear the crucial role of appetite (119–121).

E. Possible Biochemical Basis of Vitamin B_{12} Deficiency Symptoms in Ruminants

A reduced capacity of vitamin B_{12}-deficient liver tissue to convert methylmalonyl coenzyme A into succinyl CoA was first detected in vitamin B_{12}-deficient rats (126). It followed the demonstration in 1958 that liver homogenates from vitamin B_{12}-deficient sheep were severely impaired in their ability to oxidize propionate compared with livers from control animals treated with vitamin B_{12} (119,127). Identification of the specific sheep liver enzyme involved as methylmalonyl CoA mutase, requiring adenosyl cobalamin for its activity, followed (119), and it was shown that methylmalonyl coenzyme A accumulated in the liver of vitamin B_{12}-deficient sheep (128). Development of the symptoms of vitamin B_{12} deficiency in this series of experiments was studied in animals fed a high-roughage, whole wheaten hay diet (129). On this diet, appetite began to fail when vitamin B_{12} concentrations in liver fell below about 0.1 μg/g and plasma vitamin B_{12} levels fell to around 0.2 ng/mL (147 pmol/L). Thereafter, progressive failure of appetite accompanied an increasing impairment of the rate of clearance of propionate by the whole animal, but there was no evidence of any overall change in volatile acid production or in the ratios of volatile fatty acids in the cobalt-deficient rumen (121).

The impaired clearance of propionate was accompanied by a moderate reduction in the initial rate at which blood glucose rose after injection with propionate, but blood glucose was never found to be low in the deficient animal and there was no suggestion that impaired formation of glucose was a factor in development of the deficiency syndrome (121,130). The impairment in propionate clearance was not accompanied by any reduction in the rate of clearance of acetate when given alone, but if both were administered together, acetate clearance was severely inhibited. Such inhibition of acetate clearance by propionate was much more pronounced in the vitamin B_{12}-deficient sheep than in its pair-fed control receiving vitamin B_{12}, primarily because the propionate persisted longer in the blood (121). These findings led to the proposition that the impairment of appetite, although clearly linked to the degree to which propionate metabolism was hindered, could equally well have represented an inhibitory effect of circulating acetate on appetite. Following consumption of food by vitamin B_{12}-deficient animals, more acetate than propionate accumulated in the circulation (121).

In human vitamin B_{12} deficiency, most of the physiologic effects seem to be attributable to the depleted activity of N5-methyltetrahydrofolate:homocysteine methyltransferase (methionine synthetase). In ruminants, although neither of the two pathognomonic outcomes seen in humans (megaloblastic anemia and spinal cord degeneration) is found, there is good evidence not only of depleted activity of this enzyme in vitamin B_{12} deficient sheep tissues (137,138), but also of some secondary consequences of this lowered activity.

Subnormal levels of S-adenosylmethionine (SAM), the body's common methylating agent, and a fatty liver with a depleted content of choline, are both seen (92,93,132). Lowered levels of phosphatidyl choline in brain occurred in cobalt-deficient animals despite there being no reduction in methyl transferase activity or of SAM in brain (132). The absence of reduced levels of SAM in the central nervous system (CNS) of vitamin B_{12}-deficient sheep is consistent with the lack of CNS lesions. A lowered methionine status may contribute to the impaired nitrogen retention found in vitamin B_{12}-deficient sheep as compared with their pair-fed controls (169), but the effects of administering methionine to deficient sheep are metabolically more dramatic than restoration of generally diminished protein synthesis would suggest. In general, these effects seem to be a reflection of improved folate status, but the mechanism by which this improvement occurs is unclear.

A consequence of severe vitamin B_{12} deficiency in sheep is a very marked depletion in liver folate stores, especially of the polyglutamate forms (92). A similar effect on total folate is seen in rats (139), and in both cases the folate stores can be restored by administration of methionine (93,140). The effects of improved folate status are seen in a reduction of the urinary excretion of excess formiminoglutamate (93), a substance sometimes used as a marker for folate deficiency or even for vitamin B_{12} deficiency (141).

VI. BIOCHEMICAL FUNCTIONS OF COBALT AND VITAMIN B_{12}

A. Range of Corrinoid Functions

The reactions catalyzed by corrinoid-dependent enzymes are biochemically remarkable ones but fall clearly into two mechanistically distinct groups: those involving the donation of an activated methyl group attached to the cobalt atom, and those involving homolytic cleavage of the cobalt–carbon bond of 5′-deoxyadenosyl cobalamin to initiate reversible processes involving free radicals. The two coenzyme forms in animal tissues are those already discussed; 5′-deoxyadenosyl cobalamin will also support the bacterial ribonucleotide reductases. Other methyl corrinoids serve the rather exotic reaction sequences discovered in the past few years to underlie the synthesis of methane by the methanogens and the total synthesis of acetate from carbon monoxide by certain acetic acid bacteria, especially *Clostridium thermoaceticum.*

The latter two bacterial groups are believed to represent the survival of very ancient bacterial forms which evolved prior to the appearance of photosynthesis or of an atmosphere containing oxygen (146). These reaction groups and the corrinoids employed in them are listed in Table 5. An exhaustive examination of bacterial corrinoid metabolism is beyond the scope of this chapter, but some key references to recent literature are included in Table 5.

B. Adenosyl Cobalamin-Dependent Mutases

Mammalian mitochondrial methylmalonyl CoA mutase is one of a class of enzymes which catalyse the reversible exchange of groups attached to two adjacent carbon atoms of a

TABLE 5   Reaction Types Catalyzed by Corrinoids

Reaction type	Corrinoid coenzyme involved	Enzymes and sources
Reversible exchange of groups on two adjacent carbon atoms of a substrate. One of the groups exchanged is a hydrogen atom.	5′-Deoxyadenosyl cobalamin	Methylmalonyl CoA mutase in animal tissues and bacteria, plus a variety of mutases and isomerases (nine are known) in a range of bacteria
Reduction of ribose to form deoxyribose.	5′-Deoxyadenosyl cobalamin	Ribonucleotide reductase from certain bacteria (142,143)
Methyl group transfer.	Methyl cobalamin	Methionine synthetase from animal tissues and certain bacteria
Methanogenesis.	Methyl cobamides derived from Factor III or from pseudo-vitamin B_{12}	Coenzyme M-methyl transferase from methanogenic bacteria (144,145)
Synthesis of acetate from CO or from CO_2 and H_2.	Methyl corrinoid perhaps derived from Factor IIIm (5′-methoxy benzimidazolyl cobamide)	Corrinoid iron/sulfur protein from *Clostridium thermoaceticum* (146,147)

substrate molecule. One of these groups must be a hydrogen atom which becomes sequestered by the 5′-deoxyadenosyl radical during migration of the second group and is then redonated to the deserted carbon atom, without having exchanged with solvent hydrogen. The enzymes which make up this group are all active with 5′-deoxyadenosyl cobalamin, although 5-deoxyadenosyl forms of other cobamides may be active in some wild-type organisms. The reactions catalyzed by this group of enzymes are given in Table 6, classified by the nature of the migrating group.

The formal nature of all of these reactions catalyzed by adenosyl cobalamin is similar, and although proof of individual aspects of reaction mechanisms is lacking in many of them, it is likely that both the role of the B_{12} enzyme and the mechanism of the actual rearrangement is at least superficially similar in all cases. A simplified version of the probable course of events as suggested by Pratt (160) is as follows.

1. Homolytic splitting of the cobalt–carbon bond of adenosyl cobalamin with the generation of a 5′-adenosyl free radical and a paramagnetic Co(II) species. Labilization of the Co–C bond is promoted by steric distortion of the corrin ring brought about by the presence of enzyme and to some extent by substrate (160).
2. Abstraction of a hydrogen radical from the substrate into stable association with the adenosyl radical, a process suggested by the absence of solvent exchange with the transferred H atom of the substrate.
3. Stabilization of the radical–substrate intermediate by Co(II) to allow reversible transfer of the migrating group on the substrate. The details of this transfer are not well understood but could involve a "cobalt-promoted carbonium ion" in which the Co(II) ion withdraws electron density from the substrate radical during rearrangement (160).

4. Redonation of the H radical from the adenosyl group to the carbon atom vacated by the migrating group with dissociation of the product.
5. Re-formation of the cobalt–carbon bond from the regenerated adenosyl radical and the Co(II) atom.

C. Methyl Cobalamin and Methionine Synthesis

As shown in Figure 6, the catalytic role of methyl cobalamin in the methylation of homocysteine consists of a methylation-demethylation cycle from the donor methyltetra-hydrofolate to an acceptor homocysteine. Although the cyclic participation of methyl cobalamin in this reaction proceeds readily, at about every 100th turn the cobalamin becomes oxidatively inactivated and a vigorous reductive step is needed to restore the catalytically active species. The nature of this effect has been studied exhaustively in *E. coli*, an organism which shows both a cobalamin-dependent and a cobalamin-independent form of methionine synthetase (161). Mechanistic studies of the cobalamin-dependent *E. coli* enzyme and with chemical models reveal that the transfer of a methyl group from

TABLE 6 Migration of Groups Catalyzed by Adenosylcobalamin-Dependent Mutase Enzymes

Migration type	Group X	Enzyme	Reaction	Ref.
Migration of a relatively large group	$\overset{O}{\underset{\parallel}{-C}}$-S-CoA	Methylmalonyl coenzymeA mutase	Methylmalonyl CoA ⇔ succinyl CoA	(148) (149)
	$\overset{NH_2}{\underset{\parallel}{-C}}$-COOH	Glutamate mutase	L-Glutamate ⇔ threo-β-methylaspartate	(150) (151)
	$\overset{CH_2}{\underset{\mid}{-C}}$-COOH	α-Methyleneglutarate mutase	α-Methyleneglutarate ⇔ β-methylitaconate	(152) (153)
Migration of an amino group	-ωNH$_2$	L-β-Lysine mutase	L-β-Lysine ⇔ 3,5-diaminohexanoate	(154)
	-ωNH$_2$	D-α-Lysine mutase	D-α-Lysine ⇔ 2,5-diaminohexanoate	(154)
	-ωNH$_2$	Ornithine mutase	Ornithine ⇔ 2,4-diaminovalerate	(154)
	-αNH$_2$	Leucine 2,3-amino mutase	L-Leucine ⇔ β-leucine	(154)
Migration of a hydroxyl group or an amino group followed by elimination of water or ammonia and so irreversible	-OH	Diol dehydrase	Ethane-1,2-diol → acetaldehyde	(155) (156)
	-OH	Diol dehydrase	Propane-1,2-diol → propionaldehyde	(155) (156)
	-OH	Glycerol dehydrase	Glycerol → β-hydroxypropionaldehyde	(157)
	-NH$_2$	Ethanolamine ammonia lyase	Ethanolamine → acetaldehyde + NH$_3$	(158) (159)

N^5-methyl tetrahydrofolate, as well as requiring preliminary activation, demands a strong nucleophilic attack. This may be provided by the cobalt atom of cobalamin in its highly reduced Co(I) state (B_{12s}). Whereas methyl cobalamin has the octahedral Co(III) base-on configuration, the product of transmethylation, B_{12s}, is present in a base-off square planar configuration. Labilization of the Co–C bond is promoted by displacement of the α ligand. Cleavage of the bond is thus heterolytic rather than homolytic, and the requirement for a strong nucleophilic reactant is also met (162). The nature of this reaction makes clear its susceptibility to adventitious oxidation and the need for a vigorous cellular reducing system that will restore the cycling species. This is provided during in-vitro studies of the mammalian enzyme (as well as that from *E. coli*) by the addition of S-adenosylmethionine, which is then consumed in catalytic amounts to regenerate enzyme-bound methyl cobalamin and allow the cycle to proceed. The reductant for the in-vivo mammalian system has not yet been identified.

According to Pratt (160), the uniqueness of the cobalt atom among the biologically available transition elements capable of forming metal–carbon bonds lies not only in the thermodynamic (as distinct from the kinetic) stability of the cobalt–carbon bond, but also in its remarkable range of valencies. This is well illustrated in the nature of the trans-methylases that employ methyl corrinoids (162).

D. Noncorrinoid Cobalt

The concentration of noncorrinoid cobalt in biological tissues is extremely small, and occasional reports of cobalt as an essential component of enzymes must be regarded with caution. Thus a claim that cobalt was necessary for activation of a phosphoglycerate mutase from wheat germ has been examined and disputed (163). Others may be activated effectively by other metals likely to be found in higher concentration in the source material (164). For others, for example, an aminopeptidase from bovine cornea (165), alternative activators may in time be found.

In a few cases, however, the evidence for biological actions of noncorrinoid cobalt is more convincing. Thus, when cobalt in the medium was used to induce a nitrile hydratase in cultures of *Rhodococcus rhodochrous*, the purified enzyme contained bound cobalt and was distinct from iron-containing nitrile hydratases (166).

A case of particular interest has arisen in studies of a lysine-2,3-aminomutase from *Clostridium SB4*. Apart from substrate specificity, the action of the enzyme is similar to that of the adenosyl cobalamin amino transferases mentioned in Table 6, but it does not contain a corrinoid. The lysine-2,3-aminomutase from *Clostridium SB4* contains iron and sulfide in equimolar amounts, as well as cobalt, zinc, and copper. Enzyme-bound cobalt (about 3.5 g-atoms/mol) was found to be a cofactor in the activity of the enzyme and the EPR signal indicated the presence of high-spin Co(II). In addition to a requirement for pyridoxal phosphate, the enzyme required S-adenosylmethionine (167). Further evidence supports the conclusion that the rearrangement involves a free-radical mechanism and suggests the involvement of a 5′-deoxyadenosyl moiety arising from S-adenosylmethionine (168). The analogies with the cobalamin-dependent amino mutases are obvious and intriguing.

VII. TOXICOLOGY OF COBALT

Although environmental concentrations of cobalt are low, significant industrial exposure may occur (169). Industrial uses of cobalt include the manufacture of hard alloys, catalysts, ceramics, and pigments. Occupational air exposure limits vary from 0.05 mg/m^3 in the United States to 0.5 mg/m^3 in the former USSR.

Cobaltous chloride is toxic at high concentration, with an LD_{50} in rats of 150–500 mg/kg (170). Cardiovascular effects have been reported in humans, but long industrial exposure was not clearly associated with cardiomyopathy (171). Workers exposed to cobalt-containing metal dust (0.1–2.00 mg Co/m^3 air) developed bronchial symptoms, emphysema, and fibrosis (170), while diamond polishers exposed to dust from cobalt-containing polishing disks developed fibrosing alveolites and decreased pulmonary function (172). Exposure to airborne soluble Co(II) has been followed by cytotoxic effects in bronchial tissues thought to be associated with oxidative stress (173,174).

VIII. PERSPECTIVES AND FUTURE RESEARCH NEEDS

The recognition that cobalt is an essential nutrient for some animals and that it is a component of vitamin B_{12} constitutes a distinctive chapter in trace element research. These observations were followed by studies on metabolic requirements and elucidation of the biochemical processes that underlie the physiologic effects of deficiency. Although some aspects of these inquiries are incomplete (see below), the search for new knowledge to explain biochemical mechanisms involving vitamin B_{12} is now centered on the techniques of molecular biology and protein structure. A recent publication (175) describes a superb X-ray crystallographic analysis of methylcobalamin bound to a trypsin fragment of methionine synthase from *E. coli*. This illustrates how a time-honored technique may be allied with the newer knowledge of protein sequence and structure to shed new light on what was formerly an imponderable: How may an enzyme modulate the properties of the cobalt atom in vitamin B_{12} to effect a homolytic split of the cobalt–carbon bond in mutase reactions but a heterolytic split during methyl transfer?

The new insight arises from the unexpected finding that methylcobalamin, when bound to the enzyme, undergoes a major and significant conformational change. The α-ligand, 5,6-dimethylbenzimidazole, is displaced by a histidine ligand donated by the protein and is accommodated within a specific polypeptide pocket, where it acts as an "anchor" for the cobamide. Histidine and the pocket polypeptide sequence are strongly conserved not only in methionine synthase from different sources but also in methylmalonyl CoA mutases from human and bacterial sources, suggesting that such displacement and mode of binding are common to those disparate enzymatic activities. The authors advanced a plausible mechanism based on local structure and involving reversible proton donation to account for the heterolytic split during methyl transfer, and they speculate on the alternatives needed to secure homolytic splitting in the case of the mutases. The development of this new line of inquiry will be made possible by the techniques of molecular biology.

Some outstanding and unresolved areas of inquiry that relate to the more physiologic phases of vitamin B_{12} research include:

> Understanding the cellular and subcellular mechanisms that regulate the retention of vitamin B_{12} in the body at the gastric, hepatic, and renal levels
>
> The processes responsible for the massive depletion of tissue folates that occur in severe vitamin B_{12} deficiency and the related question of how administered methionine restores folate levels
>
> The mechanisms underlying the development of myelinopathy in severe vitamin B_{12} deficiency in some species but not in others.

REFERENCES

1. Clarke FW. The data of geochemistry. US Geol Surv Bull 1916; 616.
2. Young RS, ed. Cobalt: Its Chemistry, Metallurgy and Uses. Am Chem Soc Mono. New York: Reinhold, 1960.
3. Poston JM. Leucine 2,3-aminomutase: a cobalamin-dependent enzyme present in bean seedlings. Science 1976; 195:301–302.
4. Dickman SR. Ribonucleotide reduction and the possible role of cobalamin in evolution. J Mol Evol 1977, 10:251–260.
5. Wood HG. Life with CO or CO_2 and H_2 as a source of carbon and energy. FASEB J 1991; 5:156–163.
6. Gould SJ. The Panda's Thumb, London: Penguin, 1980: 181–188.
7. Marston HR, Lines EW. Problems associated with "coast disease" in South Australia. J CSIRO 1935; 8:111–119.
8. Rickles EL, Brink NG, Koniuszy FR, Wood TR, Folkers K. Crystalline vitamin B_{12}. Science 1948; 107:396–397.
9. Underwood EJ, Filmer JF. The determination of a biological potent element (cobalt) in limonite. Austral Vet J 1935; 11:84–92.
10. Smith RM. Cobalt. In: Mertz W. ed. Trace Elements in Human and Animal Nutrition. Vol. 1. 5th ed. New York: Academic Press, 1987: 143–183.
11. Marston HR, Allen SH, Smith RM. Production within the rumen and removal from the bloodstream of volatile fatty acids in sheep given a diet deficient in cobalt. Br J Nutr 1972; 27:1147–1157.
12. Pauling L. The Nature of the Chemical Bond. Ithaca, NY: Cornell University Press, 1948.
13. Nyholm RS. Complex compounds of the transition elements. Report to Tenth Solvay Council, Brussels, 1956.
14. Orgil LE. Some applications of crystal field theory to some problems in transition metal chemistry. Report to Tenth Solvay Council, Brussels, 1956.
15. Busch DH. Coordination compounds of cobalt. In Young RS, ed. Cobalt. New York: Reinhold, 1960: 88–156.
16. IUPAC-IUB. Commission on Biochemical Nomenclature. Biochemistry 1974; 13:1555–1560.
17. Lenhert PG. The structure of vitamin B_{12} part 7. The X-ray analysis of the vitamin B_{12} coenzyme. Proc Roy Soc 1968; A303:45–84.
18. Pratt JM. Coordination chemistry of the B_{12}-dependent isomerase reactions. In Dolphin D, ed. B_{12}. Vol. 1. New York: John Wiley, 1982; 325–392.
19. Anderson I, Hegetveit AC. Analysis of cobalt in plasma by electrothermal atomic absorption spectrometry. Fresenius Z Anal Chem 1984; 318:41–48.
20. Baruthio F, Pierre F. Cobalt determination in serum and urine by electrothermal atomic absorption spectrometry. Biol Trace Elem Res 1993; 39:21–31.
21. Lavi N, Alfassi ZB. Determination of trace amounts of cadmium, cobalt, chromium, iron, molybdenum, nickel, selenium, titanium, vanadium and zinc in blood and milk by neutron activation analysis. Analyst 1990; 115:817–822.
22. Linnell JC. In Babior BM, ed. Cobalamin: Biochemistry and Pathophysiology. New York: Wiley-Interscience, 1986: 287.
23. Beck WS. Biological and medical aspects of vitamin B_{12}. In Dolphin D., ed. B_{12}. Vol. 2, Biochemistry and Medicine. New York: Wiley-Interscience, 1982: 1–30.
24. Kolhouse JF, Kondo H, Allen NC, Podell E, Allen RH. Cobalamin analogues are present in human plasma and can mask cobalamin deficiency because current radioisotope dilution assays are not specific for true cobalamin. N Engl J Med 1978; 229:785–792.
25. Kanazawa S, Herbert V. Noncobalamin vitamin B_{12} analogues in human red cells, liver and brain. Am J Clin Nutr 1983; 37:774–777.
26. Shaw S, Jayatilleke E, Meyers S, Colman H, Hertzlich B, Herbert V. The ileum is the major site of absorption of vitamin B_{12} analogues. Am J Gastroenterol 1989; 84:22–26.

27. O'Sullivan JJ, Leeming RJ, Lynch SS, Pollock A. Radioimmunoassay that measures serum vitamin B_{12}. J Clin Pathol 1992; 45:328–331.

28. Kennedy DG, O'Harte FPM, Blanchflower WJ, Rice DA. Development of a specific radio-immunoassay for vitamin B_{12} and its application in the diagnosis of cobalt deficiency in sheep. Vet Res Commun 1990; 14:255–265.

29. Khanna PL, Dworschack RT, Manning WB, Harris JD. A new homogeneous enzyme immuno-assay using recombinant enzyme fragments. Clin Chim Acta 1989; 185:231–240.

30. Kelleher BP, Broin SDO. Microbiological assay for vitamin B_{12} performed in 96-well micro-titre plates. J Clin Pathol 1991; 44:592–595.

31. Rasmussen K, Moelby L, Jensen MK. Studies on methylmalonic acid in humans: II. Relation-ship between concentrations in serum and urinary excretion and the correlation between serum cobalamin and accumulation of methylmalonic acid. Clin Chem 1989; 35:2277–2280.

32. Allen RH, Stabler SP, Savage DG, Lindenbaum J. Diagnosis of cobalamin deficiency I: usefulness of serum methylmalonic acid and total homocysteine concentrations. Am J Hematol 1990; 34:90–98.

33. O'Harte FPM, Kennedy GD, Blanchflower WJ, Rice DA. Methylmalonic acid in the diagnosis of cobalt deficiency in barley-fed lambs. Br J Nutr 1989; 62:729–738.

34. Fisher GEJ, MacPherson A. Serum vitamin B_{12} and methylmalonic acid determinations in the diagnosis of cobalt deficiency in pregnant ewes. Br Vet J 1990; 146:120–128.

35. McMurray CH, Blanchflower WJ, Rice DA, McLaughlin M. Sensitive and specific gas chromatographic method for the determination of methylmalonic acid in the plasma and urine of ruminants. J Chromatogr 1986; 378:201–207.

36. McGhie TK. Analysis of serum methylmalonic acid for the determination of cobalt deficiency in cattle. J Chromatogr 1992; 566:215–222.

37. Stabler SP, Marcell PD, Podell ER, Allen RH. Quantitation of total homocysteine, total cysteine and methionine in normal serum and urine using capillary gas chromatography–mass spectrometry. Anal Biochem 1987; 1162:185–196.

38. Lindenbaum J, Savage DG, Stabler SP, Allen RH. Diagnosis of cobalamin deficiency II. Relative sensitivities of serum cobalamin, methylmalonic acid and total homocysteine concen-trations. Am J Hematol 1990; 34:99–107.

39. Toskes PP, Smith GW, Conrad ME. Cobalt absorption in sex-linked anemic mice. Am J Clin Nutr 1973; 26:435–437.

40. Engel RW, Price NO, Miller RF. Copper, manganese, cobalt and molybdenum balance in pre-adolescent girls. J Nutr 1967; 92:197–204.

41. Harp MJ, Scoular FI. Cobalt metabolism of young college women on self selected diets. J Nutr 1952; 47:67–72.

42. Looney JW, Gille G, Preston RL, Graham ER, Pfander WH. Effects of plant species and cobalt intake upon cobalt utilization and ration digestibility by sheep. J Anim Sci 1976; 42:693–698.

43. Monroe RA, Sauberlich HE, Comar CL, Hood SL. Vitamin B_{12} biosynthesis after oral and intra-venous administration of inorganic Co^{60} to sheep. Proc Soc Exp Biol Med 1952, 80:250–257.

44. Smith RM, Marston HR. Production, absorption, distribution and excretion of vitamin B_{12} in sheep. Br J Nutr 1970; 24:857–877.

45. Thomson ABR, Valberg LS, Sinclair DG. Competitive nature of the intestinal transport system for cobalt and iron in the rat. J Clin Invest 1971; 50:2384–2394.

46. Valberg LS. In Skoryna SC, Waldron-Edwards D, eds. Intestinal Absorption of Metal Ions, Trace Elements and Radionuclides. Oxford: Pergamon, 1971: 257.

47. Lee CC, Wolterink LF. Blood and tissue partition of cobalt 60 in dogs. Am J Physiol 1955; 1983:173–177.

48. Onkelinx C. Compartment analysis of cobalt(II) metabolism in rats of various ages. Toxicol Appl Pharmacol 1976; 38(2):425–438.

49. International Commission of Radiological Protection No. 23. Report of the Task Group on Reference Man. Oxford: Pergamon, 1975: 300–301.

50. Schroeder HA, Nason AP, Tipton IH. Essential trace elements in man: cobalt. J Chronic Dis 1967; 20:869–890.

51. Yalberg LS, Ludwig J, Olatunbosun D. Alteration in cobalt absorption in patients with disorder of iron metabolism. Gastroenterology 1969; 56:241–251.

52. Comar CL. Radio isotopes in nutritional trace element studies—11. Nucleonics 1948; 3:30–42.

53. Heyssel RM, Bozian RC, Darby WJ, Bell MC. Vitamin B_{12} turnover in man: the assimilation of vitamin B_{12} from natural food stuff by man and estimates of minimal daily dietary requirements. Am J Clin Nutr 1966; 18:176–181.

54. Adams JF. In Heinrich HC, ed. Vitamin B_{12} und Intrinsic Factor 2. Europaisches Symposium, Hamburg. Stuttgart: Ferdinand Enke, 1962: 628.

55. Green R, Jacobsen DW, Vantonder SV, Kew MC, Metz J. Enterohepatic circulation cobalamin in the non-human primate. Gastroenterology 1981; 81:773–776.

56. Seetharam B, Ramanujam KS, Seetharam S, Li N, Fyfe JC. Normal and abnormal physiology of intrinsic factor mediated absorption of cobalamin. Indian J Biochem Biophys 1991; 28: 324–330.

57. Gibson RS. Principles of Nutritional Assessment. Oxford: Oxford Univ. Press, 1990: 139.

58. Lowick MRH, Schrijver J, Odink J, van den Berg H, Wedel M. Long-term effects of a vegetarian diet on the nutritional status of elderly people (Dutch nutrition surveillance system). J Am Coll Nutr 1990; 9:600–609.

59. Hall CA. Long term excretion of Co^{57}-vitamin B_{12} and turnover within the plasma. Am J Clin Nutr 1964; 14:156–162.

60. Smith SE, Loosli JK. Cobalt and vitamin B_{12} in ruminant nutrition. a review. J Dairy Sci 1957; 40:1215–1227.

61. Smith RM, Marston HR. Production, absorption, distribution and excretion of vitamin B_{12} in sheep. Br J Nutr 1970; 24:857–877.

62. Hedrich MF, Elliot JM, Lowe JE. Response in vitamin B_{12} production and absorption to increasing cobalt intake in the sheep. J Nutr 1973; 103:1646–1651.

63. Smith SE, Becker DE, Loosli JK, Beeson KC. Cobalt deficiency in New York State. J Animal Sci 1950; 9:221–230.

64. Marston HR. The requirement of sheep for cobalt or for vitamin B_{12}. Br J Nutr 1970; 24: 615–633.

66. El Kholty S, Gueant J-L, Bressler L, et al. Portal and biliary phases of enterohepatic circulation of corrinoids in humans. Gastroenterology 1991; 101:1399–1408.

67. Stupperich E, Nexø E. Effect of cobalt-N coordination on the cobamide recognition by the human vitamin B_{12} binding proteins intrinsic factor transcobalamin and heptocorrin. Eur J Biochem 1991; 199:299–303.

68. Nexø E, Olesen H. Intrinsic factor, transcobalamin and heptocorrin. In Dolphin D, ed B_{12}. Vol. 2. New York: John Wiley, 1982; 87–104.

69. Hewitt JE, Gordon MM, Taggart RT, Mohandas TK, Alpers DH. Human gastric intrinsic factor: characterization of cDNA and genomic clones and localization to human chromosome 11. Genomics 1991; 10:432–440.

70. Johnston J, Yang-Feng T, Berliner N. Genomic structure and mapping of the chromosomal gene for transcobalamin 1: comparison to human intrinsic factor. Genomics 1992; 12:459–464.

71. Arwert F, Porck HT, Frater-Schroder M, et al. Assignment of human transcobalamin 11 to chromosome 22 using somatic cell hybrids and monosomic meningioma cells. Hum Genet 1986; 73:378–381.

72. Platica O, Zaneczko R, Quadros EV, Regec A, Romain R, Rothenbereg SP. The cDNA sequence and the deduced amino acid sequence of human transcobalamin II show homology with rat intrinsic factor and human transcobalamin I. J Biol Chem 1991; 266:7860–7863.

73. Newman GE, O'Brien JRP, Spray GH, Witts LJ. Distribution of vitamin B_{12} in rat liver cell factors. In Heinrich HC, ed. Vitamin B_{12} und Intrinsic Factor 2. Stuttgart: Ferdinand Enke, 1962; 424–432.

74. Lindemans J, van Kapel J, Abels J. Uptake of transcobalamin II-bound cobalamin by isolated rat kidney tubule cells. Scand J Clin Lab Invest 1986; 46:223–232.

75. Ramanujam KS, Seetharam S, Ramasamy M, Seetharam B. Renal brush border membrane bound intrinsic factor. Biochim Biophys Acta 1990; 1030:157–164.

76. McRae TD, Freedman ML. Why vitamin B_{12} deficiency should be managed aggressively. Geriatrics 1989; 44:70–73.

77. Thompson WG, Freedman ML. Vitamin B_{12} and unanswered questions. Acta Haematol 1989; 82:169–174.

78. Goodman KI, Salt, WB. Vitamin B_{12}-deficiency: important new concepts in recognition. Postgrad Med 1990; 88:147–158.

79. Herbert V. The folate and vitamin B_{12} paradigm. Am J Clin Nutr 1987; 46:387–402.

80. Thompson WG, Cassino C, Babitz L, et al. Hypersegmented neutrophils and vitamin B_{12} deficiency. Acta Haematol 1989; 81:186–191.

81. Hines JD, Hoffbrand AV, Mollin DL. The hematological complications following partial gastrectomy: a study of 292 patients. Am J Med 1967; 43:555–569.

82. Simon SR, Zemel R, Betancourt S, Zidar BL. Hematologic complications of gastric bypass for morbid obesity. Southern Med 1989; 82:1108–1110.

83. Skidmore MD, Shenker N, Kliegman RM, Shurin S, Allen R. Biochemical evidence of asymptomatic vitamin B_{12} deficiency in children after ileal resection for necrotizing enterocolitis. J Pediatr 1989; 115:102–105.

84. Suter PM, Golner BB, Goldin BR, Morrow FD, Russell RM. Reversal of protein bound vitamin B_{12} malabsorption with antibiotics in atrophic gastritis. Gastroenterology 1991; 101:1039–1045.

85. Abe S, Wakabayashi Y, Hirose S. Megaloblastic anemia associated with intestinal Crohn's disease. Rinsho Ketsueki 1989; 30:51–55.

86. Stabler SP, Allen RH, Savage DG, Lindenbaum J. Clinical diagnosis of cobalamin deficiency. Blood 1990; 76:871–881.

87. Carmel R. Nutritional vitamin B_{12} deficiency. Ann Intern Med 1978; 88:647–649.

88. Cheron G, Girot R, Zittoun J, Mouy R, Schmitz J, Rey J. Anémie mégaloblastique sévère chez une enfant des six mois allaitée par une mère végétarienne. Arch Fr Pediatr 1989; 46:205–207.

89. Kühne T, Bubl R, Baumgartner R. Maternal vegan diet causing a serious infantile neurological disorder due to vitamin B_{12} deficiency. Eur J Pediatr 1991; 150:205–208.

90. Dagnelie PC, Van Staveren WA, Hautvast JGAJ. Stunting and nutrient deficiencies in children on alternative diets. Acta Paediatr Scand Suppl 1991; 374:111–118.

91. Kondo H, Iseki T, Isawa S, et al. Cobalamin-dependent replication of L1210 leukemia cells and effects of cobalamin analogues. Acta Haematol 1989; 81:61–69.

92. Smith RM, Osborne-White WS. Folic acid metabolism in vitamin B_{12}-deficient sheep. Depletion of liver folates. Biochem J 1973; 136:279–293.

93. Smith RM, Osborne-White WS, Gawthorne JM. Folic acid metabolism in vitamin B_{12}-deficient sheep. Effects of injected methionine on liver constituents associated with folate metabolism. Biochem J 1974; 142:105–117.

94. Agamanows DP, Victor M, Harris JW. An ultrastructural study of subacute combined degeneration of the spinal cord in vitamin B_{12} deficient rhesus monkeys. J Neuropathol Exp Neurol 1978; 37:273–299.

95. Goodman AM, Harris JW, Kiraly D. Studies in B_{12}-deficient monkeys with combined system disease. 1. B_{12}-deficient patterns in bone marrow deoxyuridine suppression tests without morphologic or functional abnormalities. J Lab Clin Med 1980; 96:722–733.

96. Green R, Van Tonder SV, Oettle GJ, Cole G, Metz J. Neurological changes in fruit bats deficient in vitamin B_{12}. Nature 1975; 254:148–150.

97. Duffield MS, Phillips JI, Viera-Makings E, Van der Westhuyzen J, Metz J. Demyelinisation in the spinal cord of vitamin B_{12} deficient fruit bats. Comp Biochem Physiol 1990; 96:291–297.

98. Scalabrino G, Monzio-Compagnoni B, Ferioli ME, Lorenzini EC, Chiodini E, Candiani R.

Subacute combined degeneration and induction of ornithine decarboxylase in spinal cords of totally gastrectomised rats. Lab Invest 1990; 62:297–304.

99. Beck WS. Neuropsychiatric consequences of cobalamin deficiency. Adv Intern Med 1991; 36:33–56.

100. Barley FW, Sato GH, Abeles RH. An effect of vitamin B_{12} deficiency in tissue culture. J Biol Chem 1972; 247:4720–4726.

101. Frenkel EP, Kitchens RL, Hersh LB. Effect of vitamin B_{12} deprivation on the in vivo levels of coenzyme A intermediates associated with propionate metabolism. J Biol Chem 1974; 249:6984–6991.

102. Rosenberg LE, Fenton WA. Disorders of propionate and methylmalonate metabolism. In Scriver CR, et al. eds. The Metabolic Basis of Inherited Disease, 5th ed. New York: McGraw-Hill, 1989; 821–844.

103. Green R, Jacobsen DW, Sommer C. Effect of nitrous oxide on methionine synthetase activity in brain and kidney of vitamin B_{12} deficient fruit bats. Abstr 148, Proc. 18th Cong Int Soc Hematol. Montreal, Canada, 1980.

104. Freeman AG. Optic neuropathy and chronic cyanide intoxication: a review. J R Soc Med 1988; 81:103–106.

105. Robertson JSR, Batten FE, Collier J. Subacute combined degeneration of the spinal cord. No association with vitamin B_{12} deficiency. Arch Neurol 1971; 24:203–209.

106. Lever EG, Elwes RDC, Williams A, Reynolds EH. Subacute combined degeneration of the cord due to folate deficiency: response to methyl folate treatment. J Neurol Neurosurg Psych 1986; 49:1203–1207.

107. Clayton PT, Smith I, Harding B, Hyland K, Leonard JV, Leeming RJ. Subacute combined degeneration of the spinal cord, dementia and parkinsonism due to an inborn error of folate metabolism. J Neurol Neurosurg Psychiat 1986; 49:920–927.

108. Dayan AD, Ramsay RB. An inborn error of vitamin B_{12} metabolism associated with cellular deficiency of coenzyme forms of the vitamin. Pathological and neurochemical findings in one case. J Neurol Sci 1974; 23:117–128.

109. Surtees R, Leonard J, Austin S. Association of demyelination with deficiency of cerebrospinal-fluid S-adenosylmethionine in inborn errors of methyl transfer pathway. Lancet 1991; 338: 1550–1554.

110. Cooper BA, Rosenblatt DS. Inherited defects of vitamin B_{12} metabolism. Annu Rev Nutr 1987; 7:291–320.

111. Raff ML, Crane AM, Jansen R, Ledley FD, Rosenblatt DS. Genetic characterisation of a mut-locus invitation discriminating heterogeneity in mut° and mut_ methylmalonic aciduria by interallelic complementation. J Clin Invest 1991; 87:203–207.

112. Crane AM, Jansen R, Andrews ER, Ledley ED. Cloning and expression of a mutant methyl-malonyl coenzyme A mutase with altered cobalamin affinity that causes methylmalonic aciduria. J Clin Invest 1992; 89:385–391.

113. Chalmers RA, Bain MD, Mistry J, Tracey BM, Weaver C. Enzymological studies on patients with methylmalonic aciduria. Basis for a clinical trial of deoxyadenosyl cobalamin in a hydroxocobalamin-unresponsive patient. Ped Res 1991; 30:560–563.

114. Russo P, Doyon J, Sonsino E, Ogier H, Saudu Bray J-M. A congenital anomaly of vitamin B_{12} metabolism. Hum Pathol 1992; 23:504–512.

115. Byck S, Rosenblatt DS. Metabolic cooperation among cell lines from patients with inborn errors of vitamin B_{12} metabolism: differential response of cblC and cblD. Clin Invest Med 1991; 14:153–159.

116. Watkins D, Rosenblatt DS. Functional methionine synthase deficiency (cblE and cblG): clinical and biochemical heterogeneity. Am J Med Genet 1989; 34:427–434.

117. Shih VE, Axel SM, Tewksbury JC, Watkins D, Cooper BA, Rosenblatt DS. Defective lyso-somal release of vitamin B_{12} (cblF): a hereditary cobalamin metabolic disorder associated with sudden death. Am J Med Genet 1989 ; 33:555–563.

119. Marston HR, Allen SH, Smith RM. Primary metabolic defect supervening on vitamin B_{12} deficiency in sheep. Nature 1961; 190:1085–1091.

120. Smith RM, Marston HR. Some metabolic aspects of vitamin B_{12} deficiency in sheep. Br J Nutr 1970; 24:879–891.

121. Marston HR, Allen SH, Smith RM. Production within the rumen and removal from the bloodstream of volatile fatty acids in sheep given a diet deficient in cobalt. Br J Nutr 1972; 27:147–157.

126. Smith RM, Monty KJ. Vitamin B_{12} and propionate metabolism. Biochem Biophys Res Commun 1959; 1:105–109.

127. Smith RM. Oxidation and metabolism of propionic acid by liver homogenates of normal and vitamin B_{12} deficient sheep. M.Sc. thesis, University of Adelaide, Australia, 1958.

128. Smith RM, Osborne-White WS, Russell GR. Methylmalonic acid and coenzyme A concentrations in the livers of pair-fed vitamin B_{12}-deficient and vitamin B_{12}-treated sheep. Biochem J 1969; 112:703–707.

129. Marston HR, Smith RM. Cobalt in the nutrition of ruminants. Control of cobalt deficiency in sheep by injection of vitamin B_{12}. Nature 1952, 170:791.

130. Smith RM, Marston HR. Metabolism of propionate by pair-fed vitamin B_{12}-deficient and vitamin B_{12}-treated sheep. Br J Nutr 1971; 26:41–53.

137. Kennedy DG, Cannavan A, Molloy A, et al. Methylmalonyl-CoA mutase (EC2.1.1.13) in the tissues of cobalt-vitamin B_{12}-deficient sheep. Br J Nutr 1990; 64:721–732.

138. Gawthorne JM, Smith RM. Folic acid metabolism in vitamin B_{12}-deficient sheep. Effects of injected methionine on methotrexate transport and the activity of enzymes associated with folate metabolism in liver. Biochem J 1974; 142:110–126.

139. Kutzbach C, Galloway E, Stokstad ELR. Influence of vitamin B_{12} and methionine on levels of folic acid compound and folate enzymes in rat liver. Proc Soc Exp Biol Med 1967; 124:801–805.

140. Gawthorne JM, Stokstad ELR. The effect of vitamin B_{12} and methionine on folic acid uptake by the rat liver. Proc Soc Exp Biol Med 1971; 136:42–46.

141. Russel AJF, Whitelaw A. Urinary formiminoglutanic acid in lambs (letter). Vet Rec 1983; 112:418.

142. Blakley RL. Cobalamin-dependent ribonucleotide reductases. In Dolphin D, ed. B_{12}. Vol. 2. New York: John Wiley, 1982; 381–418.

143. Sitjes J, Ysern P, Barbe J, Llagostera M. Induction of ribonucleoside diphosphate reductase gene transcription by chemicals in *Escherichia coli*. Mutagenesis 1992; 7:47–49.

144. Di Marco AA, Bobik TTA, Wolfe RS. Unusual coenzymes of methanogens. Annu Rev Biochem 1990; 59:355–394.

145. Kengen SWM, Daas PJH, Duits EFG, Keltjens JT, van der Drift C, Vogels GD. Isolation of a 5-hydroxybenzimidazolyl cobamide-containing enzyme involved in the methyltetrahydromethanopterin: coenzyme M methyl transferase reaction in *Methanobacterium thermoantotrophicum*. Biochim Biophys Acta 1992; 1118:249–260.

146. Wood, HG. Life with CO or CO_2 and H_2 as a source of carbon and energy. FASEB J 1991; 5:156–163.

147. Lu WP, Ragsdale SW. Reductive actuation of the coenzyme A/acetyl CoA isotopic exchange reaction catalysed by carbon monoxide dehydrogenase from *Clostridium thermoaceticum* and its inhibition by nitrous oxide and carbon monoxide. J Biol Chem 1991; 266:3554–3564.

148. Retey J. Methylmalonyl-CoA mutase. In Dolphin D, ed. B_{12}. Vol. 2. New York: John Wiley, 1982: 357–378.

149. McKie N, Keep NH, Patchett ML, Leadlay PF. Adenosylcobalamin-dependent methymalonyl-CoA mutase from *Propionibacterium shermanii*. Biochem J 1990: 269–298.

150. Switzer RL. Glutamate mutase. In Dolphin D, ed. B_{12}. Vol. 2. New York: John Wiley, 1982: 289–305.

151. Leutbecher V, Böcher R, Linder D, Buckel W. Glutamate mutase from *Clostridum cohclearium*. Eur J Biochem 1992; 2005:759–765.

152. Michel C, Hartrampf G, Buckel W. Assay and purification of the adenosyl cobalamin-

dependent α-methyl glutarate mutase from *Clostridium barkerii*. Eur J Biochem 1989; 184:103–107.

153. Michel C, Albracht PJ, Buckel W. Adenosyl cobalamin and Cob (II) alamin as prosthetic groups of 2-methyleneglutarate mutase from *Clostridium barkerii*. Eur J Biochem 1992; 205: 767–773.

154. Baker JJ, Stadtman TC. Amino mutases. In Dolphin D, ed. B_{12}. Vol. 2. New York: John Wiley, 1982: 203–232.

155. Toraya T, Fukui S. Diol dehydrase. In Dolphin D, ed. B_{12}. Vol. 2. New York: John Wiley, 1982: 234–262.

156. Toraya T, Ishida A. Acceleration of cleavage of the carbon-cobalt bound of sterically hindered alkyl cobalamins by binding to apoprotein of diol dehydrase. Biochemistry 1988; 27:7677–7681.

157. Forage RG, Foster AM. Glycerol dehydrase. Biochim Biophys Acta 1979; 569:249–255.

158. Babior BM. Ethanolamine ammonia-lyase. In Dolphin D, ed. B_{12}. Vol. 2. New York: John Wiley, 1982: 263–288.

159. Faust LP, Babior BM. Overexpression, purification and some properties of the AdoCbl-dependent ethanolamine ammonia lyase from *Salmonella typhimurium*. Arch Biochem Biophys 1992; 294:50–54.

160. Pratt JM. Coordination chemistry of the B_{12}-dependent isomerase reactions. In Dolphin D, ed. B_{12}. Vol. 2. New York: John Wiley, 1982: 325–392.

161. Gonzalez JC, Banerjee RV, Huang S, Sumner JS, Matthews RG. Comparison of cobalamin-independent and cobalamin-dependent methionine syntheses from *Escherichia coli*: Two solutions to the same chemical problem. Biochemistry 1992; 31:6045–6056.

162. Matthews RG, Banerjee RV, Ragsdale SW. Cobamide-dependent methyltransferases. Biofactors 1990; 2:147–153.

163. Johnson CM, Price NC. Do metal ions promote the re-action of the 2,3-biphosphoglycerate-independent phosphoglycerate mutase. Biochem J 1988; 252:111–117.

164. Ganson RJ, Jensen RA. The essential role of cobalt in the inhibition of the cytosolic isozyme of 3-deoxy-D-arabino-heptulosonate-7-phosphate synthase from *Nicotiana silvestris* by glyphosphate. Arch Biochem Biophys 1988; 260:85–93.

165. Sharma KK, Ortwerth BJ. Purification and characterisation of an amino peptidase from bovine cornea. Exp Eye Res 1987; 45:117–126.

166. Nagasawa T, Takeuchi K, Yamada H. Characterisation of a new cobalt-containing nitrile hydratase purified from urea-induced cells of *Rhodococcus rhodochrous* J 1. Eur J Biochem 1991; 196:581–589.

167. Petrovich RM, Ruzicka FJ, Reed GH, Frey PA. Metalcofactors of lysine-2,3-amino mutase. J Biol Chem 1991; 266:7656–7660.

168. Ballinger MD, Reed GH, Frey PA. An organic radical in the lysine-2,3-amino mutase reaction. Biochemistry 1992; 31:949–953.

169. Beyersmann D, Hartwig A. The genetic toxicology of cobalt. Tox Appl Pharmacol 1992; 115: 137–145.

170. Elinder CG, Friberb L. Cobalt. In Friberg L, Nordberg GF, Vouk V, eds. The Industrial Toxicology of Metals. Amsterdam: Elsevier, 1986: 211–232.

171. Horowitz SF, Fischbein A, Matza D, et al. Effects of chronic exposure to soluble salts of cobalt. Br J Ind Med 1988; 45:742–746.

172. Nemery B, Casier P, Roosels D, La Haye D, Demedts M. Survey of cobalt exposure and respiratory health in diamond polishers. Am Rev Respir Dis 1992; 145:610–616.

173. Lewis CPL, Demedts M, Nemery B. Indices of oxidative stress on hamster lung following exposure to cobalt (II) ions: in vivo and in vitro studies. Am J Respir Cell Mol Biol 1991; 5:163–169.

174. Lewis CPL, Demedts M, Nemery B. The role of thiol oxidation in cobalt (II)-induced toxicity in hamster lung. Biochem Pharmacol 1992; 43:519–525.

175. Drennan CL, Huang S, Drummond JT, Matthews RG, Ludwig ML. How a protein binds B_{12}: A 3.0Å X-ray structure of B_{12}-binding domains of methionine synthase. Science 1994; 266: 1669–1674.

12
Chromium

Esther G. Offenbacher and F. Xavier Pi-Sunyer
St. Luke's-Roosevelt Hospital Center, New York, New York

Barbara J. Stoecker
Oklahoma State University, Stillwater, Oklahoma

I. INTRODUCTION AND HISTORY

Trivalent chromium was identified in 1959 as the active element in a substance needed to potentiate insulin action and to maintain normal glucose metabolism (1). During the 1960s and 1970s, evidence accumulated that marginal or deficient chromium intakes may predispose to maturity-onset diabetes mellitus and atherosclerotic disease (2–5). In 1977, chromium supplementation relieved diabetic signs in a patient receiving total parenteral nutrition (6). Chromium supplementation trials in malnourished children, the elderly, and subjects with abnormal glucose tolerance generally supported the association between chromium and glucose metabolism, but a few did not, resulting in controversy regarding the role of chromium in human nutrition.

Disagreements abound in the literature for several reasons. First, chromium could not be measured accurately before 1978; second, the composition and structure of the biologically active form(s) of chromium remain uncertain; third, basic knowledge of the mechanism(s) of chromium action is rudimentary; and, fourth, there still is no clinical test to identify chromium deficiency in orally fed people, making it impossible to select for study only those subjects who are chromium deficient.

In this chapter, the focus is primarily on studies conducted in the 1980s and 1990s, when reliable methods were developed that now enable analysts to make accurate chromium measurements in animal tissues, in human blood serum and plasma, in hair, and in foods (7–18).

II. CHEMICAL PROPERTIES OF CHROMIUM

A. Oxidative States

Chromium, a transition series element, $3d^5$, occurs most commonly in oxidation states 0, $2+$, $3+$, and $4+$. Trivalent chromium (Cr^{3+}) is the most stable oxidation state of chromium in the food supply; any adventitious amounts of Cr^{6+} are rapidly reduced to Cr^{3+} under physiologic conditions. In contrast to Cr^{6+}, Cr^{3+} is poorly absorbed and has low oral toxicity, with a margin of safety well beyond the quantities in the food supply or in dietary supplements. In the hexavalent (Cr^{6+}) form, chromium is a strong oxidant that can easily penetrate cell membranes and cause tissue damage. The radioactive isotope ^{51}Cr, with a half-life of 27.8 days, is used as a red cell marker and in tracer studies (19).

B. Chelating and Binding Properties

At neutral or basic pH, inorganic Cr^{3+} occurs as the hexaquo ion $[Cr(H_2O)_6]$, which readily polymerizes to form macromolecules. This process, known as olation, causes the chromium to precipitate, reducing its already poor rate of absorption and preventing it from binding to biologically useful ligands. Once Cr^{3+} is absorbed, it tends to form one or more biologically active molecules. At acid pH, several amino acids and pyrophosphate form coordination compounds or chelates and prevent olation (20); these retain solubility at the pH of intestinal contents.

C. Bioactive Molecule

The most widely postulated model is an octahedral coordination complex containing two molecules of nicotinic acid with four coordination sites linked to glutamic acid, glycine, and cysteine (21–23). A possible structure for a biologically active chromium molecule is depicted in Fig. 1.

Nicotinic acid may act as an independent cofactor in chromium metabolism or as a constituent of a biologically active chromium molecule (25). As such, nicotinic acid, rather than nicotinamide, the more common dietary form of niacin, is postulated as a substrate for the synthesis of the biologically active chromium molecule (25). To date the molecular composition of the putative biologically active chromium-containing molecule earlier designated "glucose tolerance factor" is uncertain (9), and whether or not chromium as found in brewer's yeast and in some other naturally occurring and synthetic complexes is better utilized than inorganic chromium (26,27) remains to be clarified.

Efforts to extract or synthesize a biologically active chromium compound have yielded several complexes of varied biological activity (measured as a product of glucose oxidation either in yeast systems or in adipose tissue) (22,23,26,28–30). However, when purified, none of these molecules has retained fully the activity of the source material.

Okada et al. (31) identified a 70-kDa, high-molecular-weight protein with 5–6 atoms of chromium per molecule that was formed in regenerating rat liver following the intraperitoneal administration of trivalent chromium. This molecular species bound to nucleolar chromatin and stimulated RNA synthesis. Yamamoto et al. (29) isolated a low-molecular-weight (approximately 1500-kDa) chromium-binding substance from mouse liver, kidney, plasma, erythrocytes, urine, and feces following an intraperitoneal injection of hexavalent chromium. The substance contained trivalent chromium, aspartic acid, glutamic acid, glycine, and cysteine. Nicotinic acid was not detected, but there was a constituent that had an absorption maximum at 260 nm, which is the peak for nicotinic acid. Yamamoto

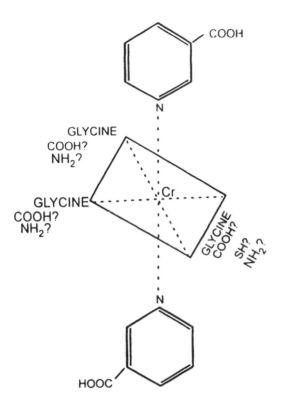

STEREO CHEMISTRY: CIS-TRANS?
CO-ORDINATION TO FUNCTIONAL GROUPS OF AA?
DISTRIBUTION OF CHARGES?

FIGURE 1 Proposed structure of the glucose tolerance factor, a biologically active molecule. (Reproduced from Ref. 24, with permission.)

postulated that this substance plays an important role in the incorporation of chromium into liver cells and in the release of chromium to the circulation, urine, and feces.

III. ANALYTIC METHODOLOGY

The reported chromium concentrations in body tissues or fluids and in foods have decreased over the years by several orders of magnitude (Table 1) as analytic methods improved. Until 1978 (32), analysts were unaware that they had been measuring both background and environmental contamination in amounts that far exceeded the true nanomole and picomole quantities of chromium in body tissues and fluids and in foods. Therefore, the literature reporting these measures has been unreliable and is largely of historical interest. Even some measurements made recently without the benefit of strict quality control are still orders of magnitude too high.

Three types of modern instrumentation, dual-label isotope spectrometry, radiochemical neutron activation analysis, and Zeeman graphite furnace atomic absorption spectrome-

TABLE 1 Reported Mean Values for Serum Chromium in Normal, Fasted Subjects, 1962–1987

Year	nmol/L	Number of subjects	Reference
1962	10,000	5	5
	3,269	3	5
1968	446	16	33
1973	90	10	34
1973	30	15	35
1978	3.08	17	36
1985	2.50	76	37
1987	2.88	52	38

try, now enable accurate measurements (36,39–45). Accurate chromium assays require, in addition, dedicated "clean room" facilities to control environmental contamination, filtered air and water, ultrapure reagents, suitable reference materials (i.e., serum for measuring serum, urine for measuring urine) (42), and trained technical personnel with "useful paranoia" (46). The daily use of appropriate reference materials is essential to verify analytic accuracy. Graphite furnace atomic absorption spectrometry with appropriate background correction is the method of choice for routine and relatively rapid chromium measurement. However, chromium measurement taxes the sensitivity even of modern instrumentation. The detection limit for chromium in biological fluids is approximately 1 nmol/L (47,48).

A. Chromium in Blood and Urine

The collection and processing of blood and urine samples requires the utmost care to avoid contamination. Blood is drawn through siliconized needles into plastic, chromium-free syringes, and the process of preparing and analyzing samples is accompanied by "blanks" throughout. Values of <3.8 nmol/L in human serum and urine are now verified as normal (37,41), with most studies finding serum chromium concentrations <2.9 nmol/L (7,10,12). Plasma values are higher but are still <5.8 nmol/L (47). Red and white blood cells, the most readily available body tissues, are not now amenable to contamination-free methods of sample preparation for electrothermal atomic absorption spectrometry.

Urinary chromium typically ranges from 1.0 to 20.0 nmol/L, with group means of approximately 3.9 nmol/L (0.2 to 0.3 ug/d) (37,49,50). Detailed protocols for methods of sample collection, preparation, and analysis are available (36,39–45,51).

B. Tissue Chromium

The reported chromium concentration in liver of Finnish accident victims from 0 to 4 months of age was 179 pmol/g (dry weight) and 138 pmol/g at 3 to 8 years of age (52). In spleen, values averaged 269 pmol/g. Chromium concentrations in blood serum or plasma are not in equilibrium with tissue concentrations and so are not reflective of body stores.

Hair measurements are currently of little value in individuals (53). Variables associated with trace mineral analyses in hair include age, sex, health status, site and rate of growth, hair color, hair treatment, water supplies, binding of exogenous materials, and the removal of endogenous materials by chelating agents during sample preparation (53).

Randall and Gibson (54) reported median chromium hair levels of 2.4 nmol/g, ranging from 1.5 to 4.0 nmol/g, but despite careful collection and analysis, hair chromium measurements often are not reproducible (53), and the use of hair to assess chromium status remains unreliable.

C. Chromium in Foods

Procedures for measuring chromium in foods require the same care as for body tissues and fluids. No stainless steelware can be used (55) and equipment for homogenization of samples must be fitted with low-chromium or chromium-free blades. The chromium content of typical Western diets ranges from 13 to 28 μg/1000 kcal (60 to 129 nmol/1000 kJ) (11). A table listing the chromium in a variety of common foods (56) is presented in Section VII.

IV. METABOLISM

A. Absorption

Chromium is one of the most poorly absorbed of the essential trace minerals. In 22 free-living elderly subjects, net chromium absorption averaged 2.3% (57). On a constant diet containing 37 μg chromium/day, two men in a metabolic unit absorbed a net of 2.4% and 1.4%, respectively (58).

1. Site

The jejunum is reported to be the most active intestinal segment for chromium absorption in the rat (59) and in humans (60). In the absence of amino acids, the retention of chromium by the intestinal cells may shift from the proximal to the distal region (61). In rats intubated with $^{51}CrCl_3$, 85% had ^{51}Cr below the cecum 4 h after intubation, indicating its rapid transit. ^{51}Cr seemed to accumulate with pools of water at ligatures placed at various points in the intestine; this may indicate that chromium is moving through the lumen with water (62).

2. Mechanism

The mechanism of chromium absorption is poorly understood. Chromium is absorbed by passive diffusion in rats, but mediated or active transport appear also to be involved (63). The presence of transferrin or albumin in the blood stream enhances chromium absorption (64), suggesting that passive diffusion is augmented by these transport molecules. Also, amino acids in the intestinal perfusate enhance both chromium absorption and its release from the mucosal cells to the blood (61).

In mice, previous chromium intake did not affect ^{51}Cr absorption (65). However, guinea pigs fed chromium-depletion diets had more ^{51}Cr in liver and blood 3 h after a dose of $^{51}CrCl_3$ than did animals fed adequate dietary chromium (66). Absorption in humans appears to decrease with increasing chromium intake: Based on estimates from urinary excretion, about 2% was absorbed at a daily dietary intake of 10 μg (0.19 μmol), and only 0.5% at intakes above 40 μg (0.77 μmol) (37). The latter observations support the concept that a higher percentage of absorption occurs in chromium depletion.

3. Dietary Factors

Interactions between chromium and other components of the diet could be important, because chromium absorption is usually low. There is evidence that other dietary constituents affect chromium absorption and utilization.

Amino acids, ascorbic acid, and oxalate (which is widely distributed in vegetables, plants, and feeds) enhance chromium uptake. Absorption may be enhanced by formation of chelates that prevent chromium from precipitation at the alkaline pH of the intestine (21,59).

Ascorbic acid may increase the solubility of inorganic chromium, permitting the formation of more readily absorbable complexes of chromium. In rats, concurrent dosing with $^{51}CrCl_3$ and ascorbic acid increased total urinary ^{51}Cr excretion without significantly reducing ^{51}Cr in tissues, suggesting that ascorbic acid enhanced ^{51}Cr absorption (67,68). In a human trial, three women were given 1 mg (19.2 μmol) Cr^{3+} plus 100 mg (568 μmol) ascorbic acid and, on another day, the same chromium dose without ascorbic acid. The plasma chromium was consistently greater in each of the women when the Cr^{3+} was accompanied by ascorbic acid (69).

Excesses of other trace elements may interfere with chromium absorption and/or utilization. When oral Zn was given with a dose of ^{51}Cr to zinc-deficient rats, chromium absorption was decreased (70). Zinc and chromium may share a common absorptive pathway. An inverse relationship between dietary chromium and iron status was found in which chromium absorption was higher in iron-deficient mice than in iron-replete animals (26). Thus, the implications of supplementation with zinc and other trace minerals need further exploration.

Phytate (a component of dietary fiber), at high (59) but not low (71,72) levels, may have adverse effects on chromium absorption. The effect of carbohydrate was measured in mice. A carbohydrate load of starch generally increased the ^{51}Cr absorption from $^{51}CrCl_3$ compared with carbohydrate loads of sucrose, fructose, and glucose (65).

The habitual consumption of therapeutic agents such as antacids (67,68), appears likely to impair chromium absorption and/or retention. In rats, large doses of calcium carbonate reduced ^{51}Cr in blood 3 h after dosing (67). An antacid containing magnesium hydroxide given with a dose of $^{51}CrCl_3$ reduced ^{51}Cr in blood, urine, and several tissues (68).

B. Transport

Transferrin was identified in 1964 as the plasma transport protein for chromium (73). Chromium showed an affinity for transferrin that approached that of iron (73). Transferrin may bind newly absorbed chromium, while albumin assumes the role of acceptor and transporter of chromium if the transferrin-binding sites are unavailable. In addition, other plasma protein fractions, including gamma- and beta-globulins and lipoproteins, bind chromium and may have a role in chromium metabolism (20). The binding of chromium to apotransferrin is increased by citric acid and decreased by iron (74). A mechanism has not yet been determined.

Hemochromatosis serves as a ready model for the study of effects of iron on chromium transport and retention. In hemochromatosis, transferrin becomes saturated with iron, and many of the patients develop diabetes mellitus with liver involvement. A hypothesis is that the high frequency of diabetes in hemochromatosis is due not only to pancreatic damage by iron but also to exclusion of chromium from the tissues due to the saturation of the common transport system (75), inducing a chromium deficit.

Chromium, except in pharmacologic doses, would not seem likely to impair iron binding to transferrin because the absorbed amounts of chromium are so low. However, when human serum was incubated with different concentrations of iron up to 40 μM in the absence or presence of 19.2 nmol/L chromium (the situation reported in dialysis patients), there was significant interference with iron binding by chromium (76). Rats injected intraperitoneally for 45 days with high doses of chromium (19.2 μmol/kg body weight) had reduced serum iron, total iron-binding capacity, ferritin, hemoglobin, and hematocrit (76).

C. Retention and Tissue Distribution

1. Models

Mertz and co-workers (77) injected rats intravenously with $^{51}CrCl_3$ and used whole-body counting to determine ^{51}Cr retention. On the basis of retention rates, they proposed at least three body chromium compartments with half-lives estimated at 0.5, 5.9, and 83.4 days. Onkelinx (78) also proposed a three-compartment model but suggested different characteristics for the third compartment. A rapidly exchanging chromium pool and an "inner" pool with "sinklike" characteristics have also been suggested (79).

In humans the distribution of intravenous $^{51}Cr^{3+}$ was observed with whole-body scanning and counting in three normal subjects (80), resulting in a model with a plasma pool in equilibrium with fast ($T_{1/2}$ = 0.5–12 h), medium (1–14 days), and slow (3–12 months) compartments. However, chromium-exposed workers had consistently lower serum chromium values than those predicted by this model (81).

2. Pregnancy

In pregnant rats injected with ^{51}Cr the placentofetal tissue extracted large amounts of ^{51}Cr at the expense of serum and nonfetal tissue (82), suggesting that maternal chromium may be depleted during gestation. Several investigators have suggested human chromium depletion during pregnancy based on hair analyses (83–85), but these hair analyses are not reliable.

3. Aging

A number of animal studies indicate different tissue distribution of chromium in older than in younger animals. Younger rats injected with ^{51}Cr had more ^{51}Cr in bones and less in the spleen, kidney, and testes compared to mature animals (86). Others have found that chromium declined in most tissues of aging rats (78,87). Tissue concentrations in the 9- to 10-month-old rats were lower in several tissues, including liver, heart, fat, muscle, and skeleton. Spleen and serum (or plasma) ^{51}Cr increased.

There are no data on the tissue distribution of chromium in aging humans (11), but no differences were found in the absorption or excretion of ^{51}Cr between elderly subjects and younger individuals (88). There is no information on whether aging impairs the ability to convert inorganic chromium to a biologically active form.

4. Diabetes

In rats with experimentally induced diabetes mellitus, there was a significant reduction in total body retention of ^{51}Cr that could be partially restored toward normal with insulin (89). Also, the fractional distribution of ^{51}Cr in liver of diabetic rats and in rats fed a high-fat diet differed from control animals (90). The relevance of these studies to humans is uncertain.

D. Excretion

Once it is in the bloodstream, chromium is excreted rapidly via the urine. Very small losses are thought to occur in sweat, bile, and hair (86).

1. Mechanism

Some uncertainty surrounds the mechanism of chromium excretion. Glomerular filtration without reabsorption has been postulated. Ultrafilterable ^{51}Cr was in a ratio of approximately 1 with creatinine in dogs given ^{51}Cr by gavage and intravenously (91). This ultrafilterable chromium was 9–19% of total plasma chromium when given by gavage and 2–3% when given i.v., indicating that the ultrafilterable ^{51}Cr and the glomerular filtration rate are the primary determinants of ^{51}Cr excretion. However, in rats, diuresis did not affect body retention of chromium, suggesting that there may be reabsorption of chromium in the proximal tubules (92).

2. Normal Losses

Average urinary chromium excretion in humans ranges from about 4 to 8 nmol/d (0.2–0.4 μg) (37,57,58). In a study in which normal subjects were given a dose of $^{51}CrCl_3$, a mean of 0.69% of the dose (range = 0.3–1.3%) was found in the urine within 72 h (60). Five- to ten-fold increases occur after oral doses of 200 μg (3.85 μmol) (49). Baseline levels are restored about 6 h later. Moderate exercise does not significantly increase urinary chromium losses (93), while strenuous exercise did increase urinary excretion on the day of a 6-mile run (94).

   The urinary excretion of chromium by an individual varies little from day to day, assuming consistent patterns of diet and exercise (58). During a 12-day period, chromium excretion was 5.77 nmol/day for one man and 5.38 nmol/day for the other with standard deviations of ±0.58 and ±0.96 nmol/day, respectively. Other investigators reported similar daily urinary chromium excretions (37,57). Because the kidney is the major route of excretion of absorbed chromium, measures of urinary chromium are suggestive, but not precise, indicators of chromium absorption. Several lines of evidence point to increased urinary losses of chromium associated with moderate increases in circulating insulin (95).

3. Excessive Losses

Chromium losses were stimulated by consumption of diets that were high in simple sugars (65,96). Urinary chromium losses were related to the insulinogenic properties of carbohydrates (95). Urinary chromium increased in trauma patients (50) and in diabetic patients (93). After an orally administered dose of $^{51}CrCl_3$, insulin-requiring diabetic patients excreted a mean of 1.9% (0.9–3.2%); this excretion was two- to threefold higher than excretion from nondiabetic subjects (88). Also, urinary ^{51}Cr excretion was increased in guinea pigs when they were depleted of ascorbic acid (66).

E. Metabolic Balance

Metabolic chromium balance is possible on diets containing <40 μg (<0.77 μmol) chromium/day. Two men, studied for 12 days in a metabolic ward (58), were fed nutritionally adequate diets containing 37 μg (0.71 μmol) chromium/day. While the subjects were in apparent balance (+11.5 nmol/day and +3.8 nmol/day), dermal and hair losses were not measured. These data concur with those of a 5-day balance study in free-living subjects (57). Such balances may become precarious during illness and physiologic stress. Much work remains in order to understand the effects that exogenous and endogenous constituents may have on chromium balance and to relate the chemical form of the dietary chromium to the metabolic processes.

V. PHYSIOLOGIC FUNCTIONS

A. Metabolic Roles

1. Insulin Action

Chromium has been reported to potentiate insulin action, promoting glucose uptake by the cells, but the mechanism remains elusive (97). An early report indicated that hepatic sensitivity to insulin increased in chromium-supplemented rats (98). When insulin together with methionine was injected into chromium-supplemented rats, hepatic protein synthesis increased. Several in vitro and in vivo animal studies, conducted to investigate the biochemical function of chromium, have been reviewed (7–13,16–18).

A deficiency of chromium or an impairment of its metabolism may limit the potentiation of insulin action and adversely affect the metabolism of carbohydrate, protein, and lipid. Circulating levels of glucose, insulin, and glucagon in response to a glucose load were decreased by chromium supplementation in subjects with mildly impaired glucose tolerance who were being fed a low-chromium diet (99). The difficulty in interpreting these data relates to the lack of information on the chromium status of the patients and thus whether the response was physiologic.

Glucose utilization and beta-cell sensitivity, measured by a hyperglycemic clamp technique, improved modestly with chromium supplementation in five glucose-intolerant people (100). These subjects, mean age 66 years, were fed 200 μg (3.85 μmol) of chromium for 12 weeks. The small improvement in glucose economy was attributed to the higher insulin levels, caused either by an increased beta-cell sensitivity to glucose or a decreased insulin clearance. Normal subjects showed an inverse relationship between plasma chromium and insulin during and 24 h after a glucose load (101). Increased urinary losses did not fully account for the removal of chromium from the plasma, suggesting that the chromium was taken up or bound possibly by the insulin-sensitive tissues. The clinical relevance of this remains to be established.

Three studies have indicated that chromium affects the pancreas directly. In pregnant rats, chromium supplementation began on day 1 of gestation and continued for 50 days after conception. Chromium supplemented adults had lower pancreatic insulin concentrations. Neonates whose dams received chromium had basal serum insulins of 77 ± 40 pmol/L, while control neonates had 131 ± 67 pmol insulin/L. Insulin secretion of neonates' islets was not different in this study, but insulin biosynthesis increased significantly in the islets from the +Cr neonates (102). In a second study, insulin secretion by perfused rat pancreata from chromium-supplemented rats was higher than in controls (103). In a third, chromium-deprived rats had greater pancreas weight than rats supplemented with 1 μg chromium/kg of diet (104).

2. Lipid Metabolism

A link has been suspected between chromium and lipid metabolism at least since 1962 (5). In rats, chromium supplementation reduced serum cholesterol and aortic plaque (21,105). In rabbits fed a high-cholesterol diet, atherosclerotic plaques regressed after the rabbits received chromium (106). In obese mice, hepatic lipid concentration decreased in chromium-supplemented animals (107). In another study, the combination of chromium and ascorbate deprivation increased serum cholesterol of guinea pigs (108). Several human trials are described in Section V.C, but neither animal nor human studies have provided a basis for proposing and testing a mode of action.

3. Interactions with Nucleic Acids

Chromium has been administered to mice as $CrCl_3$, 0.1–96 µmol/kg body weight (109). About 20% of the dose remained in the nuclei of liver cells 48 h after the intraperitoneal injection, and RNA synthesis was enhanced. The effect of the chromium was dose dependent. The chromium dose in this experiment was high, but results confirmed earlier studies noting the association of chromium with nucleic acids. A second experiment investigated hepatic nucleolar RNA synthesis in partially hepatectomized rats (110). Synthesis was enhanced and the RNA was processed to rRNA. To test the hypothesis that chromium which accumulates in nucleoli may participate in nucleolar gene expression, the investigators studied a chromatin-chromium complex prepared from mouse liver chromatin and $CrCl_3$ (111). The results of this in-vitro experiment suggested the Cr^{3+} was bound preferentially to DNA in chromatin and caused an increase in initiation sites, thus enhancing RNA synthesis. Nielsen (16) hypothesizes an indirect role for Cr on insulin action, regulating gene expression of a molecule that potentiates insulin action. Further work will be necessary to support this hypothesis.

4. Other Proposed Targets for Chromium Action

Investigators have proposed the involvement of chromium in the lens (112,113) and in the thyroid gland (114). One study found that supplementation of growing feeder pigs with chromium picolinate increased longissimus muscle area and percentage of muscling and decreased tenth-rib fat (115), while another study found no improvement in growth rate or composition of gain with chromium picolinate supplementation (116).

Mertz (8) has noted that the slow reaction rate at which Cr^{3+} tends to form coordination compounds "suggests that chromium would exert a structural function rather than one as an active site in an enzyme. Consistent with this suggestion, no chromium-containing enzymes have been identified" (8).

B. Signs of Deficiency

1. Animals

Impaired glucose tolerance has been attributed to chromium depletion in a number of species (7,21). Schroeder and co-workers reported increased serum cholesterol and plaque formation with chromium deficiency in rats (117); accumulation of hepatic lipid also has been observed in obese mice (107). Reduced ability to incorporate glycine, serine, and methionine into protein was noted in chromium-deficient rats (98). However, investigators today have difficulty in producing a clear-cut chromium deficiency syndrome in most animal species. Animals must be housed in plastic cages, and exposure to any adventitious chromium must be controlled. Semipurified laboratory diets must be formulated to contain <1.0 µmol/kg to demonstrate chromium depletion (65). Furthermore, an additional metabolic stress may be required for symptoms of chromium deficiency to be apparent (118). Whether the early investigators of chromium deficiency actually produced the syndrome remains a mystery, particularly since they had no accurate way to measure it.

2. Humans

Patients Receiving Total Parenteral Nutrition

In 1977, Jeejeebhoy et al. (6) described a patient who developed hyperglycemia, weight loss, ataxia, and peripheral neuropathy after receiving total parenteral nutrition (TPN) without chromium for 3½ years. After 250 μg (4.81 μmol) of chromium as $CrCl_3$ were added, without insulin, to the daily infusate for 2 weeks, glucose tolerance and neurologic function returned to normal and the lost body weight was regained. Normal glucose tolerance was then maintained on an intravenous dose of 0.38 μmol (20 μg) of chromium daily. The clinical course of the patient is shown in Fig. 2.

A second and third report of successful chromium therapy in TPN patients followed in 1979 (119) and 1986 (120). In the second case, severe hyperglycemia occurred 5 months after the beginning of TPN therapy without added chromium. In this case the rapid development of symptoms of chromium deficiency and the patient's prior rapid weight loss suggest that the chromium deficit may have antedated the TPN therapy (119). The third patient developed unexplained hyperglycemia, glycosuria, and weight loss with no signs of mental changes or peripheral neuropathy after almost 7 months of TPN containing 0.115 μmol (6 μg) of chromium/day (120). The investigators postulated that the rapid development of chromium depletion, despite the chromium in the daily infusate, was possible because this patient suffered excessive jejunostomy losses during hospitalization.

Although these cases document that chromium deficiency can be identified retrospectively in patients whose unexplained hyperglycemia is corrected by chromium supplementation, they provide no correlation between levels of chromium in body tissues or fluids and the signs of chromium deficiency. This is because the chromium methodology in these cases generated measurements that were 20 to 100 times too high.

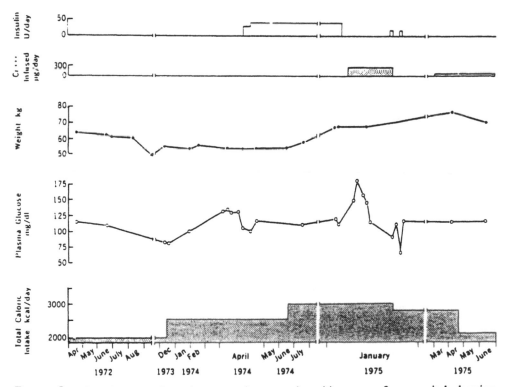

FIGURE 2 Clinical course of a patient on total parenteral nutrition over a 3-year period, showing caloric intake (kcal/day), plasma glucose (mg/dL), body weight (kg), and amounts of Cr^{3+} (μg) and insulin (U) infused per day during treatment periods. (Reproduced from Ref. 6, with permission.)

These TPN studies, accidental experiments, made apparent the following: (1) Inorganic chromium given intravenously can, in a matter of days, reverse the abnormality in glucose metabolism; (2) if conversion to a biologically active form is necessary, this conversion can occur quite rapidly, (3) chromium is an essential nutrient in the human; and (4) 0.38 μmol (20 μg) of inorganic chromium per day is a quite adequate intravenous dose for maintenance of normal carbohydrate physiology. A recent review of trace element recommendations for parenteral nutrition summarizes current recommendations (121).

Subjects Fed Orally

Documenting chromium deficiency and its sequelae in orally fed people has been very difficult. Severe chromium deficiency is most unlikely, because the very small amounts of dietary chromium needed are found not only in a variety of foods, but also as a contaminant from cookware (55). While habitually unsound eating habits with consequent deficits or excesses of other dietary or therapeutic elements may contribute to marginal chromium deficiencies, the absence of a reliable laboratory marker to diagnose chromium deficiency is a serious impediment to establishing causality.

C. Clinical Significance

1. Malnourished Children

Malnourished children in Jordan suffering from diverse types of undernutrition were given varying amounts of $CrCl_3$ under disparate conditions. Improvement in glucose removal followed in a number of children, but because preexisting chromium deficiency states were not documented in these studies and other therapeutic interventions were being carried out, it is not certain that the chromium was responsible for the improvement in glucose tolerance in those children who showed a change (122).

2. Pregnancy

Animal work lends credence to the suggestion that maternal chromium depletion may be a factor in the prevalence of glucose intolerance and transient diabetes of pregnancy (82). While a study in pregnant women supports this thesis (85), no measurements of deficiency were done by hair analysis, a very inaccurate technique.

3. Maturity-Onset Diabetes Mellitus

Chromium deficiency was suggested early to be an etiologic factor in some cases of maturity-onset diabetes mellitus (2). There might be more chromium lost in the urine due to the increased diuresis common in uncontrolled diabetes; in an animal study, however, diuresis was not a major factor in chromium loss (123). In human diabetes, there has been inconsistency in the reported changes in glucose tolerance following supplementation with inorganic chromium or chromium in brewer's yeast (10).

Major problems in the design and evaluation of the supplementation studies have been the uncertainty of the biologic activity of inorganic chromium and the lack of a purified, biologically active chromium compound. Consequently, a number of different types of chromium supplements have been used, including different strains and quantities of brewer's yeast, synthetic chromium compounds, and inorganic Cr^{3+}. Thus, the possible role of chromium in diabetes mellitus is unclear. This is not surprising when we consider the heterogeneity of the diabetic population, the diversity of etiological factors, and the fact that there is no way of separating for study those diabetics whose diets might be chromium deficient from those who might suffer from impaired chromium absorption, faulty chromium conversion to the biologically active molecule, a metabolic defect, or excessive urinary excretion of chromium. There is need for careful research using better methodology.

To identify a group of subjects having a high likelihood of abnormal chromium status, Anderson et al. (99) selected as hyperglycemic subjects eight adults whose glucose values 90 min after a glucose load were >5.56 but <11.1 mmol/L. Controls had 90-min glucose values <5.56 mmol/L. After a 4-week pretest period, the subjects were given one tablet daily of 200 μg (3.85 μmol) chromium as $CrCl_3$, or placebo, in a double-blind, 14-week crossover design. Four-hour oral glucose tolerance tests were performed after weeks 1, 4, 9, and 14. The subjects were fed a low-chromium diet of <20 μg (<0.38 μmol) chromium. The diet was nutritionally adequate, and a multivitamin supplement was added. The glucose tolerance of the control subjects did not change regardless of whether they were on the low-chromium diet or whether they received the chromium supplement. The hyperglycemic subjects had increasingly elevated 60-min glucose values during the 9 weeks on the low-chromium diet. During chromium supplementation, their glucose values were equal to or lower than the corresponding placebo values. Insulin values followed a similar course for hyperglycemic and control subjects. Serum immunoreactive glucagon sums from 0 to 120 min and 0 to 240 min were also lower after supplementation in the hyperglycemics. Whether the hyperglycemic subjects fed a low-chromium diet became chromium depleted is unclear.

4. Elderly Persons

Because the incidence of impaired glucose tolerance is age related, there have been a number of supplementation trials in elderly groups. In studies in the 1960s and 1970s, improved glucose disposal rates were reported in about half of the elderly subjects given inorganic chromium or brewer's yeast supplements for periods of several weeks to 4 months (11,13). More recent supplementation trials have been better designed but still have provided seemingly contradictory data. Two groups of investigators found that glucose tolerances improved after they fed $CrCl_3$ or brewer's yeast supplements to elderly subjects deemed to be "at risk" (124,125). In another study of healthy, free-living subjects who were given brewer's yeast, or 200 μg (3.85 μmol) of Cr as $CrCl_3$, or placebo, there were no changes in glucose, insulin, or lipid values (126). Perhaps the latter group, though elderly, was not chromium deficient. In one study, glucose tolerance improved only when 200 μg (3.86 μmol) chromium as $CrCl_3$ was given together with 100 mg (812 μmol) nicotinic acid (25). In other groups of supplemented middle-aged and older adults, glucose tolerance improved little, but some improvement in insulin levels was reported (127,128).

Interpretation of these data, as well as the data obtained in studies of diabetics, is hampered by the multifactorial nature of abnormal glucose and insulin metabolism. The studies may have been done on the wrong target populations, so that supplementation was given either to subjects with normal glucose tolerance who were therefore unlikely to suffer from chromium deficiency, or to subjects who, while showing abnormal glucose tolerance, had normal chromium status and thus would not be expected to respond to supplementary chromium. The confusion concerning who is and who is not chromium deficient makes it difficult to interpret the supplementation studies. Also, an adequate effect might not be obtained with inorganic chromium in individuals who might have problems absorbing or converting the inorganic chromium to the active form.

5. Cardiovascular Disease

Chromium has been positively correlated with a decrease in the risk of cardiovascular disease (2,3); several studies have focused on the role of chromium in increasing high-density lipoprotein cholesterol (HDL-C) (128–130) or on other favorable lipid responses to chromium supplementation (130–134). Additional larger-scale studies are needed to confirm these effects of chromium on risk factors for cardiovascular disease.

VI. NUTRITIONAL ASSESSMENT AND REQUIREMENTS

A. Recommended Intakes Compared with Customary Intakes

Based on the dietary intakes of healthy subjects and on the experimental data available in the 1970s, the Food and Nutrition Board of the National Academy of Sciences established the first dietary recommendations for chromium in 1980. These estimated safe and adequate daily dietary intakes (ESADDI) were not changed in 1989 (135) and are 10–40 μg/day (0.19–0.77 μmol/day) in infancy, increasing to 50–200 μg (0.96–3.85 μmol) after age 7.

However, customary diets of many people, varying in age, geographic, ethnic, and socioeconomic status, in the United States and elsewhere contain only 20–40 μg (0.38–0.77 μmol) chromium/day (11,37,57,126,136). Some are as low as 15–20 μg/day. Diets consumed by two different groups of free-living, well-nourished elderly volunteers contained an average of 37 μg/day (range 15–55 μg) (126) and 25 μg/day (range 14–48 μg) (57). A group of healthy young adults averaged 39 μg/day (range 11–84 μg) (47), similar to a 7-day average chromium intake of 33 μg/day (range 22–48 μg) for men and 25 μg/day (range 13–36 μg) for women. Chromium in most of the diets was between 20 and 25 μg/1000 kcal (91 and 115 nmol/1000 kJ) (11), similar to the 15 μg/1000 kcal chromium content of 22 daily diets designed by nutritionists (56). Diets that were high in fat were lower in chromium than diets that were lower in fat (137).

B. Sources of Dietary Chromium

1. In Infant Feedings

The chromium concentration of human milk is reported to range from 2.3 to 10.2 nmol/L (0.12 to 0.53 ng/mL), with a mean and standard deviation of 5.2 ± 1.9 nmol/L (138). The mean daily intake of fully breast-fed infants for 31 days postpartum was 150 ng (2.88 nmol)/day. Other workers found a mean chromium concentration in breast milk of 3.54 ± 0.40 nmol/L (139). Assuming a breast milk intake of 715 mL/d, exclusively breast-fed babies would receive <2% of the 10-μg lower limit of the ESADDI. Others report infant intakes of from 100 ng (1.92 nmol) chromium/day (140) to 270 ng (5.2 nmol)/day (141), with no decline in chromium content as lactation progresses (141). Three-month-old Belgian babies fed cow's milk received 0.5 μg (9.6 nmol) chromium/day, compared with 0.1 μg (1.9 nmol) through breast milk (140). Similar intakes are reported for a large number of infants from widely varied geographic regions (142). If human milk is accepted as the desirable standard for infant feeding (139), the current ESADDI for infants (some 50–350 times greater) needs to be reassessed.

2. In Foods and Beverages

Only recently have reliable data on the chromium content of a wide variety of foods become available, due notably to the Food Research Programme of the FAO European Research Network on Trace Elements (141) and the analyses of commonly consumed foods and beverages by Anderson et al. (56) at the United States Department of Agriculture laboratories.

As shown in Table 2, dairy products contain little chromium. Meats, poultry, and fish vary widely, with much of the chromium attributable to its introduction during the transport, processing, and fortification of foods (56). The use of stainless steel equipment in food processing adds measurable amounts of chromium (55), especially to acidic foods, salted foods, and foods that are in close contact to stainless steel while being heated, ground, or chopped.

Chromium varies widely in grain products, fruits, and vegetables, probably for the reasons cited above. While some condiments and spices have generous amounts of chromium, most normally contribute trivial amounts to the total diet because very small amounts are customarily consumed.

C. Are Intakes Too Low or Recommendations Too High?

The balance studies described in Section IV (57,58) raise the question of whether the low chromium intakes that have been reported are adequate for positive metabolic balance. If dietary chromium is marginal and the diet contains factors that reduce chromium absorption and/or increase chromium losses, or if needs increase, chromium balance could be compromised. That is, dietary chromium below 50 µg/day (1 µmol/day) may indeed be marginal and metabolic penalties may result.

However, because many elderly subjects are able to maintain apparent good health on even lower chromium intakes than those reported in the metabolic balance studies, several possibilities are suggested: (a) Utilization is materially enhanced by the form of the dietary chromium (inorganic versus organically complexed) or by the presence of compounds that promote absorption; (b) human chromium requirements are not as high as previously thought in healthy individuals; or (c) low chromium intakes are a risk to health only if dietary factors that inhibit chromium absorption are present, or when illness, aging, or other stresses increase chromium needs or losses.

From the available data, it would seem that the most likely cause of a chromium deficit in healthy people is the combination of a low-chromium diet with (a) the habitual underconsumption of nutrients that enhance its absorption and utilization, and/or (b) overconsumption of nutrients or other food factors that impair chromium absorption or retention, and/or (c) the chronic ingestion of therapeutic agents that adversely affect chromium. This casts doubt on the ability of individuals to sustain positive metabolic balance under adverse conditions when their customary diets contain only enough chromium for balance under ideal conditions. Whether or not the 50–200-µg (0.96–3.85-µmol) estimate of a safe and adequate daily chromium intake is higher than necessary should be reexamined in light of the more recent studies that correlate actual chromium intakes with concomitant dietary constituents and with the indirect health effects now being studied. However, precise recommendations await the development of a clinically feasible measure of chromium status. These information gaps have not inhibited the promotion of chromium supplements as a panacea for weight loss. Recently chromium picolinate has been promoted in tabloids

TABLE 2 Chromium Content of Selected Foods

	Cr, ng/g[a]	μg/serving
Dairy products		
Milk, 1 cup = 244 g	<0.50	<0.12
Margarine, 1 pat = 5 g	3 ± 1	0.02
American cheese, 1 oz = 28 g	20 ± 1	0.56
Meats, poultry, fish and eggs		
Eggs, 1 egg = 50 g	4 ± 1	0.20
Beef cubes, 3 oz = 85 g	24 ± 1	2.0
Chicken breast, 3 oz = 85 g	6 ± 1	0.50
Turkey breast 3 oz = 85 g	20 ± 1	1.7
Turkey ham, 3 oz = 85 g	122 ± 19	10.4
Ham, 3 oz = 85 g	42 ± 4	3.6
Haddock, baked, 3 oz = 85 g	7 ± 1	0.60
Grain products		
Waffles, 1 waffle = 75 g	89 ± 6	6.7
Whole wheat bread, 1 slice = 25 g	39 ± 1	0.98
English muffin, whole wheat, 1 muffin = 100 g	36 ± 1	3.6
Rye bread, 1 slice = 25 g	37 ± 6	0.92
Bagel egg, 1 bagel = 55 g	46 ± 7	2.5
Spaghetti, 1 cup = 140 g	2 ± 1	0.28
Fruits and vegetables		
Banana, peeled, 1 med = 126 g	8 ± 2	1.0
Grapes, 10 grapes = 50 g	2 ± 0	0.10
Apple, unpeeled, 1 med = 150 g	9 ± 1	1.4
Juice, grape, 1 cup = 250 g	30 ± 1	7.5
Juice, orange, 1 cup = 248 g	9 ± 2	2.2
Peas, 1 cup = 160 g	5 ± 1	0.80
Tomato, 1 med = 135 g	7 ± 1	0.94
Green beans, 1 cup = 135 g	16 ± 0	2.2
Potatoes, mashed, 1 cup = 210 g	18 ± 1	2.7
Broccoli, 1 cup = 185 g	118 ± 0	22.0
Condiments		
Pepper, 1 packet = 0.25 g	145 ± 15	0.04
Mustard, 1 tsp = 5 g	48 ± 6	0.24
Ketchup, 1 tbsp = 17 g	58 ± 0	0.99
Barbecue sauce, 1 tbsp = 16 g	108 ± 8	1.73

[a]Based on wet weight, "as served."
Source: Adapted from Ref. 56.

and featured in popular books as an appetite suppressant and muscle builder that can increase metabolism and decrease body fat. While several studies (142,144) have suggested that it may be better absorbed than $CrCl_3$, the results with chromium picolinate have been inconsistent. Nevertheless, it continues to sell briskly over-the-counter, through distributors and mail-order houses, and even via pyramid-type selling schemes in what one writer (145) has characterized as "the scam of the hour."

VII. PHARMACOLOGY AND TOXICITY

Hexavalent chromium, Cr^{6+}, not trivalent chromium, Cr^{3+}, poses a health hazard (146). Exposure to chromate dust is correlated with an increased incidence of lung cancer and is a known cause of dermatitis (147). The occupational exposure to Cr^{6+} compounds is potentially carcinogenic, and experiments indicate that these compounds may be genotoxic and mutagenic. Inside cells, Cr^{6+} is reduced to Cr^{3+} via intermediates that can react with protein and nucleic acids. For this reason, some salts of hexavalent chromium are cytotoxic and pose an industrial problem (148).

The mechanism by which Cr^{6+} exerts its toxic effects is uncertain. Recent evidence implicates the reduction of Cr^{6+} to Cr^{5+} and the subsequent formation of hydroxyl radicals ($\cdot OH$). Direct evidence using electron spin resonance indicates that NADPH in the presence of glutathione reductase (GRx) is involved in the reduction of Cr^{6+} to the Cr^{5+} species (149). Thus, at least one of the initial steps in the Cr^{6+} reduction involves a one-electron transfer process. Hexavalent chromium caused DNA–protein crosslinks in some cell lines, while trivalent chromium compounds caused no damage to DNA (148).

The body burden of chromium due to occupational exposure may decrease rapidly after the exposure ends. Workers in the leather tanning industry in Ontario exhibited significantly elevated levels of chromium in hair, serum, and urine, but hair and serum chromium had declined to levels comparable to control subjects by 9 months or more following cessation of employment (81). The health consequences from cessation of the occupational exposure are not known.

VIII. FUTURE RESEARCH NEEDS

Future research needs include: (a) A clinical test to identify individuals who are chromium deficient and those who have a problem converting inorganic chromium to its active form; (b) identification, purification, and/or synthesis of a biologically active molecule; (c) elucidation of mechanisms for chromium's role in insulin/glucose metabolism and in lipid metabolism and the clinical relevance; (d) identification of factors in the diet that may affect absorption/distribution of chromium thus affecting the needs of people; (e) evaluation of the proper recommendations for ESADDI, especially for infants, and of recommendations for TPN; and (f) evaluation of effects of disease states on the requirements for chromium.

REFERENCES

1. Schwartz K, Mertz W. Chromium(III) and the glucose tolerance factor. Arch Biochem Biophys 1959; 85:292–295.
2. Schroeder HA, Nason AP, Tipton IH. Chromium deficiency as a factor in atherosclerosis. J Chron Dis 1970; 23:123–128.
3. Mertz W. Trace minerals and atherosclerosis. Fed Proc 1982; 41:2807–2812.
4. Newman HAI, Leighton RF, Lanese RR, Freedland NA. Serum chromium and angiographically determined coronary artery disease. Clin Chem 1978; 24:541–544.
5. Schroeder HA, Balassa JJ, Tipton IH. Abnormal trace metals in man—chromium. J Chron Dis 1962; 15:941–964.
6. Jeejeebhoy KN, Chu RC, Marliss EB, Greenberg GR, Bruce-Robertson A. Chromium deficiency, glucose intolerance, and neuropathy reversed by chromium supplementation, in a patient receiving long-term total parenteral nutrition. Am J Clin Nutr 1977; 30:531–538.

7. Anderson RA. Chromium. In: Mertz W, ed. Trace Elements in Human and Animal Nutrition. Vol. 5. New York: Academic Press, 1987:225–244.

8. Mertz W. Chromium: History and nutritional importance. Biol Trace Elem Res 1992; 32:3–8.

9. Mertz W. Chromium in human nutrition: a review. J Nutr 1993; 123:626–633.

10. Offenbacher EG, Pi-Sunyer FX. Chromium in human nutrition. In: Olson RE, Beutler E, Broquist HP, eds. Annual Reviews of Nutrition. Vol. 8. Palo Alto, CA: Annual Reviews, 1988: 543–563.

11. Offenbacher EG. Chromium in the elderly. Biol Trace Elem Res 1992; 32:123–131.

12. Stoecker B. Chromium. In: Brown M, ed. Present Knowledge in Nutrition. Vol. 6. Washington, DC: International Life Sciences Institute, Nutrition Foundation, 1990:287–293.

13. Wallach S. Clinical and biochemical aspects of chromium deficiency. J Am Coll Nutr 1985; 4:107–120.

14. Gibson RS, Ferguson EF, Vanderkooy PDS, Macdonald AC. Seasonal variations in hair zinc concentrations in Canadian and African children. Sci Total Envir 1989; 84:291–298.

15. Anderson RA. Recent advances in the clinical and biochemical effects of chromium deficiency. Prog Clin Biol Res 1993; 380:221–234.

16. Nielsen FH. Chromium. In: Shils ME, Olson JA, Shike M, eds. Modern Nutrition in Health and Disease. Vol. 8. Philadelphia: Lea & Febiger, 1994:264–268.

17. Anderson RA. Nutritional and toxicologic aspects of chromium intake: an overview. In: Mertz W, Abernathy CO, Olin SS, eds. Risk Assessment of Essential Elements. Washington, DC: ILSI Press, 1994:187–196.

18. Stoecker BJ. Derivation of the estimated safe and adequate daily dietary intake for chromium. In: Mertz W, Abernathy CO, Olin SS, eds. Risk Assessment of Essential Elements. Washington, DC: ILSI Press, 1994:197–205.

19. Emsley J. The Elements. Oxford: Oxford University Press, 1992:1–251.

20. Ducros V. Chromium metabolism: a literature review. Biol Trace Elem Res 1992; 32:65–77.

21. Mertz W. Chromium occurrence and function in biological systems. Physiol Rev 1969; 49: 163–239.

22. Toepfer EW, Mertz W, Polansky MM, Roginski EE, Wolf WR. Preparation of chromium-containing material of glucose tolerance factor activity from brewer's yeast extracts and by synthesis. J Agric Food Chem 1977; 25:162–166.

23. Yamamoto A, Wada O, Suzuki H. Purification and properties of biologically active chromium complex from bovine colostrum. J Nutr 1988; 118:39–45.

24. Mertz W, Toepfer EW, Roginski EE, Polansky MM. Present knowledge of the role of chromium. Fed Proc 1974; 33:2275–2280.

25. Urberg M, Zemel MB. Evidence for synergism between chromium and nicotinic acid in the control of glucose tolerance in elderly humans. Metabolism 1987; 36:896–899.

26. Gonzalez-Vergara E, DeGonzalez BC, Hegenauer J, Saltman P. Chromium coordination compounds of pyridoxal and nicotinic acid: synthesis, absorption and metabolism. Israel J Chem 1981; 21:18–22.

27. Stoecker BJ, Li Y-C, Wester DB, Chan S-B. Effects of torula and brewer's yeast diets in obese and lean mice. Biol Trace Elem Res 1987; 14:249–254.

28. Mirsky N, Weiss A, Dori Z. Chromium in biological systems, I. Some observations on glucose tolerance factor in yeast. J Inorg Biochem 1980; 13:11–21.

29. Yamamoto A, Wada O., Manabe S. Evidence that chromium is an essential factor for biological activity of low-molecular-weight, chromium-binding substance. Biochem Biophys Res Commun 1989; 163:189–193.

30. Kienle KH, Ditschuneit HH, Opferkuch R, Seeling W. The synthesis of GTF-like chromium coordination compounds and their in vitro action on the fat cell. In: Shapcott D, Hubert J, eds. Chromium in Nutrition and Metabolism. Amsterdam: Elsevier/North-Holland Biomedical Press, 1979:189–197.

31. Okada S, Tsukada H, Tezuka M. Effect of chromium(III) on nuclear RNA synthesis. Biol Trace Elem Res 1989; 21:35–39.

32. Guthrie BE, Wolf WR, Veillon C. Background correction and related problems in the determination of chromium in urine by graphite furnace atomic absorption spectrometry. Anal Chem 1978; 50:1900–1902.

33. Levine RA, Streeten DHP, Doisy RJ. Effects of oral chromium supplementation on the glucose tolerance of elderly human subjects. Metabolism 1968; 17:114–125.

34. Davidson IWF, Burt RL. Physiologic changes in plasma chromium of normal and pregnant women: effect of a glucose load. Am J Obstet Gynecol 1973; 116:601–608.

35. Pekarek RS, Hauer EC, Wannemaker RW, Beisel WR. The direct determination of serum chromium by an atomic absorption spectrophotometer with a heated graphite atomizer. Anal Biochem 1973; 59:283–292.

36. Versieck J, Hoste J, Barbier F, Steyaert H, De Rudder J, Michels H. Determination of chromium and cobalt in human serum by neutron activation analysis. Clin Chem 1978; 24:303–308.

37. Anderson RA, Kozlovsky AS. Chromium intake, absorption and excretion of subjects consuming self-selected diets. Am J Clin Nutr 1985; 41:1177–1183.

38. Randall JA, Gibson RS. Serum and urine chromium as indices of chromium status in tannery workers. Proc Soc Exp Biol Med 1987; 185:16–23.

39. Veillon C, Wolf WR, Guthrie BE. Determination of chromium in biological materials by stable isotope dilution. Anal Chem 1979; 51:1022–1024.

40. Veillon C, Patterson KY, Bryden NA. Chromium in urine as measured by atomic absorption spectrometry. Clin Chem 1982; 28:2309–2311.

41. Veillon C, Patterson KY, Bryden NA. Determination of chromium in human serum by electrothermal atomic absorption spectrometry. Anal Chim Acta 1984; 164:67–76.

42. Veillon C. Trace element analysis of biological samples. Anal Chem 1986; 58:851A–858A.

43. Veillon C. Analytical chemistry of chromium. Sci Total Envir 1989; 86:65–68.

44. Versieck J, Vanballenberghe L, De Kesel A, et al. Certification of a second generation biological reference material (freeze-dried human serum) for trace element determinations. Anal Chim Acta 1988; 204:63–75.

45. Versieck J. Trace elements in human body fluids and tissues. CRC Crit Rev Clin Lab Sci 1985; 22:97–184.

46. Wolf WR. Nutrient trace element composition of foods: Analytical needs and problems. Anal Chem 1978; 50:190A–194A.

47. Offenbacher EG, Dowling HJ, Rinko CJ, Pi-Sunyer FX. Rapid enzymatic pretreatment of samples before determining chromium in serum or plasma. Clin Chem 1986; 32:1383–1386.

48. Veillon C, Patterson KY, Bryden NA. Determination of chromium in human serum by electrothermal atomic absorption spectrometry. Anal Chim Acta 1984; 164:67–76.

49. Anderson RA, Polansky MM, Bryden NA, Patterson KY, Veillon C, Glinsmann WH. Effects of chromium supplementation of urinary Cr excretion of human subjects and correlation of Cr excretion with selected clinical parameters. J Nutr 1983; 113:276–281.

50. Borel JS, Majerus TC, Polansky MM, Moser PB, Anderson RA. Chromium intake and urinary chromium excretion of trauma patients. Biol Trace Elem Res 1984; 6:317–326.

51. Versieck J. Trace element analysis–a plea for accuracy. Trace Elem Med 1984; 1:2–12.

52. Vuori E, Kumpulainen J. A new low level of chromium in human liver and spleen. Trace Elem Med 1987; 4:88–91.

53. Hambridge KM. Hair analysis: worthless for vitamins, limited for minerals. Am J Clin Nutr 1982; 36:943–949.

54. Randall JA, Gibson RS. Hair chromium as an index of chromium exposure of tannery workers. Br J Ind Med 1989; 46:171–175.

55. Offenbacher EG, Pi-Sunyer FX. Temperature and pH effects on the release of chromium from stainless steel into water and fruit juices. J Agric Food Chem 1983; 31:89–92.

56. Anderson RA, Bryden NA, Polansky MM. Dietary chromium intake: freely chosen diets, institutional diets, and individual foods. Biol Trace Elem Res 1992; 32:117–121.

57. Bunker VW, Lawson MS, Delves HT, Clayton B. The uptake and excretion of chromium by the elderly. Am J Clin Nutr 1984; 39:797–802.

58. Offenbacher E, Spencer H, Dowling HJ, Pi-Sunyer FX. Metabolic chromium balances in men. Am J Clin Nutr 1986; 44:77–82.

59. Chen NSC, Tsai A, Dyer IA. Effect of chelating agents on chromium absorption in rats. J Nutr 1973; 103:1182–1186.

60. Doisy RJ, Streeten DHP, Souma ML, Kalafer ME, Rekant SI, Dalakos TG. Metabolism of chromium-51 in human subjects. In: Mertz W, Cornatzer WE, eds. Newer Trace Elements in Nutrition. New York: Marcel Dekker, 1971:155.

61. Dowling HJ, Offenbacher EG, Pi-Sunyer FX. Effects of amino acids on the absorption of trivalent chromium and its retention by regions of the small intestine. Nutr Res 1990; 10:1261–1271.

62. Oberleas D, Li Y-C, Stoecker BJ, Henley SA, Keim KS, Smith JC Jr. The rate of chromium transit through the gastrointestinal tract. Nutr Res 1990; 10:1189–1194.

63. Dowling HJ, Offenbacher EG, Pi-Sunyer FX. Absorption of inorganic, trivalent chromium from the vascularly perfused rat small intestine. J Nutr 1989; 119:1138–1145.

64. Dowling HJ, Offenbacher EG, Pi-Sunyer FX. Effects of plasma transferrin and albumin on the absorption of trivalent chromium. Nutr Res 1990; 10:1251–1260.

65. Seaborn CD, Stoecker BJ. Effects of starch, sucrose, fructose, and glucose on chromium absorption and tissue concentrations in obese and lean mice. J Nutr 1989; 119:1444–1451.

66. Seaborn CD, Stoecker BJ. Effects of ascorbic acid depletion and chromium status on retention and urinary excretion of ^{51}chromium. Nutr Res 1992; 12:1229–1234.

67. Seaborn CD, Stoecker BJ. Effects of antacid or ascorbic acid on tissue accumulation and urinary excretion of ^{51}chromium. Nutr Res 1990; 10:1401–1407.

68. Davis ML, Seaborn CD, Stoecker BJ. Effects of over-the-counter drugs on ^{51}chromium retention and urinary excretion in rats. Nutr Res 1995; 15:202–210.

69. Offenbacher EG. Promotion of chromium absorption by ascorbic acid. Trace Elem Elect 1994; 11:178–181.

70. Hahn CJ, Evans GW. Absorption of trace metals in the zinc-deficient rat. Am J Physiol 1975; 228:1020–1023.

71. Keim KS, Holloway CL, Hegsted M. Absorption of chromium as affected by wheat bran. Cereal Chem 1987; 64:352–355.

72. Keim KS, Stoecker BJ, Henley S. Chromium status of the rat as affected by phytate. Nutr Res 1987; 7:253–263.

73. Hopkins LL Jr, Schwarz K. Chromium(III) binding to serum proteins, specifically siderophilin. Biochim Biophys Acta 1964; 90:484–491.

74. Moshtaghie AA, Ani M, Bazrafshan MR. Comparative binding study of aluminum and chromium to human transferrin: effect of iron. Biol Trace Elem Res 1992; 32:39–46.

75. Sargent T III, Lim TH, Jenson RL. Reduced chromium retention in patients with hemochromatosis, a possible basis of hemochromatotic diabetes. Metabolism 1979; 28:70–79.

76. Ani M, Moshtaghie AA. The effect of chromium on parameters related to iron metabolism. Biol Trace Elem Res 1992; 32:57–64.

77. Mertz W, Roginski EE, Reba RC. Biological activity and fate of trace quantities of intravenous chromium(III) in the rat. Am J Physiol 1965; 209:489–494.

78. Onkelinx C. Compartment analysis of metabolism of chromium(III) in rats of various ages. Am J Physiol 1977; 232:E478–E484.

79. Jain R, Verch RL, Wallach S, Peabody RA. Tissue chromium exchanges in the rat. Am J Clin Nutr 1981; 34:2199–2204.

80. Lim TH, Sargent T III, Kusubov N. Kinetics of trace element chromium(III) in the human body. Am J Physiol 1983; 244:R445–R454.

81. Simpson JR, Gibson RS. Hair, serum, and urine chromium concentrations in former employees of the leather tanning industry. Biol Trace Elem Res 1992; 32:155–159.

82. Wallach S, Verch RL. Placental transport of chromium. J Am Coll Nutr 1984; 3:69–74.

83. van de Werve G, Assimacopoulos-Jeannet F, Jeanrenaud B. Altered liver glycogen metabolism in fed genetically obese mice. Biochem J 1983; 216:273–280.

84. Saner G. The effect of parity on maternal hair chromium concentration and the changes during pregnancy. Am J Clin Nutr 1981; 34:853–855.

85. Aharoni A, Tesler B, Paltieli Y, Tal J, Dori Z, Sharf M. Hair chromium content of women with gestational diabetes compared with nondiabetic pregnant women. Am J Clin Nutr 1992; 55: 104–107.

86. Hopkins LL Jr. Distribution in the rat of physiological amounts of injected Cr-51(III) with time. Am J Physiol 1965; 209:731–735.

87. Wallach S, Verch RL. Radiochromium distribution in aged rats. J Am Coll Nutr 1986; 5:291–298.

88. Doisy RJ, Streeten DHP, Freiberg JM, Schneider AJ. Chromium metabolism in man and biochemical effects. In: Prasad AS, Oberleas D, eds. Trace Elements in Human Health and Disease. Vol. 2. Essential and Toxic Elements. New York: Academic Press, 1976:79.

89. Kraszeski JL, Wallach S, Verch RL. Effect of insulin on radiochromium distribution in diabetic rats. Endocrinology 1979; 104:881–885.

90. Mathur RK, Doisy RJ. Effect of diabetes and diet on the distribution of trace doses of chromium in rats. Proc Soc Exp Biol Med 1972; 139:836–838.

91. Donaldson DL, Smith CC, Yunice AA. Renal excretion of chromium-51 chloride in the dog. Am J Physiol 1984; 246:F870–F878.

92. Wallach S, Verch RL. Radiochromium distribution during saline diuresis. J Am Coll Nutr 1986; 5:299–304.

93. Anderson RA. Chromium metabolism and its role in disease processes in man. Clin Physiol Biochem 1986; 4:31–41.

94. Anderson RA, Polansky MM, Bryden NA, Roginski EE, Patterson KY, Reamer DC. Effect of exercise (running) on serum glucose, insulin, glucagon, and chromium excretion. Diabetes 1982; 31:212–216.

95. Anderson RA, Bryden NA, Polansky MM, Reiser S. Urinary chromium excretion and insulinogenic properties of carbohydrates. Am J Clin Nutr 1990; 51:864–868.

96. Kozlovsky AS, Moser PB, Reiser S, Anderson RA. Effects of diets high in simple sugars on urinary chromium losses. Metabolism 1986; 35:515–518.

97. Evans GW, Roginski EE, Mertz W. Interactions of the glucose tolerance factor (GTF) with insulin. Biochem Biophys Res Commun 1973; 50:718–722.

98. Roginski E, Mertz W. Effects of chromium(III) supplementation on glucose and amino acid metabolism in rats fed a low protein diet. J Nutr 1969; 97:525–530.

99. Anderson RA, Polansky MM, Bryden NA, Canary JJ. Supplemental-chromium effects on glucose, insulin, glucagon, and urinary chromium losses in subjects consuming controlled low-chromium diets. Am J Clin Nutr 1991; 54:909–916.

100. Potter JF, Levin P, Anderson RA, Freiberg JM, Andres R, Elahi D. Glucose metabolism in glucose-intolerant older people during chromium supplementation. Metabolism 1985; 34: 199–204.

101. Morris BW, Blumsohn A, MacNeil S, Gray TA. The trace element chromium—a role in glucose homeostasis. Am J Clin Nutr 1992; 55:989–991.

102. Hubner G, Noack K, Zuhlke H, Hartmann K. Influence of trivalent chromium on the beta-cell function. Exp Clin Endocrinol 1989; 93:293–298.

103. Striffler JS, Polansky MM, Anderson RA. Dietary chromium enhances insulin secretion in perfused rat pancreas. J Trace Elem Exp Med 1993; 6:75–81.

104. Campbell WW, Polansky MM, Bryden, Soares JHJ, Anderson RA. Exercise training and dietary chromium effects on glycogen, glycogen synthase, phosphorylase and total protein in rats. J Nutr 1989; 119:653–660.

105. Schroeder HA. The role of chromium in mammalian nutrition. Am J Clin Nutr 1968; 21: 230–244.

106. Abraham AS, Brooks BA, Eylath U. Chromium and cholesterol-induced atherosclerosis in rabbits. Ann Nutr Metab 1991; 35:203–207.

107. Li Y-C, Stoecker BJ. Chromium and yogurt effects on hepatic lipid and plasma glucose and insulin of obese mice. Biol Trace Elem Res 1986; 9:233–242.

108. Stoecker BJ, Oladut WK. Effects of chromium and ascorbate deficiencies on glucose tolerance and serum cholesterol of guinea pigs. Nutr Rep Int 1985; 32:399–405.

109. Okada S, Suzuki M, Ohba H. Enhancement of ribonucleic acid synthesis by chromium(III) in mouse liver. J Inorg Biochem 1983; 19:95–103.

110. Okada S, Tsukada H, Ohba H. Enhancement of nucleolar RNA synthesis by chromium(III) in regenerating rat liver. J Inorg Biochem 1984; 21:113–124.

111. Ohba H, Suketa Y, Okada S. Enhancement of in vitro ribonucleic acid synthesis on chromium(III)-bound chromatin. J Inorg Biochem 1986; 27:179–189.

112. Pineau A, Guillard O, Risse JF. A study of chromium in human cataractous lenses and whole blood of diabetics, senile, and normal population. Biol Trace Elem Res 1992; 32:133–138.

113. Pineau A, Guillard O, Chauvelon F, Risse J-F. Total chromium in the human lens: determination with Zeeman electrothermal atomic absorption spectrometry following mineralization in a mini-autoclave. Biol Trace Elem Res 1992; 32:139–143.

114. Lifschitz ML, Wallach S, Peabody RA, Verch RL, Agrawal R. Radiochromium distribution in thyroid and parathyroid deficiency. Am J Clin Nutr 1980; 33:57–62.

115. Page TG, Southern LL, Ward TL, Thompson DL Jr. Effect of chromium picolinate on growth and serum and carcass traits of growing-finishing pigs. J Anim Sci 1993; 71:656–662.

116. Evock-Clover CM, Polansky MM, Anderson RA, Steele NC. Dietary chromium supplementation with or without somatotropin treatment alters serum hormones and metabolites in growing pigs without affecting growth performance. J Nutr 1993; 123:1504–1512.

117. Schroeder HA, Balassa JJ. Influence of chromium, cadmium, and lead on rat aortic lipids and circulating cholesterol. Am J Physiol 1965; 209:433–437.

118. Nielsen FH. Nutritional significance of the ultratrace elements. Nutr Rev 1988; 46:337–341.

119. Freund H, Atamian S, Fischer JE. Chromium deficiency during total parenteral nutrition. JAMA 1979; 241:496–498.

120. Brown RO, Forloines-Lynn S, Cross RE, Heizer WD. Chromium deficiency after long-term total parenteral nutrition. Dig Dis Sci 1986; 31:661–664.

121. Frankel DA. Supplementation of trace elements in parenteral nutrition: rationale and recommendations. Nutr Res 1993; 13:583–596.

122. Hopkins LL Jr, Ransome-Kuti O, Majaj AS. Improvement of impaired carbohydrate metabolism by chromium(III) in malnourished infants. Am J Clin Nutr 1968; 21:203–211.

123. Wallach S, Verch RL. Radiochromium conservation and distribution in diuretic states. J Am Coll Nutr 1983; 2:163–172.

124. Martinez OB, Macdonald AC, Gibson RS, Bourn D. Dietary chromium and effect of chromium supplementation on glucose tolerance of elderly Canadian women. Nutr Res 1985; 5:609–620.

125. Offenbacher EG, Pi-Sunyer FX. Beneficial effect of chromium-rich yeast on glucose tolerance and blood lipids in elderly subjects. Diabetes 1980; 29:919–925.

126. Offenbacher E, Rinko C, Pi-Sunyer FX. The effects of inorganic chromium and brewer's yeast on glucose tolerance, plasma lipids, and plasma chromium in elderly subjects. Am J Clin Nutr 1985; 42:454–456.

127. Liu VJK, Morris JS. Relative chromium response as an indicator of chromium status. Am J Clin Nutr 1978; 31:972–976.

128. Riales R, Albrink MJ. Effect of chromium supplementation on glucose tolerance and serum lipids including high-density lipoprotein of adult men. Am J Clin Nutr 1981; 34:2670–2678.

129. Mossop RT. Effects of chromium III on fasting blood glucose, cholesterol and cholesterol HDL levels in diabetics. Central Afr J Med 1983; 29:80–82.

130. Abraham AS, Brooks BA, Eylath U. The effects of chromium supplementation on serum

glucose and lipids in patients with and without non-insulin-dependent diabetes. Metabolism 1992; 41:768–771.

131. Urberg M, Benyi J, John R. Hypocholesterolemic effects of nicotinic acid and chromium supplementation. J Fam Practice 1988; 27:603–606.

132. Hermann J, Arquitt A, Stoecker BJ. Effect of chromium supplementation on plasma lipids, apolipoproteins, and glucose in elderly subjects. Nutr Res 1994; 14:671–674.

133. Press RI, Geller J, Evans GW. The effect of chromium picolinate on serum cholesterol and apolipoprotein fractions in human subjects. West J Med 1990; 152:41–45.

134. Roeback JR Jr, Hla KM, Chambless LE, Fletcher RH. Effects of chromium supplementation on serum high-density lipoprotein cholesterol levels in men taking beta-blockers. Ann Intern Med 1991; 115:917–924.

135. National Research Council. Recommended Dietary Allowances. Washington, DC: National Academy Press, 1989:241–243.

136. Gibson RS, Scythes CA. Chromium, selenium, and other trace element intakes of a selected sample of Canadian premenopausal women. Biol Trace Elem Res 1984; 6:105–116.

137. Kumpulainen JT, Wolf WR, Veillon C, Mertz W. Determination of chromium in selected United States diets. J Agric Food Chem 1979; 27:490–494.

138. Casey CE, Hambidge KM, Neville MC. Studies in human lactation: zinc, copper, manganese and chromium in human milk in the first month of lactation. Am J Clin Nutr 1985; 41:1193–1200.

139. Anderson RA, Bryden NA, Patterson KY, Veillon C, Andon MB, Moser-Veillon PB. Breast milk chromium and its association with chromium intake, chromium excretion, and serum chromium. Am J Clin Nutr 1993; 57:519–523.

140. Deelstra H, Van Schoor O, Robberecht H, Clara R, Eylenbosch W. Daily chromium intake by infants in Belgium. Acta Paediatr Scand 1988; 77:402–407.

141. Kumpulainen JT. Chromium content of foods and diets. Biol Trace Elem Res 1992; 32:9–18.

142. Iyengar V, Woittiez J. Trace elements in human clinical specimens: evaluation of literature data to identify reference values. Clin Chem 1988; 34:474–481.

143. Evans GW, Pouchnik DJ. Composition and biological activity of chromium-pyridine carboxylate complexes. J Inorg Biochem 1993; 49:177–187.

144. Evans GW. Effect of chromium picolinate on insulin controlled parameters in humans. Int J Biosocial Med Res 1989; 11:163–180.

145. Berg FM. Chromium picolinate: scam of the hour. Obesity and Health 1993; 7:54.

146. Baruthio F. Toxic effects of chromium and its compounds. Biol Trace Elem Res 1992; 32:145–153.

147. Paustenbach DJ, Sheehan PJ, Paull JM, Wisser LM, Finley BL. Review of the allergic contact dermatitis hazard posed by chromium-contaminated soil: identifying a "safe" concentration. J Toxicol Environ Health 1992; 37:177–207.

148. Witmer CM, Park H-S. Mutagenicity and disposition of chromium. Sci Total Envir 1989; 86:131–148.

149. Coudray C, Faure P, Rachidi S, et al. Hydroxyl radical formation and lipid peroxidation enhancement by chromium: in vitro study. Biol Trace Elem Res 1992; 32:161–170.

13
Molybdenum

JEAN L. JOHNSON
Duke University Medical Center, Durham, North Carolina

I. INTRODUCTION AND HISTORY

Molybdenum has been recognized as an essential component of the animal enzyme xanthine oxidase since 1953 (1) and was identified in sulfite oxidase in 1971 (2). The essential nature of sulfite oxidase in humans is documented by the identification of more than 100 patients who lack this enzyme function, either as the result of a defect in the gene coding for the sulfite oxidase protein or as the result of a genetic deficiency in the molybdenum cofactor required for proper function of the metal in the enzyme. In addition, the molybdoenzymes nitrate reductase and nitrogenase function in plants and microorganisms, catalyzing reactions that are essential to the global nitrogen cycle.

Similarities between molybdenum and tungsten allow both to function with an identical organic cofactor that was first identified (3) in molybdoenzymes and termed molybdopterin (see Fig. 1). Subtle but critical differences between the two metals dictate that they fill unique, nonoverlapping roles. Functional tungsten enzymes have been identified in numerous microoroganisms; however, in animal systems, molybdopterin-containing enzymes function exclusively with molybdenum. In animals, tungsten serves as a molybdenum antagonist at many levels (transport, uptake, and utilization), and as such it can prevent molybdenum incorporation into the target proteins or in some cases be substituted in its place, yielding nonfunctional enzymes in both cases.

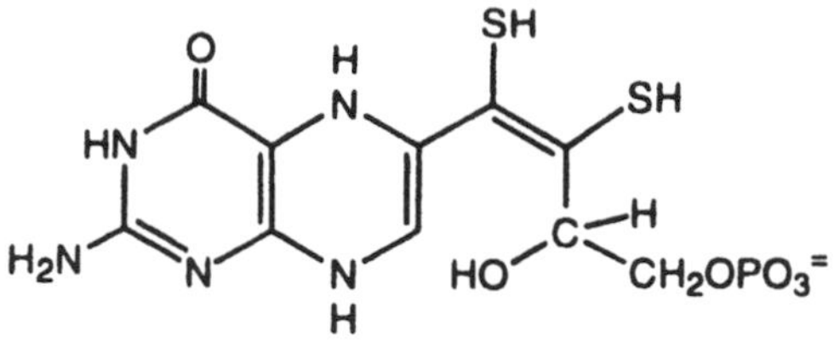

FIGURE 1   Structure of molybdopterin, the organic component of the molybdenum and tungsten cofactors.

II. CHEMICAL PROPERTIES

A. Oxidative States

The most common form of inorganic molybdenum is the oxyanion molybdate, MoO_4^{2-}. However, the numerous other stable oxidation states of the metal underlie its versatility as a biological redox catalyst. Valence states ranging from $+2$ to $+6$ are known, although in biological systems, the $+6$, $+5$, and $+4$ states are most commonly encountered.

B. Chelating and Binding Properties

In biological systems, molybdenum is generally found with oxygen and sulfur ligands. Molybdopterin contains a unique dithiolene structure borne on the side chain of a pterin ring system. As shown in Fig. 2, the vicinal sulfhydryl groups of molybdopterin chelate molybdenum or tungsten. The metal centers contain, in some cases, protein ligands to the metal as well as terminal oxo or sulfido ligands. One class of molybdoenzymes, the xanthine dehydrogenases and aldehyde oxidases, contains one oxo and one terminal sulfido ligand. Chemical studies showed that removal of this terminal sulfur ligand by cyanide (as thiocyanate) produced nonfunctional enzyme (4), and spectroscopic studies (X-ray absorption fine structure analysis) documented that cyanide treatment generated a molybdenum center with the dioxo structure (5). In contrast, the dioxo structure is present in the active forms of sulfite oxidase, nitrate reductase, and related enzymes. These proteins, as expected, are insensitive to cyanide.

A dinucleotide variant of the molybdenum cofactor, with GMP in pyrophosphate linkage with the terminal phosphate ester of molybdopterin, was identified in dimethyl sulfoxide reductase from *Rhodobacter sphaeroides* (6), and shortly thereafter pterin dinucleotides containing CMP, AMP and IMP were discovered (7,8). The role of the nucleotide portion of the cofactor in these enzymes has not yet been established. The first three-dimensional analysis of the molybdopterin-metal center of an enzyme has recently been accomplished and has revealed yet another variant. Chan et al. (9) have solved the structure of aldehyde ferredoxin oxidoreductase, a tungsten protein from a hyperthermophilic archaeon, *Pyrococcus furiosus*. In this enzyme a single tungsten atom is liganded by the dithiolene functions of two molybdopterin groups, forming a dimeric pterin cofactor. Two additional ligands, oxo groups or bound glycerol from the storage buffer, complete the tungsten center in this enzyme. The possible presence of dimeric pterins in molybdenum or tungsten enzymes from other sources is currently being investigated. All animal enzymes examined to date contain the monomeric molybdopterin form of the cofactor.

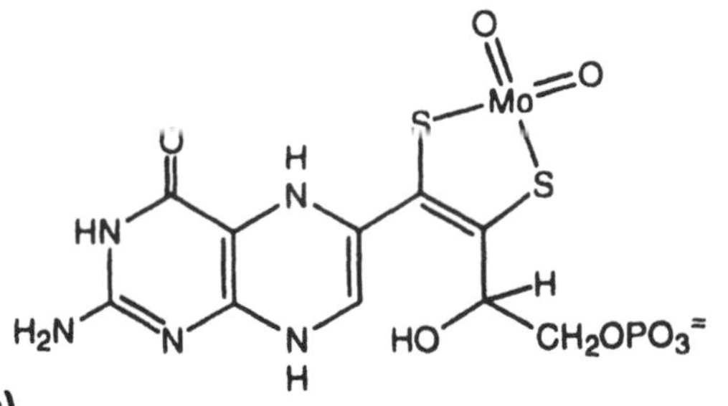

(a)

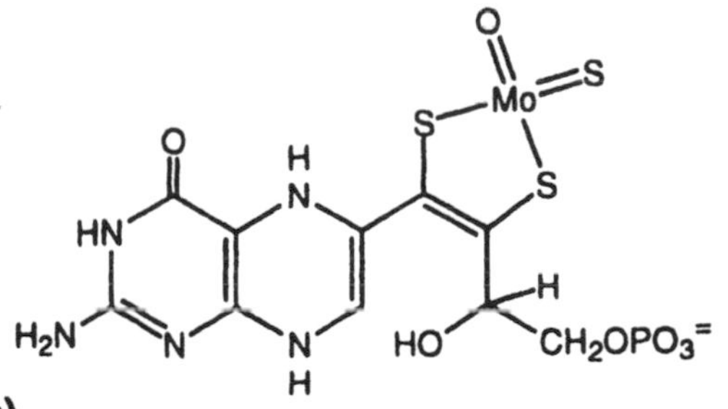

(b)

FIGURE 2 Structures of the (a) dioxo and (b) oxo/sulfido forms of the molybdenum cofactor. The dioxo form of the molybdenum cofactor is present in sulfite oxidase and nitrate reductase, while the oxo/sulfido form is found in xanthine dehydrogenase and aldehyde oxidase. The dithiolene sulfurs and additional ligands, perhaps provided by the protein, complete the metal coordination sphere.

III. ANALYTICAL METHODOLOGY

A. Colorimetric Methods

The most common colorimetric procedure for analysis of molybdenum uses 4-methyl-1,2-dimercaptobenzene, also referred to as toluene-3,4-dithiol, as a metal complexing agent (10). The molybdenum–mercaptide complex is formed under acidic conditions and then extracted into an organic solvent for quantitation of absorbance at 680 nm. Biological samples must be wet-ashed by heating in concentrated sulfuric acid or dry-ashed in a muffle furnace prior to metal complexation. Interference from ferric iron is eliminated by reduction with KI prior to addition of the dithiol reagent, and tungsten interference is prevented by inclusion of a large excess of tartrate.

The method has been adapted to the quantitation of tungsten in biological samples. Although the absorption properties of the tungsten–dithiol complex differ only slightly from those of the molybdenum–dithiol chromophore, the pH and ionic strength conditions required for formation of the tungsten–dithiol complex are more stringent. Thus, the strategy for analysis of samples that contain both metals is to prepare duplicate samples, measuring molybdenum and tungsten in one and molybdenum only in the second. A method for quantitation of both metals in a single sample has been described (11). The approach in this case is first to complex and extract the molybdenum, then to alter the conditions to allow tungsten complexation.

B. Atomic Absorption Spectroscopy

Molybdenum can be conveniently detected at the picomole level by heated graphite furnace atomic absorption spectroscopy (10). Molybdenum is somewhat refractory to atomization, and even at high furnace temperatures molybdenum carbides can accumulate on the walls of the graphite furnace and cause memory effects. This problem can be minimized by ashing at lower temperatures and including a burnoff cycle between analyses. Tungsten is not amenable to analysis by atomic absorption, since it is even less volatile than molybdenum, but both tungsten and molybdenum can be quantitated by inductively coupled plasma emission spectroscopy.

C. Electron Paramagnetic Resonance Spectroscopy

Electron paramagnetic resonance (EPR) has been widely applied to the study of molybdoenzymes. The metal center is paramagnetic in its $+5$ state, and this has been exploited to gain an understanding of the nature of the molybdenum center in a wide variety of molybdoenzymes both in the resting state and during catalysis (12). Specific incorporation of tungsten into the molybdenum center of sulfite oxidase from livers of tungsten-fed rats was demonstrated by documenting the line shape and g values of the tungsten center of the inactive, tungsten-substituted enzyme (13).

D. Identification and Quantitation of Molybdopterin

Methods have been developed that allow the quantitation of molybdopterin, the organic component of the molybdenum cofactor. The pterin in its native state is nonfluorescent but is readily oxidized to several fluorescent derivatives. To direct the oxidation to a single fluorescent species, it is convenient to acidify the sample and add a mixture of iodine/KI as oxidant. Upon heating to 100°C, molybdopterin is released from its protein environment and oxidized to the fluorescent species form A (see Fig. 3). After centrifugation, the pH of the supernatant fraction is adjusted to 11 and the fluorescence monitored with excitation at 380 nm and emission at 455 nm. The yield of form A is quantitated by comparison to an appropriate standard. Careful pH adjustment is critical when using this procedure, since the fluorescent properties of form A are extremely pH dependent. For more accurate quantitation, particularly if additional fluorescent compounds are present in the sample, the form A can be dephosphorylated with alkaline phosphatase and chromatographed on a C-18 reversed-phase high-performance liquid chromatography (HPLC) column. The conversion of molybdopterin to form A is not quantitative, but if proper precautions are taken, a consistent yield of 50% is observed which allows accurate assessment of molybdopterin levels (14).

Procedures have been reported for analysis of molybdopterin and molybdopterin guanine dinucleotide by acid-iodine oxidation to form A and form A-GMP (see Fig. 3), respectively, at room temperature (15). This milder method, incorporating sodium dodecyl sulfate as protein denaturant, preserves the labile diphosphate linkage in the dinucleotide derivatives and is applicable to purified enzymes or to less purified systems. It is also

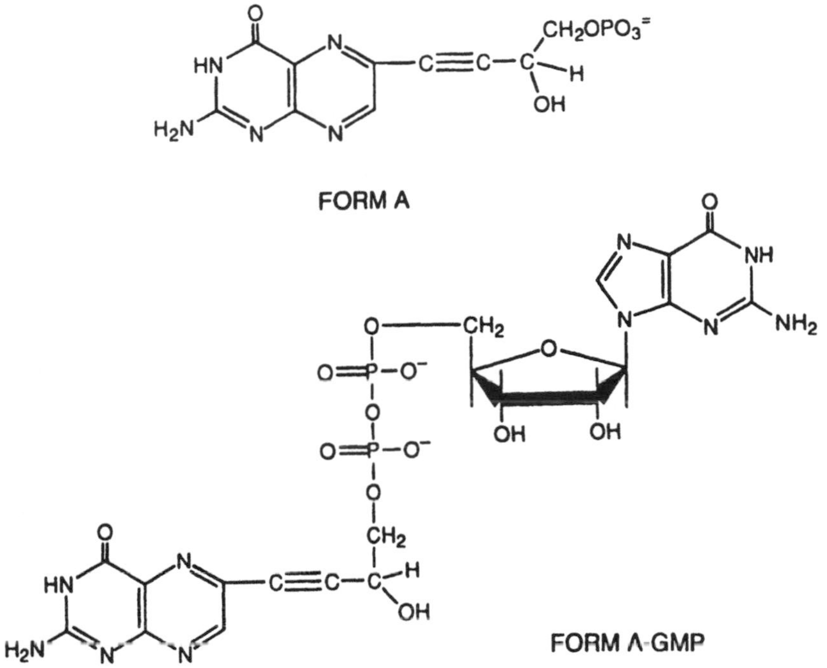

FIGURE 3 Structures of form A, the oxidized derivative of molybdopterin, and of form A-GMP, the oxidized derivative of molybdopterin guanine dinucleotide.

possible to prepare and quantitate by absorption spectroscopy the carboxamidomethyl derivatives of molybdopterin and molybdopterin dinucleotides (6,16). However, the absence of fluorescence in these derivatives makes them somewhat more difficult to purify and requires more starting material.

IV. METABOLISM

A. Absorption

Molybdenum appears to be very efficiently absorbed under conditions of both low (22 mg/day) and high (467 mg/day) dietary levels (17). This suggests that molybdenum absorption is exclusively passive and not saturable, in contrast to observations with copper and zinc, which are absorbed most efficiently at lower intakes, with absorption efficiency declining as intake increases (18,19).

B. Transport

Molybdenum is transported in the blood, attached primarily to proteins in the red blood cells. Concentrations in whole blood range from 30 to 700 nmol/L and vary with dietary intake (20). Serum contains approximately 5 nmol/L, mostly as molybdate (21). Specific carrier proteins that transport the metal as molybdate or as the assembled molybdenum cofactor have not yet been identified.

C. Tissue Concentration and Storage

Molybdenum is present at highest concentrations in the liver, kidney, adrenal gland, and bone (0.1–1 mg/g wet weight) and at lower levels in lung, spleen, and muscle (22). The metal is stored in the tissues primarily as a component of the molybdenum cofactor. The cofactor occurs bound to molybdoenzymes in the soluble cell fraction (xanthine dehydrogenase and aldehyde oxidase) or in the mitochondrial intermembrane space (sulfite oxidase); the release of cofactor and metal from the molybdoenzymes requires vigorous denaturing conditions. An additional pool of molybdenum cofactor has been identified bound to the mitochondrial outer membrane (23). This form of the cofactor is readily transferred from the membrane to apomolybdoenzymes, without harsh conditions or addition of detergents, and may represent a storage form of the cofactor for assembly of nascent molybdoenzymes. Liver tissue from molybdenum cofactor-deficient patients is extremely low in molybdenum content (24,25), suggesting that the metal is sequestered in the tissues primarily by means of its association with molybdopterin.

D. Excretion

Excretion of molybdenum is primarily in the urine. Very little molybdenum is excreted into the gastrointestinal tract. Molybdenum uptake is essentially unregulated; thus, control of molybdenum levels appears to occur exclusively by regulation of urinary excretion, with mechanisms to conserve molybdenum (such as increased molybdopterin biosynthesis) acting to reduce urinary excretion when dietary intake is low. These observations are in contrast to those with copper and zinc, which are excreted at low levels in the urine and in amounts that are not strongly influenced by dietary intake levels (26,27).

E. Interactions

The chemical similarities between molybdenum and tungsten that result in competition between the two metals at the levels of uptake and utilization have been mentioned earlier. However, since tungsten is rarely found at high levels in the environment, interference with molybdenum metabolism by this trace element is rare. In contrast, interactions of molybdenum with copper and sulfate are more widespread and have important consequences in humans and other animals. Antagonism between molybdenum and copper has long been recognized from studies of grazing animals. Excess molybdenum induces copper deficiency, which can be alleviated by increasing copper in the diet (28). Molybdenum-induced copper deficiency is particularly common in ruminants (29–31), but is also seen in nonruminants grazing on molybdenum-poisoned pastures (31). Molybdenum absorption is also inhibited by high levels of dietary sulfate; molybdate and sulfate may compete for the same or similar uptake systems (32).

V. BIOCHEMICAL FUNCTION

A. Molybdoenzyme Function

In animals, molybdenum is found as a component of three enzymes, sulfite oxidase, xanthine dehydrogenase, and aldehyde oxidase. All of these enzymes catalyze oxidative hydroxylations of substrate molecules at the molybdenum center and subsequently transfer electrons to other redox active cofactors and ultimately to the electron acceptors cytochrome c, molecular oxygen, or NAD^+. The reactions catalyzed by these enzymes are diagrammed in Fig. 4. Sulfite oxidase, the molybdoenzyme most crucial for human health, catalyzes the last step in the pathway of degradation of sulfur amino acids. Xanthine dehydrogenase and aldehyde oxidase hydroxylate various heterocyclic substrates as indicated in Fig. 4. Electron transfer to acceptor molecules produces variable amounts of NADH, superoxide anion radical, and hydrogen peroxide, depending on the source of the enzyme and substrate availability.

Plants and microorganisms contain numerous molybdoenzymes that catalyze redox reactions involving a wide range of substrates. The most well characterized plant molybdoenzyme is nitrate reductase, which catalyzes the reductive dehydroxylation of nitrate to form nitrite (the reverse of the typical reaction catalyzed by animal molybdoenzymes). This assimilatory form of nitrate reductase is crucial to the global nitrogen cycle. Bacteria use molybdoenzymes to support growth on various substrates, catalyzing electron transfer to alternative, non-oxygen acceptors including nitrate (dissimilatory nitrate reductase), or in the metabolic degradation of heterocyclic substrates for energy.

B. The Molybdenum Cofactor

Molybdoenzymes from this diverse range of sources contain, with one exception, a pterin-containing molybdenum cofactor. The unique case, which will not be considered further in this chapter, is nitrogenase, which contains an iron-molybdenum-homocitrate cofactor (33). While this enzyme is crucial to the global nitrogen cycle because of its ability to return N_2 to the biosphere in the form of ammonia, it is found only in a limited number of bacterial species and in the root nodules of nitrogen-fixing plants and has no direct involvement in metabolism in humans and other animals.

On the other hand, an understanding of the nature and role of the pterin-containing molybdenum cofactor is essential for analyzing the function of molybdenum in the animal molybdoenzymes. The proposed structure of the molybdenum cofactor is shown in Fig. 2. Neither the metal-free form of the cofactor (molybdopterin) not the metal-pterin complex (the molybdenum cofactor) has been isolated in the native state, since the cofactor, separated from its protective protein environment, is extremely labile. To circumvent this problem, the structure of the cofactor was deduced from a study of selective degradation products, as outlined in Figs. 3 and 5.

It was noted many years ago that acidification of molybdoenzymes from diverse sources released a labile but transferable entity or cofactor that could reconstitute nitrate reductase activity in vitro when incubated with extracts of a mutant of *Neurospora crassa*, *nit-1* (34). The reconstitution assay is shown in Fig. 6. This functional assay for molybdenum cofactor provided support for the existence of such a species originally postulated from the reports of bacterial mutants with pleiotropic loss of several molybdoenzymes (35), and remains an important means of semiquantitative analysis of the molybdenum cofactor. The assay can also be used to measure the presence of molybdopterin, since the inclusion of 10 mM molybdate leads to nonenzymatic, in-vitro production of molybdenum cofactor from molybdopterin and metal during the course of the reconstitution procedure.

The same conditions that led to the release of the transferable, *nit-1*-reconstituting cofactor from sulfite oxidase, xanthine dehydrogenase, and nitrate reductase were noted to result in a gradual evolution of fluorescent material in the denatured enzyme solution (3). The appearance of fluorescence appeared to be negatively correlated with the retention of active cofactor in the solution, and the difficult task of keeping the cofactor in an active state during purification and subsequent chemical characterization was abandoned in favor of

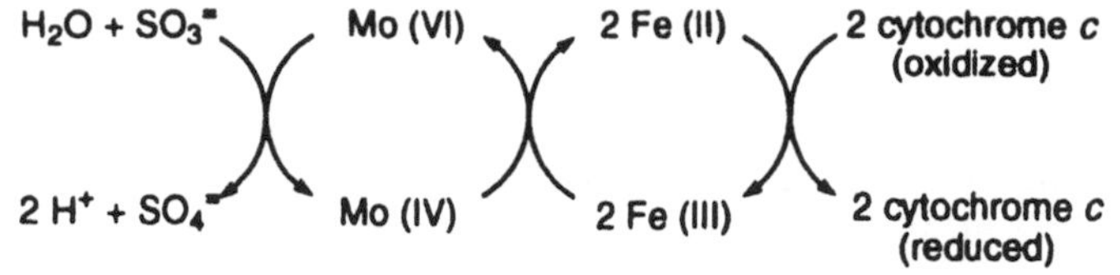

$$H_2O + SO_3^- \quad \quad Mo\,(VI) \quad \quad 2\,Fe\,(II) \quad \quad 2\ \text{cytochrome } c\ (\text{oxidized})$$

$$2\,H^+ + SO_4^- \quad \quad Mo\,(IV) \quad \quad 2\,Fe\,(III) \quad \quad 2\ \text{cytochrome } c\ (\text{reduced})$$

A. Reaction scheme of sulfite oxidase

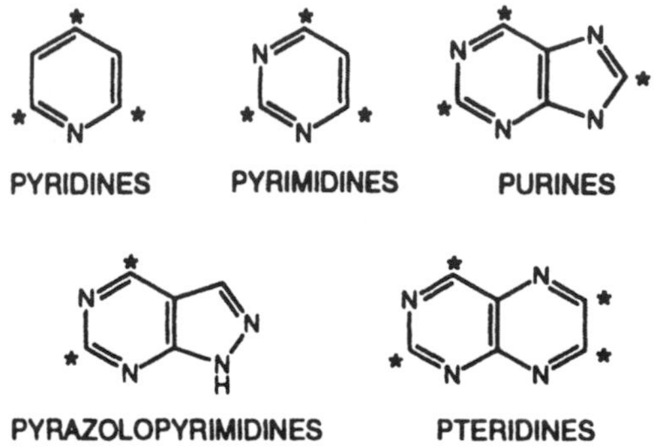

PYRIDINES   PYRIMIDINES   PURINES

PYRAZOLOPYRIMIDINES   PTERIDINES

B. Substrates hydroxylated by xanthine dehydrogenase and aldehyde oxidase

$$AH + H_2O + E \rightarrow AOH + EH_2$$

$$EH_2 + NAD^+ \rightarrow E + NADH + H^+$$

$$EH_2 + 2\,O_2 \rightarrow E + 2\,O_2^- + 2\,H^+$$

$$EH_2 + O_2 \rightarrow E + H_2O_2$$

C. Reaction scheme of xanthine dehydrogenase and aldehyde oxidase

FIGURE 4 Reactions catalyzed by molybdoenzymes in animals. Sulfite oxidase (A) oxidizes sulfite to sulfate with concomitant reduction of molybdenum VI to molybdenum IV. The electrons are transferred sequentially to the heme iron center in the enzyme and then to cytochrome *c* on the mitochondrial inner membrane. Xanthine dehydrogenase and aldehyde oxidase hydroxylate various heterocyclic substrates in the positions indicated by asterisks (B) according to reaction scheme (C). The specific sites of hydroxylation vary with the source of the xanthine dehydrogenase or aldehyde oxidase and are further defined by the presence or absence of substituents already present on the substrate.

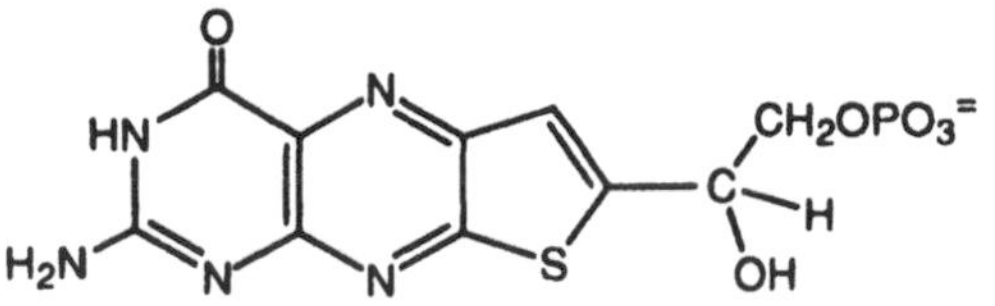

FORM B

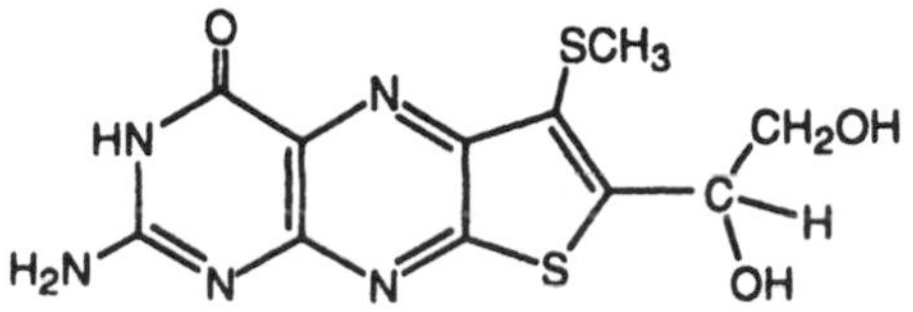

UROTHIONE

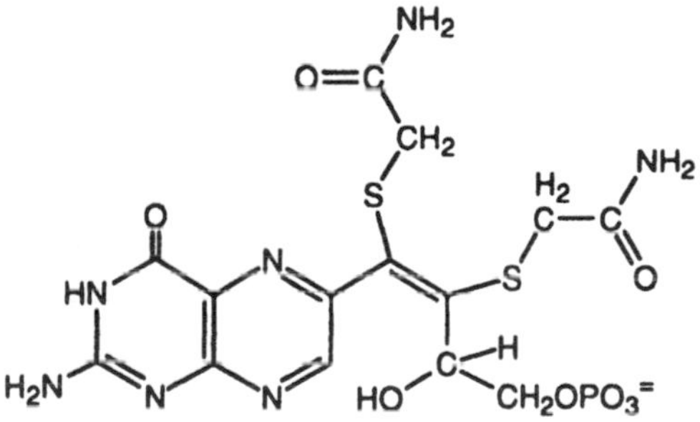

DICARBOXAMIDOMETHYL MOLYBDOPTERIN

FIGURE 5 Structures of form B, urothione, and dicarboxamidomethyl molybdopterin.

promoting decay to two stable, fluorescent derivatives. With fluorescence as a convenient marker, it was possible to purify and characterize these cofactor derivatives, form A and form B (see Figs. 3 and 5) (14). The presence of a pterin with a four-carbon side chain was apparent from both derivatives, and the presence of sulfur in form B suggested that the cofactor contains at least one sulfur atom. A search of the pterin literature for relevant sulfur-containing pterins brought to light an unusual urinary pterin of unknown metabolic origin termed urothione (36). From an inspection of the structure, it was apparent that this thienopterin contained the correct number of side chain carbon atoms with a sulfur on the C-2′ in thiophene linkage as in form B. The presence of a second sulfur on C-1′ was particularly intriguing, since opening the thiophene ring produced a linear four-carbon side chain with vicinal sulfhydryl groups positioned as potential molybdenum ligands. Further studies (37) demonstrated a metabolic as well as a structural link between the molybdenum cofactor and urothione. Patients with molybdenum cofactor deficiency failed to excrete detectable levels of urothione, suggesting that the latter was the metabolic degradation

RECONSTITUTION REACTION

apo nitrate reductase + molybdenum cofactor → holo nitrate reductase

NITRATE REDUCTASE ASSAY–NITRITE FORMATION

NADPH + NO$_3^-$ → NADP$^+$ NO$_2^-$ + H$_2$O

NITRATE REDUCTASE ASSAY–NITRITE DETECTION

NO$_2^-$ + sulfanilamide → diazotized amine

diazotized amine + N-(1-napthyl)ethylenediamine → colored complex

FIGURE 6   The *nit-1* reconstitution assay for molybdenum cofactor. The assay consists of three steps, all carried out in a single tube. For *reconstitution*, a source of molybdenum cofactor to be quantitated is incubated with an extract of mycelia of the *N. crassa nit-1* mutant (containing inactive apo nitrate reductase) and molybdate for 20 min at room temperature or overnight at 4°. For the *nitrate reductase assay-nitrite formation* step, the substrates for the newly reconstituted nitrate reductase (NADPH and nitrate) are added, and the mixture is incubated at room temperature for 20 min. For *nitrite detection*, sulfanilamide in HCl is added to diazotize the newly formed nitrite, followed by N-(1-napthyl)ethylenediamine. After 20 min of incubation at room temperature, the mixture is centrifuged, and the absorbance of the colored complex in the supernatant fraction is determined at 540 nm.

product of molybdopterin. Additional evidence in support of the proposed structure for molybdopterin came from structural studies on a fourth nonfunctional derivative, selectively produced by alkylation of both sulfhydryls to prevent their elimination and/or cyclization to the thienopterin form (16).

C.   Molybdenum Cofactor Biosynthesis

The complete pathway of molybdenum cofactor biosynthesis has not yet been elucidated; however, early and late steps as carried out by microorganisms are known, and late steps in the pathway in animals appear to be similar to those in lower species. The description of the metabolic pathway has been greatly facilitated by the existence of *mol* mutants (38) in *Escherichia coli* and by studies carried out with cells from the human molybdenum cofactor-deficient patients. Without question, an understanding of the biosynthetic pathway in humans is essential to an understanding of the specific defects resulting in the syndrome(s) known collectively as molybdenum cofactor deficiency and in ultimately gaining access to potential therapeutic agents to correct the defect or alleviate the devastating clinical symptoms.

Molybdopterin biosynthesis in *E. coli* is outlined in Fig. 7, with the reactions carried out by the various *mol* gene products indicated. The *mol* mutants were initially isolated as chlorate-resistant mutants with the designation *chl*. Chlorate resistance is associated with

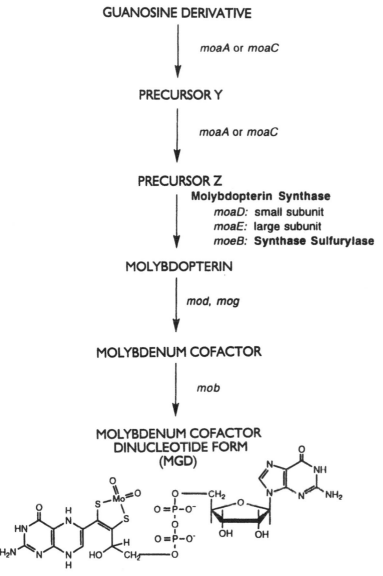

GUANOSINE DERIVATIVE

↓ *moaA* or *moaC*

PRECURSOR Y

↓ *moaA* or *moaC*

PRECURSOR Z

Molybdopterin Synthase
moaD: small subunit
moaE: large subunit
moeB: **Synthase Sulfurylase**

↓

MOLYBDOPTERIN

↓ *mod, mog*

MOLYBDENUM COFACTOR

↓ *mob*

MOLYBDENUM COFACTOR
DINUCLEOTIDE FORM
(MGD)

FIGURE 7 Molybdenum cofactor biosynthesis in *E. coli*. Guanosine or a phosphorylated derivative thereof is converted to precursor Z by the action of the product of *moaA* and *moaC* genes. The conversion of precursor Z to molybdopterin is catalyzed by molybdopterin synthase, a heterodimeric protein coded for by the *moaD* and *moaE* genes. Regeneration of the sulfur on molybdopterin synthase required for the next catalytic cycle is achieved through the action of MoeB (synthase sulfurylase). The molybdate uptake system is encoded by the *mod* genes, and the product of the *mog* locus is necessary for processing or incorporation of molybdate into the molybdenum cofactor. Addition of GMP to form the dinucleotide form of the molybdenum cofactor requires the *mob* gene product(s). At present, the functions of MoaB and MoeA have not been identified.

the absence of nitrate reductase activity, since this molybdoenzyme also uses chlorate as a substrate, reducing it to the highly toxic chlorite. Many of the chlorate-resistant mutants showed a pleiotropic loss of other molybdoenzyme activities as well, as a consequence of mutations in the molybdopterin biosynthetic pathway (39).

Molybdopterin in *E. coli*, like other pterins in bacteria, plants, and animals, is derived from a guanosine species. The guanine ring and a portion of the ribose ring constitute the pterin ring, while the remaining ribose carbons contribute to the pterin side chain. Unlike classical pathways, however, in which the C-8 of the guanine ring is eliminated as formate (40), in molybdopterin biosynthesis, this carbon is fully retained as C-1' of the molybdopterin side chain (41).

Other details of the structure of the first intermediate in the pathway remain to be elucidated. The enzyme catalyzing the reaction is presumably the product of the *moaA* or the *moaC* gene. These gene products have not been characterized as yet, but the gene sequence of *moaA* predicts a protein of 37.3 kDa (42) with a GTP-binding motif. Similarly, the role of the *moaB* gene product has yet to be defined, along with its substrates and products.

A major advance toward the understanding of molybdopterin biosynthesis came with the identification of a late intermediate in the pathway, precursor Z (43,44). Historically, the identification of precursor Z was the fortuitous result of studies aimed at quantitating the molybdenum cofactor in the various *mol* mutants. As illustrated in Fig. 8, quantitation of cofactor in the *moaA* mutant by two different procedures gave contradictory results: While extracts of this mutant were able to generate nitrate reductase activity when combined with extracts of *N. crassa nit-1* (45,46), quantitation of molybdopterin by conversion to the fluorescent form A derivative indicated that there was no molybdopterin in the *moaA* mutant (46). This apparent paradox was resolved by the demonstration that nitrate reductase activity was generated, not by the presence of molybdopterin in the *moaA* mutant, but as a result of the presence of precursor Z in the *nit-1* extract (47). Separation of this

PARADOX–

moaA extract + *nit-1* extract → nitrate reductase activity

moaA extract + acid/iodine → no Form A

HYPOTHESIS–

nit-1 extract has precursor form of molybdopterin

moaA extract has activity that converts precursor to molybdopterin

VERIFICATION–

nit-1 extract fractionated on gel filtration column

moaA extract + *nit-1* high molecular weight fraction → no nitrate reductase activity

moaA extract + *nit-1* high *and* low molecular weight fractions → activity restored

FIGURE 8 Identification of a molybdopterin precursor in extracts of *N. crassa nit-1* and molybdopterin synthase in *E. coli moaA*.

precursor from the extract by fractionation on a gel filtration column prevented the activation of the apo nitrate reductase by the *moaA* extract, while adding back the low-molecular-weight fraction restored this activity. Conversion of precursor Z to molybdopterin was accomplished in the combined crude extracts by the action of an enzyme provided by the *moaA* mutant. Thus, it appeared that the *moaA* locus coded for a protein required early in the biosynthetic pathway such that the *moaA* mutant was unable to make precursor Z, but retained the function(s) necessary to convert precursor Z to molybdopterin. Screening of additional *mol* mutants revealed that several, like *nit-1*, were blocked later in the pathway and accumulated high levels of precursor Z (see below). From these studies, it was then possible to devise assays for precursor Z and for the enzyme that converts it to molybdopterin and to isolate and characterize both from appropriate source materials.

The processing of precursor Z to molybdopterin is carried out by an enzyme termed molybdopterin synthase (converting factor). Molybdopterin synthase is a two-subunit protein, the small and large subunits of which are coded for by the *moaD* and *moaE* genes, respectively (48). Mutants in *moaD* or *moaE* or in a separate genetic locus, *moeB*, have nonfunctional molybdopterin synthase and accumulate and excrete into the culture medium high levels of precursor Z. The structures of precursor Z and its oxidized degradation product, compound Z, have been determined (43,44) and are shown in Fig. 9. The cyclic phosphate moiety of precursor Z is of particular interest, suggesting that the constrained ring system, decyclized concomitant with sulfur addition, could serve as an internal source of energy for molybdopterin synthesis. The sulfur for molybdopterin dithiolene formation is borne by the small subunit of molybdopterin synthase, and must be regenerated in order for the protein to engage in an additional cycle of precursor Z-to-molybdopterin conversion. An investigation into the mechanism of sulfur regeneration led to the characterization of another cofactor biosynthetic enzyme, molybdopterin synthase sulfurylase, encoded by the *moeB* locus. The synthase sulfurylase gene has been cloned and sequenced (49); characterization of the recombinant protein revealed that the enzyme contains stoichiometric zinc which contributes to a strong shoulder at 320 nm in the absorption spectrum (Bali and Rajagopalan, unpublished). The metal is tightly bound, but is released by 6 M guanidine-HCl with loss of the 320-nm absorption band. Sulfhydryl ligation to the metal is highly likely, since release is effected when the protein is treated with mercurials. Zinc binding may be accomplished through the cysXXcys motif that occurs twice in the MoeB sequence. The predicted amino acid sequence also shows the presence of a distinct nucleotide-binding motif at the amino terminus (50) and a possible ATP-binding site near the carboxyl terminus (51).

Significant sequence similarities between MoeB and a number of other proteins have been identified and are illustrated in Fig. 10. A highly interesting and potentially informa-

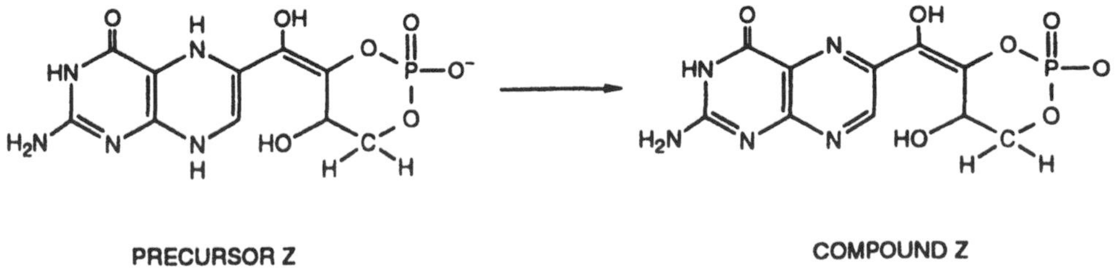

PRECURSOR Z   COMPOUND Z

FIGURE 9 Structures of precursor Z and compound Z.

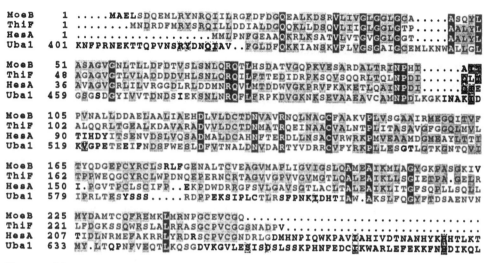

```
MoeB     1  .....MAELSDQEMLRYNRQIILRGFDFDGQEALKDSRVLIVGLGGLGCA.....ASQYL
ThiF     1  ...MNDRDFMRYSRQILLDDIALDGQQKLLDSQVLIICLGGLGTP.....AALYL
HesA     1  ...................MMLPNFGEAAQKRLKSATVLVTGVGGLGT.....AALYL
Uba1   401  KNFPRNEKTTQPVNSRYDNQIAV..FGLDFQKKIANSKVFLVGSCAIGCEMLKNWALLGL

MoeB    51  ASAGVCNLTLLDFDTVSLSNLQRQTLHSDATVGQPKVESARDALTRINPHI......A
ThiF    48  AGAGVCTLVLADDDDVHLSNLQRQILFTTEDIDRPKSQVSQQRLTQLNPDI......QLI
HesA    36  AVAGVCRLILVRGGDLRLDDMNRQVLMTDDWVGKPRVFKAKETLQAINPDI......QME
Uba1   459  GSGSDCYIVVTDNDSIEKSNLNRQFLFRPKDVGKNKSEVAAEAVCAMNPDLKGKINAKED

MoeB   105  PVNALLDDAELAALIAEHDLVLDCTDNVAVRNQLNAGGFAAKVPLVSGAAIRMEGQITVF
ThiF   102  ALQQRLTGEALKDAVARADVVLDCTDNMATRQEINAACVALNTPLITASAVGFGGQLMVL
HesA    90  TIHDYITSENVDSLVQSADMALDCAHNFTERDLLNSACVRWRKPMVEAAMDGMEAYLTTI
Uba1   519  KYGPETEEIFNDSFWESLDFVTNALDNVDARTYVDRRCVFYRKPLLESGTLGTKGNTQVI

MoeB   165  TYQDGEPCYRCLSRLFGENALTCVEAGVMAPLIGVIGSLQAMEAIKMLAGYGKPASGKIV
ThiF   162  TPPWEQGCYRCLWPDNQEPERNCRTAGVVGPVVGVMGTLQALEAIKLLSGIETPA.GELR
HesA   150  I.PGVTPCLSCIFP..EKPDWDRRGFSVLGAVSGTLACLTALEAIKLITGFSQFLLSQLL
Uba1   579  IPRLTESYSSS.....RDPPEKSIPLCTLRSFPNKIDHTIAW.AKSLFQGYFTDSAENVN

MoeB   225  MYDAMTCQFREMKFMRNPGCEVCGQ..............................
ThiF   221  LFDGKSSQWRSLALRRASGCPVCGGSNADPV..........................
HesA   207  TIDLNRMEFAKRRLYRDRSCPVCGNDRLGDMHNPIQWKPAVIAHIVDTNANHYKHHTLKT
Uba1   633  MY.LTQPNFVEQTLKQSGDVKGVLESISDSLSSKPHNFEDCIKWARLEFEKKFNHDIKQL
```

FIGURE 10 Sequence similarities between MoeB, ThiF, HesA, and Uba1.

tive homology is that between *moeB* and *UBA1*, the gene coding for ubiquitin activating enzyme E1 (52). The amino acid sequences of MoeB and the yeast-activating enzyme show 23% identity. Similar levels of identity are noted with the activating enzymes from wheat and humans, with MoeB showing 50% identity to the sequences of the activating enzymes from the three sources as a group. The sequence similarity to ubiquitin-activating enzymes has direct implications as to the sulfur transfer mechanism of the sulfurylase, since ATP-dependent thioester formation is an essential aspect of the ubiquitin-dependent protein degradation system as outlined in Fig. 11. To initiate the process by which ubiquitin is attached to a protein targeted for degradation, the free carboxyl of ubiquitin's carboxy-terminal glycine residue is linked to a cysteine of the activating enzyme E1, forming a thioester. Ubiquitin is a highly conserved protein of 76 amino acids. Its sequence bears little similarity to any of the known *mol* gene sequences, with the notable exception that its carboxy terminal Gly-Gly sequence is identical to that of the small subunit of molybdopterin synthase. Thus, using the same chemistry, it could be postulated that a thioester is formed between the glycine on molybdopterin synthase and a cysteine sulfur of the sulfurylase (Fig. 11). Generation of the active thiocarboxylate of the synthase could then be accomplished by the metal center and a low-molecular-weight sulfur source (sulfide). Additional systems in which this mechanism may be invoked for sulfur transfer reactions are suggested by the homologies between MoeB and other protein sequences. Both the ThiF protein in the *E. coli* thiamine biosynthetic pathway (53) and the HesA protein in the *nif* gene region of *Anabaena* (54) show significant homology with MoeB. In *Anabaena*, a protein with a carboxyl terminal di-glycine (HesB) is coded for by an adjacent open reading frame and would be a likely target for thiocarboxylate generation.

The molybdoenzymes nitrate reductase, formate dehydrogenase (55), and dimethyl sulfoxide reductase (56) in *E. coli* contain molybdopterin guanine dinucleotide which is generated from molybdopterin and a source of GMP. The formation of the dinucleotide is catalyzed by the product of the *mob* locus: Wild-type cells were shown to contain both molybdopterin and MGD, while *mob* cells contained elevated levels of molybdopterin but no detectable MGD (15). The *mob* gene has recently been cloned (57,58), and the Mob

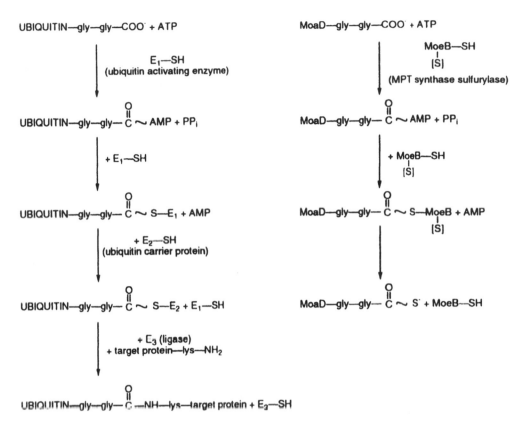

FIGURE 11 The ubiquitin-dependent protein-degradation system (left) and a proposed mechanism for sulfurylation of molybdopterin synthase by molybdopterin synthase sulfurylase (right).

protein purified to homogeneity (58). A computer search of the predicted amino acid sequence failed to reveal any specific sequence motifs; by visual inspection, however, a nucleotide binding site could be identified.

Molybdenum cofactor assembly requires that molybdenum, in the correct oxidation state, be made available at the site of molybdopterin biosynthesis. The *mod* and *mog* loci in *E. coli* are involved in some manner in these aspects of molybdenum metabolism; both phenotypes are repaired to some degree by culture on high levels of the metal (39). Cloning and sequencing of a portion of the *mod* operon revealed two open reading frames, *modB* and *modC*. Their deduced amino acid sequences suggested that these gene products are membrane permease proteins and account for two of a predicted four-protein molybdate uptake system (59). Further study of the DNA region upstream from these genes revealed another open reading frame, designated *modA*, that appears to encode the periplasmic binding protein of the molybdate uptake system (60). Regulation of expression of the *mod* operon by molybdenum is discussed in Section VII.

It is not known whether metal incorporation to form the molybdenum cofactor is enzyme catalyzed. Certainly, at high levels of the metal, as in the in vitro *nit-1* reconstitution assay, molybdenum incorporation can occur nonenzymatically. However, since in vivo levels of the metal are much lower, it is likely that assembly is enzyme dependent. One possible candidate for the molybdenum insertion enzyme is Mog. A significant difference between *mod* and *mog* mutants is that the former are repaired completely by growth on 0.1–1 mM molybdate, while the latter show incomplete restoration of molybdoenzyme activities even at the near-toxic 10-mM level. These observations would be consistent with a requirement of exceptionally high extracellular levels of molybdenum to force the elevated intracellular levels needed to overcome a defective molybdenum insertion enzyme in *mog*. The *mog* gene has been cloned and sequenced; the predicted protein sequence contains three cysteine residues that may serve as molybdenum ligands (61).

In a study of molybdenum cofactor levels in the *mod* and *mog* mutants, Miller and Amy (62) reported that the *mod* mutant cells produce very low levels of molybdenum cofactor and molybdopterin when grown on 1 mM molybdenum, but near-wild-type levels of both in the presence of higher levels of the metal (1 mM). In contrast, the *mog* mutant cells produced near-wild-type levels of molybdopterin under conditions of low molybdate in the culture medium and near-wild-type levels of molybdenum cofactor in the presence of 1 mM molybdate. Recent studies (Joshi and Rajagopalan, in preparation) have shown that the measurements of molybdopterin levels in *mog* were subject to the same artifact identified in studies of the *moaA* mutant (see above); that is, the presence of rather high levels of molybdopterin synthase in the *mog* mutant generates high levels of molybdopterin from precursor Z in unfractionated extracts of *nit-1*. Assay of molybdopterin in *mog* using only the high-molecular-weight fraction of *nit-1* or by quantitation as the form A derivative showed that very low levels of molybdopterin and molybdenum cofactor are present under these growth conditions, consistent with the observation that only very low levels of molybdoenzyme activity are generated.

Our understanding of the steps in molybdenum cofactor biosynthesis in eukaryotes is less well advanced than that just described for bacterial systems. However, several lines of evidence indicate that a similar pathway is involved. Precursor Z and compound Z have been demonstrated in the urine of certain molybdenum cofactor-deficient patients (see below) (63), and molybdopterin synthase has been partially purified from human liver (64). None of the human molybdenum cofactor biosynthetic genes has yet been cloned, but recently the *cin* locus in *Drosophila melanogaster*, essential for cofactor biosynthesis, has been sequenced and analyzed for sequence similarities to the bacterial genes (65). The *cin* gene product is related to three bacterial proteins; the amino-terminal portion is homologous to MoaB and Mog, while the carboxyl portion has strong sequence similarities to MoeA. Although the homologies identified involve three *mol* genes whose functions are yet to be defined, further characterization of the *Drosophila cin* mutant may be the key to identification of the roles of these gene products in bacterial and eukaryotic systems. An additional intriguing relationship between Cin and other known eukaryotic protein sequences was the similarity, across the entire length of the Cin protein, to a rat synaptosomal protein called gephyrin. Gephyrin has been implicated in the mobilization of glycinergic receptors and has been shown to bind to tubulin (66).

VI. PHYSIOLOGIC FUNCTIONS AND PATHOLOGY OF DEFICIENCY

A. Signs of Deficiency

1. Animals

Molybdenum deficiency in experimental animals has been induced by administration of tungsten. Early studies on the effect of this antagonist on xanthine dehydrogenase activity indicated that chickens were somewhat more affected than rats by impaired xanthine dehydrogenase activity, owing to the importance of this enzyme in purine metabolism and nitrogen excretion in birds (67). After the discovery of molybdenum as a component of sulfite oxidase, studies were carried out to determine the effect of tungsten treatment on the functioning of this enzyme in rats. Sulfite oxidase levels were decreased to less than 3% of normal without outward effects on the health of the animals; however, challenges with parenteral sulfite or inhaled SO_2 revealed that the treated animals were significantly more sensitive to these agents (68–70).

2. Humans

One clear case of molybdenum deficiency in humans has been documented (71). A patient with Crohn's disease was supported exclusively by total parenteral nutrition (TPN) for 18 months. During the last 6 months of TPN he developed a syndrome characterized by tachycardia, tachypnea, severe headache, night blindness, nausea, vomiting, and central scotomas leading to coma. His symptoms disappeared with discontinuation of the adminis- tered amino acid solutions, and metabolic studies suggested disturbances in sulfite oxidase and xanthine dehydrogenase functions. Treatment with ammonium molybdate at 300 mg/ day improved the clinical condition and normalized molybdoenzyme metabolite levels.

There have been scattered reports of nutritional deficiency of molybdenum in humans and associated increased incidence of cancer or other diseases (see, for example, Refs. 72 and 73). In many cases, however, decreased levels of other trace elements are also noted, and it is difficult to assess which effects can be attributed specifically to a deficiency of molybdenum.

B. Clinical Significance

Except in very rare instances, molybdenum deficiency in humans due to insufficient intake of the metal is essentially unknown. However, because the metal functions only in associa- tion with molybdopterin, in the form of the molybdenum cofactor, any disturbance of molybdenum cofactor metabolism can disrupt molybdoenzyme function, with severe clini- cal consequences. Inborn errors of metabolism resulting in sulfite oxidase deficiency have been identified in the human population with increasing frequency, in the form of both isolated sulfite oxidase deficiency and molybdenum cofactor deficiency (see below). Al- though currently identified in a relatively small number of individuals, both forms of the deficiency are quite newly discovered syndromes and are not often included in differential diagnoses of acutely ill newborns. Thus, their true incidence and effect on the human population remain to be established.

C. Inborn Errors of Metabolism

1. Isolated Sulfite Oxidase Deficiency

The first case of sulfite oxidase deficiency was described in 1967 (74) in a young child suffering from seizures, mental retardation, and dislocated ocular lenses. The identification of an unusual amino acid, S-sulfocysteine, in the plasma and urine from this patient, along with abnormally high levels of sulfite, thiosulfate, and taurine, suggested a defect in the enzyme that normally eliminates sulfite. Assays of sulfite oxidase in tissues obtained postmortem confirmed a deficiency in the activity of this molybdoenzyme and provided the first evidence of the essential nature of this enzyme in humans (75). The initial studies on this patient were carried out before it had been determined that sulfite oxidase was a molybdoenzyme. Thus the nature of the defect was assumed to be in the sulfite oxidase protein, and the possibility that a defect in the molybdenum cofactor could have been the underlying cause was not investigated until some years later (76). This study showed that xanthine dehydrogenase activity and molybdenum cofactor levels were normal in this individual, and led to the conclusion that this was indeed a case of isolated sulfite oxidase deficiency.

Since the description of the first patient, at least 20 additional cases of isolated sulfite oxidase deficiency have been identified (77). The severity of clinical symptoms and age of onset show considerable variation, but the most common picture is one of intractable seizures appearing within hours or days of birth and death at an early age. Symptoms associated with sulfite oxidase deficiency are summarized in Table 1.

The rat and human liver sulfite oxidase genes have been cloned (78,79), and their sequences have been compared to those of other molybdoenzymes. A single invariant cysteine has been identified in sulfite oxidases from three animal species and in nitrate reductases from 10 species of plants and fungi, and has been proposed to be a ligand of molybdenum (79). The amino acids flanking the invariant cysteine are highly conserved and may be required for molybdopterin binding (see Fig. 12). Specific mutation of the invariant cysteine in sulfite oxidase (Garrett and Rajagopalan, in preparation) and in nitrate reductase from *Aspergillus nidulans* (80) has been accomplished, and expression of the mutant proteins has confirmed the essential nature of this cysteine residue for enzyme activity. Fibroblasts are available from many of the sulfite oxidase-deficient patients, and molecular analysis of the specific defects in each individual case is in progress.

2. Molybdenum Cofactor Deficiency

An inborn error of metabolism that is clinically closely related to sulfite oxidase deficiency (see Table 1) and more prevalent in the human population is molybdenum cofactor deficiency (77). In this disease syndrome, the activities of all molybdoenzymes are affected owing to a lack of functional molybdopterin, the organic component of the molybdenum

TABLE 1   Clinical Symptoms and Metabolic Changes Associated with Sulfite Oxidase Deficiency

Clinical symptoms	Seizures	
	Mental retardation	
	Dislocated lenses	
	Brain atrophy/lesions	
	Death at early age	
Metabolite changes	Sulfite	Increased
	Sulfate	Decreased
	Thiosulfate	Increased
	S-sulfocysteine	Increased
	Taurine	Increased
	Xanthine[a]	Increased
	Hypoxanthine[a]	Increased
	Uric acid[a]	Decreased

[a]Oxypurine changes in cases of molybdenum cofactor deficiency; unchanged in cases of isolated sulfite oxidase deficiency.

human sulfite oxidase	204	**TLQCAGNRR**SEMTQVKEVKGLEWRTGAI**ST**
rat sulfite oxidase	204	**TLQCAGNRR**SEMNKVKEVKGLEWRTGAI**ST**
chicken sulfite oxidase	183	**TLQCAGNRR**SEMSRVRPVKGLPWDIGAI**ST**
N. crassa nitrate reductase	237	**TLVCAGNRR**KEQNVLRKSKGFSWGAGGL**ST**

FIGURE 12 Sequence similarities between sulfite oxidase from various sources and nitrate reductase from *N. crassa* in the region of the conserved cysteine (207 in the human and rat numbering schemes).

cofactor. Molybdenum cofactor deficiency can result from a defect at any of a number of steps in the molybdopterin biosynthetic pathway. At this time, two complementation groups, designated A and B, have been identified based on fibroblast co-culture experiments. Patients in the A complementation group appear to exhibit a block early in the pathway but retain the later enzyme(s), while those in the B complementation group have an defect later in the pathway (63). The possibility that group B patients were defective in an enzyme activity comparable to the molybdopterin synthase of *E. coli* was investigated by assaying for the presence of accumulated precursor Z in urine samples. Both precursor Z and its fluorescent degradation product, compound Z, were detected in urine samples from group B patients, but not from group A patients. Further studies showed that fibroblasts from group A patients contained an activity identical to molybdopterin synthase that could convert precursor Z to molybdopterin; this activity was not present in fibroblasts from group B patients (63). These results suggested that the late steps in molybdopterin biosynthesis in humans are the same as those in microorganisms and raised the possibility that precursor Z could serve as a therapeutic agent to correct molybdenum cofactor deficiency in group A patients.

The final stages of molybdenum cofactor assembly in humans, involving absorption, transport, and incorporation of the metal, are poorly understood at this point, and no patients have been identified that make molybdopterin but fail to generate the functional molybdenum complex. However, one may anticipate that defects in molybdenum uptake, transport, or processing could occur and that these would result in molybdenum cofactor deficiency (analogous to *mod* or *mog*). Since many of these defects could potentially be overcome by administration of higher levels of the metal by appropriate routes, it is important to be alert for those variants of cofactor deficiency that might respond to molybdate administration.

Patients with molybdenum cofactor deficiency lack the activities of sulfite oxidase, xanthine dehydrogenase, and aldehyde oxidase. Of these, the absence of sulfite oxidase is clearly the most devastating. Quite a number of individuals have been identified with xanthinuria (specific loss of xanthine dehydrogenase), and the resultant clinical symptoms are generally mild and seldom life threatening (81). A smaller class of patients has more recently been described with deficiencies in xanthine dehydrogenase and aldehyde oxidase, and even in these individuals, the clinical symptoms are mild (82). On the other hand, isolated sulfite oxidase deficiency and molybdenum cofactor deficiency are severely debilitating, often resulting in death at an early age. From these considerations, it would appear that the pathological sequelae in these cases must arise from altered levels of the substrate and/or product of sulfite oxidase. Sulfite oxidase-deficient patients exhibit progressive encephalopathy, with atrophy of brain tissue and enlarged ventricles evident by computed tomography or magnetic resonance imaging. Dislocated ocular lenses often develop at an age of 3–4 years, possibly as a result of sulfite attack on critical disulfide bonds in fibrillin, the major component of the suspensory ligament (83).

At present no therapy or treatment is available for either form of sulfite oxidase deficiency. Prenatal diagnosis is possible by assay of sulfite oxidase activity in cultured amniocytes or directly in chorionic villus biopsy material (84).

VII. REGULATION OF GENE EXPRESSION BY MOLYBDENUM

The finding that Mod is important in molybdate uptake by *E. coli* led Miller et al. (85) to investigate the effects of metal concentration in the culture medium on *mod* transcription. Using *mod-lac* operon fusions, they showed that Mod expression was strongly influenced by molybdate concentrations. The fusion protein was highly expressed at levels of molybdate less than 10 nM. Increasing concentrations of molybdate led to a steep decline in expression, with less than 5% of the activity present at 500 nM molybdate. This work was recently extended by Rech et al. (60), who identified a regulatory motif at the *moaD* promoter that is required for the molybdate-dependent control of the *modABCD* operon. A similar sequence occurs near the start of transcription of the *moa* operon, suggesting that it may also serve as a binding site for a molybdenum-responsive regulatory protein. The proposed regulatory protein(s) have not been identified, and it is not known whether molybdate uptake and molybdopterin synthesis are coordinately controlled by the same protein or whether they are regulated independently. A low-molecular-weight molybdenum-pterin-binding protein (mop) has been identified in *Clostridium pasteruianum* (86) with an amino-terminal helix-turn-helix motif characteristic of DNA-binding proteins; a similar protein may function in *E. coli* to regulate *mod* and/or *moa* expression.

VIII. NUTRITIONAL ASSESSMENT AND REQUIREMENTS

Molybdenum is required in the diet in very low amounts, and over the last 20 years the recommended dietary allowance has been progressively revised in a downward direction. In the 10th edition of the *Recommended Dietary Allowances* (87), the estimated safe and adequate daily dietary intake (ESADDI) is given as 0.075–0.250 mg/day. A recent balance study by Turnlund et al. (17), however, concludes that the minimum daily molybdenum requirement is approximately 25 μg/day or possibly less.

Several studies have been conducted to estimate the average daily intake of molybdenum. The usual dietary intake was estimated in 1970 to be 0.36 mg/day (22). A study in 1980 suggested that the daily average was 0.18 mg (88), and a study reported in 1987 found a daily intake of 0.076 mg for females and 0.109 mg for males (89). All of these values exceed the lower end of the range of recommended intake, with the consequence that molybdenum deficiency in humans is a rare occurrence. Even molybdenum deficiency resulting from long-term parenteral nutrition, although documented in one instance (71), appears also to be an unlikely event, since TPN solutions often contain adequate amounts of the metal (90).

IX. FUTURE RESEARCH NEEDS

The greatest impact on human health associated with disturbances in molybdenum metabolism lies in the area of inborn errors of metabolism, rather than frank deficiency or toxicity of molybdenum. What appeared initially to be a rare disorder, affecting only a limited number of individuals, has now been classified into two distinct syndromes, each with a rapidly increasing number of identified patients. The number of affected individuals far exceeds the number of cases of molybdenum deficiency or toxicity identified worldwide in the last 50 years. Consequently, it is critical that future research be directed toward a further understanding of the molecular mechanism underlying these genetic diseases. Pathways of biosynthesis have been partially deciphered, and different cofactor complementation groups have been identified. Further studies should reveal the precise enzymes and the defects therein in the two classes. Progress has already been made in identification of molecular defects in isolated sulfite oxidase deficiency. Extension of this work should bring to light interesting mutations that will key in on specific residues essential for catalytic activity, giving more insight into the nature of the molybdenum center and its catalytic mechanism.

The early steps in the biosynthesis of molybdopterin in humans have yet to be established. It will be important to determine whether guanosine conversion with retention of the C-8, as recently documented in *E. coli*, occurs in animals as well. The possibility remains that humans may not have the ability to catalyze this unusual reaction, and that a molybdopterin precursor is required in the diet as a vitamin. Such a finding would have important ramifications, since dietary molybdopterin requirements may pose an entirely new set of problems than are raised by requirements for metal only.

Screening procedures for sulfite oxidase and molybdenum cofactor deficiency need to be improved. Recently, a HPLC method for quantitation of urinary S-sulfocysteine, a metabolic marker of sulfite oxidase deficiency, has been reported (91). The availability of this and other diagnostic tests will aid in more widespread detection of the disease and allow prenatal screening of future pregnancies in affected families. The development of a screening test that could detect heterozygous carriers of the genetic disease would be highly desirable.

Further studies are needed to understand the pathogenesis of sulfite oxidase deficiency. A significant number of sulfite oxidase-deficient patients has been reported presenting with mild or transient lactic acidemia (92–95). Dysmorphic facial features described in some of these patients (24,94,96,97), including narrowed head, frontal bossing, wide nasal bridge, long filtrum and flared nostrils, as well as cortical atrophy, ventricular enlargement, and cerebral cystic lesions, are reminiscent of features associated with pyruvate dehydrogenase deficiency (98). Although sulfite oxidase-deficient patients are not overtly deficient in pyruvate dehydrogenase, the long-recognized susceptibility of thiamine to destruction by sulfite (99) raises the possibility that limited thiamine and pyruvate dehydrogenase deficiencies could occur (especially in the brain), which could account for some of these observations. Certainly, further research into these areas is warranted.

ACKNOWLEDGMENTS

The research studies described from this laboratory were supported by National Institutes of Health grants GM00091 and GM44283. Encouragement and advice from Dr. K. V. Rajagopalan in the preparation of this chapter are gratefully acknowledged.

REFERENCES

1. Richert DA, Westerfeld WW. Isolation and identification of the xanthine oxidase factor as molybdenum. J Biol Chem 1953; 203:915–923.
2. Cohen HJ, Fridovich I, Rajagopalan KV. Hepatic sulfite oxidase. A functional role for molybdenum. J Biol Chem 1971; 246:374–382.
3. Johnson JL, Hainline BE, Rajagopalan KV. Characterization of the molybdenum cofactor of sulfite oxidase, xanthine oxidase and nitrate reductase. Identification of a pteridine as a structural component. J Biol Chem 1980; 255:1783–1786.
4. Massey V, Edmondson D. On the mechanism of inactivation of xanthine oxidase by cyanide. J Biol Chem 1970; 245:6595–6598.
5. Cramer SP, Wahl R, Rajagopalan KV. Molybdenum sites of sulfite oxidase and xanthine dehydrogenase—a comparison by EXAFS. J Am Chem Soc 1981; 103:7721–7727.
6. Johnson JL, Bastian NR, Rajagopalan KV. Molybdopterin guanine dinucleotide: a modified form of molybdopterin identified in the molybdenum cofactor of dimethyl sulfoxide reductase from *Rhodobacter sphaeroides* forma specialis *denitrificans*. Proc Natl Acad Sci USA 1990; 87:3190–3194.
7. Johnson JL, Rajagopalan KV, Meyer O. Isolation and characterization of a second molybdopterin dinucleotide: molybdopterin cytosine dinucleotide. Arch Biochem Biophys 1990; 283: 542–545.
8. Börner G, Karrasch M. Thauer RK. Molybdopterin adenine dinucleotide and molybdopterin hypoxanthine dinucleotide in formylmethanofuran dehydrogenase from *Methanobacterium thermoautotrophicum* (Marburg). FEBS Lett 1991; 290:31–34.
9. Chan MK, Mukund S, Kletzin A, Adams MWW, Rees DC. Structure of a hyperthermophilic tungstopterin enzyme, aldehyde ferredoxin oxidoreductase. Science 1995; 267:1463–1469.
10. Johnson JL. Molybdenum. Meth Enzymol 1988; 158:371–382.
11. Cardenas J, Mortenson LE. Determination of molybdenum and tungsten in biological materials. Anal Biochem 1974; 60:372–381.
12. Bray RC. The inorganic biochemistry of molybdoenzymes. Q Rev Biophys 1988; 21:299–329.
13. Johnson JL, Rajagopalan KV. Electron paramagnetic resonance of the tungsten derivative of rat liver sulfite oxidase. J Biol Chem 1976; 251:5505–5511.
14. Johnson JL, Hainline BE, Rajagopalan KV, Arison BH. The pterin component of the molybdenum cofactor. Structural characterization of two fluorescent derivatives. J Biol Chem 1984; 259:5414–5422.
15. Johnson JL, Indermaur LW, Rajagopalan KV. Molybdenum cofactor biosynthesis in *Escherichia coli*. Requirement of the *chlB* gene product for the formation of molybdopterin guanine dinucleotide. J Biol Chem 1991; 266:12140–12145.
16. Kramer SP, Johnson JL, Ribeiro AA, Millington DS, Rajagopalan KV. The structure of the molybdenum cofactor. Characterization of di-(carboxamidomethyl)molybdopterin from sulfite oxidase and xanthine oxidase. J Biol Chem 1987; 262:16357–16363.
17. Turnlund JR, Keyes WR, Peiffer GL, Chiang G. Molybdenum absorption, excretion, and retention studied with stable isotopes in young men during depletion and repletion. Am J Clin Nutr 1995; 61:1102–1109.
18. Turnlund JR, Keyes WR, Anderson HL, Acord LL. Copper absorption and retention in young men at three levels of dietary copper by use of the stable isotope ^{65}Cu. Am J Clin Nutr 1989; 49:870–878.
19. Kung JC, Turnlund JR. Human zinc requirements. In: Mills CF, ed. Zinc in Human Biology. Berlin: Springer-Verlag, 1989:335–350.
20. Allaway WH, Kubota J, Losee F, Roth M. Selenium, molybdenum, and vanadium in human blood. Arch Environ Health 1968; 16:342–348.
21. Versieck J, Hoste J, Vanballenberghe L, Barbier F, Cornelis R, Waelput I. Serum molybdenum in diseases of the liver and biliary system. J Lab Clin Med 1981; 97:535–544.

22. Schroeder HA, Balassa JJ, Tipton IH. Essential trace metals in man: molybdenum. J Chron Dis 1970; 23:481–499.
23. Johnson JL, Jones HP, Rajagopalan KV. *In vitro* reconstitution of demolybdosulfite oxidase by a molybdenum cofactor from rat liver and other sources. J Biol Chem 1977; 252:4994–5003.
24. Johnson JL, Waud WR, Rajagopalan KV, Duran M, Beemer FA, Wadman SK. Inborn errors of molybdenum metabolism: combined deficiencies of sulfite oxidase and xanthine dehydrogenase in a patient lacking the molybdenum cofactor. Proc Natl Acad Sci USA 1980; 77:3715–3719.
25. Roesel RA, Bowyer F, Blankenship PR, Hommes FA. Combined xanthine and sulphite oxidase defect due to a deficiency of molybdenum cofactor. J Inher Metab Dis 1986; 9:343–347.
26. Turnlund JR, Keen CL, Smith RG. Copper status and urinary and salivary copper in young men at three levels of dietary copper. Am J Clin Nutr 1990; 51:658–664.
27. Turnlund JR, Costa F, Durkin N, Margen S. Stable isotope studies of zinc absorption and retention in young and elderly men. J Nutr 1986; 116:1239–1247.
28. Underwood EJ. Molybdenum in animal nutrition. In: Chappell WR, Petersen KK, eds. Molybdenum in the Environment. New York: Marcel Dekker, 1976:9–31.
29. Faye B, Grillet C, Tessema A, Kamil M. Copper deficiency in ruminants in the Rift Valley of East Africa. Trop Anim Health Prod 1991; 23:172–180.
30. Liu ZP, Ma Z, Zhang YJ. Studies on the relationship between sway disease of bactrian camels and copper status in Gansu province. Vet Res Commun 1994; 18:251–260.
31. Ladefoged O, Sturup S. Copper deficiency in cattle, sheep and horses caused by excess molybdenum from fly ash: a case report. Vet Hum Toxicol 1995; 37:63–65.
32. Mills CF, Bremner I. Nutritional aspects of molybdenum in animals. In: Coughlan MP, ed. Molybdenum and Molybdenum-Containing Enzymes. Oxford: Pergamon Press, 1980:517–542.
33. Allen RM, Chatterjee R, Madden MS, Ludden PW, Shah VK. Biosynthesis of the iron-molybdenum cofactor of nitrogenase. Crit Rev Biotechnol 1994; 14:225–249.
34. Nason A, Lee K-Y, Pan S-S, Ketchum PA, Lamberti A, DeVries J. *In vitro* formation of assimilatory reduced nicotinamide adenine dinucleotide phosphate: nitrate reductase from a *Neurospora* mutant and a component of molybdenum-enzymes. Proc Natl Acad Sci USA 1971; 68:3242–3246.
35. Pateman JA, Cove DJ, Rever BM, Roberts DB. A common cofactor for nitrate reductase and xanthine dehydrogenase which also regulates the synthesis of nitrate reductase. Nature 1964; 201:58–60.
36. Goto M, Sakurai A, Ohta K, Yamakami H. Die Struktur des Urothions. J Biochem 1969; 65:611–620.
37. Johnson JL, Rajagopalan KV. Structural and metabolic relationship between the molybdenum cofactor and urothione. Proc Natl Acad Sci USA 1982; 79:6856–6860.
38. Shanmugam KT, Stewart V, Gunsalus RP, et al. Proposed nomenclature for the genes involved in molybdenum metabolism in *Escherichia coli* and *Salmonella typhimurium*. Mol Microbiol 1992; 6:3452–3454.
39. Stewart V. Nitrate respiration in relation to facultative metabolism in enterobacteria. Microbiol Rev 1988; 52:190–232.
40. Brown GM. The biosynthesis of pteridines. Adv Enzymol 1971; 35:35–77.
41. Wuebbens MM, Rajagopalan KV. Investigation of the early steps of molybdopterin biosynthesis in *Escherichia coli* through the use of *in vivo* labeling studies. J Biol Chem 1995; 270:1082–1087.
42. Rivers SL, McNairn E, Blasco F, Giordano G, Boxer DH. Molecular genetic analysis of the *moa* operon of *Escherichia coli* K-12 required for molybdenum cofactor biosynthesis. Mol Microbiol 1993; 8:1071–1081.
43. Johnson JL, Wuebbens MM, Rajagopalan KV. The structure of a molybdopterin precursor. Characterization of a stable, oxidized derivative. J Biol Chem 1989; 264:13440–13447.
44. Wuebbens MM, Rajagopalan KV. Structural characterization of a molybdopterin precursor. J Biol Chem 1993; 268:13493–13498.

45. Amy NK. Identification of the molybdenum cofactor in chlorate-resistant mutants of *Escherichia coli*. J Bacteriol 1981; 148:274–282.

46. Johnson ME, Rajagopalan KV. Involvement of *chlA, E, M*, and *N* loci in *Escherichia coli* molybdopterin biosynthesis. J Bacteriol 1987; 169:117–125.

47. Johnson ME, Rajagopalan KV. *In vitro* system for molybdopterin biosynthesis. J Bacteriol 1987; 169:110–116.

48. Pitterle DM, Rajagopalan KV. The biosynthesis of molybdopterin in *Escherichia coli*. Purification and characterization of the converting factor. J Biol Chem 1993; 268:13499–13505.

49. Nohno T, Kasai Y, Saito T. Cloning and sequencing of the *Escherichia coli chlEN* operon involved in molybdopterin biosynthesis. J Bacteriol 1988; 170:4097–4102.

50. Wierenga RK, Terpstra P, Hol WGJ. Prediction of the occurrence of the ADP-binding βαβ-fold in proteins, using an amino acid sequence fingerprint. J Mol Biol 1986; 187:101–107.

51. Saraste M, Sibbald PR, Wittinghofer A. The P-loop—a common motif in ATP- and GTP-binding proteins. Trends Biochem Sci 1990; 15:430–434.

52. McGrath JP, Jentsch S, Varshavsky A. *UBA1*: an essential yeast gene encoding ubiquitin-activating enzyme. EMBO J 1991; 10:227–236.

53. vander Horn PB, Backstrom AD, Stewart V, Begley TP. Structural genes for thiamine biosynthetic enzymes (*thiCEFGH*) in *Escherichia coli* K-12. J Bacteriol 1993; 175:982–992.

54. Borthakur D, Basche M, Buikema WJ, Borthakur PB, Haselkorn R. Expression, nucleotide sequence and mutational analysis of two open reading frames in the *nif* gene region of *Anabaena* sp. strain PCC 7120. Mol Gen Genet 1990; 221:227–234.

55. Axley MJ, Grahame DA, Stadtman TC. *Escherichia coli* formate-hydrogen lyase. Purification and properties of the selenium-dependent formate dehydrogenase component. J Biol Chem 1990; 265:18213–18218.

56. Rothery RA, Simala Grant JL, Johnson JL, Rajagopalan KV, Weiner JH. Association of molybdopterin guanine dinucleotide with *Escherichia coli* dimethyl sulfoxide reductase: effect of tungstate and a *mob* mutation. J Bacteriol 1995; 177:2057–2063.

57. Plunkett G III, Burland V, Daniels DL, Blattner FR. Analysis of the *Escherichia coli* genome. III. DNA sequence of the region from 87.2 to 89.2 minutes. Nucleic Acids Res 1993; 21:3391–3398.

58. Palmer T, Vasishta A, Whitty PW, Boxer DH. Isolation of protein FA, a product of the *mob* locus required for molybdenum cofactor biosynthesis in *Escherichia coli*. Eur J Biochem 1994; 222:687–692.

59. Johann S, Hinton SM. Cloning and nucleotide sequence of the *chlD* locus. J Bacteriol 1987; 169:1911–1916.

60. Rech S, Deppenmeier U, Gunsalus RP. Regulation of the molybdate transport operon, *modABCD*, of *Escherichia coli* in response to molybdate availability. J Bacteriol 1995; 177:1023–1029.

61. Hinton SM, Dean D. Biogenesis of molybdenum cofactors. Crit Rev Microbiol 1990; 17:169–188.

62. Miller JB, Amy NK. Molybdenum cofactor in chlorate-resistant and nitrate reductase-deficient insertion mutants of *Escherichia coli*. J Bacteriol 1983; 155:793–801.

63. Johnson JL, Wuebbens MM, Mandell R, Shih VE. Molybdenum cofactor biosynthesis in humans. Identification of two complementation groups of cofactor-deficient patients and preliminary characterization of a diffusible molybdopterin precursor. J Clin Invest 1989; 83:897–903.

64. Johnson JL, Rajagopalan KV. Molybdopterin biosynthesis in man. Properties of the converting factor in liver tissue from a molybdenum cofactor deficient patient. Adv Exp Med Biol 1993; 338:379–382.

65. Kamdar KP, Shelton ME, Finnerty V. The *Drosophila* molybdenum cofactor gene *cinnamon* is homologous to three *Escherichia coli* cofactor proteins and to the rat protein gephyrin. Genetics 1994; 137:791–801.

66. Prior P, Schmitt B, Grenningloh G, et al. Primary structure and alternative splice variants of gephyrin, a putative glycine receptor-tubulin linker protein. Neuron 1992; 8:1161–1170.
67. Higgins ES, Richert DA, Westerfeld WW. Molybdenum deficiency and tungstate inhibition studies. J Nutr 1956; 59:539–559.
68. Johnson JL, Rajagopalan KV, Cohen HJ. Molecular basis of the biological function of molybdenum. Effect of tungsten on xanthine oxidase and sulfite oxidase in the rat. J Biol Chem 1974; 249:859–866.
69. Johnson JL, Cohen HJ, Rajagopalan KV. Molecular basis of the biological function of molybdenum. Molybdenum-free sulfite oxidase from livers of tungsten-treated rats. J Biol Chem 1974; 249:5046–5055.
70. Cohen HJ, Drew RT, Johnson JL, Rajagopalan KV. Molecular basis of the biological function of molybdenum. The relationship between sulfite oxidase and the acute toxicity of bisulfite and SO_2. Proc Natl Acad Sci USA 1973; 70:3655–3659.
71. Abumrad NN, Schneider AJ, Steel D, Rogers LS. Amino acid intolerance during prolonged total parenteral nutrition reversed by molybdate therapy. Am J Clin Nutr 1981; 34:2551–2559.
72. Luo XM, Lu SM, Liu YY. Correlative studies of the contents of chemical elements in drinking water and cereals consumed by 50 commune members and the mortality of esophageal carcinoma. Chin J Epidemiol 1982; 3:91–96.
73. Szabo G, Balint S, Nyeste E, Medgyesi I, Tamaskovics A, Podmaniczky G. [Trace element deficiency in healthy subjects based on multi-element analysis of serum and plasma]. Orv Hetil 1991; 132:395–400.
74. Irreverre F, Mudd SH, Heizer WD, Laster L. Sulfite oxidase deficiency: studies of a patient with mental retardation, dislocated ocular lenses, and abnormal urinary excretion of S-sulfo-L-cysteine, sulfite, and thiosulfate. Biochem Med 1967; 1:187–217.
75. Mudd SH, Irreverre F, Laster L. Sulfite oxidase deficiency in man: demonstration of the enzymatic defect. Science 1967; 156:1599–1602.
76. Johnson JL, Rajagopalan KV. Human sulfite oxidase deficiency. Characterization of the molecular defect in a multicomponent system. J Clin Invest 1976; 58:551–556.
77. Johnson JL, Wadman SK. Molybdenum cofactor deficiency and isolated sulfite oxidase deficiency. In: Scriver CR, Beaudet AL, Sly WS, Valle D, eds. The Metabolic and Molecular Bases of Inherited Disease. 7th ed. New York: McGraw-Hill, 1995:2271–2283.
78. Garrett RM, Rajagopalan KV. Molecular cloning of rat liver sulfite oxidase. Expression of a eukaryotic Mo-pterin-containing enzyme in *Escherichia coli*. J Biol Chem 1994; 269:272–276.
79. Garrett RM, Bellissimo DB, Rajagopalan KV. Molecular cloning of human liver sulfite oxidase. Biochim Biophys Acta 1995; 1262:147–149.
80. Garde J, Kinghorn JR, Tomsett AB. Site-directed mutagenesis of nitrate reductase from *Aspergillus nidulans*. Identification of some essential and some nonessential amino acids among conserved residues. J Biol Chem 1995; 270:6644–6650.
81. Simmonds HA, Reiter S, Nishino T. Hereditary xanthinuria. In: Scriver CR, Beaudet AL, Sly WS, Valle D, eds. The Metabolic and Molecular Bases of Inherited Disease. 7th ed. New York: McGraw-Hill, 1995:1781–1797.
82. Reiter S, Simmonds HA, Zöllner N, Braun SL, Knedel M. Demonstration of a combined deficiency of xanthine oxidase and aldehyde oxidase in xanthinuric patients not forming oxipurinol. Clin Chim Acta 1990; 187:221–234.
83. Sakai LY, Keene DR, Glanville RW, Bächinger HP. Purification and partial characterization of fibrillin, a cysteine-rich structural component of connective tissue microfibrils. J Biol Chem 1991; 266:14763–14770.
84. Johnson JL, Rajagopalan KV, Lanman JT, et al. Prenatal diagnosis of molybdenum cofactor deficiency by assay of sulphite oxidase activity in chorionic villus samples. J Inher Metab Dis 1991; 14:932–937.
85. Miller JB, Scott DJ, Amy NK. Molybdenum-sensitive transcriptional regulation of the *chlD* locus of *Escherichia coli*. J Bacteriol 1987; 169:1853–1860.

86. Hinton SM, Freyer G. Cloning, expression and sequencing the molybdenum-pterin binding protein (mop) gene of *Clostridium pasteruianum* in *Escherichia coli*. Nucleic Acids Res 1986; 14:9371–9380.

87. National Research Council. Recommended Dietary Allowances. 10th ed. Washington, DC: National Academy Press, 1989.

88. Tsongas TA, Meglen RR, Walravens PA, Chappell WR. Molybdenum in the diet: an estimate of average daily intake of the United States. Am J Clin Nutr 1980; 33:1103–1107.

89. Pennington JAT, Jones JW. Molybdenum, nickel, cobalt, vanadium, and strontium in total diets. J Am Diet Assoc 1987; 87:1644–1650.

90. Pinna K. Determination of Molybdenum in Human Samples and Diets by Electrothermal Atomic Absorption Spectroscopy. Berkeley: University of California, 1987.

91. Johnson JL, Rajagopalan KV. An HPLC assay for detection of elevated urinary S-sulphocysteine, a metabolic marker of sulphite oxidase deficiency. J Inher Metab Dis 1995; 18:40–47.

92. Brown GK, Scholem RD, Croll HB, Wraith JE, McGill JJ. Sulfite oxidase deficiency: clinical, neuroradiologic, and biochemical features in two new patients. Neurology 1989; 39:252–257.

93. Boles RG, Ment LR, Meyn MS, Horwich AL, Kratz LE, Rinaldo P. Short-term response to dietary therapy in molybdenum cofactor deficiency. Ann Neurol 1993; 34:742–744.

94. Arnold GL, Greene CL, Stout JP, Goodman SI. Molybdenum cofactor deficiency. J Pediatr 1993; 123:595–598.

95. Rupar CA, Gillett J, Gordon BA, et al. Isolated sulfite oxidase deficiency. Neuropediatrics 1995; in press.

96. Endres W, Shin YS, Günther R, Ibel H, Duran M, Wadman SK. Report on a new patient with combined deficiencies of sulphite oxidase and xanthine dehydrogenase due to molybdenum cofactor deficiency. Eur J Pediatr 1988; 148:246–249.

97. Hansen LK, Wulff K, Dorche C, Christensen E. Molybdenum cofactor deficiency in two siblings: diagnostic difficulties. Eur J Pediatr 1993; 152:662–664.

98. Robinson BH. Lactic acidemia (disorders of pyruvate carboxylase, pyruvate dehydrogenase). In: Scriver CR, Beaudet AL, Sly WS, Valle D, eds. The Metabolic and Molecular Bases of Inherited Disease. 7th ed. New York: McGraw-Hill, 1995:1479–1499.

99. Til HP, Feron VJ, de Groot AP. The toxicity of sulphite I. Long-term feeding and multigeneration studies in rats. Food Cosmet Toxicol 1972; 10:291–310.

14
Nickel

K. Eder and M. Kirchgessner
Technische Universität München,
Freising-Weihenstephan, Germany

I. INTRODUCTION AND HISTORY

The first biological studies of nickel, conducted at the beginning of the nineteenth century, were concerned with its toxicity (1). In 1890, nickel carbonyl, a highly toxic nickel compound, was detected, and in 1912, nickel contact dermatitis in industrial workers was described for the first time. The first reports about carcinogenicity of nickel compounds were published in 1932 (1,2). By 1926 it was observed that nickel influences the metabolism of glucose, and in 1929 it was observed that nickel has a positive effect on anemia (3). Although these findings implied that nickel might be an essential element for animals, it was not until 1970 that the first possible signs of nickel deprivation were described (4). However, these first nickel deficiency signs, and others that were described shortly thereafter, were obtained under conditions that produced suboptimal growth in the experimental animals, and some signs of nickel deprivation appeared inconsistent (5). Since 1974, diets have been used which allowed production of nickel deficiency signs, and the essentiality of nickel has been confirmed in several studies in rats (6,7), chicks (8), pigs (9), goats (10), sheep (11), and cows (12). Although the biochemical functions of nickel in animals are not yet clear, today there is no doubt that nickel plays an important role in metabolism (3,5,13–15).

II. CHEMICAL PROPERTIES

Nickel, atomic number 28 and atomic weight 58.71, is a silvery white metal. It has a density of about 8.9 g/cm^3, a melting point of 1725 K, and a boiling point of about 3170 K. Like iron and cobalt, nickel belongs to the first transition series of the Periodic Table. Nickel occurs in several oxidative states, $-I$, 0, I, II, III, and IV, of which state II plays the most important role in general, and in physiology. Bivalent nickel resembles $Co(II)$ in its general behavior (1,16–18).

III. ANALYSIS OF NICKEL IN BIOLOGICAL MATERIALS

The analysis of nickel in biological materials requires several steps, including sample collection, sample storage, sample decomposition, separation and enrichment, and finally determination. For these steps, various methods have been applied and described in detail (16,19). In general, it should be noted that nickel concentrations in biological samples are in most cases very low, although nickel and its alloys with other metals are widespread. Thus, contamination during analysis is a severe problem. In order to avoid contamination, all materials and chemicals coming into contact with the sample should be selected with regard to possible contamination.

For determination of nickel in organic samples, it is necessary to eliminate the organic constituents by digestion procedures such as dry or wet ashing. Dry ashing in muffle furnaces is the method of choice for digestion of biological materials. It is very simple, large numbers of samples can be treated at the same time, and a large quantity of the sample can be ashed. The ash is dissolved in ultrapure diluted acid. In the wet ashing method, the organic constituents of the sample are eliminated by oxidizing agents such as nitric acid, hydrochloric acid, or hydrogen peroxide, and the ash remains in the solution.

If the concentration of nickel is very low or if accompanying substances would interfere with the determination, separation and/or enrichment may be necessary. For separation or enrichment, nickel is complexed with ligands to form stable water insoluble complexes which are extracted by organic solvents. For the analysis of nickel, electrothermal atomic absorption spectrometry (ETAAS) and voltammetry (VA) are the most effective methods. ETAAS is the most widely used method for determination of nickel in biological materials. It permits the quantitation of Ni below the nanogram-per-gram range. Adsorption differential pulse voltammetry (ADPV) is more sensitive than ETAAS and allows the determination of nickel down to the picogram-per-gram range. Voltammetric methods are highly reproducible and the equipment is inexpensive compared to that of the AAS. However, voltammetric methods are very time consuming and require complete mineralization. Other methods for determination of nickel include flame atomic absorption spectrometry and colorimetry. However, these methods can be used only for materials with a rather high nickel content or after enrichment.

IV. METABOLISM OF NICKEL

A. Body Burden and Composition

Nickel occurs in all animal tissues and fluids in low concentrations. Relatively high nickel concentrations have been found in scalp hair (1700 ng/g), lymph nodes (810 ng/g), and testis (549 ng/g); lower nickel concentrations have been found in kidney (100 ng/g), liver (80 ng/g), muscle (100 ng/g), and skin (100 ng/g) (5). Nickel concentrations in tissues depend on sex, age, and nickel intake. In one experiment (20), rats were fed diets with a nickel concentration between 0.06 and 600 mg/kg. Nickel concentrations in tissues increased as the dietary nickel content rose, but the relative retention rates of nickel decreased from 22% to 0.14%. Similar results were obtained for calves (21). This means that there are mechanisms for the homeostatic regulation of nickel concentrations in tissues, as has been demonstrated for other essential trace elements (22).

In human plasma, the mean nickel concentration is 2.6 μg/L; dogs, rats, goats, cats, and guinea pigs have similar plasma nickel concentrations, ranging between 2 and 5 μg/L, whereas rabbits have higher concentrations (9.3 μg/L) (5). In humans, high plasma concentrations have been observed under pathologic conditions, for example, after acute myocardial infarction, stroke, and severe burns (5).

B. Absorption

The gastrointestinal absorption rate of dietary nickel is rather low and ranges under normal circumstances between 1% and 5% (23). However, the rate of absorption can be regulated depending on the nickel supply (20). This enables the body to compensate for under- or oversupply. In general, the absorption rate of trace elements is influenced by other dietary factors, and this might be true also for nickel (22). The most important nutritional factors which might influence absorption of nickel, apart from nickel concentration in the gut, are concentrations of other divalent ions and cation ligands. Moreover, physiologic factors such as sex, gravidity, lactation, growth rate, and age can influence nickel absorption. For example, nickel absorption was reported to be higher in nickel-deficient gravid animals (24), and in iron-deficient animals (5). Absorption of orally consumed nickel salts is also depressed by simultaneous intake of solid food (25). The absorption rate of nickel also depends on the solubility of the nickel compound consumed (18). With regard to the mechanism of nickel absorption there is little information. Nickel may be taken up biphasically (18). The first step involves crossing of the brush border. It seems that this step is saturable and is influenced by other cations such as zinc and calcium. The second step, the transfer of nickel from the mucosa into the blood, seems to be passive, with ion flow occurring in both directions. Likely, the absorption of nickel is an active process; nickel ions may be absorbed by the iron absorption system (26). Highest nickel concentrations in blood have been found between 2 and 3 h after oral intake of nickel sulfate (27–29).

C. Transport

In plasma, nickel does not occur in free form, but is bound to carriers, the most important being albumin. In rabbit serum, approximately 40% is bound to albumin, in human serum approximately 34% (30). Another high-molecular-mass protein that binds nickel is nickeloplasmin. Nickeloplasmin has been characterized as an α_2-macroglobulin with an estimated molecular weight of 7×10^5 (30). Nickeloplasmin contains 0.9 g of nickel per mole. In rabbit, 44% of the total nickel in serum is bound to nickeloplasmin, and 26% in human. Apart from albumin and nickeloplasmin, low-molecular binding ligands play an important role in extracellular nickel transport. Forty percent of the nickel in human serum was associated with an ultrafiltrable fraction (30). It is likely that these low-molecular-mass, ultrafiltrable ligands are amino acids. Reports suggest that L-histidine might be the most important amino acid in physiologic binding of nickel (31), but nickel might also be complexed by cysteine and aspartic acid (5). In the cell, nickel might be bound predominantly to low-molecular-mass ligands (32–34). In in vivo and in vitro studies, nickel was also bound to proteins and nucleic acids (33,35,36). Nickel induces metallothionin in liver but not or only to a small extent in kidney (37,38). Moreover, binding of nickel to metallothionein was observed only in vitro, not in vivo (35,38,39).

D. Excretion

Of orally consumed nickel, more than 90% is excreted in the feces. The main excretion pathway of absorbed nickel is renal. In human, nickel is reabsorbed in the renal tubular system, likely in the proximal tubule. Like urea and other solutes, nickel excretion increases with urinary flow (18). Besides renal excretion, some nickel is also excreted via bile (5,18). Sweat contains a relatively high concentration of nickel. Thus, by excessive sweating losses of nickel are relatively high (5).

E. Interaction

Nickel has been reported to interact with several elements, including calcium, chromium, cobalt, copper, iodine, iron, magnesium, manganese, molybdenum, phosphorus, potassium, sodium, and zinc. A comprehensive overview is given by Nielsen (40). Interactions between nickel and iron, zinc, and copper might be of primary importance, and are emphasized here. In 1959, Kirchgessner (41) showed that the retention of nickel correlates with the retention of iron and cobalt in heifers. Later, Schnegg and Kirchgessner (42,43) showed that nickel deficiency impairs absorption of iron, and decreases the iron concentration in liver, spleen, and kidneys. Nielsen and co-workers (44,45) reported changes in iron metabolism during nickel deficiency. During iron deficiency, nickel absorption was increased, and it was suggested that there is a common intestinal transport system (26). In spite of these interactions between nickel and iron, high nickel supply did not change biliary iron secretion (46). On the other hand, high dietary iron intake prevents toxicity of high nickel doses in chicks (47). In nickel deficiency, the tissue zinc concentrations in rats (43), goats (48), lambs (49), and pigs (9) have been observed to be decreased. Kirchgessner and co-workers conducted a two-factorial experiment with variable zinc and nickel concentrations in the diet, and it was shown that growth, protein concentration, and contents of nickel, zinc, iron, copper, manganese in several organs, hematologic parameters, and activities of some enzymes were influenced by interactions between dietary zinc and nickel (50–54). High zinc intake also was reported to prevent toxicity of high nickel doses, likely by depressing nickel absorption (55). Interrelations have also been observed for nickel and copper. Schnegg and Kirchgessner (43) observed reduced copper contents in liver, spleen, and kidney of rats in nickel deficiency. On the other hand, Spears et al. (56) reported that nickel supplementation reduced tissue copper concentrations in rats fed a copper-deficient diet. Nickel supplementation also exacerbated copper deficiency symptoms (15). Antagonistic interactions between copper and nickel in rats were also observed by Nielsen and Zimmerman (57). Nickel also interacts with calcium, magnesium, and phosphorus, since Kirchgessner and co-workers found that the contents of these elements in rat femurs were changed by nickel deprivation (58).

V. ESSENTIALITY AND SIGNS OF DEPRIVATION

A. Clinical Signs of Deficiency

In general, essential trace elements perform crucial physiologic and biochemical functions in the body, and insufficient intake causes signs of deficiency. Clinical signs of deficiency have been observed in animal experiments in which diets with very low nickel contents were fed. Table 1 lists the gross clinical signs of deficiency observed in experiments with some species. Nickel deficiency has not been described in humans (13).

In general, reduced growth rate due to deficient intake of a trace element is consid-

TABLE 1 Clinical Signs of Nickel Deprivation in Selected Species

Clinical sign	Rat	Chick	Pig	Goat
Growth rate decreased	+ (6, 7)	−	+ (9)	+ (48)
Reproduction decreased	+ (7)	−	+ (9)	+ (48)
Anemia	+ (59)	+ (8)	−	+ (48)
Structural changes[a]	+ (7)	+ (4, 8)	+ (9)	+ (48)
Ultrastructural changes[b]	+ (7)	+ (4, 8)	−	−

+ indicates that clinical sign has been observed
[a]Bones, joints, skin.
[b]Liver.

ered evidence for its essentiality. Reduced growth caused by nickel deprivation has been observed in rats (6,7), pigs (9), and goats (48). As an example, Schnegg and Kirchgessner (6) observed growth reduction in rats during the whole experimental period, that was reproduced in several experiments. In these studies, the weight difference between 30-day-old rats given 15 ng/g versus 20 μg/g dietary nickel averaged 16% in the second generation and 26% in the third generation (Fig. 1).

Nickel deprivation also has been shown to affect reproduction in rats, pigs, and goats. In rats, nickel deprivation caused a higher mortality rate in the offspring of nickel-deficient rats and reduced activity of nickel-deficient young animals (7). In chicks fed a nickel-deficient diet for a few weeks, there was gross pathology, including changes in shank skin pigmentation, thicker bones, swollen joints, and ultrastructural changes in the liver (8). Moreover, nickel deprivation caused rough coat and uneven hair development in rats (7), and a scaly and crusty skin, similar to parakeratosis in zinc-deficient piglets (9).

Also, iron metabolism and blood parameters have been shown to be changed by

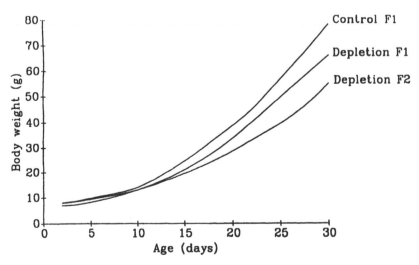

FIGURE 1 Body weights of neonatal rats whose dams were fed diets of different nickel contents. F1 refers to second generation and F2 to third generation (6).

TABLE 2 Chemical and Biochemical Changes Caused by Nickel Deprivation

Parameter	Tissue	Change[a]	Species	Ref.
Glucose-6-phosphate dehydrogenase	Liver	89%	Rat	(66)
Lactate dehydrogenase	Liver	67%	Rat	(66)
Isocitrate dehydrogenase	Liver	73%	Rat	(66)
Malate dehydrogenase	Liver	59%	Rat	(66)
Glutamate dehydrogenase	Liver, kidney	67%, 34%	Rat	(66)
Alanine aminotransferase	Liver, kidney	65%, 55%	Rat	(66)
Aspartate aminotransferase	Liver, kidney	67%, 70%	Rat	(66)
α-Amylase	Pancreas	57%	Rat	(67)
Sorbitol dehydrogenase	Liver, serum	36%, 65%	Goat	(68)
Urease	Rumen	>80%	Lamb, goat	(69,70)
Urea	Serum	23%	Rat	(65)
Triacylglycerols	Liver	37%	Rat	(65)
Phospholipids	Liver	6%	Chick	(8)
Glucose	Liver, serum	90%/64%	Rat	(65)
Glycogen	Liver	87%	Rat	(65)
ATP	Serum	25%	Rat	(65)

[a]Change refers to percent decrease.

nickel deprivation in the rat. Schnegg and Kirchgessner (43,59) observed anemia, characterized by reduced erythrocyte count, hemoglobin, and hematocrit levels, and reduced iron concentrations in liver, spleen, and kidney. These changes have been shown to be due to impaired iron absorption. Nielsen and co-workers (44,45,60–62) found that the effect of nickel deficiency on iron metabolism might relate to the form of iron source, and on iron status.

B. Chemical and Biochemical Pathology

Nickel deprivation in animals has been shown to change the activity of several enzymes and concentrations of various metabolites (Table 2). Most of the enzymes which have been shown to be affected by nickel deficiency are involved in glycolysis, the citrate cycle, and the metabolism of amino acids. This indicates that several important metabolic functions are disturbed in the state of nickel deficiency. Since nickel deficiency was shown to impair iron metabolism, it was important to investigate whether the changes of enzyme activities and substrate concentrations are due to the induced iron deficiency. However, additional studies (63–65) showed that various enzymes (catalase, GOT, GPT, and various dehydrogenases), as well as substrates (glucose, glycogen), are affected distinctively by iron and nickel deprivation. This means that the changes of these enzyme activities and substrate concentration are due to nickel deficiency per se, rather than to an induced iron deficiency.

VI. FUNCTIONS

Nickel plays in an important role as a constituent or activator of some bacterial enzymes. The first evidence for biological functions of nickel was presented by Bartha and Ordal in 1965 (71). They showed that "Knallgas" bacteria require nickel for their growth. Later, nickel was shown to be required for the synthesis of some hydrogenases, carbon monoxide dehydrogenase, methyl coenzyme M reductase, urease, and some other bacterial enzymes (for an overview, see Ref. 5).

Hydrogenases play an important role in bacteria that derive energy from the conversion of H_2 and CO_2 to CH_4 and H_2O (methanogenic bacteria). All hydrogenases contain iron, some contain additional nickel, and some need nickel for activation (68,72). Cammack (73) suggested that nickel might center in some hydrogenases, coordinated to cysteine sulfur, histidine nitrogen, and probably other ligands from the protein. At this site, nickel appears to undergo redox interconversion between two oxidation levels, Ni(III) and Ni(II). This redox-sensitive nickel probably is the binding site for H_2. Kovacs et al. (74) reported that hydrogenases isolated from photosynthetic bacteria contain 7 ± 1 iron atoms and 1 nickel atom per native enzyme molecule. Their studies indicate that iron atoms are located on the large subunit and the nickel atom on the small subunit of these hydrogenases.

Carbon monoxide dehydrogenase is another nickel-containing enzyme which is of central importance for metabolism in acetogenic bacteria. It catalyzes the reduction of CO_2 to CO and mediates the formation of acetyl CoA in a carbonylation reaction (72). Carbon monoxide dehydrogenase is thought to be an iron–sulfur protein with a nickel-containing prosthetic group (5). More than 50% of nickel taken up by methanogenic bacteria is incorporated into factor F 430, which has been identified as prosthetic group of methyl coenzyme M reductase. This enzyme catalyzes the reduction of methyl coenzyme M into methane (68).

Nickel also has been demonstrated to be an essential component of jackbean (72) and ruminal urease (75). The urease protein is composed of six subunits, of which each contains 2 mol nickel at the active site (72). Lee et al. (76) proposed a model of the bi-nickel active site of *Klebsiella aerogenes* urease in which ligands to nickel are nonsulfurous. Other plants, algae, and fungi have also been reported to require nickel for growth on urea as sole nitrogen source and/or for synthesis of urea (72). Although Chlorophyceae do not contain urease, growth of two *Chlorella* species was stimulated by nickel. However, the function of nickel in *Chlorella* is not yet known.

Although nickel deprivation experiments clearly demonstrated that nickel is essential for animals, to date there is no firmly established biological function of nickel in humans or animals (13). From the results of the nickel deficiency studies it can be concluded that nickel might play a role in activation of enzymes. Since the activity of several dehydrogenases and transaminases has been shown to be decreased in nickel-deprived rats (66–68), it is likely that nickel acts as activator or structural component in some of these enzymes. Nickel might play an important role in energy and protein metabolism.

On the other hand, since nickel deprivation impairs intestinal iron absorption, nickel might play a role in the intestinal absorption of iron or in iron metabolism in general. Nickel may be a bioligand cofactor facilitating absorption of iron(III) (5).

VII. REQUIREMENTS

The nickel requirements of humans and animals are not known. In order to assess nickel requirements, all data obtained from nickel deficiency experiments have to be considered. Results from several studies suggest that the nickel requirement for monogastric animals might be between 50 and 200 ng/g food (5,68,77). For ruminants, the nickel requirement might be higher than for monogastric animals, because ruminal urease requires nickel. Anke and co-workers suggested that the nickel requirement for ruminants might be in the range of 300 to 350 ng/g food (5,77). Since nickel has been shown to be essential in various animal species, it is highly probable that it is also essential for humans, although nickel deficiency has not been described in humans. By extrapolation from animal data, Nielsen (5) suggested that the nickel requirement of humans might be approximately 35 μg daily.

Nickel intake in humans depends on the composition of the diet, especially on the amount and proportion of foods of animal and plant origin. As a rule, foods of animal origin contain less nickel than those of plant origin. The dietary nickel intake might be in the range between 150 and 700 μg daily (5). Thus, the hypothetical requirement of nickel seems to be met in humans. However, as for other essential trace elements, the requirement of nickel might be influenced by other dietary factors (the chemical form of the nickel compound, supply with other interacting trace elements, amount and form of organic ligands) and physiologic factors (sex, gravidity, lactation, growth rate, age). It is possible that such factors make the requirement for nickel higher than is supplied by some dietary regimens (78).

VIII. TOXICITY

As a rule, nickel toxicity is caused by inhalation of nickel-containing particulates in workplace environments. The toxicity of oral nickel is low, and thus toxicity occurs only at very high nickel intake. Acute toxicity of nickel is in most cases caused by nickel carbonyl. Nickel carbonyl and other nickel forms are also known to be carcinogenic and genotoxic and to cause miscellaneous health effects. Moreover, nickel is one of the most common skin allergens in the general population (79).

A. Oral Toxicity

It has been found that there are mechanisms for the homeostatic regulation of nickel concentrations, and large oral doses of nickel salts are necessary to overcome the homeostatic control (17). Thus, acute and chronic toxicity of oral nickel is low. The oral nickel LD_{50} ranges between 100 and 1000 mg nickel salt per kilogram body weight, depending on the chemical form of the nickel compound. In contrast, parenteral LD_{50} intake ranges between 5 and 100 mg nickel salt per kilogram body weight (23). Main signs of acute oral nickel toxicity are gastrointestinal irritations (5,23).

Chronic effects of high oral nickel doses have been investigated in numerous studies with rats, mice, rabbits, dogs, chicks, piglets, and calves (23). In most of the studies, chronic ingestion of high nickel doses caused weight loss in adult animals, and growth retardation in growing animals. Typically, nickel doses between 5 and 50 mg/kg body weight were required to induce growth retardation in various species. Toxic effects of nickel might depend on the solubility of the nickel salt used, on the species, on the composition of the diet, and on the sex of the animal (23). In rats, 1 mg nickel/g diet caused reduced food intake and growth retardation, as well as changes in physiologic and biochemical parameters such as blood parameters, activities of enzymes, and concentrations of various trace elements (80). In piglets, growth retardation occurred in animals which were fed 0.375 mg nickel/g diet and more (81). Nickel toxicity caused by high oral nickel intake has been shown to be influenced by several dietary factors, such as intake of iron, copper, and zinc (5).

If animal data are extrapolated to humans, a daily dose of 250 mg of soluble nickel is required to produce toxic symptoms in humans (17). Thus, oral nickel toxicity plays an insignificant role in humans. In contrast, nickel toxicity might be a greater problem in parenteral nutrition, because replacement solutions are often contaminated with nickel.

Infusion of solutions that are highly contaminated with nickel could affect cardiac and uterine function and could cause allergic reactions (5).

B. Carcinogenesis and Contact Dermatitis

Several epidemiologic studies have shown that workers in the nickel-producing industry have a higher risk of nasal and lung cancer (79,82). In animal experiments, parenteral application of various nickel compounds such as nickel powder, -carbonyl, -acetate, -bisulfide, -hydroxide, -fluoride, Ni(II) and Ni(III) oxides, and nickelocene has been found to be carcinogenic in at least one species. The activity of parenteral applied nickel compounds might be related to their solubility—the least soluble are the most cancerogenic. Nickel subsulfide might be the most cancerogenic compound, whereas the most soluble compounds, such as nickel chloride and nickel sulfate, are less active (23,82). In contrast, oral applied nickel did not increase tumor rate in animal experiments (23,83).

Nickel has been reported to interact with the immune system (79). Dermal contact with sources of nickel such as jewelry, coins, clothing fasteners, tools, cutlery, cosmetics, detergents, or surgical and medical instruments can cause nickel contact dermatitis. Clinically, nickel contact dermatitis tends to be chronic and persistent, and different types of lesions occur. Hand eczema is a common finding in patients with nickel contact allergy. Typically, nickel dermatitis spreads from the primary area, which is in direct contact with the allergen, to secondary sites such as elbow flexures, eyelids, and the sides of the neck (79). In provocation studies, oral nickel doses provoked hand eczemia in patients with nickel dermatitis. Thus, some dermatologists advise their patients with nickel dermatitis to avoid the ingestion of foodstuffs with very high nickel contents, such as nuts and cocoa products (84).

IX. FUTURE RESEARCH

Nickel is involved in two aspects of human and animal nutrition: the toxic and the essential. Toxicity of nickel, because of its important practical meaning, is the subject of considerable research. On the other hand, nickel deficiency plays practically no role in human nutrition, since intake has been reported to be far higher than assessed requirements (see above). However, nickel interacts with other essential trace elements such as iron, copper, and zinc. Thus, future research should include biochemical mechanisms of interactions between nickel and other essential elements. Moreover, another aim should be to identify nickel functions by searching for nickel-containing and nickel-dependent enzymes. This would clarify the role of nickel in metabolism.

REFERENCES

1. Nriagu JO. Global cycle and properties of nickel. In: Nriagu JO, ed. Nickel in the Environment. New York: Wiley Interscience, 1980: 1–26.
2. Reichlmayr-Lais AM, Kirchgessner M. Nickel (Ni). In: Zumkley H, ed. Spurenelemente: Grundlagen—Ätiologie—Diagnose—Therapie. Stuttgart, New York: Thieme Verlag, 1983: 167–173.
3. Schnegg A, Kirchgessner M. Nickel—ein neues essentielles Spurenelement. Übers Tierernährg 1979; 7:179–184.
4. Nielsen FH, Sauberlich HE. Evidence of a possible requirement for nickel in the chick. Proc Soc Exp Biol Med 1970; 134:845–859.

5. Nielsen FH. Nickel. In: Mertz W, ed. Trace Elements in Human and Animal Nutrition, Vol. I. 5th ed. San Diego, CA: Academic Press, 1987: 245–273.

6. Schnegg A, Kirchgessner M. Zur Essentialität von Nickel für das tierische Wchstum. Z Tierphysiol Tierernaehrg Futtermittelkde 1975; 36:63–74.

7. Nielsen FH, Myron DR, Givand SH, Zimmerman TJ, Ollerich DA. Nickel deficiency in rats. J Nutr 1975; 105:1620–1630.

8. Nielsen FH, Myron DR, Givand SH, Ollerich DA. Nickel deficiency and nickel-rhodium interaction in chicks. J Nutr 1975; 105:1607–1619.

9. Anke M, Grün M, Dittrich D, Groppel B, Hennig A. Low nickel rations for growth and reproduction in pigs. In: Hoekstra WG, Sutte JW, Ganther HE, Mertz W, eds. Trace Element Metabolism in Animals. Vol. II. Baltimore, MD: University Park Press, 1974: 715–718.

10. Anke M, Hennig A, Grün M, Partschefeld M, Groppel B, Lüdke H. Nickel—ein essentielles Spurenelement. Arch Tierernährg 1977; 27:25–38.

11. Spears JW, Hatfield EE, Forbes RM, Koeing SE. Studies on the role of nickel in the ruminant. J Nutr 1978; 108:313–320.

12. Spears JW, Hatfield EE. Role of nickel in ruminant nutrition. In: Anke M, Schneider HJ, Brückner C, eds. 3. Spurenelement Symposium, Nickel. Jena: Friedrich Schiller Universität, 1980: 47–53.

13. Kirchgessner M, Schnegg A. Biochemical and physiological effects of nickel deficiency. In: Nriagu JO, ed. Nickel in the Environment. New York: Wiley-Interscience, 1980: 635–659.

14. Anke M, Groppel B, Kronemann H. Significance of newer essential trace elements (like Si, Ni, As, Li, V ...) for the nutrition of man and animal. In: Brätter P, Schramel P, ed. Trace Element Analytical Chemistry in Medicine and Biology. Vol. 3. Berlin: De Gruyter, 1984: 421–464.

15. Spears JW. Nickel as a "newer trace element" in the nutrition of domestic animals. J Animal Sci 1984; 59:823–835.

16. Stoeppler M. Analysis of nickel in biological materials and natural waters. In: Nriagu JO, ed. Nickel in the Environment. New York: Wiley Interscience, 1980: 661–821.

17. Nielsen FH. Nickel. In: Frieden E, ed. Biochemistry of the Essential Ultratrace Elements. New York: Plenum Press, 1984: 293–308.

18. Nieboer E, Rickey TT, Sanford WE. Nickel metabolism in man and animals. In: Sigel H, ed. Nickel and Its Role in Biology. New York: Marcel Dekker, 1988: 91–121.

19. Seiler HG. Analysis of nickel in biological materials. In: Sigel H, ed. Nickel and Its Role in Biology. New York: Marcel Dekker, 1988: 403–428.

20. Kirchgessner, M, Reichlmayr-Lais AM, Maier R. Ni-Retention und Ni-Gehalte in Organen und Geweben nach unterschiedlicher Ni-Versorgung bei Ratten. Z Tierphysiol Tierernährg Futter-mittelkde 1984; 52:27–34.

21. O'Dell GD, Miller WJ, Moore SL, King WA, Ellers JC, Jureck H. Effect of dietary nickel level on excretion and nickel content of tissues in male calves. J Animal Sci 1971; 32:769–773.

22. Kirchgessner M, Schwarz FJ, Schnegg A. Interactions of essential metals in human physiology. In: Prasad AS, ed. Clinical, Biochemical, and Nutritional Aspects of Trace Elements. New York: Alan R. Liss, 1982; 477–512.

23. Zimmerli B, Candrian U, Schlatter C. Vorkommen und toxikologische Bedeutung von Nickel in der Nahrung. Mitt Gebiete Lebensm Hyg 1987; 78:344–396.

24. Kirchgessner M, Roth-Maier DA, Schnegg A. Progress of nickel metabolism and nutrition research. In: Howell, J McC, Gawthorne JM, White CL, eds. Trace Elements in Man and Animals (TEMA-4). Canberra: Australian Academy of Science, 1981: 621–624.

25. Solomons NW, Viteri F, Shuler TR, Nielsen FH. Bioavailability of nickel in man: effect of foods and chemically-defined dietary constituents on the absorption of inorganic nickel. J Nutr 1982; 112:39–50.

26. Becker G, Dorstelman U, Frommberger V, Forth W. On the absorption of cobalt(II) and nickel (II) ions by isolated intestinal segments in vitro of rats. In: Anke M, Schneider HJ, Brückner C, eds. 3. Spurenelement Symposium, Nickel. Jena: Friedrich Schiller Universität, 1980: 79–86.

27. Cronin E, Di Michiel AD, Brown SS. Oral challenge in nickel-sensitive women with hand eczema. In: Brown SS, Sunderman WF Jr, eds. Nickel Toxicology. London: Academic Press, 1980: 149–152.

28. Christensen OB, Möller H, Andrasko L, Lagesson V. Nickel concentration of blood, urine and sweat after oral administration. Contact Dermatitis 1979; 5:312–316.

29. Christensen OB, Lagesson V. Nickel concentration of blood and urine after oral administration. Ann Clin Lab Sci. 1981; 11:119–125.

30. Sunderman FW, Jr. A review of the metabolism and toxicology of nickel. Ann Clin Lab Sci 1977; 7:377–398.

31. Lucassen M, Sarcar B. Nickel(II)-binding constituents of human blood serum. J Toxicol Environm Health 1979; 5:897–905.

32. Eaton DL, Stacey NH, Wong KL, Klaassen CD. Dose-response effects of various metal ions on rat liver metallothionin, glutathione, heme oxygenase, and cytochrome P-450. Toxicol Appl Pharmacol 1980; 55:393–402.

33. Sunderman FW Jr, Costa ER, Fraser C, Hui G, Levine JJ, Tse TPH. (63)Nickel-constituents in renal cytosol of rats after injection of (63)nickel chloride. Ann Clin Lab Sci 1981; 11:488–496.

34. Sunderman FW Jr, Zaharia O, Reid MC, Belliveau JF, O'Leary GP Jr, Griffin H. Effects of diethyldithiocarbamate and nickel chloride on glutathione and trace metal concentrations in rat liver. Toxicology 1984; 32:11–21.

35. Okarsson A, Tjälve H. Binding of (63)nickel by cellular constituents in some tissues of mice after the administration of (63)nickel chloride and (63)nickel carbonyl. Acta Pharmacol Toxicol 1979; 45:306–314.

36. Ciccarelli RB, Wetterhahn KE. Nickel-bound chromatin, nucleic acids, and nuclear proteins from kidney and liver of rats treated with nickel carbonate in vivo. Cancer Res 1984; 44:3892–3897.

37. Piotrowski JK, Szymanska A. Influence of certain metals on the level of metallothionein-like-proteins in the liver and kidneys of rats. J Toxicol Environm Health 1976; 1:991–1002.

38. Sunderman FW Jr, Fraser CB. Effects of nickel chloride and diethyldithiocarbamate on metallothionein in rat liver and kidney. Ann Clin Lab Sci 1983; 13:489–495.

39. Waalkes MP, Kasprzak KS, Oshima M, Poirier LA. Relative in vitro affinity of hepatic metallothionein for metals. Toxicol Lett 1984; 20:33–39.

40. Nielsen FH. Interactions of nickel with essential minerals. In: Nriagu JO, ed. Nickel in the Environment. New York: Wiley Interscience, 1980: 611–634.

41. Kirchgessner M. Wechselbeziehungen zwischen Spurenelementen in Futtermitteln und tierischen Substanzen sowie Abhängigkeitsverhältnisse zwischen einzelnen Elementen bei der Retention. Z Tierphysiol Tierernährg Futtermittelkde 1959; 14:270–277.

42. Schnegg A, Kirchgessner M. Zur Absorption and Verfügbarkeit von Eisen bei Nickel-Mangel. Int Z Vit Ern Forschung 1976; 46:96–99.

43. Schnegg A, Kirchgessner M. Zur Interaktion von Nickel mit Eisen, Kupfer und Zink. Arch Tierernährung 1976; 26:543–549.

44. Nielsen FH, Zimmerman TJ, Collings ME, Myron DR. Nickel deprivation in rats: nickel-iron interactions. J Nutr 1979; 109:1623–1632.

45. Nielsen FH. Effect of form of iron on the interaction between nickel and iron in rats: growth and blood parameters. J Nutr 1980; 110:965–973.

46. Kirchgessner M, Kulig W, Kreuzer M. Biliary flow rate and concentration of Fe, Cu and Mn as affected by enteral or parenteral Ni supply. J Trace Elem Electrolytes Health Dis 1990; 4:175–182.

47. Hill CH. The effect of iron and zinc on metal toxicities in the chick. Fed Proc 1981; 40:715.

48. Anke M, Kronemann H, Groppel B, Hennig A, Meissner D, Schneider HJ. The influence of nickel deficiency on growth, reproduction, longevity and different parameters of goats. In: Anke M, Schneider HJ, Brückner C, eds. 3. Spurenelement Symposium, Nickel. Jena: Friedrich Schiller Universität, 1980: 3–10.

49. Spears JW, Hatfield EE, Fahey GC Jr. Nickel depletion in the growing ovine. Nutr Rep Int 1978; 18:621–628.

50. Mathur AK, Reichlmayr-Lais AM, Kirchgessner M. Wachstum, Futterverwertung und Proteingehalt einzelner Organe bei unterschiedlicher Zink- und Nickelversorgung. Z Tierphysiol Tierernährg Futtermittelkde 1982; 47:101–109.

51. Reichlmayr-Lais AM, Kirchgessner M, Mathur AK. Zn- und Ni-Konzentrationen in Organen und Geweben von Ratten nach unterschiedlicher Zn- und Ni-Versorgung. Z Tierphysiol Tierernährg Futtermittelkde 1985; 53:207–213.

52. Kirchgessner M, Reichlmayr-Lais AM, Mathur AK. Fe-, Cu- und Mn-Konzentrationen in ausgewählten Organen und Geweben von Ratten nach unterschiedlicher Zn- und Ni-Versorgung. Z Tierphysiol Tierernährg Futtermittelkde 1985; 53:214–222.

53. Reichlmayr-Lais AM, Kirchgessner M, Mathur AK. Hämatologische Veränderungen bei Ratten nach unterschiedlicher Ni- und Zn-Versorgung. Z Tierphysiol Tierernährg Futtermittelkde 1985; 53:279–284.

54. Kirchgessner M, Reichlmayr-Lais AM, Mathur AK. Aktivität ausgewählter Enzyme nach unterschiedlicher Zn- und Ni-Versorgung von Ratten. Z Tierphysiol Tierernährg Futtermittelkde 1985; 54:6–14.

55. Hill CH. Studies of a nickel-zinc interaction in chicks. Fed Proc 1977; 36:1106.

56. Spears JW, Hatfield EE, Forbes RM. Nickel-copper interrelationship in the rat. Proc Soc Exp Biol Med 1977; 156:140–146.

57. Nielsen FH, Zimmerman TJ. Interactions among nickel, copper and iron in rats. Biol Trace Element Res 1981; 3:83–98.

58. Kirchgessner M, Perth J, Schnegg A. Mangelnde Ni-Versorgung und Ca-, Mg- und P-Gehalte im Knochen wachsender Ratten. Arch Tierernährung 1980; 30:805–810.

59. Schnegg A, Kirchgessner M. Veränderungen des Hämoglobingehaltes, der Erythrozytenzahl und des Hämatokrits bei Nickelmangel. Nutr Metabol 1975; 19:268–278.

60. Nielsen FH, Shuler TR. Effect of dietary nickel and iron on the trace element content of rat liver. Biol Trace Element Res 1979; 1:337–346.

61. Nielsen FH, Shuler TR. Effect of form of iron on nickel deprivation in the rat. Liver content of copper, iron, manganese, and zinc. Biol Trace Element Res 1981; 3:245–256.

62. Nielsen FH, Shuler TR, Zimmerman TJ, Collings ME, Uthus EO. Interactions between nickel and iron in the rat. Biol Trace Element Res 1979; 1:325–335.

63. Schnegg A, Kirchgessner M. Alkalische und Saure Phosphatase- Aktivität in Leber und Serum bei Ni- bzw. Fe-Mangel. Int Z Vit Ern Forschung 1977; 47:274–276.

64. Schnegg A, Kirchgessner M. Zur Differentialdiagnose von Fe- und Ni-Mangel durch Bestimmung einiger Enzymaktivitäten. ZBl Vet Med A 1977; 24:242–247.

65. Schnegg A, Kirchgessner M. Konzentrationsänderungen einiger Substrate in Serum und Leber bei Ni- bzw. Fe-Mangel. Z Tierphysiol Tierernährg Futtermittelkde 1977; 39:247–251.

66. Schnegg A, Kirchgessner M. Aktivitätsänderungen von Enzymen der Leber und Niere im Nickel- bzw. Eisen-Mangel. Z Tierphysiol Tierernährg Futtermittelkde 1977; 38:200–205.

67. Kirchgessner M, Schnegg A. Alpha-Amylase und Dehydrogenasenaktivität bei suboptimaler Ni-Versorgung. Ann Nutr Metab 1981; 25:307–310.

68. Anke M. Nickel als essentielles Spurenelement. In: Gladtke E, Heimann G, Lombeck I, Eckert I, eds. Spurenelemente. Stuttgart: Thieme Verlag, 1984: 106–125.

69. Spears JW, Smith CJ, Hatfield EE. Rumen bacterial urease requirement for nickel. J Dairy Sci 1977; 60:1073–1076.

70. Hennig A, Jahreis G, Anke M, Partschefeld M, Grün M. Nickel-ein essentielles Spurenelement. Arch Tierernährung 1978; 28:267–268.

71. Bartha R, Ordal EJ. Nickel-dependent chemo-lithotropic growth of two Hydrogenomonas strains. J Bacteriol 1965; 89:1015–1019.

72. Ankel-Fuchs D, Thauer RK. Nickel in biology: nickel as an essential trace element. In: Lancaster JR Jr, ed. Chemistry of Nickel. New York: VCH, 1988: 93–109.

73. Cammack R. Nickel centres in hydrogenase and other enzymes. J Inorg Biochem 1991; 43:650.
74. Kovacs KL, Szökefalvi-Nagy Z, Demeter I, Bagyinka CS. Location of metals in NiFe hydrogenases and its relevance to the protein conformation forms. J Inorg Biochem 1991; 43:651.
75. Fishbein WN, Smith MJ, Nagarajan K, Scurzi W. The first natural nickel metalloenzyme: urease. Fed Proc 1976; 35:1680.
76. Lee MH, Mulrooney SB, Todd MJ, Hausinger RP. Biosynthesis and characterization of the Binickel center in *Klebsiella aerogenes* urease. J Inorg Biochem 1991; 43:660.
77. Anke M, Grün B, Groppel B, Kronemann H. Nutritional requirements of nickel. In: Sarkar B, ed. Biological Aspects of Metals and Metal-Related Diseases. New York: Raven Press, 1983: 89–105.
78. Nielsen FH. Possible future implications of ultratrace elements in human health and disease. In: Prasad AS, ed. Essential and Toxic Trace Elements in Human Health and Disease. New York: Alan R. Liss, 1988: 277–292.
79. Nieboer E, Rossetto FE, Menon CR. Toxicology of nickel compounds. In: Sigel H, ed. Nickel and Its Role in Biology. New York: Marcel Dekker, 1988: 359–402.
80. Schnegg A, Kirchgessner M. Zur Toxizität von alimentär verabreichtem Nickel. Landwirtsch Forschung 1976; 29:177–185.
81. Kirchgessner M, Schnegg A, Roth FX. Zur Wirkung hoher alimentärer Nickel-Zulagen. In: Anke M, Schneider HJ, Brückner C, eds. 3. Spurenelement Symposium, Nickel. Jena: Friedrich Schiller Universität, 1980: 309–313.
82. Furst A, Radding SB. An update of nickel carcinogenesis. In: Nriagu JO, ed. Nickel in the Environment. New York: Wiley Interscience, 1980: 585–600.
83. Schroeder HA, Balassa JJ, Vinton WH. Chromium, lead, cadmium, nickel and titanium in mice: effect on mortality, tumors and tissue levels. J Nutr 1964; 83:239–250.
84. Spruit D, Bongaarts PJM, Malten KE. Dermatological effects of nickel. In: Nriagu JO, ed. Nickel in the Environment. New York: Wiley Interscience, 1980: 585–600.

15
Boron

FORREST H. NIELSEN
U.S. Department of Agriculture, Grand Forks, North Dakota

I. BRIEF INTRODUCTION AND HISTORY

In the 1870s, it was discovered that pharmacologic amounts of borax and boric acid could be used to preserve foods. For about the next 50 years, borates were considered some of the best preservatives for extending the palatability of foods such as fish, meat, cream, and butter. In 1904, however, Wiley (1) reported that human volunteers consuming over 500 mg of boric acid per day for 50 days displayed disturbed appetite, digestion, and health. Subsequent to his report, the opinion that boron posed a risk to health gained momentum; by the middle 1950s, boron was essentially forbidden throughout the world as a food preservative.

In 1923, Warington (2) showed that boron is an essential element for plants. About 15 years later, attempts to demonstrate boron essentiality for higher animals began; these attempts (3–7) were unsuccessful. Thus, before 1980, students of biochemistry and nutrition were taught that boron was a unique element because it was essential for plants but not for higher animals. In 1981, it was reported that boron stimulated growth and partially prevented leg abnormalities present in cholecalciferol-deficient chicks (8). Since then, evidence has been accumulating which suggests that boron has an essential biochemical role in higher animals including humans.

II. CHEMICAL PROPERTIES OF BORON

Boron exists in biological material mainly bound to oxygen. Thus, boron biochemistry is essentially that of boric acid. Dilute aqueous boric acid solutions are comprised of $B(OH)_3$

and $B(OH)_4^-$ species at the pH of blood (7.4); because the pK_a of boric acid is 9.2, the abundance of these two species should be 98.4% and 1.6%, respectively.

Boric acid forms ester complexes with hydroxyl groups of organic compounds; this preferably occurs when the hydroxyl groups are adjacent and cis (9). The structures of the complexes believed to be formed between hydroxyl-containing compounds and tetraborate are shown in Figure 1. The importance of the proper hydroxyl arrangement is demonstrated by the fact that polysaccharides made of carbohydrates such as glucose, glucuronic acid, and xylose as generally encountered in plants do not react with borate because they do not have the required paired hydroxyl groups. Hydroxyl groups distorted from a single plane also do not react well with borate. Among the many substances of biological interest with which boron complexes are adenosine 5-phosphate, pyridoxine, riboflavin, dehydroascorbic acid, and pyridine nucleotides. Formation of these complexes may be biologically important because, in vitro, it results in the competitive inhibition of some enzymes (11). These include oxidoreductases which require cis-hydroxyl containing pyridine or flavin nucleotides as cofactors. Figure 2 shows the complex between borate and nicotinamide adenine dinucleotide (NAD^+) which prevents it from functioning as a coenzyme.

The added stabilization of hydrogen bonding between hydroxyls bound to boron and hydrogen of imidazole or amido groups allows complexes to be formed between borate and compounds containing single hydroxyl groups. Through forming this type of complex, borate and boronic acid derivatives can form transition-state analogs that inhibit the activity of some enzymes (13). For example, serine hydrolases are inhibited when a tetrahedral complex is formed between the serine hydroxyl group and boron, with hydrogen bonding to an imidazole ring of an adjacent histidine adding stabilization; a visualization of this complex is shown in Figure 2.

To date, two naturally occurring organoboron compounds have been identified; they contain boron bound to four oxygen groups. These compounds are aplasmomycin (14), a novel ionophoric macrolide antibiotic isolated from strain SS-20 of *Streptomyces griseus*, and boromycin (15), an antibiotic synthesized by *Streptomyces antibioticus*. The structures of boromycin and aplasmomycin are shown in Figure 3. Boromycin has the ability to encapsulate alkali metal cations and increase the permeability of the cytoplasmic membrane to potassium ions.

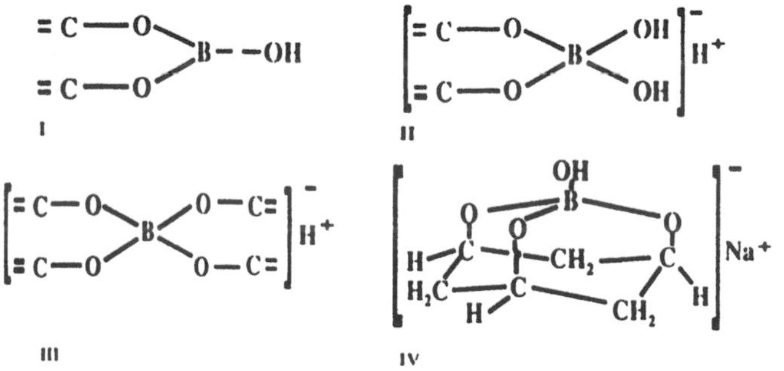

FIGURE 1 Structures of the types of complexes formed between hydroxyl-containing compounds and tetraborate. Boron forms complexes with hydroxyl groups of organic compounds, preferably when the groups are adjacent and cis. (From Ref. 10.)

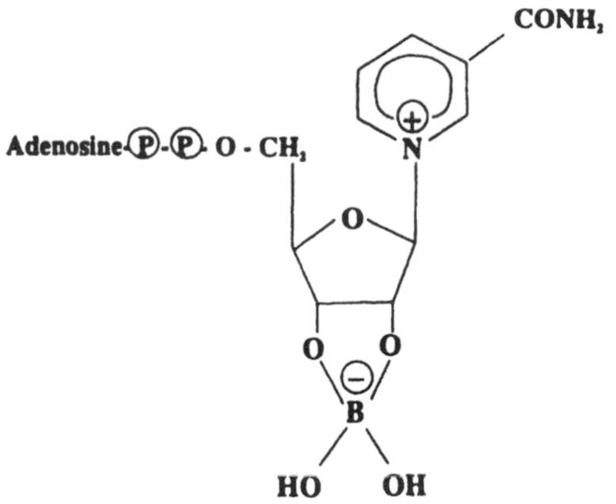

FIGURE 2 Examples of boron complexes that inhibit enzyme action. Complex I illustrates inhibition of a coenzyme. Borate complexes with the ribose moiety of nicotinamide adenine dinucleotide (NAD$^+$) and inhibits its function. Complex II illustrates a tetrahedral borate complex involving a serine hydroxyl, an imidazole ring of histidine, and other amino acid residues in a serine hydrolase. This is an example of a transition-state analog complex with borate that inhibits the activity of some enzymes. (From Ref. 12.)

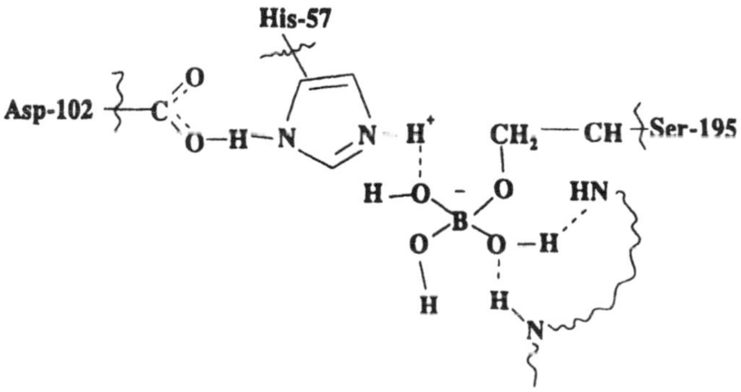

III. BORON ANALYTICAL METHODS

Only recently have methods been developed which can determine low concentrations of boron in biological substances with acceptable accuracy. Development of boron analytical methods has been difficult because many boron compounds volatilize at temperatures far below those required for most dry or wet ashing procedures, and most forms of glassware and chemical reagents contain significant amounts of boron. Procedures that have been developed to digest biological substances with minimal boron loss or contamination include a low-temperature wet digestion in semiclosed Teflon tubes (16), and a Teflon bomb digestion in a microwave oven (17). Inductively coupled argon plasma spectroscopy is generally used to determine the boron content of the digestates (16,17).

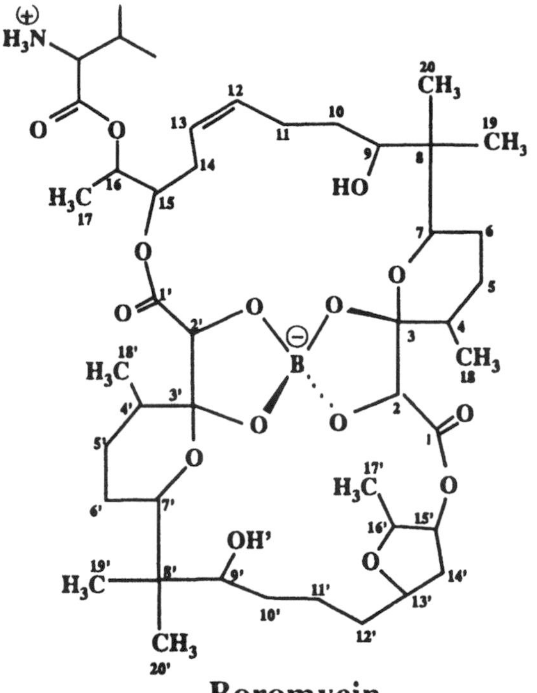

Boromycin

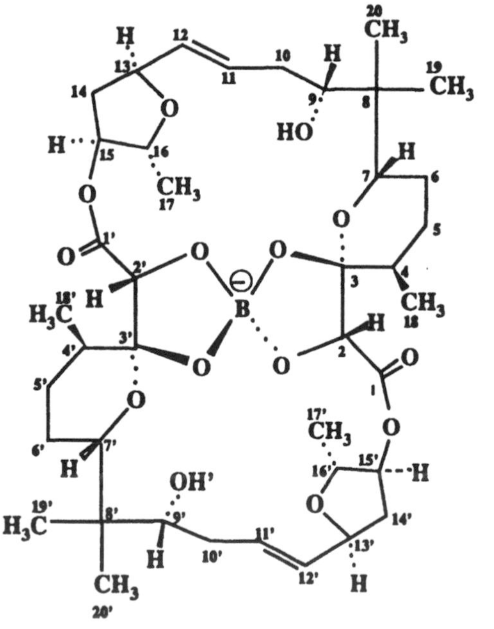

Aplasmomycin

FIGURE 3 Structures of two known naturally occurring organoboron compounds, boromycin and aplasmomycin. These compounds contain boron bound to four oxygen ligands. Aplasmomycin is a novel ionophoric macrolide antibiotic isolated from strain SS-20 of *Streptomyces griseus*, and boromycin is an antibiotic produced by *Streptomyces antibioticus*. (From Ref. 10.)

Prompt gamma-activation analysis and neutron activation-mass spectrometry (NA-MS) techniques have been developed which can accurately measure the usual or normal concentration of boron in biomaterials (18). One major advantage of these techniques is that they do not require the destruction of the organic matrix containing boron. For example, with NA-MS a freeze-dried sample is irradiated to generate ^{4}He from ^{10}B; the ^{4}He is measured by mass spectrometry. The sophistication and cost of the equipment precludes either of these methods from being of general laboratory use.

IV. METABOLISM OF BORON

A. Absorption and Excretion

Sodium borate, boric acid, and possibly food boron are rapidly absorbed and are excreted largely in the urine. Because there is no usable radioisotope of boron, the study of its metabolism has been made difficult. However, it is likely that most ingested boron is converted into $B(OH_3)$, the normal end product of hydrolysis of most boron compounds and the dominant inorganic species at the pH of the gastrointestinal tract. It is postulated that boron is absorbed and excreted mainly as undissociated $B(OH_3)$. The mechanism by which boron is transported through the body has not been defined. This lack of knowledge may be overcome shortly because, recently, inductively coupled plasma-mass spectrometry was used to establish a method using the ratio of the two stable isotopes, ^{11}B/^{10}B, to study boron metabolism (19). This method was used to show that boron in broccoli, intrinsically enriched with ^{10}B, was absorbed as well as extrinsic boron ^{10}B in boric acid from a test meal by rats. When 20 μg of ^{10}B isotope were fed to rats, 95% of this isotope was detected in the urine and 4% in the feces after 3 days. This agrees with other urinary recovery findings indicating that more than 90% of ingested boron is usually absorbed.

B. Tissue Concentration and Storage

Boron is distributed throughout soft tissues and fluids of animals and humans at concentrations mostly between 0.015 and 0.6 μg/g fresh tissue (20–25). Bone, fingernails, hair, and teeth usually contain several times these concentrations. Disease can modify organ concentrations. For example, thalassemia/hemoglobin E disease elevates boron in brain, heart, kidney, and spleen (24). Boron concentrations were found reduced in brains of schizophrenic patients (26), and in arthritic bones (21,23). .

Evidence showing that boron is homeostatically controlled includes the rapid urinary excretion of absorbed boron, the lack of accumulation of boron in tissues, and the relatively narrow range of boron concentrations in blood of apparently healthy individuals. In a group of 50 blood samples collected from hospitals and clinics in the United Kingdom, the serum boron concentration ranged from 8.4 to 48.1 ng/mL with a median of 22.3 ng/mL (25). In postmenopausal women, an increase in dietary boron from 0.36 mg/day (probably deficient) to 3.3 mg/day (luxuriant) did not increase plasma boron concentrations when dietary magnesium was 340 mg/day; only a 2.4-fold increase occurred when dietary magnesium was 109 mg/day (CD Hunt, unpublished data). Increasing dietary boron from 0.465 (deficient) to 3.465 (luxuriant) mg/kg diet increased the plasma boron concentration by only 50% in cholecalciferol-deficient chicks (27). As with other mineral elements, overcoming apparent homeostatic mechanisms by high boron intakes will elevate tissue boron concentrations.

V. SIGNS OF BORON DEFICIENCY

A. Animals

The signs of boron deficiency in animals have not been clearly defined. The response to boron deprivation is affected by parameters that affect macromineral metabolism. In other words, the response to boron deprivation varies as the diet varies in its content of nutrients such as calcium, phosphorus, magnesium, potassium, and cholecalciferol (28). However, although the nature and severity of the changes may vary with dietary composition, many findings indicate that boron deprivation impairs calcium and energy metabolism. For example, a boron supplement of 3 μg/g to a basal diet containing 0.465 μg boron/g alleviated the cholecalciferol deficiency-induced distortion of marrow sprouts of chick proximal tibial epiphyseal plate, and elevated the number of osteoblasts within the marrow sprouts (27). Boron also was found to substantially alleviate or correct cholecalciferol deficiency-induced elevations in plasma glucose, changes in energy substrate utilization and depressions in growth (11).

Brain composition and function are also affected by dietary boron. Boron deprivation was found to systematically influence brain electrical activity assessed by an electrocorticogram in mature rats; the principal effect was on the frequency distribution of electrical activity (29). In this study, brain copper concentrations were higher in boron-deprived than in boron-supplemented rats. Furthermore, calcium concentrations in total brain and in brain cortex, as well as the phosphorus concentration in the cerebellum, were found to be higher in boron-deprived than in boron-supplemented rats fed a cholecalciferol-deficient diet (30).

Some of the preceding findings may reflect an effect of dietary boron on macromineral metabolism. The apparent absorption and balance of calcium, magnesium, and phosphorus were found to be higher in boron-supplemented (2.72 μg/g diet) than in boron-deprived (0.158 μg B/g diet) rats fed a cholecalciferol-deficient diet (30).

B. Humans

Findings involving boron deprivation of humans have come mainly from two studies (31–37) in which men over the age of 45, postmenopausal women, and postmenopausal women on estrogen therapy were fed a boron-low diet, or about 0.25 mg/2000 kcal for 63 days and then fed the same diet supplemented with 3 mg of boron per day for 49 days. These dietary intakes were near the low and high values in the range of dietary boron intakes (0.5–3.1 mg/day) found in a limited number of surveys (38). In the first experiment (31,32), the diet was low in magnesium, 115 mg/2000 kcal, and marginally adequate in copper, 1.6 mg/2000 kcal, throughout the study. In the second experiment (33,34), the diet provided only 1.7 mg copper/2000 kcal for the first 32 days; from day 33 onward, the diet was supplemented to contain 2.4 mg of copper/2000 kcal. Also at the intake of 2000 kcal, the diet provided 300 mg of magnesium. Thus, the major differences between the two experiments were the intakes of copper and magnesium; in one experiment they were marginal or inadequate, in the other they were adequate. Among the effects of boron supplementation in these experiments after 63 days of boron depletion were the following: (a) an effect on macromineral and electrolyte metabolism evidenced by increased serum 25-hydroxycholecalciferol (32,34), decreased serum calcitonin (with low dietary magnesium and copper) (32), and increased serum magnesium (with adequate magnesium and copper) (37); (b) an effect on energy substrate metabolism suggested by decreased serum glucose (with low dietary magnesium and copper) (31) and increased serum triglycerides

TABLE 1 Examples of Boron Effects in Humans[a]

Dietary boron (mg/day)	Serum 25-OH-cholecalciferol[b] (ng/ml)	Urinary-OH proline[c] (mmol/day)	Erythrocyte superoxide dismutase[d] (units/g Hb)	Platelets[e] (10^9/L)	Serum 17β-estradiol[b] (pg/mL)
Men over the age of 45 ($n = 4$)					
0.25	18	0.0418	3091	280	20
3.25	26	0.0470	3231	256	17
p value	0.34	0.36	0.79	0.008	0.12
Postmenopausal women ($n = 4$)					
0.25	18	0.0546	2666	312	11
3.25	20	0.0706	3169	278	11
p value	0.75	0.06	0.04	0.007	0.86
Postmenopausal women on estrogen therapy ($n = 5$)					
0.25	18	0.0520	2520	297	99
3.25	30	0.0609	3327	268	157
p value	0.06	0.05	0.03	0.007	0.02
Above combined plus one premenopausal woman ($n = 14$)					
0.25	18	0.0495	2735[f]	297	48[f]
3.25	25	0.0601	3243[f]	269	69[f]
p value	0.04	0.001	0.04	0.0001	0.06

[a]After an equilibration period of 14 days when dietary boron was about 3.25 mg/day, there was a depletion period of 63 days when dietary boron was 0.25 mg/2000 kcal followed by a repletion period of 49 days when the basal diet was supplemented with 3 mg boron/day as sodium borate. Dietary magnesium and copper were adequate, 300 mg and 2.4 mg/2000 kcal, respectively.
[b]From Ref. 34.
[c]From Ref. 37.
[d]From Ref. 35.
[e]From Ref. 33.
[f]Values do not include the premenopausal woman.

(with adequate dietary magnesium and copper) (34); (c) an effect on nitrogen metabolism indicated by decreased blood urea nitrogen (31,33), serum creatinine (31,34), and urinary urea excretion (37) and increased urinary hydroxyproline excretion (35); (d) an effect on oxidative metabolism indicated by increased erythrocyte superoxide dismutase (31,35) and serum ceruloplasmin (31,35); and (e) an effect on erythropoiesis and hematopoiesis suggested by (all with adequate dietary magnesium and copper) increased blood hemoglobin and mean corpuscular hemoglobin content, but decreased hematocrit, platelet number, and red blood cell number (33). Boron supplementation after depletion also enhanced the elevation in serum 17β-estradiol and plasma copper caused by estrogen ingestion (34), altered electroencephalograms such that they suggested improved behavioral activation (e.g., less drowsiness) and mental alertness (36,37), and improved psychomotor skills and the cognitive processes of attention and memory (36,37). Some examples of the nature of the changes caused by dietary boron are shown in Table 1.

VI. BIOCHEMICAL FUNCTION OF BORON

A biochemical function for boron has not been elucidated, even for plants, for which boron has been known to be essential for 70 years, and where its deficiency also has a multiplicity of effects (39). At least 15 hypotheses have been advanced as to the specific essential function of boron in plants (39,40). These hypotheses have boron involved in sugar transport, cell wall synthesis and lignification, cell wall structure, carbohydrate metabolism, RNA metabolism, respiration, indole acetic acid metabolism, phenol metabolism, membrane function, and DNA synthesis. The hypotheses receiving the most attention at present are those that have boron with a function with a cascade effect; that is, in cell wall structure or in membrane function. The evidence that boron is involved in lignin biosynthesis and cell wall cross-linking, including the finding that plants grown on sufficient boron media bend easily while plants grown on low-boron media are brittle, has been reviewed (39). The hypothesis that is of more interest here, because the role may be similar to that in the animal kingdom, is that of boron having a regulatory role involving plant hormones such as auxin, gibberellic acid, and cytokinin, and the control of a second messenger such as calcium at the cell membrane level (41). This hypothesis is supported by findings that boron influences membrane potential and proton movement through membranes of plant cells (42). Suggestions for the nature of the role of boron in plant membranes include an influence on cell lipid biosynthesis (43), the bridging of lipids via hydroxyl groups similar to structure 3 in Figure 1 (43), and the formation of complexes similar to structure IV in Figure 1 with messenger molecules containing inositol (42). Neither boron–lipid nor boron–inositol complexes have been isolated from plant membranes.

Another hypothesis is that boron is involved in ascorbate metabolism in the plant plasmalemma (43). Plasmalemma NADH oxidase is stimulated by boron (44). The role of NADH oxidase in plant metabolism is unknown, but it has been speculated to be involved in the reduction of ascorbate-free radical (AFR) to ascorbate, and thus has been referred to as AFR reductase (43). Perhaps the basis for a boron effect on this reaction is that boron forms a complex with dehydroascorbate but not with ascorbate (9). Through an effect on ascorbate metabolism, boron possibly affects cell wall formation by influencing proline hydroxylation, or membrane transport through influencing redox reactions. Evidence that boron affects ascorbate metabolism includes the finding that ascorbate supplementation restores growth of the squash root meristem retarded by boron deprivation (43).

Two hypotheses recently have been advanced for the biochemical function of boron in higher animals which also accommodate a large and varied response to boron deprivation and the known biochemistry of boron. Hunt (11) has proposed that boron is a metabolic regulator through complexing with a variety of substrate or reactant compounds in which there are hydroxyl groups in favorable positions. Based on the knowledge that two classes of enzymes are competitively inhibited in vitro by borate or its derivatives, and on his findings that show dietary boron can alter the in-vivo activity of a number of these enzymes, Hunt has hypothesized that the metabolic regulation by boron is mainly negative; that is, boron controls a number of metabolic pathways by competitively inhibiting some key enzyme reactions. Nielsen (45) has hypothesized that boron has a role in cell membrane function or stability such that it influences the response to hormone action, transmembrane signaling, or transmembrane movement of regulatory cations or anions. This hypothesis is supported by the recent finding that boron influences the transport of extracellular calcium into rat platelets activated by thrombin (46). This hypothesis is based on the concept that boron reacts with hydroxyl groups of phosphoinositides and glycolipids of membranes. It also could be based on the hypothesis put forward for plants; that is, boron influences redox reactions involved in membrane transport. Evidence that boron influences redox reactions in higher animals includes findings that dietary boron affects urinary hydroxyproline and erythrocyte superoxide dismutase concentrations in humans (see Table 1).

VII. ASSESSMENT OF BORON STATUS

The lack, until recently, of good analytical techniques for boron, the lack of radioisotopes to study boron metabolism, the lack of a known biochemical function, and the recency of the suggestion that boron is of nutritional importance have contributed to the lack of established indices of inadequate boron status. Also, because boron is not a particularly toxic element, indices for chronic excessive boron intake are not well defined. Elevated blood boron and urinary excretion of boron may be indicators of acute and possibly chronic excessive intake of boron (47).

VIII. PHARMACOLOGY AND TOXICOLOGY OF BORON

Simple borates were used as mild antiseptics in the past, but relatively high concentrations were required to be effective. Borates act more as a bacteriostat, not as a bacteriocide; thus, they are not effective enough for most modern medical applications and have been replaced by superior alternatives. Recently, however, a number of amine-carboxyborane derivatives have been synthesized that show promising beneficial pharmacologic properties (48). Animal studies show these compounds, which apparently need to contain boron for activity, have hypolipidemic, antiobesity, antiinflammatory, antiosteoporotic, and antineoplastic actions (48). It has been suggested that these boron compounds act by affecting the interleukins, leukotrienes, and other chemical mediators.

Boron has a low order of toxicity when administered orally. Toxicity signs in animals generally occur only after dietary boron exceeds 100 μg/g. When boron was 150 mg/L in drinking water, rats exhibited depressed growth, lack of incisor pigmentation, aspermia, and impaired ovarian development (49). When boron was 300 mg/L in drinking water, rats exhibited depressed plasma triglycerides, protein, and alkaline phosphatase, and depressed bone fat and calcium (50). Pigs fed 8 mg boron/kg body weight per day exhibited an osteoporosis associated with a reduction in parathyroid activity (51).

In humans, the signs of acute toxicity include nausea, vomiting, diarrhea, dermatitis, and lethargy (52). In addition, high boron induces riboflavinuria (53). The signs of chronic boron toxicity through dietary intake have not been clearly defined. As mentioned previously, Wiley (1) found that humans consuming over 500 mg of boric acid per day for 50 days displayed disturbed appetite, digestion, and health. Two infants who had their pacifiers dipped into a preparation of borax and honey for a period of several weeks exhibited scanty hair, patchy dry erythema, anemia, and seizure disorders (54). The seizures stopped and the other abnormalities were alleviated when the use of the borax-and-honey preparation was discontinued.

IX. FUTURE RESEARCH NEEDS

Knowledge about boron nutrition, biochemistry, and metabolism is very limited; thus, future research needs are immense. However, the primary research need is the elucidation of a biochemical function for boron. A defined function would facilitate research in other areas such as the determination of boron status indicators and whether boron is of importance in some clinical situations. Realistically, unless a function is found for boron, it is unlikely that this element will be generally accepted as being an essential nutrient requiring a recommended dietary intake.

However, findings to date show that boron is a dynamic trace element which, in physiologic amounts, can affect the metabolism or utilization of numerous substances involved in life processes, including calcium, magnesium, nitrogen, glucose, triglycerides, oxygen, and estrogens. Through these effects, boron can affect the function or composition of several body systems, including blood, brain, and skeleton generally in a beneficial fashion. Thus, even though boron has not been established as essential, its beneficial actions suggest that an intake of over 1 mg/day (but probably not over 10 mg/day) is desirable; diets low in fruits, vegetables, legumes, and nuts may not supply this amount of boron. Thus, boron may be of more practical nutritional importance than is currently acknowledged.

REFERENCES

1. Wiley HW. Influence of Food Preservatives and Artificial Colors on Digestion and Health. I. Boric Acid and Borax. Washington, DC: U.S. Department of Agriculture Bull. No. 84, Pt. 1, 1904: 477 pp.
2. Warington K. The effect of boric acid and borax on the broad bean and certain other plants. Ann Bot 1923; 37:629–672.
3. Hove E, Elvehjem CA, Hart EB. Boron in animal nutrition. Am J Physiol 1939; 127:689–701.
4. Orent-Keiles E. The role of boron in the diet of the rat. Proc Soc Exp Biol Med 1941; 44:199–202.
5. Teresi JD, Hove E, Elvehjem CA, Hart EB. Further study of boron in the nutrition of rats. Am J Physiol 1944; 140:513–518.
6. Skinner JT, McHargue JS. Response of rats to boron supplements when fed rations low in potassium. Am J Physiol 1945; 143:385–390.
7. Follis RH Jr. The effect of adding boron to a potassium-deficient diet in the rat. Am J Physiol 1947; 150:520–522.
8. Hunt CD, Nielsen FH. Interaction between boron and cholecalciferol in the chick. In: Howell JMcC, Gawthorne JM, White CL, eds. Trace Element Metabolism in Man and Animals (TEMA-4). Canberra: Australian Academy of Science, 1981: 597–600.
9. Zittle CA. Reaction of borate with substances of biological interest. In: Nord FF, ed. Advances in Enzymology and Related Subjects of Biochemistry. New York: Interscience, 1951; XII: 493–527.
10. Hunt CD. Boron. In: Macrae R, Robinson RK, Sadler MJ, eds. Encyclopaedia of Food Science, Food Technology and Nutrition. Vol. 1. London: Academic Press, 1993: 440–447.
11. Hunt CD. The biochemical effects of physiologic amounts of dietary boron in animal nutrition models. Environ Health Perspect 1994; 102 (Suppl 7):35–43.
12. Woods WG. An introduction to boron—history, sources, uses and chemistry. Environ Health Perspect 1994; 102 (Suppl 7):5–11.
13. Lindquist R, Terry C. Inhibition of subtilisin by boronic acids, potential analogs of tetrahedral reaction intermediates. Arch Biochem Biophys 1974; 160:135–144.
14. Chen TSS, Chang C-J, Floss HG. Biosynthesis of the boron-containing antibiotic aplasmomycin. Nuclear magnetic resonance analysis of aplasmomycin and desboraplasmomycin. J Antibioticus 1980; 33:1316–1322.
15. Dunitz JD, Hawley DM, Miklos D, et al. Structure of boromycin. Helv Chim Acta 1971; 54: 1709–1713.
16. Hunt CD, Shuler TR. Open-vessel, wet-ash, low-temperature digestion of biological materials for inductively coupled argon plasma spectroscopy (ICAP) analysis of boron and other elements. J Micronutr Anal 1989; 6:161–174.

17. Ferrando AA, Green NR, Barnes KW, Woodward B. Microwave digestion preparation and ICP determination of boron in human plasma. Biol Trace Elem Res 1993; 37:17–25.

18. Clarke WB, Koekebakker M, Barr RD, Downing RG, Fleming RF. Analysis of ultratrace lithium and boron by neutron activation and mass spectrometric measurement of ^{3}He and ^{4}He. Appl Radiat Isot 1987; 38:735–743.

19. Vanderpool RA, Hoff D, Johnson PE. Use of inductively coupled plasma mass spectrometry in boron-10 stable isotope experiments with plants, rats and humans. Environ Health Perspect 1994; 102 (Suppl 7):13–20.

20. Iyengar GV, Clarke WB, Downing RG. Determination of boron and lithium in diverse biological matrices using neutron activation-mass spectrometry (NA-MS). Fresenius J Anal Chem 1990; 338:562–566.

21. Havercroft JM, Ward NI. Boron and other elements in relation to rheumatoid arthritis. In: Momčilović B, ed. Trace Elements in Man and Animals 7. Zagreb: IMI 1991:8.2–8.3

22. Hamilton EI, Minski MS, Cleary JJ. The concentration and distribution of some stable elements in healthy human tissues from the United Kingdom. An environmental study. Sci Total Environ 1972/73; 1:341–374.

23. Ward NI. The determination of boron in biological materials by neutron irradiation and prompt gamma-ray spectrometry. J Radioanalyt Nuclear Chem 1987; 110:633–639.

24. Shuler TR, Pootrakul P, Yarnsukon P, Nielsen FH. Effect of thalassemia/hemoglobin E disease on macro, trace, and ultratrace element concentrations in humans tissues. J Trace Elem Exp Med 1990; 3:31–43.

25. Abou-Shakra FR, Havercroft JM, Ward NI. Lithium and boron in biological tissues and fluids. Trace Elem Med 1989; 6:142–146.

26. Corrigan FM, Reynolds GP, Ward NI. Multi-element analysis of the frontal cortex, temporal cortex and basal ganglia in schizophrenia. Trace Elem Med 1990; 7:1–7.

27. Hunt CD. Dietary boron modified the effects of magnesium and molybdenum on mineral metabolism in the cholecalciferol-deficient chick. Biol Trace Elem Res 1989; 22:201–220.

28. Nielsen FH. The saga of boron in food: From a banished food preservative to a beneficial nutrient for humans. Curr Top Plant Biochem Physiol 1991; 10:274–286.

29. Penland JG. Dietary boron affects brain function in mature Long-Evans rats. Proc ND Acad Sci 1990; 44:78.

30. Hegsted M, Keenan MJ, Siver F, Wozniak P. Effect of boron on vitamin D deficient rats. Biol Trace Elem Res 1991; 26:243–255.

31. Nielsen FH. Dietary boron affects variables associated with copper metabolism in humans. In: Anke M, Baumann W, Bräunlich H, Brückner C, Groppel B, Grün M, eds. 6th Int. Trace Element Symp. 1989. Vol. 4. Jena: Friedrich-Schiller-Universitat, 1989: 1106–1111.

32. Nielsen FH, Mullen LM, Gallagher SK. Effect of boron depletion and repletion on blood indicators of calcium status in humans fed a magnesium-low diet. J Trace Elem Exp Med 1990; 3:45–54.

33. Nielsen FH, Mullen LM, Nielsen EJ. Dietary boron affects blood cell counts and hemoglobin concentrations in humans. J Trace Elem Exp Med 1991; 4:211–223.

34. Nielsen FH, Gallagher SK, Johnson LK, Nielsen EJ. Boron enhances and mimics some effects of estrogen therapy in postmenopausal women. J Trace Elem Exp Med 1992; 5:237–246.

35. Nielsen FH. Biochemical and physiological consequences of boron deprivation in humans. Environ Health Perspect 1994; 102 (Suppl 7):59–63.

36. Penland JG. Dietary boron, brain function and cognitive performance. Environ Health Perspect 1994; 102 (Suppl 7):65–72.

37. Nielsen FH, Penland JG. Clinical and biochemical consequences of boron deprivation in humans. In: Abdulla M, Vohora SB, Athar M, eds. Trace and Toxic Elements in Food. New Delhi: Jamia Hamdard & Wiley Eastern, 1995:361–374.

38. Nielsen FH. The ultratrace elements. In: Smith KT, ed. Trace Minerals in Foods. New York: Marcel Dekker, 1988: 357–428.

39. Loomis WD, Durst RW. Boron and cell walls. Curr Top Plant Biochem Physiol 1991; 10: 149–178.
40. Gauch HG, Duggar WM Jr. The physiological action of boron in higher plants: A review and interpretation. Bulletin A-80 (Technical). College Park, MD: Agric. Exp. Stat. 1954: 43 pp.
41. Parr AJ, Loughman PC. Boron and membrane function in plants. Annu Proc Phytochem Soc Eur 1983; 21:87–107.
42. Blaser-Grill J, Knoppik D, Amberger A, Goldbach H. Influence of boron on the membrane potential in *Elodea densa* and *Helianthus annuus* roots and H^+ extrusion of suspension cultured *Daucus carota* cells. Plant Physiol 1990; 90:280–284.
43. Blevins DG, Lukaszewski KM. Proposed physiologic functions of boron in plants pertinent to animal and human metabolism. Environ Health Perspect 1994; 102 (Suppl 7):31–33.
44. Barr R, Crane FL. Boron stimulated NADH oxidase of plasma membranes. Curr Top Plant Biochem Physiol 1991; 10:290.
45. Nielsen FH. Nutritional requirements for boron, silicon, vanadium, nickel and arsenic: current knowledge and speculation. FASEB J 1991; 5:2661–2667.
46. Nielsen FH, Poellot RA. Changes in resting and activated platelet $[Ca^{2+}]_i$ in response to boron deprivation. FASEB J 1993; 7:A204.
47. Weeth JH, Speth CF, Hanks DR. Boron content of plasma and urine as indicators of boron intake in cattle. Am J Vet Res 1981; 42:474–477.
48. Hall IH, Chen SY, Rajendran KG, Kottakkatta G, Sood A, Spielvogel BF, Shih J. Hypo-lipidemic, anti-obesity, anti-inflammatory, anti-osteoporotic, and anti-neoplastic properties of amine carboxyboranes. Environ Health Perspect 1994: 102 (Suppl 7):21–30.
49. Green GH, Lott MD, Weeth HJ. Effects of boron-water on rats. Proc West Sec Am Soc Anim Sci 1973; 24:254–258.
50. Seal BS, Weeth HJ. Effect of boron in drinking water on the male laboratory rat. Bull Environ Contam Toxicol 1980; 25:782–789.
51. Franke J, Runge H, Bech R, et al. Boron as an antidote to fluorosis? Part 1. Studies on the skeletal system. Fluoride 1985; 18:187–197.
52. Linden CH, Hall AH, Kulig KW, Rumack BH. Acute ingestions of boric acid. Clin Toxicol 1986; 24:269–279.
53. Pinto J, Huang YP, McConnell RJ, Rivlin RS. Increased urinary riboflavin excretion resulting from boric acid ingestion. J Lab Clin Med 1978; 92:126–134.
54. Gordon AS, Prichard JS, Freedman MH. Seizure disorders and anemia associated with chronic borax intoxication. Can Med Assoc J 1973; 108:719–721.

16

Lithium

MANFRED ANKE, W. ARNHOLD, M. MÜLLER, H. ILLING, U. SCHÄFER, AND M. JARITZ
Friedrich Schiller University, Jena, Germany

I. INTRODUCTION

The discovery of lithium in 1817 took place at a time when only 49 chemical elements were known and half a century before the Periodic System came into being. The lightest of all elements, silvery lithium, was discovered in the laboratories of the famous Swedish scientist Berzelius (1). Other scientists tried very early to use lithium in medicine and agriculture. Since lithium urate is the most soluble urate compound (2), lithium salts were used for the treatment of gout in 1850. Due to unpleasant side effects, this method disappeared in the course of time (3). Almost 100 years passed before lithium again played a role in medicine and the science of nutrition. Lithium chloride was used as a substitute for cooking salt in the United States at the end of the 1940s, until the U.S. Food and Drug Administration prohibited its use after four deaths (4) and the occurrence of heart and kidney disorders. At about the same time, Cade (5) used lithium urate to test the effect of uric acid on the toxicity of urea in animals. Lithium injected into guinea pigs made them lethargic and less susceptible to stimuli. Cade then tested the effect of orally administered lithium preparations in patients with mental diseases and observed improvements in manic-depressed patients. In spite of side effects (6,7), lithium therapy was introduced as an effective treatment for acute psychic states of agitation (8–12) when coupled with careful monitoring of the lithium blood level. Experience with lithium therapy of endogenous depression and mania soon showed that the therapeutic range of lithium compounds is very small (13).

Investigations into the possible essentiality of lithium for fauna started with rats and goats in 1976, and the results support the concept of essentiality (14,15). Lithium-dependent enzymes, proteins, hormones, or other essential functions of lithium are not known.

II. PHYSICAL AND CHEMICAL PROPERTIES

Lithium with an atomic weight of 6.94 consists of the two natural isotopes, ^7Li (92.5%) and ^6Li (7.5%). There are also radioactive isotopes ($^5Li–^{11}Li$) with half-life periods of between 8.5 ms and 0.85 s, periods too short to be useful in biological research and medicine (16). However, the enriched stable isotopes ^6Li and ^7Li have been used as tracers (17,18). Lithium is the least reactive of the alkali metals, resembling calcium and magnesium more than sodium. The atomic and ionic radii of lithium and magnesium are similar. For these reasons, lithium may interact with magnesium and calcium in physiologic processes that depend on the latter ions (19).

III. DISTRIBUTION IN THE ENVIRONMENT

On average, 50–65 mg/kg lithium are found in the upper layer of the earth's 16-km-thick crust. Thus, it occupies the 27th position in abundance of the elements. Lithium is concentrated in acid igneous rocks and sedimentary aluminosilicates. Lithium concentration varies from 1.3 ppm in light organic soils to 56 ppm in calcareous soils. Lower lithium concentrations are reported for light sandy soils, especially for those derived from glacial drift in a humid climate (20). As a rule, the water from all acid soils is lithium-poor and has a mean lithium content of < 15 µg/L, whereas > 25 µg/L are found in the water of slightly acid and neutral sites (7). The water from lowland moors has the highest lithium content. The drinking water in Germany has a mean lithium content of 10µg/L. Even more striking variations of the lithium content of the water (1–2500 µg Li/L) have been described (6).

  Since the soluble lithium in soils is readily absorbed by plants, the lithium content of plants is a good indicator of the available lithium status of the soil (21). There are considerable differences in the tolerance of various plant species to lithium concentrations as well as in their ability to absorb them. Solanaceae are able to store very high amounts of lithium. Some plants of this family accumulate > 1000 ppm Li (22). However, lithium is not an essential plant nutrient (20).

IV. METABOLISM

A. Tissue Distribution

The organs of children store more lithium than those of adults (23). The lithium variation in human organs due to age and sex is accentuated in babies and young children. This age dependence of the lithium concentration disappears in the kidneys at age 10, whereas it had vanished in liver and ribs by age 5. The normal lithium content of the serum varies between 7 and 21 µg/L. Values of 1 to 7 µg/L have been reported (24). The lithium content of the organs of several animals is species- and site-specific (25). The distribution of lithium among rat tissues is shown by the data in Table 1 (26). It is notable that bone has the highest concentration of lithium and that it loses most of its lithium when lithium consumption is restricted. It is also of interest that pituitary and thyroid are high in lithium.

B. Absorption

A number of studies on the mucosal mechanisms of lithium absorption in the gastrointestinal tract have shown that lithium transfer across the tract occurs, not by passage through the cell, but by paracellular transport via the tight junctions and pericellular spaces (19). The

TABLE 1 Lithium Concentration in Tissues of Rats Fed Low and Adequate Levels of Lithium and a Normal Sodium Level[a]

Tissue	Adequate Li	Low Li
	ng/g dry tissue	
Adrenal	20 ± 9.9 (14)	8.2 ± 5.1 (10)
Blood, whole	35 ± 12 (12)	0.9 ± 0.6 (8)
Blood, serum	67 ± 26 (8)	2.3 ± 2.1 (8)
Bone (tibia)	304 ± 33 (12)	<7
Cerebellum	20 ± 6.0 (14)	2.8 ± 2.0 (12)
Cerebrum	26 ± 8.2 (14)	2.0 ± 1.1 (11)
Heart	25 ± 8.1 (13)	2.3 ± 1.6 (11)
Hippocampus	26 ± 8.3 (12)	4.8 ± 4.2 (12)
Hypothalamus	21 ± 5.0 (11)	5.6 ± 5.9 (9)
Liver	12 ± 5.3 (13)	1.6 ± 1.2 (9)
Pancreas	6.4 ± 1.5 (14)	1.8 ± 1.2 (12)
Pituitary	44 ± 19 (13)	14 ± 10 (8)
Thyroid	66 ± 20 (14)	8.1 ± 5.6 (6)

[a] Data from Ref. 26 showing means ± SD. The low-lithium diet contained 0.6 ng/g and the adequate-lithium diet, 500 ng/g.

absorption of a single oral dose occurs within an 8-h period with the appearance of peak serum levels within 2–4 h after dosing (first phase). The balance is excreted over a period of 10 to 14 days (second phase). The half-life of the first phase is approximately 7 h, and that of the second phase about 14–20 h. Potassium, sodium, and calcium can have an effect on lithium utilization and influence the toxicity of high Li intake (27). Lithium absorption into red blood cells and fibroblasts, and lithium-induced leukocytosis and transport mechanisms, are comprehensively described by Gallicchio (28,29).

C. Transport

Lithium transport in the body is carried out via blood, and it is distributed to all tissues. Blood lithium concentration best reflected the lithium status in goats that consumed lithium-poor rations; hair and milk were also good indicators of lithium consumption, whereas cardiac muscle, pancreas, skeleton muscles, and brain did not reflect the lithium status significantly (7,30,31).

D. Excretion

Lithium is excreted mainly renally in animals and humans, and the excretion depends on the sodium and potassium intake. Young rats (5 days old) excrete 50% of the lithium renally and 50% fecally. At the age of 15 and 105 days, respectively, the rats excreted 80% and 90% renally. In young and adult rats, only one-fifth of the lithium found in the feces reaches the intestine via bile. It is supposed that the main part of lithium reaches the feces through the intestinal wall (32–38). The renal lithium excretion of men and women varied between 19 and 700 μg/day (39).

V. PHYSIOLOGIC FUNCTION

The essentiality of lithium in goats has been investigated by two different research teams, one in Germany and one in Hungary, with 15 repetitive experiments over a 15-year period (6,7,14,40–43). Work with rats has been done in the United States (15,44–46) and Japan (47). Bach (48) summarized the results with the comment: "There are animal studies which support lithium's role as a sine qua non for physical health in the case of goats and rats." The influence of a lithium-poor ration on the reproductive and growth performance of goats is summarized in Table 2. The kids of lithium-deficient dams had a 9% lower birth weight than those of controls (49), the difference amounting to 15% by the end of the suckling period, 91 days. The lithium intake of kids is essentially determined by the lithium content of the milk, and the lithium-deficient kids received only one-third as much lithium (49). During the following 168 experimental days, the effect of lithium on growth was insignificant (49).

The consumption of lithium-poor rations by female goats did not have an effect on the intensity of estrus behavior. However, the first mating resulted in a significantly lower rate of conception in these animals. The conception rate with repeated services at the following ovulations was improved, but the difference between the groups remained significant. There was also a higher abortion rate among the lithium-deficient goats. The effect of lithium deficiency on the sex ratio was most surprising (Table 2). As a rule, hornless goats give birth to more male than female kids. Lithium-deficient goats, however, gave birth to significantly more female kids.

Long-term lithium-deficiency experiments with female goats allowed the analysis of the influence of the lithium-poor nutrition on life expectancy. The data showed that 41% of the lithium-deficient goats and 7% of the control animals died during the 2-year experiment. The oldest Li-deficient goats suffered from a disturbed hematopoiesis. Gallicchio et al. (50) have described the influence of high lithium intake on hematopoiesis.

Lithium deficiency did not affect the biochemical blood profile, but it lowered the serum lithium concentration and the activity of several serum enzymes, mainly those concerned with the citrate cycle (ICDH, MDH), with glycolysis (ALD), and with nitrogen metabolism (GLDH). There were significant differences in enzyme activities between control and lithium-deficient goats. Only creatine kinase, a stress indicator enzyme, was

TABLE 2   Effects of Lithium-Poor Diets on Goat Performance (7,51)

Parameter	Control animals	Deficiency animals	Percent of control	p value
Live weight, 1st day, kg	2.86	2.60	91	<0.01
Live weight, 91st day, kg	17.4	14.8	85	<0.001
Success of 1st insemination, %	77	51	—	<0.001
Conception rate, %	86	74	—	<0.05
Abortion rate, %	1	14	—	<0.001
Matings per gravidity	1.3	2.0	—	<0.001
Male:female ratio	1.6	0.70	—	<0.001
Mortality 1st and 2nd year, %	7	41	—	<0.001
Creatine kinase, U/L	20.1	35.1	175	<0.05
ICDH, U/L	4.0	1.4	35	<0.05
MAO, liver, mmol/mg/h	36	26	72	<0.01

significantly increased in lithium-deficient goats. Owing to the particular role of mono-amine oxidase (MAO) in manic-depressive disease, chronic schizophrenia, and unipolar depression, this enzyme was also investigated in the liver of control and lithium-deficient goats. The MAO activity in the hepatic tissue of the latter group was reduced by 28%. These findings are in good agreement with the results obtained in rats. Ono et al. (47) found behavioral disturbances in animals with lithium-poor rations, which disappeared after lithium supplementation. The biochemical effect of lithium on the behavior of rats needs further clarification (52).

There is good agreement with regard to the effects of lithium-poor nutrition on reproduction and survival in rats and goats. In his first study, Pickett (15,46) found that the first generation of rats fed a low-lithium diet had a 2-week longer period for conception than controls fed a diet with added lithium. Overall, fertility was impaired in second- and third-generation dams, but the growth rate of the offspring was not impaired. In a subsequent study (26), low lithium intake decreased litter size and litter weight of rats in the third-generation dams when the dietary sodium was maintained at the usual level, 1160 mg/kg diet. Additional sodium (4660 mg/kg) aggravated the effect of low lithium on reproductive performance.

VI. LITHIUM IN HUMAN FOODS

The lithium contents of foods consumed in Germany are presented in Table 3. As shown by the high standard deviation of the mean values, the lithium content of foodstuffs and beverages varies extraordinarily. Sugar- and starch-rich cereals, pasta, bread, cakes, and pastries generally contain little lithium unless they are supplemented with spices, milk, or eggs. The lithium content of several vegetables, e.g., tomatoes, mushrooms, cucumbers, and the cabbage family, is relatively high. Apples and bananas supply relatively little lithium.

Compared to plant foodstuffs, foods derived from animals are generally lithium-rich. Beef, pork, mutton, and milk contain > 3000 µg/kg lithium, the concentrations increase in the same order. The lithium of milk is lost via whey in the making of cheese so that cheese contains < 3000 µg/kg, as do fish and poultry. Eggs and milk supply the highest concentration of lithium to humans, > 7000 µg/kg dry matter.

Weiner (24) estimated human lithium intake at 660 in the case of a low, and at 3420 µg/day in the case of a rich lithium diet. This estimate is too high for Central Europe. The lithium intake of adults in Germany before (1988) and after (1991) reunification was investigated using 10 test populations—each consisting of seven men and women—on 7 subsequent days (53). The two sexes consumed about the same groups of foodstuffs and beverages, and there was no sex preference for a particularly lithium-rich group of foodstuffs. The lithium intake was influenced by the dry-matter intake of the individual person, and the latter may reflect local influences. Since men consume 25% more dry matter, they take in more lithium than women. On the average, the lithium consumption of the women and men in the test populations varied between 371 and 990 µg Li/day. Of the 70 test women, 40% consumed 375 µg/day based on the weekly average. The daily lithium consumption of both sexes showed that women and men consumed only 125 µg Li on 35–40% of the days studied. The extreme variation was caused in part by the drinking water and beverages consumed.

The lithium content of the dry matter consumed doubled after the reunification of Germany, and this led to the approximate doubling of lithium intake, as shown in Table 4.

TABLE 3 Lithium Content of Selected Foodstuffs (μg/kg dry matter) and Beverages (μg/L) (53)

Variety	$\bar{x}$	s	Variety	$\bar{x}$	s
Cereals, pasta			Vegetables, fruit		
Sugar (15)	199	197	Bananas (6)	383	180
Honey (15)	527	351	Apples (15)	1449	1176
Semolina (15)	538	458	Potatoes (15)	1592	1262
Noodles (15)	628	611	White cabbage (15)	1874	870
Vanilla pudding (15)	639	592	Asparagus ((6)	2217	1224
Lentils (6)	748	771	Kohlrabi (15)	2966	2160
Wheat flour (15)	905	817	Cauliflower (6)	3462	2165
Pearl barley (6)	995	753	Red cabbage (15)	3579	2447
Rice (6)	1260	1392	Cucumbers (15)	5017	2685
Oat flakes (15)	1391	880	Mixed mushrooms (6)	5788	4687
Ready-to-serve soups (15)	2513	2141	Tomatoes (15)	6707	4185
Luxury food, spices			Animal foodstuffs		
Milk chocolate (15)	372	217	Butter (15)	1070	1079
Coffee (15)	874	716	Herring fillet (15)	1734	1192
Cinnamon (15)	1046	658	Soft cheese (15)	2276	1640
Cocoa (15)	1728	2419	Poultry meat (15)	2379	2272
Cooking salt (6)	1748	607	Beef (15)	3428	3682
Marjoram (15)	2289	999	Pork (15)	3844	2279
Paprika, highly seasoned (15)	2316	515	Eggs (15)	7373	6500
Black tea (6)	3737	2639	Milk (15)	7533	8510
Bread and confectionery			Beverages (μg/L)		
Rolls (5)	317	168	Brandy (6)	85	87
Wheat and rye bread (15)	474	294	Coca Cola (6)	122	90
Crispbread (15)	517	557	Pilsner (6)	296	149
Toasted bread (15)	819	949	White wine (6)	305	125
Rusk (15)	935	1226	Red wine (6)	329	285

The question arises as to why the lithium content doubled after reunification. It appears that local foodstuff production and consumption had a significant effect on lithium intake. This might be due to the diluvial and alluvial soil formations dominating in East Germany, which deliver less lithium than other weathering soils. There may also have been a change in the type of foods consumed.

TABLE 4 Lithium Intake of Adults Depending on Sex and Time of Testing (μg/day) (54)

Year (n)	Women		Men		Fp	%
	s	$\bar{x}$	$\bar{x}$	s		
1988 (392)	446	371	417	434	<0.01	112
1991 (588)	732	706	990	1065		140
Fp		<0.001			—	
%		190		237		

VII. TOXICITY OF LITHIUM

The effects of high lithium intake have been systematically investigated in pigs, chickens, cattle, sheep, and rats (55–59). It was demonstrated that lithium supplements of > 100 mg/kg ration dry matter reduced feed consumption in all experiments. This was particularly true for growing animals, including calves, pigs, and chickens. Growing broilers were highly sensitive, and pigs responded to this lithium supplementation with an 8% lower feed consumption (55). High lithium consumption by pigs reduced the feed intake drastically, and induced a thirst response that led to an enormous water consumption.

As a consequence of high lithium intake, the physiologic performance was impaired; e.g., broilers with a supplement of 100 mg Li/kg ration gained 13% less weight than the corresponding control animals, and hens exposed to the same amount of lithium laid 14% fewer eggs. Furthermore, the eggs laid by hens with 100- or 150-mg Li/kg rations were lighter than those of control animals (57). On average, fattening bulls fed 100 mg Li/kg dry matter gained 18% less weight than corresponding control bulls. The aggressivity and sexual activity of the bulls were significantly decreased by high lithium intake (55). These advantages of high lithium could not compensate for the negative effects on growth and adipose deposition. In pigs, supplementation of 500 mg Li/kg dry matter led to a drastic reduction of daily weight gain and to an enormous water consumption. All pigs with 1000-mg Li/kg ration dry matter died within 92 days. One of the six animals with 500-mg Li/kg ration died during the same period (55). These findings are important in the consideration of lithium therapy for patients with manic depressions insofar as they illustrate the necessity of minimizing the dose.

This statement is supported by the considerable deviations from normal values of serum enzymes and the blood sodium status of lithium-treated pigs (60,61). Lithium selectively interferes with the phosphoinositide cycle, and this is the basis for the proposed unifying hypothesis for lithium's biochemical effects. Administration of lithium to rats resulted in a reduction of brain myoinositol and an increase in the reaction substrate, inositol-1-phosphate. Lithium reduces the cell concentration of myoinositol, which would otherwise be converted to phosphatidylinositol, and this reduction attenuates the response to external stimuli (19,62).

The enzymatic measurement of the GABA (gamma-aminobutyric acid) cycle after chronic lithium treatment shows a marked inhibition of GABA-transaminase activity, but there was no effect on the succinate semialdehyde dehydrogenase and glutamate dehydrogenase behavior. This may mean that GABA accumulates in the brain during chronic lithium treatment and is responsible for the tranquilizing effect. The MAOB isoenzyme is also involved in behavioral effects (63).

The major clinical application of lithium therapy is in the prevention of the major changes in mood which are characteristic of affective disorders. In mania the patient exhibits excitement, high activity, talkativeness, aggression, flights of ideas, speed of thought, grandiosity, eloquence, humor, and overindulgence of many kinds. In depressions the converse is true, with low self-esteem, suicidal thoughts, inactivity, indecisiveness, inability to formulate action plans or ideas, and general inertia (19). Clinical control of bipolar disease is achieved by the administration of lithium carbonate at doses of 900–1500 mg/day or 169–282 mg Li/day. The requirement for the therapeutic effectiveness of lithium necessitates an elevation of the normal serum lithium level of 2–20 μg/L to a level of from 2,180 to 55,550 μg/L (0.4 to 0.8 in Eq/L) serum. The 12-h serum lithium level serves as an accurate method for evaluating therapeutic effectiveness and monitoring toxic responses.

Higher lithium levels in the blood serum may be associated with toxic side effects, which can include tremor, dizziness, drowsiness, and diarrhea (24).

Lithium is almost exclusively eliminated from the body by a renal mechanism. After the intake of most lithium preparations, urinary recovery of the lithium ion is almost 100% (64).

VIII. EFFECTS OF LITHIUM IN DRINKING WATER

Johnson (65) concluded that human exposure to the lithium level found in drinking water is not an obvious development hazard. Triffleman and Jefferson (66) summarized the effects of lithium-rich drinking water on animals and humans without demonstrating a positive or negative effect.

Dawson (67) reported that, in Texas, there was a significant inverse relationship between the lithium content of tap water, and urine lithium, with state mental hospital admissions that resulted in the diagnosis of psychosis, neurosis, schizophrenia, and personality problems and homicide. Schrauzer (68) demonstrated that the incidence rates of suicide, homicide, and rape were significantly higher in counties whose drinking water supplies contain low lithium than in counties in which the lithium levels of water ranged from 70 to 170 μg/L; the differences were statistically significant ($p < 0.01$). The results suggest that lithium at low dosage levels has a generally beneficial effect on human behavior (68).

IX. PERSPECTIVES AND FUTURE RESEARCH NEEDS

Lithium supplementation has been shown to improve the reproductive performance of two species, the goat and the rat. The biochemical basis of the reproductive impairment is unknown but deserves study. Elucidation of a metabolic pathway dependent on lithium would greatly strengthen the classification of lithium as a dietary essential. Without such evidence the beneficial effect of lithium might be due to a pharmacologic action, including interaction with another nutrient.

BIBLIOGRAPHY

Anderson CE. Lithium in plants. In: Bach RO, Gallicchio VS, eds. Lithium and Cell Physiology. New York: Springer Verlag, 1990: 25–46.

Angelow L. Rubidium in der Nahrungskette. Habilitationsarbeit, Friedrich-Schiller-Universität Jena, Biol.-Pharm. Fakultät, 1994.

Angelow L, Anke M. Rubidium in der Nahrungskette. Mengen- und Spurenelemente 1994; 14: 285–300.

Anke M, Arnhold W, Glei M, Schäfer U. Lithiumverzehr, Lithiumausscheidung und Lithiumbilanz Erwachsener Deutschlands. Mengen- und Spurenelemente 1995; 15:17–24.

Anke M, Krämer K, Illing H, Müller M, Glei M. Der Kupfergehalt der Lebensmittel und Getränke Deutschlands. Mengen- und Spurenelemente 1994; 14:301–316.

Arfvedson A. Afhandlinger i Fysik. Kemi och Mineralogi 1818; 6:145. Zitiert von Berzelius, 1822.

Bagchi N, Brown TR. Hypothalamicpituitary regulation of thyroid function. In: Johnson FN, ed. Lithium Therapy Monographs. Vol. 2, Lithium and the Endocrine System. Basel: S. Karger, 1988: 99–106.

Banerji TK. Luteinizing hormone, follicle-stimulating hormone, prolactin and testosterone. In: Johnson FN, ed. Lithium Therapy Monographs. Vol. 2, Lithium and the Endocrine System. Basel: S. Karger, 1988: 51–62.

Bardot PM. Possible mechanisms of action of lithium in plants. Lithium, 1992; 3:155–167.

Börtitz S, Dässler HG. Aus zeitgenössischen Berichten der Entdeckung von Li, Rb und Cs. In: Anke M, Baumann W, Bräunlich H, Brückner Chr, eds. 4. Spurenelementsymposium—Lithium, Universität Leipzig, Universität Jena, 1983: 10–17.

Christensen St. Vasopressin and renal concentrating ability. In: Johnson FN, ed. Lithium Therapy Monographs. Vol. 2, Lithium and the Endocrine System. Basel: S. Karger, 1988: 20–34.

Dietzel M, Lesch OM. Monoamine oxidase inhibitors. In: Johnson FN, ed. Lithium Therapy Monographs. Vol. 1, Lithium Combination Treatment. Basel: S. Karger, 1987: 32–42.

Drummond AH, Joels LA, Hughs PJ. Thyrotropin-releasing hormone. In: Johnson FN, ed. Lithium Therapy Monographs. Vol. 2, Lithium and the Endocrine System. Basel: S. Karger, 1988: 107–122.

Germain DL. Thyroid hormone metabolism. In: Johnson FN, ed. Lithium Therapy Monographs. Vol. 2, Lithium and the Endocrine System. Basel: S. Karger, 1988: 123–133.

Hansen HE, Amdisen A. Lithium intoxication and acute renal failure. In: Johnson FN, ed. Lithium Therapy Monographs. Vol. 3, Lithium and the Kidney. Basel: S. Karger, 1987: 134–142.

Hart DA. Modulation of immune system elements by lithium. In: Bach RO, Gallicchio VS, eds. Lithium and Cell Physiology. New York: Springer Verlag, 1990: 58–81.

Hassman RA, McGregor AM. Lithium and autoimmune thyroid disease. In: Johnson FN, ed. Lithium Therapy Monographs. Vol. 2, Lithium and the Endocrine System. Basel: S. Karger, 1988: 134–146.

Horrobin DF. Effects of lithium on essential fatty acid and prostaglandin metabolism. In: Bach RO, Gallicchio VS, eds. Lithium and Cell Physiology. New York: Springer Verlag, 1987: 137–149.

Horrobin DF. Lithium and dermatological disorders. In: Bach RO, Gallicchio VS, eds. Lithium and Cell Physiology. New York: Springer Verlag, 1990: 158–167.

Horrobin DF. Lithium effects on fatty acid metabolism and their role in therapy of seborrhoeic dermatitis and herpes infections. In: Schrauzer GH, Klippel KF, eds. Lithium in Biology and Medicine. Weinheim: VHC, 1991: 67–72.

Jackson BA, Dousa TP. Lithium-induced nephrogenic diabetes insipidus. In: Johnson FN, ed. Lithium Therapy Monographs. Vol. 3, Lithium and the Kidney. Basel: S. Karger, 1987: 126–133.

Jones KL, Johnson KA, Chambers CC, Reed KL, Sahn DJ. Pregnancy outcome in women treated with lithium. In: Schrauzer GH, Klippel KF, eds. Lithium in Biology and Medicine. Weinheim: VHC, 1991: 115–119.

Joyce RA. Murine hematopoietic response of normal and hypoplastic marrow to lithium administration. In: Schrauzer GH, Klippel KF, eds. Lithium in Biology and Medicine. Weinheim: VHC, 1991: 1–14.

Källen AJB. Lithium therapy and congenital malformations. In: Schrauzer GH, Klippel KF, eds. Lithium in Biology and Medicine. Weinheim: VHC, 1991: 123–130.

Kehr G. Study of the prophylactic effect of lithium in radiogenic leucocytopenia. In: Schrauzer GH, Klippel KF, eds. Lithium in Biology and Medicine. Weinheim: VHC, 1991: 49–63.

Kirchhoff G, Bunsen R. Chemische Analyse durch Spektralbeobachtungen. Annalen d. Chemie und Pharmacie 1861; 118:349–361.

Kopp H. *Geschichte der Chemie.* Vol. 4. Braunschweig: Theil, 1847: 41.

Kushner JP, Wartofsky L. Lithium-thyroid interactions. An overview. In: Johnson FN, ed. Lithium Therapy Monographs. Vol. 2, Lithium and the Endocrine System. Basel: S. Karger, 1988: 74–98.

Liebig J. *Handbuch der Chemie.* Vol. 1. Heidelberg: Abth, 1843, 1909: 402.

Mitchell SW. Quoted from Coldwell AE. History of psychopharmacology. In: Clark WG, del Giudice J, eds. Principles of Psychopharmacology. New York: Academic Press, 1978 (1870): 9.

Olesen OV, Thomsen K. Effects of lithium on sodium excretion. In: Johns FN, ed. Lithium Therapy Monographs. Vol. 3, Lithium and the Kidney. Basel: S. Karger, 1987: 106–113.

Salm-Horstmar, Fürst zu. Ueber die Notwendigkeit des Lithions und des Fluorkaliums zur Fruchtbildung der Gerste. J prakt Chem 1861; 84:140.

Shou M. Lithium treatment and kidney function, clinical observations. In: Johnson FN, ed. Lithium Therapy Monographs. Vol. 3, Lithium and the Kidney. Basel: S. Karger, 1987: 143–154.

Szentmihályi S, Regius A, Lokay D, Anke M. Der Lithiumgehalt der Vegetation in Abhängigkeit von der geologischen Herkunft des Standortes. In: Anke M, Baumann W, Bräunlich H, Brückner Chr, eds. 4. Spurenelementsymposium—Lithium, Universität Leipzig, Universität Jena, 1983: 18–24.

Wöhler F. Lithion in Meteoriten. Annalen d. Chemie und Pharmacie 1861; 120:253–254.

REFERENCES

1. Berzelius J. Jahresbericht über die Fortschritte der physischen Wissenschaften, 1822; 1:39–52.
2. Garrod AB. Gout and Rheumatic Gout. London: Walton and Maberley, 1859.
3. Luff AP. The treatment of gout in its various forms. Practitioner 1909; 83:26.
4. Corcoran AC, Taylor RD, Page I. Lithium poisoning from the use of salt substitutes. JAMA 1949; 139:685.
5. Cade JFJ. Lithium salts in the treatment of psychotic excitement. Med J Austral 1949; 2:349.
6. Arnhold W. Die Versorgung von Tier und Mensch mit dem lebensnotwendigen Spurenelement Lithium. Diss. Universität Leipzig, Sektion Tierprod. und Vet.-med., 1989.
7. Anke M, Arnhold W, Groppel B, Krause U. The biological importance of lithium. In: Schrauzer GH, Klippel GH, eds. Lithium in Biology and Medicine. Weinheim: VHC, 1991: 149–167.
8. Schou M. Special review. Lithium in psychiatric therapy and prophylaxis. J Psychiat Res 1968; 6:177.
9. Schou M. Possible mechanism of action of lithium salts: approaches and perspectives. Biochem Soc Trans 1973; 1:81.
10. Schou M, Baastrup PC, Grof P, Weis P, Angst J. Pharmacological and clinical problems of lithium prophylaxis. Br J Psychiat 1970; 116:615.
11. Johnson FN. The psychopharmacology of lithium. Neurosci Biobehav Rev 1979; 3:15.
12. Johnson FN. Depression and mania-modern lithium-therapy. Oxford, Washington, DC: IRL Press, 1987.
13. Brückner Chr, Holzapfel G, Hanf G. History and importance of lithium. In: Anke M, Baumann W, Bräunlich H, Brückner Chr, eds. 4. Spurenelementsymposium—Lithium, Universität Leipzig, Universität Jena, 1983: 6–9.
14. Anke M, Groppel B, Kronemann H, Grün M. Evidence for the essentiality of lithium in goats. In: Anke M, Baumann W, Bräunlich H, Brückner Chr, eds. 4. Spurenelementsymposium—Lithium, Universität Leipzig, Universität Jena, 1983: 58–65.
15. Pickett EE. Evidence for the essentiality of lithium in the rat. In: Anke M, Baumann W, Bräunlich H, Brückner Chr, eds. 4. Spurenelementsymposium—Lithium, Universität Leipzig, Universität Jena, 1983: 66–70.
16. Falbe J, Regitz U. Römpp Chemie Lexikon, H–L. Stuttgart, New York: Georg Thieme. 1990.
17. Thellier MC, Wissocq JC, Heurteaux C. Quantitative microlocation of lithium in the brain by a nuclear reaction. Nature 1980; 283:299.
18. Thellier M, Heurteaus C, Garrec JP, Alexandre J, Wissocq JC. Use of a tonic probe and of the stable ^{6}Li and ^{7}Li isotopes to perform unidirectional Li-flux measurements: application to compartmental analysis of lithium in the serum of Li-treated mice. In: Anke M, Baumann W, Bräunlich H, Brückner Chr, eds. 4. Spurenelementsymposium—Lithium, Universität Leipzig, Universität Jena, 1983: 134–138.

19. Birch NJ, Padghom C, Hughes MS. Lithium. In: Seiler HG, Sigel A, Sigel H, eds. Handbook on Metals in Clinical and Analytical Chemistry. New York: Marcel Dekker, 1994: 441–450.

20. Kabata-Pendias A, Pendias H. Trace Elements in Soils and Plants. 2d ed. Boca Raton, FL: CRC Press, 1992.

21. Gough LP, Shacklette HT, Case AA. Element concentrations toxic to plants, animals, and man. US Geol Surv Bull 1979; 1466:80.

22. Sievers ML, Cannon HL. Disease patterns of Pima Indians of the Gila River Indian Reservation of Arizona in relation to the geochemical environment. In: Hemphill DD, ed. Trace Subst. Environ. Health 7, Univ. of Missouri, Columbia, 1973; 57.

23. Baumann W, Stadie G, Anke M. Der Lithiumstatus des Menschen. In: Anke M, Baumann W, Bräunlich H, Brückner Chr, eds. 4. Spurenelementsymposium—Lithium, Universität Leipzig, Universität Jena, 1983: 180–185.

24. Weiner ML. Overview of lithium toxicology. In: Schrauzer GH, Klippel KF, eds. Lithium in Biology and Medicine. Weinheim: VHC, 1991: 83–99.

25. Arnhold W, Anke M. Der Lithiumstatus verschiedener Wiederkäuerarten in Mitteleuropa. Mengen- und Spurenelemente 1987; 7:283–288.

26. Pickett EE, O'Dell BL. Evidence for dietiary essentiality of lithium in the rat. Biol Trace Elem Res 1992; 34:299–319.

27. Klemfuss H, Greene KE. Cations affecting lithium toxicity and pharmacology. In: Schrauzer GH, Klipel KF, eds. Lithium in Biology and Medicine. Weinheim: VHC, 1991: 133–145.

28. Gallicchio VS. Transport of the lithium ion. In: Bach RO, Gallicchio VS, eds. Lithium and Cell Physiology. New York: Springer Verlag, 1990: 47–57.

29. Gallicchio VS. Lithium and granulopoiesis: mechanism of action. In: Bach RO, Gallicchio VS, eds. Lithium and Cell Physiology. New York: Springer Verlag, 1990: 83–93.

30. Arnhold W, Anke M. Möglichkeiten der Identifizierung des Lithiumstatus. Z Pharm Pharmakother Lab Diagn 1988; 127:243–244.

31. Anke M. Lithium. In: Macrae R, Robinson RK, Sadler MJ, eds. Encyclopaedia of Food Science, Food Technology and Nutrition. Vol. 4. 1992: 2779–2781.

32. Bokori J, Tölgyesi G. Influence of lithium on sodium and potassium metabolism in the bovine. In: Anke M, Baumann W, Bräunlich H, Brückner Chr, eds. 4. Spurenelementsymposium—Lithium, Universität Leipzig, Universität Jena, 1983: 174–179.

33. Bräunlich H, Kersten L. Mechanisms of renal lithium transport in rats. In: Anke M, Baumann W, Bräunlich H, Brückner Chr, eds. 4. Spurenelementsymposium—Lithium, Universität Leipzig, Universität Jena, 1983: 195–201.

34. Kersten L. The pharmacokinetics of lithium in rats of different ages. In: Anke M, Baumann W, Bräunlich H, Brückner Chr, eds. 4. Spurenelementsymposium—Lithium, Universität Leipzig, Universität Jena, 1983: 209–214.

35. Kersten L, Barth A. Age-dependent differences in the excretion routes of lithium in rats. In: Anke M, Baumann W, Bräunlich H, Brückner Chr, eds. 4. Spurenelementsymposium—Lithium, Universität Leipzig, Universität Jena, 1983: 215–218.

36. Kersten L, Fleck Ch, Bräunlich H. Evidence for an intestinal lithium excretion in rats. In: Anke M, Baumann W, Bräunlich H, Brückner Chr, eds. 4. Spurenelementsymposium—Lithium, Universität Leipzig, Universität Jena, 1983: 219–225.

37. Mormede P, Ledoux JM. Comparative pharmakinetics of lithium consequences in its therapeutic use in humans and animals. In: Anke M, Baumann W, Bräunlich H, Brückner Chr, eds. 4. Spurenelementsymposium—Lithium, Universität Leipzig, Universität Jena, 1983: 202–208.

38. Schäfer M, Uhlig A, Anke M, Kirbach H. Der Gehalt an Lithium sowie Natrium, Kalium, Kalzium und Magnesium in verschiedenen Körperflüssigkeiten der Milchkuh nach Applikation von Glukokortikoiden. In: Anke M, Baumann W, Bräunlich H, Brückner Chr, eds. 4. Spurenelementsymposium—Lithium, Universität Leipzig, Universität Jena, 1983: 186–194.

39. Lehmann K. Endogenous lithium levels. Pharmacopsychiat 1994; 27:130–132.

40. Anke M, Groppel B, Grün M, Kronemann H, Riedel E. Effects of Li-poor rations in ruminants. In: Szentmihályi S, ed. Conference on Feed Additives, Budapest, Hungary, 1981: 245–248.

41. Anke M, Grün M, Groppel B, Kronemann H. The biological importance of lithium. Mengen- und Spurenelemente 1981: 217–239.

42. Szentmihályi S, Anke M, Regius A. The importance of lithium for plant and animal. In: Pais I, ed. Nes Results in the Research of Hardly Known Trace Elements. Univ. of Horticulture, Budapest, 1985: 136–151.

43. Szilágyi M, Anke M, Balogh I, Regius-Mócsényi A, Suri A. Lithium status and animal metabolism. In: Anke M, et al., eds. 6th International Trace Element Symposium. Vol. 4, University Leipzig, University Jena 1989: 1249–1261.

44. Burt JL. The essentiality of lithium in the rat. Ph.D. dissertation, University of Missouri, Columbia, 1982.

45. Burt J, Dowdy RP, Pickett EE, O'Dell BL. Effect of low dietary lithium on tissue lithium content in rats. Fed Proc 1982; 41:460.

46. Patt EL, Pickett EE, O'Dell BL. Effect of dietary lithium level on tissue lithium concentration, growth rate and reproduction in the rat. Bioinorg Chem 1978; 9:299–310.

47. Ono T, Wada O, Yamamoto M. Study on the essentiality of lithium. Biomed Res Trace Elem, 1992: 41–47.

48. Bach JO. Some aspects of lithium in living systems. In: Bach RO, Gallicchio VS, eds. Lithium and Cell Physiology. New York: Springer Verlag, 1990: 1–15.

49. Anke M, Arnhold W, Groppel B, Kräuter U. Die biologische Bedeutung des Lithiums als Spurenelement. Erfahrungsheilkunde 1991; 10:656–664.

50. Gallicchio VS, Messino MJ, Hulette BC, Hughes NK. Lithium enhances recovery of hemato-poiesis and lengthens survival in an allogeneic transplant model. In: Schrauzer GH, Klippell KF, eds. Lithium in Biology and Medicine. Weinheim: VHC, 1991: 33–46.

51. Anke M, Illing H, Müller M, et al. Die Bedeutung der Ultraspurenelemente Aluminum, Arsen, Brom, Cadmium, Fluor, Lithium, Rubidium und Vanadium für das Tier. REKASAN J 1995; 3:5–7.

52. Belmaker RH, Schreiber-Avissar S, Schreiber G, et al. Does the effect of lithium on G-proteins have behavioral correlates? In: Bach RO, Gallicchio VS, eds. Lithium and Cell Physiology. New York: Springer Verlag, 1990: 94–101.

53. Anke M, Angelow L, Müller M. Der Lithiumgehalt der Lebensmittel und Getränke Deutsch-lands. Mengen- und Spurenelemente 1995; 15:1–16.

54. Anke M, Arnhold W, Glei M, Müller M, Illing H, Schäfer U, Jaritz M. Essentiality and toxicity of lithium. In: Košla T, ed. Lithium. Warszawa, Warsaw Agricultural University, 1995: 17–42.

55. Anke M, Groppel B, Kühnert E, Angelow L. Der Einfluß des Lithiums auf Futterverzehr, Wachstum und Verhalten von Schwein und Rind. Mengen- und Spurenelemente 1984; 6: 537–544.

56. Anke M, Richter G, Meixner B, Arnhold W, Angelow L. Der Einfluß des Lithiums auf den Futterverzehr, das Wachstum bzw. die Eiproduktion des Broilers und der Legehenne. Mengen- und Spurenelemente 1985; 5:412–419.

57. Anke M, Arnhold W, Groppel B, Richter G, Meixner B, Angelow L. Influence of lithium on feed-intake, growth and egg production of broilers and laying hens. In: Pais I, ed. New Results in the Research of Hardly Known Trace Elements. Budapest: University of Horticulture and Food Industry, 1986: 41–55.

58. Opitz K, Schäfer G. The effect of lithium on food intake in rats. Pharmacopsychiat 1976; 11:197–201.

59. Regius A, Anke M, Sardi J, Mucsy I. Effect of lithium supplementation on performance of ewes and growing lambs. Trace Elem Man and Animals 1983; 8:603–604.

60. Szilágyi M, Anke M, Balogh I, Regius-Mócsényi A, Suri A. Lithium status and animal metabolism. In: Yüregir T, Donma O, Kayrin L, eds. Proc Third Int. Congress on Trace Elements in Health and Disease at Adana, Turkey 1989: 107–118.

61. Szilágyi M, Súri A, Balogh I, Anke M, Borka G. Líthiumadagolást követö biokémiai és morfológiai változások malacokon. Magyar Állatorvosok Lapja 1990; 45:231–236.
62. Ragan CI. The effect of lithium on inositol phosphate metabolism. In: Bach RO, Gallicchio VS, eds. Lithium and Cell Physiology. New York: Springer Verlag, 1990: 102–120.
63. Ribas B. Lithium. In: Merian E, ed. Metals and Their Compounds in the Environment. Weinheim: VHC, 1991: 1015–1023.
64. Alexander BP, Perry J. Diuretics. In: Johnson FN, ed. Lithium Therapy Monographs. Vol. 1, Lithium Combination Treatment. Basel: S. Karger, 1987: 179–200.
65. Johnson EM. A summary review and human perspective for developmental toxicity evaluations of lithium in laboratory animals. In: Schrauzer GH, Klippel KF, eds. Lithium in Biology and Medicine. Weinheim: VHC, 1991: 103–112.
66. Triffleman EG, Jefferson JW. Naturally occurring lithium. In: Bach RO, Gallicchio VS, eds. Lithium and Cell Physiology. New York: Springer Verlag, 1990; 16–24.
67. Dawson EB. The relationship of tap water and physiological levels of lithium to mental hospital admission and homicide in Texas. In: Schrauzer GH, Klippel KF, eds. Lithium in Biology and Medicine. Weinheim: VHC, 1991: 171–187.
68. Schrauzer GN, Shrestha KP. Lithium in drinking water and the incidences of crimes, suicides, and arrests related to drug addictions. In: Schrauzer GH, Klippel KF, eds. Lithium in Biology and Medicine. Weinheim: VHC, 1991: 191–203.

17

Lead

A. M. REICHLMAYR-LAIS AND M. KIRCHGESSNER
Technische Universität München, Freising-Weihenstephan, Germany

I. INTRODUCTION

The element lead is ubiquitous in nature. In recent decades the natural concentrations have been supplemented by anthropogenic burden. Because of lead's widespread use, lead intoxication is common and has been known since ancient times.

Recently, scientific interest has concentrated on lead metabolism and the biochemical changes caused by toxic lead intake. The reason for the interest in toxic reactions is to prevent lead intoxication and to enable diagnosis, even of latent forms, so as to start an expedient therapy as early as possible.

Despite its toxicity, for centuries lead has been administered by many physicians for almost every illness. Altogether, the notable effects were of pharmacologic nature. Indications of a positive effect of lead on metabolic processes and the high affinity of lead toward biological ligands gave way to the supposition in recent years that lead might also be an essential element.

II. CHEMICAL PROPERTIES OF LEAD

A. Oxidative States

The element lead is a heavy metal and belongs to the Group 4 elements of the Periodic Table. The atomic weight of lead is 207.2. There are four stable (204, 206, 207, 208) and more than 20 radioactive isotopes (^{194}Pb–^{214}Pb). Lead is bivalent and quadrivalent. The lead(II) salts are the most common and form the most stable compounds, whereas the lead-organic compounds are mostly derived from lead(IV).

B. Chelating and Binding Properties

Generally, the binding sites for lead are macromolecules, mainly proteins. Proteins with several free SH groups tightly bind lead in vivo and in vitro. Metallothionein, which has a high cysteine content, can also bind lead in vitro and in vivo (1). Lead forms not only mercaptides with SH groups of cysteine but also much less stable complexes with other side chains of amino acids (2), for example, with the ε-amino group of lysine, the carboxyl group of glutamic and aspartic acids, the phenoxyl group of tyrosine, and the imidazole group of histidine (3).

III. ANALYTICAL METHODOLOGY

The following methods are applied for the determination of lead in biological materials.

> Colorometric and spectrophotometric methods (e.g., the dithizone method)
> Atomic absorption spectrophotometry (AAS)
> Electrochemical methods (e.g., differential pulse stripping voltammetry)
> Emission spectroscopy
> X-ray fluorescence analysis
> Mass spectrophotometry

The analytical detection limits and the sensitivity of the methods are not only dependent on the kind of the method but also markedly on the sample preparation and the sample matrix. Especially for the determination of low doses of lead, extreme methodological care is necessary. Generally the detection of lead in biological material requires continuous internal and external quality control with standard reference materials.

IV. METABOLISM

A. Absorption

Humans and animals take in lead with food, water, and air. Under normal conditions, the lead content in foodstuffs, as recorded in the literature, ranges from 0.02 to 3 mg/kg fresh matter, in drinking water from 0.01 to 0.03 mg/L, and in air from 0.03 to 0.3 $\mu g/m^3$. These values could be far higher, depending on environmental pollution (see Ref. 4).

The total lead intake of humans has been estimated at 0.3–0.6 mg/day. The intake is predominantly oral, with a minor amount taken in through the respiratory track or absorbed through the skin. The provisional tolerable weekly intake established by the FAO-WHO Expert Committee on Food Additives in 1972 (5) is 3 mg per person.

1. Pulmonary Absorption

Pulmonary lead absorption depends on the state of aggregation (gas, solid particles), particle size of the lead-containing dust, respiratory volume, concentration in the air, and distribution within the respiratory tract. Particles of < 0.5 μm in average mass media equivalent diameter especially are retained in the nasopharynx and tracheobronchial tree, including the terminal bronchioles. Larger particles are removed by the activity of the ciliated cells of the respiratory epithelium. Lead can be retained by the pulmonary macrophages (6), but both the mechanism and the quantity of this clearance are largely unknown.

2. Gastrointestinal Absorption

The gastrointestinal absorption of lead depends on many factors, such as the amount of intake, chemical form, dietary composition, intraluminal interactions with other dietary constituents, presence of bile acids, and age. According to the literature, the absorbability of lead falls into the range of 5–15% (7).

The absorbability depends critically on the solubility of lead compounds. Lead, as the acetate, chloride, oxide, and tetraethyl, is readily absorbed. Less soluble yet fairly absorbable are chromates, sulfides, sulfates, and carbonates. Delwaide et al. (8) suspect that part of the lead is converted by the action of the digestive secretions to lead chloride and complexes with bile acids and is then absorbed in these forms. Conrad and Barton (9) also pointed out that bile stimulates the transport of lead across the intestinal mucosal cells and, subsequently, into the body. Ascorbic acid (7) and amino acids with sulfhydryl groups (9) improve solubility and hence absorbability of lead compounds. Lead absorption is increased in the absence of food or during food restriction (10). The intake of calcium, iron, magnesium, phosphate, ethanol, and high-fat diets lower the absorption of lead (11–13). The decrease in lead absorption by various elements is attributed mainly to their competition for carrier systems in the intestinal epithelium. In the case of children and young animals, lead absorption is higher than in adults (14). This may at least partially explain their high sensitivity to lead.

At present, little is known about the mechanism of lead absorption; some studies implicate active transport. In the case of high lead doses, diffusion processes might predominate.

B. Transport and Distribution

Kinetic studies of radiolabeled lead disappearance from tissues and organs indicate the presence of roughly three compartments. Blood shows the shortest half-life for lead compounds. Soft tissues, including the skeletal muscle, represent a pool of medium half-life (weeks), and the skeleton represents a pool of very long half-life (months up to years) (15). Goyer and Mahaffey (7) distinguished between a diffusible or mobile form and a nondiffusible or fixed form of lead in the body. The diffusible part is defined as the transport forms of lead in blood and intracellular lead that can be mobilized and transported through membranes. Lead in blood is to a large extent exchangeable with that in tissues and organs. The distribution between tissues and organs is a function of time, dose, supply state, and turnover rates of the particular compounds. During normal exposure, relatively high lead concentrations were found in bones, and somewhat lower levels were found in liver and kidneys (16).

In blood, more than 90% of the lead is associated with erythrocytes (see e.g., Ref. 15). This erythrocyte-bound lead probably represents, in part, a transport form, since lead disappears from red cells at a rate greater than explained by their life span (9). Studies by Kaplan et al. (17) indicate that lead occurs mainly in the cellular constituents of the erythrocytes and to a lesser extent in the stroma. It is assumed that lead is bound mainly to hemoglobin. Lead may, however, also be present in low-molecular compounds (18).

The plasma lead concentration appears to remain constant over a wide range of whole-blood concentration (19,20). Plasma lead, as the studies by Kochen and Greener (21) have shown, is bound predominantly to transferrin and at the same binding sites as iron. Saturation of the total iron-binding capacity suppresses the uptake of plasma lead by red cells and increases the uptake of lead by the liver. With respect to soft tissues, the subcellular distribution of lead has been studied especially in liver and kidneys (see e.g., Refs. 15 and 22). Fractionation of organ homogenates into nuclei, mitochondria, lysosomes, microsomes, and soluble fraction have shown that lead is bound to all fractions. Its distribution between the individual fractions, however, depends largely on the state of supply and the dose applied. The major part of lead doses is recovered in the nuclei and the soluble fraction. In the nuclear fraction, lead seems to be bound in particular to membrane components. Sabbioni and Marafante (22) could not detect lead in high-molecular-weight components, comprising RNA-membranes combined with nuclear pore complexes, nor in low-molecular-weight phospholipids of cell nuclei. The binding of lead in cell nuclei does not seem to be restricted to membranes, but may also involve intranuclear chromatin components, predominantly a histone fraction. The intramitochondrial distribution of lead shows a marked localization in the heavy subfractions consisting of inner membranes and part of the matrix. There lead is bound to proteins of the membranes. Walton (23) and Barltrop et al. (24) showed that pretreatment of experimental animals with lead diminishes mitochondrial lead uptake, indicating saturation of binding sites. They also found impaired respiratory and phosphorylative abilities and, accordingly, impaired active transport. This may explain the morphologic and functional changes observed in the mitochondria. In the endoplasmic reticulum, lead is associated with both membranous and ribosomal components. In the cytosol, lead may be bound to high-molecular-weight components.

Ruessel (25) demonstrated that, in the case of toxic doses, lead in kidneys, liver, and spleen is bound partially to ferritin and partially to an insoluble ferric hydroxide. Whether this holds true also for normal lead metabolism needs to be investigated. In the brain, lead concentration differs in various regions. The highest concentrations are found in cortical gray matter and basal ganglia (26). Subcellularly, lead is located especially within the neural mitochondria, perhaps at calcium-binding sites.

More than 90% of the lead in the body is located in bones even under normal conditions. Seventy percent of this occurs in cortical bones (27). The lead concentration is higher in dense cortical bones than in the spongy hemopoietic trabecular bone (27). In bones, lead is deposited at first in labile form, later as triphosphate (28). Lead metabolism in bones is very similar to that of calcium. In certain metabolic situations that cause demineralization, lead may be mobilized from the bones and even cause a lead crisis under certain circumstances (29). The lead concentration in teeth is higher than in bone. Lead in teeth appears to be firmly bound (27).

C. Excretion

Lead can be excreted via feces, urine, sweat, and saliva. Fecal excretion is particularly high because of the high percentage of unabsorbed lead and may average approximately 0.2 mg/day. By comparison, urinary excretion amounts to an average of 30 μg/day. In the kidneys, lead is excreted usually by glomerular filtration. In the case of high blood lead concentration, tubular secretion also occurs (30). Excretion through sweat, reported by Schroeder and Tipton (31), appears to be sizable, averaging 60 μg/day.

D. Interactions

Elements with similar physicochemical properties can influence each other during absorption, intermediary metabolism, and excretion. In the case of lead, such interactions are known to occur especially with calcium and iron, but also with zinc, copper, magnesium, and cadmium (see, e.g., Ref. 88). These interactions are dependent on the concentrations of the respective elements.

V. ESSENTIALITY

The first indices of a possible essentiality of lead came from studies with microorganisms, in which low lead concentrations stimulated heme synthesis and growth (32–34). Later, Schwarz (35) found the growth of rats was improved when a diet with 0.5 ppm lead was supplemented to provide 1 or 2.5 ppm.

In our laboratory a series of experiments were done with rats fed a synthetic diet that contained selected and purified components with an extremely low lead content. Signs of lead deficiency were seen in the f_1 generation from lead-depleted mothers. Besides growth depression (36) a microcytic hypochromic anemia was observed (37, see Table 1). The anemia was associated with disturbances in iron metabolism (38–42). As further evidence of disturbances in metabolism, especially the lipid metabolism, changes in enzyme activities and metabolite concentrations were determined (43–47).

In more recent studies the activities of Na, K-ATPase and Mg, Ca-ATPase in red cell membranes of the offspring of lead-depleted mothers were reduced by about 30% in comparison to control animals (48). Besides these reduced enzyme activities, the concentration of free Ca^{2+} in erythrocytes was increased (49). These results could explain the smaller volume of erythrocytes in offspring from lead-depleted mothers. The increase of free Ca^{2+} in the erythrocyte may result from reduced activity of the calcium pump, Ca,Mg-ATPase, and it may induce K^+ leakage that cannot be fully compensated because of the reduced Na,K-ATPase in the membrane. The K^+ leakage leads to a reduction of erythrocyte volume.

Other changes resulting from lead depletion include a decreased concentration of certain elements in milk, including Ca, Na, K, Fe, Cu, Zn, and Mn (50). Table 2 shows the concentration of these elements at day 10 of lactation. This observation may explain the reduced body mass and development of the offspring from depleted mothers.

Reduced growth rate and disturbances in lipid metabolism were observed in piglets which were separated from their mothers immediately after birth and fed a synthetic lead-poor diet (51,52).

In the most recent lead depletion experiments, growth reduction and clinical signs caused by extreme lead depletion were produced in rats of the f_0 generation (90). During the growth phase of the breeding mothers, those fed the lead-depleted diet had a reduced growth rate, as shown in Figure 1. The reduction of growth was associated with changes of coat color, loss of hair, and eczema. In addition, reproduction was impaired dramatically by lead depletion; 35% of the newborns died within the first few days after birth. Survivors

TABLE 1 Blood Parameters for Anemia Assessment in 24-Day Offspring of Lead-Depleted Rats Compared to Controls (Means ± SD)

Treatment	Erythrocytes ($10^6/\mu L$)	Hematocrit (%)	Hemoglobin (g/100 ml)	MCV (μ^3)
Depleted (20 ppb Pb)	5.1 ± 0.3	27.8 ± 1.5[a]	7.0 ± 0.3[a]	54 ± 2[a]
Control (800 ppb Pb)	4.9 ± 0.5	35.5 ± 4.0[b]	9.3 ± 0.9[b]	70 ± 4[b]

[a,b]Different superscript letters indicate significantly different means ($p < 0.05$).

TABLE 2 Concentration of Selected
Elements in the Milk of Lead-Deficient
and Control Rats at Day 10 of Lactation
(Means ± SD)

Element	Deficient (μg/g)	Control (μg/g)
Ca	3722 ± 855[a]	5645 ± 879[b]
Na	777 ± 171[a]	1228 ± 126[b]
K	1627 ± 317[a]	2669 ± 429[b]
Fe	11.0 ± 1.8[a]	14.7 ± 2.5[b]
Cu	4.0 ± 0.7[a]	6.6 ± 1.8[b]
Zn	17.8 ± 4.4[a]	29.2 ± 6.1[b]
Mn	467 ± 110[a]	979 ± 363[b]

[a,b]Different superscript letters indicate significantly
different means (p < 0.05).

among the f_1 generation showed reduced growth during the suckling period, as demonstrated in Figure 2. The reduced growth was accompanied by a thin coat and a scaly skin, as illustrated by the photograph in Figure 3.

Because of the consistent evidence of disturbed lipid metabolism, in recent studies further parameters of lipid metabolism have been determined. The first results show that lead depletion induces changes in the fatty acid composition of erythrocyte membranes and liver from mothers and offspring as well as in milk and mammary glands (86,87).

In conclusion, lead depletion induces signs of lead deficiency in rats and pigs that can be prevented or abolished by lead supplementation. The signs of lead deficiency are summarized in Table 3. Further experiments are necessary in order to explore the exact role of lead in the metabolism.

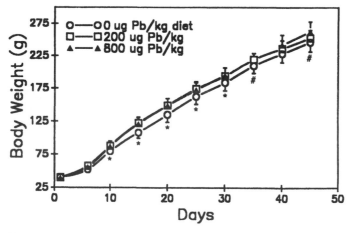

FIGURE 1 Body mass during the growth phase of f_0-generation female rats fed diets supplemented with variable concentrations of lead. The points represent the means ± SD, and the asterisks indicate significant ($p < .05$) differences between both treatment groups and the unsupplemented group (0 μg Pb/kg). # indicates a difference between the 0 and 800-μg levels only.

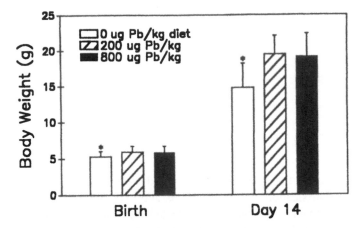

FIGURE 2 Body mass of the offspring of the f_0-generation females (Fig. 1) at birth and 14 days of age. The dams consumed diets supplemented with 0, 200, or 800 μg Pg/kg, and the numbers of offspring at birth were 77, 100, and 103, and at 14 days, 26, 59, and 90, respectively. The bars and extensions represent means and standard deviations, and asterisks significance at $p < .05$.

VI. TOXICITY

The toxicity of lead is dependent mainly on dose and chemical compound. Symptoms of lead toxicity have been reviewed in detail by many authors (see, e.g., Refs. 4 and 53); therefore, only the main symptoms are described here.

Lead intoxication is generally divided into acute and chronic forms. Chronic poisoning describes a prolonged exposure. Manifestations, however, are often acute. Depending

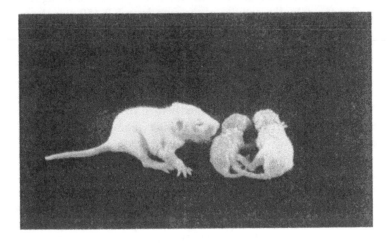

FIGURE 3 Offspring from a lead-depleted mother, on the right, compared to a control offspring at 14 days of age.

TABLE 3 Signs of Experimental
Lead Deficiency in Rats

Growth depression
High mortality of offspring
Anemia, hypochromic and microcytic
Disturbance in iron metabolism
Loss of hair and eczema
Disturbance in lipid metabolism

on duration and severity of exposure, the effects range from lead colic to encephalopathy and death. Early symptoms of intoxication include headache, anorexia, fatigue, nervousness, tremor, and constipation. Later, colic occurs at repeated intervals. Frequently, a marked fatigue of the extensor muscles may accompany the distinct state of tremor.

Clinical signs are manifested mainly in the blood (anemia), nervous system (encephalopathy and neuropathy), and kidneys (renal dysfunction).

A. Hematologic Effects of Toxic Lead Doses

Acute and chronic lead intoxications cause anemia associated with reticulocytosis and basophilic stippling of the erythroblastic cells (54). The anemia results from diminished hemoglobin synthesis, hemolysis of immature erythrocytes, and direct hemolysis of mature erythrocytes in conjunction with a shortened life span.

The reduced hemoglobin synthesis following lead intoxication may be attributed primarily to an inhibition of heme synthesis (55). Toxic lead doses adversely affect several enzymes of the heme pathway: δ-aminolevulinic acid synthetase (δ-ALAS), δ-aminolevulinic acid dehydratase (δ-ALAD) (56), heme synthetase (ferrochelatase) (57), and uroporphyrinogen I synthetase (58).

Because of the defective heme formation, disturbances other than the impaired synthesis of hemoglobin must also be expected in the case of enzymes possessing heme as the prosthetic group. For example, the activity of the cytochrome P-450 complexes has been shown to be reduced, especially in acute lead poisoning, while there was only a mild inhibition in chronic cases (59,60).

Apart from the defects in the heme pathway, the synthesis of hemoglobin may also be diminished by a reduced globin synthesis following lead poisoning (61). Piddington and White (62) postulated that the in-vivo inhibition of globin synthesis is caused secondarily by the inhibition of heme synthesis. It has been observed both in vivo with children (61) and in vitro (62) that the synthesis of the α-chains of hemoglobin is inhibited to a greater extent than that of the β-chains.

The anemia due to lead poisoning is caused not only by impaired hemoglobin synthesis, but also by a shortened life span of the erythrocytes. Toxic lead levels exert a direct hemolytic effect on mature erythrocytes (63). The cause may be found in the high affinity of erythrocytes for lead, especially of their membranes; this results in a decrease of the osmotic resistance and mechanical fragility (64). The consequence is that potassium is released from the erythrocytes into the plasma (65). This could also be associated with a reduced activity of the Na^+,K^+-ATPase (18).

Another phenomenon, which can be observed soon after the first days of lead exposure, is the basophilic stippling of the polychromatic erythroblasts and reticulocytes in the cytoplasm because of changes in the ultrastructure of these cells (66). This change concerns the mitochondria and, especially, the ribosomes of the erythroblasts and reticulo-blasts. Furthermore, lesions of the nuclear membrane and swelling of the Golgi apparatus occur. The basophilic stippling represents essentially aggregations of undergraded and partially degraded ribosomes (67). The cause might be an inhibition of the erythrocyte pyrimidine-5'-nucleotidase, with the consequence that large amounts of pyrimidine nu-cleotides accumulate intracellularly and bring about retardation of ribosomal RNA degra-dation, similar to hereditary nucleotidase deficiency. These defects ultimately result in pre-mature erythrocyte hemolysis.

B. Neurotoxic Effects of Lead

Among all organ symptoms, the brain reacts most sensitively to higher lead doses (68). Depending on the exposure level, lead toxicity may result in lead encephalopathy and neuropathy. Children and young animals appear to be especially sensitive, according to the ontogenic differences in neural tissue susceptibility or because of a greater accessibility to lead of the nervous system in the young (69).

Lead affects the functions of both the central and peripheral nervous system. Early lead exposure of children correlates with decreased IQ, symptoms of hyperkinesis or minimal brain dysfunction, poor learning, or defects in specific neuromotor tasks (70,71). It has been claimed that infants may suffer cerebral damage perhaps even at blood lead levels of about 1 μmol/L (200 μg/L). However, this is controversial, not least because of the methodological difficulties (see Ref. 89). Higher loads cause depressed behavior, lethargy, mental regression, coma, and seizure (68).

Cerebral edema resulting from lead poisoning is often associated with a rise of cerebrospinal fluid pressure. Other changes observed include proliferation and swelling of the endothelial cells, accompanied by dilatation of the arterioles and capillaries, prolifera-tion of the glial cells, focal necrosis, and neural degeneration. Severe cases manifest as acute communicating hydrocephalus because of inflammation of the pia arachnoid or choroid plexus (72). Another symptom of lead encephalopathy is a diffuse astrocytic proliferation in the gray and white matter (73). Peripheral signs are segmental demyelina-tion resulting from the degeneration of Schwann cells and axons (74).

At the molecular level, the biochemical changes of lead poisoning may be explained by interactions with other elements, for example, with Ca, Na, and Mg. Calcium is involved in neurotransmitter function (e.g., the stimulus-coupled release of transmitters, the regula-tion of some enzymes in neurotransmitter synthesis, the storage of transmitter, and the regulation of hormone-sensitive cyclases) (75). Higher lead concentrations reduce the calcium concentrations in bathing or superfusing media, possibly because of interactions at the site of the transmembrane calcium transport leading to defects in calcium functions (76). Lead–sodium interactions may explain the accumulation of calcium and the enhanced dopanine release from CNS synaptosomes (77). Interactions between lead and Mg might play a role in mitochondrial binding and in oxidative phosphorylation. Another cause of the neurotoxicity of lead may be related to a direct inhibition of the activity of myelin-synthesizing enzymes, as demonstrated by in vitro studies. Also, inhibition of heme synthesis resulting in an increase of δ-aminolevulinic acid and porphobilinogens may be involved as a cause of the encephalopathy. In vitro, δ-aminolevulinic acid can displace Γ-aminobutyric acid in its binding to the synaptic membranes and block its reuptake by the synaptosomes because of their structural similarity.

C. Renal Effects of Toxic Lead

Functional, metabolic, and morphological abnormalities of the kidneys have been reported in the case of lead intoxication. The vessels and tubules are affected especially. Tubular lesions dominate in acute poisoning, while in the case of chronic poisoning vascular lesions also occur and may sometimes be progressive, with the ultimate development of nephrosclerosis. These morphologic changes bring about impairment of the reabsorptive mechanisms, with the effect of aminoaciduria, glycosuria, hyperphosphaturia, and acidosis (78). Newer experimental studies also report on an increased urinary excretion of K, Na, and Ca (79). These functional defects of the kidney caused by lead poisoning may be explained by the influence of lead on the mitochondria (80). Accordingly, active transport mechanisms may be impaired because of the resulting deficiency of ATP. Other explanations concern changes in the tubular permeability or interference with carrier molecules.

Apart from the toxic effects of lead on the tubular lining cells, there are also indications that excessive doses of lead interfere with the metabolism of the juxtaglomerular apparatus, with the consequence of a transient decrease in the synthesis or release of renin (81), followed by a prolonged increase (79). The effects of lead on the renin–angiotensin–aldosterone system might also explain the hypertension encountered during lead exposure (83).

VI. CONCLUSION AND FUTURE RESEARCH NEEDS

Because of new experimental reports, we can say that lead is not only a toxic metal but also an essential one, at very low dietary levels. For future research in both fields, essentiality and toxicity, further analytical work is necessary to determine reliable lead concentrations in biological materials.

Concerning lead toxicity, it is necessary to find out the molecular mechanisms responsible for the pathologic disturbances in order to prevent or treat lead toxicity.

In the field of lead essentiality, it is necessary to determine the role of lead in metabolism. For this purpose, further studies with extreme depletion are necessary. We believe that a role of lead may be in the metabolism of lipids, particularly phospholipids.

REFERENCES

1. Ulmer DD, Vallee BL. Effects of lead on biochemical systems. Proc. 2nd. Missouri Conf. Trace Substances Environ. Health 1968: 7.
2. Vallee BL, Ulmer DD. Biochemical effects of mercury, cadmium and lead. Annu Rev Biochem 1972; 41:91.
3. Wong PRS, Silverberg BA, Chan YK, Hodson PV. In: Nriagu JO, ed. The Biogeochemistry of Lead in the Environment. Amsterdam: Elsevier/North Holland, 1978: 279.
4. Quaterman J. Lead. In: Mertz W, ed. Trace Elements in Human and Animal Nutrition. Orlando, FL: Academic Press, 1986: 281.
5. Joint FAO/WHO Expert Committee on Food Additives. FAO Nutr Met Rep Ser No. 51. Rome: FAO/UN, 1972.
6. Bingham E, Pfitzer EA, Barkley W, Radford EP. Alveolar macrophages: reduced number in rats after prolonged inhalation of lead sesquioxide. Science 1968; 162:1297.
7. Goyer RA, Mahaffey KR. Susceptibility to lead toxicity. Environ Health Perspect, 1972; 2:73.
8. Delwaide PC, Hensghem C, Noirfalise A. Le saturnisme: lésions biochimiques et sémeiologie biologique. Ann Biol Clin 1968; 26:987.

9. Conrad ME, Barton JC. Factors affecting the absorption and excretion of lead in the rat. Gastroenterology 1978; 74:731.

10. Rabinowitz MB, Kopple JD, Wetherill GW. Effect of food intake and fasting on gastrointestinal lead absorption in humans. Am J Clin Nutr 1980; 33:1784.

11. Fine B, Barth A, Sheffet A, Levenhar M. Influence of Mg on the intestinal absorption of lead. Environ Res 1976; 12:224.

12. Barltrop D, Kehoe HE. The influence of nutritional factors on lead absorption. Post-grad Med J 1975; 51:795.

13. Ragan H. Effects of iron deficiency on the absorption and distribution of lead and cadmium in rats. J Lab Clin Med 1977; 90:700.

14. Kostial K, Simonovic L, Pisonic M. Lead absorption from the intestine in newborn rats. Nature 1971; 233:564.

15. Castellino N, Aloj S. Kinetics of the distribution and excretion of lead in the rat. Br J Ind Med 1964; 21:308.

16. Kehoe RA. Normal metabolism of lead. Environ Health 1964; 8:232.

17. Kaplan ML, Jones AG, Davis MA, Kopito L. Inhibitory effect of iron on the uptake of lead by erythrocytes. Life Sci 1975; 16:1545.

18. Raghavan SRV, Culver BD, Gonick HC. Erythrocyte lead-binding protein after occupational exposure. II. Influence on lead inhibition of membrane Na^+,K^+-adenosinetriphosphatase. J Toxicol Environ Health 1981; 7:561.

19. Rosen JF, Trinidad EE. Significance of plasma lead levels in normal and lead-intoxicated children. Environ Health Perspect Exp Issue 1974; 7:139.

20. Rosen JF, Zarate-Salvador C, Trinidad EE. Plasma blood levels in normal and lead intoxicated children. J Pediatr 1974; 84:45.

21. Kochen J, Greener Y. Interaction of ferritin with lead and cadmium. Ped Res 1975; 9:323.

22. Sabbioni E, Marafante E. Identification of lead-binding components in rat liver: in vivo study. Chem Biol Interactions 1976; 15:1.

23. Walton, JR. Intranuclear inclusions in the lead-poisoned cultured kidney cells. J Pathol 1973; 112:213.

24. Barltrop D, Barrett AJ, Dingle JT. Subcellular distribution of lead in the rat. J Lab Clin Med 1971; 77:705.

25. Ruessel HA. Über die Bindung von Blei an eisenhydroxyhaltige Stoffe in Leber, Niere und Milz vergifteter Rinder. Bull Environ Contam Toxicol 1970; 5:115.

26. Klein M, Namer R, Harpur E, Corbin R. Earthenware containers as a source of fatal lead poisoning. Case study and public-health considerations. N Engl J Med 1970; 283:669.

27. Barry PSF. A comparison of concentrations of lead in human tissues. Br J Ind Med 1975; 32:119.

28. Ligeois FJ, Derivaux J, Depelchin A. L'Intoxication saturnine chez les animaux. Ann Med Vet 1961; 2:57.

29. Six KM, Goyer RA. Experimental enhancement of lead toxicity by low dietary calcium. J Lab Clin Med 1970; 76:933.

30. Vostal J, Heller J. Renal excretory mechanisms of heavy metals. I. Transtubular transport of heavy metal ions in the avian kidney. Environ Res 1968; 2:1.

31. Schroeder HA, Tipton IH. The human body burden of lead. Arch Environ Health 1968; 17:965.

32. Pecora L, Fati S, Mole R, Pesaresi C. Azione del piombo sul metaboism porfirinico nel midollo osseo. Folia Med 1965; 48:33.

33. Devigne JP. Geomicrobiologie—precipation du sulfure de plomb par un micrococcus tellurique. CR Acad Sci D 1968: 267:935.

34. Devigne JP. Arch Inst Pasteur Tunis 1968; 45:341.

35. Schwarz K. New essential trace elements (Sn, V, F, Si): progress report and outlook. In: Hoekstra WG, Suttie JW, Ganther HE, Mertz W, eds. Trace Elements in Man and Animals—2. Baltimore, MD: University Park Press, 1974: 355.

36. Reichlmayr-Lais AM, Kirchgessner M. Aktivitäts-Veränderungen verschiedener Enzyme im alimentären Blei-Mangel. Z Tierphysiol Tierernähr Futtermittelkunde 1981; 46:145.

37. Reichlmayr-Lais AM, Kirchgessner M. Hämatologische Veränderungen bei alimentärem Bleimangel. Ann Nutr Metabol 1981; 25:281.

38. Reichlmayr-Lais AM, Kirchgessner M. Eisen-, Kupfer- und Zinkgehalte in Neugeborenen sowie in Leber und Milch wachsender Ratten bei alimentärem Blei-Mangel. Z Tierphysiol Tierernähr Futtermittelkunde 1981; 46:8.

39. Kirchgessner M, Reichlmayr-Lais AM. Retention, Absorbierbarkeit und intermediäre Verfügbarkeit von Eisen bei alimentärem Bleimangel. Int Z Vit Ern Forschung 1981; 51:421.

40. Kirchgessner M, Reichlmayr-Lais AM. Changes of iron concentration and iron binding capacity in serum resulting from alimentary lead deficiency. Biol Trace Elem Res 1981; 3:279.

41. Kirchgessner M, Reichlmayr-Lais AM. In vitro-Absorption von Eisen bei Nachkommen von an Blei depletierten Ratten. J Animal Physiol Animal Nutr 1986; 55:24.

42. Reichlmayr-Lais AM, Kirchgessner M. Fe-Retention bei Nachkommen von an Blei depletierten Ratten. J Animal Physiol Animal Nutr 1986; 55:77.

43. Reichlmayr-Lais AM, Kirchgessner M. Zur Essentialität von Blei für das tierische Wachstum. Z Tierphysiol Tierernähr Futtermittelkunde 1981; 46:1.

44. Reichlmayr-Lais AM, Kirchgessner M. Katalse- und Coeruloplasmin-Aktivität im Blut bzw. Serum von Ratten im Blei-Mangel. Zbl Vet Med A 1981; 28:410.

45. Kirchgessner M, Reichlmayr-Lais AM. Konzentrationen verschiedener Stoffwechselmetaboliten im experimentellen Bleimangel. Ann Nutr Metabol 1982; 26:50.

46. Reichlmayr-Lais AM, Kirchgessner M. Aktivität der Enzyme Lipase, Amylase und Carboxypeptidase A im Pankreas von Ratten bei Blei-Mangel. J Animal Physiol Animal Nutr 1986; 56:123.

47. Reichlmayr-Lais AM, Kirchgessner M. Effects of lead deficiency on lipid metabolism. Z Ernährungswiss 1986; 25:165.

48. Eder K, Reichlmayr-Lais AM, Kirchgessner M. Activity of Na-K-ATPase and Ca-Mg-ATPase in red blood cell membranes of lead-depleted rats. J Trace Elem Electrolytes Health Dis 1990; 4:21.

49. Loipführer AM, Reichlmayr-Lais AM, Kirchgessner M. Concentration of free calcium in erythrocytes of lead—depleted rats. J Trace Elem Electrolytes Health Dis 1993; 7:27.

50. Reichlmayr-Lais AM, Kirchgessner M. Konzentrationen verschiedener Mengen- und Spurenelemente in der Milch von Ratten nach Depletion an Blei. J Animal Physiol Animal Nutr 1990; 64:80.

51. Plass DL, Reichlmayr-Lais AM, Kirchgessner M. Depletionsstudien an Ferkeln zur Essentialität des Elements Blei. Agribiol Res 1991; 44:133.

52. Kirchgessner M, Plass DL, Reichlmayr-Lais AM. Untersuchungen zur Essentialität von Blei an post partum abgesetzten Ferkeln. J Animal Physiol Animal Nutr 1991; 66:94.

53. Reichlmayr-Lais AM, Kirchgessner M. Lead. In: Frieden E, ed. Biochemistry of the Essential Ultratrace Elements. New York: Plenum Press, 1984: 367.

54. Goyer RA, Rhyne BC. Pathological effects of lead. In: Richter GW, Epstein EA, eds. Int. Rev. Exp. Path. 12. New York: Academic Press, 1973: 1.

55. Goldberg A. Lead poisoning. As a disorder of heme synthesis. Sem Hematol 1968; 9:424.

56. Dresel EIB, Faulk JE. Studies on the biosynthesis of blood pigments. II. Haem and porphyrin formation in intact chicken erythrocytes. Biochem J 1956; 63:72.

57. Goldberg A, Ashenbrucker H, Cartwright GE, Wintrobe MM. Studies on the biosynthesis of heme in vitro by avian erythrocytes. Blood 1956; 11:821.

58. Piper WN, Tephly TR. Differential inhibition of erythrocyte and hepatic uroporphyrinogen I synthetase activity by lead. Life Sci 1974; 14:873.

59. Alvares AP, Fischbein A, Sassa S, Anderson KE, Kappas A. Lead intoxication: effects of cytochrome P-450 mediated hepatic oxidations. Clin Pharmacol Ther 1976; 19:193.

60. Fischbein A, Alvares AP, Anderson KE, Sassa S, Kappas A. Lead intoxication among demoli-

tion workers, the effect of lead on the hepatic cytochrome P-450 system in humans. J Toxicol Enviorn Health 1977; 3:431.

61. White JM, Harvey DR. Defective synthesis of α- and β-globin chains in lead poisoning. Nature 1972; 236:71.

62. Piddington SK, White JM. The effect of lead on total globin and α- and β-chain synthesis; in vitro and in vivo. Br J Haematol 1974; 27:415.

63. Berk PD, Tschundy DP, Shepley LA, Waggoner JG, Berlin NI. Hematological and biochemical studies in a case of lead poisoning. Am J Med 1970; 48:137.

64. Griggs RC. Lead poisoning: hematologic aspects. Prog Hematol 1964; 4:117.

65. Hasan J, Hernberg SL, Metsälä P, et al. Enhanced potassium loss in blood cells from men exposed to lead. Arch Environ Health 1967; 14:309.

66. Albahary C. Lead and hemopoiesis. The mechanism and consequences of the oerythropathy of occupational lead poisoning. Am J Med 1972; 52:367.

67. Jansen WN, Moreno GD, Bessis MC. An electron microscopic description of basophilic stippling in red cells. Blood 1965; 25:933.

68. Silbergeld EK. Neurochemical and ionic mechanisms of neurotoxicity. In: Prasad KN, Vernadakis A; eds. Mechanism of Actions in Neurotoxic Substances. New York: Raven Press, 1982: 1.

69. Keller CA, Doharty RA. Distribution and excretion of lead in young and adult female mice. Environ Res 1980; 21:217.

70. Landrigan PJ, Baker E, Whitworth R, Feldman RG. Neuroepidemiologic evaluation of children with chronic increased lead absorption. In: Needleman HI., ed. Low Level Lead Exposure. The Clinical Implementation of Current Research. New York: Raven Press, 1980: 17.

71. Needleman HL. Human lead exposure: difficulties and strategies in the assessment of neuropsychological impact. In: Singhal R, Thomas JA, eds. Lead Toxicity. Baltimore, MD: Urban Schwarzenberg, 1980: 1.

72. Mirando EH, Ranasinghe L. Lead encephalopathy in children. Uncommon clinical aspects. Med J Austral 1970; 2:966.

73. Pentschew A. Morphology and morphogenesis of lead encephalopathy. Acta Neuropathol 1965; 5:133.

74. Fullerton PM. Chronic peripheral neuropathy produced by lead poisoning in guinea pigs. J Neuropathol Exp Neurol 1966; 25:214.

75. Rubin RP. The role of calcium in the release of neurotransmitter substances and hormones. Pharmacol Rev 1970; 22:289.

76. Kober TE, Cooper GP. Lead Competitively inhibits calcium-dependent synaptic transmission in the bullfrog sympathetic ganglion. Nature 1976; 262:704.

77. Silbergeld EA, Adler HS. Subcellular mechanisms of lead toxicity. Brain Res 1978; 148:451.

78. Morgan JM. Hyperkalemia and acidosis in lead nephropathy. South Med J 1976; 69:881.

79. Mouw DR, Vander AJ, Cox J, Fleischer N. Acute effects of lead on renal electrolyte excretion and plasma renin activity. Toxicol Appl Pharmacol 1978; 46:435.

80. Goyer RA. The renal tubule in lead poisoning: I: Mitochondrial swelling and aminoaciduria. Lab Invest 1968; 19:71.

81. McAllister RG, Michelakis AM, Sandstead HH. Plasma renin activity in chronic plumbism. Arch Intern Med 1971; 127:919.

82. Moore JF, Goyer RA. Lead-induced inclusion bodies: composition and probable role in lead metabolism. Environ Health Perpect Exp Issue 1974; 7:121.

83. Beevers DG, Erskine E, Robertson M. Blood-lead and hypertension. Lancet 1976; 2:1.

84. Locatelli C, Fagioli F, Bighi C, Scanavini L. Simultaneous determination of trace metals in vegetable materials by alternating current anodic stripping voltammetry and atomic absorption spectroscopy. In: Brätter P, Schramel P, eds. Element Analytical Chemistry in Medicine and Biology—3. Berlin, New York: Walter de Gruyter, 1984: 529.

85. Schulze H. Neue Anwendungsmöglichkeiten der Graphitrohr-Atom-Absorptions-Spektro-

skopie durch den Einsatz von mikrocomputergesteuerten Programmen. GIT Fachz Lab 1979; 23: 42.

86.   Reichlmayr-Lais AM, Eder K, Kirchgessner M. Fatty acid composition of erythrocyte membranes, liver and milk of rats depending on different alimentary lead supply. J Animal Physiol Animal Nutr 1993; 70:109.

87.   Eder K, Reichlmayr-Lais AM, Kirchgessner M. The effect of lead supply on liver phospholipids of lactating rats. J Animal Physiol Animal Nutr 1993; 70:104.

88.   Petering HG. Some observations on the interaction of zinc, copper, and iron metabolism in lead and cadmium toxicity. Environ Health Perspect 1978; 25:141.

89.   Skerfving S. Toxicology of inorganic lead. In: Prasad AS, ed. Essential and Toxic Trace Elements in Human Health and Disease. New York: Alan R. Liss, 1988: 611.

90.   Reichlmayr-Lais AM, Kirchgessner M. Bleimangel bei an Blei depletierten Ratten und deren Nachkommen. J Animal Physiol Animal Nutr 1993; 70:246.

18
Selenium

ROGER A. SUNDE
University of Missouri, Columbia, Missouri

I. INTRODUCTION AND HISTORY

Selenium, with atomic number 34, has been enigmatic since its discovery in 1817 by the Swedish chemist Jons Jakob Berzelius. Its chemistry has proved to be novel and has stimulated chemical research leading to modern developments such as the telephone, transistor, and photocopying machine. In biology, it was initially known to be toxic and later shown to be essential, and first identified as a carcinogen and later shown to be anticarcinogenic. The biochemistry of selenium was elusive, as a biochemical function evaded intense research until in 1972, when selenium was identified as a component of the enzyme glutathione peroxidase (1). Research to unravel the full biochemistry of selenium, however, continues to identify new aspects involving the molecular biology of selenium incorporation into proteins and selenium's role as a regulator of gene expression. This chapter provides a background on selenium history, chemistry, and analysis and then discusses the salient features of the nutritional biochemistry and molecular biology of selenium. The reader is encouraged to seek additional information in a number of recent reviews (2–6) as well as research papers that are cited in the text.

The chemist Berzelius identified selenium in the flue dust of iron pyrite burners in association with tellurium, which had been discovered 35 years before and named after the Latin, *tellus*, for earth. Thus Berzelius named this new element after the Greek, *selene*, for moon; this was a prophetic name choice considering selenium's future use as a photoconductor. The remainder of the nineteenth century saw limited use of selenium in the coloring of glass. Modest doses of cadmium selenite (CdSe) remove the green tint in glass, and additional CdSe and CdS result in the ruby red glass coloring which is still useful today. Selenium's notoriety as a toxic element emerged in the 1930s with the identification as selenium as the causative agent of blind staggers and alkali disease, two different versions

493

of selenium toxicity due to the ingestion of high-selenium-containing plants. These signs of toxicity were very similar to those reported by Marco Polo in his travels to China, dated 1295, where native lore described the loss of mane, tail hair, and hooves in horses due to the ingestion of certain poisonous plants. In 1943, Nelson et al. (7) reported the development of neoplasms in liver of rats ingesting 5 μg Se/g diet, thus earmarking selenium as a carcinogenic agent. Thus it was quite surprising when Klaus Schwarz in 1957 (8) reported that liver necrosis in rats could be prevented by inorganic selenium, leading to the demonstration that selenium is a nutritionally essential trace element. In the 1960s and 1970s, epidemiological data and animal research began to demonstrate that selenium also possesses anticarcinogenic activity. Since the discovery that glutathione peroxidase is a selenoenzyme, at least nine additional selenoenzymes have been identified in higher animals. Reexamination of the report (9) that media selenium is necessary to observe formate dehydrogenase activity in *Escherichia coli* resulted in demonstration that bacterial formate dehydrogenase is a selenoenzyme. At least seven additional selenoenzymes in bacteria have now been discovered, showing that there is a clear biochemical value in employing selenium for certain enzymatic reactions. In the past decade, ongoing research in selenium biochemistry and in disparate areas has identified unique and novel molecular biology in both prokaryotes and eukaryotes for incorporating selenium into proteins. With this kind of history, it is hard to predict what additional novel features will be identified with this trace element named for the moon.

II. CHEMISTRY

Selenium is the third member of Group VIA in the elements in the Periodic Table, following oxygen and sulfur and preceding tellurium and polonium (10). The 34 electrons are distributed with 18 in the argon shell, ten $3d$ electrons, and six electrons in the $4s$ and $4p$ orbitals (see Table 1). These latter electrons can be lost to give the common +6 and +4 oxidation states, whereas a two-electron addition to the $4p$ orbitals completes the octet to yield the −2 oxidation state. This position in the Periodic Table classifies selenium as a metalloid element with both metallic and nonmetallic properties, resulting in its unique chemistry and biochemistry. The natural-abundance molecular weight of selenium is 78.96, and there are six naturally occurring stable isotopes of selenium (isotope, natural abundance %): ^{74}Se, 0.87; ^{76}Se, 9.02; ^{77}Se, 7.58; ^{78}Se, 23.52; ^{80}Se, 49.82; and ^{82}Se, 9.19. ^{74}Se and to a lesser extent ^{76}Se and ^{82}Se have potential for use as stable isotopic tracers in studying selenium metabolism. ^{77}Se has a nuclear spin of ½ and thus has potential use in physical studies of selenium-containing proteins using NMR or EPR analysis. ^{75}Se is a modestly strong γ-emitter with a half-life of 120.4 days and thus is especially suitable for radioactive tracer analysis. ^{75}Se is produced via thermal neutron irradiation of ^{74}Se [$^{74}Se(n,\gamma)^{75}Se$] over 18–24 weeks, and can result in specific activities > 500 Ci/g.

Selenium's position in the Periodic Table thus confers a series of chemical properties (10) that impact strongly on selenium biology. (a) The element undergoes catenation; that is, it forms bonds with itself like carbon, silicon, and sulfur, such that catenated species up to Se_8 can form. Elemental selenium exists in three different forms: the gray-black form of metallic hexagonal selenium, an amorphous white form, and a monoclinic red Se_8 form. Common inorganic forms include selenic acid, H_2SeO_4, with selenium in the +6 oxidation state; selenious acid, H_2SeO_3, in the +4 oxidation state; and H_2Se, hydrogen selenide, in the −2 oxidation state. The faint pink colloidal selenium that forms in neutralized selenocystine-containing solutions is Se_8, indicating decomposition and loss of organic

TABLE 1 Atomic Properties, Electronic Configurations, and Reduction Potentials of Sulfur and Selenium[a]

	S	Se
Atomic weight	32.06	78.96
Atomic number	16	34
Electronic configuration	$[Ne]3s^23p^4$	$[Ar]3d^{10}4s^24p^4$
Van der Waals radius, Å	1.85	2.00
Covalent radius, –M–, Å	1.03	1.17
Ionic radius, M^{2-}, Å	1.90	2.02
Common oxidative states		
−2 M^{2-}	Sulfide	Selenide
0 M^0	Sulfur	Selenium
+4 MO_3^{2-}	Sulfite	Selenite
H_2MO_3	Sulfurous acid	Selenious acid
+6 MO_4^{2-}	Sulfate	Selenate
H_2MO_4	Sulfuric acid	Selenic acid
Bond energy (M–M), kJ/mol	226	172
Bond energy (M–H), kJ/mol	467	276
Bond energy (M–C), kJ/mol	336	243
Ionization potential, eV	10.36	9.75
Electron affinity, eV	2.07	4.21
Electronegativity	2.44	2.48
pK_a: H_2MO_3 (pK_1)	1.81	2.46
HMO_3^{1-} (pK_2)	6.91	7.31
HMO_4^{1-} (pK_2)	1.92	1.92
$H[M]CH_2C(NH_3^+)COO^-$, (pK_2)	8.25	5.24
$H_2MO_3 \rightarrow M^0$, eV	0.45	0.74
$MO_4^{2-} \rightarrow H_2MO_3$, eV	0.17	1.15

[a]From Cotton and Wilkenson (10).

selenium. (b) The empty $d\pi$ orbitals of selenium can be filled by $p\pi$ electrons of oxygen, resulting in multiple "$d\pi-p\pi$ bonds" similar to sulfur, thus permitting the formation of more than four σ bonds to other atoms. The shortness of the Se–O bonds suggests that there must be considerable multiple-bond character to these bonds. (c) Selenium and sulfur have similar radii, such that the ionic radii are 1.9 and 2.0 and the covalent radii are 1.03 and 1.07 Å for sulfur and selenium, respectively. This means that sulfur and selenium compounds cannot be readily distinguished based on bond length. (d) They also have similar electronegativities of 2.44 and 2.48, respectively, giving them similar chemical reactivities. Two aspects of selenium and sulfur chemistry are significantly different, however, permitting ready separation of selenium and sulfur under physiologic conditions. (e) H_2Se is a much stronger acid than $H_2 S$ and at physiologic pH, selenocysteine (Sec) has a pK of 5.24 and is predominantly deprotonated while cysteine, with a pK of 8.25, is largely protonated (11). (f) The reduction potentials of selenious and selenic acid are much greater than those of the analogous sulfur acids, such that in a mixture of sulfite and selenite, selenite is reduced to elemental selenium and sulfite is oxidized to sulfate. The chemistry of selenium thus has important implications for its biochemistry.

A. Photochemistry

Two nonbiological uses of selenium deserve comment. The available $4d$ orbitals and unfilled $4p$ orbitals of selenium convey photochemical properties to selenium. Thus an atomic layer of selenium on a metalloid creates a photocell that can be used in a light meter. The photoconductivity of selenium increases by three orders of magnitude when in the light versus dark because the electrons are stimulated by light to occupy these higher orbitals. Selenium is the photoconductor on photocopying drums; light reflecting from the white surface on a sheet of paper causes the selenium on the drum to become a photoconductor and discharge that region, whereas areas corresponding to dark images are not discharged. Thus charged ink sticks to the drum only corresponding to the dark characters and is applied to paper, resulting in photocopying. Lastly, selenium is used in rectifiers, p-type semiconductors, and superconductors, showing the value of selenium's unique chemistry in electronic and solid-state devices (10).

B. Geochemistry

Selenium appears to be present in the earth's crust at 0.000009% and thus ranks 69th on the list of abundances. The origin in the crust is thought to be principally volcanic and thus selenium can also be present in sedimentary rock arising from weathering of igneous rock (12). Typical rock values are 0.05–0.09 μg Se/g as compared to approximately 300 μg S/g. The principal industrial selenium sources today are as a by-product of electrolytic refining of copper, with selenium building up on the anode slime in this process. Seleniferous rocks containing levels of selenium generally from 2 to 50 μg Se/g can be found from all years and periods, although most seleniferous rocks arise from the cretaceous period ($63–135 \times 10^6$ years ago). Uranium ores can contain as much as 600 μg Se/g selenium. Soils in the Dakotas contain considerably higher concentrations of selenium than in the Midwest, such as Ohio. This selenium in the Dakotas is of volcanic origin, and it has been estimated that there is as much as 0.1 g Se/cm² reaching down to a thickness of 800 m (12). Rainfall of less than 20 in./yr does not leach the soil sufficiently, resulting in soil concentrations of selenium that give rise to alkali disease and the equine problems that were identified in 1860, near Fort Randall. In these areas there are four types of primary indicator plants that actually require selenium, found in the genuses *Astragalus* (vetches), *Xylorhiza* (woody asters), *Oonopsis* (golden weeds), and *Stanleya* (princess plumes). Thus *Astragalus rasemosis* grows well on 9 μg Se/g, whereas *Astragalus succulentus* is adversely affected under the same conditions. Because the sulfides and selenides from magma tend to crystallize and separate out prior to the crystallization of uranium-containing crystals, these selenium indicator plants actually form halos around uranium deposits and have been used to prospect for uranium. The nature of the growth-enhancing effect of selenium in these indicator plants, however, is unknown.

III. ANALYSIS

Literature values for selenium content of tissues and foods tend to be in good agreement, primarily because methods for selenium analysis are not trivial and thus depend on a great deal of expertise, specialized methods and instruments, use of NBS standards, and careful pretreatment of samples prior to analysis. Today the vast majority of selenium analyses are conducted by one of three methods, fluorometric analysis, neutron activation analysis, and specialized atomic absorption spectroscopy using graphite furnace or hydride generation. The first two of these methods will be discussed briefly to illustrate the techniques used.

A. Fluorometric Determination of Selenium

Fluorometric determination of selenium is based on the original work published by J. H. Watkinson in 1966 (13) as modified and described briefly by Oh (14). Samples are predigested overnight in nitric acid, and then digested in a mixture of nitric, sulfuric, and perchloric acids (8 HNO_3:3 H_2SO_4:1 $HClO_4$) in Kjeldahl flasks. Temperatures are slowly increased and never allowed to exceed 200°C, because selenium is volatile above 217°C. The nitric acid and then the white perchloric acid fumes are slowly evolved, leaving the remaining 3 mL of sulfuric acid so that the danger due to explosive dry perchlorates is minimized. Se(VI) is reduced by perchlorate ($HClO_4$) to Se(IV). Subsequent addition of hydrogen peroxide oxidizes any remaining selenide and elemental selenium to Se(IV). Selenium is actually detected by the formation of piazselenol using 2,3-diaminonaphthalene (DAN) under mildly acidic conditions (pH ~ 2.0). Selenious acid reacts with DAN and forms the selenodiazole five-member ring, which can be excited at 365 nm and read at 525 nm. To increase sensitivity, the piazselenol can be quantitatively extracted into a small volume of distilled cyclohexane, resulting in a detection limit of approximately 10 ng selenium. EDTA is included in the reaction mixture prior to cyclohexane extraction to chelate iron, copper, and vanadium, which interfere with this analysis.

B. Neutron Activation Analysis of Selenium

Neutron activation analysis is, by its nature, limited to collaboration with scientists at research reactors for irradiation of samples and subsequent detection of the 162-keV γ rays from [77m]Se, which has a half-life of 17.5 s. The method is described by McKown and Morris (15), and we continue to conduct the analysis following their procedures with minor modifications. Typically, 200–400 mg of sample such as liver are placed in a quartz cuvette and irradiated for 5 s followed by a 15-s decay to let short-lived contaminates decay, and then the sample is counted on the face of a germanium lithium detector for 25 s. The integrated 162-keV peak area correlates linearly with selenium content up to 30 nmol of selenium, with a detection limit of approximately 0.5 nmol for liver. Morris and colleagues use this method routinely to analyze toenails for selenium in epidemiology studies. Diets must be digested because of the interference due to the added minerals; 3–4 g of diet are subjected to nitric acid/percholoric acid digestion, filtered, and then subjected to a reduction/precipitation step using arsenic and hypophosphorous acid (H_3PO_2) to increase specificity.

C. Other Methods

Older gravimetric and titration methods are well reviewed (2). Methods for selenium analysis using graphite furnace atomic absorption spectroscopy (16) or hydride generation and atomic absorption spectroscopy (17) are described. Hydride generation can also be used with inductively coupled mass spectroscopy for isotopic analysis (18). Routine analysis of blood samples by Zeeman atomic absorption spectroscopy is also being proposed (19). Quantitation of inorganic and low-molecular-weight organic selenium compounds may also be of interest. Thin-layer chromatography techniques have been very useful in the past for separation of selenide, selenite, and selenate (20). More recent approaches include simultaneous determination of selenate and trimethylselenonium [Se(CH$_3$)$^+$] by ion-exchange chromatography (21) and/or HPLC-based chromatography to separate selenate and selenite (22).

IV. TISSUE DISTRIBUTION

A. Rats

The selenium concentration and distribution in animals fed selenium-deficient and selenium-adequate diets has been reviewed extensively (2). Estimated total body selenium in the male rat is shown in Table 2. Female rats fed 0.3 µg Se/g diet in commercial rat chow were estimated to contain 49 µg Se (180 µg Se/kg rat) (23). Similar selenium concentrations were found in male rats fed a torula-yeast diet and supplemented with a 0.25-µg Se/g diet as Na$_2$SeO$_3$ (24), except that muscle selenium concentration in the selenite-fed rats was 75% of the level in the female rats fed a commercial diet (which is

TABLE 2 Estimated Total Body Selenium

Tissue or organ	Human[a] Se[b] (mg/kg)	Human[a] Se (mg)	Rat[g] Se[d] (mg/kg)	Rat[g] Se (µg)	R$_f$[h]
Muscle	0.24	6.984	0.12[e]	16.61	1.8
Fatty tissue	0.04	0.504	0.04[f]	0.99	
Skeleton	0.42	4.662	0.15	1.73	
Blood plasma	0.13[c]	0.435	0.52[e]	5.16	1.7
Erythrocytes	0.29[c]	0.670	0.54[e]	4.57	0.6
Brain	0.13	0.221	0.13	0.27	51.9
Liver	0.54	0.864	0.78[e]	10.66	0.9
GI tract	0.21	0.267	0.21[f]	1.26	
Lungs	0.15	0.150	0.38	0.67	
Heart	0.28	0.092	0.37	0.39	1.9
Kidneys	1.09	0.294	1.50	3.28	
Spleen	0.34	0.044	0.45	0.56	
Pancreas	0.30	0.030	0.41[e]	0.36	
Adrenals	—	—	0.70[e]	0.05	21.9
Thymus	—	—	0.23	0.06	
Testes	0.30	0.009	0.92[e]	1.84	22.5
Total		15.2		48.5	

[a]Estimated for a 70-kg male and accounting for 92.6% of the body weight.
[b]From Schroeder et al. (30) unless noted.
[c]Calculated from Levander (197) assuming a 40% hematocrit.
[d]From Behne et al. (23) unless noted.
[e]From Behne et al. (24)
[f]From human data.
[g]Estimated for 309-g male rat fed 0.25 mg Se/kg as Na$_2$SeO$_3$; accounts for 72.8% of body weight but not skin, hair, etc.
[h]Retention factors from Behne et al. (32). The R_f is the percentage of the ^{75}Se retained in each tissue in Se-deficient rats relative to the ^{75}Se retained in Se-adequate rats, when expressed on a per-gram tissue basis.

likely to contain a significant portion of the selenium as selenomethionine). In addition, liver selenium in male rats was 60.5% of the level found in female rats, similar to what we observe (25) due to the higher level of GPX1 in female versus male rat liver (26). These values are comparable to values determined using a combination of direct analysis and stable isotope kinetics (27–29). In selenium-adequate male rats, kidney, testes, and liver contain the highest concentrations of Se. A second group of tissues consisting of adrenal, erythrocytes, spleen, pancreas, plasma, lungs, and hearts contain intermediate selenium concentrations. A third group consisting of thymus, muscle, and brain contained < 0.23 μg Se/g, respectively. Muscle, liver, blood, kidney, and testes contain 83% of the estimated total body selenium.

B. Humans

Estimates of total body content of selenium have been made from cadavers and range between 13.0 and 20.3 mg (30) (see Table 2). Metabolic stable-isotope methodology models predict that total body selenium asymptotically approaches 30 mg, but these studies are based on subjects dosed with 200 μg of Se as the tracer (33). Individuals living in New Zealand or China with considerably lower selenium intakes thus would be presumed to have a much lower total body burden of selenium. Muscle, liver, blood, and kidneys contain 61% of the estimated total body selenium in humans; if skeleton is included, this increases to 91.5%.

C. Selenium Retention

Long-term ^{75}Se tracer studies conducted by Behne and colleagues (32) have made a significant contribution to our understanding of selenium distribution. Multiple-generation selenium-deficient and selenium-adequate rats were fed a selenium-deficient diet containing 2 ng of Se/g of diet or a selenium-adequate diet containing 300 ng of Se/g of diet as of Na_2SeO_3. Adult rats were injected with 30 μCi of [^{75}Se]selenite and killed 42–45 days later. Retention of ^{75}Se when expressed per gram of tissue was highest in erythrocytes, testes, adrenals, and liver, and lowest in muscle and brain. When the ratios of retention of ^{75}Se/g tissue in selenium-deficient rats versus selenium-adequate rats was determined, the highest relative retention (R_f) was found in brain, thyroid, pituitary, and corpora lutea (see Table 2). Approximately half of that level of retention was found in testes, adrenals, and ovaries, and then an order-of-magnitude lower retention was found in heart, muscle, plasma, liver, and erythrocytes. Intermediate retention was observed in eyes, epididymis, femur, hair, kidneys, lungs, thymus, and uterus. When the authors examined retention of total selenium in similarly treated animals, liver in selenium-deficient rats retained only 1% of the level of selenium found in selenium-adequate rats. Muscle was 5%, but pituitary was 35%, testes was 20%, and adrenals was 19%. Behne hypothesized a hierarchy for the long-term distribution of selenium such that brain, endocrine, and reproductive organs have priority over heart, muscle, and liver for selenium in selenium-deficient conditions. The search for the biochemical mechanism to explain this phenomenon is ongoing, but partial solutions are now at hand.

D. Models of Selenium Distribution

Janghorbani and co-workers (28) have hypothesized that whole-body selenium can be divided into two heterogenous biochemical pools. One pool, called the selenite-exchangeable metabolic pool, can be labeled with administered selenite. A second pool, consisting of all compounds present as selenomethionine, will not be labeled with selenite. The underlying rationale for this work was to develop a model for accurate determination of selenium status in humans using in-vivo isotope dilution. The concept was to use stable isotopes and oral administration of the tracer and take a single blood sample close to the time of isotope administration. In rats fed diets with selenium from natural sources, total-body selenium was approximately 54–66 μg; in weanling rats fed diets supplemented with selenite, the estimates were approximately 23 μg of Se in rats weighing ~143 g (29), indicating comparable total-body stores of selenium on a weight basis with the data in Table 2. The measured selenite exchangeable pool for the total animal accounted for about 36% of the endogenous selenium in animals fed selenite. Other important aspects were that skeletal muscle contributed 41% of the endogenous total selenium, but only 17% of the selenite exchangeable pool, whereas liver contributed 10% of the endogenous selenium but 19% of the selenite exchangeable pool. The same numbers for kidneys were 5 and 12, and plasma numbers were 7 and 13, respectively, showing that muscle selenium is far less exchangeable than selenium in other tissues (29).

In humans, Patterson and colleagues (33–35) have conducted some careful modeling experiments with humans given a single oral 200-μg dose of ^{74}Se and have developed a model of selenium metabolism that estimates the flux of selenium among tissue compartments (see below). Selenium absorption was nearly complete in these subjects, 84% for selenite and 98% for selenomethionine. After 12 days of dosing, about 35% and 15% of the administered selenite and selenomethionine was excreted, respectively, suggesting that the decreased selenomethionine excretion was caused by a higher reutilization of selenium from the peripheral tissues.

V. METABOLISM

A. Dietary Form of Selenium

The form of selenium in foods and feeds arises from metabolic components of plant and animal origin, although we cannot discount the inorganic forms which are commonly used to supplement animal feeds and to provide inexpensive selenium in "vitamin" pills. Numerous references including Ref. 2 have summarized the older literature in this field, and thus we shall only briefly review this information. In large part, most of the concern about the particular dietary form of selenium is a moot academic point, because selenium absorption from most sources is very high; homeostasis at the organism level does not occur via regulation of absorption.

The majority of selenium in non-selenium-accumulator plants is selenomethionine. Literature reports suggest that at least 50% of the selenium in wheat (36) and up to 70% of the selenium in alfalfa (37) is present as selenomethionine. More recent chromatographic analysis of selenium in plant-derived feedstuffs confirms that the majority of the selenium is present as selenomethionine (230). In selenium-accumulator plants, the selenium is accumulated as a detoxification product as selenium analogs of intermediates in sulfur amino acid metabolism, such as selenocystathionine and methylselenocysteine.

The most common inorganic form of selenium used historically in animal diets has been sodium selenite (Na_2SeO_3), although selenate is increasingly being used because without the free electron pair, selenate is far less likely than selenite to oxidize other components of the diet. The majority of the selenium in animal products from animals fed usual levels of dietary selenium will be present as selenoproteins and thus mostly seleno-cysteine (38). Thomson et al. (39) injected rabbits with selenomethionine and then used rabbit kidney selenium to study the metabolism of selenium in rats. They found that the kidney selenium was metabolized more like selenite than selenomethionine. Only elemen-tal selenium, dimethylselenide, and the mercury-selenium complex in tuna are forms of selenium that are basically not available for conversion to biologically active selenium forms. Acid digestion of tuna meal makes its selenium equivalent to selenite (40).

B. Absorption

Thomson and Stewart (41) found that rats absorb 95–98% of an oral dose of seleno-methionine and 91–93% of an oral dose of selenite. Monogastric animals are reported to have higher percentage absorption than ruminants (42). In humans, high rates of absorption of both selenite and selenomethionine are also reported (43,44); selenite and seleno-methionine absorption were 84% and 98% in kinetic modeling experiments (33,34) with doses of 200 μg, illustrating that this high absorption rate is not a microtracer phenomenon. Thus, under physiologic conditions, selenium homeostasis is clearly not regulated by absorption and thus is likely to be regulated by urinary excretion of selenium (45).

C. Transport

Selenomethionine is actively transported by the same system that transports methionine, as would be expected because the covalent radii of selenium and sulfur are virtually identical, so these species cannot be distinguished by the participating enzymes. Similarly, selenate is actively absorbed in common with sulfate and is dependent on the sodium gradient maintained by Na^+K^+-ATPase (46). In contrast, selenocysteine and selenite are not ac-tively transported and uptake is not inhibited by the corresponding sulfur analog (47,48).

In summary, we know very little about the selenium-specific transport mechanisms involved in selenocysteine and selenite uptake from intestine, but it is clear that they are not rate limiting under normal conditions. A recent rat experiment by Boza et al. (49) used intrinsically labeled ^{76}Se in yeast, extrinsically labeled ^{74}Se in a test meal, or tracer ^{75}Se as selenite in a test meal, and found retention values ranging from 76% to 83% under the same conditions. This clearly indicates that the dietary form of selenium has minimal overall biological impact on selenium uptake under normal conditions.

D. Excretion

Early workers identified expired dimethylselenide, urinary trimethylselenonium ion, and an unidentified urinary selenium compound as the usual excretory forms of selenium (50). Both the size of the dose as well as the selenium status of the animal influences the form and amount of urinary selenium excretion (51). Thus trimethylselenonium constitutes only 10% of urinary selenium in rats of low selenium status, whereas it is the major urinary selenium form in animals ingesting supernutritional levels of selenium (52). More recent studies (27) showed that in animals fed 0.25 μg Se/g diet, trimethylselenonium ion constituted only 2% of urinary selenium; administration of additional selenium in the water (4 μg Se/mL) increased trimethylselenonium ion to 35–45% of urinary selenium within 3 days of selenium supplementation. In humans, trimethylselenonium ion also is a minor component of urine, with estimates that between 7% and 17% of urinary selenium is present as trimethylselenonium ion (53). Twelve days after administration of 200 μg of selenium to selenium-adequate adult humans, 17% of tracer selenite and 11% of tracer seleno-methionine appears in the urine (34). When pharmacologic doses of selenium are injected into rats, selenium is expired in the breath as dimethylselenide; 50% of selenite selenium and 35% of selenomethionine selenium is expired as dimethylselenide in the first 24 h after rats are injected with 5 mg Se/kg body weight (54).

E. Kinetic Models

Numerous researchers have conducted elegant studies using tracer ^{75}Se or stable isotopes to monitor selenium flux in metabolism. Pioneering work was done by Marion Robinson and colleagues (43) in both rats and humans. Later, additional modeling in humans and rats culminated in the definition of the selenite exchangeable pool (29,53), as reviewed above. An elegant full application of this technique has been demonstrated by Patterson and colleagues (33–35). Their current model is summarized in Figure 1, with a gastrointestinal tract compartment, four plasma compartments, a liver/pancreas compartment, and one or two tissue compartments that differ in turnover rate of selenium. The percentages between

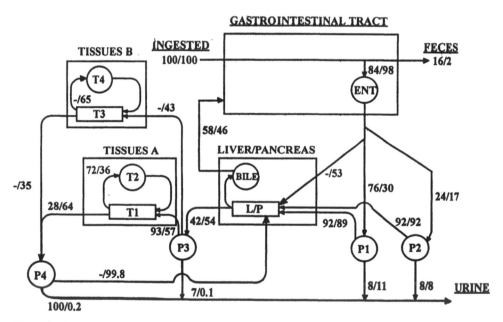

FIGURE 1 Kinetic model of human selenium metabolism. This model is modified from that of Swanson et al. (34) and Patterson et al. (33), showing the following compartments: gastrointestinal tract, enterocyte, four plasma compartments P1, P2, P3, and P4, liver-pancreas, and two tissue compartments, A (faster turnover) and B (slower turnover). Arrows between the compartments represent pathways of fractional transport; numbers indicate the fractional flux (in percent) moving from one compartment to the next as calculated from the fractional rate of flow from the preceding compartment to the next given. The first number indicates the fractional flux for selenite selenium, and the second the fractional flux for selenomethionine selenium. Subjects were fed normal diets with adequate concentrations of selenium and given 200 μg of stable isotopic tracer, and kinetic disappear-ance was determined over a 4-week period on plasma, urine, and fecal samples.

organs indicate the flux from the proceeding component to the indicated compartment or subcompartment as calculated by the percentage rate for that route relative to all routes arising from the compartment or subcompartment.

For selenite selenium, 84% of selenite selenium is absorbed, and a cumulative 18% is excreted in the feces over 12 days after ingestion. An additional 17% is excreted in the urine, with the maximum rate of excretion within the first 2 h after ingestion. Of absorbed selenium, the majority (76%) moves into the plasma P1 compartment, which peaks about 2 h after ingestion and disappears with a $t_{1/2}$ of ~20 min. The remainder of the absorbed selenium has a delayed appearance in plasma P2 with a peak at about 10 h and a disappearance $t_{1/2}$ of ~3 h. In the model, more than 90% of P1 and P2 selenium moves into the liver. In humans, some 58% of the liver selenium from selenite returns to the GI tract via the bile, whereas selenium flux through the bile is much reduced in the rat (33). Liver selenium is released to the plasma P3 compartment, which peaks 13 h after dosing but has a slow disappearance $t_{1/2}$ of 12 h. Virtually all P3 selenium moves into a single tissue compartment in the selenite model. Some 72% of the tissue selenium is recycled within the tissue; all of the selenium released from the tissue compartment enters the plasma P4 compartment (peak at > 50 h and $t_{1/2}$ of 6.6 days). With selenite, the model indicates that P4 selenium is not recycled but is excreted in the urine.

For selenomethionine selenium, there are several distinct differences in the model as compared to selenite (34). Absorption is 98%, with only 4% of the dose released in the feces and 15% of the dose released in the urine within the 12 days following ingestion. Unlike selenite, just over half of the selenomethionine appearing in the portal circulation is immediately cleared by the liver, as would be expected for an amino acid. The model also requires a large second tissue B compartment that represents tissues such as muscle, with slow selenium turnover. Less than half of the P3 selenium is taken up by the tissue B compartment, but 65% of that selenium is recycled within the compartment whereas only 36% of the tissue A selenium is recycled within the compartment. Lastly, virtually all of the selenium in the P4 compartment from selenomethionine is recycled back to the liver, whereas all of the selenite-derived selenium is released to the urine. The recycling pathway and the second tissue compartment were necessary to account for whole-body turnover of selenomethionine selenium, which was 2.5 times slower than for selenite selenium ($t_{1/2}$ of 252 days versus 102 days, respectively).

The relationship between these modeling compartments and the real tissues/organs is clearly not established. Disappearance $t_{1/2}$ for selenomethionine was more rapid for P1 and P3, but slower for P2 and P4 as compared to selenite (10 min, 4 h, 6 h, and 0.76 day for P1, P2, P3, and P4, respectively, for selenomethionine, versus 20 min, 3 h, 12 h, and 6.6 days, respectively, for selenite). The rapid clearance of P4 [Se]Met by liver suggests that the preponderance of this species is selenomethionine, whereas P4 selenite appears to be a low-molecular-weight (inorganic?) form destined for urinary secretion. Plasma selenoprotein P, secreted from liver and heart, has a $t_{1/2}$ of 4 h (55), suggesting that the P2 compartment represents selenoprotein P. This suggests that selenium in this compartment is also taken up rapidly by liver but then nearly quantitatively excreted as selenoprotein P. The secreted P3 component thus could readily represent plasma GPX3, which is secreted from human liver as well as kidney (56). The nature of the P1 compartment is least readily assigned; a combination of selenide release following selenite reduction in either the enterocyte or erythrocyte might generate this species, which then disappears with a $t_{1/2}$ of 10–20 min.

This kinetic model clearly demonstrates the potential and the limitations of using modeling to unravel the metabolism of a mineral element. It does provide very useful information about selenium flux among various compartments. Additional work to better characterize the nature of the plasma components will make these models stronger and more useful.

VI. METABOLIC PATHWAYS OF SELENIUM

Because of the similarities of sulfur and selenium chemistry, selenium metabolism was initially assumed to follow the pathways of sulfur metabolism. While the covalent radius and the ability to use $d\pi-p\pi$ multiple bonding make selenium and sulfur similar metabolically, the lower reduction potential of sulfur versus selenium means that selenium tends to

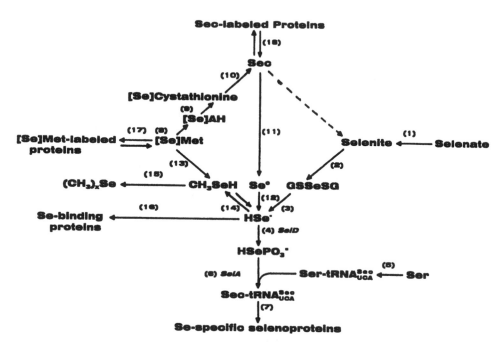

FIGURE 2 Proposed metabolic pathways of selenium: path 1, selenate reduction to selenite via APSe or PAPSe; path 2, GSH nonenzymatic reduction of selenite; path 3, glutathione reductase-catalyzed reduction; path 4, selenophosphate synthase or SELD; path 5, seryl-tRNA synthase; path 6, selenocysteine synthase or SELA; path 7, translational selenocysteine insertion, mediated by tRNA[Sec] and SELB at position specified by UGA codon; path 8, transmethylation resulting in Se-adenosyl homocysteine (SeAH); path 9, cystathionine β-synthetase; path 10, cystathionine γ-lyase; path 11, selenocysteine lyase; path 12, nonenzymatic reduction via GSH; path 13, transamination pathway resulting in methane selenol; path 14, S-methyltransferase; path 15, thioether S-methyltransferase; path 16, hypothetical selenide binding to proteins; path 17, selenomethionine acylation of tRNA[Met] followed by incorporation at positions specified by an AUG codon; path 18, selenocysteine incorporation into tRNA[Cys] by the regular synthetases followed by incorporation in place of cysteine at UGU and UGC codons.

be reduced in biological metabolism whereas sulfur tends to be oxidized. Thus, there are some dramatic differences in sulfur and selenium metabolism as well. The known selenium-specific pathways can be combined with sulfur pathways into the diagram of selenium metabolism shown in Figure 2. This is an updated version of earlier diagrams (4,47,57–60).

A. Inorganic Selenium Metabolism

Little is known about the selenate-to-selenite conversion shown in path 1, but by analogy to sulfur metabolism, it is thought to involve APSe- or PAPSe-activated intermediates (61). One of the best-characterized pathways of selenium metabolism is that of selenite reduction. Ganther, in 1966 (62), provided clear evidence that mouse liver synthesizes dimethylselenide. Selenite is reduced nonenzymically (path 2) by glutathione to elemental Se^0 in the form of seleno-diglutathione (GS-Se-SG), which in the absence of oxygen is further reduced by glutathione reductase (path 3) to selenide (63). Selenide can be methylated (path 14) using SAM by either microsomal or cytosolic methyl transferases in liver to form methaneselenol and (path 15) dimethylselenide or trimethylselenonium ion (64). Carrithers and Hoffman (65) have recently identified specific thio S-methyltransferases (E.C. 2.1.1.9) and thioether S-methyltransferases (E.C. 2.1.1.96), which will catalyze this sequential methylation of selenols as well as thiols. It is clear that liver is able to catalyze these reactions, but lung and kidney may also have activities.

Selenide is proposed to be the species that binds to selenium-binding proteins (path 16) such as the 14-kDa fatty acid-binding protein and the 56-kDa selenium-binding protein. Alternatively, it is the substrate for selenophosphate synthetase (path 4) for tRNA-mediated synthesis of selenoproteins (paths 5, 6, and 7). These latter two steps (paths 6 and 7) are the transitional steps that convert inorganic selenium back to the organic forms of selenium that are found in mammalian tissues.

The selenite reduction pathway is an important pathway because erythrocytes rapidly take up and metabolize selenite using GSH, and then transport the selenium back to the plasma (66). The selenium that leaves the erythrocytes has been shown to be selenide (67); interestingly, this selenide binds with cadmium to a 130-kDa plasma protein that has been otherwise unidentified.

B. Organic Selenium Metabolism

Dietary selenomethionine in higher animals is readily incorporated into protein (path 17) (160) as selenomothionine is esterified to methioninyl-tRNA by the methioninyl-tRNA synthase at rates only slightly less favorable than for methionine itself (K_m 11 μM for [Se]Met versus 7 μM for Met) (68). Selenomethionine is readily metabolized to [Se]-adenosyl methionine (SeAM) (69) and SeAM is reported to be a better methyl donor than SAM in mammalian systems (path 8) (70). [Se]-adenosyl homocysteine (SeAH) is a ready substrate for cystathionine β-synthase and cystathionine γ-lyase (paths 9 and 10) and is thus readily converted to selenocysteine in mammalian tissues. Selenocysteine may be degraded with release of selenite, analogous to sulfur metabolism, but because of the reductive nature of selenium metabolism, selenide release is far more likely. Soda and coworkers have identified a selenocysteine-specific enzyme, selenocysteine lyase (path 11), which releases elemental selenium directly, which is then reduced nonenzymatically to selenide (path 12) by glutathione or other thiols (71). Lastly, the methionine transamination pathway (path 13) reported by Benevenga and co-workers (72) should readily be able to metabolize selenomethionine; selenium is a better leaving group in the γ-lyase-catalyzed α,γ elimination, which releases methaneselenol (73).

Yeast and bacteria assimilate sulfur using *o*-acetyl serine and ATP-activated sulfur, and it is likely that organisms with this system also assimilate selenium via the sulfur pathways. In addition, there is clear evidence for unique selenium assimilation pathways in bacteria and in mammals. Careful nutritional experiments as well as use of sulfur metabolism mutations, however, indicate that selenium assimilation by yeast may simply follow sulfur metabolism (74). Figure 2 organizes what we do know about selenium metabolism and suggests additional areas that need to be considered in proposed modeling and nutritional evaluation of selenium metabolism in humans. As can be seen, there appears to be specific and perhaps ready interconversion between organic and inorganic forms of selenium, thus permitting reutilization of selenium.

C. Selenomethionine Metabolism

Schwarz and Foltz (75) reported that selenite and selenomethionine have equivalent abilities to prevent liver necrosis in rats. The above diagram of selenium metabolism (Fig. 2) suggests that there is strong interaction between methionine and selenomethionine in terms of incorporation into proteins as methionine analogs. In a series of experiments we have demonstrated that insufficient levels of dietary methionine result in decreased availability of dietary selenomethionine for synthesis of GPX1 and that there is as much as a 3.5-fold increase in muscle selenium in these animals as compared to animals fed adequate or high levels of dietary methionine (100% or 200% of the dietary sulfur amino acid requirement). Under the same conditions, GPX1 activity was decreased after 20 days to about half of that in methionine-supplemented animals in plasma, liver, and muscle (60,76). Even in animals supplemented with adequate or high levels of dietary methionine, the stored selenium, presumably present as selenomethionine, only provides transient protection against selenium deficiency in animals fed a selenium-deficient diet (60). These experiments suggest that selenomethionine may not be the optimal form of selenium to be used for selenium supplementation in humans, because conversion of selenomethionine to biochemically active selenium may be impaired under conditions of inadequate dietary methionine intake or of increased protein synthesis and/or catabolism, such as in burn patients.

VII. SELENIUM INCORPORATION INTO SELENOPROTEINS

Early workers studying selenium metabolism recognized that the analogous sulfur amino acid forms were present in both bacteria and in higher animals, and that these selenoamino acids are incorporated into proteins in place of the sulfur residues. Even after the identification of GPX1 as a selenium-containing enzyme in 1973, researchers were unable to identify the nature of the selenium moiety in GPX1. Rotruck and colleagues (1) noted that selenium was not dialyzed out of the enzyme, nor would dialysis with inorganic selenium restore GPX1 activity when selenium-deficient hemolysates were incubated with selenite alone or with selenite and glutathione or dithiothreitol. A breakthrough occurred when Stadtman and colleagues (61) identified the selenium moiety in protein A of clostridial glycine reductase as selenocysteine, leading Tappel and colleagues (77) and Wendel and colleagues

(78) to identify selenocysteine in GPX1. In 1979, Hawkes (79) reported preliminary results suggesting that selenocysteine is incorporated directly into GPX1 using a Sec-specific tRNA. This apparent translational process for incorporating selenium into GPX1 was in conflict with the data from isotope dilution experiments (57), which indicated that selenite and selenide are more readily incorporated into GPX1 than was preformed selenocysteine. Thus, a posttranslational or cotranslational modification of an amino acid already present in the peptide backbone appeared to be the mechanism that was used to synthesize the selenocysteine moiety in GPX1. Contributions from three research laboratories provided the answer to this conundrum.

A. tRNA

Textbook assignment of the 64 codons involved in protein translation designates 61 of the possible 64 triplet codons as encoding the 20 amino acids. Three codons, UAA (ochre), UAG (amber), and UGA (opal), serve as stop or nonsense codons. It is obvious that the genetic code is degenerate, with six codons specifying leucine, arginine, and serine. It is also clear that codons can have dual functions, as AUG specifies N-formyl methionyl-tRNA for chain initiation and methionyl-tRNA for methionine incorporation. In addition to the usual tRNAs, a number of nonsense suppressor tRNAs have been characterized extensively in bacteria and yeasts, and are also found in higher eukaryotes (80). These rarer tRNAs cause readthrough of termination codons, resulting in larger polypeptides. Research in this area was predicated on the possibility that human disease might result from nonsense mutations which could be elevated by gene therapy. This concept remains exciting, with potential selenium roles in the process. One of the most interesting naturally occurring nonsense suppressor tRNAs comprises about 1–3% of the total seryl tRNAs in mammalian avian and *Xenopus* tissues; see Figure 3. The mammalian suppressor tRNAs are 90 nucleotides long as compared to the usual 76 nucleotide tRNAs (81). They have extra base

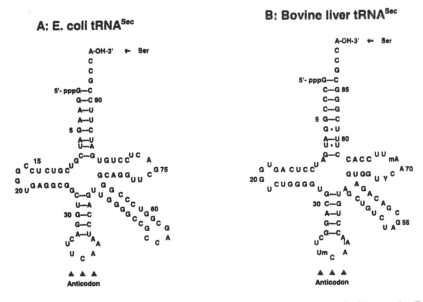

FIGURE 3 Prokaryotic (A) and eukaryotic (B) selenocysteinyl-tRNA$_{UCA}$. A. *E. coli* tRNA[sec] consisting of 76 nucleotides (227); B. Bovine liver tRNA[sec] consisting of 90 nucleotides (81).

pairs in the acceptor stem of the tRNA (8–9 versus the usual 7 base pairs) and a longer *d* loop (with approximately 16 bases and 5 base pairs as compared to the usual 5 bases and 0 base pairs), and a UCA anticodon. These suppressor tRNAs read the UGA codon in protein synthesis and some have the unique characteristic of forming phosphoseryl-tRNA in the presence of a kinase from bovine mammary tissue (80).

B. Serine as the Selenocysteine Precursor

Sunde and Evenson perfused isolated rat liver with ^{14}C and ^{3}H-labeled amino acids to study the mechanism used to incorporate selenium into GPX1 (59). After 4 h of labeling, GPX1 was purified to homogeneity and derivitized to form carboxymethyl selenocysteine, the proteins hydrolyzed, and then the specific activity of the amino acids in purified GPX1, including selenocysteine, was determined. They found that [^{14}C]cystine labeled GPX1 without incorporation into selenocysteine. [U-^{14}C]serine or [3-^{3}H]serine resulted in specific incorporation of labeled serine into serine residues and into selenocysteine residues in GPX1. The nearly equal specific activity of serine and selenocysteine indicated that the serine pool was used both to acylate seryl tRNA and to synthesize selenocysteine, further suggesting that the selenocysteine moiety of GPX1 is formed cotranslationally.

C. UGA Codon Specifies Selenocysteine

At the Beatson Cancer Institute in Glasgow, P. H. Harrison was studying erythroid cell differentiation in a model for regulation of gene expression. In 1986 this group reported that they had cloned and sequenced a 19-kDa protein from murine erythroblasts because it was expressed at higher levels in mouse erythroblasts than in erythroid stem cells. Initial attempts to identify the cloned gene by nucleotide sequence or amino acid sequence homology did not identify any related sequences. When GPX1 amino acid sequences were added to the database, it revealed that they had serendipitously cloned GPX1. The mouse gene encoded a 201-amino acid polypeptide including a UGA codon at the position of the selenocysteine at residue 47 in the middle of the open reading frame in the first of two exons making up the gene (82). Chambers and colleagues puzzled over the implied mechanism for a termination UGA codon specifying translational insertion of selenocysteine into a growing polypeptide chain, and they noted Hatfield's serine suppressor tRNA (80) as a potential player in this mechanism. Sunde and Evenson's (59) discovery that serine provided the carbon skeleton for the selenocysteine moiety, in combination with the UGA codon and the suppressor tRNA, suggested a mechanism of cotranslational selenocysteine incorporation at the UGA codon mediated by one of these unique tRNAs. These tRNAs are now designated tRNA$_{UCA}^{Ser \rightarrow Sec}$ or tRNA$_{UCA}^{Sec}$. Confirmation that selenocysteines in selenoproteins are specified by UGA was rapid. Bock, Stadtman, and co-workers reported that the selenocysteine in formate dehydrogenase was specified by UGA in the open reading frame of the *E. coli* gene (83), extending this apparent mechanism to prokaryotes.

D. Cotranslational Selenium Incorporation

The mechanism used to insert selenium as selenocysteine at the position specified by UGA can be inferred from the corresponding prokaryotic mechanisms used to insert selenium to formate dehydrogenase and glycine reductase. This area has been reviewed recently by Stadtman (84). Four unique genes have been identified in prokaryotes that are essential for selenium incorporation; these genes are designated selA, selB, selC, and selD. The starting reactants are selenide, serine, and ATP.

The first unique player is the sel C gene product, which is tRNA$^{Sec}_{UCA}$ (85), which is a 90-nucleotide tRNA with a UCA anticodon. Serine, the source of the carbon skeleton, is esterified to this novel tRNA by the usual cellular seryl-tRNA syntheses (path 5). The major mammalian tRNA^{Sec}s apparently are not edited as previously reported and exist as shown in Figure 3, including a methylcarboxy-methylated uridine at the 5' position of the UCA anticodon, as well as partial ribosylmethylation on the same residue (81).

Selenide, arising from the selenite reduction pathway or selenocysteine lyase or the methionine transamination pathway, is converted to selenophosphate by the selD gene product, selenophosphate synthetase (path 4). In bacteria this is a 37-kDa species (86). Selenophosphate is very labile, but its nature was identified by ^{31}P-NMR (87), and seleno-phosphate is a substrate for both synthesis of selenocysteinyl-tRNA and for formation of rare, 2-selenouridine bases found in tRNAs. The reaction appears to proceed with initial formation of an enzyme pyrophosphate intermediate with liberation of AMP. Subsequent addition of selenide forms selenophosphate containing the γ-phosphate of ATP and libera-tion of orthophosphate arising from the β-phosphate group (84). Human selD has been cloned as well, and has only 30% sequence identity with the bacterial protein (88). It has an apparent molecular weight of 45 kDa, and alignment with the E. coli peptide reveals that both contain a conserved ATP/GTP-binding consensus sequence.

Selenocysteine is actually synthesized by a novel mechanism catalyzed by the selA gene product, selenocysteine synthase (path 6). In E. coli it has a subunit molecular weight of 51 kDa, has a native weight of approximately 600 kDa, and contains pyridoxal phos-phate. It catalyzes dehydration of L-serine while attached to the tRNA to form aminoacrylyl-tRNA^{Sec}, followed by a 2–3 addition of selenium to form the selenocysteine moiety still esterified to the tRNA (89).

The fourth required element is a 68-kDa selB gene product, SELB, that is similar to elongation factor EF-Tu. Native EF-Tu has a molecular weight of 43 kDa. The SELB protein is very specific for Sec-tRNA and for the stem loop structure, thus serving to increase the concentration of the Sec-tRNA on the mRNAs. The formation of a quaternary SELB-GTP-Sec tRNA-mRNA complex is hypothesized to tether the selenocysteine at just the appropriate position to facilitate the specificity of selenocysteine insertion. Removal of an extra base pair in the acceptor stem, or a decrease in the size of the d loop, drastically reduces the specificity.

Recognition of UGA as a selenocysteine codon rather than a stop codon in bacteria requires a fifth element, a stem-loop secondary structure in the RNA immediately down-stream from the UGA (90). The stable secondary structure is called a pSECIS or prokary-otic selenocysteine insertions sequence (see Fig. 4). It allows the SELB-binding site to protrude into the channel between the ribosomal units, thus placing the SELB-GTP-Sec-tRNA^{Sec} in a favorable position to interact with the approaching ribosomal A site; see Figure 5 (91). The pSECIS secondary structure consists of 38 nucleotides immediately following the UGA arranged in a stem loop with a 4-base pair GGUC sequence in the loop. Mutation of the second G to a C disrupts binding to SELB. Various bulges (unpaired bases) distort the α-helix and give rise to two domains that are important for formation of the quaternary complex. The first domain comprises the UGA codon, and the second domain is located within the apical loop of the mRNA hairpin structure. The primary structure of the pSECIS in a second formate dehydrogenase is vastly different, but it folds into an almost

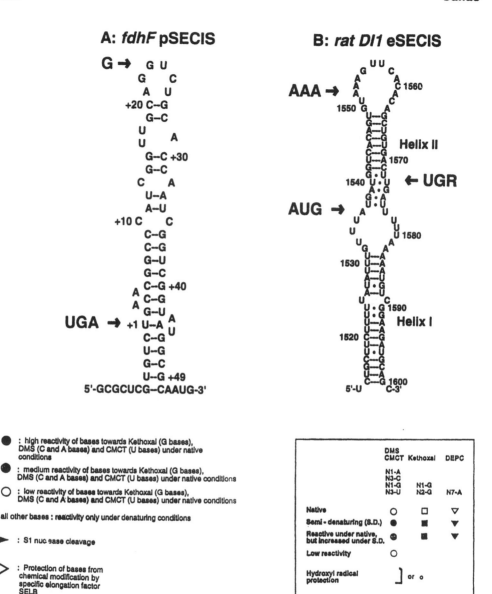

FIGURE 4 *Seleno*Cysteine *I*nsertion *S*equence (SECIS) elements. A. Prokaryotic pSECIS element that resides just 3′ of the UGA within the *E. coli fdhF* coding region (92). B. Eukaryotic eSECIS element that resides in the 3′UTR of rat DI1 (95).

identical pSECIS, illustrating the importance of secondary structure in the function of the pSECIS element. The K_d of the pSECIS for SELB is approximately 30 nM (92).

The fifth element required for selenium insertion into mammalian selenoproteins is a stemloop structure in the 3′UTR (untranslated region) of the messenger RNAs (93) (Fig. 4). Working with fusion chimera of GPX1 and selenium-dependent type 1 5′ deiodinase (DI1), Berry and Larsen found that the rat GPX1 3′UTR is equally effective as the native DI1 3′UTR in catalyzing insertion of selenium into DI1. An 8-base deletion in the loop of the

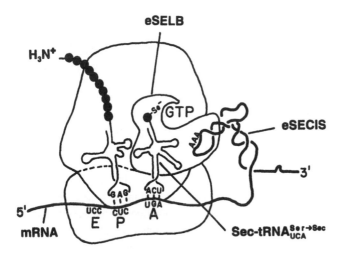

FIGURE 5 Model for the ribosomal-mRNA-SECIS-SELB complex, modified from (91).

stem loop was sufficient to eliminate selenocysteine insertion. Thus Berry identified and named this 3'UTR structure a eSECIS element, for *SelenoCysteine Insertion Sequence* (93), and in mammalian cells, the eSECIS element is necessary for incorporation of selenium. Subsequent analysis indicates that two similar 3'UTR eSECIS elements are present in plasma selenoprotein P mRNA (94) and one eSECIS is present in GPX4.

The consensus eSECIS element is a stem loop structure with a variable loop consisting of 7–10 unpaired bases including a consensus AAA sequence (Fig. 4). 5' to the loop is a consensus AUG sequence, and 3' to the loop is a consensus UGR sequence. The second and third As in the AAA sequence appears to be especially important, as do the AUG and UGR sequences, but base-pair changes in the intervening stem do not affect efficacy for mediating selenium incorporation (94). The distance between the UGA codon and the loop of the eSECIS ranges from 548 bases for rat GPX to 1145 for rat DI1, 1409 for human DI1, and 1239/1272 nucleotides from the first UGA to the midpoint of the first stem loop in human/rat Sel-P and 1638/1653 nucleotides to the second stem loop, respectively; the shortest distance is 303 nucleotides between the tenth UGA and the first Sel-P stem loop. Mutations which inserted an additional 1.5 kb between the eSECIS and the UGA do not impair selenium incorporation relative to wild-type expression (94).

The specific secondary structure of these eSECIS elements can have an impact on relative rates of selenocysteine insertion. When different eSECIS elements are fused to the same DI1 coding region and expressed in transfected cells, the resulting DI1 activity permits direct comparisons. Relative to DI1 (relative activity 1.0), rat GPX1 eSECIS has an activity of 0.46, Sel-P eSECIS1 has an activity of 2.9, Sel-P eSECIS2 has an activity of 0.9, and the full-length 3' UTR of Sel-P containing both eSECIS elements has an activity of 3.7. Detailed experimental study of the secondary structure of the eSECIS elements using RNase protection and chemical probing has resulted in a model eSECIS (Fig. 4) characterized by a stem-loop structure with two helical regions separated by an internal loop. The top helical region ends in a quartet motif of non-Watson-and-Crick base pairs, containing the AUG and UGR sequences, which results in a more than >90° kink in the stem loop. The α-helix continues and ends with an apical loop containing the AAA triad (95). This interesting model awaits confirmation but is an exciting step forward in our understanding of the molecular biology of selenium insertion.

The search for a eukaryotic elongation factor analogous to prokaryotic SELB has not yet been successful. Shen et al. (96) and Hubert et al. (97) have used mobility-shift assays to find proteins that have some specificity for binding to eSECIS element. Shen et al. have identified two proteins with molecular weights of 55 kDa and 65 kDa that appear to bind specifically to the eSECIS element. Hubert et al. have identified a single 60- to 65-kDa protein with preliminary data suggesting that this eSECIS-binding protein binds to either DI1 mRNA as well as GPX1 mRNA. Identification of the protein(s) involved in this process in eukaryotes will be exciting.

In prokaryotes, optimum insertion of selenocysteine requires a UGA immediately 5′ to the established loop structure to recode the termination codon to a selenocysteine insertion codon. The primary structure must concomitantly encode the necessary amino acid residues immediately downstream of the selenocysteine, thus dramatically curtailing the ability to conserve pSECIS secondary structure. This strongly suggests that there is a great deal of diversity in primary structure of pSECIS elements. In contrast, eukaryotes have adapted a 3′UTR eSECIS element which has as high as 37% sequence identity between two distinct selenoproteins. This also suggests that there are few or no additional requirements for selenocysteine insertion beyond the in-frame UGA in the open reading frame of a mRNA for a protein. There is, however, very limited evidence to suggest that this is the case. Shen and colleagues (98) chose an unrelated 25-kDa GTP-binding protein, mutated it to contain an in-frame UGA, and fused it to the 3′UTR of GPX1. Separation of immunoprecipitated, labeled GTP-binding proteins revealed that the fusion constructs incorporated ^{75}Se into appropriately sized polypeptide product, implying that an in-frame UGA and eSECIS stem loop are all that is necessary and sufficient in a particular mRNA to specify selenocysteine incorporation. Care must be taken in interpreting these results, however, as nonspecific insertion of selenocysteine at UGA may be mediated by a tRNA^{Cys}, as has been shown in *E. coli* SELD mutants (84). Considerable difficulty in expressing wild-type selenoproteins in expression vectors, as well as unrelated proteins containing an in-frame UGA fused to a 3′UTR-GPX eSECIS element, suggests that there is considerably more complexity in this process (R. A. Sunde, unpublished results).

VIII. MAMMALIAN SELENOPROTEINS

The nature of mammalian selenoproteins has been reviewed recently at the 5th International Symposium on Selenium in Biology in Medicine (6). These proteins are listed in Table 3 and reviewed below. All confirmed selenoenzymes to date catalyze redox reactions, showing that evolution is taking advantage of the unique chemistry of selenium.

A. Classical Glutathione Peroxidase (GPX1)

GPX (glutathione:H_2O_2 oxidoreductase, E. C. 1.11.1.9) was discovered by Mills in 1957 (99) in a search for factors that protect erythrocytes against oxidative hemolysis. GPX1 is unique with respect to many other peroxidases because it is not inhibited by azide or cyanide, and hyperperoxides as well as H_2O_2 are substrates for the enzyme. The enzyme catalyzes the following reaction:

$$2GSH + ROOH \rightarrow GSSG + ROH + HOH \tag{1}$$

TABLE 3 Selenoenzymes, Selenoproteins, and Related Proteins

Abrev.	Name	Se moiety
Mammalian		
GPX1	Classical glutathione peroxidase (classical GSH-Px)	Sec
GPX2	Gastrointestinal glutathione peroxidase (GPX-GI)	Sec
GPX3	Plasma glutathione peroxidase (plasma GPX)	Sec
GPX4	Phospholipid hydroperoxide GPX (PHGPX or GPX-II)	Sec
GPX5	Androgen-regulated epididymal secretory protein	Cys
GPX6	Odorant-metabolizing protein	Cys
DI1	Iodothyronine 5'-deiodinase-1 (type I DI)	Sec
DI2	Iodothyronine 5'-deiodinase-2 (type II DI)	Sec
DI3	Iodothyronine 5-deiodinase-3 (type III DI)	Sec
Sel-P	Plasma selenoprotein P	ten Sec
Sel-W	Muscle selenoprotein W (formerly selenoprotein G)	Sec
Bacterial		
FDH_H	Formate dehydrogenase, hydrogenase linked (80 kDa)	Sec
FDH_N	Formate dehydrogenase, nitrate reductase linked (110 kDa)	Sec
[W]FDH	Formate dehydrogenase, tungsten containing	Sec
GR	Glycine reductase protein A (12 kDa)	Sec
NAH	Nicotinic acid hydroxylase	??
XDH	Xanthine dehydrogenase	??
	[NiFeSe]hydrogenasse	Sec

GPX1 is very specific for glutathione as the donor substrate, and no other substrate has more than 30% of the activity relative to GSH. In contrast, GPX1 is not specific at all for the acceptor substrate, and thus destroys hydroperoxides at rates very similar to H_2O_2. Only cholesterol 25- and cholesterol-7-α hydroperoxide, and phospholipid hydroperoxides such as phosphatidylcholine hydroperoxide are poor substrates for GPX1. Because almost all hydroperoxide substrates have similar maximum velocities, ternary enzyme complexes are not likely to be formed during catalysis (100,101). The enzyme reaction is a ter-uni ping-pong mechanism as shown below.

$$
\begin{array}{ccccccc}
\text{ROOH} & \text{ROH} & & \text{GSH} & \text{HOH} & & \text{GSH} & \text{GSSG} \\
\downarrow & \uparrow & & \downarrow & \uparrow & & \downarrow & \uparrow \\
\hline
\text{E-Se}^- & & \text{E-Se-OH} & & \text{E-Se-SG} & & \text{E-Se}^-
\end{array}
\tag{2}
$$

The lack of formation of any ternary complexes results in inability to saturate the enzyme with both substrates, such that there are no fixed K_m's or V_{max}'s for either glutathione or the peroxide substrate. Instead, kinetic analysis yields an apparent peroxide K_m and an apparent V_{max} at a given concentration of glutathione, but changing the glutathione concentration changes the V_{max} as well as the K_m for the peroxide substrate. Table 4 shows the effective second-order rate constants of GPX1 for various hydroperoxide substrates.

B. GPX1 Assay

Early assays for GPX1 incubated the enzyme with a fixed concentration of glutathione, and then added an excess of hydrogen peroxide and determined the decrease in glutathione over

TABLE 4 Apparent Second-Order Rate Constants for Reaction Between GPX1 or GPX4 and Hydroperide Substrates[a]

Substrate	K^b (mM^{-1} min^{-1})	
	GPX1	GPX4
Hydrogen peroxide	2.9×10^6	1.9×10^5
Cumene hydroperoxide	1.0×10^6	1.3×10^5
tert-Butyl hydroperoxide	7.1×10^5	7.1×10^4
Linoleic acid hydroperoxide	2.3×10^6	1.8×10^6
Phosphatidylcholine hydroperoxide	—	7.0×10^5

[a]From Maiorino et al. (114).
[b]Determined at 1 mM GSH.

time using Elman's reagent to quantify GSH concentration (102). The more convenient coupled assay procedure is now much more commonly used, as shown below:

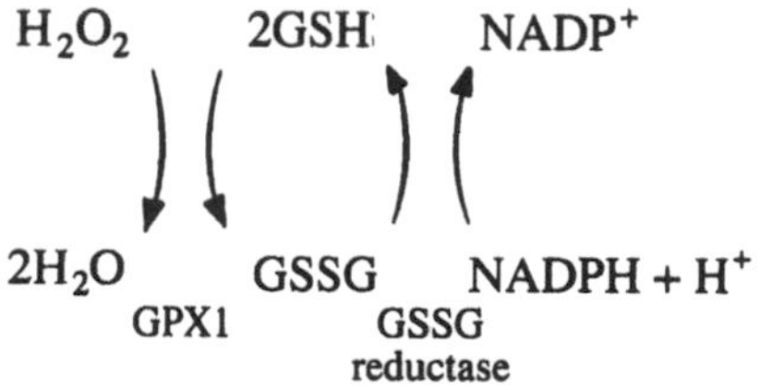

$$H_2O_2 \qquad 2GSH \qquad NADP^+$$

$$2H_2O \qquad GSSG \qquad NADPH + H^+ \tag{3}$$
$$\quad GPX1 \qquad GSSG$$
$$\qquad\qquad reductase$$

Typically (103), a reaction mixture contains 100 mM potassium phosphate, 3 mM EDTA, 1 mM NaN$_3$ (to inhibit catalase), 0.1 mM NADPH, 2 mM GSH, and 1 enzyme unit glutathione reductase in a 1-mL reaction cuvette. Diluted tissue homogenate or supernatant is added, and the cuvette is incubated for 5 min at 37°C to exhaust any non-GPX1 enzyme reactions and to allow the GSH to fully reduce GPX1, so the enzyme present will have maximum activity. The reaction is started with 10 uL of H$_2$O$_2$, resulting in a final H$_2$O$_2$ concentration of 0.12 mM. The enzyme reaction followed at A_{340} for 3 min because glutathione reductase rapidly re-reduces any oxidized glutathione so a constant concentration of GSH is maintained. The peroxide concentration is well above the apparent K_m for H$_2$O$_2$, resulting in a linear reaction rate (ΔA_{340}/time) for A_{340} values between 0.6 and 0.05 unit. Under these conditions, a sample blank must be run because at pH 7.0 there is considerable nonenzymatic reaction between glutathione and H$_2$O$_2$. This nonenzymatic rate is subtracted from the sample reaction rate to obtain the rate due to GPX1 in the sample. Using the molar extinction coefficient for NADPH of 6.22×10^3 M^{-1} cm^{-1} and a stoichiometry of two glutathione oxidized per NADPH reduced, one enzyme unit is defined as that amount of GPX1 that will oxidize 1 μmol of GSH per minute under the conditions specified. As described, this assay uses H$_2$O$_2$ and thus is specific for selenium-dependent GPX1, as the non-selenium-dependent GPX does not react with H$_2$O$_2$. The assay is conducted at pH 7.0, which is more than 1 pH unit below the pK of cysteine, so as to reduce the nonenzymatic reaction between GS$^-$ and H$_2$O$_2$. The careful reader of the literature must pay attention to specific reaction conditions (temperature, glutathione concentration, etc.) to compare one enzyme assay with another. Using these units, purified GPX1 has 853 enzyme units per milligram of protein (59), which is equivalent to a turnover number of 159 per second per selenium at 2 mM glutathione using H_2O_2 as the acceptor substrate.

GPX1 is a tetrametric protein with four identical subunits, each with a molecular weight of approximately 23 kDa and each containing one selenium per subunit. The amino acid sequence is shown in Figure 6. A tetrapeptide NVAS one residue before selenocysteine and a GXT immediately following the selenocysteine are conserved in the GPX family members with peroxidase activity. The bovine erythrocyte GPX1 has been crystallized (104), and it consists of four spherical subunits each with a diameter of 3.8 nm arranged in an almost flat square planar configuration ($9 \times 11 \times 6$ nm). Selenium atoms located in slight depressions are no closer than 2 nm, strongly suggesting that each selenium functions independently. The selenocysteine moiety is located 47 residues from the N-terminal end of the protein, and at the end of an α-helix associated with two parallel β sheets on a βαβ structure. The active site is actually comprised of sequences from two subunits, and charged amino acids within the active site apparently confer specificity for glutathione as well as permit iodoacetate to alkylate the fully reduced GPX1, whereas uncharged iodoacetamide

```
RATGPX1                         MSAARLSAVAQSTVYAFSARPLAG   24
HUMGPX2                          MAFIAKSFYDLSAISLD-        17
RATGPX3  MSRILRASCLLSLLLAGFVPPGRGQEKSKTDC------HGGMSGTIYEYGALTIDG   50
RATGPX6  MTQQFWGPCLFSLFMAVLAQETLDPQKSKVDC------NKGVAGTVYEYGANTLDG   50
RATGPX5  MAIQLRVFYLVPLLLASYVQTTPRLEKMKMDC------YKDVKGTIYNYEALSLNG   50
RATGPX4                          MCASRDDWRCARSMHEFAAKDIDG   24
          *        .      *. *..*      .* * **    ... .*   . *

RATGPX1  GEPVSLGSLRGKVLLIENVASLUGTTTRDYTEMNDLQKRLGPRGLVVLGF   74
HUMGPX2  GEKVDFNTFRGRAVLIENVASLUGTTTRDFTQLNELQCRF-PRRLVVLGF   66
RATGPX3  EEYIPFKQYAGKYILFVNVASYUGLTD-QYLELNALQEELGPFGLVILGF   99
RATGPX6  GEYVQFQQYAGKHILFVNVASFCGLTA-TYPELNTLQEELRPFNVSVLGF   99
RATGPX5  KERIPFKQYAGKHVLFVNVATYCGLTI-QYPELNALQDDLKQFGLVILGF   99
RATGPX4  -HMVCLDKYRGCVCIVTNVASQUGKTDVNYTQLVDLHARYAECGLRILAF   73
          .  .       *   .   *** .* .  . .  .*.   . .*.*

RATGPX1  PCNQFGHQENGKNEEILNSLKYVRPGGGFEPNFTLFEKCEVNGEKAHPLF   124
HUMGPX2  PCNQFGHQENCQNEEILNSLKYVRPGGGYQPTFTLVQKCEVNGQNEHPVF   116
RATGPX3  PCNQFGKQEPGENSEILPSLKYVRPGGGFVPNFQLFEKGDVNGEKEQKFY   149
RATGPX6  PCNQFGKQEPGKNSEILLGLKYVRPGGGFVPNFQLFEKGDVNGDNEQKVF   149
RATGPX5  PCNQFGKQEPGDNTEILPGLKYVRPGKGFLPNFQLFAKGDVNGEKEQEIF   149
RATGPX4  PCNQFGRQEPGSNQEIKE---F---AAGYNVRFDMYSKICVNGDDAHPLW   117
          ******.**  * **   .  *.   * .  ***....

RATGPX1  TFLRNALPAPSDDPTALMTDPKYIIWSPVCRNDISWNFEKFLVGPDGVPV   174
HUMGPX2  AYLKDKLPYPYDDPFSLMTDPKLIIWSPVRRSDVAWNFEKFLIGPEGEPF   166
RATGPX3  TFLKNSCPPTAE----LLGSPGRLFWEPMKIHDIRWNFEKFLVGPDGIPI   195
RATGPX6  SFLKSSCPPTSE----LLGSPEHLFWDPMKVHDIRWNFEKFLVGPDGAPV   195
RATGPX5  TFLKRSCPHPSE----TVVTSKHTFWEPIKVHDIRWNFEKFLVGPNGVPV   195
RATGPX4  KWMKVQ-----PKGRGMLGNA-----------IKWNFTKFLIDKNGCVV   150
          ...            . ..         . ***.***.. .*

RATGPX1  RRYSRRFRTIDIEPDIEALLSKQPS----NP   201
HUMGPX2  RRYSRTFPTINIEPDIKRLLK---V----AI   190
RATGPX3  MRWYHRTTVSNVKMDILSYMRRQAALGARGK   226       U = Sec
RATGPX6  MRWFHQTPVRVVQSDIMEYLNQ-----TRTQ   221
RATGPX5  MRWFHQAPVSTVKSDILAYLNQ-----FKTI   221       ▼ = Sec or Cys
RATGPX4  KRYGPMEEPQVIEKDLPCYL-----------   170
          .*. .    .. *.   .
```

FIGURE 6 Alignment of amino acid sequences of GPX family sequences. Rat GPX1 (228), human GPX2 (107), rat GPX3 (229), rat GPX4 (L24896, 3), rat GPX5 (123), and rat GPX6 (124) were aligned using PCGENE Multiple Sequence Alignment program. A "*" indicates that a position is the alignment is perfectly conserved, and a "•" indicates that the position is well conserved. Overall the sequences had 16% sequence identity and 20% sequence similarity. Pairwise sequence identities with GPX1 were 60%, 42%, 30%, 40%, and 41% for GPX2–GPX6, respectively. U47, Q82 and W160 are important for catalytic activity, and R52, R98 and R179 are important for GSH binding (117).

does not. Fully reduced GPX1 that is then treated with a 10-fold excess of hydrogen peroxide is insensitive to iodoacetate and insensitive to cyanide. GPX1 reduced with [^{14}C]GSH will bind [^{14}C]GSH; it is insensitive to iodoacetate but will be completely inhibited by cyanide (105). Recombinant analogs of murine GPX1 with cysteine or serine replacing the selenocysteine moiety have been prepared. The serine moiety is completely without activity, whereas the cysteine mutant has 1/1000th the activity of the wild-type enzyme (106). The functions of GPX1 will be discussed in Section XII.

C. GPX-GI or GPX2

Using probes based on the GPX1 sequence, a cDNA from a human liver cDNA library was isolated that encoded a protein with 66% amino acid sequence identity and 61% nucleotide sequence identity to GPX1. This member of the GPX family is properly identified as GPX2 because it was the second member sequenced, although it was the fourth GPX to be described. GPX2 is also designated as GPX-GI because Northern blotting identified this species only in gastrointestinal cells in the rat (107), and GPX2 has been overexpressed in transfected MCF-7 cells. Northern blotting demonstrates expression of GPX2 in human liver and colon, but not in kidney, heart, lung, placenta, or uterus. Recently, preliminary evidence indicated that more than 70% of the total GPX activity in the rat small bowel is due to GPX2, although there is also a low level of GPX1 (108). The discovery of this fourth GPX (third intracellular GPX) might at first glance suggest that these activities are redundant. Further reflection, however, suggests that evolution has apparently crafted multiple GPXs with apparently unique niches. Future work will be needed to define the corresponding biochemical roles.

D. Plasma Glutathione Peroxidase or GPX3

A comprehensive review of the extracellular GPX3 has been written recently (109). Virtually all cells and animal sera seem to contain GPX, GPX activities decrease in plasma and cells in selenium deficiency, and selenium supplementation restores these activities to normal. Thus it was believed initially that plasma GPX activity originated nonspecifically from tissues and reflected the selenium status of the tissues, and thus could be used as a general parameter of selenium status in animals and humans. The plasma enzyme is specific for glutathione as the donor substrate and oxidizes both organic hydroperoxides and hydrogen peroxide, and thus it was thought that these two peroxidases were identical.

Almost immediately after the discovery that GPX1 is a selenium-dependent enzyme, researchers observed that plasma GPX activity responds more quickly to selenium deficiency and to selenium resupplementation (110). GPX activity in the plasma cannot be accounted for by red blood cells hemolysis, and the relative rate of increase of plasma GPX in selenium repletion is comparable to the increase observed in liver when expressed as a percent of selenium-adequate values (111). Cohen and colleagues (112) observed that plasma GPX can be increased within 6 h after selenium supplementation in patients with low initial GPX activities. Preparation of antibodies against erythrocyte GPX1 also precipitated liver GPX1 but would not precipitate plasma GPX. Purification and characterization of human plasma GPX demonstrated that it is a distinct enzyme. The enzyme has an apparent molecular weight of 92 kDa, a subunit molecular weight of 23 kDa with one selenium per subunit, and it is glycosylated. The specific activity of the purified plasma enzyme, however, is only 10% of GPX1. In 1990 Takahashi (113) isolated cDNA clones for human plasma GPX from a human placenta cDNA library, conferring plasma GPX as GPX3. The sequence encoded a 226-amino acid polypeptide with a molecular weight of

25,389 and with 44% homology with human GPX1, including a selenocysteine residue encoded by a UGA at residue 73. Northern blot analysis indicated that this gene is not expressed in human liver. Additional Northern blot analysis as well as immunoblot analysis revealed that the kidney is the major source of circulating GPX3, with low levels also detected in the lungs. Human patients undergoing chronic dialysis due to renal failure have low levels of plasma GPX3 in spite of normal plasma selenium content. After renal transplantation, plasma GPX3 increased up to 200% of normal (109). GPX3 is a secreted enzyme, and thus it is not surprising in hindsight that 90% of human milk GPX activity is precipitated by anti-GPX3 antibodies, demonstrating the genetic origin of milk GPX activity. The expression of GPX3 in milk may have evolved specifically to maintain milk selenium levels rather than to protect milk from peroxidation in the (short) trip from breast to infant stomach.

The role of GPX3 is unknown. It is logical to predict that GPX3 is an important antioxidant in the plasma, but low levels of reduced glutathione in plasma challenge this hypothesis because glutathione is well below half-saturating concentrations. Circulating reduced GPX3, however, can encounter and reduces a hydroperoxide, thus blocking initiation of prooxidant attack, and then awaits re-reduction at a later place and time when it next encounters GSH. Alternatively, Cohen and Avissar have suggested that the site of action may be in renal extracellular space (109).

E. Phospholipid Hydroperoxide Glutathione Peroxidase or GPX4

Several recent reviews of phospholipid hydroperoxide glutathione peroxidase are available (3,114). In 1982 Ursini and colleagues purified a 20-kDa protein with GPX activity which could use phosphatidyl choline hydroperoxide as a substrate, but which is not a substrate for GPX1 (115). In 1985, Ursini and co-workers reported that this protein is a selenium-dependent phospholipid hydroperoxide GPX (E.C. 1.11.1.12). The enzyme is a monomer, however, and it catalyzes the reduction of hydroperoxides as well as H_2O_2 to the corresponding alcohol, using glutathione as the reducing substrate (116). The specificity for the peroxide substrate is even broader than for the other glutathione peroxidases, as the enzyme will reduce all phospolipid hydroperoxides as well as cholesterol hydroperoxides, which are not substrates for GPX1 (114). Thiol reagents which do not reduce GPX1 react readily with selenocysteine in GPX4, and the arginine residues in GPX1 that are thought to be integral for binding glutathione are mutated or deleted in GPX4. This suggests that GPX4 may be misnamed as a *glutathione* peroxidase. So far no alternative thiol substrate has proved to be a better donor substrate than glutathione, and the physiologic availability of glutathione suggests that this is the primary donor substrate. The enzyme uses a ter-uni ping-pong mechanism, the same as GPX1, and addition of detergents such as Triton X-100 stimulates the activity of this enzyme. This suggested to the discoverers that this enzyme may work the interface between the membrane and the aqueous phase of the cell. Table 4 shows the relative second-order rate constants for GPX4 and GPX1. Note that GPX1 has 15-fold higher activity against hydrogen peroxide than does GPX4, nearly equivalent activities against linoleic acid hydroperoxide, and no activity against phosphatidyl choline hydroperoxide. The rate constant of GPX4 for phosphatidyl choline hydroperoxide is over 3.5 times that of hydrogen peroxide. Several useful experimental consequences emerge from this data. First, in tissues with low GPX1 activity, a substantial amount of the H_2O_2 activity may be due to GPX4. Second, H_2O_2 can be used effectively as an inexpensive alternative substrate in the assay for GPX4 when GPX1 is not present.

GPX4 appeared to be distinct from GPX1 because the amino acid composition is different, the monomer is active, and iodoacetimide will inhibit the enzyme (114). Irrefutable evidence that GPX4 is distinct from GPX1 emerged in 1991 with a partial cDNA sequence that included an estimated 75% of the coding region plus approximately 200 base pairs of the 3'UTR, and that included a UGA at the appropriate point in the coding sequence (117). Sunde et al. (118) isolated a full-length cDNA clone of pig GPX4 from a pig embryo cDNA using degenerate primers prepared from the published partial nucleotide sequence. Resulting pig and rat sequences matched with the C-terminal portion of the sequence, and included an apparent 15-amino acid N-terminal portion. This gave a full-length GPX4 polypeptide of 170 amino acids with a calculated molecular weight of 19,492 kDa, and the selenocysteine residue located 46 amino acids from the N-terminal end. The full-length nucleotide and amino acid sequences have 39% identity with rat GPX1. GPX4 is the least similar of all the proteins in the family (Fig. 6), and it varies considerably from the other members in the C-terminal portion, with several deleted regions with a total of 23 residues as compared to GPX1. These are regions that in this monomer are not necessary for subunit assembly. An apparent 3'UTR eSECIS element is located 461 base pairs downstream from the UGA. The GPX4 gene has been cloned and sequenced from the pig (119) with 7 exons and 600 base pairs of 5'UTR, including several potential estrogen-responsive and progesterone/glucocorticoid-responsive elements which might be important in testes-specific expression of GPX.

Recently, Pushpa-Rekha and colleagues (120) isolated a full-length cDNA clone from rat testes. Sequence analysis indicated that the cDNA encodes a protein of 197 amino acids including an additional 27 amino acids at the N-terminal end featuring a mitochondrial targeting sequence. In-vitro translation suggested that the GPX4 mRNA initiates predominantly at the AUG that yields the 197-amino acid polypeptide. The leader sequence contains a bipartite targeting signal with basic residues at the N-terminus followed by a hydrophobic stretch of approximately 20 amino acids. This suggests that the positively charged N-terminal sequences are cleaved by a mitochondrial peptidase after import of the protein into the mitochondrial matrix, and then the remaining hydrophobic residues direct export of the protein back to the mitochondrial intermembrane space, consistent with recent localization information (121). It has been suggested that GPX4 rolls along membrane surfaces in the cytosol and in the mitochondrial intermembrane space and protects the membrane components by detoxifying hydroperoxides that would otherwise damage or impair membrane function.

F. Other Glutathione Peroxidases

In addition to GPX1–4, a number of other glutathione peroxidases have been identified. The fifth in the sequence of cloned GPX-related proteins is the androgen-regulated epididymal secretory proteins GPX5 (122,123). GPX5 has 67% identity to the GPX1 coding region, but these secretory proteins retain a cysteine codon in place of UGA and possess a 21-amino acid signal peptide-directing secretion. The sixth sequenced member of the GPX family is the odorant/metabolizing protein (GPX6) identified by Dear et al. in 1991 (124). It has about 40% amino acid sequence identity to GPX1, but retains a cysteine codon in place of UGA. It appears to be expressed only in Bohman's gland of the olfactory system.

In addition, several other members of the GPX family have been identified. A TGA-containing GPX gene in the parasitic worm *Schistosoma mansoni* has 38% amino acid sequence identity with GPX1 (125). A secreted homolog of GPX with cysteine substituting for selenocysteine in the nematoid *Brugia pahangi* shows GPX activity with a range of organic hydroperoxides including PCOOH, but no activity against H_2O_2 (126). A tetrameric selenium-containing GPX from *Chlamydomonas reinhardtii* has been found with a subunit molecular weight of 17 kDa (127). Lastly, a selenium-independent GPX with enzyme activity is reported in *Euglena gracilis* (128). The retention of intracellular and secreted GPX-like proteins with activity suggests strongly that this is one of evolution's solutions to an oxidant-filled environment.

G. Glutathione-S-Transferase or Non-Selenium-Dependent GPX

A non-selenium-dependent GPX activity in the liver of selenium-deficient animals was discovered in 1976 (129), and the activity was shown to be due to several of the glutathione -S-transferases (E.C. 2.5.1.18) (138). The enzyme normally catalyzes GHS conjugation to hydroxylated species as part of the phase II detoxification mechanism for compounds such as aromatic hydrocarbons, which are then targeted for excretion via the bile. The enzyme does not catalyze the reduction of H_2O_2, however, so enzyme assays using H_2O_2 will just measure the true selenium-dependent GPX if properly conducted to avoid catalase and/or hemoglobin-mediated peroxidase activity. The apparent K_m's for typical hydroperoxide substrates are 10- to 34-fold higher than the apparent K_m's for GPX1, suggesting that GPX1 is physiologically more important under normal conditions than is the non-selenium-dependent GPX activity of glutathione-S-transferase (130).

The reaction catalyzed by glutathione-S-transferase is zero order with respect to glutathione, and in contrast to GPX1, the initial velocity patterns indicate an ordered sequential mechanism:

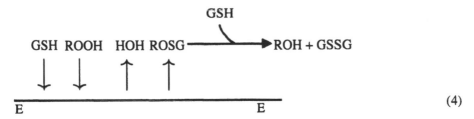

$$(4)$$

By analogy with the phase II conjugation reaction glutathione binds to the enzyme, followed by addition of hydroperoxide which effectively causes enzyme-bound glutathione attack on the electrophilic oxygen of the hydroperoxide. Water is released and then the hydroperoxide conjugate reacts nonenzymatically with a second molecule of GSH to complete the reaction (130). In almost a premonition of things yet to be discovered, Wendel and colleagues in 1984 reported the multiple enzymatic changes that occur in liver, both up and down, only after liver glutathione peroxidase is fully depleted (131); glutathione-S-transferase activity increases twofold under these conditions (see below). The selenium changes in glutathione-S-transferase were important in focusing on the role of selenium in deiodinases.

H. Thyroxine 5'-deiodinase-1 or DI1

Several excellent reviews have appeared recently, including the proceedings of a 1993 workshop on the interrelationships among selenium deficiency, iodine deficiency, and thyroid hormones (132,133). Thyroxine 5'-deiodinase-1 (E.C. 2.8.1.4) is often referred to in the literature as type I 5'-DI. The identification of DI1 as a selenium-containing enzyme illustrates the confluence of three distinctly separate approaches to understanding a biochemical problem. Arthur and colleagues were studying the impact of severe selenium deficiency in rats and observed elevated glutathione-S-transferase activity, elevated plasma pyruvate kinase activity, elevated thyroxine (T_4) levels, and reduced triiodothyronine (T_3) levels (134). Injection of 10 μg Se/kg rat reduced the elevated GST levels and pyruvate kinase activity with negligible effect on GPX1 activity. Higher doses of selenium completely reversed the effects on T_3 and T_4 metabolism, with marginal effect on GPX1 activity. Concurrently, Behne and co-workers used ^{75}Se labeling to discover a 28-kDa selenoprotein at high concentrations in thyroid, liver, and kidney, and proposed a role for selenium in thyroid hormone metabolism (32). In 1990, Arthur (135) and Behne (136) independently identified DI1 as a selenoenzyme. Also independently, Berry and Larsen (137) used expression cloning to isolate and sequence the DI1 from rat liver poly (A)$^+$ RNA and isolated a full-length clone for a 257-amino acid polypeptide with a UGA-encoding selenocysteine at residue 126. Expression of the cDNA clone in a wheat germ system resulted in a protein of approximately 14 kDa, corresponding to termination at the UGA codon, but translation in a reticulocyte lysate system resulted in both 14-kDa and 27-kDa proteins. Conversion of the UGA codon to a cysteine UGU by site-directed mutagenesis resulted in a protein with approximately 10% of the activity of the selenocysteine-containing protein. Subsequent studies by Berry et al. led to the discovery of the eSECIS element as discussed previously.

DI1 catalyzes both outer- and inner-ring deiodination of thyroxine, but the preferred reaction is removal of the outer-ring 5' iodine from either T_4 or reverse T_3 (rT_3), leading to T_3 or T_2, respectively. Formation of T_3 is thought to be the most important physiologic role for DI1, but production of T_2 from rT_3 may also be of biological importance in the elimination of excess thyroid hormone from circulation (132). The catalyzed reaction in very analogous to the glutathione peroxidase reaction:

$$
\begin{array}{cccccc}
T_4 & T_3 & GSH & I^- & GSH & GSSG \\
\downarrow & \uparrow & \downarrow & \uparrow & \downarrow & \uparrow \\
\end{array}
$$

$$
\text{E-Se}^- \qquad\quad \text{E-SeI} \qquad\quad \text{E-Se-SG} \qquad\quad \text{E-Se}^- \tag{5}
$$

$$
\begin{array}{ll}
\quad\downarrow \text{Au}^+ & \text{PTU}\downarrow \\
\text{E-SeAu} & \text{E-SePTU}
\end{array}
$$

The enzyme is assayed using dithiothreitol as the substrate, but reduced GSH is the likely physiologic substrate, and thus the mechanism can be best described as a bi-uni ping-pong mechanism for DTT and as a ter-uni mechanism with GSH. Two inhibitors have also proved to be very helpful in characterizing the enzyme activity of the selenocysteine in the enzyme. Gold thioglucose reacts readily with the deprotoinated selenol in the enzyme, and the thiourea compound, 6-*n*-propylthiouracil (PTU) inhibits T_4-to-T_3 conversion by interacting noncompetitively with the E-SeI form of the enzyme to form the E-Se-PTU adduct. Consistent with the chemistry, the cysteine enzyme is about 300-fold less sensitive to 6-*n*-

propylthiouracil. DI1 is localized in the membrane and copurifies with microsomal markers from liver, but with the basolateral membrane of kidney-proximal convoluted tubule cells. The single transmembrane segment of the protein is located at the N terminus of the protein with the catalytic portion oriented toward the cytoplasm. In kidney, the N terminus is found on the external cell surface with the catalytic portion facing the interior of the cell. Physical and chemical studies suggest that DI1 may function as a homodimer with a molecular weight of approximately 55 kDa. Liver DI1 is thought to be responsible for most of the circulating plasma T3 levels.

More than 90% of plasma T_3 is produced by DI1 in liver, kidney, and muscle. Pituitary and brain in the central nervous system and brown adipose tissue contain DI2 and DI3, which catalyze the 5'- and 5-deiodination, respectively. Selenium deficiency alone has no effect on thyroid weight in rats, whereas iodine deficiency results in a 60% increase in thyroid weight and combined iodine and selenium deficiency results in thyroid weights that are 148% above those in controlled animals. Changes in T_4 and T_3 concentration mirror those changes with the usual dramatic effects with iodine deficiency, which are further altered away from normal values with combined deficiency, but are only modestly affected with selenium deficiency alone (139). DI2 is found in much lower activities in brain, pituitary, brown adipose tissue, placenta, and skin, and its principal physiologic role is for local, intracellular production of T_3. DI2 is also a selenocysteine-containing enzyme. DI3 catalyzes the inner-ring 5-deiodination, and activity levels are highest in adult brain, skin and placenta, and in fetal liver, muscle, brain, and the central nervous system. The role of DI3 has been proposed to protect fetal tissue from high levels of T_3 and T_4 during development by converting them to the inactive rT_3 and T_2, respectively. A DI3 cDNA has recently been cloned and reveals the presence of an inframe TGA codon encoding seleno-cysteine as DI1 (132).

This array of three deiodinases may confer additional regulation on iodine metabolism. In iodine deficiency, downregulation of DI1 conserves precious iodine by limiting DI1's conversion of T_4 to circulating T_3, thus making the limited T_4 available for intracellular conversion by DI2 in important endocrine organs. It has been proposed that combined selenium as well as an iodine deficiency may contribute to the etiology of endemic myxedematous cretinism in populations in Zaire. Administration of selenium alone appears to aggravate this disease by restoring DI1 activity leading to increased production of plasma T_3, which in turn further reduces T_4 substrate for DI2 in critical endocrine tissues. This lowers intracellular T_3 even more (140).

Bermano et al. (141) have conducted a series of experiments showing that in severe selenium deficiency, GPX1 activity and mRNA in liver and heart are reduced dramatically. DI1 activity and mRNA are decreased by 95% and 50%, respectively, in liver, but in the thyroid DI1 activity is increased by 15% and mRNA by 95%. Nuclear runoff assays demonstrated that transcription cannot explain these effects. GPX4 activity and mRNA are little changed. These studies suggest that the decrease in thyroid GPX1 activity of about 50% might provide the selenium to restore or even increase DI1 activity in thyroid. The authors have postulated (141) that the thyroid is protected against loss of selenium in selenium deficiency relative to liver, and that there may be specific mechanisms which channel selenium to the synthesis of DI1 in thyroid during deficiency. The continued increase in DI1 mRNA levels after selenium repletion may reflect intracellular selenium stores that are sufficient to stabilize mRNA but are insufficient to fully maintain elevated selenoenzyme activity.

I. Plasma Selenoprotein P or Sel-P

The nature and characterization of selenoprotein P has recently been reviewed by Burk and Hill (55). Following the discovery that GPX1 is a selenoenzyme, the antioxidant activity of this enzyme was logically (142) and generously used to explain the biochemical role for selenium. A number of investigators, however, continued to search for critical roles of selenium that lay outside the realm of GPX1. Burk (143) found that injecting selenium-deficient rats with 50 μg of selenium protected rats early on against diquat toxicity with virtually no change in GPX1 activity 10 h after injection, indicating that GPX1 is not responsible for selenium's protective role under these conditions. Further work revealed a fast-responding plasma selenoprotein that is rapidly labeled with ^{75}Se by 3–4 h after selenium injection. This protein was named plasma selenoprotein P or Sel-P (144).

Initial attempts to characterize this protein further were unsuccessful because the protein lost its selenium during purification and the apparent molecular weight changed. An alternative approach of preparing monoclonal antibodies against partially purified Sel-P followed by affinity chromatography resulted in purification of the native Sel-P (145). Mature Sel-P is a 366-amino acid protein in rats (362 amino acids in humans) with approximately 70% nucleotide and amino acid sequence identity, with a molecular weight of 41 kDa (146). In addition, a cDNA sequence indicates a secretion signal peptide (MWRSLGLALALCLLP), and five glycosylation sites (six in humans) resulting in a deduced native molecular weight of approximately 57 kDa during SDS-PAGE. Selenium analysis of purified Sel-P reveals that it contains 7.5 ± 1 Se atoms per molecule, whereas the cDNA sequence has 10 open reading frame TGAs. The first selenocysteine is located at residue 40 from the N-terminal end of the mature protein, and the remaining nine seleno-cysteines are in N-terminal 122 amino acids along with an additional 10 cysteines. Notably, the 3′UTR contains two eSECIS elements. Sequence comparison between the human and rat shows complete conservation of eight of the selenocysteines, and cysteine in the homologous position for three of the four remaining selenocysteines. This suggests that either amino acid may be able to meet the functional requirement at several of the positions in the sequence (55). In addition, under limited selenium conditions, early termination at one of the UGAs might reduce the selenium content of Sel-P and result in a smaller circulating protein.

Sel-P is a basic protein, and it has two heavy concentrations of histidine (146) that may potentiate interaction with membranes, or function as an as yet unidentified metal-binding motif. It is estimated that selenium-adequate rats have 25–30 mg Sel-P/L plasma, but that this can fall in selenium deficiency to less than 3 mg/L. The half-life of ^{75}Se and Sel-P is 3–4 h, indicating rapid turnover. Sel-P is estimated to contain 60–65% of the plasma selenium. Northern blot analysis indicates that mRNA for Sel-P is highest in concentration in kidney and liver, with smaller amounts in heart, testis, and some in lung, suggesting that kidney and liver are major secretors of Sel-P (55).

The physiologic role of Sel-P is unknown. The initial hypothesis was that Sel-P might be a selenium transport protein (147). Burk and co-workers injected ^{75}Se-labeled Sel-P into selenium-deficient and selenium-adequate rats, and only observed an effect of selenium status on ^{75}Se uptake in brain compatible with a Sel-P receptor in brain (148). A second postulated function is as an antioxidant defense protein. Follow-up studies to the original diquat toxicity studies have shown that selenium incorporation into Sel-P correlates well with protection against diquat toxicity (148), suggesting to Burk and colleagues that secretion of this putative antioxidant protein into the interstitial space may be the function of Sel-P. An attractive third hypothesis based solely on the high cysteine-plus-selenocysteine content suggests a role for Sel-P in disulfide exchange or related biochemistry. Sel-P concentrations in selenium-deficient Chinese were 10–20% of U.S. levels (55), showing that this protein decreases in human populations as well, and may be associated with the onset of selenium deficiency disease.

J. Muscle Selenoprotein W or Sel-W

The search for mammalian selenoproteins to explain selenium deficiency diseases has been successful in several areas of research. Focusing on white muscle disease, Pedersen reported existence of a 10-kDa selenoprotein that was lacking in lambs suffering from white muscle disease (149). Subsequent attempts to purify and identify this protein were not successful, although the selenium in this species was reported to be selenocysteine (150). Classical as well as modern protein purification techniques have now been successful in purifying the protein 1200-fold to about 95% purity, which was sufficient to determine a molecular weight of approximately 9.8 kDa and a selenium content of 1 g-atom Se per mole (151). The selenium has been shown to be present as selenocysteine, and a partial N-terminal sequence has been determined. Degenerate PCR primers were prepared from this sequence, and RT/PCR was used to screen a rat muscle cDNA library. Sequence analysis revealed 50 bp of 5'UTR, 267 nucleotides encoding an 89-amino acid polypeptide including selenocysteine at residue 12, and 370 bp of the 3'UTR. In rat muscle, selenium-adequate levels (0.1 μg Se/g diet) increased muscle Sel-W RNA fourfold relative to selenium-deficient rat muscle (152). The role of this low-molecular-weight protein in protecting muscle against white muscle disease is unknown.

K. Other Selenoproteins

In the 1970s and early 1980s a number of groups used column chromatography to examine ^{75}Se labeling of selenoproteins in various mammalian tissues (4,58). The chromatographic procedures, however, had several problems that limited further advances, such as inability to resolve various selenoproteins from one another, inability to separate selenoproteins from proteins with weak affinity for selenium, and inability to distinguish low-molecular-weight proteins from inorganic or nonprotein forms of selenium. SDS-PAGE proved to be far more useful because it would electrophoretically strip selenium from proteins that bind selenium only weakly, and thus distinguish proteins that are "well labeled" with selenium, and evaluate the apparent subunit molecular weight of these species. Where previous sephadex G-150 chromatography revealed four ^{75}Se-labeled peaks (153), SDS-PAGE showed that selenium-deficient liver cytosol contains two major ^{75}Se proteins of 65 and 23 kDa as well as minor ^{75}Se-labeled proteins of 77, 58, 20, 14, and 10 kDa (154). More important, cychoheximide pretreatment completely eliminated ^{75}Se labeling of any of these selenoproteins, demonstrating that protein synthesis is required for selenium incorporation. In 1988 Behne (32) listed 13 selenium-containing polypeptides with molecular weights of 12.1, 15.6, 18.0, 19.7, 22.2, 23.7, 28.7, 33.3, 55.5, 59.9, 64.9, 70.1, and 75.4 kDa, which were detected in tissue homogenates. At that time only the 23.7-kDa protein was positively identified as a GPX1 subunit. It is now clear that the 19.7-kDa protein is GPX4, the 27.8-kDa protein found in thyroid is DI1, and one of the 55.5 and 59.9 proteins is likely Sel-P. The other important concept to emerge from their studies is that in selenium deficiency, selenoproteins other than GPX1, especially in brain, endocrine, and reproductive organs, appear to have priority for the selenium. Subsequent estimates for the number of selenium-containing proteins in higher animals range from 30 to 50 selenoproteins (3,5,155). The nature of some of these additional potential selenoproteins is discussed below.

L. 17-kDa Sperm Mitochondria Capsule Protein or [Se]MCP

Whether or not this protein is a true selenocysteine-containing protein is yet again unclear. This area has recently been reviewed by Kleene 1994 (156), but recent discussion at meetings suggest that this protein may be a cysteine- rather than a selenocysteine-containing protein. This apparent 17-kDa sperm selenoprotein has been isolated both from rat (157) and cattle (158). It is found in the mitochondria capsule in the midpiece region of the sperm in association with mitochondria helix, and Calvin (159) gave this species the name mitochondria capsule protein ([Se]MCP). This protein is thought to be a cysteine-rich protein, so it was unclear whether this protein is a true selenoprotein, or whether it contains selenocysteine inserted in place of cysteine inserted by cysteinyl, tRNAs or is the [Cysteine] MCP that copurified with an unknown selenoprotein of the same molecular weight. Kleene (156) reported the cloning of a cDNA from a mouse testis cDNA library which encoded 197-amino acid protein containing three in-phase UGAs that presumably encode selenocysteine, and with a predicted molecular weight of 21.1 kDa. The selenocysteines are located at residues 7, 17, and 34, and appear as three selenocysteine-cysteine dipeptides. Reports of the molecular weight of this species, however, range from 15 to 31 kDa, and the isoelectric point also varies. The report is that MCP is a selenoprotein is attractive because it readily explains early reports of midpiece breakage (51). High levels of GPX4 in rat testis, however, suggest that [Se]MCP might be GPX4. Thus it remains unclear whether the impact of selenium deficiency in rat testis is due to diminished selenium in [Se]MCP, decreased amounts of GPX4, or another selenoprotein. It is clear that testis has unique and specific accumulation of selenium, especially in selenium-deficient animals. Evenson and Sunde observed that in selenium-deficient rats, the 17-kDa selenoprotein in testis was the second most labeled ^{75}Se protein in deficient rats 24 and 72 h after selenium administration (154).The high content of GPX4 activity as well as mRNA suggests that [Se]MCP in testes (187) may well be due to contamination of a non-selenium-containing MCP by GPX4, the major selenoprotein in testis.

M. Selenium-Binding Proteins

Several additional apparent selenium-binding proteins have been identified (4). Bansal et al. purified a 14-kDa selenoprotein from mouse liver and determined the amino acid sequence of 75% of the polypeptide. Comparison of the resulting sequence with other sequences revealed a 92% amino acid sequence with rat liver fatty acid-binding protein (161). Fatty acid-binding protein, however, has been cloned and sequenced, and does not contain an open reading frame UGA or a 3'UTR eSECIS, suggesting that selenium is not incorporated into fatty acid-binding protein by the usual tRNA-mediated mechanism. This species is undoubtedly one of the low-molecular-weight selenoproteins detected by Behne and by Evenson and Sunde. Labeling is blocked with cychoheximide (154), suggesting that fatty acid-binding protein is labeled cotranslationally by selenocysteine incorporation, or by binding of selenium to sites that are exposed only as the nascent polypeptide is synthesized, or ^{75}Se labeling of a contaminating selenoprotein is blocked by cycloheximide.

A second series of apparent selenium-binding proteins with a molecular weight corresponding to 56–58 kDa are also putative selenium-binding proteins. Medina and co-workers were studying the impact of increased selenium concentrations on mouse mammary epithelial cells in culture as a means to study selenium in an attenuation of chemical carcinogenesis, and identified a 58-kDa selenoprotein (SP58) that was increasingly labeled with anticarcinogenic concentrations of selenium (5 μM), but also labeled at 0.05 μM (162). Partial amino acid sequences of the SP58 revealed homology with the thiol protein disulfide oxidoreductase with a 100% sequence identity (163). A second 56-kDa selenium-binding species (SP56) was also identified, and the cDNA sequence from mouse liver predicted a 472-amino acid polypeptide. This sequence matched with the amino acid sequences of eight internal peptides for a 56-kDa acetaminophen-binding protein (AP56) (164). The nucleotides sequence lacks any TGA codons for selenocysteine. In 1993, isolation of genomic DNA recombinants from a cosmid genomic library showed that SP56 and AP56 are separate genes that differ only in 14 residues of the deduced amino acid sequence, and neither sequence contains a UGA (165).

The nature of selenium incorporation into these proteins is unclear, and overexpression of the first three-quarters of the AP56 clone does not result in ^{75}Se labeling of a recombinant protein in spite of dramatic increases in corresponding mRNA levels in stably transfected CHO cells (Beveridge and Sunde, unpublished). This work suggests either that a hypothetical true selenoprotein with high specific activity is a contaminate, resulting in the misidentification of these proteins as selenium-binding proteins, or that, during translation, preformed selenocysteine is being incorporated into these proteins in a disulfide-exchange reaction.

IX. PROKARYOTIC SELENOENZYMES

The first suggestion of a specific role of selenium in an enzyme was made by Pincent (9), who observed that addition of selenium and molybdenum is necessary for optimum formate dehydrogenase (FDH) activity when *E. coli* is grown anaerobically in nitrate-free media. Selenium-dependent enzymes are observed in strict anaerobes such as *Clostridia* or under anaerobic conditions in facultative anaerobes such as *E. coli*. This suggests that specialized processes may be necessary to incorporate selenium discriminately into protein when oxygen is present. The following is an overview of prokaryotic selenoproteins to illustrate the diversity of the selenoproteins in lower forms of life. These examples are also likely to serve as models for additional new roles for selenium in higher organisms. Several insightful reviews and references cited herein provide additional information (61,166,167).

Formate dehydrogenase (FDH$_H$), which is observed in nitrate-free media, passes electrons to a hydrogenase in the following reaction, where A is the electron acceptor:

$$HCOOH + A \rightarrow CO_2 + AH_2 \tag{6}$$

H$_2$ is liberated in vivo. FDH$_H$ is a 120-kDa protein consisting of an 80-kDa selenocysteine-containing α subunit and a 40-kDa β subunit with FeS centers and Mo. In nitrate-containing media, a different formate dehydrogenase (FDH$_N$) is induced instead. FDH$_N$ also catalyzes reaction (6), and it passes electrons to nitrate reductase. FDH$_N$ is an approximately 600-kDa protein with three subunits present in a $\alpha_4\beta_4\gamma_{2 \text{ or } 4}$ structure containing 1 selenium as selenocysteine in each of the 4 110-kDa α subunits. Other components are 4 g-atoms of Mo, 56 nonheme Fe, 52 acid-labile sulfide, and 4 B-type heme groups. The molybdenum is present as molybdenum cofactor (168). Additional non-selenium-containing formate dehydrogenases are present in other species (61). A novel formate dehydrogenase in *Clostridium thermoaceticum* is a 340-kDa enzyme with $\alpha_2\beta_2$ structure that contains 2 g-atoms of Se and 2 g-atoms of tungsten rather than molybdenum (61).

Glycine reductase from *Clostridia* was the second bacterial enzyme identified as a selenoenzyme, and it has 3 subunits including an apparent 12-kDa protein A subunit that contains a UGA-encoded selenocysteine (61). The true molecular weight now appears to be 17 kDa (169). Glycine reductase catalyzes a substrate-level phosphorylation of ATP:

$$NH_2-CH_2-COOH + R(SH)_2 + ADP + Pi \rightarrow CH_3COOH + NH_3 + RS_2 + ATP \quad (7)$$

Dithiothreitol is the usual in-vitro electron donor, and GSH is the likely in-vivo donor. The reaction proceeds through a carboxymethylselenocysteine intermediate, and then forms a mixed selenodisulfide (ESeS) intermediate when a high-energy acetylthiol intermediate is formed on the C subunit, leading to formation of ATP and acetate.

Nicotinic acid hydroxylase from *Clostridium barkeri* catalyzes the following reaction:

$$\text{Nicotinic acid} + H_2O + NADP^+ \rightarrow 6-OH-\text{nicotinic acid} + NADPH + H^+ \quad (8)$$

The enzyme has four different types of subunits, 5–7 Fe, 1 FAD, and 1 Mo per 160-kDa protein promoter. The selenium is present in a low-molecular-weight form that is readily lost, suggesting that it may not be present as selenocysteine or is very labile; perhaps the selenium is a selenium analog of a FeS center or a Se ligand rather than S as an outer ligand of the molybden cofactor. The Mo is present as molybdenum cofactor, which now appears to be coordinated to the Se (170).

Xanthine dehydrogenase from clostridial species catalyzes the following reaction where A is an electron acceptor:

$$\text{Uric acid} + AH_2 \rightleftharpoons \text{xanthine} + H_2O + A \quad (9)$$

The enzyme has a molecular weight of 300 kDa, and also reacts with purines and aldehydes. The chemical reactivity suggests that the selenium moiety is very similar to that in nicotinic acid hydroxylase (61,166).

[NiFeSe]hydrogenases containing nickel and selenium have been isolated from *Methanococcus* and *Desulfovibrio* species. An 8-hydroxy-5-deazaflavin cofactor (F_{420}) is the natural electron acceptor for these hydrogenases, which is then used to generate NADPH. This reaction is

$$H_2 + F_{420} \rightarrow F_{420}H_2 \quad (10)$$

The selenium is present as selenocysteine, and is encoded by a UGA in at least some species. The enzymes typically have an $\alpha_2\beta_4\gamma_2$ or similar structure, and contain the selenocysteine in the β subunit. These selenoenzymes also contain 2 g-atoms of Ni/mole and several FAD and FeS clusters per mole, but not all Ni-hydrogenases contain selenium (61,166).

X. SELENIUM DEFICIENCY

T. E. Weichselbaum (171) discovered that rats maintained on a cystine-free diet develop a degenerative liver disease which causes death. This disease, liver necrosis, is distinct from fatty liver, and liver cirrhosis and could be prevented by either cystine or vitamin E. In 1951, Klaus Schwarz demonstrated the existence of a third factor present in American's brewer's yeast which would prevent liver necrosis in rats fed a torula yeast-based diet unsupplemented with cystine or vitamin E (172). This water-soluble "factor-3" was stable to acid hydrolysis and could not be replaced by any known vitamin. In 1957, Schwarz and Foltz discovered that factor-3 isolated from pig kidney contained selenium, and that a variety of inorganic as well as organic forms of selenium prevent liver necrosis in rats (8). The exact chemical nature of factor-3 remains elusive, but some diseleno, dicarboxylic acids such as diseleno-dipropionate as well as longer-chained species with 9 or 11 carbons have activity equivalent to factor-3. Schwarz later found that the ability of cystine to protect against liver necrosis is due in part to selenium contamination of the cysteine, and this remains a problem today for those of us formulating crystalline amino acid diets. [Use of methionine alone tends to alleviate this problem (Sunde, unpublished).]

In 1969, McCoy and Weswig (173) demonstrated that selenium is essential in a diet containing adequate levels of vitamin E and the sulfur amino acids. Selenium-deficient female rats fed a selenium-deficient diet from weaning grew normally, but their offspring were devoid of hair, grew slowly, and failed to reproduce, thus demonstrating that selenium is an essential element in the rat, and that selenium cannot be completely spared by another nutrient.

A. Selenium Deficiency in Other Species

The effect of selenium and vitamin E deficiency varies among species. In contrast to the rat, which develops primarily liver necrosis and to a lesser extent degeneration of some other tissues during combined selenium and vitamin E deficiency, the mouse develops a multiple neurotic degeneration of skeletal muscle, heart, kidney, liver, and pancreas (174). Swine develop a syndrome called "mulberry heart," which includes coronary capillary degeneration, liver and skeletal muscle degeneration, skin lesions, gastric ulcers, and gastric keratosis (175). Lambs develop a nutritional muscular dystrophy which can be prevented by selenium alone, although dietary unsaturated fatty acid supplementation and other unknown conditions produce a muscular dystrophy which is prevented only by vitamin E. Note that significant hepatic lesions are not observed in selenium-deficient sheep. In cattle, deficiency of selenium and vitamin E also causes a nutritional myopathy which affects skeletal and heart muscle with sudden onset of death when the heart is involved, especially in young calves. Attempts to induce these disease signs experimentally are often unsuccessful, whereas they are often observed under practical conditions (176). Additions of polyunsaturated fatty acids tend to exacerbate the condition in experimental trials, but it is clear that high polyunsaturated fat is only one factor along with selenium and vitamin E deficiency that predisposes cattle to develop nutritional myopathy.

Chickens develop one of four disease states, depending on which nutrient is missing. Chicks develop muscular dystrophy when fed diets deficient in vitamin E and the sulfur amino acids, and develop encephalomalacia, a degenerative change in the cerebellum, when fed a vitamin E-deficient, sulfur amino acid-adequate diet containing high polyunsaturated fatty acid content. Selenium may sometimes delay but will never prevent nutritional muscular dystrophy or encephalomalacia in chicks. Chick diets are supplemented with methionine and low levels of ethoxyquin, a synthetic antioxidant to prevent these diseases, thus allowing researchers to study selenium and/or vitamin E deficiency in the chick. Either selenium or vitamin E supplementation prevents exudative diathesis, which is diagnosed as an accumulation of blue/green viscus fluid under the ventral skin of the chick. Chicks fed a selenium-deficient diet supplemented with vitamin E and methionine grow poorly, show poor feathering, and develop a pancreatic degeneration sometimes called pancreatic fibrosis or pancreatic atrophy. Thus in the chick there are four disease syndromes that result from vitamin E and/or selenium deficiency (2,58,177).

B. Human Selenium Deficiency

Clear-cut evidence for the essentiality of selenium in humans did not develop until two decades after the demonstration that selenium was essential for rats and chickens. In 1979, VanRij et al. (178) made the first report of human selenium deficiency symptoms in a New Zealand patient undergoing total parenteral nutrition (TPN). The patient lived in a rural area with low-selenium soils in which endemic white muscle disease in sheep was controlled by selenium dosing. Following surgery, she received TPN for 20 days and developed dry, flaky skin, and after 30 days she developed bilateral muscular discomfort and muscle pain. Plasma selenium had dropped to 9 ng Se/mL versus 25 ng/mL immediately before the start of TPN. The muscle pain was sufficient to aggravate walking, and a generalized muscular wasting occurred. The patient was then infused intravenously with a 100 μg Se/day as selenomethionine, and within the next week, muscle pain disappeared and she returned to full mobility. TPN-associated selenium deficiency in humans is not restricted to countries with low soil selenium content. A similar TPN-induced case of muscle pain and cardio-myopathy leading to death has been reported in the United States (179). These cases are associated with very low plasma and red blood cell selenium and GPX1 activity, and with elevated plasma marker enzymes indicative of tissue damage. A fourth sign of selenium deficiency, white nail beds, has also been reported associated with TPN (180), although this may be due to an associated liver necrosis rather than a specific function of selenium.

The dramatic impact of selenium deficiency in humans is revealed in the descriptions of Keshan disease and endemic cardiomyopathy that occurred until the 1980s in China. Keshan disease affected primarily children under 15 years of age and women of child-bearing age. Incidence rates prior to the start of selenium supplementation were of the order of 6.5–13.5 per thousand, and the disease was localized primarily in the peasant popula-tions in certain hilly and mountainous regions associated with low soil selenium. Urban inhabitants and families of the managerial classes living in the same area are unaffected (due to an improved diet with more animal products and with products from a more diverse geographic range). The main pathologic feature is a multiple focal myocardial necrosis scattered throughout the heart muscle. Criteria for diagnosis include acute or chronic heart function insufficiency, heart enlargement, gallop rhythm or arrhythmia, ECG changes, and pulmonary edema. Subacute cases may also have facial edema. The demonstration that selenium is essential for laboratory animals and livestock in the 1960s, and the observations that the cardiomyopathy associated with Keshan disease was similar to that observed in Se-deficient mice and swine, suggested trials with selenium. Encouraging preliminary results indicated that selenium might be preventive. All affected areas were found to be invariably poor in selenium, and thus a large-scale study was begun in 1974 with all children in 119 production teams in three communes. Half the children were given weekly sodium selenite tablets orally, and the other half were given a placebo. Children 1–5 years old received 0.5 mg, and children 6–9 received 1 mg of sodium selenite (0.23 and 0.46 mg Se/week, respectively); a total of 46,033 children were in this study. The last two years of the study, the control group was omitted. In the first two years, there were 53 deaths in the control group (5.6/1000) versus 0.08/1000 in the treatment group. Total cases in the selenium-treatment group were not immediately eliminated, but progressively declined through the

4-year period, suggesting that more than restoration of selenium status alone is involved in the disease. The average hair selenium in nonaffected sites was above 0.2 μg Se/g; the average in all affected sites was below 0.12 μg Se/g. GPX1 activity in blood of peasant children was two-thirds of that observed in staff children. Average daily selenium intake for women in these affected areas was estimated to be 12 μg Se/day, which is considerably lower than the New Zealand estimate of 20 μg Se/day necessary for maintenance of normal human health (43,181). The disease has now virtually been eliminated by selenium supplementation, but troubling questions remain about the etiology. The ineffectiveness in completely eradicating the disease in one season following selenium supplementation, and a seasonal prevalence of the disease, both suggest that other factors are involved. A cardiotoxic virus has been isolated from the hearts of individuals who died from Keshan disease.

C. Selenium Deficiency and Virus Resistance

Recent exciting studies by Beck (182) have demonstrated that a virulent coxsackie virus B3 (CVB3/20), which induces myocardial lesions in the hearts of mice, is more virulent in Se-deficient than in Se-supplemented mice. The lesions occur more quickly, more severely, and with higher virus titer in heart and liver of selenium-deficient mice versus selenium-adequate mice. In addition, a cloned and sequenced benign amyocarditic coxsackie virus B3 (CVB3/0), which causes no pathology in the hearts of selenium-adequate mice, induces extensive cardiac pathology in selenium-deficient mice. Most interestingly, the "CVB3/0" virus recovered from the hearts of selenium-deficient mice and inoculated into selenium-adequate mice now induces significant heart damage, suggesting that the mutation of the virus to a virulent genotype is predisposed by culturing in the selenium-deficient mice (183). Taylor (184) has suggested a novel hypothesis that selenium deficiency may potentiate mutation of viruses including HIV and other retroviruses. The foundation of the hypothesis is the presence of highly conserved alternate reading frames in viral genomes, which are accessed by formation of a thermodynamically stable "pseudo-knot" secondary structure in the mRNA. The pseudo-knot is a stem loop structure with 3′ sequences after the stem adding additional stability by forming Watson-Crick base pairs with bases in the loop. In viruses, Taylor has found that putative alternate reading frames often contain UGA codons and eSECIS elements such that selenocysteine might be inserted in a Se-adequate host, thus sustaining survival pressure to retain the native sequence. As the hypothesis goes, in selenium deficiency these alternate frame-shift proteins would not be made, thus promoting and selecting for mutations of the virus which do not require selenium. The hypothesis is intriguing, but remains untested (184). An alternative hypothesis is simply that in selenium deficiency there may be increased reactive oxygen species, resulting in altered immune response that allows the virus a chance to achieve higher titers or persist longer (183). Explanation of selenium biochemistry in other organisms, such as viruses, promises to be most interesting and may yield novel solutions to current problems.

XI. SELENIUM REQUIREMENTS

Numerous methods have been used to assess selenium requirements. Excellent reviews in this area can be found in Refs. 2, 3, 185, 186. This review focuses on the use of laboratory rats to set requirements, and then discusses the implications for setting human requirements. Schwarz, in his early work (75), determined the effective dose that would prevent 50% of the animals from dying from liver necrosis within 30 days, and found that selenite, selenocysteine, selenomethionine, selenocystathionine, and KSeCN are approximately equivalent in their protection. Here we are not concerned about small, ~10% differences in requirements, because animal-to-animal variation and homeostasis clearly negate closer approximation in spite of our increased ability to interpolate between data points.

Hafeman and colleagues were the first to use GPX1 activity as an indicator of selenium status and requirements (102). Animals from a commercial supplier (purchased in 1971) were fed a torula yeast-based diet containing 8 µg Se/kg diet. This is the diet of Schwarz and colleagues, based on 30% low-selenium torula yeast and supplemented with 0.3% D,L-methionine to raise the methionine content to 0.54%—which, along with the cysteine content of 0.18%, makes the diet just adequate in sulfur amino acids. The diet also contained 5% stripped lard and 3% cod liver oil, but was supplemented with 50 mg of all-rac-α-tocopherol so that just selenium deficiency was being evaluated. In this 1971 experiment, there was a significant effect of feeding the selenium-deficient diet on growth as rats fed the deficient diet grew at 85% of the rate of animals supplemented with 0.1 µg Se/g diet. Supplementation with 0.05 µg Se/g or more raised growth to that of selenium-supplemented animals, indicating that 0.05 µg Se/g diet is sufficient for adequate growth. Experiments conducted with commercially available weanling rats in the 1990s do not show any effect of feeding selenium-deficient torula yeast diet (187) or crystalline amino acid diet (2–3 ng Se/g) on growth rate through 28 days. Pups from selenium-deficient dams, however, grow at 53% of the rats fed 0.1 µg Se/g diet (188).

Erythrocyte GPX1 activity decreased exponentially in rats fed a selenium-deficient diet with $t_{1/2}$ of 30 days, reaching 21% of initial levels 66 days after the start of the experiment (102). Approximately 0.1 µg Se/g diet was sufficient to maintain erythrocyte GPX activity at initial levels, but excess selenium increased GPX activity in erythrocytes, making the parameter less useful for determining selenium requirements. Behne (24) found that erythrocyte selenium in selenium-deficient rats was 11% of that found in rats fed 0.25 µg Se/g diet. Plasma selenium similarly decreased to 15% of selenium-adequate levels. Levander and colleagues (189) found that plasma selenium in deficient animals was approximately 4% of plasma selenium found in animals fed 0.25 µg Se/g diet for 4 weeks. This concentration of selenium was sufficient to raise platelet GPX as well as plasma, heart, and liver GPX1 to selenium-adequate levels after 2 weeks of selenium supplementation, whereas 0.1 µg Se/g diet was not. Hafeman et al. showed graded responses in repletion of erythrocyte GPX1 activity. Sixty days were required for 0.5 µg Se/g diet to raise erythrocyte GPX activity to initiate levels, and 5µg Se/g diet resulted in overshooting the initial erythrocyte GPX1 concentrations (102,190). When weanling rats are supplemented with graded levels of selenium there is a linear increase in plasma GPX3 and plasma Sel-P up to 0.1 µg Se/g diet (191). Plasma GPX3 activity appears to plateau between 0.1 and 2 µg Se/g diet, but Sel-P levels are unchanged between 0.1 and 0.5 µg Se/g diets, and then show a 40% increase between 0.1 and 2 µg Se/g diets. This indicates that Sel-P may not be especially effective in assessing selenium requirements, unless the plateau region is clearly known. Thus, blood selenium, erythrocytes GPX1 activity, and plasma Sel-P level do not appear to be especially effective for routine determination of selenium requirements because they continue to increase beyond usual adequate levels of dietary selenium.

Assessment of selenium status using liver parameters has been very useful, although it is relatively inconvenient. In commercially available rats fed a crystalline amino acid diet containing 2 ng Se/g, liver selenium is 3% of adequate animals and plasma GPX3 activity is 2% of selenium-adequate levels. In contrast, in second-generation selenium-deficient rats raised under otherwise identical conditions, liver selenium content falls to as low as 0.06

nmol Se/g wet weight, or 1% of selenium-adequate values (188), illustrating that the influence of maternal selenium stores on body stores extends more than 7 weeks after birth. Hafeman and colleagues found that liver GPX1 activity is especially effective in determining selenium status (102), and a clear plateau was demonstrated in liver GPX activity in animals fed 0.1 μg Se/g diet or higher at times ranging from 10 days to 134 days after weaning, thus establishing the dietary selenium requirement for rats at 0.1 μg Se/g diet. Liver GPX activity in male rats seems to somewhat increase with age, so the age of the rats should be considered for careful studies.

In the intervening two decades since the demonstration that GPX1 activity is a most useful parameter for the determination of selenium requirements, selenium requirements have been established for a wide variety of animals (see Table 5). Unlike the dietary nutrient requirements for almost all of the other trace elements, it is immediately apparent that the selenium requirement is virtually the same for all species identified, ranging from humans to laboratory animals to domestic animals to poultry, and even fish. This similarity of requirement is undoubtedly based in part on the early conclusive evidence for dietary selenium requirement of 0.1 μg Se/g diet in the laboratory rat. This fixed value would not have remained in the face of solid conflicting experimental data or conflicting data from analysis of diets or food consumption data. Specific molecular mechanisms must be maintaining the dietary requirement across this range of species.

Discussion on a couple of specific points also needs to be added. First the shown dietary requirements for the rat, hamster, and guinea pig are the National Research Council (NRC) 1978 requirements (192). In 1995, the NRC raised the requirement for the rat to 0.15 μg Se/g (193) as well as using this requirement as a basis to raise the requirement for the hamster, guinea pig, and mouse. This more recent recommendation includes a safety factor to ensure that the diets are adequate in selenium. Also important, it is based in part on the need for levels of selenium higher than 0.1 μg Se/g to protect against microvascular lesions

TABLE 5 Selenium Requirements of Various Species[a]

Species	Requirement (μg/g diet)	Reference	Species	Requirement (μg/g diet)	Reference
Rat	0.1	NRC, 1978[b]	Cat	0.1	NRC, 1978
Mouse	0.1	NRC, 1978[b]	Dog	0.11	NRC, 1985
Hamster	0.1	NRC, 1978[b]	Rabbit	—	NRC, 1977
Guinea pig	0.1	NRC, 1978[b]	Chick	0.1	NRC, 1977[c]
Cattle	0.1	NRC, 1978	Turkey	0.2	NRC, 1977[c]
Sheep	0.1–0.2	NRC, 1985	Primates	0.07	NRC, 1978
Horse	0.1	NRC, 1989	Human	0.10	RDA, 1989[d]
Pig	0.1–0.3	NRC, 1988	Fish	0.09	NRC, 1978

[a]The values in this table are minimum nutrient requirements, and are discussed in the indicated references. Most recent, full requirements are given for some of these values in the notes.

[b]The NRC 1995 rat requirement now includes a margin of safety and is increased to 0.15 μg Se/g. The pregnant and lactating rat requirement is 0.4 μg Se/g, and may be an overestimate, as discussed in the text. Mouse, hamster, and guinea pig requirements are based on the rat recommendations.

[c]The NRC 1994 chick requirement for the chick is 0.1–0.15 μg Se/g. The NRC 1994 turkey requirement is 0.20–0.28 μg Se/g.

[d]Calculated from the 1989 RDA excluding the 0.3 safety factor, based on the recommended energy, protein, and fat intake of adult humans.

of the retina (194). These experiments were conducted with male rats fed high levels of sucrose, under conditions that induce insult to the microvascular system. In these experiments, 0.2 μg Se/g diet results in a halving of the indicators of microvascular damage relative to rats fed 0.1 μg Se/g, suggesting that the minimum requirement for selenium are more than 0.1 μg/g. Similarly, studies by Smith and Picciano (195) suggest that pregnant female rats may require between 0.2 and 0.5 μg Se/g diet to allow liver GPX1 activity to reach a plateau level and so that nursing pups will have adequate selenium for GPX1 activity. Female rats in these studies, however, were fed selenium-deficient diets prior to the start of the experiment, and potential other changes in the selenium regulation due to pregnancy and/or lactation (steroid hormone modulations of transcription of GPX1) may be modulating these effects. In summary, the minimum dietary selenium requirement based on GPX1 activity appears to be at or very close to 0.1 μg Se/g diet. The recent studies, suggesting that a higher level of dietary selenium may be protective of the microvascular of the eye under certain stressful conditions or during pregnancy and lactation point out that we need to identify the underlying molecular biology and biochemistry of nutritional regulation so that isolated reports can be interpreted within the full framework of our understanding of selenium biochemistry, rather than calling for an entire new round of experimentation.

Several additional comments need to be made with regard to the higher selenium requirements of several domestic livestock species. The tight range of dietary selenium requirements for sheep, cattle, and pigs indicates first that these animals are quite similar to the other organisms in terms of their selenium regulation, and second, careful study of the supporting experiments indicates that the initial selenium status of the animal and the choice of main parameter used to set the requirement must be made carefully. Choice of tissue selenium levels, for instance, which continue to rise with increasing dietary selenium well beyond saturation of selenium incorporation into known biochemical functions, does not appear to be the most reliable indicator of minimum dietary requirement. In addition, the initial selenium status of the animals needs to be well defined when conducting these experiments, and any choice of margin of safety should be clearly documented to separate out the minimum dietary requirement and the margin of safety. Thus for our purposes here, we have retained the more conservative estimates of minimal dietary Se requirements. In contrast, the selenium requirement for the turkey appears to be twice that of other species. These higher selenium requirements are set for protection against gizzard myopathy or hatchability problems. It is quite clear that $\geq$0.2 μg Se/g diet is necessary for the prevention of gizzard myopathy in turkey poults fed diets that are marginal in vitamin E. Recent preliminary work in our laboratory suggests that GPX1 activity requires between 0.2 and 0.3 μg Se/g diet in rapidly growing turkey poults for maximum activity (196). This suggests that the molecular mechanism for determining the selenium requirement in the turkey is distinctly modified relative to that for other animal species.

The selenium requirement for humans is presently set in the United States at 70 and 55 μg/day for North American males and females, respectively (185). Notably, this is the only one of the human dietary requirements for mineral elements that is based on a biochemical parameter as opposed to diet assessment, balance studies, etc., showing the importance of GPX1 in establishing selenium requirements. Attempts to use balance effectively to determine selenium requirements were of little help because of selenium's homeostatic mechanisms (197). Comparison of dietary selenium intakes in adult Chinese in areas susceptible to Keshan disease versus areas seemingly protected, and comparison with New Zealand estimates of daily selenium intakes that are not associated with any selenium deficiency symptoms, suggests that 33 and 23 μg/day for men and women, respectively, are minimally adequate. Similarly, selenium repletion studies in China suggested that 40 μg Se/day for adult Chinese male subjects might be adequate. Adjustments for body weight and factoring in a 30% safety factor results in values of 70 and 55 μg Se/day, respectively, for males and females. Thus it appears that rats and other animals with the exception of the turkey are good models for understanding human selenium metabolism requirements. This also suggests that careful human work such as modeling of selenium metabolism can be extrapolated effectively to animals.

A. Parameters for Determining Selenium Requirements

By now it should be clear that a number of direct as well as indirect measures can be used to assess selenium status of animal and humans, and can be used to determine selenium requirements. Death and the development of overt disease are obviously the most stringent as well as clear cut. Careful work by Reiter and Wendel (131) examined changes in over 20 enzyme parameters in liver associated with drug-metabolizing enzymes during selenium depletion and selenium repletion. They found that virtually all of these enzyme changes were restored in mice injected with 10 μg Se/kg body weight, whereas GPX1 required 250 μg Se/kg body weight to restore 50% of the GPX1 activity. Glutathione-S-transferase was one of these enzymes and can be a useful marker in this set of selenium-dependent parameters. These effects are clearly indirect and occur in a concerted fashion, suggesting that the primary event may be controlled by a common selenium-sensitive process; some enzyme changes are up and some are down, and the number as well as the quantity of enzymes responsible excludes stoichiometric involvement of selenium in these enzymes themselves. They concluded that a dietary selenium concentration of around 35 ng Se/g diet will maintain these enzyme activities at normal conditions. Rises in circulating pyruvate kinase activity, indicative of tissue damage, reported by Arthur and colleagues (134) also should fit into this category. This concept is also consistent with that proposed by Behne (32) that endocrine tissues have a higher priority for selenium than tissues such as liver and kidney, and that within these tissues non-GPX functions have higher priority than GPX for activity.

The term *parameter* arises mostly in a mathematical setting and is often defined as "an arbitrary constant each of whose values characterizes a member of a system, such as a family of curves" or "a quantity or constant whose value varies with the circumstances of its application." This means that this is a constant with variable values which can be used for determining other factors. Thus, in nutrient status assessment, we define *parameter* as a "measured concentration, rate, or level whose value can vary with the nutrient status of the subject, and which is used as a referent for determining nutrient status." Thus a vast set of parameters indicates the nature of some aspect of the selenium status of the subject. Examples are: alive or dead, body weight, liver glutathione-S-transferase activity, GPX1 activity, GPX1 mRNA, DI1 activity, DI1 mRNA, GPX4 activity and mRNA, tissue selenium concentration, etc. In general, these parameters vary in a consistent or linked pattern, but they don't have to. For instance, rats fed selenomethionine in a methionine-deficient diet will have much higher tissue selenium values than is indicated by GPX1 activity. Rats that were initially selenium deficient and then repleted for short periods of time with limiting doses of selenium may show restoration of some parameters back to Se-adequate levels, while other parameters lag due to flux of selenium to more critical biochemical functions or to the slow turnover of selenium in the deficient tissues, such as muscle, brain, or red blood cells. The implication is that the overall nutrient status of a subject will be a functional sum of these individual parameters used to assess selenium status. The challenge of nutrition research today is to identify which parameter is most useful under the appropriate conditions for assessing nutrient status.

XII. SELENIUM REGULATION OF GPX1 EXPRESSION

Thus we set out to examine the underlying mechanism responsible for the constancy of dietary selenium requirements shown in Table 5. Our first approach was to examine selenium regulation of GPX1 protein as well as mRNA levels. It makes sense that GPX1 activity will decline when selenium is lacking, because selenium is the integral cofactor necessary for activity. We found, however, that weanling rats placed on a selenium-deficient diet showed a rapid exponential decline in GPX1 protein as well as GPX1 activity, with half-lives in liver of 5.2 days and 2.8 days, respectively, indicating that more than just loss of cofactor is responsible for this decrease in activity (198). For selenium repletion, GPX1 protein as well as activity requires larger doses and longer time periods than for maintenance. This is likely occurring because the other selenoproteins have first priority for selenium in selenium-deficient rat liver. The cloning of GPX1 next gave us the opportunity to assess the impact of selenium status on GPX1 mRNA levels. We found that selenium deficiency has a dramatic effect on GPX1 mRNA levels in liver (199), falling to approximately one-tenth of those found in selenium-adequate animals. In progressive selenium deficiency we saw a coordinated dramatic exponential drop in GPX1 mRNA ($T_{1/2}$ = 3.2 days) as well as GPX1 activity ($T_{1/2}$ = 3.3 days) and GPX1 protein ($T_{1/2}$ = 5.0 days) (190). These experiments thus begin to reveal that an underlying molecular mechanism is likely to be responsible for selenium regulation of GPX1 mRNA levels (4).

A series of experiments has carefully evaluated the effect of dietary selenium status on GPX1 and GPX4 activity and mRNA levels in male and female rats (Fig. 7). In selenium-deficient male rats (187), liver GPX1 activities were 1% of selenium-adequate animals. Between 0.002 and 0.033 μg Se/g diet there was little increase in GPX1 activity, and then there was a sharp increase between 0.033 and 0.065 μg Se/g diet. The plateaus are reached after 0.1 μg Se/g diet. Graphical analysis can be used to determine a break point between the steepest part of the response curve and the plateau for each of the parameters. The intersection of the line tangent to the steepest slope and a line through the plateau region can be defined as a *plateau break point* and used as a quantitative means to determine the minimum dietary selenium required for maximal response (see Fig. 7). The plateau break point for GPX1 occurs at 0.1 μg Se/g diet. Similar response curves also appear in heart, kidney, and lung (187). In contrast, GPX4 activity decreases only to 41% of selenium-adequate GPX4 activities in liver. The sharpest increase in GPX4 activity was seen between 0.013 and 0.65 μg Se/g diet in liver, and was at the plateau by 0.065 μg Se/g diet with a plateau break point occurring at 0.065 μg Se/g diet. Again, similar response curves were observed in other tissues for GPX4. These experiments show clearly that there is differential regulation of GPX1 and GPX4 in the same tissue. When mRNA levels were quantitated, GPX1 mRNA was reduced to 7% of selenium-adequate levels and also responded sigmoidally to increasing dietary selenium concentration such that GPX1 mRNA levels in liver reached the break point at 0.065 μg Se/g diet. In contrast, liver GPX4 mRNA was not affected significantly by dietary selenium, but was decreased to 61% of the levels found in selenium-adequate animals. Similar response curves were observed for the other tissues as well. It is clear that the plateau break point for GPX4 mRNA in male

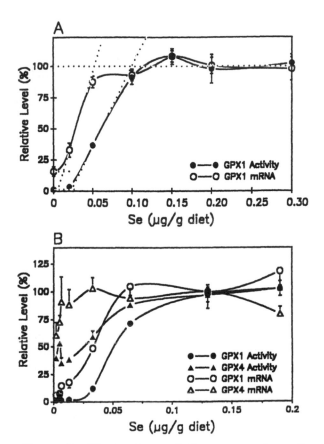

FIGURE 7 Effective dietary selenium concentration on liver GPX1 and GPX4 activity and mRNA in female (top) and male (bottom) rats. Top: Female weanling rats were fed graded levels of dietary Se from 0 to 0.3 μg Se/g diet for 32 days and GPX1 activity and mRNA determined (25). Bottom: Male weanling rats were fed graded levels of dietary Se from 0 to 0.19 μg Se/g diet for 28 days and GPX1 activity, GPX1 mRNA levels, GPX4 activity, and GPX4 mRNA levels determined (187).

rat liver and other tissues occurs before 0.013 μg Se/g diet. In rat testes, the plateau break point for GPX activity determined using either H_2O_2 or PCOOH occurs at approximately 0.025 μg Se/g diet, suggesting that this activity is not due to GPX1 or that GPX1 is regulated differently in testes compared to other tissues.

In females rats which have more than two and a half times the level of GPX1 mRNA as well as activity, the selenium regulation curves are very similar (25). Liver selenium concentration in rats fed a torula yeast-based selenium-deficient diet was 4% of selenium-adequate values, and the plateau break point for liver selenium was 0.1 μg Se/g diet. Erythrocyte GPX1 activity in selenium-deficient rats was 40% of selenium-adequate levels. While erythrocyte GPX1 activity continues to increase with increasing selenium, a plateau break point could be identified for this activity as well at 0.1 μg Se/g diet. Interestingly, plasma GPX3 activity in selenium-deficient plasma was 8% of the levels found in selenium-adequate animals, and reached a plateau break point at 0.07 μg Se/g diet, showing an altered response curve for this kidney-derived plasma activity. Liver GPX1 activity in selenium-deficient female rats was 2% of the level found in females fed selenium-adequate diets, and the plateau break point was 0.1 μg Se/g diet. Se-deficient liver GPX mRNA levels were 11–17% of selenium-adequate levels, and the plateau break point was reached at 0.05 μg Se/g diet. In this experiment (25), plotting the change in GPX1 activity in liver as a function of liver GPX1 mRNA levels shows that GPX1 mRNA levels respond to increasing selenium status before GPX1 activity, such that GPX1 mRNA reached half-maximum at 0.27 μg Se/g diet whereas half-maximal GPX1 activity requires 0.75 μg Se/g diet. At concentrations greater than 0.1 μg Se/g diet, this relationship breaks down, showing that above 0.1 μg Se/g diet, selenium is no longer rate limiting for either GPX1 mRNA or GPX1 activity.

Similar experiments have been conducted to evaluate the effect of dietary selenium on DI1 activity in mRNA and liver. Arthur and colleagues (141) saw similar effects on GPX1 and GPX4 activity and mRNA levels in male hooded Wister rats fed diets containing 3 ng Se/g diet. Liver DI1 activity in selenium-deficient animals was 5% of that observed in selenium-adequate animals, and DI1 mRNA levels were 50% of that observed in selenium-adequate animals. As dietary selenium increased, the increases in DI1 activity were parallel to the increases in GPX1 mRNA levels. The DI1 mRNA response curve was hyperbolic rather than sigmoidal, with a plateau break point at about half of that observed for GPX4 activity, GPX1 mRNA, and DI1 activity. Thus it appears that GPX1 mRNA levels reach maximum only when selenium incorporation into DI1 as well as GPX4 are maximized.

Se deficiency in rats causes a decrease in plasma Sel-P concentration to less than 10% of that in Se-adequate animals (55), and selenium supplementation of deficient rats results in an increase in Sel-P concentration ahead of the increases in plasma GPX3 activity and liver GPX1 activity (when expressed on a percentage basis relative to rats supplemented with 0.5 μg Se/g diet). At 4.5 weeks after feeding selenium-deficient diet to rats, GPX1, DI1, and Sel-P mRNA levels in liver had all decreased (200). The impact of selenium deficiency on Sel-P mRNA levels was that Sel-P mRNA levels fell to 67% of the levels found in selenium-adequate animals, whereas liver GPX1 mRNA levels were 19% of adequate levels. The magnitude of the decrease in liver Sel-P mRNA after feeding a Se-deficient diet for 4.5 weeks was 40% of the drop in liver GPX1 mRNA level; the drop in DI1 mRNA was 80% of the fall in GPX1 mRNA. These studies indicate that in selenium deficiency, Sel-P mRNA is less affected than DI1 mRNA, which is less affected than GPX1 mRNA.

The discovery that selenium is a component of GPX1 logically explained the antioxidant functions of selenium (142). The discovery of multiple GPX enzymes and genes, however, indicates that this perception was clearly an oversimplification. The hierarchy of protection of these enzymes against decreases due to dietary selenium deficiency shows that GPX4, Sel-P, and DI1 all are protected from selenium deficiency relative to GPX1. Second, when mRNA changes are carefully compared relative to the mRNA changes in GPX1, it is clear that GPX1 mRNA levels fall by an order of magnitude or more, whereas these mRNA levels for GPX4, DI1, and Sel-P typically do not change or decrease by only a factor of 2–3. The unique and specific regulation of GPX1 mRNA suggests that this may be an important aspect of the physiologic role of GPX1.

The important role of GPX1 in the liver, and perhaps other tissues, may be as part of the homeostatic mechanism that keeps free concentration of selenium low, diverts selenium to more important biological functions during times of selenium deficiency, and absorbs excess selenium over the deficient-to-adequate range. In other words, the major role of GPX is to serve as a *biological selenium buffer* (3). This suggests that the effect of this buffering capacity provides an expansion of the dietary range between selenium deficiency and selenium toxicity. This function is more appropriately "biological selenium" buffer, rather than a "selenium store" or "selenium sink," because it indicates the dynamic homeostatic nature and indicates GPX1's active role in modulating selenium flux between incorporation into other selenoenzymes and incorporation into GPX1. The model, as originally proposed, consists of a system that contains a 1-μM high-affinity protein (effective $K_m = 0.005$ μM) a 5-μM lower-affinity protein ($K_m = 0.5$ μM), and a free or labile selenium pool that rises only after selenium incorporation into these other processes is saturated. The K_m values describe processes, presumably mediated by binding or incorporation, that are half-saturated at the indicated K_m concentrations of selenium. The resulting distribution of selenium as the total system concentration increases is shown in Figure 8: (a) Initially, selenium associates only with the high-affinity protein; (b) selenium begins to associate with the low-affinity protein only after the high-affinity protein is saturated; (c) the labile selenium pool rises only after the low-affinity protein is saturated. This results in a dramatic increase in the labile selenium, just as selenium incorporation into the low-affinity protein is maximized. The rapid increase in labile selenium would occur a full order of magnitude lower without the low-affinity protein. This model suffers, however, because it is a closed system, and yet in vivo it is clear that selenium in liver and other tissues does not increase linearly as dietary selenium increases.

To test the selenium buffer hypothesis directly, GPX1 mRNA levels were set in rats by feeding diets ranging between 0 and 0.2 μg Se/g diet to rats for 35 days, and then the rats were injected intraperidoneally with 100 μCi of ^{75}Se as selenite and killed 6 h later (3). Selenium incorporation into selenoproteins was determined using SDS-PAGE. In addition, the free or labile selenium in the cytosol was quantitated by determining the ^{75}Se that was no longer bound to protein after SDS/PAGE (Fig. 8B). Under these conditions, ^{75}Se incorporation into GPX4 was maximized between 0.02 and 0.05 μg Se/g diet; at higher dietary selenium concentrations, the dietary selenium diluted ^{75}Se incorporation into GPX4. In contrast, there was little ^{75}Se incorporation into GPX1 below 0.02 μg Se/g, ^{75}Se incorporation was maximized at 0.1 μg Se/g, and it declined at higher dietary levels, indicating dilution. Labile or free selenium in the cytosol increased only above 0.1 μg Se/g, showing that this pool is elevated in liver only after ^{75}Se incorporation into GPX1 is maximized. Note, however, that this labile selenium pool falls above 0.15 μg Se/g, suggesting that an additional hypothetical process is transporting the ^{75}Se out of the liver. This might be a detoxification mechanism (3).

Bermano and colleagues recently found new evidence that supports the selenium buffer hypothesis (141). We have previously discussed the regulation of DI1 in this experiment. The novel observation in this experiment was that selenium regulation of selenoproteins in thyroid is in many ways contrary to what is observed in liver and heart. This shows that there is a tissue specificity as well as selenoprotein specificity to selenium regulation. In thyroid, GPX1 activity in selenium deficiency decreased to about 50% of that found in selenium-adequate animals, but GPX1 mRNA levels were not affected significantly, suggesting that free selenium concentrations in the thyroid never dropped to the extent necessary to decrease the stability of GPX1 mRNA. GPX4 activity was unaffected, but GPX4 mRNA increased by 50% in selenium deficiency. Most strikingly, DI1 activity increased slightly and DI1 mRNA increased 40% in selenium deficiency, suggesting that TSH upregulates transcription of DI1 as part of the feedback mechanisms to maintain thyroid T_3 levels. The decrease in GPX1 activity apparently releases sufficient selenium to provide selenium for DI1 and GPX4. These other, more critical selenium functions are

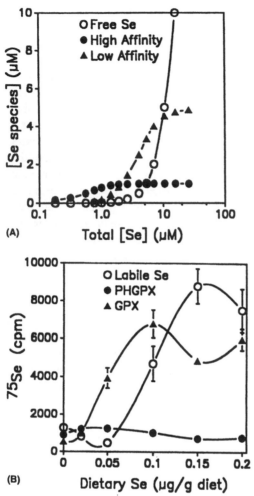

(A)

(B)

FIGURE 8 Hypothetical (A) and experimental (B) illustrations of the hypothesis that GPX1 functions as a biological selenium buffer. A. Distribution of selenium among a high-affinity component (K_m 0.005 μM) and a lower-affinity component (K_m 0.5 μM), and free labile selenium, as total selenium increases from 0.1 to 100 μM. B. Distribution of the ^{75}Se in rat liver cytosol among GPX4, GPX1, and the labile selenium pool, as determined by SDS PAGE. Rats were fed the indicated levels of selenium and injected with 100 μCi [^{75}Se]selenite 6 h prior to sacrifice (3).

preserved at the expense of GPX1. Clearly, whether or not GPX1 has a major function as a biological selenium buffer, it nonetheless readily accomplishes this task in thyroid.

XIII. MECHANISM OF SELENIUM REGULATION

The mechanism for the specific downregulation of GPX1 mRNA in selenium deficiency, as well as the more modest downregulation in liver and other tissues of the mRNA for other selenoproteins, has not been established. It is clear that this regulation is posttranscriptional, as the use of nuclear runoff transcription assays shows clearly that there is no effect of selenium deficiency on the levels of initiated transcripts. In selenium-deficient rats selenium status has no effect on in-vitro [^{32}P]UTP incorporation into total RNA, and isolation of hnRNA shows equivalent levels of GPX1 mRNA in the nuclei of selenium-adequate and selenium-deficient rat liver (201). This indicates that selenium deficiency does not impair transcription, nor does it impair translocation of GPX1 RNA from the nucleus. Christensen and Burgener (202), Burk and Hill (55), and Toyoda (203) have demonstrated clearly that selenium deficiency has no effect on transcription for any of the selenium-dependent enzymes and proteins. Thus this regulation must occur posttranscriptionally.

Presently, the most logical mechanism is that the intracellular concentration of one particular selenium species, such as selenite or selenophosphate or selenocysteinyl-tRNA, specifically regulates GPX1 mRNA stability, in a manner analogous to iron regulation of transferrin receptor mRNA stability as mediated by the iron-regulatory protein. This convenient model suggests that the binding of a putative selenium-dependent binding factor to the mRNA regulates its stability (see Fig. 5).

Weiss and Sunde (204) have recently used site-directed mutagenesis to alter the 3'UTR of GPX1 mRNA and express these transcripts in CHO cells to monitor selenium regulation of GPX1 mRNA stability. Both the regulation of the endogenous GPX1 mRNA as well as regulation of the larger transfected GPX1 mRNA can be determined at the same time in the same cells. Under these conditions, transfection with wild-type GPX1 results in at most a fivefold increase in GPX1 activity, and a two- to threefold increase in GPX1 mRNA relative to endogenous GPX1 levels. Transfection with non-Se-dependent reporter genes, in contrast, results in dramatic overexpression of mRNA and protein, demonstrating clearly that the necessary factors for selenium incorporation are limiting or kinetically dampened such that translation of selenocysteine-containing polypeptides is reduced by a factor of 100 or more. Nonetheless, it is clear that overexpression of GPX1 does not alter the break point for regulation of GPX1 activity which occurs at 50–100 nM Se. Endogenous GPX1 mRNA is decreased to as low as 33% of selenium-adequate GPX1 mRNA levels when CHO cells are grown in low-selenium media. Transfected GPX1 mRNA levels are decreased significantly, to 66% of the levels observed in selenium-supplemented cells, and the plateau break point for the regulation of GPX1 mRNA levels occurs at approximately 4 nM Se. This demonstrates that intracellular selenium has differential effects on GPX1 mRNA stability and translation. More important, deletion of portions of the 3'UTR completely eliminates selenium regulation of GPX1 mRNA; point mutations that alter the structure of the eSECIS element also result in loss of selenium regulation of GPX1 mRNA, but additional mutations that restore the stem base pairing of the eSECIS restore selenium regulation. This provides strong evidence that selenium-specific regulation of GPX1 mRNA steady-state levels is mediated via the 3'UTR and message stability. Several preliminary reports have identified SELB-like eukaryotic proteins which bind to the eSECIS element of the 3'UTR (96,205). It is possible that one or more of these proteins also regulates mRNA levels. Sufficient selenium to saturate a hypothetical selenium-dependent regulatory factor which binds GPX1 mRNA would thus fully protect GPX1 mRNA from degradation and result in the plateau break points observed in cultured cells and in animal tissues. The increase in mRNA for selenoproteins prior to the increase in the corresponding protein suggests that this is a regulatory process that does not readily drain selenium away from this pool, whereas selenium incorporation into selenoproteins does drain selenium away, thus yielding sigmoidal selenium response curves with plateau break points for GPX1 activity that occur at higher selenium concentrations than for GPX1 mRNA levels.

The downregulation of mRNA levels for selenoprotein-P, DI1, and even GPX4 may be explained by pausing that must occur if selenocysteinyl tRNA concentrations are limiting for protein synthesis. The competition between termination factors and fully active tRNA complexes would predispose translation for early termination, and early termination of translation often might be accompanied by increased mRNA degradation. This suggests that two components are involved in selenium regulation of mRNA levels: (a) nonspecific effects relative to whether or not sufficient selenium (as selenocysteinyl-tRNA) is available for translation; (b) GPX1 mRNA-specific effects mediated by one or more protein factors. Differential regulation of selenoprotein mRNAs promises to be an exciting area of future research.

XIV. SELENIUM AND VITAMIN E

Vitamin E and selenium have been inexorably linked since the discovery that selenium prevents liver necrosis. Hoekstra (142) affirmed the antioxidant theory of the function of vitamin E, and noted that the role of selenium in GPX1 provides a logical antioxidant function for the nutrient selenium. In his careful way, he pointed out that this discovery did not "clarify whether or not there are other roles for both vitamin E and selenium," and he presented a model illustrating a role for vitamin E in quenching the production of hydroperoxides which would otherwise lead to lipid peroxidation, malondialdehyde formation, and cell damage. In this model, the role for GPX1 was to rapidly convert to the corresponding alcohol any hydroperoxides that slipped past vitamin E and any H_2O_2 produced as a by-product of necessary biochemical reactions, thus minimizing peroxidative damage. Unfortunately, we are really no closer today to identifying the specific biochemical mechanism for vitamin E. It is clear, however, that we have found additional roles for selenium and a number of additional specific peroxidase roles for selenium as well.

The current model for vitamin E function and its role as an antioxidant were reviewed recently by Sies and Stahl (206). They conclude that tocopherols and tocotrienols along with ascorbic acid and the carotenoids react with free radicals, notably peroxyradicals and singlet molecular oxygen, and that this is the basis for the function as an antioxidant. Specifically α-tocopherol is the major peroxyradical scavenger in biological membranes and in low-density lipoproteins; these antioxidants protect against a shift toward the proxidant side in the prooxidant–antioxidant balance that characterizes the normal metabolic state in living organisms. Peroxyradicals (LOO·) are generated from polyunsaturated fats in membrane phopholipids after abstraction of a proton and addition of molecular oxygen. Peroxyradicals are estimated to have a half-life of 7 s, whereas hydroxy radical has a half-life estimated at 1×10^{-9} s and singlet oxygen at 1×10^{-6} s (206). Thus α-tocopherol, with high reactivity against these species, is the major lipid-soluble antioxidant in membranes and microsomes, and it determines the susceptibility to damage by these various oxidants. Part of the protective action for ascorbate and glutathione may be to regenerate reduced α-tocopherol from the tocopherol radical that is formed in free-radical quenching. Expanding this model, selenium's antioxidant role is mediated all or in part via one or more of the peroxidases that rapidly metabolize the resulting products of the α-tocopherol reaction to the corresponding alcohols, before these dangerous but less reactive species cause membrane or protein cell damage (206).

The relative roles for vitamin E and selenium in this process are grudgingly being revealed. Studies in the 1970s showed that ethane and pentane evolution in the breath of rats due to peroxidative breakdown of unsaturated fatty acids is minimized by vitamin E alone, and partially reduced to 40% of the rate in doubly deficient rats by 0.2 μg Se/g diet (207). More recent studies by Awad et al. (208) report the development of a new marker of in-vivo lipid peroxidation using mass spectroscopy to quantitate a series of prostaglandin F_2-like compounds which result from the free radical-catalyzed peroxidation of arachidonic acid in vivo. These F_2 isoprostanes are esterified to phospholipids in tissues and are also found as free F_2 isoprostanes in plasma. Rats were depleted of selenium and vitamin E by feeding a doubly deficient diet for 12 weeks, and then divided into four groups: rats continued with the doubly deficient diet, rats supplemented with 0.25 μg Se/g diet alone, rats supplemented with 100 mg of all-rac-α-tocopheryl acetate alone, and rats supplemented with both (control). Plasma F_2 isoprostanes in rats continued with the doubly deficient diet were fivefold higher than in animals refed the control diet. Selenium deficiency alone was not associated with any excess production of F_2 isoprostanes, but plasma F_2 isoprostane level was twice control rats in the vitamin E-deficient alone group. F_2 isoprostanes present in phospholipids in various tissues also showed similar results, with selenium deficiency exacerbating vitamin E deficiency in most tissues, whereas selenium deficiency alone was without effect compared to doubly supplemented rats. Nine of 16 rats that were continued on the doubly deficiency diet died within 16 days, apparently due to liver necrosis. One of the strengths of this technique is that F_2 isoprostanes esterified to phospholipids can be assessed in specific tissues. F_2 isoprostanes in liver were doubled by the combined deficiency, but vitamin E supplementation completely blocked these changes. Selenium deficiency in the face of adequate vitamin E resulted in F_2 isoprostanes that were about 40% of the levels seen in the doubly deficient animals. Similar effects were also seen in muscle and heart, suggesting that myodegeneration is most likely occurring in the vitamin E-deficient animals, and that selenium can partially but not totally prevent this occurrence.

Thus a model to explain the relative roles of vitamin E and selenium would need to make vitamin E the primary antioxidant molecule that can intercept and detoxify damaging prooxidants before these species cause detectable damage. Selenium-dependent functions appear to be an important, second arm of the overall protective mechanism. Under different conditions or stressors, such as the mix of metabolic by-products in the chick pancreas, selenium may have the more critical role, while in sheep liver selenium's role is less important. The specific molecular role(s) for selenium are unclear, but it appears that selenium-dependent functions other than GPX1 are the major components of this protective mechanism, either because of compartmentalization or because GPX1 can fall to near-zero levels without appreciable damage while these other selenium-dependent enzymes or proteins are still at effective strength. Circulating GPX3 or selenoprotein P, GPX4 rolling along membranes in the plasma, microsomal or mitochondrial intermembrane space, Sel-W in muscle, or another as yet undiscovered selenoprotein could be the major selenium-dependent antioxidant agent. This model illustrates that evolution appears to have dispatched duplicate protective mechanisms to defend against prooxidant species. Knockout cell and animal models will most certainly prove to be critical in unraveling this duplication.

XV. SELENIUM TOXICITY

The historical cases of selenium toxicity have already been reviewed. There is quite a narrow range of dietary selenium concentrations that are adequate and yet not toxic. The minimum dietary requirement is 0.1 μg Se/g diet, and dietary levels above 2 μg Se/g diet are chronically toxic, resulting in a factor of 20 between the dietary selenium requirement and the onset of selenium toxicity. In rats, hydrogen selenide is the most toxic form of selenium, and exposure to 0.02 mg H_2Se/L air for 60 min results in death in 25 days. The relative toxicities of various low-molecular-weight selenium compounds are illustrated by the following LD_{50} or LD_{75} values in rats given intraperitoneal injections (in mg Se/kg body weight): sodium selenite, 3.25–3.5; sodium selenate, 5.5–5.8; D,L-selenocysteine, 4; D,L-selenomethionine, 4.3; diseleno-dipropionic acid, 25–30; dimethyl selenide, 1600; tri-methylselenonium chloride, 49 (209). Dimethyl selenide is readily excreted in the breath, resulting in the garliclike odor that one detects on the breath of humans several hours after ingestion of 200 or 400 μg Se in pills used as anticancer nutriceuticals. Chronically, dietary selenium levels of 4–5 μg Se/g are sufficient to cause growth inhibition and result in tissue damage, as shown by elevated levels of marker enzymes (102). Liver toxicity and hyper-plastic hepatocytes have been reported in rats receiving 0.5–2 μg Se/g diet for 30 months, and higher concentrations between 4 and 16 μg Se/g diet cause edema and poor hair quality as well as short life spans (210,211).

In humans, chronic exposure to high dietary concentrations of selenium can arise due to water supplies with high concentrations of selenium. For instance, populations in Wyoming were found to consume selenium in drinking waters at levels approximately 50 times the U.S. drinking standard of 10 μg Se/L. Valentine and colleagues (212) found that selenium concentration in urine increased as water supply selenium increased, but selenium concentration in blood did not reflect the increased selenium exposure. When erythrocyte GPX1 activity was plotted relative to blood selenium, a negative correlation was observed, thus precluding use of erythrocyte GPX1 activity as an indicator of toxic exposure.

Abernathy and colleagues (213) have recently carefully reviewed the literature to help in the evaluation of a reference dose (RfD) for determining a safe upper level that will not cause deleterious effects over a lifetime of exposure. The underlying assumption is that there is a threshold of selenium toxicity, and that below this level selenium intakes will not in all probability cause adverse effects. This safe upper level is referred to as a NOAEL, that is, a *no-observed-adverse-effect level*. Early selenium toxicity in humans is associated with nausea, weakness, and diarrhea. With continuous intakes of excess selenium these symp-toms lead to loss of hair, changes in nail structure, lesions of the skin and nervous system, and mottling of the teeth. These toxicity symptoms are present with selenium intakes ranging from 3200 to 6700 μg Se/day. Later evaluation reported morphologic changes in the fingernails of individuals consuming an average of 1260 μg Se/day, whereas there was no evidence of selenium poisoning in 142 subjects in seleniferous areas of South Dakota and Wyoming who were consuming as much as 724 μg Se/day. Additional epidemiology data was provided from 400 Chinese living in an area with high dietary selenium concentra-tion who were evaluated for clinical and biochemical indices of selenosis. Regression analysis evaluated blood selenium levels relative to selenium intoxication, indicating a NOAEL of 853 μg Se/day, which results in blood selenium levels of ≤1 mg Se/L. At this blood selenium level, mildly prolonged prothrombin times and reduced glutathione con-centrations are observed, but these changes are not considered reliable indicators of selenium toxicity. Dividing this level of ingestion by the average weight of Chinese subjects (55 kg) yields a value of 15.5 μg Se/kg/day, which is thought to be without prolonged impact on human health. This compares with the current U.S. RDA of 0.9 μg Se/kg/day (70 μg Se/day divided by 79 kg, which is the average weight of American males) (213). Thus in humans, there is about a 17-fold difference between the recommended daily dietary allowance for selenium and the NOAEL, which results in a factor that is virtually identical to this factor for rats.

An interesting case of U.S. selenium intoxication occurred in 13 people who were taking an over-the-counter, improperly formulated dietary supplement that contained 27.3 mg Se per tablet (182 times higher than the amount specified on the label). Symptoms included nausea, abdominal pain, diarrhea, nail and hair changes, peripheral neuropathy, fatigue, and irritability. One individual took one tablet a day for a 2.5-month period in spite of these symptoms (214). This incident has numerous lessons: it demonstrates that ingestion of nutrients above the requirement is not the benign process that the public and even physicians often assume; it demonstrates the need for quality control in the manufacturing of nutritional supplements; it illustrates how easily an individual's faith in the health-promoting aspects of their supplements can overshadow a negative impact as well as lack of benefit on their health.

The biochemical mechanism underlying selenium toxicity is completely unknown, but is often postulated to be mediated by interaction with critical protein thiols. The only known specific biochemical reaction with regard to selenium toxicity is inactivation of eukaryotic initiation factor-2 (eIF-2) in reticulocyte lysates by selenite. The mechanism appears to be accompanied by an increase in the phosphorylation of eIF-2α, and 10 μM Se as selenite and above inhibits reinitiation of translation in this in-vitro assay. Selenite-inhibited lysates show an increase in ^{32}P incorporation into eIF-2α. This inactivation, however, does not appear to be direct, and it may involve either nonenzymatic oxidation of unpaired cysteine residues or inactivation of eIF-2α kinases (215). To date, this specific toxicity mechanism has not been exploited to learn more about how selenium impairs biochemistry as well as health.

A. Kesterson Reservoir

The Kesterson Reservoir is a 1280-acre reservoir located about 90 miles southeast of San Francisco and is part of the Kesterson National Wildlife Refuge. This artificially developed wetland, completed in 1978, was designed to collect subsurface drainage from tile drainage systems that are used to irrigate the agriculture land of the San Joaquin Valley. Fish began dying in the reservoir in 1981, and in 1983 field observation showed a high incidence of dead and deformed newborn waterfowl as well as adult coots. Selenium was identified as the probable cause of the deformities in the chicks. The selenium content of high-selenium soils in the San Joaquin Valley may be greater than 2000 ng Se/g, and drainage water may contain an average of 350 ng Se/g and occasionally as much as 1350 ng Se/g. Mosquito fish in the reservoir had reported selenium accumulations 36–72 times higher than the national average selenium concentrations. Toxicity studies in aquatic organisms (the algae *Ankistrodesmus falcatus*) have suggested that selenium as selenate may show signs of selenium toxicity at concentrations as low as 10 ng Se/g. Adding theoretical bioaccumulation factors, whereby aquatic organisms accumulate higher concentrations of selenium than that found in their environment and then magnify or increase this concentration as organisms at the lower levels of the food chain pass the selenium up the food chain, conservative water quality goals have been suggested as low as 1.0 ng Se/g (216). These goals are not based on experimental data, and there is little consideration that microorganisms as well as higher animals all show homeostatic regulation of selenium, which is decidedly different than for DDT or mercury. Organisms have evolved with molecular biochemical regulatory mechanisms to handle selenium deficiency and to tolerate selenium excess. Mathematical application of bioconcentrations and biomagnification factors should not be done without demonstration that these factors are accurate and predictive of what happens in the living setting.

This remains an exciting opportunity for research both in terms of basic selenium bio-chemistry and as justification for continued responsible nutritional supplementation of animals and protection of the environment.

The specific toxicity to waterfowl bears additional mention. Chronically toxic levels of selenium (3–5 μg Se/g), which generally do not have the same degree of adverse effects on other species, routinely result in decreased hatchability and deformed embryos in birds (217). These concentrations of selenium may be more toxic to birds because, unlike embryos sustained in utero and supplied by a maternal blood supply, the developing chick embryo is unable to release or exchange toxic metabolites. The leaching of selenium from San Joaquin soils is accompanied by the leaching of other minerals such as cadmium and other heavy metals, which may also be playing a role in the toxic conditions that developed at Kesterson Reservoir. Recent studies examining the impact of 30 days of administration of up to 300 μg Se/kg body weight as selenomethionine to macaque monkeys showed no deleterious effects on neonates (218). This demonstrates that care must be taken in extrapolating between species, or between one situation and another. Nonetheless, the coots of Kesterson should serve as canaries to remind us that the best intentions can go awry and that previous as well as ongoing basic science will be necessary to solve these problems.

XVI. CANCER

Selenium and cancer is a topic sufficiently broad and deep to merit a chapter of its own to receive thorough coverage. The following will serve to introduce the area and to make several biochemical comments relative to the material in the rest of the chapter. The reader is encouraged to consult several excellent reviews on the subject (219,220). The story begins in 1943 with the early work of Nelson (7), who fed female rats up to 10 μg Se/g diet for up to 24 months. There were no effects in rats that died or were killed before 18 months, but in rats with liver cirrhosis, 11 of 43 rats developed liver cell adenoma or low-grade carcinoma without metastasis. This study clearly identified selenium as a carcinogen. Some 24 years later, Tinsley and Harr (210,211) reported a repeat of these experiments with larger numbers of animals that did not find hepatic tumors, suggesting that selenium is merely toxic. The results of Nelson (7) may have been complicated by the marginal protein content of the diet. Epidemiologic studies conducted in the late 1960s and 1970s began to provide solid evidence of an inverse relationship between selenium intake and cancer mortality. Schrauzer and co-workers (219) correlated the per-capita selenium intake with cancer mortality rate in more than 20 countries based on international food disappearance data, and found an inverse relationship between selenium intake and leukemia as well as with cancers of the colon, rectum, pancreas, breast, ovaries, prostate, bladder, lung (males), and skin. Pooled blood samples from healthy donors in 19 U.S. states and 22 countries also showed an inverse correlation between blood selenium levels and cancer mortality rates, and there were significant inverse relationships for most of these within the same site as well across the collective 19 states and 22 countries (219). Thus it became clear that selenium is potentially anticarcinogenic.

A. Antitumorigenic Effects

In a number of systems, selenium supplementation at levels that are chronically toxic (2–5 μg Se/g diet) will decrease the tumor incidence in animals treated with chemical carcino-gens such as 7,12-dimethylbenz(a)anthracene (DMBA), animals infected with virally-transmitted spontaneous mammary tumors, or animals given intraperitoneal injected *Ascites* tumor cells. For these studies, the level of carcinogenic agent is generally set to just result in a 100% tumor incidence, and the dietary selenium supplementation above adequate levels generally reduces tumor incidence around 50% within the period of study. Selenium must be provided during both the initiation and the promotional stages of tumor formation for maximal effectiveness. Near maximal inhibition is obtained when selenium is provided 1–2 weeks after administration of the carcinogen, indicating that the major role of selenium may be to inhibit proliferation of tumors (221,222). This situation is not completely clear cut, as illustrated by the fact that animals fed a selenium-deficient diet relative to animals fed a 0.1 μg Se/g diet have equal susceptibility to DMBA-induced mammary tumors except when fed diets high in polyunsaturated fat (25% corn oil). Selenium deficiency here results in a marked enhancement of tumorigenesis (221). The 1982 NRC review, *Diet, Nutrition and Cancer* (219) suggested three potential mechanisms of action that could account for the antitumorigenic effect of selenium. The first proposed mechanism is that selenium alters the activity of enzymes that activate procarcinogens such as hydroxylating enzymes or enzymes that detoxify carcinogens such as glucoronyl transferase or GSH-S-transferase. Alterations and activation of detoxification enzymes have been reported for selenium deficiency in mice, but the effects of high levels of selenium supplementation are less clear cut. This type of antitumoriginic activity would presumably affect the initiation phase of tumorigenesis. Studies with chemically induced tumor models, however, indicate that selenium is most effective if it is provided throughout both the initiation and the promotional stages, but is almost as effective when provided only after initiation (221). This strongly suggests that the major antitumorigenic effect of high levels of selenium is to inhibit tumor proliferation rather than initiation. The second listed mechanism for the antitumorigenic action was as a component of GPX1. This hypothesis is based on the belief that GPX1 is an important cytosolic and mitochondrial matrix enzyme that destroys peroxides and, thus, along with superoxide dismutase and vitamin E, protects cells against free-radical attack. GPX1 activity, however, tends to plateau at 0.1 μg Se/g diet, whereas higher levels of dietary selenium (2–5 μg Se/g diet) result in decreased numbers of tumor, delayed appearance of the first tumor, and decreased percent incidence of the tumors. These results suggest that the potent antitumorigenicity of selenium supplementation at 20- to 50-fold higher than the requirement is not associated directly with GPX1. The third stated possible mechanism for selenium's antitumorigenic activity was that selenium protects against heavy metal-catalyzed tumorigenicity by sequestering the toxic heavy metals in a nontoxic form. Selenium, however, protects in experimental cases without heavy metal involvement. A fourth possible role not mentioned in the NRC review would be enhanced rate of DNA repair, stimulated by high levels of dietary selenium (223). Unfortunately, these hypotheses remain basically unproved.

Excitement about selenium's anticarcinogenic role rose when Willet and colleagues (224), in 1983, presented the results of a retrospective study that used prediagnostic serum selenium concentrations. Patients who developed cancer had a serum selenium concentration of 0.129 μg Se/mL versus noncancer individuals with a concentration of 0.136 μg Se/mL. Those in the lowest quintile of serum selenium concentration had a risk twice as high as those in the highest quintile. This early excitement, however, has now been modulated, as Willet now cites six case control and prospective studies looking at tissue selenium and breast cancer which quite consistently provided no evidence of a protective effect of selenium (220). With regard to breast cancer, a Finnish study is consistent with the hypothesis that there is a threshold below which low selenium intake increases breast cancer risk, but selenium intake is not likely to be associated with breast cancer in countries with moderate or high levels of selenium intake.

Early studies found reduced plasma selenium concentration in patients with skin cancer that were not melanomas; thus Clark and colleagues (225) initiated a randomized trial with 1312 patients with histories of basal cell or squamous cell carcinomas of the skin, and provided them with either an oral supplement of 200 μg Se/day or a placebo. Selenium treatment did not significantly affect the primary end points of incidence of new basal or squamous cell carcinoma of the skin. Selenium treatment was, however, associated with a statistically significant reduction in several secondary end points that were not the focus of the study: total and lung cancer mortality; total cancer incidence; colon-rectal cancer; and prostate cancer incidence. Total cancer incidence was 42% lower in the selenium group ($p < 0.001$).

Two randomized nutrition intervention trials were conducted in a rural county in northcentral China which has some of the highest rates of cancer found in the world, including more than 85% of the malignancies appearing primarily in the esophagus and stomach (226). This population historically has a low intake of several nutrients and so was selected for these trials which were begun in the mid-1980s. Nearly 30,000 participants were randomly assigned to eight groups and continued for 5 years. Small but significant reductions in total mortality were observed in subjects receiving a combination of 15 mg β-carotene, 50 μg Se as selenized yeast, and 30 mg α-tocopherol, whereas no appreciable effects were found for other supplements, which included retinol, zinc, riboflavin, niacin, ascorbate, and molybdenum. The reduction was more pronounced in this study for women than for men, and for younger rather than older individuals, but these differences were not significant (226). The mechanism is unclear, but it is likely that vitamin E in particular may be one of the potent components in this trial because this population is thought to be relatively deficient in vitamin E relative to other treatments. These studies continue to excite our interests in modifying dietary habits to improve human health. Many important questions remain, and it is not clear whether or not supplements themselves, or food choices that emphasize frequent consumption of fruits and vegetables, will protect against cancer. The tools of molecular biology are beginning to help unravel the interaction between diet and genetics. Identification of markers of genetic predisposition to a specific disease such as cancer will be necessary if dietary intervention is without effect in 999 of 1000 individuals, but can dramatically shift the susceptibility of the remaining one individual to the disease.

REFERENCES

1. Rotruck JT, Pope AL, Ganther HE, Swanson AB, Hafeman DG, Hoekstra WG. Selenium: biochemical role as a component of glutathione peroxidase. Science 1973; 179:588–590.
2. National Research Council. Selenium in Nutrition. Washington, DC: National Academy Press, 1983.
3. Sunde RA. Intracellular glutathione peroxidases—structure, regulation and function. In: Burk RF, ed. Selenium in Biology and Human Health. New York: Springer-Verlag, 1994:45–77.
4. Sunde RA. Molecular biology of selenoproteins. Annu Rev Nutr 1990; 10:451–474.
5. Burk RF, Hill KE. Regulation of selenoproteins. Annu Rev Nutr 1993; 13:65–81.
6. Burk RF. Selenium in Biology and Human Health. New York: Springer-Verlag, 1994:1–221.
7. Nelson AA, Fitzhugh OG, Calvery HO. Liver tumors following cirrhosis caused by selenium in rat. Cancer Res 1943; 3:230–236.

8. Schwarz K, Foltz CM. Selenium as an integral part of factor 3 against dietary necrotic liver degeneration. J Am Chem Soc 1957; 79:3292–3293.

9. Pinsent J. The need for selenite and molybdate in the formation of formic dehydrogenase by members of the coli-aerogenes group of bacteria. Biochem J 1954; 57:10–16.

10. Cotton FA, Wilkinson G. Advanced Inorganic Chemistry. New York: John Wiley, 1972:421–457.

11. Huber RE, Criddle RS. Comparison of the chemical properties of selenocysteine and selenocystine with their sulfur analogs. Arch Biochem Biophys 1967; 122:164–173.

12. Rosenfeld I, Beath OA. Selenium: Geobotany, Biochemistry, Toxicity and Nutrition. New York: Academic Press, 1964.

13. Watkinson JH. Fluorometric determination of selenium in biological material with 2,3-diaminoaphthalene. Anal Chem 1966; 38:92–96.

14. Oh SH, Ganther HE, Hoekstra WG. Selenium as a component of glutathione peroxidase isolated from ovine erythrocytes. Biochemistry 1974; 13:1825–1829.

15. McKown DM, Morris JS. Rapid measurement of selenium in biological samples using instrumental neutron activation analysis. J Radioanal Chem 1978; 43:411–420.

16. Henn EL. Determination of selenium in water and industrial effluents by flameless atomic absorption. Anal Chem 1975; 47:428.

17. Hahn MH, Kuennen RW, Caruso JA, Fricke FL. Determination of trace amounts of selenium in corn, lettuce, potatoes, soybeans, and wheat by hybrid generation of condensation and flame atomic absorption spectrometry. J Agric Food Chem 1981; 29:792.

18. Janghorbani M, Ting BT. Comparison of pneumatic nebulization and hybrid generation inductively coupled plasma mass spectrometry for isotopic analysis of selenium. Anal Chem 1989; 61:701–708.

19. Morisi G, Patriarca M, Menotti A. Improved determination of selenium in serum by zeeman atomic absorption spectrometry. Clin Chem 1988; 34(1):127–130.

20. Ganther HE. Reduction of the selenotrisulfide derivative of glutathione to a persulfide analog by glutathione reductase. Biochemistry 1971; 10:4089–4098.

21. Blotcky AJ, Hansen GT, Borkar N, Ebrahim A, Rack EP. Simultaneous determination of selenite and trimethylselenonium ions in urine by anion exchange chromatography and molecular neutron activation analysis. Anal Chem 1987; 59:2063–2066.

22. Mehra HC, Frankenberger WT. Simultaneous analysis of selenate and selenite by single-column ion chromatography. Chromatography 1988; 25:585–588.

23. Behne D, Wolters W. Distribution of selenium and glutathione peroxidase in the rat. J Nutr 1983; 113:456–461.

24. Behne D, Hofer-Bosse T. Effects of a low selenium status on the distribution and retention of selenium in the rat. J Nutr 1984; 114:1289–1296.

25. Weiss SL, Evenson JK, Thompson KM, Sunde RA. The selenium requirement for glutathione peroxidase mRNA level is half of the selenium requirement for glutathione peroxidase activity in female rats. J Nutr 1996; 126:2260–2267.

26. Prohaska JR, Sunde RA. Comparison of liver glutathione peroxidase activity and mRNA in female and male mice and rats. Comp Biochem Physiol [B] 1993; 105:111–116.

27. Janghorbani M, Rockway S, Mooers CS, Roberts EM, Ting BT, Sitrin MD. Effect of chronic selenite supplementation on selenium excretion and organ accumulation in rats. J Nutr 1990; 120:274–279.

28. Janghorbani M, Lynch NE, Mooers CS, Ting BT. Comparison of the magnitude of the selenite-exchangeable metabolic pool and whole body endogenous selenium in adult rats. J Nutr 1990; 120:190–199.

29. Janghorbani M, Mooers CS, Smith MA, Hazell T, Blanock K, Ting BT. Correlation between the size of the selenite-exchangeable metabolic pool and total body or liver selenium in rats. J Nutr 1991; 121:345–354.

30. Schroeder HA, Frost DV, Balassa JJ. Essential trace metals in man: selenium. J Chron Dis 1970; 23:227–243.

31. Janghorbani M, Kasper LJ, Young VR. Dynamics of selenite metabolism in young men: studies with the stable isotope tracer method. Am J Clin Nutr 1984; 40:208–218.

32. Behne D, Hilmert H, Scheid S, Gessner H, Elger W. Evidence for specific selenium target tissues and new biologically important selenoproteins. Biochim Biophys Acta 1988; 966:12–21.

33. Patterson BH, Levander OA, Helzlsouer K, et al. Human selenite metabolism: a kinetic model. Am J Physiol 1989; 257:R556–R567.

34. Swanson AB, Patterson BH, Levander OA, et al. Human selenomethionine metabolism: a kinetic model. Am J Clin Nutr 1991; 54:917–926.

35. Patterson BH, Zech LA. Development of a model for selenite metabolism in humans. J Nutr 1992; 122:709–714.

36. Olson OE, Novacek EJ, Whitehead EI, Palmer IS. Investigations on selenium in wheat. Phytochemistry 1970; 9:1181–1188.

37. Allaway WH, Cary EE, Ehlig CF. The cycling of low levels of selenium in soils, plants and animals. In: Muth OH, ed. Selenium in Biomedicine. Westport, Conn: AVI, 1967; 273–296.

38. Hawkes WC, Wilhelmsen EC, Tappel AL. Abundance and tissue distribution of selenocysteine-containing proteins in the rat. J Inorg Biochem 1985; 23:77–92.

39. Thomson CD, Stewart RDH, Robinson MF. Metabolic studies in rats of [75Se]selenomethionine and 75Se incorporated in vivo into rabbit kidney. Br J Nutr 1975; 33:45–54.

40. Cantor AH, Scott ML, Noguchi T. Biological availability of selenium in feedstuffs and selenium compounds for prevention of exudative diathesis in chicks. J Nutr 1975; 105:106–111.

41. Thomson CD, Stewart RDH. Metabolic studies of [75Se]selenomethionine and [75Se]selenite in the rat. Br J Nutr 1973; 30:139–147.

42. Wright PL, Bell MC. Comparative metabolism of selenium and tellurium in sheep and swine. Am J Physiol 1966; 211:6–10.

43. Robinson MF, Thomson CD. The role of selenium in the diet. Nutr Abstr Rev 1983; 53:3–26.

44. Martin RF, Janghorbani M, Young VR. Experimental selenium restriction in healthy adult humans: changes in selenium metabolism studied with stable-isotope methodology. Am J Clin Nutr 1989; 49:854–861.

45. Burk RF. Selenium in man. In: Prasad AS, ed. New York: Academic Press, 1976:105–133.

46. Arduser F, Wolffram S, Scharrer E. Active absorption of selenate by ileum. J Nutr 1985; 115:1203–1208.

47. Sunde RA, Hoekstra WG. Structure, synthesis and function of glutathione peroxidase. Nutr Rev 1980; 38:265–273.

48. McConnell KP, Cho GJ. Active transport of L-selenomethionine in the intestine. Am J Physiol 1967; 213:150–156.

49. Boza JJ, Fox TE, Eagles J, Wilson PDG, Fairweather-Tait SJ. The validity of extrinsic stable isotopic labeling for mineral absorption studies in rats. J Nutr 1995; 125:1611–1616.

50. Palmer IS, Fischer DD, Halverson AW, Olson OE. Identification of a major selenium excretory product in rat urine. J Pharm Soc 1969; 58:1279–1280.

51. Burk RF, Brown DG, Seely RJ, Scaief CC. Influence of dietary and injected selenium on whole-body retention, route of excretion, and tissue retention of 75SeO2 in the rat. J Nutr 1972; 102:1049–1055.

52. Nahapetian AT, Janghorbani M, Young VR. Urinary trimethylselenonium excretion by the rat: effect of level and source of selenium-75. J Nutr 1983; 113:401–411.

53. Janghorbani M, Young VR. Selenium metabolism in North Americans: studies based on stable isotope tracers. In: Combs GFJ, Spallholz JE, Levander OA, Oldfield JE, eds. Selenium in Biology and Medicine. New York: AVI, 1987:450–471.

54. McConnell KP, Roth DM. Respiratory excretion of selenium. Proc Soc Exp Biol Med 1966; 123:919–921.

55. Burk RF, Hill KE. Selenoprotein P. A selenium-rich extracellular glycoprotein. J Nutr 1994; 124:1891–1897.

56. Chu FF, Esworthy RS, Doroshow JH, Doan K, Liu XF. Expression of plasma glutathione peroxidase in human liver in addition to kidney, heart, lung, and breast in humans and rodents. Blood 1992; 79:3233–3238.

57. Sunde RA, Hoekstra WG. Incorporation of selenium from selenite and selenocystine into glutathione peroxidase in the isolated perfused rat liver. Biochem Biophys Res Commun 1980; 93:1181–1188.

58. Sunde RA. The biochemistry of selenoproteins. J Am Oil Chem Soc 1984; 61:1891–1900.

59. Sunde RA, Evenson JK. Serine incorporation into the selenocysteine moiety of glutathione peroxidase. J Biol Chem 1987; 262:933–937.

60. Waschulewski IH, Sunde RA. Effect of dietary methionine on the utilization of tissue selenium from dietary selenomethionine for glutathione peroxidase in the rat. J Nutr 1988; 118: 367–374.

61. Axley MJ, Stadtman TC. Selenium metabolism and selenium-dependent enzymes in microorganisms. Annu Rev Nutr 1989; 9:127–137.

62. Ganther HE. Enzymic synthesis of dimethyl selenide from sodium selenite in mouse liver extracts. Biochemistry 1966; 5:1089–1098.

63. Hsieh HS, Ganther HE. Acid-volatile selenium formation catalyzed by glutathione reductase. Biochemistry 1975; 14:1632–1636.

64. Hsieh HS, Ganther HE. Biosynthesis of dimethyl selenide from sodium selenite in rat liver and kidney cell-free systems. Biochim Biophys Acta 1977; 497:205–217.

65. Carrithers SL, Hoffman JL. Sequential methylation of 2-mercaptoethanol to the dimethyl sulfonium ion, 2-(dimethylthio)ethanol, in vivo and in vitro. Biochem Pharmacol 1994; 48: 1017–1024.

66. Sandholm M. The initial fate of a trace amount of I.V. administered selenite. Acta Pharmacol Toxicol 1973; 33:1–5.

67. Gasiewicz TA, Smith JC. Properties of the cadmium and selenium complex formed in rat plasma in vivo and in vitro. Chem Biol Interact 1978; 23:171–183.

68. Hoffman JL, McConnell KP, Carpenter DR. Aminoacylation of *Escherichia coli* methionine tRNA by selenomethionine. Biochim Biophys Acta 1970; 199:531–534.

69. Markham GD, Hafner EW, Tabor CW, Tabor H. Adenosylmethionine synthetase from *Escherichia coli*. J Biol Chem 1980; 255:9082–9092.

70. Bremer J, Natori Y. Behavior of some selenium compounds in transmethylation. Biochim Biophys Acta 1960; 44:367–370.

71. Esaki N, Nakamura T, Tanaka H, Soda K. Selenocysteine lyase, a novel enzyme that specifically acts on selenocysteine. J Biol Chem 1982; 257:4386–4391.

72. Steele RD, Benevenga NJ. The metabolism of 3-methylthiopropionate in rat liver homogenates. J Biol Chem 1979; 254:8885–8890.

73. Esaki N, Tanaka H, Uemura S, Suzuki T, Soda K. Catalytic action of L-methionine-γ-lyase on selenomethionine and selenosis. Biochemistry 1979; 18:407–410.

74. Batley BL, Sunde RA. Selenium incorporation into proteins follows sulfur amino acid incorporation in yeast. FASEB J 1989; 3:A781.

75. Schwarz K, Foltz CM. Factor 3 activity of selenium compounds. J Biol Chem 1958; 233: 245–251.

76. Waschulewski IH, Sunde RA. Effect of dietary methionine on tissue selenium and glutathione peroxidase activity in rats fed selenomethionine. Br J Nutr 1988; 60:57–68.

77. Forstrom JW, Zakowski JJ, Tappel AL. Identification of the catalytic site of rat liver GSH-Px as selenocysteine. Biochemistry 1978; 17:2639–2644.

78. Wendel A, Kerner B, Graupe K. The selenium moiety of glutathione peroxidase. In: Sies H, Wendel A, eds. Functions of Glutathione in Liver and Kidney. Berlin: Springer-Verlag, 1978:107–113.

79. Hawkes WC, Lyons DE, Tappel AL. Identification and purification of a rat liver selenocysteine-specific transfer RNA. Fed Proc 1979; 38:820.

80. Hatfield D. Suppression of termination codons in higher eukaryotes. Trends Biochem Sci 1985; 10:201–204.

81. Amberg R, Urban C, Reuner B, et al. Editing does not exist for mammalian selenocysteine tRNAs. Nucleic Acids Res 1993; 21:5583–5588.

82. Chambers I, Frampton J, Goldfarb P, Affara N, McBain W, Harrison PR. The structure of the mouse glutathione peroxidase gene: the selenocysteine in the active site is encoded by the "termination" codon, TGA. EMBO J 1986; 5:1221–1227.

83. Zinoni F, Birkmann A, Stadtman TC, Böck A. Nucleotide sequence and expression of the selenocysteine-containing polypeptide of formate dehydrogenase (formate-hydrogen-lyase-linked) from *Escherichia coli*. Proc Natl Acad Sci USA 1986; 83:4650–4654.

84. Stadtman TC. Selenocysteine. Annu Rev Biochem 1996; 65:83–100.

85. Leinfelder W, Zehelein E, Mandraand-Berthelot M, Böck A. Genes for a novel tRNA species that accepts L-serine and cotranslationally inserts selenocysteine. Nature (Lond.) 1988; 331:723–725.

86. Ehrenreich A, Forchhammer K, Tormay P, Veprek B, Böck A. Selenoprotein synthesis in *E. coli*—purification and characterisation of the enzyme catalysing selenium activation. Eur J Biochem 1992; 206:767–773.

87. Veres Z, Tsai L, Scholz TD, Politino M, Balaban RS, Stadtman TC. Synthesis of 5-methyl-aminomethyl-2-selenouridine in tRNAs: ^{31}P NMR studies show the labile selenium donor synthesized by the selD gene product contains selenium bonded to phosphorus. Proc Natl Acad Sci USA 1992; 89:2975–2979.

88. Low SC, Harney JW, Berry MJ. Cloning and functional characterization of human seleno-phosphate synthetase, an essential component of selenoprotein synthesis. J Biol Chem 1995; 270:21659–21664.

89. Forchhammer K, Leinfelder W, Boesmiller K, Veprek B, Böck A. Selenocysteine synthase from *Escherichia coli*: nucleotide sequence of the gene (selA) and purification of the protein. J Biol Chem 1991; 266:6318–6323.

90. Heider J, Baron C, Böck A. Coding from a distance: dissection of the mRNA determinants required for the incorporation of selenocysteine into protein. EMBO J 1992; 11:3759–3766.

91. Ringquist S, Schneider D, Gibson T, Baron C, Böck A, Gold L. Recognition of the mRNA selenocysteine insertion sequence by the specialized translational elongation factor SELB. Genes and Development 1994; 8:376–385.

92. Huttenhofer A, Westhof E, Böck A. Solution structure of mRNA hairpins promoting seleno-cysteine incorporation of *Escherichia coli* and their base-specific interaction with special elongation factor SELB. RNA 1996; 2:354–366.

93. Berry MJ, Banu L, Chen Y, et al. Recognition of a UGA as a selenocysteine codon in Type I deiodinase requires sequences in the 3′ untranslated region. Nature 1991; 353:273–276.

94. Berry MJ, Banu L, Harney JW, Larsen PR. Functional characterization of the eukaryotic SECIS elements which direct selenocysteine insertion at UGA codons. EMBO J 1993; 12: 3315–3322.

95. Walczak R, Westhof E, Carbon P, Krol A. A novel RNA structural motif in the selenocysteine insertion element of eurkaryotic selenoprotein mRNAs. RNA 1996; 2:367–379.

96. Shen Q, McQuilkin PA, Newburger PE. RNA-binding proteins that specifically recognize the selenocysteine insertion sequence of human cellular glutathione peroxidase mRNA. J Biol Chem 1995; 270:30448–30452.

97. Hubert N, Walczak R, Carbon P, Krol A. A protein binds the selenocysteine insertion element in the 3′-UTR of mammalian selenoprotein mRNAs. Nucleic Acids Res 1996; 24:464–469.

98. Shen Q, Chu F-F, Newburger PE. Sequences in the 3′-untranslated region of the human cellular glutathione peroxidase gene are necessary and sufficient for selenocysteine incorporation at the UGA codon. J Biol Chem 1993; 268:11463–11469.

99. Mills GC. Hemoglobin catabolism. I. Glutathione peroxidase, an erythrocyte enzyme which protects hemoglobin from oxidative breakdown. J Biol Chem 1957; 229:189–197.

100. Flohé L, Loschen G, Günzler WA, Eichole E. Glutathione peroxidase. V. The kinetic mechanism. Hoppe-Seylers Z Physiol Chem 1972; 353:987–999.

101. Günzler WA, Vergin H, Muller I, Flohé L. Glutathione-peroxidase. VI. Die Reaktion der Glutation-peroxidase mit verschiedenen Hydroperosiden. Z Physiol Chem 1972; 353:1001–1004.

102. Hafeman DG, Sunde RA, Hoekstra WG. Effect of dietary selenium on erythrocyte and liver glutathione peroxidase in the rat. J Nutr 1974; 104:580–587.

103. Lawrence RA, Sunde RA, Schwartz GL, Hoekstra WG. Glutathione peroxidase activity in rat lens and other tissues in relation to dietary selenium intake. Exp Eye Res 1974; 18:563–569.

104. Epp O, Ladenstein R, Wendel A. The refined structure of the selenoenzyme glutathione peroxidase at 0.2-nm resolution. Eur J Biochem 1983; 133:51–69.

105. Prohaska JR, Oh S-H, Hoekstra WG, Ganther HE. Glutathione peroxidase: inhibition by cyanide and release of selenium. Biochem Biophys Res Commun 1977; 74:64–71.

106. Rocher C, Lalanne JL, Chaudiere J. Purification and properties of a recombinant sulfur analog of murine selenium-glutathione peroxidase. Eur J Biochem 1992; 205:955–960.

107. Chu FF, Doroshaw JH, Esworthy RS. Expression, characterization, and tissue distribution of a new cellular selenium-dependent glutathione peroxidase, GSH-Px-GI. J Biol Chem 1993; 268:2571–2576.

108. Esworthy RS, Chu FF. Glutathione peroxidase-GI(GPX-GI) is the major glutathione peroxidase activity of the mucosal epithelium of the rat small bowel. FASEB J 1996; 10:A558.

109. Cohen HJ, Avissar N. Extracellular glutathione peroxidase: a distinct selenoprotein. In: Burk RF, ed. Selenium in Biology and Human Health. New York: Springer-Verlag, 1994:81–91.

110. Chow CK, Tappel AL. Response of glutathione peroxidase to dietary selenium in rats. J Nutr 1974; 104:444–451.

111. Sunde RA, Gutzke GE, Hoekstra WG. Effect of dietary methionine on the biopotency of selenite and selenomethionine in the rat. J Nutr 1981; 111:76–86.

112. Cohen HJ, Brown MR, Hamilton D, Lyons-Patterson J, Avissar N, Liegey P. Glutathione peroxidase and selenium deficiency in patients receiving home parenteral nutrition: time course for development of deficiency and repletion of enzyme activity in plasma and blood cells. Am J Clin Nutr 1989; 49:132–139.

113. Takahashi K, Akasaka M, Yamamoto Y, Kobayashi C, Mixoguchi J, Koyama J. Primary structure of human plasma glutathione peroxidase deduced from cDNA sequences.. J Biochem (Tokyo) 1990; 108:145–148.

114. Maiorino M, Gregolin C, Ursini F. (47) Phospholipid hydroperoxide glutathione peroxidase. Meth Enzymol 1990; 186:448–457.

115. Maiorino M, Ursini F, Leonelli M, Finato N, Gregolin C. A pig heart peroxidation inhibiting protein with glutathione peroxidase activity on phospholipid hydroperoxides. Biochem Int 1982; 5:575–583.

116. Ursini F, Maiorino M, Gregolin C. The selenoenzyme phospholipid hydroperoxide glutathione peroxidase. Biochim Biophys Acta 1985; 839:62–70.

117. Schuckelt R, Brigelius-Flohé R, Maiorino M, et al. Phospholipid hydroperoxide glutathione peroxidase is a selenoenzyme distinct from the classical glutathione peroxidase as evident from cDNA and amino acid sequencing. Free Rad Res Commun 1991; 14:343–361.

118. Sunde RA, Dyer JA, Moran TV, Evenson JK, Sugimoto M. Phospholipid hydroperoxide glutathione peroxidase: full-length pig blastocyst cDNA sequence and regulation by selenium status. Biochem Biophys Res Commun 1993; 193:905–911.

119. Brigelius-Flohé R, Aumann KD, Blocker H, et al. Phospholipid hydroperoxide glutathione peroxidase. Genomic DNA, cDNA and deduced amino acid sequence. J Biol Chem 1994; 269:7342–7348.

120. Pushpa-Rekha TR, Burdsall AL, Oleksa LM, Chisolm GM, Driscoll DM. Rat phospholipid-hydroperoxide glutathione peroxidase: cDNA cloning and identification of multiple transcription and translation start sites. J Biol Chem 1995; 270:26993–26999.

121. Godeas C, Sandri G, Panfili E. Distribution of phospholipid hydroperoxide glutathione perox-idase (PHGPx) in rat testis mitochondria. Biochim Biophys Acta 1994; 1191:147–150.

122. Ghyselinck NB, Jimenez C, Dufaure JP. Sequence homology of androgen-regulated epididy-mal proteins with glutathione peroxidase in mice. J Reprod Fertil 1991; 93:461–466.

123. Perry CF, Jones R, Niang LSP, Jackson RM, Hall L. Genetic evidence for an androgen-regulated epididymal secretory glutathione peroxidase whose transcript does not contain a selenocysteine codon. Biochem J 1992; 285:863–870.

124. Dear TN, Campbell K, Rabbitts TH. Molecular cloning of putative odorant-binding and odorant-metabolizing proteins. Biochemistry 1991; 30:10376–10382.

125. Williams DL, Pierce RJ, Cookson E, Capron A. Molecular cloning and sequencing of gluta-thione peroxidase from *Schistosoma mansoni*. Mol Biochem Parasitol 1991; 52:127–130.

126. Tang L, Gournaris K, Griffiths C, Selkirk ME. Heterologous expression and enzymatic properties of a selenium-independent glutathione peroxidase from the parasitic nematode *Brugia pahangi*. J Biol Chem 1995; 270:18313–18318.

127. Shigeoka S, Takeda T, Hanaoka T. Characterization and immunological properties of selenium-containing glutathione peroxidase induced by selenite in *Chlamydomonas rein-hardtii*. Biochem J 1991; 275:623–627.

128. Overbaugh JM, Fall R. Characterization of a selenium-independent glutathione peroxidase from *Euglena gracilis*. Plant Physiol 1985; 77:437–442.

129. Lawrence RA, Burk RF. Glutathione peroxidase activity in selenium-deficient rat liver. Bio-chem Biophys Res Commun 1976; 71:952–958.

130. Lawrence RA, Parkhill LK, Burk RF. Hepatic cytosolic nonselenium-dependent glutathione peroxidase activity: its nature and the effect of selenium deficiency. J Nutr 1978; 108:981–987.

131. Reiter R, Wendel A. Selenium and drug metabolism—II: independence of glutathione perox-idase and reversibility of hepatic enzyme modulations in deficient mice. Biochem Pharmacol 1984; 33:1923–1928.

132. Larsen PR, Berry MJ. Nutritional and hormonal regulation of thyroid hormone diodinases. Annu Rev Nutr 1995; 15:323–352.

133. Arthur JR. Interrelationships between selenium deficiency, iodine deficiency, and thyroid hormones. Am J Clin Nutr 1992; 57:235S–318S.

134. Beckett GJ, Beddows SE, Morrice PC, Nicol F, Arthur JR. Inhibition of hepatic deiodination of thyroxine is caused by selenium deficiency in rats. Biochem J 1987; 248:443–447.

135. Arthur JR, Nicol F, Beckett GJ. Hepatic iodothyronine 5'deiodinase: the role of selenium. Biochem J 1990; 272:537–540.

136. Behne D, Kyriakopoulos A, Meinhold H, Kohrle J. Identification of type I iodothyronine 5'-deiodinase as a selenoenzyme. Biochem Biophys Res Commun 1990; 173:1143–1149.

137. Berry MJ, Banu L, Larsen PR. Type I iodothyronine deiodinase is a selenocysteine-containing enzyme. Nature 1991; 349:438–440.

138. Prohaska JR, Ganther HE. Glutathione peroxidase activity of glutathione-S-transferases puri-fied from rat liver. Biochem Biophys Res Commun 1977; 76:437–445.

139. Beckett GJ, Nicol F, Rae PWH, Beech S, Guo Y, Arthur JR. Effects of combined iodine and sele-nium deficiency on thyroid hormone metabolism in rats. Am J Clin Nutr 1993; 57:240S–243S.

140. Vanderpas JB, Contempre B, Duale NL, et al. Selenium deficiency mitigates hypothyrox-inemia in iodine-deficient subjects. Am J Clin Nutr 1993; 57:271S–275S.

141. Bermano G, Nicol F, Dyer JA, et al. Tissue-specific regulation of selenoenzyme gene expres-sion during selenium deficiency in rats. Biochem J 1995; 311:425–430.

142. Hoekstra WG. Biochemical function of selenium and its relation to vitamin E. Fed Proc 1975; 34:2083–2089.

143. Burk RF, Lawrence RA, Lane JM. Liver necrosis and lipid peroxidation in the rat as the result of paraquat and diquat administration. Effect of selenium deficiency. J Clin Invest 1980; 65:1024–1031.

144. Burk RF, Gregory PE. Characteristics of 75Se-P, a selenoprotein found in rat liver and plasma and comparison of it with selenoglutathione peroxidase. Arch Biochem Biophys 1982; 213:73–80.

145. Yang JG, Morrison-Plummer J, Burk RF. Purification and quantitation of a rat plasma selenoprotein distinct from glutathione peroxidase using monoclonal antibodies. J Biol Chem 1987; 262:13372–13375.

146. Hill KE, Lloyd RS, Yang JG, Read R, Burk RF. The cDNA for rat selenoprotein P contains 10 TGA codons in the open reading frame. J Biol Chem 1991; 266:10050–10053.

147. Motsenbocker MA, Tappel AL. A selenocysteine-containing selenium-transport protein in rat plasma. Biochim Biophys Acta 1982; 719:147–153.

148. Burk RF, Hill KE, Read R, Bellew T. Response of rat selenoprotein P to selenium administration and fate of its selenium. Am J Physiol 1991; 261:E26–E30.

149. Pedersen ND, Whanger PD, Weswig PH, Muth OH. Selenium binding proteins in tissues of normal and selenium-responsive myopathic lambs. Bioinorg Chem 1972; 2:33–45.

150. Beilstein MA, Whanger PD. Evidence for selenocysteine in ovine tissue organelles. J Inorg Biochem 1981; 15:339–347.

151. Vendeland SC, Beilstein MA, Chen CL, Jensen ON, Barofsky E, Whanger PD. Purification and properties of selenoprotein W from rat muscle. J Biol Chem 1993; 268:17103–17107.

152. Vendeland SC, Beilstein MA, Yeh JY, Ream W, Whanger PD. Rat skeletal muscle selenoprotein W: cDNA clone and mRNA modulation by dietary selenium. Proc Natl Acad Sci USA 1995; 92:8749–8753.

153. Sunde RA, Hoekstra WG. Incorporation of selenium into liver glutathione peroxidase in the Se-adequate and Se-deficient rat. Proc Soc Exp Biol Med 1980; 165:291–297.

154. Evenson JK, Sunde RA. Selenium incorporation into selenoproteins in the Se-adequate and Se-deficient rat. Proc Soc Exp Biol Med 1988; 187:169–180.

155. Arthur JR, Beckett GJ. Roles of selenium in type I iodothyronine 5'-deiodinase and in thyroid hormone and iodine metabolism. In: Burk RF, ed. Selenium in Biology and Human Health. New York: Springer-Verlag, 1994:95–115.

156. Kleene KC. The mitochondrial capsule selenoprotein—a structural protein in the mitochondrial capsule of mammalian sperm. In: Burk RF, ed. Selenium in Biology and Human Health. New York: Springer-Verlag, 1994:135–149.

157. Calvin HI. Selective incorporation of selenium-75 into a polypeptide of the rat sperm tail. J Exp Zool 1978; 204:445–452.

158. Pallini V, Bacci E. Bull sperm selenium is bound to a structural protein of mitochondria. J Submicrosc Cytol 1979; 11:165–170.

159. Calvin HI, Cooper GW, Wallace E. Evidence that selenium in rat sperm is associated with a cysteine-rich structural protein of the mitochondrial capsule. Gamete Res 1981; 4:139–149.

160. McConnell KP, Hoffman JL. Methionine-selenomethionine parallels in rat liver polypeptide chain synthesis. FEBS Lett 1972; 24:60–62.

161. Bansal MP, Cook RC, Danielson KG, Medina D. A 14-kilodalton selenium-binding protein in mouse liver is fatty acid-binding protein. J Biol Chem 1989; 264:13780–13784.

162. Morrison DG, Dishart MK, Medina D. Intracellular 58-kd selenoprotein levels correlate with inhibition of DNA synthesis in mammary epithelial cells. Carcinogenesis 1988; 9:1801–1810.

163. Sinha R, Bansal MP, Ganther H, Medina D. Significance of selenium-labeled proteins for selenium's chemopreventive functions. Carcinogenesis 1993; 14:1895–1900.

164. Pumford NR, Martin BM, Hinson JA. A metabolite of acetaminophen covalently binds to the 56 kDa selenium binding protein. Biochem Biophys Res Commun 1992; 182:1348–1355.

165. Lanfear J, Fleming J, Walker M, Harrison P. Different patterns of regulation of the genes encoding the closely related 56 kDa selenium- and acetaminophen-binding proteins in normal tissues and during carcinogenesis. Carcinogenesis 1993; 14:335–340.

166. Stadtman TC. Selenium biochemistry. Annu Rev Biochem 1990; 59:111–127.

167. Stadtman TC. Biosynthesis and function of selenocysteine-containing enzymes. J Biol Chem 1991; 266:16257–16260.

168. Gladyshev VN, Boyington JC, Khangulov SV, Grahame DA, Stadtman TC,Sun PD. Characterization of crystalline formate dehydrogenase H from *Escherichia coli*. J Biol Chem 1996; 271:8095–8100.

169. Kimura Y, Stadtman TC. Glycine reductase selenoprotein A is not a glycoprotein: the positive periodic acid-Schiff reagent test is the result of peptide bond cleavage and carbonyl group generation. Proc Natl Acad Sci USA 1995; 92:2189–2193.

170. Gladyshev VN, Khangulov SV, Stadtman TC. Properties of the selenium- and molybdenum-containing nicotinic acid hydroxylase from *Clostridium barkeri*. Biochemistry 1996; 35: 212–223.

171. Weichselbaum TE. Cystine deficiency in the albino rat. Quart J Exp Physiol 1935; 25:363–367.

172. Schwarz K. A hitherto unrecognized factor against dietary necrotic liver degeneration in American yeast (factor 3). Proc Soc Exp Biol Med 1951; 78:852–856.

173. McCoy KEM, Weswig PH. Some selenium responses in the rat not related to vitamin E. J Nutr 1969; 98:383–389.

174. Schwarz K. Development and status of experimental work on factor 3-selenium. Fed Proc 1961; 20:666–673.

175. Bengtsson G, Hakkarainen J, Jönsson L, Lannek N, Lindberg P. Requirements for selenium (as selenite) and vitamin E (as α-tocopherol) in weaned pigs. II. The effect of varying selenium levels in a vitamin E deficient diet on the development of the VESD syndrome. J Animal Sci 1978; 46:153–160.

176. Arthur JR. Nutritional inter-relationships between selenium and vitamin E. Rep Rowett Inst 1982; 38:124–135.

177. Thompson JN, Scott ML. Impaired lipid and vitamin E absorption related to atrophy of the pancreas in selenium-deficient chicks. J Nutr 1970; 100:797–809.

178. van Rij AM, Thomson CD, McKenzie JM, Robinson MF. Selenium deficiency in total parenteral nutrition. Am J Clin Nutr 1979; 32:2076–2085.

179. Johnson RA, Baker SS, Fallon JT, Cohen HJ. An Occidental case of cardiomyopathy and selenium deficiency. N Engl J Med 1981; 304:1210–1212.

180. Kien CL, Ganther HE. Manifestations of chronic selenium deficiency in a child receiving total parenteral nutrition. Am J Clin Nutr 1983; 37:319–328.

181. Chen X, Yang G, Chen J, Wen Z, Ge K. Studies on the relations of selenium and Keshan disease. Biol Trace Element Res 1980; 2:91–107.

182. Beck MA, Kolbeck PC, Shi Q, Rohr LH, Morris VC, Levander OA. Increased virulence of a human enterovirus (Coxsackievirus B3) in selenium-deficient mice. J Infect Dis 1994; 170: 351–357.

183. Beck MA, Kolbeck PC, Rohr LH, Shi Q, Morris VC, Levander OA. Benign human enterovirus becomes virulent in selenium-deficient mice. J Med Virol 1994; 43:166–170.

184. Taylor EW, Ramanathan CS, Jalluri RK, Nadimpalli RG. A basis for new approaches to the chemotherapy of AIDS: novel genes in HIV-1 potentially encode selenoproteins expressed by ribosomal frameshifting and termination suppression. J Med Chem 1994; 37:2637.

185. National Research Council. Recommended Dietary Allowances. Washington, DC: National Academy Press, 1989.

186. Levander OA. Considerations in the design of selenium bioavailability studies. Fed Proc 1983; 42:1721–1725.

187. Lei XG, Evenson JK, Thompson KM, Sunde RA. Glutathione peroxidase and phospholipid hydroperoxide glutathione peroxidase are differentially regulated in rats by dietary selenium. J Nutr 1995; 125:1438–1446.

188. Thompson KM, Haibach H, Sunde RA. Growth and plasma triiodothyronine concentrations are modified by selenium deficiency and repletion in second-generation selenium-deficient rats. J Nutr 1995; 125:864–873.

189. Levander OA, DeLoach DP, Morris VC, Moser PB. Platelet glutathione peroxidase activity as an index of selenium status in rats. J Nutr 1983; 113:55–63.

190. Sunde RA, Saedi MS, Knight SAB, Smith CG, Evenson JK. Regulation of expression of glutathione peroxidase by selenium. In: Wendel A, ed. Selenium in Biology and Medicine. Heidelberg, Germany: Springer-Verlag, 1989:8–13.

191. Yang JG, Hill KE, Burk RF. Dietary selenium intake controls rat plasma selenoprotein P concentration. J Nutr 1989; 119:1010–1012.

192. National Research Council. Nutrient Requirements of the Laboratory Rat. Washington, DC: National Academy Press, 1978:7–37.

193. National Research Council. Nutrient Requirements of Laboratory Animals. Washington, DC: National Academy Press, 1995:1–173.

194. Eckhert CD, Lockwood MK, Shen B. Influence of selenium on the microvasculature of the retina. Microvasc Res 1993; 45:74–82.

195. Smith AM, Picciano MF. Evidence for increased selenium requirement for the rat during pregnancy and lactation. J Nutr 1986; 116:1068–1079.

196. Hadley KB, Sunde RA. The effect of dietary selenium on glutathione peroxidase activity in turkey poults. FASEB J 1996; 10:A557.

197. Levander OA, Sutherland B, Morris VC, King JC. Selenium balance in young men during selenium depletion and repletion. Am J Clin Nutr 1981; 34:2662–2669.

198. Knight SAB, Sunde RA. The effect of progressive selenium deficiency on anti-glutathione peroxidase antibody reactive protein in rat liver. J Nutr 1987; 117:732–738.

199. Saedi MS, Smith CG, Frampton J, Chambers I, Harrison PR, Sunde RA. Effect of selenium status on mRNA levels for glutathione peroxidase in rat liver. Biochem Biophys Res Commun 1988; 153:855–861.

200. Hill KE, Lyons PR, Burk RF. Differential regulation of rat liver selenoprotein mRNAs in selenium deficiency. Biochem Biophys Res Commun 1992; 185:260–263.

201. Sugimoto M, Sunde RA. In vivo and in vitro nuclear transcription indicates selenium regulation of glutathione peroxidase occurs post-transcriptionally. FASEB J 1992; 6:A1366.

202. Christensen MJ, Burgener KW. Dietary selenium stabilizes glutathione peroxidase messenger RNA in rat liver. J Nutr 1992; 122:1620–1626.

203. Toyoda H, Himeno S, Imura N. Regulation of glutathione peroxidase mRNA level by dietary selenium manipulation. Biochim Biophys Acta 1990; 1049:213–215.

204. Weiss SL, Sunde RA. Mutations within the glutathione peroxidase 3′ untranslated region can eliminate selenium regulation of glutathione peroxidase mRNA levels. FASEB J 1996; 10: A557.

205. Hubert N, Walczak R, Carbon P, Krol A. A protein binds the selenocysteine insertion element in the 3′-UTR of mammalian selenoprotein mRNAs. Nucleic Acids Res 1996; 24:464–469.

206. Sies H, Stahl W. Vitamins E and C, B-carotene, and other carotenoids as antioxidants. Am J Clin Nutr 1995; 62:1315s–1321s.

207. Hafeman DG, Hoekstra WG. Protection against carbon tetrachloride-induced lipid peroxidation in the rat by dietary vitamin E, selenium, and methionine as measured by ethane evolution. J Nutr 1977; 107:656–665.

208. Awad JA, Morrow JD, Hill KE, Roberts LJ, Berk RF. Detection and localization of lipid peroxidation in selenium- and vitamin E-deficient rats using F2-isoprostanes. J Nutr 1994; 124:810–816.

209. Wilber CG. Toxicology of selenium: a review. Clin Toxicol 1980; 17:171–230.

210. Harr JR, Bone JF, Tinsley IJ, Weswig PH, Yamamoto RS. Selenium toxicity in rats. Histopathology 1967; 153–178.

211. Tinsley IJ, Harr JR, Bone JF, Weswig PH, Yamamoto RS. Selenium toxicity in rats. I. Growth and longevity. Selenium in Biomedicine 1967; 141–152.

212. Valentine JL, Faraji B, Kang HK. Human glutathione peroxidase activity in cases of high selenium exposures. Environ Res 1988; 45:16–27.

213. Abernathy CO, Cantilli R, Du JT, Levander OA. Essentiality versus toxicity: some considerations in the risk assessment of essential trace elements. In: Saxena J, ed. Hazard Assessment of Chemicals. Washington, DC: Taylor and Francis, 1993:81–113.

214. Helzlsouer K, Jacobs R, Morris S. Acute selenium intoxication in the United States. Fed Proc 1985; 44:1670(abstr).

215. Safer B, Jagus B, Crouch D. Indirect inactivation of eukaryotic initiation factor 2 in reticulocyte lysate by selenite. J Biol Chem 1980; 255:6913–6917.

216. Davis EA, Maier KJ, Knight AW. The biological consequences of selenium in aquatic ecosystems. Calif Agric 1988; 18–29.

217. National Research Council. Mineral Tolerance of Domestic Animals. Washington, DC: National Academy of Sciences, 1980:392–420.

218. Hawkes WC, Willhite CC, Omaye ST, Cox DN. Selenium kinetics, placental transfer, and neonatal exposure in cynomolgus macaques (*Macaca fascicularis*). Teratology 1994; 50: 148–159.

219. National Research Council. Diet, Nutrition, and Cancer. Washington, DC: 1982:163–169.

220. Hunter DJ, Willett WC. Diet, body build, and breast cancer. Annu Rev Nutr 1994; 14:393–418.

221. Ip C. Selenium inhibition of chemical carcinogenesis. Fed Proc 1985; 44:2573–2578.

222. Milner JA. Effect of selenium on virally induced and transplantable tumor models. Fed Proc 1985; 44:2568–2572.

223. Lawson T, Birt DF. Enhancement of the repair of carcinogen-induced DNA damage in the hamster pancreas by dietary selenium. Chem Biol Interact 1983; 45:95–104.

224. Willett WC, Polk BF, Morris JS. Prediagnostic serum selenium and risk of cancer. Lancet 1983; ii:130–134.

225. Clark LC, Combs GF Jr, Turnbull BW. The nutritional prevention of cancer with selenium 1983–1993: a randomized clinical trial. FASEB J 1996; 10:A550.

226. Taylor PR, Wang GQ, Dawsey SM, et al. Effect of nutrition intervention on intermediate endpoints in esophageal and gastric carcinogenesis. Am J Clin Nutr 1995; 62:1420S–1423S.

227. Böck A, Forchhammer K, Heider J, Baron C. Selenoprotein synthesis: an expansion of the genetic code. Trends Biochem Sci 1991; 16:463–467.

228. Ho Y, Howard AJ, Crapo JD. Nucleotide sequence of a rat glutathione peroxidase cDNA. Nucl Acids Res 1988; 16:5207.

229. Yoshimura S, Watanabe K, Suemizu H, et al. Tissue specific expression of the plasma glutathione peroxidase gene in rat kidney. J Biochem (Tokyo) 1991; 109:918–923.

230. Beilstein MA, Whanger PD. Deposition of dietary organic and inorganic selenium in rat erythrocyte proteins. J Nutr 1986; 116:1701–1710.

19
Iodine

BASIL S. HETZEL
International Council for Control of Iodine Deficiency Disorders, Adelaide, Australia

MAURICE L. WELLBY
The Queen Elizabeth Hospital, Adelaide, Australia

I. HISTORY

Iodine is an essential constituent of the thyroid hormones, 3,5,3′,5′-tetraiodothyronine (T_4, thyroxine) and 3,5,3′-triiodothyronine (T_3). The major role of iodine in nutrition arises from the importance of thyroid hormones to growth and development (1–5).

Iodine was discovered by Courtois in 1811 during the course of making gunpowder. Some seaweed ash was being used, from which the iodine vaporized as a violet vapor. The element was discovered in the thyroid gland by Baumann in 1895.

The relation of iodine deficiency to enlargement of the thyroid gland, or goiter, was first shown by David Marine, who found that hyperplastic changes occurred regularly in the thyroid when the iodine concentration fell below 0.1% (3). Subsequently, Marine and Kimball in 1922 demonstrated in school children in Akron, Ohio, that endemic goiter could be prevented and substantially reduced by administration of small amounts of iodine (5).

Mass prophylaxis of goiter with iodized salt was first introduced in Switzerland and in Michigan (5). In Switzerland the widespread occurrence of a severe form of mental deficiency and deaf mutism (endemic cretinism) was a heavy toll on public funds. However, following the introduction of iodized salt in 1922, goiter incidence fell rapidly and new cretins were no longer born. Goiter also disappeared from Army recruits (5).

A further major development was the administration of injections of iodized oil in Papua New Guinea for people living in inaccessible mountain villages. The successful prevention of goiter and subsequently cretinism was shown in controlled trials over the period 1959–1972 (1–5).

Major attention is now focused on the effects of iodine deficiency on brain development in the fetus and in infancy. Iodine deficiency is now accepted as the most common cause of preventable mental defects in the world today (6). More details on the historical aspects of iodine can be found in the reviews which have been cited (1–5).

II. THE ECOLOGY OF IODINE DEFICIENCY

There is a geologic recycling of iodine in nature. Most of the iodine resides in the ocean. It was present during the primordial development of the earth, but large amounts were leached from the surface soil by glaciation, snow, or rain and were carried by wind, rivers, and floods into the sea. Iodine occurs in the deeper layers of the soil and is found in oil well and natural gas effluents. Water from such deep wells can provide a major source for iodine.

In general, the older an exposed soil surface is, the more likely it is to be leached of iodine (1,5), and the most likely to be leached are the mountainous areas. The most severely deficient regions are those of the Himalayas, the Andes, the European Alps, and the vast mountains of China. But iodine deficiency is likely to occur in all elevated regions subject to glaciation and high rainfall, with runoff into rivers. However, it also occurs in flooded river valleys such as the Ganges in India.

Iodine occurs in soil and the sea as the iodide. Iodide ions are oxidized by sunlight to elemental iodine, which is volatile, so that every year some 400,000 tons of iodine escape from the surface of the sea. The concentration of iodide in the sea water is about 50–60 μg/L; in the air it is approximately 0.7 μg/m^3. The iodine in the atmosphere is returned to the soil by rain, which has concentrations in the range 1.8–8.5 μg/L. In this way the cycle is complete.

However, the return of the iodine is slow and small in amount compared to the original loss of iodine, and subsequent repeated flooding ensures the continuity of iodine deficiency in the soil. Hence no "natural correction" can take place and iodine deficiency persists in the soil indefinitely. All crops grown in these soils will be iodine deficient. As a result, human and animal populations which are totally dependent on food grown in such soil become iodine deficient. The iodine content of plants grown in iodine-deficient soils may be as low as 10 μg/kg, compared to 1 mg/kg dry weight in plants in a non-iodine-deficient soil. This accounts for the occurrence of severe iodine deficiency in vast populations in Asia who live within systems of subsistence agriculture in flooded river valleys (India, Bangladesh, Burma).

An indication of the iodine content of the soil is given by the local drinking-water concentration. In general, iodine-deficient areas have water iodine levels below 2 μg/L, as in Nepal and Sub-Himalayan India (0.1–1.2 μg/L), compared with levels of 9.0 μg/L in the city of Delhi, which is not iodine deficient.

Iodine deficiency in the human population will persist unless supplementation is provided, or alternatively, diversification of the diet occurs, with increase in iodine intake derived from food sources outside the iodine-deficient areas. This occurred progressively in Europe during the nineteenth century. However, substantial areas of iodine deficiency remain in some countries (Germany, Italy, and Spain), as well as in more localized areas in others (see below).

In developing countries, the WHO (6) estimated in 1990 that 1 billion were at risk of iodine deficiency disorders (IDD), of which 220 million are suffering from goiter, more than 5 million are suffering from mental retardation as gross cretins, while three to five

TABLE 1 Prevalence of Iodine Deficiency Disorders in Developing Countries and Numbers of Persons at Risk (in millions)

	At risk	Goiter	Overt cretinism
Africa	227	39	0.5
Latin America	60	30	0.3
Southeast Asia	280	100	4.0
Asia (other countries including China)	400	30	0.9
Eastern Mediterranean	33	12	—
Total	1000	211	5.7

Source: Ref. 6.

times this number suffer from lesser degrees of mental defect (Table 1). More recently (1993), the WHO has increased the estimate of the population at risk to 1.6 billion (7).

III. CHEMISTRY AND PHYSIOLOGY OF THE THYROID HORMONES

A. Chemistry and Biosynthesis of Thyroid Hormones

The normal daily dietary intake of iodine approximates 100 μg, which is readily absorbed from the gut into the plasma. Because of its remarkable concentrating power, the thyroid gland takes up much of this iodine, achieving a steep gradient of up to 20 times the plasma level. The normal human adult thyroid contains about 70–80% of the total body stores of 15–20 mg of iodine. Apart from some other minor sites of uptake, iodide not used by the thyroid gland is excreted by the kidneys. Virtually all biological effects of iodide are expressed by the thyroid hormones, L-thyroxine (T_4) and L-triiodothyronine (T_3), synthesized in the thyroid gland. See Fig. 4, below, for structures.

Histologically, the functional cells of the thyroid are arranged in follicles, which surround a central lumen containing a colloid in which T_3 and T_4 are stored in the form of thyroglobulin (Tg), a 660-kDa glycoprotein (Fig. 1). The follicular cells extract iodine from the blood, which is transported rapidly through the cell into the colloid. Trapping of iodide is dependent on the adenylate cyclase system activated by thryotropin, i.e., thyroid-stimulating hormone (TSH) produced in the anterior pituitary gland. Trapped iodide is oxidized to iodine by iodide peroxidase (thyroid peroxidase in Fig. 1) at the luminal cell surface. The latter diffuses into the lumen and iodinates tyrosyl residues within Tg ("organification") to form the thyroid hormone precursors mono- and diiodotyrosine (MIT and DIT), respectively, which subsequently undergo oxidative condensation ("coupling") to form T_4 T_3, and small amounts of 3,3′,5′-triiodothyronine (reverse T_3, r-T_3).

The Tg in the lumen is synthesized in the follicular cell as prethyroglobulin, which undergoes glycosylation and sialylation before exocytosis into the lumen (8). Fully iodinated Tg is subject to pinocytosis into the cell under TSH control, with subsequent proteolysis and resultant release of all iodinated compounds. The precursors, MIT and DIT, are deiodinated rapidly by a microsomal deiodinase, the resultant iodide and tyrosine being reutilized for iodination and Tg synthesis, respectively. By contrast, insignificant amounts of T_3 and T_4 are deiodinated, and both are secreted into the blood.

Other anions taken up by the thyroid gland include perchlorate, thiocyanate, and

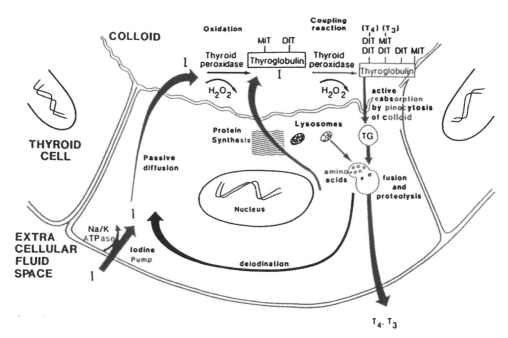

FIGURE 1 Diagram of the steps in thyroid hormone biosynthesis and secretion. See text for details. (Modified from Ref. 39, with permission.)

pertechnetate ($^{99m}TcO_4$), but these are not processed further. Perchlorate and thiocyanate discharge trapped iodide and thus are goiterogenic. Thiocyanate occurs in significant concentration in most of the brassica family, and cyanide, which occurs in cassava, is converted to thiocyanate in the liver (more later). Thyroid uptake of the synthetic tracer pertechnetate ($^{99m}TcO_4$) is a useful test of thyroid function.

B. Control of Thyroid Biosynthesis and Secretion

The control of thyroid function and secretion is effected mostly within the hypothalamic-pituitary region, as well as at the level of the thyroid gland (autoregulation). TSH, the key mediator of the hypothalamic-pituitary axis, is a glycoprotein composed of (alpha) and (beta) subunits produced by pituitary thyrotropic cells (Fig. 2) that stimulates all phases of T_3 and T_4 biosynthesis including their release from the gland. The hypothalamic neuropeptide thyrotropin-releasing hormone (TRH) is formed in the paraventricular and supraoptic neurons and binds to the thyrotrope cell membrane, leading to increase in TSH synthesis and secretion. All phases of biosynthesis and secretion of thyroid hormones are stimulated by TSH. Additionally, increased TSH secretion, which accompanies falling thyroid function from various causes—such as, for example, iodine deficiency—leads to hyperplasia of the follicular cells and enlargement of the thyroid gland, i.e., goiter.

The thyroid hormones in the plasma affect both hypothalamic and anterior pituitary function. The effect on hypothalamic TRH release is mainly inhibitory, but this effect is overshadowed by the marked negative effect on the thyrotropic function effected by T_3 derived mostly by deiodination of T_4 within the pituitary (9). The key negative factor opposing the TRH stimulation of TSH secretion is the intrapituitary T_3 concentration (10), and the probable role of TRH is to alter the T_3 setpoint (above which inhibition occurs).

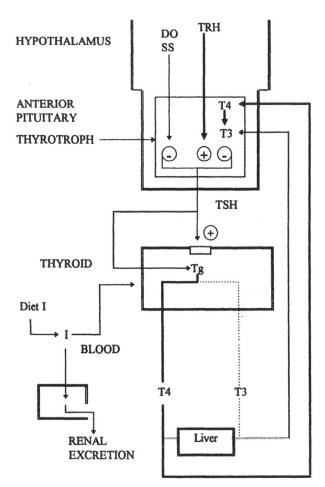

FIGURE 2 Diagram of the interrelationships among the secretions of the hypothalamus, anterior pituitary, and negative feedback by thyroid hormones in the control of thyroid hormone synthesis and secretion. See text for details. DO, dopamine; SS, somatostatin; TRH, thryotopin-releasing hormone.

Other neurotransmitters affecting the balance between the positive TRH and negative T_3 effects include the inhibitory effect of dopamine, which is estrogen mediated (11), and of somatostatin (12).

Autoregulation of thyroid function by various means has been postulated, the most effective being the Wolff-Chaikoff effect, according to which excess intrathyroidal organic iodine renders the gland insensitive to TSH, thus impeding iodine uptake and transport.

C. Thyroid Hormone Transport in Blood and Free Hormone Hypothesis

Over 99% of plasma T_3 and T_4 are transported from the thyroid gland to other tissues bound to proteins (13). In humans the thyroid-binding proteins (TBP) include T_4-binding globulin (TBG) and transthyretin (TTR). Nonspecific low-affinity binding to albumin also occurs. Some properties of the TBPs are shown in Table 2.

TABLE 2 Physicochemical Properties of Human Thyroid-
Binding Proteins

	TBG[a]	TTR[a]	Albumin
Molecular mass (Da)	54,000	55,000	66,000
Concentration	20 mg/L	300 mg/L	40 g/L
Association constant (M^{-1})			
T_4	1.0×10^{10}	7.0×10^7	7.0×10^5
T_3	4.6×10^8	1.4×10^7	1.0×10^3
Dissociation rate, T/2 (s)			
T_4	39	7.4	—
T_3	4.2	1.0	—
Binding sites/molecule	1	2	6

[a]TBG, T_4-binding globulin; TTR, transthyretin.

TBG is comprised of a single polypeptide and four oligosaccharide chains, and its carbohydrate content is approximately 15%. Variations in amino acid and sialic acid content lead to significant microheterogeneity, one example being "slow TBG" (14), a relatively desialylated form which is characteristic of the TBG seen in severe systemic illnesses (SSI) (15) and which binds T_4 with one-tenth of the affinity of native TBG. TTR, by contrast, is a stable, mostly invariable molecule of four polypeptide chains bound covalently. Two identical sites for binding T_3 and T_4 exist. Each molecule of TTR can bind also four molecules of retinol-binding protein and the ligand, retinol. The binding of T_3 and T_4 by albumin is of low affinity and is similar to its binding of ligands such as bilirubin, calcium, nonesterified fatty acids, and many drugs. Albumin binding of T_3 and T_4 becomes more relevant in low-TBG states.

With greater than 99% of T_3 and T_4 being bound to TBP, the question arises about the physiologic function of unbound hormone. The free hormone hypothesis, first propounded by Robbins and Rall (16), states that the miniscule amounts of unbound ("free") T_3 and T_4 bathing the tissues determine the physiologic status of the individual. Although it appears logical that only the comparatively small and unhindered T_3 and T_4 molecules can be taken up by tissues, and that those bound to proteins are excluded, this concept has been challenged on both logical and mathematical grounds (17). Even if or where the free hormone concept holds, the carriage of T_3 and T_4 by TBP must be considered important in delivering a reservoir of hormone to the tissue, such that when some T_3 and T_4 is taken up by the cell, more becomes immediately available by dissociating from TBP.

Differing mechanisms of uptake between tissues seems a plausible proposition. For example, hormone delivery in short-transit-time tissues is more likely to depend on unbound moieties, whereas in low-transit-time tissues such as hepatic sinusoids, greater opportunity exists for the slower exchange of plasma protein-bound T_4 with intracellular binding proteins (18).

D. Cellular Uptake and Transport of T_3 and T_4

Nuclear T_3 and T_4 receptors, of acidic nonhistone nature and closely related to steroid hormone receptors (see Fig. 3), have been identified in most tissues and are of higher density in the more T_3-reactive tissue such as liver and anterior pituitary. Nuclear uptake of

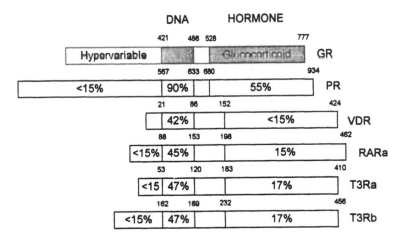

FIGURE 3 Schematic comparison of the thyroid receptors to those of the steroid and retinoic acid superfamily. The primary amino acid sequences are numbered above the structures, and the percentage identity in each domain to the sequence in the glucocorticoid receptor (GR) are indicated. The DNA- and hormone-binding domains are indicated at the top. Represented, in addition to the GR, are the progesterone receptor (PR), the vitamin D_3 receptor (VDR), the retinoic acid receptor alpha (RARa), and two T_3 receptors, alpha and beta (T3Ra and T3Rb). (Modified from Ref. 55.)

thyroid hormones mandates both a nuclear membrane uptake mechanism and active cytoplasmic transport. Nuclear membrane uptake may be either via saturable membrane-binding sites such as have been described for many tissues, or by passive diffusion effected through the lipophilic property of T_3 and T_4.

After traversing the plasma membrane, T_3 and T_4 are mostly bound to cytosolic proteins, leaving some hormone in the free state. This unbound intracellular hormone is available to bind to either mitochondrial sites or to the nuclear receptors.

E. Metabolic Effects of Thyroid Hormones

It is a reasonable assumption that thyroid hormones influence the growth, maturation, and metabolism of all tissues, although some, such as adipose tissue, are relatively insensitive. Other tissues, for example, neural tissue, are very sensitive, especially when very actively growing as in early fetal life. T_3 stimulates metabolic rate or thermogenesis through increased mitochondrial oxidative metabolism, not so much by increasing activity as by synthesizing new enzymes, particularly Na^+,K^+-ATPase.

The many metabolic actions of T_3 and T_4 include stimulatory effects on protein synthesis, especially certain enzymes. Some plasma proteins of hepatic origin, however, are not thyroid hormone dependent. The underlying processes whereby T_3 and T_4 influence protein synthesis are uncertain, but include effects at the nucleus to modify genomic expression as well as effects on the membrane to alter transmembrane flux of precursors. T_3 and T_4 also affect many postreceptor events quite significantly.

F. Metabolism of Thyroid Hormones: Deiodination

In-vitro conversion of T_4 to $3,5,3,'$-T_3, the metabolically active form in humans, was first demonstrated by Albright and Larson (19) in 1959, i.e., some seven years after the discovery of T$_3$ by Gross and Pitt-Rivers. However, the role of the nonmetabolically active, "reverse" T$_3$ (3,3'5'-T$_3$, r-T$_3$), in deiodinative processes was not appreciated for another decade and was due largely to Chopra and his co-workers. For a review, see (20).

It is now known that T$_4$ which has a daily production rate in man of 110 nmol, is deiodinated in a wide range of tissues to T$_3$ and r-T$_3$ by deiodinases that are relatively specific for the outer ring (β or 5'-position) or the inner ring (α or 5-position), respectively (Fig. 4). The daily production rate of r-T$_3$ is 36 compared to 33 nmol for T$_3$. Plasma concentration of T$_3$ is 6 to 10 times that of r-T$_3$, however. This reflects the normally more rapid clearance of r-T$_3$ relative to T$_3$, both being subject to further deiodination to the T$_2$ series (Fig. 4) and beyond.

Deiodination is catalyzed by three different deiodinases, whose properties are shown in Table 3. They occur in the endoplasmic reticulum and plasma membranes and are activated by thiol (SH) groups. Peripheral (i.e., extrathyroidal) production of T$_3$ accounts for about 75% of the plasma T$_3$, the remainder coming from the thyroid gland, mostly by coupling of MIT and DIT and some by deiodination. Very little thyroidal production of r-T$_3$ occurs. The relative concentrations of T$_3$ and r-T$_3$ in plasma, which are normally similar, are altered in favor of r-T$_3$ in a variety of situations, such as in the normal fetus, and for older individuals in states such as malnutrition in severe systemic illnesses. Such alteration arises from inhibition of β-deiodination. The inhibition of β-deiodination of T$_4$ leads to a marked decrease in plasma T$_3$ concentration, and the inhibition of β-deiodination of r-T$_3$, which is its main clearance mechanism causes an accumulation of r-T$_3$ in the plasma. These changes have implications for the testing of thyroid function in the clinical situations listed. One obvious example is that plasma T$_3$ measurement is not a suitable test to perform in hospital inpatients.

Deiodinase 1 (type I), found largely in the liver, is a selenium-containing enzyme, and

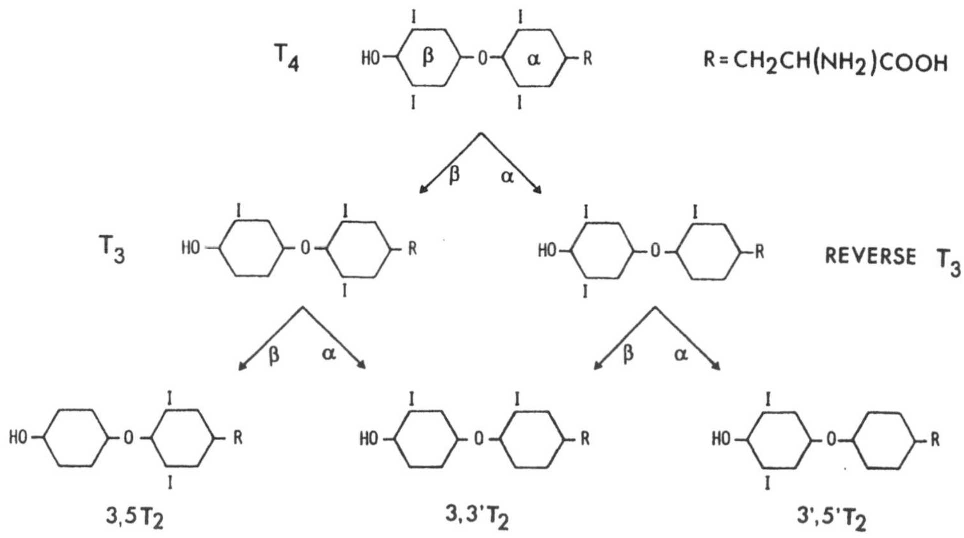

FIGURE 4 Pathways of inner or α ring, i.e., the 5-position, and of outer or β ring, i.e., the 5'-position, deiodination of T$_4$ through r-T$_3$ and T$_3$, respectively, to the diiodothryonine (T$_2$). These reactions are catalyzed by the deiodinases described in Table 3.

TABLE 3 Characteristics of Iodothyronine Deiodinases

	Deiodinase 1	Deiodinase 2	Deiodinase 3
Ring preferences	$\beta > \alpha$	β only	α only
Tissue sources	Liver, kidney, thyroid	Pituitary, brain, placenta, adipose	Ubiquitous
Substrate preference	$r\text{-}T_3 > T_4$	$T4 > r\text{-}T_3$	$T_3 > T_4$
Propyl thiouracil	Inhibits	Insensitive	Insensitive
SH	Activates	Activates	Activates
Selenocysteine	Yes	?	Yes

selenium deficiency to some extent protects against the subnormal plasma T_4 and the low brain T_3 observed in simple iodine deficiency. As less T_4 is deiodinated in the liver during selenium deficiency, more becomes available for brain metabolism and local conversion to T_3 by deiodinase 2 (type II). Selenium deficiency appears to cause a block in the thyroid feedback-control system. In rat experiments, combined iodine and selenium deficiency exacerbated the thyroid enlargement associated with iodine deficiency, resulting in a further 50% increase in thyroid weight above the 57% increase induced by iodine deficiency alone (56). However, compensatory increases in deiodinase 2 activity in combined deficiency may partially reduce the impact of hypothyroidism. For example, selenium supplementation (50 mg Se per day as selenomethionine) of cretins in Zaire significantly reduced plasma T_4 levels that were already low (57). This might further aggravate conversion of T_4 to T_3 in extrahepatic tissues such as brain and accentuate the effect of iodine deficiency. The authors (57) postulated that combined selenium and iodine deficiency may be the cause of pronounced (myxedematous) cretinism of northern Zaire; elevated H_2O_2 production in thyroid gland in these doubly deficient individuals would be without the protection of the selenium-dependent peroxidases, leading to the progressive involution of thyroid function that is characteristic of cretinism. In combined iodine and selenium deficiency, it is expeditious to correct iodine deficiency before correcting selenium status.

G. Metabolism of Thyroid Hormones: Alternative Pathways

Conjugation of iodothyronines, particularly by hepatic glucuronidation and sulfation, accounts for most of their disposal other than by primary deiodination. Most of the conjugated products are secreted into the bile and excreted in the feces, the degree of their enterohepatic circulation being probably insignificant. Possibly up to 20% of T_3 and T_4 and derived iodothyronines are accounted for by fecal excretion.

Glucuronate derivatives of iodothyronine are not metabolized further before biliary excretion, but sulfated forms are deiodinated. This may be an important mechanism of control of deiodination, particularly for T_3, as T_3 sulfate is deiodinated far more rapidly than is T_3 itself. Furthermore, as α-ring deiodination of T_4 (nonmetabolic pathway) is enhanced and β-ring (metabolic pathway) is retarded by prior sulfation, sulfation would appear to be an irreversible mechanism of inactivation of thyroid hormone.

Hepatic transamination of T_4 followed by oxidation of the product to tetraiodothyroacetic acid (TRIAC) is an alternative degradation pathway, particularly as TRIAC itself has some intrinsic metabolic activity. Finally, T_4 may be degraded to its precursors, MIT and

DIT, by cleavage of the ether (–O–) link under some conditions in humans, a finding which is relevant to earlier findings of MIT and DIT in plasma in states of thyroid stimulation.

IV. TESTS OF THYROID FUNCTION

An overview of testing thyroid function in relation to iodine nutrition disorders will be presented with emphasis on the principles rather than details of the underlying technologies employed.

Thyroid tests may be divided into

1. Tests that confirm the level of thyroid hormone secretion
2. Tests that help to elucidate the cause of any dysfunction

A. Tests of Thyroid Hormone Secretion (Table 4)

1. Principles of Measurement

The introduction of automated, computerized, multichannel analytical systems into clinical chemistry laboratories has led to the production of multiple results speedily and economically. The automation of immunoassay and related assays has also been developed and applied to thyroid-associated analytes. The quality of the analytical result, although improved in terms of reproducibility and accuracy, can be subject to interference and artefact.

Radioimmunoassay (RIA) has been succeeded by immunometric assay (IMA), which eliminates some of the errors arising from separating bound and free antigen systems in RIA. The radioactive labels are being replaced by nonisotopic signals which prevent autodestruction of labeled antibody.

2. Plasma T_4 Measurements

Although over 99% of plasma T_4 is bound to TBP, it is generally considered that the minute portion in the unbound form, i.e., free $T_4(FT_4)$, best indicates the metabolic status of tissues. Reference methods of measuring FT_4 are available (22). Routine FT_4, when measured by a suitable IMA system, has high throughput, acceptable analytical reliability, and corrects for the increased TBG status of pregnancy and estrogen treatment, as for a variety of low-TBP states.

TABLE 4 Normal Levels for Human Plasma or Serum Hormones (T_3, T_4), and Pituitary Thyroid-Stimulating Hormone (TSH) Together with Variations in Common Thyroid Disorders

	Normal[a]	Primary hypothyroidism	Hyperthyroidism
Free T_4	16 pmol/L	Low	High
Free T_3	5 pmol/L	Normal or low	High
TSH	2 μg/L	High	Low

[a]Representative mid-normal values.

3. Plasma TSH Measurements

Plasma TSH competes with FT_4 as the single most important thyroid function test and has recently undergone much refinement, particularly in terms of sensitivity. In general, plasma TSH is increased in primary hypothyroidism and suppressed (i.e., unmeasurable) in hyperthyroidism.

4. First-Line Testing of Thyroid Function

The combination of FT_4 and TSH as the first line of testing should achieve about 95% accuracy in determining the status of thyroid function.

V. COMMON THYROID DISORDERS

The thyroid gland is subject to a variety of disorders which occur with iodine deficiency. The epidemiology and prevention of these various conditions is discussed in the next sections. At this stage we discuss the symptoms and signs, and the common causes of these conditions in addition to iodine deficiency. Three conditions will be considered: endemic or nontoxic goiter, hypothyroidism, and hyperthyroidism.

A. Endemic Goiter

Goiter is defined as enlargement of the thyroid gland from any cause. In endemic goiter, which is usually multinodular, the cause of the enlargement is usually iodine deficiency. Patients are clinically euthyroid, and usually have normal thyroid function tests. Occasional patients with single thyroid nodules may become hyperthyroid.

B. Hypothyroidism

Hypothyroidism is defined as the clinical and biochemical state resulting from a failure of the thyroid to synthesize sufficient T_3 and T_4 to maintain normal thyroid function. In subclinical hypothyroidism the failure is insufficient to produce clinical symptoms, compensation being effected through preferential secretion of T_3. Common symptoms are fatigue, slowing of all bodily functions, slowing of mental processes, and increase in weight and cold intolerance. All of these effects are due to slowing of the metabolic rate. The first signs are those of slowing of mental processes particularly evident in iodine deficiency. Common causes of hypothyroidism are listed in Table 5.

TABLE 5 Common Causes of Hypothyroidism (Other than Iodine Deficiency)

Primary hypothyroidism (autoimmune)
Iatrogenic; arising from the treatment with radioactive iodine (^{131}I), or by thyroid surgery, or overtreatment with antithyroid drugs
Congenital hypothyroidism due to disorders of biosynthesis and thyroid dysgenesis
Chronic thyroiditis (Hashimoto's disease)
Secondary hypothyroidism from anterior pituitary or hypothalamic dysfunction

1. Primary Hypothyroidism

The most common cause of hypothyroidism is due to a chronic autoimmune thyroiditis arising from autoantibody-induced injury and is not associated with goiter. A goiterous variant occurs, namely, Hashimoto's disease (see below). Elevated antibodies directed against the biosynthetic enzyme, thyroid peroxidase, cause the gland to shrink, with progressive functional failure. Plasma T_3 and T_4 levels consequently decrease and TSH levels increase because of removal of the inhibitory effect on the thyrotroph (Fig. 2). Antibodies, which compete with TSH on its thyroid receptors, prevent the compensatory enlargement of the gland.

Plasma TSH is the most sensitive indicator of primary hypothyroidism. Treatment is with T_4, increasing the dose until plasma TSH returns into the reference range. This treatment is usually dramatically successful. Supplementary treatment of other organ systems may be required where these have been affected by long-term hypothyroidism.

2. Iatrogenic Hypothyroidism

Iatrogenic hypothyroidism is a complication of treatment of hyperthyroidism; diagnosis and treatment is the same as for primary hypothyroidism.

3. Congenital Defects in Biosynthesis

Congential defects in biosynthesis (dyshormono-genetic goiter) may occur at any site in the biosynthetic sequence, and these are listed in the previous section. These defects are relatively rare, and elucidating the exact site, although complex, may be useful in relation to genetic counseling. This subject is reviewed by Lever el al. (26).

4. Thyroid Dysgenesis

Thyroid dysgenesis may be either partial or complete. In partial dysgenesis the thyroid gland frequently appears sublingually. Prevalence of thyroid dysgenesis and of homozygous dyshormonogenesis is 1 in 3500 of new births in the absence of iodine deficiency and is detected with neonatal blood spot TSH, which is now a routine screening procedure for all neonates in many industrialized countries. Early treatment is essential to prevent progressive damage to the rapidly developing brain (see below). Persistence of hypothyroidism will lead to severe mental defect and dwarfism.

5. Chronic Thyroiditis

Chronic thyroiditis (Hashimoto's disease) is an autoimmune disease associated with goiter related to primary hypothyroidism and to Graves' disease. The antibody/antigen reaction causes the thyroid dysfunction. Slowly reducing thyroid reserve leads to progressive increase in plasma TSH and goiter. Hashimoto's disease frequently coexists with other autoimmune diseases, e.g., rheumatoid arthritis.

6. Secondary Hypothyroidism

Secondary hypothyroidism is due to TSH deficiency, arising either in the pituitary or the hypothalamus. Destruction of thyrotropes by tumors and postpartum necrosis are among the common causes. Hypothalamic hypothyroidism may also be due to neoplastic infiltration. Low plasma T_4 and low TSH levels are found. Diagnosis and treatment of iatrogenic hypothyroidism is the same as for primary hypothyroidism.

C. Hyperthyroidism (Thyrotoxicosis)

Hyperthyroidism is defined as an overactivity of thyroid function of sufficient magnitude to cause symptoms and signs due to the elevated T_3 and T_4 levels in the plasma. Common symptoms are nervousness, irritability, tremor, excess sweating, and loss of weight due to the elevated levels of thyroid hormones.

Graves' disease is an autoimmune disorder with the following features: hyper-thyroidism, goiter, ophthalmopathy (prominent eyes), and infiltrative dermopathy (thickened skin). The pathogenesis may be simplified as follows. Autoantibodies against the TSH receptor on the thyroid membrane, which are capable of binding to the receptor and stimulating biosynthesis, are produced in excess. Most of these autoantibodies stimulate thyroid function, although some are inhibitory and block thyroid function. Graves' disease can thus present with a spectrum of thyroid function ranging from hyperthyroidism to hypothyroidism.

Graves' disease is confirmed by testing thyroid function and finding elevated plasma levels of T_3 and T_4 and suppressed TSH. Treatment of Graves' disease depends on various factors such as age and sex of the patient and the size of the goiter. The treatments available are subtotal thyroidectomy, ^{131}I, and oral antithyroid drugs. Supplementary treatments of other organ systems, e.g., the cardiovascular system, are frequently necessary.

Toxic nodular goiter occurs in older patients as a result of long-standing iodine deficiency. The goiter is usually multinodular in structure but may be uninodular. The thyroid has become autonomous. This condition usually develops following increasing iodine intake in previous long-standing iodine deficiency. This may occur sporadically in patients given iodine-containing medicines or in areas of endemic iodine deficiency when measures to increase the iodine intake in the population such as salt iodization are undertaken. Treatment of toxic nodular goiter is either surgery or radioactive iodine.

VI. THE IODINE DEFICIENCY DISORDERS

The effects of iodine deficiency on growth and development are now denoted by the term iodine deficiency disorders (IDD). These effects are evident at all stages, including particularly the fetus, the neonate, and in infancy, which are the periods of rapid growth. The term "goiter" has been used for many years to describe the effect of iodine deficiency. Goiter is indeed the obvious and familiar feature of iodine deficiency, but knowledge has greatly expanded in the last 25 years so that it is not surprising that a new term is needed (Table 6) (3–5).

A. The Fetus

Iodine deficiency of the fetus is the result of iodine deficiency in the mother. The condition is associated with a greater incidence of stillbirths, abortions, and congenital abnormalities, which can be reduced by iodization. The effects are similar to those observed with maternal hypothyroidism, which can be reduced by thyroid hormone replacement therapy (27). Controlled trials with iodized oil have revealed a significant reduction in recorded fetal and neonatal deaths in the treated group, which is consistent with animal evidence indicating the effect of iodine deficiency on fetal survival (3–5).

Further data from Papua New Guinea indicate a relationship between the level of maternal thyroxine with the outcome of current and recent past pregnancies, including

TABLE 6 The Spectrum of Iodine Deficiency Disorders (IDD)

Fetus	Abortions
	Stillbirths
	Congenital anomalies
	Increased perinatal mortality
	Increased infant mortality
	Neurological cretinism (mental deficiency, deaf mutism, spastic diplegia, squint)
	Hypothyroid cretinism (dwarfism, mental deficiency)
	Psychomotor defects
	Increased susceptibility of the thyroid gland to nuclear radiation (after 12 weeks)
Neonate	Neonatal goiter
	Neonatal hypothyroidism
	Increased susceptibility of the thyroid gland to nuclear radiation
Child and adolescent	Goiter
	Juvenile hypothyroidism
	Impaired mental function
	Retarded physical development
	Increased susceptibility of the thyroid gland to nuclear radiation
Adult	Goiter with its complications
	Hypothyroidism
	Impaired mental function
	Iodine-induced hyperthyroidism
	Increased susceptibility of the thyroid gland to nuclear radiation

mortality and the occurrence of cretinism. The rate of perinatal deaths was twice as high among mothers (36.0%) with very low serum concentrations of total thyroxine compared to 16.4% as in the women with levels about 25 μg/mL (27,28).

These data, indicating the importance of maternal thyroid function to fetal survival and development, are complemented by extensive animal data (3).

A major effect of fetal iodine deficiency is the condition of endemic cretinism, which is quite distinct from the condition of sporadic cretinism (1–3,28). This condition, which occurs with an iodine intake of below 25 μg/day in contrast to a normal intake of 80–150 μg/day, is still widely prevalent, affecting, for example, up to 10% of the populations living in severely iodine-deficient areas in India, Indonesia, and China (28, 29) (Fig. 5). In its most common form, it is characterized by mental deficiency, deaf mutism, and spastic diplegia, which is referred to as the "nervous" or neurologic type in contrast to the less common "hypothyroid" type characterized by hypothyroidism with dwarfism.

Apart from its prevalence in Asia and Oceania (Papua New Guinea), cretinism also occurs in Africa (Zaire) and in South America in the Andean region (Eucador, Peru, Bolivia, and Argentina) (28). In all these situations, with the exception of Zaire, neurologic features are predominant. In Zaire the hypothyroid form is more common, probably due to the high intake of cassava (30). However, there is considerable variation in the clinical manifestations of neurologic cretinism, including isolated deaf mutism and mental defect of varying degrees. In China the term "cretinoid" is used to describe these individuals (29).

The apparent spontaneous disappearance of endemic cretinism in Italy and Switzerland raised doubts as to the relation of iodine deficiency to the condition (1,3,5). However,

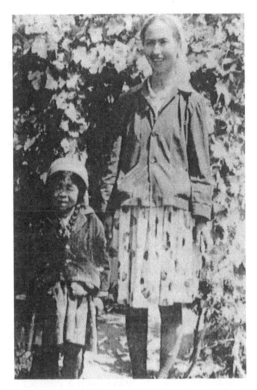

FIGURE 5 A hypothyroid cretin dwarf from Sinjiang, China, who is also deaf mute. This condition is completely preventable by prevention of iodine deficiency. Right: the barefoot doctor of her village. Both are about 35 years of age. (Photograph courtesy of Prof. T. Ma, Tianjin, People's Republic of China.)

a controlled trial in the Western Highlands of Papua New Guinea revealed that endemic cretinism could be prevented by correction of iodine deficiency with iodized oil before pregnancy (1,3,31).

The value of iodized oil injection in the prevention of endemic cretinism has been confirmed in Zaire and in South America. Mass injection programs were carried out in New Guinea in 1971–1972 and in Zaire, Indonesia, and China. Recent evaluations of these mass programs in Indonesia and China indicate that endemic cretinism has been prevented where correction of iodine deficiency has been achieved.

The apparent spontaneous disappearance of the condition is now attributed to increase in iodine intake due to dietary diversification as a result of social and economic development affecting more remote rural areas.

B. The Neonate

Increased perinatal mortality due to iodine deficiency has been shown in Zaire from the results of a controlled trial of iodized oil injections given in the latter half of pregnancy, alternately with a control injection (3,4). There is a substantial fall in perinatal and infant mortality with improved birth weight. Low birth weight, whatever the cause, is generally associated with a higher rate of congenital anomalies and higher risk through childhood.

Apart from the question of mortality, the importance of the state of thyroid function in the neonate relates to the fact that at birth the brain of the human infant has reached only about one-third of its full size and continues to grow rapidly until the end of the second year (32). The thyroid hormone, dependent on an adequate supply of iodine, is essential for normal brain development, as has been confirmed by animal studies (3,33).

Recently, data on iodine nutrition and neonatal thyroid function in Europe have been published. These data confirm the continuing presence of severe iodine deficiency affecting neonatal thyroid function and hence constituting a threat to early brain development (34).

There is similar evidence from neonatal observations in Zaire, where rates of 10% of chemical hypothyroidism have been found (35). In Zaire it has been observed that this hypothyroidism persists into infancy and childhood if the deficiency is not corrected, with resultant retardation of physical and mental development. These observations indicate a much greater risk of mental defect in severely iodine-deficient populations than is indicated by the presence of classical cretinism.

C. The Child

Iodine deficiency in children is characteristically associated with goiter. The classification of goiter which has been standardized by the World Health Organization is discussed in the next section. The goiter rate increases with age and reaches a maximum with adolescence. Girls have a higher prevalence than boys. Observations of goiter rates in school children from ages 8 to 14 provides a convenient indication of the presence of iodine deficiency in a community.

Recent studies in school children living in iodine-deficient areas from a number of countries indicate impaired school performance and IQs in comparison with matched groups from noniodine-deficient areas. These studies are difficult to set up because of the problem of the control group. There are many possible causes for impaired school performance, and impaired performance on an IQ test, which may be operating, and so make difficult the interpretation of any difference that might be observed. The iodine-deficient area is likely to be more remote, suffer more social deprivation, with a disadvantage in school facilities, a lower socioeconomic status, and poorer general nutrition. All such factors have to be taken into account in evaluating the effects of iodine deficiency, in addition to the problem of adapting tests developed in Western countries for use in Third World countries.

The results of a number of studies have been brought together in a meta-analysis in which a comparison has been made between iodine-deficient and normal children from a total of 18 studies. The results indicate a difference in the mean scores of 13.5 IQ points (34,36).

D. The Adult

Iodine administration in the form of iodized salt, iodized bread, or iodized oil have all been demonstrated to be effective in the prevention of goiter in adults. Iodine administration may also reduce existing goiter in adults. This is particularly true of iodized oil injections (1,4,5). This obvious effect leads to ready acceptance of the measure by people living in iodine-deficient communities. A rise in circulating thyroxine can be readily demonstrated in adult subjects following iodization by various means.

The major determinant of brain (and pituitary) triiodothyronine (T_3) concentration is serum thyroxine (T_4) and not T_3 (as is true of the liver, kidney, and muscle) (37). Low levels of brain T_3 have been demonstrated in the iodine-deficient rat, in association with reduced levels of serum T_4, and these have been restored to normal with correction of iodine deficiency (38).

These findings provide a rationale for suboptimal brain function in subjects with endemic goiter and lowered serum T_4 levels and its improvement following correction of iodine deficiency.

In Northern India, a high degree of apathy has been noted in populations living in iodine-deficient areas. This may even affect domestic animals such as dogs! It is apparent that reduced mental function is widely prevalent in iodine-deficient communities, with effects on their capacity for initiative and decisionmaking. This means that iodine deficiency is a major block to the human and social development of communities living in an iodine-deficient environment. Correction of the iodine deficiency is indicated as a major contribution to development. Correction of iodine deficiency will also reduce susceptibility to iodine-nuclide radiation, including reduction of the risk of thyroid cancer.

E. The Effects of Iodine Deficiency in Animals

Observations on naturally occurring iodine deficiency have been made on farm animals, in which reproductive failure and thyroid insufficiency have been fully reported in the older literature (39). In areas of iodine deficiency, development of the fetus has been retarded or arrested at some stage in gestation, resulting in early death or resorption, abortion, and stillbirth, or the birth of weak, hairless offspring associated with prolonged gestation and parturition and retention of placental membranes. Subnormal thyroid hormone levels in herds of cattle have been accompanied by a high incidence of aborted, stillborn, and weak calves (39).

An important new dimension has been provided by recent experimental work with animal models (3,33,39). Severe iodine deficiency has been established prior to and during pregnancy and then the effects on fetal development studied. Iodine deficiency in the sheep (5–8 µg/day for sheep weighing 40 kg) is associated with an increased incidence of abortions and stillbirths. At the end of pregnancy the fetus shows a reduced body weight, complete absence of wool growth, deformation of the skull, and retardation of bone development (Fig. 6). There is retardation of brain development as indicated by reduced brain weight and a reduced number of cells (as measured by DNA). Similar effects have been observed in the marmoset monkey (0.3 µg/day for a 340-g animal).

In the light of the available data and observations on the animal models, it may be concluded that the effects of severe iodine deficiency on fetal development are mediated by a combination of maternal and fetal hypothyroidism, the effect of maternal hypothyroidism being earlier than the onset of fetal thyroid secretion. This would infer an effect on neuroblast multiplication, which occurs from 40–80 days of gestation in the sheep and 11–18 weeks in the human (3,33,40). In the rat (a postnatal brain in which neuroblast multiplication occurs in the last one-third of fetal life), an effect of the maternal thyroid early in pregnancy is indicated by reduced weight and number of embryos, reduced brain weight, and reduced transfer of maternal T_4 (3,33).

The findings suggest that iodine deficiency has an early effect on neuroblast multiplication and, if so, this could be important in the pathogenesis of the neurologic form of endemic cretinism (3,33,40).

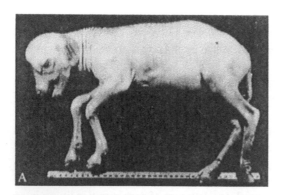

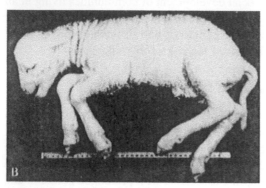

FIGURE 6 Effect of severe iodine deficiency during pregnancy on lamb development. A 140-day-old lamb fetus (A) was subjected to severe iodine deficiency through feeding the mother an iodine-deficient diet (5–8 μ/day) for 6 months prior to and during pregnancy (full term 150 days). Compared to a control lamb (B) of the same age fed the same diet with the addition of an iodine supplement. The iodine-deficient lamb showed absence of wool coat, subluxation of the leg joints, and a smaller brain. (From Ref. 5, with permission.)

VII. ASSESSMENT OF IODINE NUTRITIONAL STATUS

The assessment of iodine nutritional status is important in relation to public health programs in which iodine supplementation is carried out. The problem is therefore one of assessment of a population or group living in an area or region that is suspected to be iodine deficient.

The data methods recommended are

1. The goiter rate, including the rate of palpable or visible goiter classified according to accepted criteria (41)
2. The urine iodine excretion
3. The determination of the level of blood thyroid stimulating hormone (TSH)

Particular attention is now focused on the levels in the neonate because of the importance of the level of thyroid function for early brain development.

1. A new classification of goiter severity has recently been adopted by the World Health Organization (Table 7) (1,2,41). There are still minor differences in technique between different observers. In general, visible goiter is more readily verified than palpable

TABLE 7 Proposed Classification of Goiter

Grade 0	No palpable or visible goiter.
Grade 1	A mass in the neck that is consistent with an enlarged thyroid that is palpable but not visible when the neck is in the normal position. It moves upward in the neck as the subject swallows. Nodular alteration(s) can occur even when the thyroid is not enlarged.
Grade 2	A swelling in the neck that is visible when the neck is in a normal position and is consistent with an enlarged thyroid when the neck is palpated.

goiter. Recent observations in Tanzania (4) indicate that palpation of the thyroid overestimates the size of the gland as determined by ultrasonography, particularly in children. Determination of thyroid size by ultrasonography is now becoming standardized and is to be preferred when this technology is available, because it is an objective measure (24).

2. The determination of urine iodine excretion can be carried out on casual samples from a group of approximately 50 subjects. The iodine levels are expressed as micrograms per 100 mL and the range plotted as a histogram. This provides a reference point for the level of iodine excretion, which is also a good index of the level of iodine nutrition. Methods have been recently simplified so that many more samples can be processed (25).

3. The determination of the level of TSH provides an indirect measure of iodine nutritional status. The availability of radioimmunoassay and immunometric methods with automated equipment has greatly assisted this approach with the processing of large numbers of samples. TSH is now the preferred method because of better stability under tropical conditions and easier methodology. Particular attention should be given to levels of TSH in the neonate.

In an increasing number of developing countries, cord blood samples or heelprick samples from neonates (3–4 days after birth), spotted onto filter paper and dried are used for analysis. Blood levels of either T_4 or TSH or both are measured by immunoassay techniques. As already mentioned, the detection rate of neonatal hypothyroidism requiring treatment is about 1 per 3500 babies screened. This rate varies little among developed countries (42).

In developing countries, by contrast, severe biochemical hypothyroidism (T_4 concentrations less than 3 µg/dL has been reported in up to 10% of neonates (42) in northern India and in Zaire (4). These data indicate the massive threat to brain development posed by severe iodine deficiency.

To summarize, the most critical evidence for determination of iodine nutrition status comes from measurement of urine excretion of iodine in the first case. If this is adequate, then measurement blood TSH in the neonate should follow on a population basis. The results of these two determinations indicate the severity of the problem. They can also be used to assess the effectiveness of remedial measures.

VIII. IODINE REQUIREMENTS AND TOXICITY

In 1989 the Food and Nutrition Board, National Academy of Sciences, National Research Council, United States, confirmed the previous 1980 recommendations for a daily iodine intake of 40 µg for children aged 0–6 months, 50 µg from 6 to 12 months, 70–120 µg from 1 to 10 years, and 120–150 µg from 11 years onward. The recommended rates during pregnancy and lactation were, respectively, 175 and 200 μg. The recommendations applied equally to both sexes (43).

A. Toxicity

Iodine toxicity has been critically studied in humans, laboratory species, poultry, pigs and cattle.

Wolff (44) has suggested that human intakes of 2000 μg I/day should be regarded as an excessive or potentially harmful level of intake. Normal diets composed of natural foods are likely to supply as much as 2000 μg I/day and most supply less than 1000 μg I/day, except where the diets are exceptionally high in marine fish or seaweed, or where foods are contaminated with iodine from adventitious sources.

Inhabitants of the coastal regions of Hokkaido, the northern island of Japan, whose diets contain large amounts of seaweed, have remarkably high iodine intakes, amounting to 50,000–80,000 μg I/day (45). Urinary excretion in five patients exhibiting clinical signs of iodide goiter exceeded 20 mg I/day or about 100 times normal. Similar findings have been reported from two Chinese villages on the Yellow Sea coast in association with the consumption of large amounts of kelp (46).

In Japan (47) it has been shown that:

1. Normal subjects can maintain normal thyroid function states even when they are taking several milligrams per day (perhaps 30 mg/day) of dietary iodine.
2. Incidence of nontoxic diffuse goiter and toxic nodular goiter are remarkably decreased by high dietary iodine.
3. Incidence of Graves' disease and Hashimoto's disease appears not to be affected by high dietary iodine.
4. However, high dietary iodine may induce hypothyroidism in autoimmune thyroid diseases and may inhibit the effects of thionamide drugs.

Significant species differences exist in tolerance to high iodine intakes. In all species studied the tolerance is high, i.e., relative to normal dietary iodine intakes, pointing to a wide margin of safety for this element.

B. Iodine-Induced Hyperthyroidism

A mild increase incidence of hyperthyroidism has now been described following iodized salt programs in Europe and following iodized bread in Holland and Tasmania (48,49). A few cases have been noted following iodized oil administration in South America. No cases have yet been described in Asia. This is probably due to the scattered nature of the population in small villages and limited opportunities for observation (50). Natural remission also occurs. The condition is largely confined to those over 40 years of age. Detailed observations are available from the island of Tasmania (49,51).

Joseph et al. (52) have reported that iodine intakes of less than 0.100 mg/day pose no risk for patients with autonomous tissue due to iodine deficiency, but that critical amounts are probably between 0.100 and 0.200 mg/day. The iodization of bread in Tasmania resulted in thyrotoxicosis for some individuals at levels of iodine intake of about 0.200 mg/ day (49,51). Iodated bread in Holland contributed an additional 0.120–0.160 mg I/day and increased the incidence of thyrotoxicosis. The spring-summer peak of thyrotoxicosis (related to winter milk) in England occurred with average iodine intakes of 0.236 mg/day for women and 0.306 mg/day for men (53). The absence of iodine deficiency in the Japanese population accounts for the absence of iodine-induced thyrotoxicosis (47).

The condition is readily controlled with antithyroid drugs or radioiodine. Spontaneous remission also occurs. In general, iodization should be avoided in those over the age of 40 because of the risk of hyperthyroidism (1,2,4).

However, the correction of iodine deficiency prevents the formation of an autonomous thyroid and so prevents the condition of iodine-induced hyperthyroidism. Hence this condition is included as an "iodine deficiency disorder" (Table 6).

IX. CORRECTION OF IODINE DEFICIENCY

A. Iodized Salt

Iodized salt has been the major method used since the 1920s, when it was first used successfully in Switzerland (1,4,5). Since then, successful programs have been reported from a number of countries. These include the United States, Central and South America (e.g., Guatemala, Colombia), Finland, China, and Taiwan (5).

The difficulties in the production, and maintenance of quality to the millions that are iodine deficient, especially in Asia, are vividly demonstrated in India, where there was a breakdown in supply. The difficulties have led to the adoption of universal salt iodation for India to be achieved by 1995.

In Asia, the cost of iodized salt production and distribution at present is of the order of 3–5 cents per person per year (4). This must be considered cheap in relation to the social benefits that have been described in the previous section.

However, there is still the problem of the salt actually reaching the iodine-deficient subject. There may be a problem with distribution or preservation of the iodine content —it may be left uncovered or exposed to heat. It should be added after cooking to reduce the loss of iodine.

Finally, there is the difficulty of actual consumption of the salt. While the addition of iodine makes no difference to the taste of the salt, the introduction of a new variety of salt to an area where salt is already available and familiar and much appreciated as a condiment is likely to be resisted. In the Chinese provinces of Sinjiang and Inner Mongolia, the strong preference of the people for desert salt of very low iodine content led to a mass iodized oil injection program in order to prevent cretinism (29).

B. Iodized Oil by Injection

The value of iodized oil injection in the prevention of endemic goiter and endemic cretinism was first established in New Guinea with controlled trials involving the use of saline injection as a control. These trials established the value of the oil in the prevention of goiter and the prevention of cretinism (4,31). Experience in South America, Zaire, and China has confirmed the value of the measure. The quantitative correction of severe iodine deficiency by a single intramuscular injection has been demonstrated (4) for a period of over 4 years.

Iodized oil is singularly appropriate for isolated village communities so characteristic of mountainous endemic goiter areas. The striking regression of goiter following iodized oil injection ensures general acceptance of the measure. Iodized walnut oil and iodized soya bean oil are new preparations developed in China since 1980 (4).

In a suitable area the oil (1 ml contains 480 mg) should be administered to all females up to the age of 40 years and all males up to the age of 20 years. A repeat of the injection would be required in 3–5 years depending on the dose given and the age of the subject. In children the need is greater than in adults and the recommended dose should be repeated in 3 years if severe iodine deficiency persists (4). Because of the hazards associated with injections, there has been a strong recent trend toward oral administration of iodized oil.

C. Iodized Oil by Mouth

Recent studies in India and China reveal that oral iodized oil lasts only half as long as a similar dose given by injection (4). A recent study in children indicates that 1 ml (480 mg) of oral oil provides coverage of iodine deficiency for one year (23).

D. Indications for Different Methods of Iodine Supplementation

There are three grades of severity of IDD in a population, based on the urinary iodine excretion (4,5):

1. Mild IDD, with goiter prevalence in the range 5–10% (school children) and with median urine iodine levels in the range 5.0–9.9 ug/dL. Mild IDD can be controlled with iodized salt at a concentration of 10–25 mg/kg. It may disappear with economic development.
2. Moderate IDD, with goiter prevalence up to 30% and some hypothyroidism, with median urine iodine levels in the range 2.0–4.9 ug/dL. Moderate IDD can be controlled with iodized salt (25–40 mg/kg) if this can be effectively produced and distributed. Otherwise, iodized oil, either orally or by injection, should be used through the primary health care system.
3. Severe IDD, indicated by a high prevalence of goiter (30% or more), endemic cretinism (prevalence 1–10%), and median urine iodine below 2.0 μg/dL. Severe IDD requires iodized oil either orally or by injection for complete prevention of central nervous system defects.

Both iodized salt and iodized oil are the major mass supplementation measures which have been used on a large scale. In excess of 20 million injections of iodized oil have been given in Asia, with evidence of successful prevention of IDD.

X. INTERNATIONAL ACTION

The great gap between our new knowledge of IDD and the application of this knowledge in national IDD control programs, particularly in developing countries, has led to the formation of the International Council for the Control of Iodine Deficiency Disorders (ICCIDD).

The inaugural meeting of this multidisciplinary group of epidemiologists and nutritionists, endocrinologists and chemists, planners and economists, was held in Kathmandu, Nepal, in March 1986. A series of papers on all aspects of IDD control programs presented in Kathmandu has been published as a monograph (4). The ICCIDD has now established a global multidisciplinary network of some 400 people from more than 70 different countries with expertise relevant to IDD and IDD control programs. More than half of the members are from developing countries. It works closely with WHO, UNICEF, and national governments within the U.N. system in the development of national programs (4,5).

The major concentrations of population are in Asia, where there has been a major escalation of IDD control programs in the last 10 years in India, Indonesia, Nepal, Burma, and Bhutan (6). In Latin America, earlier efforts have produced a large measure of control in such countries as Argentina, Brazil, Colombia, and Guatemala. However, there is now evidence of recurrence of the problem in Colombia and Guatemala, associated with political and social unrest. Major IDD problems have persisted in Eucador, Peru, and Bolivia, but there has been significant progress in the last 5 years with the combination of national government initiative and support from international agencies (6).

In Africa there has been a lag in the development of IDD control programs by comparison with the other continents. However, new initiatives have begun following a Joint WHO/UNICEF/ICCIDD Regional Seminar held in Yaounde, Cameroon, in March 1987. This seminar set up a joint IDD task force which has now initiated comprehensive planning for the prevention and control of IDD in Africa (6).

In September 1990, the World Summit for Children, held at the United Nations in New York, was attended by 71 heads of state and 80 other government representatives. The world summit signed a declaration and approved a plan of action that included the elimination of IDD as a public health problem by the year 2000.

This was followed in October 1991 by a conference entitled "Ending Hidden Hunger." This was a policy and promotional meeting on micronutrients including iodine, vitamin A, and iron. It was attended by multidisciplinary delegations from 55 countries, with major IDD problems nominated by heads of state in response to an invitation by the director general of the World Health Organization (Dr. H. Nakajima) and the late executive director of UNICEF (Mr. James Grant). There was a firm commitment at this meeting to the elimination goal for IDD and vitamin A deficiency, with reduction of iron deficiency by one-third of 1990 levels.

These various developments encourage the hope that significant progress can be made toward the elimination of IDD within the next decade, with great benefits to the quality of life of the many millions affected (54).

REFERENCES

1. Stanbury JB, Hetzel BS. Endemic Goiter and Endemic Cretinism. New York: Wiley, 1980.
2. Dunn JT, Pretell EA, Daza CH, eds. Towards the Eradication of Endemic Goiter, Cretinism, and Iodine Deficiency. Washington, DC: Pan American Health Organization, 1986.
3. Hetzel BS, Potter BJ, Dulberg EM. The iodine deficiency disorders: nature, pathogenesis and epidemiology. World Rev Nutr Diet 1990; 62:59–119.
4. Hetzel BS, Dunn JT, Stanbury JB, eds. The Prevention and Control of Iodine Deficiency Disorders. Amsterdam:Elsevier, 1987.
5. Hetzel BS. The Story of Iodine Deficiency: An International Challenge in Nutrition. Oxford and Delhi: Oxford University Press, 1989.
6. World Health Organization Report to 43rd World Health Assembly, Geneva: WHO, 1990.
7. World Health Organization. Micronutrient Deficiency Information System (MDIS) Working Paper No. 1. Global Prevalence of Iodine Deficiency Disorders. Geneva: WHO/UNICEF/ICCIDD, 1993.
8. Dunn JT. Thyroglobulin, hormone synthesis and thyroid disease. Eur J Endocrinol 1995; 132:603–604.
9. Koenig RJ, Leonard JL, Senator D, Rappoport N, Watson AY, Larsen PR. Regulation of thyroxine 5'-deiodinase activity by 3,5,3'-triiodothyronine in cultured rat anterior pituitary cells. Endocrinology (Baltimore) 1984; 115:324–329.
10. Larsen PR, Dick TE, Markovitz BP, Kaplan MM, Gard TG. Inhibition of intrapituitary thyroxine to 3,5,3'-triiodothyronine conversion prevents the acute suppression of thyrotropin release by thyroxine in hypothyroid rats. J Clin Invest 1979; 64:117–128.
11. Scanlon MF Weightman DR, Shale DJ, et al. Dopamine is a physiological regulator of thyrotrophin (TSH) secretion in normal man. Clin Endocrinol 1979; 10:7–15.

12. Siler TM, Yen SSC, Vale W, Guillemin R. Inhibition by somatostatin on the release of TSH induced in man by thyrotropin-releasing factor. J Clin Endocrinol Metab 1974; 38:742–745.

13. Robbins J, Bartalena L. Plasma transport of thyroid hormones. In: Hennemann G, ed. Thyroid Hormone Metabolism. New York: Marcel Dekker 1986:3–38.

14. Marshall JS, Pensky J, Green AM. Studies on human thyroxine-binding globulin. VI. The nature of slow thyroxine-binding globulin. J Clin Invest 1972; 52:3173–3181.

15. Reilly CP, Wellby ML. Slow thyroxine binding globulin in the pathogenesis of increased dialysable fraction of thyroxine in nonthyroidal illness. J Clin Endocrinol Metab 1983; 57: 15–18.

16. Robbins J, Rall, JE. Hormone transport in circulation. The interaction of thyroid hormones and protein in biological fluids. Recent Prog Hormone Res 1957; 13:161–208.

17. Ekins R. The free hormone concept. In: Hennemann G, ed. Thyroid Hormone Metabolism. New York: Marcel Dekker 1986:77–106.

18. Pardridge WM. Transport of protein-bound hormones into tissues in vivo. Endocrinol Rev 1981; 2:103–123.

19. Albright EC, Larson FC. Metabolism of l-thyroxine by human tissue slices. J Clin Invest 1959; 38:1899–1903.

20. Chopra IJ. Triiodothyronines in Health and Disease. Berlin: Springer-Verlag, 1981.

21. Arthur JR, Nicol F, Beckett GJ. Selenium deficiency, thyroid hormone metabolism and thyroid hormone deiodinases. Am J Clin Nutr Suppl 1993; 57:2365–2395.

22. Wellby ML. Clinical chemistry of thyroid function testing. Adv Clin Chem 1990; 28:1–92.

23. Benmiloud M, Chaouki ML, Gutekunst R, Teichert H-M, Wood WG, Dunn JT. Oral iodised oil for correcting iodine deficiency: optimal dosing and outcome indicator selection. J Clin Endocrinol Metab 1994; 79:20–24.

24. Vitti P, Martino E, Aghini-Lombardi F, et al. Thyroid volume measurement by ultrasound in children as a tool for the assessment of mild iodine deficiency. J Clin Endocrinol Metab 1994; 79:600–603.

25. Dunn JT, Crutchfield HE, Gutekunst R, Dunn AD, eds. Methods for Measuring Iodine in Urine. The Netherlands: ICCIDD/UNICEF/WHO, 1993.

26. Lever EG, Medeiros-Neto GA, DeGroot LJ. Inherited disorders of thyroid metabolism. Endocrinol Rev 1983; 4:213–239.

27. McMichael AJ, Potter JD, Hetzel BS. Iodine deficiency, thyroid function, and reproductive failure. In: Stanbury JB, Hetzel BS, eds. Endemic Goitre and Endemic Cretinism. New York: Wiley, 1980: 445–460.

28. Pharoah POD, Delange F, Fierro Benitez R, Stanbury JB. Endemic cretinism. In: Stanbury JB, Hetzel BS, eds. Endemic Goitre and Endemic Cretinism. New York: Wiley 1980: 395–421.

29. Ma T, Lu T, Tan U, Chen B, Zhu HI. The present status of endemic goitre and endemic cretinism in China. Food Nutr Bull 1982; 4:13–19.

30. Delange F, Iteke FB, Ermans AM. Nutritional factors involved in the goitrogenic action of cassava. Ottawa: International Development Research Center, 1982.

31. Pharoah POD, Buttfield IH, Hetzel BS. Neurological damage to the fetus resulting from severe iodine deficiency during pregnancy. Lancet 1971; i:308–310.

32. Dobbing J. The later development of the brain and its vulnerability. In: Davis J, Dobbing J, eds. Scientific Foundations of Paediatrics. London: Heinemann, 1974: 565–577.

33. Hetzel BS, Chavadej J, Potter JB. The brain and iodine deficiency. Neuropathol Appl Neurobiol 1988; 14:93–104.

34. Bleichrodt N, Born M. A metaanalysis of research on iodine and its relationship to cognitive development. In: Stanbury JB, ed. The Damaged Brain of Iodine Deficiency. New York: Cognizand Communication Corporation 1994:195–200.

35. Ermans AM, Moulameko NM, Delange F, Alhuwalis R, eds. Role of Cassava in the Aetiology of Endemic Goitre and Cretinism. Ottawa: International Development Research Centre, 1980.

36. Stanbury JB, ed. The Damaged Brain of Iodine Deficiency. New York Cognizant Communication Corporation, 1994.

37. Crantz FR, Larsen PR. Rapid thyroxine to 3,5,3'-triiodothyronine conversion binding in rat cerebral cortex and cerebellum. J Clin Invest 1980; 65:935–938.

38. Obregon MJ, Santisteban P, Rodriguez-Pena A, et al. Cerebral hypothyroidism in rats with adult-onset iodine deficiency. Endocrinology 1984; 115:614–624.

39. Hetzel BS, Maberly GF. Iodine. In: Mertz W, ed. Trace Elements in Human and Animal Nutrition. Vol. 2. 5th ed. New York: Academic Press, 1986:139–208.

40. Delong R. Neurological involvement in iodine deficiency disorders. In: Hetzel BS, Stanbury JB, Dunn JT, eds. The Prevention and Control of Iodine Deficiency Disorders. Amsterdam: Elsevier, 1987:49–63.

41. World Health Organization. Indicators for Assessing Iodine Deficiency Disorders and Their Control through Salt Iodization. Geneva: WHO/UNICEF/ICCIDD, 1994.

42. Burrow, GN, ed. Neonatal Thyroid Screening. New York: Raven Press, 1980.

43. Food and Nutrition Board, National Academy of Sciences, National Research Council: Recommended Dietary Allowances. 10th ed. Washington, DC, 1989.

44. Wolff J. Iodide goiter and the pharmacologic effects of excess iodide. Am J Med 1969; 47:101.

45. Suzuki H. Etiology of endemic goiter and iodide excess. In: Stanbury JB, Hetzel BS, eds. Endemic Goiter and Endemic Cretinism. New York: Wiley, 1980:237–254.

46. Zhu XY, Lu TZ, Song XK, et al. Endemic goiter and cretinism in China with special reference to changes of iodine metabolism and pituitary-thyroid function two years after iodine prophylaxis in Gui-Zhou. In: Ui N, Torizuka K, Nagataki S, Miyai K, eds. Current Problems in Thyroid Research. Amsterdam: Excerpta Medica, 1983:13–18.

47. Nagataki S. Effects of iodide supplement in thyroid diseases. In: Vichayanrat A, Nitiyanant W, Eastman C, Nagataki S, eds. Recent Progress in Thyroidology. Bangkok: Crystal House Press, 1987:31–37.

48. Connolly RJ, Vidor GI, Stewart JC. Increase in thyrotoxicosis in endemic goiter area after iodation of bread. Lancet 1970; i:500–502.

49. Stewart JC, Vidor GI, Buttfield IH, Hetzel BS. Epidemic thyrotoxicosis in Northern Tasmania: studies of clinical features and iodine nutrition. Austral NZ J Med 1971; 1:203–211.

50. Larsen PR, Silva JE, Hetzel BS, McMichael AJ. Monitoring prophylactic programs: general consideration. In Stanbury JB, Hetzel BS, eds. Endemic Goiter and Endemic Cretinism. New York: Wiley, 1980:551–566.

51. Vidor GI, Stewart JC, Wall JR, Wangel A, Hetzel BS. Pathogenesis of iodine-induced thyrotoxicosis: studies in Northern Tasmania. J Clin Endocrinol Metab 1973; 37:901–909.

52. Joseph K, Mahlstedt J, Gonnermann R, Herbert K, Welcke U. Early recognition and evaluation of the risk of hyperthyroidism in thyroid autonomy in an endemic goitre area. J Mol Med 1980; 4:21–37.

53. Nelson M, Phillips DIW. Seasonal variations in dietary iodine intake and thyrotoxicosis. Hum Nutr Appl Nutr 1985; 39(3):213–216.

54. Hetzel BS, Pandav CS. SOS for a Billion: The Conquest of Iodine Deficiency Disorders. Delhi: Oxford University Press, 1994.

55. Pike JW. Vitamin D_3 receptors: structure and function in transcription. Ann Rev Nutr 1991; 11:189–216.

56. Beckett GJ, Nicol F, Rae PWH, Beech S, Guo Y, Arthur JR. Effects of combined iodine and selenium deficiency on thyroid hormone metabolism in rats. Am J Clin Nutr 1993; 57:240S–243S.

57. Vanderpas JB, Contempré B, Duale NL, et al. Selenium deficiency mitigates hypothyroxinemia in iodine-deficient subjects. Am J Clin Nutr Suppl 1993; 57:271S–275S.

20
Fluorine

FLORIAN L. CERKLEWSKI
Oregon State University, Corvallis, Oregon

I. INTRODUCTION

Fluorine, crudely prepared by Scheele in 1771 and named in 1812 by Ampere, was not actually isolated until 1886 by Moissan (1). Geochemically, fluorine is the 13th most abundant element in the earth's crust, occurring predominantly as the mineral salts fluorite (calcium fluoride), cryolite (sodium aluminum fluoride), and fluorapatite (2). The leaching of these minerals into the environment accounts for the fact that fluorine as the fluoride ion is a natural constituent of soils, plants, animal tissue, water, and diets. Fluoride is classified as a trace element because the total body content of fluoride is less than 5 g and it is beneficial when consumed at levels much less than 100 mg per day.

With regard to human health, the fluoride ion was first recognized as a cariostatic agent by Dean in his search for the agent responsible for mottled enamel (3). Subsequent studies confirmed that fluoride has a unique role in strengthening enamel structure of teeth by conferring a significant resistance to dissolution of enamel by acids (lactic acid, acetic acid) produced by cariogenic bacteria, particularly *Streptococcus mutans* (4–6). The observation by Dean, however, demonstrated that, like other nutrients, fluoride can have either a positive or a negative effect on metabolism, depending on the level of intake. In the case of the fluoride ion, the difference between essentiality and toxicity is narrow. The present review therefore focuses on fluoride metabolism and discusses both essential and toxic effects of fluoride with emphasis on human nutrition. Additional information about fluoride can be found in reviews by others (7–11).

II. CHEMICAL PROPERTIES

Fluorine, with an atomic weight of 18.99840 and an atomic number of 9, is one of three halogens known to have an important biological function. Because fluorine is the most

583

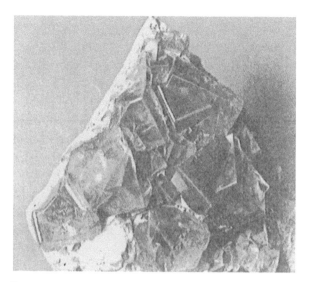

FIGURE 1 An example of the natural occurrence of fluoride as calcium fluoride (fluorite crystals). (From Ref. 13, with permission of photographer Rodolfo Crespi.)

electronegative nonmetal, with a higher oxidation potential than ozone, it does not occur in the elemental state in nature (1,2,12). Instead it exists solely as the monovalent anion fluoride (F^-). Fluoride tends to form soluble compounds with monovalent cations such as sodium and potassium and insoluble compounds with multivalent cations such as calcium, magnesium, and aluminum. An example of the natural occurrence of fluoride as calcium fluoride (fluorite) is shown in Figure 1 (13).

III. ANALYTICAL METHODOLOGY

The determination of fluoride with the fluoride-specific electrode (14) has replaced the colorimetric determination procedure. Methods to determine fluoride by gas chromatography (15) and high-performance liquid chromatography (16) have been described but are not in routine use.

For simple matrices, such as drinking water and urine, the determination of fluoride with the fluoride-specific electrode is relatively straightforward (17). More complex matrices, however, such as food, feces, and biological tissues, require separation of fluoride from the sample prior to measurement. The most common procedure for separating fluoride is to react the sample with perchloric acid at 55–60°C in a closed plastic dish such as a Conway diffusion plate that has been sealed with silicone grease (18). Hydrogen fluoride released from the sample is trapped in alkali in the center well of the diffusion plate. Fluoride can also be released, without the use of heat, by addition of hexamethyldisiloxane to the sample (19). After adjustment of pH and ionic strength, the fluoride-specific electrode can be used to determine acid-labile, ionic fluoride without interference. Although this method does not measure the nonionic fluorocarbon fraction found in some foods such as dairy products (19), the fluorocarbon fraction is unrelated to fluoride intake and is metabolically important. The procedure for isolating fluoride prior to electrode measurement has been applied to different types of samples (8,19–22).

To follow trace amounts of fluoride metabolically, isotopes of fluoride are available (12). The half-lives of the fluoride isotopes are short, however, ranging from 4 s ([22]F) to 110 min (^{18}F).

IV. METABOLISM

A. Absorption

The fate of fluoride ingested with food is summarized in Figure 2. Fluoride absorption from dietary sources is somewhat unusual compared to most other nutrients, because it can be absorbed from both the stomach and the small intestine. In the stomach, a significant proportion of fluoride uptake depends on the formation of hydrogen fluoride ($pK_a = 3.4$) prior to its assimilation into the blood as the fluoride ion (23). Conditions of higher gastric acidity therefore promote fluoride absorption from the stomach, whereas alkalinity impairs it. At least in the rat, fluoride absorption from the small intestine occurs as the fluoride ion in a non-pH-dependent event (24). Because of the large surface area for absorption along the length of the small intestine, and because food contents are in contact with the intestine for a longer period of time compared to the stomach, the majority of fluoride absorption occurs from the small intestine (25). Passage of the fluoride ion through the mucosal membrane is by passive diffusion (26), probably by way of membrane channels (10).

The efficiency of fluoride absorption is influenced by how fluoride is ingested and by other dietary components. In the fasted state, fluoride absorption from either fluoridated drinking water or from sodium fluoride tablets is essentially 100% (8,10,27). When consumed with food, fluoride absorption varies from 50% to 80% (10). At least part of this reduction in fluoride absorption from the diet is caused by insoluble complex formation with cations in the alkaline small intestine, predominately involving calcium (28–31) and magnesium (32,33). Data shown in Table 1 exemplify the effect of calcium and magnesium on fluoride absorption in the rat; Figure 3 illustrates the effect of calcium on fluoride bioavailability in women. Insoluble complex formation of calcium and fluoride largely accounts for reduced fluoride availability seen in milk, fish protein, and infant formula (8). If fluoride and the interfering cation are given separately, there is no apparent reduction in intestinal fluoride absorption (34,35). Insoluble complex formation between the dietary

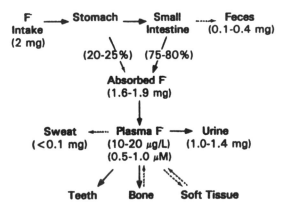

FIGURE 2 Fate of fluoride ingested with food. Dashed arrows denote minor pathway. Most of total body fluoride (> 95%) is found in bones and teeth.

TABLE 1 Influence of Dietary Calcium and Magnesium on Fecal
Fluoride Excretion in Rats Fed Diet Containing 2 mg F⁻/kg[a]

Diet variable	Fecal F⁻ (μg/5 days)	Diet variable	Fecal F⁻ (μg/5 days)
2 g/kg calcium	4 ± 2	200 mg/kg magnesium	36 ± 8
5 g/kg calcium	26 ± 4	500 mg/kg magnesium	58 ± 9
10 g/kg calcium	66 ± 5	2500 mg/kg magnesium	87 ± 7

[a]Fluoride intake in the metabolic collection averaged 192–198 μg F⁻/5 days. Values are
means ± SD. Mean differences between each group, $P < 0.05$.
Source: From Ref. 30 (calcium), with permission from Pergamon Press Ltd, Headington
Hill Hall, Oxford OX3 OBW, UK; and Ref. 32 (magnesium), with permission of the
American Institute of Nutrition.

nonessential cation aluminum (from aluminum-containing antacids) and fluoride has also
been documented (36). On the other hand, fluoride absorption is increased when either
dietary protein (37) or fat (38) is increased. Dietary protein probably increases fluoride
absorption from the stomach because high dietary protein stimulates gastric acidity. High
diet fat probably stimulates fluoride absorption from the stomach by delaying gastric
emptying time.

Absorbed fluoride ion is rapidly transferred to the plasma. The rapidity of fluoride
absorption is exemplified by an observed peak increase in plasma fluoride within 1 h of

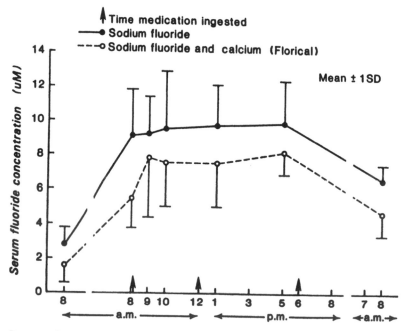

FIGURE 3 Reduction in fluoride uptake into plasma of nine healthy women when sodium fluoride
and calcium carbonate were ingested concurrently ($P < 0.05$ at all data points). (From Ref. 28, with
permission of W. B. Saunders Co.)

ingestion (27,39). At usual intake, plasma ionic fluoride ranges from 10–20 μg/L (0.5–1.0 μM) (40). Plasma fluoride concentrations reported in some of the older literature are about 10 times too high because of analytical error. Ionic fluoride in the plasma is not bound to protein, in contrast to the small, metabolically unimportant fluorocarbon fraction (9).

B. Transport and Tissue Uptake

Fluoride is quickly cleared from the plasma into tissue in exchange with other anions such as hydroxyl, citrate, and carbonate ions. At least 95% of total body fluoride (about 2600 mg in an adult) is found in bones and teeth (10), as there are high percentages of the other anions in hard tissue compared to soft tissue. A notable exception to the exchange of fluoride with other anions is that fluoride does not replace iodide in thyroid tissue (41), despite the chemical similarity of the two ions. Variation in dietary iodide was also found not to affect fluoride absorption and utilization (42).

Most of the deposition of fluoride into bones and teeth occurs during periods of rapid development. Higher concentrations of fluoride are found in surface layers of mineral structure than in deeper layers, and fluoride released during bone remodeling is largely redeposited (43). Fluoride tends to be deposited to a greater extent in cancellous than in compact bone (44), and maximum uptake occurs prior to cessation of bone growth (44–46). Fluoride deposition into bone varies directly with diet composition up until middle age (46), in contrast to soft tissue fluoride concentration which is essentially unaffected by variation in nutritional levels of dietary fluoride intake (47) and age. Deposition of fluoride into bone plateaus when net bone growth ceases at usual levels of fluoride intake, which is reflected in an increase in urinary fluoride excretion. For teeth, maximum fluoride deposition occurs during childhood (4) and, unlike bone, it is not subject to resorption because of the severed blood supply following tooth eruption (48). Low permeability within tooth structure also restricts ionic mobility within teeth.

Because the mammary (49,50) and placental (51) barriers to fluoride are formidable, fluoride supplements are not routinely recommended during either pregnancy or lactation (52). Nevertheless, because neither of these barriers is complete, it has been claimed that some degree of caries resistance in offspring can be achieved by maternal fluoride supplementation (53).

C. Excretion

Approximately 90% of total fluoride excretion occurs by way of the urine (54). Loss of fluoride in sweat is considered to be negligible except under conditions of perfuse sweating (55). Renal clearance of fluoride is linear with glomerular filtration rate, and about 60% of filtered fluoride is reabsorbed (56,57). Children appear to have a somewhat lower rate of fluoride clearance than adults, so even a moderate decrease in renal function of children could lead to unwanted fluoride retention (57).

The possibility that fluoride reabsorption is affected by factors other than urine flow rate is unclear. Whitford (9,58), for example, has summarized data indicating that reabsorption of fluoride is inversely related to tubular fluid pH and that fluoride reabsorption occurs by nonionic passive diffusion as hydrogen fluoride. Acidosis therefore would increase fluoride retention, whereas alkalosis would decrease fluoride retention. Others (56,59), however, do not support this hypothesis. Ekstrand et al. (59), for example, have disputed the possible significance of hydrogen fluoride formation in fluoride reabsorption for normal individuals because at the mildly acidic pH of urine, less than 1% of fluoride would be present as hydrogen fluoride. Indirect opposition to the Whitford hypothesis also comes from two dietary studies in rats. Feeding rats a diet containing three times the normal protein concentration significantly increased urinary fluoride excretion (37), despite the fact that high protein is known to increase urinary acidity (60). In a study of the effect of dietary chloride on fluoride bioavailability (61), chloride deficiency significantly decreased urinary fluoride excretion despite the fact that chloride deficiency causes metabolic alkalosis (62). The observed increase in fluoride reabsorption in chloride deficiency is consistent with the observation that there is some competition between ionic chloride and fluoride reabsorption (63).

Taken together, fluoride uptake into the skeleton and urinary excretion of fluoride help to prevent high levels of circulating plasma fluoride and to lessen the possible deposition of fluoride into soft tissue at the usual levels of fluoride intake. Whether this constitutes evidence for homeostasis of fluoride is open to debate. After net bone growth ceases, the deposition of fluoride into bone levels off and urinary fluoride excretion increases (55).

V. BIOCHEMICAL FUNCTION

A. Mineralized Tissue

The fluoride ion has a high affinity for mineralized tissue of bone and teeth. As illustrated in Figure 4 (64), a well-documented effect of fluoride incorporation into these tissue is an increased degree of crystallinity (mostly a measure of increased crystal size in the case of fluoride) as estimated by X-ray diffraction (65). As a reference point for Figure 4, normal human bone ash has been reported to contain $0.08 \pm 0.05\%$ F^- in the absence of fluoride supplementation and 0.24–0.67% with supplementation in the therapeutic range (30–50 mg NaF/day) (66). Increased crystallinity of bone has been shown to be associated with increased apatite crystal size, reduced crystal distortion, and reduced solubility of the apatite crystal (65).

The significance of this fluoride effect is most easily observed in teeth, where fluoride incorporation into apatite crystal significantly reduces the susceptibility of enamel to dissolution by acids produced by cariogenic bacteria (4–6). None of the other 25 trace elements found in tooth enamel (67) can duplicate fluoride's effect. Fluorapatite, formed from hydroxyapatite, is important for hardening tooth enamel and contributes to the stability of bone mineral matrix.

One reason for this apparently unique function of fluoride relates to its chemical properties (1,2). Fluoride's high degree of reactivity (electronegativity = 3.9 eV), coupled with its small ionic radius (0.133 nm), makes it possible for fluoride either to displace the larger hydroxyl ion in the apatite crystal, forming fluorapatite, or to enter spaces between the hydroxyapatite crystal, thereby increasing crystal density (68). A model for fluoride incorporation into the apatite crystal is shown in Figure 5 (11,69). A reaction equation to describe the displacement of the hydroxyl ion by fluoride in the apatite crystal is:

$$Ca_{10}(PO_4)_6(OH)_2 + 2F^- \rightarrow Ca_{10}(PO_4)_6(F)_2 + 2OH^-$$

Not all of fluoride's effect can be explained by a direct effect on the mineralized phase of tissue. Farley et al. (70), for example, found that 10 μM NaF increased osteoblast proliferation and alkaline phosphatase activity. Eanes (65) also suggests that constraints placed on apatite crystal growth by fluoride-stimulated mineralization of collagen may

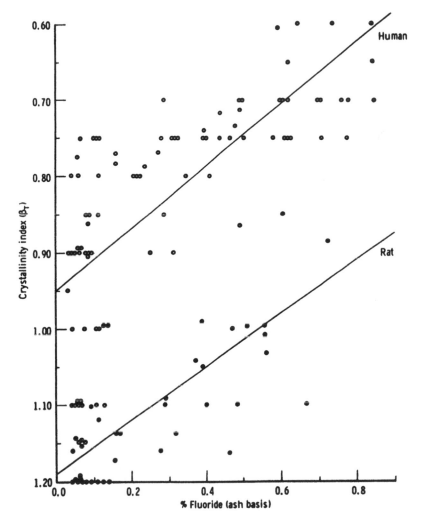

FIGURE 4 Relationship between bone crystallinity and fluoride concentration of bone. The crystallinity value, B_T, was obtained by comparing the experimental X-ray diffraction pattern to a series of bone apatite standards of varying resolution. (From Ref. 64, with permission of the New York Academy of Sciences.)

explain why fluoride has a greater effect on enamel than bone, because the enamel matrix is noncollagenous.

B. Enzyme-Related Effects of Fluoride

Although fluoride is known to have both stimulatory and inhibitory effects on many soft tissue enzymes, depending on concentration (11), its physiologic significance in this regard is doubtful because millimolar F^- is required. Fluoride, for example, can activate enzymes by way of guanine nucleotide-binding proteins (G proteins), as in the activation of adenylate cyclase and polyphosphoinositide phosphodiesterase (see Ref. 11). Both of these enzymes are involved in platelet activation and are normally activated by interaction of a

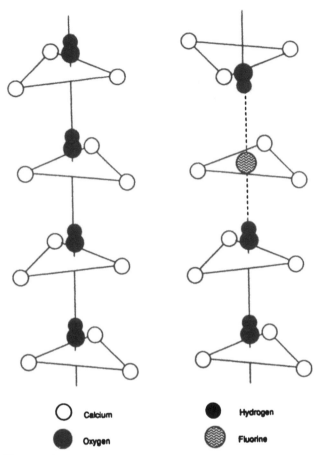

FIGURE 5 Fluoride incorporation into apatite crystal structure. This scheme suggests that the apatite crystal structure, depicted as a triangular array of calcium ions, is stabilized by the incorporation of fluoride ion, in contrast to the hydroxyl ion which is off-center from the plane of ions. (From Ref. 11, as adapted from Ref. 69, with permission from Plenum Publishing Co., New York.)

hormone, or other agonist, with its receptor (71). Fluoride stimulates platelet aggregation directly, bypassing the receptor. It is a permeant stimulant of G proteins.

The stimulatory effect of fluoride on G proteins is enhanced by the presence of micromolar concentrations of aluminum (72), possibly involving the formation of the tetrafluoroaluminate anion (AlF_4^-). Thus, AlF_4^- is the active ion that mimics the γ phosphate of GTP in the activation of G proteins. It binds with the stimulatory subunit activating the catalytic subunit of the regulatory G protein, which in turn regulates enzyme activity. Although millimolar fluoride concentration is required for platelet activation in vitro, reports of increased adenylate cyclase activity and cAMP levels in rats given fluoride in drinking water (73,74), and increased cAMP production by intact hepatocytes in the presence of 50 μM F^- (75), suggest that fluoride stimulation of enzymes via G proteins may have some physiologic relevance in vivo.

There is also evidence that fluoride can inhibit the growth of acid-producing dental plaque bacteria (76–78). Although millimolar F^- is required for a bactericidal effect, such concentrations have been found in dental plaque, the site where cariogenic bacteria are found.

VI. PATHOLOGY OF FLUORIDE DEFICIENCY

Fluoride can inhibit kidney calcification at nutritional levels of fluoride versus low fluoride intake (32,79,80). It is likely that the mechanism of this effect involves fluoride's affinity for calcium, but definitive data in this regard are lacking. Inhibition of soft tissue calcification by fluoride has also been implicated in the observed decrease in mortality due to coronary heart disease in fluoridated versus nonfluoridated cities (81). Fluoride has also been shown to lessen the effects of iron deficiency on hemoglobin and hematocrit by an unexplained mechanism (82,83), although not in all studies (84).

VII. CLINICAL SIGNIFICANCE

A. Dental Caries Resistance

Numerous studies dating back to World War II have consistently demonstrated that children growing up in an area with optimal levels of fluoride can have as many as 70% fewer dental caries than those not exposed to fluoride (4–6). In the United States, this beneficial effect of fluoride has been accomplished largely by adjusting the natural level of fluoride in the drinking water to 0.7–1.2 mg F^-/L, depending on climatic conditions (85). An increase in dental decay has been observed in children when fluoridation was halted (86). A much lower reduction in dental decay due to fluoridated drinking water occurs if the individual has been exposed to other fluoride sources (87). Nevertheless, the effectiveness of fluoridation in reducing dental decay was recently reemphasized by the observation that among 9-year-old children, the prevalence of dental caries has declined from 71% during 1971–1974 to 34% during 1985–1986 (88). Even limited exposure to fluoride has been shown to be beneficial in reducing dental decay (89).

Although it is generally believed that fluoride benefits children only during tooth formation, recent evidence suggests that lifetime benefits of fluoride are greatest when individuals are exposed to fluoride during both the preeruptive and the posteruptive life of the tooth (90). The apparent reason for this observation is that even though the blood supply to the tooth is severed upon eruption into the oral cavity, fluoride can promote remineralization of surface enamel (91,92). The current fluoridation census (85) indicates that a significant segment of the population can benefit from this fluoride effect, because 61% of the American public is served by optimally fluoridated drinking water.

Guidelines for fluoride supplementation of infants and children who do not have access to a water supply containing optimal fluoride concentration have been published (93) (Table 2). This information is intended to insure that benefits of fluoride are realized for those who need it as well as to discourage use of fluoride supplements for those who do not. Other countries that do not have a developed communal water supply system have tried other vehicles for fluoridation, most notably that involving table salt (8,92). Although chloride is chemically similar to fluoride, high levels of chloride do not impair either fluoride absorption or its uptake into bone and teeth (61), despite an earlier claim to the contrary.

TABLE 2 Fluoride Supplementation Schedule (mg F⁻/day) for Infants and Children According to Fluoride Concentration of Drinking Water

Age (years)	Concentration of fluoride in water (mg/L)		
	< 0.3	0.3–0.6	> 0.6
0.5–3	0.25	0	0
3–6	0.50	0.25	0
6–16	1.00	0.50	0

Source: From Ref. 93, courtesy of Council on Dental Therapeutics, with permission of the American Dental Association.

B. Osteoporosis

Fluoride supplementation of individuals at 30–50 mg NaF/day has been shown to promote the formation of new bone in the axial skeleton, especially in the lumbar spine (66). Calcium supplementation, usually at 1000 mg, must accompany fluoride to see increased osteoid surface, increased osteoid thickness and volume, and thickening of existing trabeculae. In only 2 months, effects can be seen in persons suffering from bone loss. The ability of fluoride to promote increased bone mass is shown in Figure 6 (66).

The successful use of fluoride as a therapeutic agent to arrest bone loss has been reported in some studies (94–96), but not all studies agree (66,97). It has been suggested

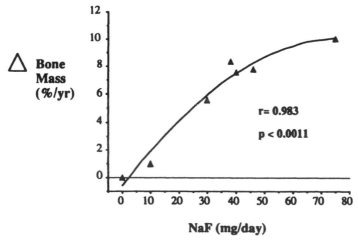

FIGURE 6 Relationship between sodium fluoride intake and change in human spinal bone mass per year. The figure represents a composite of data from several studies involving postmenopausal women as summarized in Ref. 66. (Reproduced with permission from the *Annual Review of Nutrition*, Vol. 11, copyright © 1991 by Annual Reviews, Inc.)

that part of the discrepancy in these studies is that fluoride needs to administered by slow-release sodium fluoride with calcium citrate rather than by a single F^- dose plus calcium carbonate (98).

There are problems associated with the therapeutic use of fluoride to treat osteoporosis, and this has led to questioning this use of fluoride outside the domain of controlled clinical studies (66). The problems include a response rate of only 55–75%, formation of bone that is less mechanically strong than regular bone, and failure to see a consistent reduction in vertebral fracture rate despite increased bone mass. There are suggestions that increased spinal bone mass might be accomplished at the expense of appendicular skeleton (66).

Because fluoride is known to promote mineralization, one could surmise that nutritional levels of fluoride incorporated into bone during growing periods would promote attainment of peak bone density and resistance to bone loss later in life. Evidence in support of this belief has been published (99). A report (100) to the contrary, however, suggests that further observations need to be made, especially since there are so few well-controlled studies about the relationship between fluoride in drinking water and bone health (101).

VIII. REQUIREMENT, INTAKE, AND NUTRITIONAL ASSESSMENT

A. Requirement

Although fluoride can only be classified as an essential element if a broad definition is used (102), its valuable effects on dental health have been recognized by the statement of a provisional recommended dietary allowance (103). Estimated ranges of safe and adequate intakes of fluoride by age are summarized in Table 3. The stated ranges account for the uncertainty in the overall bioavailability of fluoride from different sources, and it includes fluoride derived from both food and water.

B. Intake

Total fluoride intake has been recently estimated to be 0.9 mg/day for young adults residing in a nonfluoridated area (< 0.3 ppm F^- in water), and 1.85 mg/day for adults living in cities

TABLE 3 Estimated Safe and Adequate Daily Dietary Intake of Fluoride

Category	Age (years)	Fluoride (mg)
Infants	0–0.5	0.1–0.5
	0.5–1	0.2–1.0
Children and adolescents	1–3	0.5–1.5
	4–6	1.0–2.5
	7–10	1.5–2.5
	11+	1.5–2.5
Adults		1.5–4.0

Source: Adapted with permission from Ref. 103, copyright © 1989 by the National Academy of Sciences. Courtesy of the National Academy Press, Washington, DC.

TABLE 4 Acid-Diffusible Fluoride Content of Foods

Food	Fluoride content μg/100 g	nmol/g	Food	Fluoride content μg/100 g	nmol/g
Butter	3.8	2	Lettuce, raw	13.3	7
Milk	1.9	1	Sweet potato	20.9	11
Vanilla ice cream	13.1	7	Spinach, cooked	70.3	37
Eggs, scrambled	5.7	3	Peas, cooked	57.0	30
Beef, steak	3.8	2	Beets, pickled	26.6	14
Ham, baked	30.4	16	Apple sauce	5.7	3
Turkey, roast	20.9	11	Cranberry sauce	1.9	1
Bread, whole wheat	28.5	15	Peach, canned	7.6	4
Crackers, Ritz	26.6	14	Tomato juice	3.8	2

Source: Adapted from Ref. 20, with permission from Cambridge University Press.

served by fluoridated (> 0.7 ppm) water (104). These estimates are similar to previous reports in the older literature (8). Fluoride contributed by beverages and water will account for 70–80% of total fluoride intake, because most foods contain less than 30 μg F^-/100 g (19,20) (Table 4). Regular consumption of foods that are high in fluoride (105), such as marine fish, clams, lobster, crab, shrimp, and tea, can significantly increase fluoride intake. The higher content of fluorine in seafood versus freshwater fish is related to the fact that seawater contains 1.4 mg F^-/L (2), whereas many freshwater bodies of water contain less than half of that concentration (106). For about 130 million Americans, the fluoride content of drinking water has been adjusted to contain an average of 1 mg/L (85). Another 9 million Americans consume water that naturally contains this fluoride level or above.

Because beverages and water contribute such a high percentage of total fluoride intake of high availability, it is easy to dismiss the importance of the fluoride content of food. Preparation of food with fluoridated water at home, however, will add fluoride to a complex matrix which can significantly influence how efficiently fluoride is absorbed and utilized, as reviewed earlier. Examples of such foods include infant formulas, powdered milk, soups, cereals, juices, and vegetables (8,107).

Estimated total fluoride intake of 6-month-old infants has been reported to range from 0.2 to 0.5 mg/day (108,109). Fluoride intake for this age group is low because since 1979 manufacturers of infant formulas and other infant foods have agreed to use nonfluoridated water in the manufacturing process (109). In addition, fluoride content of cow's milk (< 2.5 μM, < 50 μg/L) and human breast milk (< 0.5 μM, < 10 μg/L) (110) is too low to have a significant impact on total fluoride intake of infants. Fluoride content of human breast milk remains low even when there is wide variation in the fluoride content of the maternal diet (49,50,111).

Infants consuming either human breast milk or cow's milk-based infant formula and living in a community that does not have fluoridated water have been shown to have a substantially lower total daily fluoride intake than those living in a fluoridated area (109,112). The importance of considering fluoride added to food for this age group is that fluoridated drinking water by itself does not become a predominant source of total fluoride intake until about 10 years of age (113). Walker et al. (114), for example, found that even among older children, daily intake of tap water rarely exceeded 500 mL. Even though total fluid intake increased with age, the proportion contributed by tap water was found to decrease.

C. Assessment

Urinary excretion of fluoride best reflects fluoride ingestion because, as discussed earlier, the kidney plays an important role in regulating internal fluoride balance. Plasma fluoride reflects fluoride content of drinking water up to 6 mg/L (40), but fluoride is rapidly cleared from plasma and plasma levels are low and difficult to detect with the fluoride-specific electrode. In addition, the significance of plasma fluoride levels is uncertain because efficiency of fluoride absorption appears to be unaffected by plasma fluoride concentration (115). Measurement of plasma fluoride has been used as an index of fluoride absorption following a test dose (27,28).

IX. TOXICITY

Like other trace elements, fluoride can be toxic (fluorosis) when consumed in excessive amounts (116). In humans, the three types of fluorosis that have been described are acute poisoning, crippling fluorosis, and mottled tooth enamel.

A. Acute Poisoning

Death is likely to result within 2–4 h when an average-size adult consumes about 5 g of sodium fluoride (103). At this high intake, fluoride is a powerful metabolic inhibitor of enzymes, especially those that are magnesium-dependent (11,116). Nausea, vomiting, and cramping are early symptoms, followed by coma and death.

B. Crippling Fluorosis

Crippling fluorosis was reported in cryolite workers who inhaled fluoride dust over a prolonged period of time (10–20 years). At a fluoride intake of 20–80 mg/day, skeletal hypermineralization, exostoses of bone, and calcification of ligaments occurred. At least part of the mechanism for abnormal calcification in crippling fluorosis may be due to an alteration in bone glycosaminoglycans (117). Today, toxic levels of airborne fluoride exposure is prevented by appropriate use of safety equipment (118). No evidence of crippling fluorosis has been attributed to controlled water fluoridation. A recent report of fluorosis in a woman consuming well water with a concentration of about 8 mg/L, however, indicates the importance of having drinking water sources tested before use (119).

C. Mottled Tooth Enamel

Mottled tooth enamel, a type of dental fluorosis which occurs when children below the age of 6 years of age ingest two to three times the recommended amount of fluoride, is characterized by white horizontal lines on the tooth surface, with yellowish to brown spots and enamel hypoplasia. The cause of mottled enamel is thought to be due to a disturbance in ameloblast activity because these enamel-forming cells appear to be the most sensitive cells in the body to fluoride (120). Although the condition is associated with caries resistance, it is cosmetically unappealing.

As shown in Figure 7 (121), there is a relatively small safety factor between beneficial effects of fluoride on dental caries reduction (122) and prevalence of dental

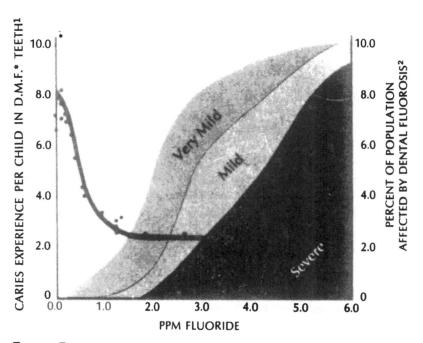

FIGURE 7 Dental caries and dental fluorosis in relation to the fluoride concentration of drinking water. D.M.F. = decayed, missing and filled. [1]Ref. 122; [2]Ref. 123. (From Ref. 121, with permission of the Upjohn Company.)

fluorosis (123). When fluoridation was first proposed, it was estimated that about 10% of children consuming fluoridated water (1 mg/L) would have some mild degree of dental fluorosis, which would be visible only to a trained dentist. Current estimates, however, place the prevalence of dental fluorosis at 22% (124).

School-age children have four potential sources of extra fluoride that could contribute to increased occurrence of dental fluorosis. These sources include school fluoridation programs, home dietary fluoride supplements, mouthrinse, and toothpaste (125). The first three of these sources of fluoride are intended for communities that do not have access to fluoridated water and are used by fewer than 20% of families surveyed. About 95% of children, however, use fluoridated toothpaste containing about 1 mg F$^-$/g. Recent studies (126,127) have in fact shown that swallowing of toothpaste by children on a daily basis can be a significant unneeded source of fluoride.

D. Fluoride and Cancer

Although preliminary reports published by the National Toxicology Program (NTP) in 1990 indicated that osteosarcoma was found in one of 50 male rats given fluoride in drinking water at 45 mg/L and in four of 80 male rats at 79 mg F$^-$/L (128), later evaluation of the data concluded that the differences were equivocal (128,129). An earlier summary of available data also found no link between fluoride and cancer (130).

X. FUTURE RESEARCH NEEDS

Although the beneficial effects of fluoride on dental health have been known for 50 years, the exact mechanism for its cariostatic effect remains unclear. Current information about fluoride content of foods and its bioavailability from different sources needs to be considered before any serious thoughts are entertained concerning a possible reduction in the level of fluoridation of drinking water. Additional observations also need to be made that relate past fluoride exposure to bone health in later years. Finally, sources of total fluoride exposure need to be defined and understood by all, so that a balance can be struck between the benefits and toxicity of fluoride.

REFERENCES

1. Greenwood NN, Earnshaw A. Chemistry of the Elements. Oxford: Pergamon Press, 1984: 920–1041.
2. Fuge R. Sources of halogens in the environment, influences on human and animal health. Environ Geochem Health 1988; 10:51–61.
3. Dean HT. Endemic fluorosis and its relation to dental caries. Public Health Reports 1938; 53:1443–1452.
4. DePaola DP, Faine MP, Vogel RI. Nutrition in relation to dental medicine. In: Shils ME, Olson JA, Shike M, eds. Modern Nutrition in Health and Disease. Vol. 2, 8th ed. Philadelphia: Lea & Febiger, 1994:1007–1028.
5. Richmond VL. Thirty years of fluoridation: a review. Am J Clin Nutr 1985; 41:129–138.
6. The Surgeon General's Report on Nutrition and Health. Dental Diseases. Washington, DC: U.S. Government Printing Office, 1988:345–380.
7. Subcommittee on Mineral Toxicity in Animals. Fluorine. In: Mineral Tolerance of Domestic Animals. Washington, DC: National Academy Press, 1980:184–226.
8. Rao GS. Dietary intake and bioavailability of fluoride. Annu Rev Nutr 1984; 4:115–136.
9. Whitford GM. The Metabolism and Toxicity of Fluoride. Monographs in Oral Science, Vol. 16. Basel: S. Karger, 1996.
10. Ophaug RH. Fluoride. In: Brown ML, ed. Present Knowledge in Nutrition. 6th ed. Washington, DC: International Life Science Institute, 1990:274–278.
11. Kirk KL. Biochemistry of the Elemental Halogens and Inorganic Halides. New York: Plenum Press, 1991:19–68.
12. Fluorine. In: Encyclopedia of Science and Technology. 7th ed. New York: McGraw-Hill, 1992:218–222.
13. Mottana A, Crespi R, Liborio G. Simon & Schuster's Guide to Rocks and Minerals. New York: Simon & Schuster, 1978:entry no. 50.
14. Frant MS, Ross JW. Electrode for sensing fluoride ion activity in solution. Science 1966; 154:1553–1555.
15. Glerum JH, Van Dijk A, Klein SW. A new and improved gas chromatographic method for the determination of fluoride in plasma and faeces. Pharm Weekblad Sci Ed 1984; 6:75–79.
16. Hannah RE. An HPLC anion exclusion method for fluoride determination in complex effluents. J Chromatogr Sci 1986; 24:336–339.
17. Tusl J. District determination of fluoride in human urine using fluoride electrode. Clin Chim Acta 1970; 27:216–218.
18. Singer L, Armstrong WD. Determination of fluoride. Procedure based upon diffusion of hydrogen fluoride. Anal Biochem 1965; 10:495–500.
19. Singer L, Ophaug RH. Determination of fluoride in foods. J Agric Food Chem 1986; 34: 510–513.
20. Taves DR. Dietary intake of fluoride ashed (total fluoride) v. unashed (inorganic fluoride) analysis of individual foods. Br J Nutr 1983; 49:295–301.
21. Gitelman HJ, Alderman FR. Automated determination of fluoride using silicone-facilitated diffusion. Anal Biochem 1990; 186:141–144.
22. van Staden JF, van Rensburg SDJ. Improvement on the microdiffusion technique for the determination of ionic and ionizable fluoride in cows' milk. Analyst 1991; 116:807–810.

23. Whitford GM, Pashley DH. Fluoride absorption: the influence of gastric acidity. Calcif Tissue Int 1984; 36:302–307.
24. Nopakun J, Messer HH, Mechanism of fluoride absorption from the rat small intestine. Nutr Res 1990; 10:771–780.
25. Nopakun J, Messer HH, Voller V. Fluoride absorption from the gastrointestinal tract of rats. J Nutr 1989; 119:1411–1417.
26. Stookey GK, Dellinger EL, Muhler JC. In vitro studies concerning fluoride absorption. Proc Soc Exp Biol Med 1964; 115:298–301.
27. Trautner K, Siebert G. An experimental study of bioavailability of fluoride from dietary sources in man. Arch Oral Biol 1986; 31:223–228.
28. Jowsey J, Riggs BL. Effect of concurrent calcium ingestion on intestinal absorption of fluoride. Metabolism 1978; 27:971–974.
29. Ekstrand J, Ehrnebo M. Influence of dietary calcium on the bioavailability of NaF tablets in man. J Dental Res 1978; 57(spec issue A):335 (abstr).
30. Cerklewski FL, Ridlington JW. Influence of type and level of dietary calcium on fluoride bioavailability in the rat. Nutr Res 1987; 7:1073–1083.
31. Cerklewski FL. Phytic acid plus supplemental calcium, but not phytic acid alone, decreases fluoride bioavailability in the rat. J Nutr Biochem 1992; 3:87–90.
32. Cerklewski FL. Influence of dietary magnesium on fluoride bioavailability in the rat. J Nutr 1987; 117:496–500.
33. Cerklewski FL, Ridlington JW. Enhanced maternal transfer of fluoride in the magnesium-deficient rat. In: Hurley LS, Keen CL, Lonnerdal B, Rucker RB, eds. Trace Elements in Man and Animals 6. New York: Plenum Press, 1988:273–274.
34. Spencer H, Osis D, Kramer L, Wiatrowski E, Norris C. Effect of calcium and phosphorus on fluoride metabolism in man. J Nutr 1975; 105:733–740.
35. Spencer H, Kramer L, Wiatrowski E, Osis D. Magnesium–fluoride interrelationships in man. II. Effect of magnesium on fluoride metabolism. Am J Physiol 1978; 234:E343–E347.
36. Spencer H, Kramer L, Norris C, Wiatrowski E. Effect of aluminum hydroxide on fluoride metabolism. Clin Pharmacol Ther 1980; 28:529–535.
37. Boyde CD, Cerklewski FL. Influence of type and level of dietary protein on fluoride bio-availability in the rat. J Nutr 1987; 117:2086–2090.
38. McGown EL, Kolstad DL, Suttie JW. Effect of dietary fat on fluoride absorption and tissue fluoride retention in rats. J Nutr 1976; 106:575–579.
39. Carlson CH, Armstrong WD, Singer L. Distribution and excretion of radiofluoride in the human. Proc Soc Exp Biol Med 1960; 104:235–239.
40. Ekstrand J. Relationship between fluoride in the drinking water and the plasma fluoride concentration in man. Caries Res 1978; 12:123–127.
41. Wallace-Durbin P. The metabolism of fluorine in the rat using ^{18}F as a tracer. J Dental Res 1954; 41:789–800.
42. Cerklewski FL, Bills N. Influence of dietary iodide on fluoride bioavailability in the rat. Nutr Rep Int 1985; 32:991–994.
43. Guo MK, Nopakun J, Messer HH, Ophaug R, Singer L. Retention of skeletal fluoride during bone turnover in rats. J Nutr 1988; 118:362–366.
44. Hodge HC, Smith FA. Biological properties of inorganic fluorides; In: Simons JH, ed. Fluorine Chemistry. Vol. 4. New York: Academic Press, 1965:137–176.
45. Suttie JW, Phillips PH. The effect of age on the rate of fluorine deposition in the femur of the rat. Arch Biochem Biophys 1959; 83:355–359.
46. Weidmann SM, Weatherell JA, Jackson D. The effect of fluoride on bone. Proc Nutr Soc 1963; 22:105–110.
47. Armstrong WD, Gedalia I, Singer L, Weatherell JA, Weidmann SM. Distribution of fluorides. In: Fluorides and Human Health. WHO Monogr Ser No 59. Geneva: World Health Organization, 1970:93–139.

48. Nizel AE. Nutrition in Preventive Dentistry: Science and Practice. Philadelphia: WB Saunders, 1981:262–286.

49. Ekstrand J, Boreus LO, De Chateau P. No evidence of transfer of fluoride from plasma to breast milk. Br Med J 1981; 283:761–762.

50. Esala S, Vuori E, Helle A. Effect of maternal fluoride intake on breast milk fluorine content. Br J Nutr 1982; 48:201–204.

51. Gedalia I, Brzezinski A, Bercovici B, Lazarow E. Placental transfer of fluorine in the human fetus. Proc Soc Exp Biol Med 1961; 106:147–149.

52. American Academy of Pediatrics Committee on Nutrition. Fluoride supplementation. Pediatrics 1986; 77:758–761.

53. Glenn FB, Glenn WD III, Duncan RC. Fluoride tablet supplementation during pregnancy for caries immunity: a study of the offspring produced. Am J Obstet Gynecol 1982; 143:560–564.

54. Maheshwari UR, McDonald JT, Schneider VS, et al. Fluoride balance studies in ambulatory healthy men with and without fluoride supplements. Am J Clin Nutr 1981; 34:2679–2684.

55. Hodge HC, Smith FA, Gedalia I. Excretion of fluorides. In: Fluorides and Human Health. WHO Monogr Ser No. 59. Geneva: World Health Organization, 1970:141–161.

56. Schiffl H, Binswanger U. Renal handling of fluoride in healthy man. Renal Physiol (Basel) 1982; 5:192–196.

57. Spak C-J, Berg U, Ekstrand J. Renal clearance of fluoride in children and adolescents. Pediatrics 1985; 75:575–579.

58. Whitford GM, Pashley DH, Stringer GI. Fluoride renal clearance: a pH-dependent event. Am J Physiol 1976; 230:527–532.

59. Ekstrand J, Ehrnebo M, Boreus MD. Fluoride bioavailability after intravenous and oral administration: importance of renal clearance and urinary flow. Clin Pharmacol Ther 1978; 23:329–337.

60. Yuen DE, Draper HH, Trilok G. Effect of dietary protein on calcium metabolism in man. Nutr Abstr Rev 1984; 54:447–459.

61. Cerklewski FL, Ridlington JW, Bills ND. Influence of dietary chloride on fluoride bioavailability in the rat. J Nutr 1986; 116:618–624.

62. Simopoulos AP, Bartter FC. The metabolic consequences of chloride deficiency. Nutr Rev 1980; 38:201–205.

63. Walser M, Rahill WJ. Renal tubular transport of fluoride compared with chloride. Am J Physiol 1966: 210:1290–1292.

64. Tannenbaum PJ, Termine JD. Statistical analysis of the effect of fluoride on bone apatite. Ann NY Acad Sci 1965; 131:743–750.

65. Eanes ED. Effect of fluoride on mineralization of teeth and bones. In: Shupe JL, Peterson HB, Leone NC, eds. Fluorides—Effects on Vegetation, Animals and Humans. Salt Lake City, UT: Paragon Press, 1983:195–198.

66. Kleerekoper M, Balena R. Fluorides and osteoporosis. Annu Rev Nutr 1991; 11:309–324.

67. Hadjimarkos DM. Trace elements and dental health. In: Hemphill DD, ed. Trace Substances in Environmental Health. Vol. VII. Columbia MO: University of Missouri Press, 1973:25–30.

68. Chandler S, Fuerstenau DW. On the dissolution and interfacial properties of hydroxyapatite. Colloids Surfaces 1982: 4:101–120.

69. Eanes ED, Reddi AH. The effect of fluoride on bone mineral apatite. Metab Bone Dis Related Res 1979; 2:3–10.

70. Farley JR, Wergedal JE, Baylink DJ. Fluoride directly stimulates proliferation and alkaline phosphatase activity of bone-forming cells. Science 1983; 222:330–332.

71. Kienast J, Arnout J, Pliegler G, Deckmyn H, Hoet B, Vermylen J. Sodium fluoride mimics effects of both agonists and antagonists on intact human platelets by simultaneous modulation of phospholipase C and adenylate cyclase activity. Blood 1987; 69:859–866.

72. Sternweis PC, Gilman AG. Aluminum: a requirement for activation of the regulatory component of adenylate cyclase by fluoride. Proc Natl Acad Sci (USA) 1982; 79:4888–4891.

73. Susheela AK, Singh M. Adenyl cyclase activity following fluoride ingestion. Toxicol Lett 1982; 10:209–212.

74. Kleiner HS, Allmann DW. The effects of fluoridated water on rat urine and tissue cAMP levels. Arch Oral Biol 1982; 27:107–112.

75. Shahed AR, Miller A, Chalker D, Allman DW. Effect of sodium fluoride on cyclic AMP production in rat hapatocytes. J Cyclic Nucleotide Res 1979; 5:43–53.

76. Maltz M, Emilson CG. Susceptibility of oral bacteria to various fluoride salts. J Dental Res 1982; 61:786–790.

77. vander Hoeven JS, Franken HCM. Effect of fluoride on growth and acid production by *S. mutans* in dental plaque. Infect Immun 1984; 45:356–359.

78. Thibodeau E, Keefe T. pH-dependent fluoride inhibition of catalase activity. Oral Microbiol Immunol 1990; 5:328–331.

79. Harrison JE, Hitchman AJW, Hasany SA, Hitchman A, Tam CS. The effect of fluoride on nephrocalcinosis in rats. Clin Biochem 1985; 18:109–113.

80. O'Dell BL, Moroni RI, Reagan WO. Interaction of dietary fluoride and magnesium in guinea pigs. J Nutr 1973; 103:841–850.

81. Taves DR. Fluoridation and mortality due to heart disease. Nature 1978; 272:361–362.

82. Cerklewski FL, Ridlington JW. Influence of zinc and iron on dietary fluoride utilization in the rat. J Nutr 1985; 115:1162–1167.

83. Wegner ME, Singer L, Ophaug RH, Magil SG. The interrelation of fluoride and iron in anemia. Proc Soc Exp Biol Med 1976; 153:414–418.

84. Tao S, Suttie JW. Evidence for lack of an effect of dietary fluoride on reproduction in mice. J Nutr 1976; 106:1115–1122.

85. Centers for Disease Control. Fluoridation Census 1989. Atlanta, GA: Centers for Disease Control, 1991.

86. Kunzel W. Effect of an interruption in water fluoridation on the caries prevalence of the primary and secondary dentition. Caries Res 1980; 14:304–310.

87. Hileman B. Fluoridation of water. Chem Eng News 1988; 66:26–42.

88. National Center for Health Statistics. Prevention Profile. Health, United States 1991. Hyattsville MD: Public Health Service, 1992.

89. Burt BA, Eklund SA, Loesche WJ. Dental benefits of limited exposure to fluoridated water in childhood. J Dental Res 1986; 61:1322–1325.

90. Grembowski D, Fiset L, Spadafora A. How fluoridation affects adult dental caries. J Am Dental Assoc 1992; 123:49–54.

91. Konttinen M-L, Hanhijarvi H. Fluoride concentrations of the surface enamel of children living in an optimally fluoridated community. Scand J Dental Res 1986; 94:427–435.

92. Stadtler P. Fluorides. Int J Clin Pharmacol Ther Toxicol 1990; 28:20–26.

93. Council on Dental Therapeutics. New fluoride schedule adopted. Am Dental Assoc News, May 16, 1994:12–14.

94. Spencer H, Kramer L, Wiatrowski E, Lender M. Fluoride therapy in metabolic bone disease. Israel J Med Sci 1984; 20:373–380.

95. Charles P, Mosekilde L, Jensen FT. The effects of sodium fluoride, calcium phosphate, and vitamin D_2 for one to two years on calcium and phosphorus metabolism in postmenopausal women with spinal crush fracture osteoporosis. Bone 1985; 6:201–206.

96. Heaney RP, Baylink DJ, Johnston CC, et al. Fluoride therapy for the vertebral crush fracture syndrome. Ann Intern Med 1989; 111:678–680.

97. Riggs BL, O'Fallon WM, Lane A, et al. Clinical trial of fluoride therapy in postmenopausal osteoporotic women: extended observations and additional analysis. J Bone Mineral Res 1994; 9:265–275.

98. Pak CYC, Sakhaee K, Piziak V, et al. Slow-release sodium fluoride in the management of postmenopausal osteoporosis—a randomized controlled trial. Ann Intern Med 1994; 120: 625–632.

99. Simonen O, Laitinen O. Does fluoridation of drinking water prevent bone fragility and osteoporosis? Lancet 1985; 2(pt 1):432–434.

100. Danielson C, Lyon JL, Egger M, Goodenough GK. Hip fractures and fluoridation in Utah's elderly population. JAMA 1992; 268:746–748.

101. Gordon SL, Corbin SB. Summary of workshop on drinking water fluoride influence on hip fracture and bone health. Osteoporosis Int 1992; 2:109–117.

102. Mertz W. The essential trace elements. Science 1981; 213:1332–1338.

103. Committee on Dietary Allowances. Fluoride. In: Recommended Dietary Allowances. 10th ed. Washington, DC: National Academy Press, 1989:235–240, 284.

104. Singer L, Ophaug RH, Harland BF. Dietary fluoride intake of 15–19-year-old male adults residing in the United States. J Dental Res 1985; 64:1302–1305.

105. Kumpulainen J, Koivistoinen P. Fluorine in foods. Residue Rev 1977; 68:37–57.

106. U.S. Dept. of Health, Education and Welfare. Natural Fluoride Content of Community Water Supplies. Washington, DC: U.S. Govern Printing Office, 1969.

107. Leverett DH. Fluorides and the changing prevalence of dental caries. Science 1982; 217:26–30.

108. Ophaug RH, Singer L, Harland BF. Estimated fluoride intake of 6-month-old infants in four dietary regions of the United States. Am J Clin Nutr 1980; 33:324–327.

109. Ophaug RH, Singer L, Harland BF. Dietary fluoride intake of 6-month and 2-year-old children in four dietary regions of the United States. Am J Clin Nutr 1985; 42:701–707.

110. Renner E. Micronutrients in Milk and Milk-Based Food Products. New York: Elsevier, 1989:212–215, 33–34.

111. Spak CJ, Hardell LI, De Chateau P. Fluorine in human milk. Acta Paediatr Scand 1983; 72:699–701.

112. Chowdhury NG, Brown RH, Shepherd MG. Fluoride intake of infants in New Zealand. J Dental Res 1990; 69:1828–1833.

113. Myers HM. Fluorides and Dental Fluorosis. Monographs in Oral Sci. Vol 7. Basel: S Karger, 1978.

114. Walker JS, Margolis FJ, Teate HL Jr, Weil ML, Wilson HL. Water intake of normal children. Science 1963; 140:890–891.

115. Whitford GM, Williams JL. Fluoride absorption: independence from plasma fluoride levels. Proc Soc Exp Biol Med 1986; 181:550–554.

116. Krishnamachari KAVR. Fluorine. In: Mertz W, ed. Trace Elements in Human and Animal Nutrition. Vol. 1. 5th ed. San Diego, CA: Academic Press, 1987:365–415.

117. Prince CW, Navia JM. Glycosaminoglycan alterations in rat bone due to growth and fluorosis. J Nutr 1983; 113:1576–1582.

118. Ehrnebo M, Ekstrand J. Occupational fluoride exposure and plasma fluoride levels in man. Int Arch Occup Environ Health 1986; 58:179–190.

119. Felsenfeld AJ, Roberts MA. A report of fluorosis in the United States secondary to drinking well water. JAMA 1991; 265:486–488.

120. Jenkins GN. Fluoride and fluoridation of water. In: Neuberger A, Jukes TH, eds. Human Nutrition: Current Issues and Controversies. Lancaster, England: MTP Press, 1982:23–72.

121. Latham MC, McGandy RB, McCann MB, Stare FJ. Fluoride. In: Scope Manual on Nutrition. 2d ed. Kalamazoo MI: Upjohn, 1972:61–63.

122. Dean HT. Epidemiological studies in the United States. In: Moulton FR, ed. Dental Caries and Fluorine. Washington, DC: American Association for the Advancement of Science, 1946:5–31.

123. Dean HT. Fluorine in the control of dental caries: some aspects of the epidemiology of the fluorine-dental caries relationship. Int Dental J 1954; 4:311–337.

124. Committee to Coordinate Environmental Health and Related Programs. Review of fluoride risks and benefits. Washington, DC: U.S. Public Health Service, 1990.

125. Wagener DK, Nourjah P, Horowitz A. Trends in childhood use of dental care products

containing fluoride: United States 1983–89. Vital and Health Statistics Advance Data No. 219. Hyattsville, MD: National Center for Health Statistics, 1992.

126.   Drummond BK, Curzon MEJ. Urinary excretion of fluoride following ingestion of MFP toothpastes by infants aged 2–6 years. J Dental Res 1985; 64:1145–1148.

127.   Naccache H, Simard PL, Trahan L, Demers M, LaPoint C, Brodeur JM. Variability in the ingestion of toothpaste by preschool children. Caries Res 1990; 24:359–363.

128.   Wei SHY. Conference report: special symposium, scientific update on fluoride and the public health. J Dental Res 1990; 69:1343–1344.

129.   Johnston J. HHS study finds no fluoride–cancer link. J NIH Res 1991; 3:46.

130.   Chilvers C, Conway D. Cancer mortality in England in relation to levels of naturally occurring fluoride in water supplies. J Epidemiol Commun Health 1985; 39:44–47.

21
Silicon

EDITH M. CARLISLE[†]
University of California—Los Angeles, Los Angeles, California

I. INTRODUCTION AND HISTORY

Among the elements required in trace amounts, silicon occupies a unique position because, next to oxygen, it is the most prevalent element on earth. It is present in a wide diversity of silicates, including crystalline silica in the form of quartz. To label silicon an ultratrace element may require some adjustment in thinking. Silicon is one of the most recent trace elements to be established as "essential," participating in the normal metabolism of higher animals. There had been little work concerned with the effect of silicon in normal metabolism until relatively recently; emphasis had been placed on the more deleterious aspects of silicon metabolism, including its effect on forage digestibility, urolithiasis, and especially silicosis caused by dust inhalation. Several important reviews on this work are available (1–3).

Silicon has generally been considered to be nonessential except for some primitive classes of organisms, notably diatoms (unicellular plants) and two groups of animals, the radiolarians (belonging to the Protozoa) and some sponges (Porifera) which utilize silica as a component of body structure. In the diatom, where silica is the major skeletal constituent, an absolute requirement for silicon has been associated with silica shell formation (4) and with the net synthesis of DNA (5). The structural relationship of silica to the organic constituents of the cell wall has also been established (6).

A series of experiments has contributed to the establishment of silicon as an essential element. The first of these were in vitro studies which showed that silicon is localized in active growth areas in bones of young mice and rats, suggesting a physiologic role of silicon in bone calcification processes. These were followed by in-vivo studies showing

---

[†]Deceased.

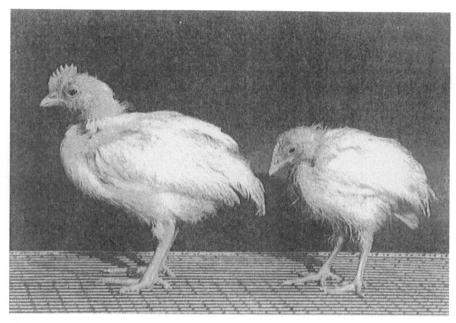

FIGURE 1 Photograph of 4-week-old chicks fed silicon-supplemented diet (left) and low-silicon basal diet (right). (From Ref. 7.)

that silicon affects the rate of bone mineralization. Most important, it was demonstrated in 1972 that silicon is required for normal growth and skeletal development in the chick (Fig. 1), and that these abnormalities could be prevented by a silicon supplement (7). During the same year, silicon deficiency in the rat was shown to result in depressed growth and skull deformations (8). Later studies, both in vitro and in vivo, emphasize silicon's importance in bone formation and connective tissue metabolism and confirm the postulate that silicon is involved in an early stage of bone formation. These observations have established silicon as an essential element.

II. CHEMISTRY

Silicon occurs in nature as the oxide, silica (SiO_2), or the corresponding silicic acids formed by the hydration of the oxide. Orthosilicic acid $[Si(OH)_4]$ is the simplest acid and the main form, soluble in water up to about 120 ppm. Supersaturation causes it to dehydrate and polymerize into less soluble forms.

Silicon belongs to group IV of the Periodic Table, along with C, Ge, Sn, and Pb, is tetravalent, and its chemistry is determined by its strong affinity to oxygen; Si–O–Si (siloxane) is very stable. The silicon atom, having the same stereochemistry as carbon, is structurally rigid and could contribute to the structural framework of connective tissue by forming links or bridges within and between individual polysaccharide chains to proteins. It is postulated that in this way silicon may aid in the development of the architecture of the fibrous elements of connective tissue and contribute to its structural integrity by providing strength and resilience. Significant here is the fact that the silicon–oxygen bond is very stable in terms of energy levels. The value reported for the bond energy of the Si–O bond is

108 kcal/mol, compared with the value of 85.5 kcal/mol for the C–O and 82.6 kcal/mol for the C–C bond (9,10).

III. ANALYTICAL METHODOLOGY

Reported silicon concentrations in serum and other tissues have declined markedly in recent years because of more attention to contamination control and better instrumentation. The most common analytical methods that can sensitively measure silicon include inductively coupled plasma emission spectrometry (11) and flameless atomic absorption spectrometry (AAS) (12). Currently the most common method employed is flameless AAS.

IV. METABOLISM

A. Absorption

It has been estimated that humans absorb 9–14 mg of silicon daily. This figure correlates well with the report of Goldwater (13) that humans excrete 9 mg of silicon in urine daily. These estimated values are in the same range as those obtained in a recent balance study in humans (14).

Balance trials in animals indicate that almost all ingested silicon is unabsorbed, passing through the digestive tract to be lost in the feces (15). Moreover, most of the small proportion absorbed is excreted in the urine. The proportion of absorbed silicon actually retained in the body is not known. Little is also known of the extent or mechanism of silicon absorption from the products entering the alimentary tract derived from food sources, such as silica, monosilicic acid, and silicon found in organic combination, such as pectin and mucopolysaccharides.

The form of dietary silicon has been shown to be an important factor affecting its absorption, appearing to correlate with the rate of production of soluble or absorbable silicon in the gastrointestinal tract (16). Silicon enters the alimentary tract from food as monsilicic acid, as solid silica, and in the organic bound forms with protein, mucopolysaccharides, and such compounds. Other factors have been reported to influence silicon absorption. The dietary fiber content of the diet has been implicated in studies with humans (17), and changes in silicon absorption in rats has been found to be related to age, sex, and the activity of various endocrine glands (18).

Silicic acid in foods and beverages has been reported to be readily absorbed across the intestinal wall of humans and to be rapidly excreted in the urine (15). In guinea pigs, absorption occurs mainly as monosilicic acid, some of which comes from the silica of the plant materials, which is partly dissolved by the fluids of the gastrointestinal tract (16).

As is the case for many other elements, silicon bioavailability is probably affected by excess amounts of certain other mineral elements in the diet. For example, interaction with aluminum or molybdenum may result in a diminution of silicon absorption. This subject is covered further in the section on mineral interactions.

B. Transport

Silicon is found to be freely diffusible throughout tissue fluids. In early studies, Baumann (15) showed that monomeric $Si(OH)_4$ penetrates all body liquids and tissues at concentrations less than its solubility (0.01%), and it is readily excreted. These findings are supported by later studies (19), which show that silicon is not protein bound in plasma and its concentration in all body fluids examined, except urine, is similar to that of normal human serum (20). This indicates that silicon is freely diffusible throughout tissue fluids, with the higher levels and wider range encountered in urine suggesting that the kidney is the main excretory organ.

C. Tissue Concentration and Storage

Earlier data on the silicon content of living tissues varied greatly, and in general, reported values were considerably higher before the advent of plastic laboratory ware and the development of suitable analytical methods. Even with more recent methods, considerable variance exists in reported tissue concentrations of silicon.

Normal human serum has a narrow range of silicon concentration, averaging 50 μg/dL (21); the range is similar to that found for most of the other well-recognized trace elements in human nutrition. The silicon is present almost entirely as free, soluble monosilicic acid (15). No correlations of age, sex, occupation, or pulmonary condition with blood silicon concentrations have been found as a result of measurements of hundreds of people, although the level increased when silicon compounds were specifically administered (22).

Connective tissues such as aorta, trachea, tendon, bone, skin, and appendages are unusually rich in silicon, as shown by studies in several animal species (23). In the rat, for example (Fig. 2), the aorta, trachea, and tendon are four to five times richer in silicon than liver, heart, and muscle. The high silicon content of connective tissues appears to arise mainly from its presence as an integral component of the glycosaminoglycans and their

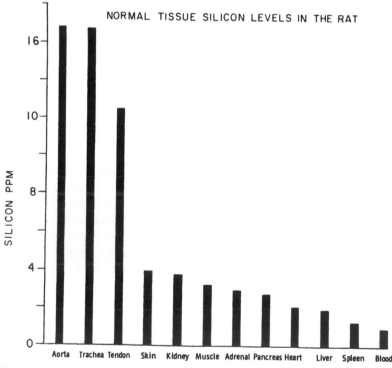

FIGURE 2   Silicon levels in tissues of normal adult male rats. Values represent mean silicon levels of 20 animals (4 months of age) expressed as parts per million wet weight of tissue. (From Ref. 23.)

protein complexes, which contribute to the structural framework of this tissue. Fractionation procedures reveal that connective tissues such as bone, cartilage, and skin yield complexes of high silicon content. Silicon is also found as a component of glycosaminoglycans isolated from these complexes (24).

The consistent low concentrations of silica in most organs do not appear to vary appreciably during life. Parenchymal tissue such as heart and muscle, for example, range from 2 to 10 μg of silicon/g dry weight. The lungs are an exception. Similar levels of silicon in rat and rhesus monkey tissues have been reported (25), where soft tissue levels in both species varied from 1 to 33 μg of silicon/g dry weight, excepting the primate lung and lymph nodes, which averaged 942 and 101 ppm, respectively. High levels in human lymph nodes have been associated with the presence of clusters and grains of quartz (26).

In order to gain information about silicon's function in soft tissues, the subcellular distribution of silicon in whole rat liver was determined in terms of percent of the total homogenate. The element was found to be equally distributed in the supernatant, mitochondrial, and nuclei/debris fractions. Little silicon was associated with the microsomal fraction (25).

D. Excretion

In humans, guinea pigs, cows, and sheep, increased urinary silicon output with increasing intake up to fairly well-defined limits has been demonstrated. The upper limits of urinary silicon excretion do not seem to be set by the ability of the kidney to excrete more, because much greater urinary excretion can occur after peritoneal injections (16). These limits are determined by the rate and extent of silicon absorption from the gastrointestinal tract into the blood. Once silicon has entered the bloodstream, it must pass rapidly into the urine and tissues, because even at widely divergent intakes, the silicon levels in the blood remain relatively constant. Fractional excretion of silicon had not been measured until recently (20). It appears that on the whole there is relatively little overall tubular reabsorption of filtered silicon, and this may indicate a mechanism for maintaining low tissue silicic acid concentrations and enabling the body to excrete much of the silicic acid absorbed from the gastrointestinal tract.

E. Mineral Interactions

A marked interaction between silicon and molybdenum occurs within normal dietary levels of these elements (27). The interaction was discovered when silicon supplementation of a diet with liver instead of casein as the source of dietary protein failed to elevate the plasma silicon concentration significantly. Plasma silicon levels were strongly and inversely affected by molybdenum intake; silicon-supplemented chicks on the diet with liver as the protein source (Mo 3 ppm) had a 348% lower plasma silicon level than chicks on a casein diet (Mo 1 ppm). Molybdenum supplementation also reduced silicon levels in those tissues examined. Conversely, plasma molybdenum levels are also markedly and inversely affected by the inorganic silicon intake. Silicon also reduced molybdenum retention in tissues. The manner in which they interact is not known.

An important interaction occurs between silicon and aluminum, which may have relevance to human conditions such as Alzheimer's disease. Studies with rats (28) showed a relationship between silicon and aluminum and indicated a protective action of silicon against aluminum neurotoxicity. A study was undertaken to further examine this silicon–aluminum interaction in brain and other body tissues (29). Two ages of rats were fed one of four diets, silicon-low and silicon-supplemented with and without the addition of aluminum over approximately a 2-year period. The silicon and aluminum concentration of the basal diet averaged 2 to 3 ppm. In the silicon-supplemented diet, silicon was supplied as sodium metasilicate at level of 600 ppm. In the aluminum-supplemented diets, aluminum was supplied as aluminum chloride at a level of 600 ppm. Aluminum supplementation was shown to have a significant effect on decreasing the silicon content of certain regions of the brain. In the brains of the younger rats, the aluminum content did not appear to be affected by aluminum supplementation. However, in the older rats an unexpected finding was that aluminum supplementation of the low-silicon diet produced a significant increase in aluminum content in certain brain regions; on the other hand, brain aluminum content was not increased in the silicon-supplemented rats. In tissues other than brain, a preferential accumulation of aluminum was also shown in rats fed the low-silicon diets. It appears that dietary silicon exerts a protective effect against aluminum accumulation. This same interaction has also been demonstrated more recently in humans (30). Isotopic ^{26}Al was administered orally to five healthy male volunteers in the presence and absence of aluminum. Dissolved silicon, at a concentration found in some water supplies (100 μmol/L), reduced the peak plasma ^{26}Al concentration to 15% of the value obtained in the absence of silicon. The results indicate that dissolved silicon is an important factor in limiting the absorption of dietary aluminum.

V. NUTRITIONAL REQUIREMENTS AND SOURCES

The minimum dietary silicon requirements in humans compatible with satisfactory growth and health are largely unknown, although there is limited evidence from experiments with rats and chicks. The silicon requirement for growth and satisfactory skeletal development in rats, using a basal ration containing ~7 μg/g silicon, was met by approximately 500 μg Si/g of diet provided as sodium metasilicate (8). In a later report it was mentioned that other silicon compounds were more effective; however, this work was not published. The basal ration used in the experiments with chicks (7) contained ~1 μg/g silicon, and a significant effect on skull formation appeared at a level of 250 μg/g of silicon supplied as sodium metasilicate. In a further experiment with chicks (23) to determine the effect of silicon on the rate of bone mineralization, silicon supplementation at the level of 250 μg/g increased the ash content of the tibia significantly more at 2 weeks than did either 25 or 10 μg/g; the difference had largely disappeared at 5 weeks.

Reliable data on the silicon content of human foods is meager. A recent paper by Pennington (31) summarizes the information currently available regarding the silicon content of foods and diets. Furthermore, little is known of the extent of silicon absorption from various sources; for example, some forms of silicon are very insoluble. Also, since silicon is ubiquitous in the environment, the likelihood of a silicon deficiency arising under natural conditions in humans or domestic animals might be questioned. Of possible significance here is the suggestion that silicon absorption might be under hormonal regulation, and if so, a decline in hormonal activity in senescence might result in decreased silicon absorption (32).

Foods of plant origin are normally much richer in silicon than those of animal origin. The foods with the highest silicon content are the unrefined grains, cereals, and vegetables. Cereal grains that are high in fiber, such as oats, are much richer than low-fiber grains such as wheat or maize (33). A human male balance study (14) indicates daily intakes of about 46 mg of silicon per day from a high-fiber diet and 21 mg from a low-fiber diet. The silicon content of adult U.S. diets, based on the Food and Drug Administration's Total Diet Study model, is 19 mg/day for women and 40 mg/day for men (34). Average daily intakes of silicon probably range from about 20 to 50 mg/day, with the lower values for animal- based diets and the higher values for plant-based diets.

Much remains to be learned about silicon requirements, consumption, and absorption. The form needed and minimum requirement have not been determined for any animal, so if there is a human requirement it probably is in the range of 10–25 mg a day.

VI. PHYSIOLOGIC FUNCTIONS AND PATHOLOGY OF DEFICIENCY

A. Calcification

1. In Vitro Studies

The first indications of a physiologic role for silicon were those reporting that silicon is involved in an early stage of bone calcification. Using electron microprobe studies (35), silicon was shown to be uniquely localized in active growth areas in young bone of mice and rats (Fig. 3). The amount present in specific very small regions within the active growth areas appeared to be uniquely related to "maturity," or degree of mineralization. In the

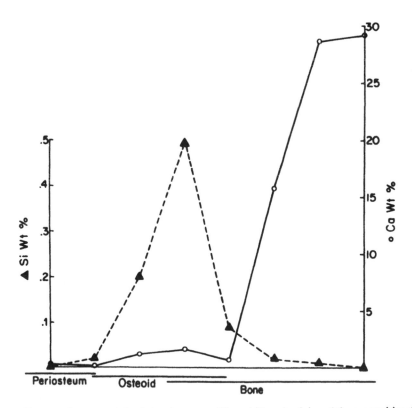

FIGURE 3   A spatial relation between silicon (▲) and calcium (○) composition (percent by weight) in a typical traverse across the periosteal region of young normal rat tibia (cross section) as obtained by electron microprobe techniques. (From Ref. 35.)

earliest stages of calcification in these regions, both the silicon and calcium contents of the osteoid tissue were found to be very low, but as mineralization progressed the silicon and calcium contents rose congruently. In a more advanced stage the amount of silicon fell markedly, so that as calcium approached the proportion present in bone apatite, the silicon was present only at the detection limit. In other words, the more "mature" the bone mineral, the smaller was the amount of measurable silicon. Further studies of the Ca/P ratio in silicon-rich regions gave values < 1.0 compared with a Ca/P ratio of 1.67 in mature bone apatite. These findings strongly suggest that silicon is involved in an organic phase during the series of events leading to calcification.

2. In Vivo Studies

Subsequent in vivo experiments showed that silicon has a demonstrable effect on in vivo calcification; that is, a relationship between the level of dietary silicon and bone mineralization was established (23). Weanling rats were maintained on diets containing three levels of calcium (0.08, 0.40, 1.20%) at three levels of silicon (10, 25, 250 ppm). Increasing silicon in the low-calcium diet resulted in a highly significant (35%) increase in the percentage ash contained in the tibia during the first 3 weeks of the experiment. Silicon was found to hasten the rate of bone mineralization. Calcium content of the bone also increased with increased dietary silicon, substantiating the theory of a relationship between mineralization and silicon intake. The tendency of silicon to accelerate mineralization was also demonstrated by its effect on bone maturity, as indicated by the Ca/P ratio. The concept of an agent that affects the speed of chemical maturity of bone is not new. Muller et al. (36) found that the chemical maturity of vitamin D-deficient bone, although inferior to control bone during the period of maximum growth, approaches the control level at the end of the experiment.

B. Bone Formation

The earliest studies suggesting a role for silicon in bone formation were those mentioned above. Most significant, however, was the establishment of a silicon deficiency state incompatible with growth and normal skeletal development (7). In the chick, this is evidenced by reduced circumference, thinner cortex, and less flexible leg bones, as well as by smaller and abnormally shaped skulls with the cranial bones appearing flatter. Silicon deficiency in rats also results in skull deformations (8).

   Recent studies further emphasize the importance of silicon in bone formation. Skull abnormalities associated with reduced collagen content have been produced in silicon-deficient chicks under conditions promoting optimal growth using a diet containing a natural protein in place of the crystalline amino acids used in earlier studies (37). The gross abnormalities of skull architecture of silicon-deficient chicks were confirmed by X-ray examination (Fig. 4). An additional finding is the striking difference in the appearance of the skull matrix between the silicon-deficient and silicon-supplemented chicks, the matrix of the deficient chicks totally lacking the normal striated trabecular pattern of the control chicks. The deficient chicks show a nodular pattern of bone arrangement, indicative of a primitive type of bone.

   Using the same conditions and by introducing three different levels of vitamin D, it has been shown that the effect exerted by silicon on bone formation is substantially independent of the action of vitamin D (38). All chicks on silicon-deficient diets, regardless of the level of dietary vitamin D, have gross abnormalities of skull architecture, and, furthermore, the silicon-deficient skulls shows considerably less collagen at each vitamin D level. As in the previous study, the bone matrix of the silicon-deficient chicks totally lacks

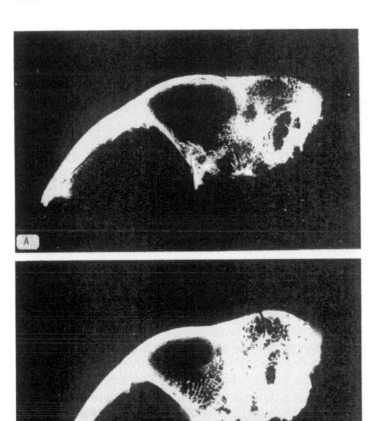

FIGURE 4 X-ray photograph of half skulls (dorsal surface view) from 4-week-old chicks fed a silicon-supplemented diet (lower) or a low-silicon basal diet (upper). Posterior end of skull on the left. Note the reduced size and reduction in height of the posterior portion of the skull of the silicon-deficient chick. (From Ref. 37.)

the normal striated trabecular pattern of the control chicks. In the rachitic groups of chicks, the appearance of the bone matrix is quite different from the groups receiving adequate vitamin D, being considerably less calcified and more transparent, enabling the cells and underlying structure to be seen more easily. The deficient chicks appear to have a marked reduction in number of osteoblasts compared with the controls. In these two studies, the major effects of silicon appears to be on the collagen content of the connective tissue matrix, and this is independent of vitamin D.

C. Cartilage and Connective Tissue Formation

In addition to bone, silicon deficiency is manifested by abnormalities involving articular cartilage and connective tissue (24). Chicks in the silicon-deficient group have thinner legs

TABLE 1 Effect of Silicon Intake on Chick Articular
Cartilage Composition[a]

Diet	Tissue (wet wt.) (mg)	Total hexosamine (wet wt.) (mg)	Percent hexosamine (wet) (%)
Low silicon	63.32 ± 8.04	0.187 ± 0.23	0.296 ± 0.009[b]
Si supplemented	86.41 ± 4.82	0.310 ± 0.031	0.359 ± 0.011

[a]There were 12 chicks per group. All values reported as mean ± SD.
[b]Significantly different from the supplemented animals at $p < .001$.

and smaller combs in proportion to their size. Long-bone tibial joints are markedly smaller and contain less articular cartilage than those of silicon-supplemented chicks. The deficient chicks also reveal a significantly lower hexosamine content in their articular cartilage (Table 1). In cock's comb also, a smaller amount of connective tissue, a lower total percentage of hexosamines, and a lower silicon content is found in the silicon-deficient group (Table 2). These findings point clearly to an involvement of silicon in glycosaminoglycan formation in cartilage and connective tissue.

Long-bone abnormalities similar to those reported have been produced in silicon-deficient chicks using a diet containing a natural protein in place of crystalline amino acids used in the earlier studies (39). Tibia from silicon-deficient chicks have significantly less glycosaminoglycans and collagen, the difference being greater for glycosaminoglycans than collagen. Tibia from silicon-deficient chicks also show rather marked pathology, profound changes being demonstrated in epiphyseal cartilage. The disturbed epiphyseal cartilage sequences resulted in defective endochondral bone growth, indicating that silicon is involved in a metabolic chain of events required for normal growth of bone.

D. Aging

Connective tissue changes are prominent in aging, so it is not surprising to find a relationship between silicon and aging in certain tissues. The silicon content of the aorta, other arterial vessels, and skin was found to decline with age, in contrast to other analyzed tissues, which showed little or no change (23). The decline in silicon content was significant and was particularly dramatic in the aorta, commencing at an early age. This relationship occurred in several animal species, including rat, rabbit, chicken, and pig.

Similarly, in human skin, the silicon content of the dermis has been reported to

TABLE 2 Effect of Silicon Intake on Comb Composition[a]

Diet	Tissue (wet wt.) (mg)	Total hexosamine (wet wt.) (mg)	Percent hexosamine (wet) (%)	Silicon (dry wt.) (ppm)
Low silicon	90.30 ± 4.99[b]	0.085 ± 0.012[b]	0.094 ± 0.003[b]	11.4 ± 0.36[b]
Si supplement	134.80 ± 10.20	0.175 ± 0.020	0.130 ± 0.009	21.2 ± 3.02

[a]There were 12 chicks per group. All values reported as mean ± SD.
[b]Significantly different from the supplemented animals at $p < .001$.

diminish with age. In contrast with an earlier finding, Loeper and Fragny (40) reported that the silicon content of the normal human aorta decreases considerably with age, and furthermore, that the level of silicon in the arterial wall decreases with the development of atherosclerosis. The potential involvement of silicon in atherosclerosis has been suggested by others (41,42). Of possible significance here, a relationship has been reported among silicon, age, and endocrine balance, and it is suggested that the decline in hormonal activity may be responsible for the changes in silicon levels in senescence (18).

VII. BIOCHEMICAL FUNCTION

The preceding in vivo studies have shown silicon to be involved in both collagen and glycosaminoglycan formation. Silicon's primary effect in bone and cartilage appears to be on formation of the matrix, although silicon appears also to participate in the mineralization process itself. The in vivo findings have been corroborated and extended by studies of bone and cartilage in organ and cell culture.

A. Metabolic Role

Studies that involved skull bones from 14-day chick embryos grown in culture (Table 3) further demonstrate the dependence of bone growth on the presence of silicon (43). Most of the increase in growth due to silicon appears to result from a rise in collagen content; silicon-supplemented (0.2 mM sodium metasilicate) bones showed a 100% higher collagen content than silicon-low bones after 12 days. Silicon is also shown to be required for formation of glycosaminoglycans; at day 6, the hexosamine content of supplemented bones is nearly 200% that of silicon-low bones, but by day 12 it is the same in both groups.

A parallel effect has been demonstrated in the growth of cartilage in culture (44) and is especially marked in cartilage from 14-day embryos as compared with 10- and 12-day embryos. Silicon's effect on collagen formation is also especially striking in cartilage from 14-day embryos (Fig. 5), appearing to parallel the rate of growth. Similarly, matrix hexosamines (glycosaminoglycans) are formed more rapidly by silicon-supplemented cartilage, the most striking difference in this case being in cartilage from 12-day embryos.

TABLE 3 Effect of Silicon on Rate of Synthesis of Bone Matrix Components in Culture

Days in culture	Silicon:	Bone chondroitin sulfate (mg)[a]		Bone collagen (mg)[b]		Bone non-collagenous protein (mg)[c]	
		Low	Suppl.	Low	Suppl.	Low	Suppl.
4		0.51	7.42*	0	62.7*	241	236
6		3.58	10.50*	64.2	117.9*	158	102
12		6.14	5.90	89.5	176.1*	200	188

[a]By hexose nitrogen × 2.65.
[b]By hydroxyproline × 7.46.
[c]As leucine by NH_2 nitrogen corrected for collagen and hexose nitrogen.
*Significantly different from the supplemented media at $p < .05$.

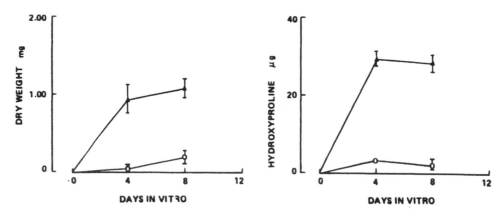

FIGURE 5 Rate of growth of tibial epiphyseal cartilage from 14-day-old chick embryos in culture, as measured by dry weight and collagen synthesis (hydroxyproline). ○, low silicon; ▲, silicon supplemented. (From Ref. 43.)

The requirement for silicon in collagen and glycosaminoglycan formation thus proves not to be limited to bone matrix but applies also to cartilage.

A role for silicon in the synthesis of proline precursors is suggested as a result of studies growing epiphyseal cartilage from 12- and 14-day embryos on a larger scale and determining proline in addition to hexosamine, hydroxyproline, and noncollagenous protein as previously (45). In 12-day cultures, the most obvious difference was in proline synthesis, large differences resulting at days 4 and 8 between deficient and silicon-supplemented media, suggesting the possibility of a role for silicon in the proline synthetic pathway.

An interaction between silicon and ascorbate (46) is also shown in cartilage. It is well established that ascorbate is required for normal cartilage growth. A study was undertaken to investigate silicon's role in cartilage formation in the presence and absence of ascorbate. Epiphyseal cartilage from 12-day-old chick embryos was grown in organ culture under Si-low and Si-supplemented conditions and 0, 150 mg/mL, or 750 mg/mL ascorbate. No significant effect on hexosamine content occurs in the absence of ascorbate. However, silicon supplementation results in significant increases in wet weight, hexosamine, and proline content in the presence of ascorbate. The greatest effect is on hexosamine content in the presence of high ascorbate, silicon-supplemented cartilage increasing by 400% at day 8 and by 272% at day 12. Furthermore, silicon and ascorbate interact to give maximal production of hexosamines. Silicon also appears to increase hydroxyproline, total protein, and noncollagenous protein beyond the effects of ascorbate.

An effect of silicon on formation of extracellular cartilage matrix components by connective tissue cells has also been demonstrated in chondrocytes isolated from chick epiphyses cultured under silicon-low and silicon-supplemented conditions (47). The major effect of silicon appeared to be on collagen. Silicon-supplemented cultures demonstrate a 243% ($p < .01$) increase in collagen, measured as hydroxyproline, over low-silicon cultures. Silicon also had a pronounced stimulatory effect on matrix polysaccharides; matrix polysaccharide content of silicon-supplemented cultures increased 152% ($p < .01$) more than that of low-silicon cultures.

A dependence on silicon for maximal bone prolyl hydroxylase activity (48) has been shown. Prolyl hydroxylase obtained from frontal bones of 14-day-old chick embryos incubated for 4 or 8 days with 0, 0.2, 0.5, or 2.0 mM Si added to a basic, low-silicon medium show lower enzyme activity in low-silicon bones with increasing enzyme activity in cultures containing 0.2, 0.5, and 2.0 mM Si in the form of sodium metasilicate. The results support the in vivo and in vitro findings of a requirement for silicon in collagen biosynthesis, the activity of prolyl hydroxylase being a measure of the rate of collagen biosynthesis. Silicon has also been found to increase the activities of prolyl 4-hydroxylase, galactosyl-hydroxylysyl transferase, and lysyl oxidase, three enzymes that catalyze post-translational modifications of collagen, in lungs of rats exposed to silica (49).

Additional support for silicon's metabolic role in connective tissue at the cellular level is provided by evidence of its presence in connective tissue cells (50,51). X-ray microanalysis of active growth areas in young bone and isolated osteoblasts show silicon to be a major ion of osteogenic cells, the amounts of silicon being in the same range as those of calcium, phosphorus, and magnesium. Moreover, silicon appears to be especially high in the metabolically active state of the cell, the osteoblast. Clear evidence that silicon occurs in the osteoblast and is localized in the mitochondria adds strong support to the proposition that silicon is required for connective tissue matrix formation.

B. Structural Role

Although the discussion above indicates that silicon plays an important metabolic role in connective tissues, a structural role has also been proposed, supported mainly by the finding that the high silicon content of connective tissue arises from its presence as an integral component of animal glycosaminoglycans and their protein complexes, which contribute to the structural framework of this tissue. In higher animals, the glycosaminoglycans, hyaluronic acids, chondroitin sulfates, and keratin sulfate, are found to be linked covalently to proteins as components of the extracellular amorphous ground substance that surrounds the collagen, elastic fibers, and the cells. By extraction and purification, silicon has been shown to be localized in the glycosaminoglycan fraction of several connective tissues. The silicon content of the glycosaminoglycan–protein complex extracted from bovine nasal septum, for example, is 87 ppm, compared with 13 ppm (dry) in the original cartilaginous tissue (24). From this complex, smaller molecules considerably richer in silicon were isolated. Silicon was found to be associated with the larger, purer polysaccharide and smaller protein moieties.

The preceding data indicate that silicon is not merely involved in glycosaminoglycan formation but that, in animal glycosaminoglycans at least, and quite probably in plant polysaccharides, silicon is a structural component.

VIII. TOXICITY

Investigations in the area of silicon toxicity are almost invariably associated with the silicosis problem. Several important reviews on this subject were mentioned in Section I (1–3). When abnormal amounts of silica enter the body by inhalation, some type of toxicity commonly results, mainly affecting the lungs and pleura.

Orally consumed silicon is generally considered to be of a relatively low order of toxicity. The ingestion of small amounts of siliceous materials and inhalation of siliceous dusts are harmless and of common occurrence for most animals. The majority of the ingested material passes unchanged through the alimentary canal. However, a small part of the silicon is absorbed and eliminated by way of the kidney, which is capable of excreting much larger doses of silicic acid than are normally absorbed. Nevertheless, occurrence of siliceous uroliths gives clear evidence that the quantity of silicon absorbed, and excreted in the urine, under conditions of excessively high intake can be harmful.

A report concerning the health aspects of using the Generally Recognized as Safe (GRAS) silicates as food ingredients concludes that although silicates vary considerably in physical properties and solubility in aqueous solvents, most of the silicates added to foods as anticaking and antifoaming agents are insoluble in water and are relatively inert (Select Committee on GRAS substances, 1979) (33). Amorphous silicates are considered safe additions in foods, therefore, and their use as anticaking agents, for example, is permitted in amounts up to 2% by weight. The water-soluble silicates are also of low toxicity; studies of the effects of feeding various silicon compounds to laboratory animals have generally shown the substances to be innocuous under the test conditions. Likewise, the available data on orally administered silicates in humans substantiate the biological inertness of these compounds.

IX. FUTURE RESEARCH NEEDS

More work is needed to clarify the consequences of silicon deficiency in animals and humans. The minimum silicon requirement compatible with human health is largely unknown, as are the dietary forms that render the mineral most available. The form needed and minimum requirement for silicon have not been determined for any animal, so there is little basis for estimating possible human requirements. The most soluble form is the metasilicate, and this has generally been the one most commonly used in supplemental studies.

Whether silicon is an essential trace element for humans remains to be determined, however, a number of human disorders have been speculated to be associated with a lack of silicon, including atherosclerosis (40–42,52,53), osteoarthritis, certain bone disorders, wound healing, and especially the aging process. The relationship between silicon and aging is probably related to glycosaminoglycan changes. These speculations demonstrate the need for study of the importance of silicon in nutrition, especially in aging humans.

REFERENCES

1. King EJ, Belt TH. The physiological and pathological aspects of silica. Physiol Rev 1938; 18:329–365.
2. Jones LHP, Handreck KA. Silica in soils, plants and animals. Adv Agron 1967; 19:107–149.
3. Carlisle EM. Silicon. In: Mertz W, ed. Trace Elements in Human and Animal Nutrition. 5th ed. New York: Academic Press, 1986:373–390.
4. Reimann BEF. Deposition of silica in a diatom cell. Exp Cell Res 1964; 34:605–608.
5. Darley WM, Volcani BE. Role of silicon in diatom metabolism. A silicon requirement for deoxyribonucleic acid synthesis in the diatom *Cylindrotheca fusiformis*. Reimann and Lewin. Exp Cell Res 1969; 58:334–342.
6. Reimann BEF, Lewin JE, Volcani BE. Studies on the biochemistry and fine structure of silica shell formation in diatoms. I. The structure of the cell wall of *Cylindrotheca fusiformis*. J Cell Biol 1965; 24:39–55.
7. Carlisle EM. Silicon an essential element for the chick. Science 1972; 178:619–621.
8. Schwarz K. Milne DB. Growth-promoting effects of silicon. Nature 239:333.
9. Needham AE. The Uniqueness of Biological Materials, Oxford: Pergamon Press, 1965.
10. Iler R. The Chemistry of Silica. New York: John Wiley, 1979.

11. Tanaka T, Yasuhisa H. Determination of silicon, calcium, magnesium and phosphorus in urine using inductively coupled plasma emission spectrometry and a matrix-matching technique. Clin Chim Acta 1986; 156:109–114.

12. Berylne GM, Caruso C. Measurement of silicon in biological fluids in man using flameless furnace absorption spectrometry. Clin Chim Acta 1983; 129:239–244.

13. Goldwater LJ. The urinary excretion of silica in non-silicotic humans. J Ind Hyg Toxicol 1936; 18:163–166.

14. Kelsay JL, Behall KM, Prather ES. Effect of fiber from fruits and vegetables on metabolic response of human subjects. II. Calcium magnesium iron and silicon balances. Am J Clin Nutr 1979; 32:1876–1880.

15. Baumann H. Verhalten der Kieselsaure in menschlichen Blut und Harn. Hoppe-Seylers Z Physiol Chem 1960; 320:11–20.

16. Sauer F, Laughland DH, Davidson WM. Silica metabolism in guinea pigs. Can J Biochem Physiol 1959; 37:183–191.

17. Benke GM, Osborn TW. Urinary silicon excretion by rats following oral administration of silicon compounds. Food Cosmet Toxicol 1978; 17:123–127.

18. Charnot Y, Pères G. Contribution à l'etude de la regulation endocrinienne du metabolisme silicique. Anal Endocrinol 1971; 32:397–402.

19. Dobbie JW, Smith MJB. Silicate nephrotoxicity in the experimental animal: the missing factor in analgesic nephropathy. Scot Med J 1982; 27:10–16.

20. Berlyne GM, Adler AJ, Ferran N, Bennett S, Holt J. Silicon metabolism. Some aspects of renal silicon handling in normal man. Nephron 1986; 43:5–9.

21. Carlisle EM. The nutritional essentiality of silicon. Nutr Rev 1982; 40:193–198.

22. Worth G. Der kieselsaürespiegel im menschlichen Blut. Klin Wochenschr 1952; 30:82–83.

23. Carlisle EM. Silicon as an essential element. Fed Proc 1974; 33:1758–1766.

24. Carlisle EM. In vivo requirement for silicon in articular cartilage and connective tissue formation in the chick. J Nutr 1976; 106:478–484.

25. Le Vier RR. Distribution of silicon in the adult rat and the rhesus monkey. Bioinorg Chem 1975; 4:109–115.

26. Hamilton EI, Minski MJ, Cleary JJ. The concentration and distribution of some stable elements in healthy human tissues from the United Kingdom. Sci Total Environment 1972–1973; 1: 341–374.

27. Carlisle EM, Curran MJ. A silicon-molybdenum interrelationship in vivo. Fed Proc 1979; 38:553.

28. Carlisle EM. A silicon aluminum relationship in aged brain. Microbiol Aging 1986; 7(6): 545–546.

29. Carlisle EM, Curran MJ. Effect of dietary silicon and aluminum on silicon and aluminum levels in rat brain. Alzheimer Disease and Associated Disorders—An International Journal 1987; 1(2):83–89.

30. Edwardson JA, Moore PB, Ferrier IN, et al. Effect of silicon on gastrointestinal absorption of aluminum. Lancet 1993; 342:211–212.

31. Pennington JAT. Silicon in foods and diets. Food Additives and Contaminants 1991; 8(1):97–118.

32. Charnot Y, Pères G. Silicon, endocrine balance and mineral metabolism. In: Bendz G, Lindquist I, Biochemistry of Silicon and Related Problems. New York: Plenum Press, 1978:269–280.

33. Bowen HJM, Peggs A. Determination of the Silicon Content of Food. J Sci Food Agric 1984; 35:1225–1229.

34. Select Committee on GRAS Substances. Evaluation of the health aspects of certain silicates as food ingredients (SCOGS-61). Bethesda, MD: Life Sciences Research Office, Federation of American Societies for Experimental Biology, 1979.

35. Carlisle EM. Silicon: a possible factor in bone calcification. Science 1970; 167:179–280.

36. Muller SA, Posner HS, Firschein HE. Effect of vitamin-D deficiency on the crystal chemistry of bone mineral. Proc Soc Exp Biol Med 1966; 121:844–846.

37. Carlisle EM. A silicon requirement for normal skull formation in chicks. J Nutr 1980; 110: 352–359.

38. Carlisle EM. A requirement in bone formation independent of Vitamin D. Calcif Tissue Int 1981; 33:27–34.

39. Carlisle EM. Biochemical and morphological changes associated with long bone abnormalities in silicon deficiency. J Nutr 1980; 110:1046–1056.

40. Loeper J, Fragny M. The physiological role of silicon and its anti-atheromatous action. In: Bendz G, Lindquist I, eds. Biochemistry of Silicon and Related Problems. New York: Plenum Press, 1978:281.

41. Schwarz K. Significance and functions of silicon in warm-blooded animals. In: Bendz G, Lindquist I, eds. Biochemistry of Silicon and Related Problems. New York: Plenum Press, 1978:207.

42. Dawson EB, Frey MJ, Moore TD, McGanity. Relationship of metal metabolism to vascular disease mortality rates in Texas. Am J Clin Nutr 1978; 31:1188–1197.

43. Carlisle EM, Alpenfels WF. A requirement for silicon for bone growth in culture. Fed Proc 1978; 37:404.

44. Carlisle EM, Alpenfels WF. A silicon requirement for normal growth of cartilage in culture. Fed Proc 1980; 39:787.

45. Carlisle EM, Alpenfels WF. The role of silicon in proline synthesis. Fed Proc 1984; 43:680.

46. Carlisle EM, Suchil C. Silicon and ascorbate interaction in cartilage formation in culture. Fed Proc 1983; 42:398.

47. Carlisle EM, Garvey DL. The effect of silicon on formation of extracellular matrix components by chondrocytes in culture. Fed Proc 1982; 41:461.

48. Carlisle EM, Berger JW, Alpenfels WF. A silicon requirement for prolyl hydroxylase activity. Fed Proc 1981; 40:866.

49. Poole A, Myllyla R, Wagner JC, Brown RC. Collagen biosynthesis enzymes in lung lesions and serum of rats with experimental silicosis. Br J Exp Pathol 1985; 66:567–575.

50. Carlisle EM. Silicon in the osteoblast. Fed Proc 1975; 34:927.

51. Carlisle EM. Silicon in bone formation. In: Simpson TL, Volani BE, eds. Silicon and Siliceous Structures in Biological Systems. New York: Springer-Verlag, 1981; 69–94.

52. Loeper J, Gay-Loeper J, Rozenztayn L, Fragny M. The antiatheromatous action of silicon. Atherosclerosis 1979; 33:397–408.

53. Najda J, Gminski J, Drod M, Danch A. Silicon metabolism. The interrelations of inorganic silicon (Si) with systemic (Fe), zinc (Zn) and copper (Cu) pools in the rat. Biol Trace Element Res 1992; 34:185–195.

22
Vanadium

FORREST H. NIELSEN
U.S. Department of Agriculture, Grand Forks, North Dakota

I. BRIEF INTRODUCTION AND HISTORY

In 1876, John Priestley of Manchester reported on the toxicity of sodium vanadate in frogs, pigeons, guinea pigs, rabbits, dogs, and cats (1). However, a paper considered to be a classic for the pharmacologic and toxicologic actions of vanadium appeared in 1912 (2). It was also at this time that high vanadium concentrations were discovered in the blood of ascidian worms (3,4). In 1977, Cantley et al. (5) reported that vanadate was the contaminant of ATP which inhibits ATPases; actually, the discovery that vanadate inhibits ATPase was made earlier (6) but was essentially ignored. In the early 1980s, vanadium was found to be an insulin-mimetic agent (7,8). The first vanadium-containing enzyme, a bromoperoxidase from the marine alga *Ascophyllum nodosum*, was isolated in 1984 (9).

The hypothesis that vanadium has an essential role in higher animals has had a long and inconclusive history. In 1950 it was stated that "we are completely ignorant of the physiological role of vanadium in animals, where its presence is constant" (10). As reviewed recently (11), findings reported between 1971 and 1974 by four different research groups led many to conclude that vanadium is an essential nutrient. However, many of these findings may have been the consequence of high vanadium supplements (10 to 50 times the amount normally found in purified or semipurified diets), which induced pharmacologic changes in animals fed imbalanced diets (11–13). The most substantive evidence for vanadium essentiality has appeared only since 1987.

II. CHEMICAL PROPERTIES OF VANADIUM

The chemistry of vanadium is complex because the element can exist in at least six oxidation states and can form polymers. In higher animals, the tetravalent and pentavalent

619

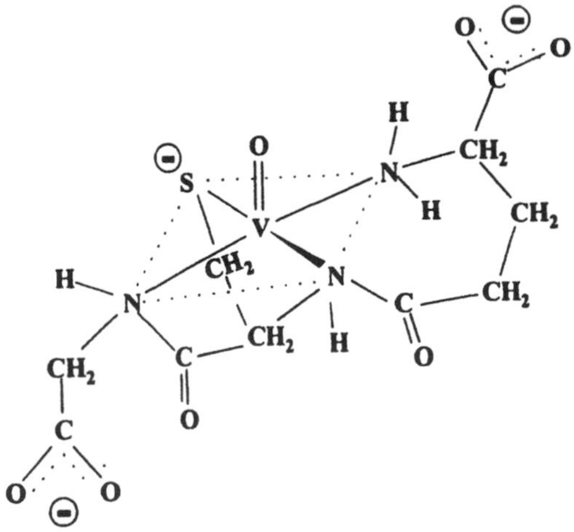

FIGURE 1 Suggested structure of the VO^{2+} or vanadyl–glutathione complex in rat adipocyte cells. Based on EPR spectroscopy, vanadate enters the cell, where it is reduced to vanadyl by glutathione. Complex formation first occurs through bonding to two carboxylate groups, the thiol group and a water molecule; this complex converts to the one illustrated, in which vanadyl is bonded through the thiol, two NH peptide groups, and a glutamyl amino group in the equational plane of the complex; in the steady state, about 90% of vanadyl is in the form of this complex. (Based on information from Refs. 15 and 17.)

valence states apparently are the most important forms of vanadium (13,14). The tetravalent state appears most simply as the vanadyl cation, VO^{2+}. The vanadyl cation behaves like a simple divalent aquo ion and competes well with Ca^{2+}, Mn^{2+}, Zn^{2+}, Fe^{2+}, etc., for ligand-binding sites. Thus, VO^{2+} easily complexes with proteins, especially those associated with iron, such as transferrin or ferritin, which stabilize vanadyl against oxidation. The pentavalent state of vanadium is known as vanadate ($H_2VO_4^-$ or more simply VO_3^-). Vanadate forms complexes with other biological substances, including those that result in it being a phosphate transition-state analog, and thus competes with phosphate in many biochemical processes. Vanadate is easily reduced by ascorbate, glutathione, or NADH. For example, with certain cells (e.g., adipocytes), vanadate enters through nonspecific anionic channels and is reduced and complexed by glutathione (15–17). The complex between glutathione and vanadyl is shown in Figure 1.

Recently, another form of vanadium has been discussed as being responsible for many biological actions of vanadium, including its insulin-mimetic action and haloperoxidase role; this is the peroxo form (18–20). Vanadate can interact with O_2^- formed by NADPH oxidase to generate peroxovanadyl [V^{4+}-OO]. Peroxovanadyl can in turn remove hydrogen from NADPH to yield vanadyl hydroperoxide [V^{4+}-OOH] (18). Peroxo (heteroligand) vandate (V^{5+}) adducts have been suggested to represent a useful model for the active-site vanadium involved in bromide oxidation in haloperoxidases (20).

III. VANADIUM ANALYTICAL METHODS

Heydorn (21) has reviewed analytical methods for the determination of vanadium in the low amounts found in tissues, blood, and urine. For this task, especially for human plasma and serum, methods using atomic emission spectrometry, particle induced X-ray emission, flame atomic absorption spectrometry, and catalysis were found to be inadequate. Methods that apparently can determine vanadium accurately in low amounts are electrothermal atomic absorption spectrometry (ETAAS) (22,23), neutron activation analysis with radiochemical separation (RNAA) (21,24,25), and neutron activation with preirradiation separation (NAA) (24,25). RNAA and NAA are methods not available to most laboratories; thus, ETAAS is the method of choice for analysis of samples that have been dry-ashed (22,25), wet-digested (23), or bomb-digested in a microwave (21). As with all trace elements, contamination of samples is a concern, but apparently for vanadium this is not as much of a concern as it is for some other trace elements (21). Biological reference materials are available for vanadium analysis (21,23–25).

IV. METABOLISM OF VANADIUM

A. Absorption

Most ingested vanadium is not absorbed and is excreted in the feces. Based on the very low concentrations of vanadium, generally less than 0.8 μg/L, found in urine (23,26), in comparison with the estimated daily intake of 12–30 μg (26,27), and the fecal content of vanadium, apparently less than 5% of vanadium ingested is normally absorbed. Byrne and Kosta (26) estimated that no more than 1% of vanadium normally ingested with the diet is absorbed. Curran et al. (28) reported that about 0.1–1.0% of vanadium in 100 mg of the very soluble diammonium oxytartratovanadate was absorbed by the human gastrointestinal tract.

Animal studies generally support the concept that vanadium is poorly absorbed (29–32). However, two studies with rats indicated that vanadium absorption can exceed 10% (33,34). These studies suggest caution in assuming that ingested vanadium always will be poorly absorbed from the gastrointestinal tract. Factors such as fasting and dietary composition probably had an influence on the percentage absorbed from the intestine in these studies.

Kinetic modeling of whole-body vanadium metabolism in sheep indicates that a significant amount of vanadium absorption occurs in the upper gastrointestinal tract (35). Most ingested vanadium probably is transformed in the stomach to VO^{2+} and remains in this form as it passes into the duodenum (36). However, in-vitro studies suggest that vanadate can enter cells through phosphate or other anion-transport systems. This may be the reason that V^{5+} is absorbed three to five times more effectively than V^{4+}. Thus, the different absorbability rates, the effect of other dietary components on the forms of vanadium in the stomach, and the speed at which it is transformed into V^{4+} apparently markedly affect the percentage of ingested vanadium absorbed (36). Supporting this concept are the findings reviewed by Nielsen (37) showing that a number of substances can ameliorate vanadium toxicity, including ascorbic acid, EDTA, chromium, protein, ferrous iron, chloride, and aluminum hydroxide.

B. Transport

Based on studies using intravenous (i.v.) or intraperitoneal (i.p.) injections of the element in animals, vanadium is rapidly removed from the blood plasma and is retained in highest amounts in the kidney, liver, testes, bone, and spleen. For example, at 96 h, 30–46% of an i.v. dose of ^{48}V was found in the urine and 9–10% in the feces of rats (39,45). Thirty minutes after an i.p. injection of ^{48}V, rats retained 7.2% in the kidney and 2.1% in bone; at 48 h, the kidney retained 1.6% and bone 3.45% of the dose (32).

Much evidence suggests that the binding of the vanadyl ion to iron-containing non-heme proteins is important in vanadium metabolism. For example, vanadium in milk of lactating rats injected with ^{48}V was found mainly in the protein fraction, and apparently was associated with a transferrinlike protein, perhaps lactoferrin (38). Nursing pups absorbed a significant amount of the ^{48}V in the milk; this suggests that a lactoferrin–vanadium complex is important in vanadium metabolism in the suckling rat pup. In older rats, vanadium apparently is converted into vanadyl–transferrin and vanadyl–ferritin complexes in plasma and body fluids (36,39–41). Vanadium (V^{5+}) in transferrin has been hypothesized to be coordinated by Tyr-426, Tyr-517, and Asp-392, with hydrogen bonding of the $V=O$ oxygens to His-585 and Arg-456 (42). The coordination geometry could be either trigonal bipyramidal, or octahedral if another ligand is coordinated (42). One study (43) showed that 1 day after intravenous administration of $^{48}VO^{2+}$, 29% of ^{48}V incorporated in rat liver cytosol existed as a vanadium low-molecular-weight complex (< 5000 mol wt). By day 9, however, the low-molecular-weight complex had disappeared and vanadium was present only as vanadyl–ferritin (15%) and vanadyl–transferrin (85%) in rat liver cytosol. It remains to be determined whether vanadyl–transferrin can transfer vanadium into cells through the transferrin receptor, or whether ferritin is a storage vehicle for vanadium.

C. Tissue Concentration and Storage

Under normal conditions, the body burden of vanadium is low—about 100 μg; most tissues contain less than 10 ng V/g wet weight (see Table 1). However, tissue vanadium is markedly elevated in animals fed high dietary vanadium. In rats, liver vanadium increased from 10 to 55 ng vanadium/g wet weight when dietary vanadium was increased from 0.1 to 25 μg/g (33). In sheep, bone vanadium increased from 220 to 3320 ng/g ash when dietary vanadium was increased from 10 to 270 μg/g (44). Thus, bone apparently is a major sink for excessive retained vanadium.

TABLE 1 Reported Mean Vanadium Concentrations in Human Fluids or Organs[a]

Fluid/organ	Vanadium (ng/g or mL)	Fluid/organ	Vanadium (ng/g or mL)
Blood	0.058[b]	Lung	30 (median)[c]
Bone	3.5[c]	Muscle	0.54[c]
Brain	0.75[c]	Serum	0.071[b]
Fat, subcutaneous	0.72[c]	Teeth	3.6[c]
Hair, scalp	40[c]	Thyroid	3.1[c]
Heart	1.1[c]	Urine	0.24[d]

[a]Fresh-weight basis.
[b]From Ref. 25.
[c]From Ref. 26 (reported individual values averaged).
[d]From Ref. 23.

D. Excretion

Based on studies in which vanadium is administered parenterally, urine is the major excretory route for absorbed vanadium (37). Both high- and low-molecular-weight complexes have been found in urine (36,39); one of these may be transferrin. A significant portion of absorbed vanadium may be excreted through the bile. Byrne and Kosta (26) found 0.65 0.55, and 1.85 ng vanadium/g of human bile. In two studies, 8–10% of an injected dose of ^{48}V was found in the feces of rats (34,45). The form of vanadium in bile apparently has not been determined.

V. DEFICIENCY SIGNS OF VANADIUM

Between 1971 and 1985, several research groups described possible signs of vanadium deficiency for some animals. These have been reviewed (11). However, most of the early studies were performed with animals fed unbalanced diets which resulted in suboptimal health and growth. The diets used often had widely varying contents of protein, sulfur-containing amino acids, ascorbic acid, iron, copper, and perhaps other nutrients that affected, or were affected by, vanadium metabolism (11). Thus, pharmacologic responses may have been induced by the high vanadium supplements fed. As a result, it is difficult to determine whether the "deficiency signs" in early experiments with questionable diets were true deficiency signs, indirect changes caused by an enhanced need for vanadium in some metabolic function, or manifestations of a pharmacologic action of vanadium. Vanadium deficiency signs for humans have not been described.

The uncertainty about vanadium deficiency signs stimulated new efforts to produce deficiency signs in animals fed diets apparently containing adequate and balanced amounts of all known nutrients. Anke and co-workers (46) found that, when compared to controls fed 2 μg vanadium/g diet, goats fed less than 10 ng vanadium/g diet exhibited a higher rate of spontaneous abortion, and those animals that delivered offspring produced less milk during the first 56 days of lactation. Forty percent of kids from vanadium-deprived goats died between days 7 and 91 of life, with some deaths preceded by convulsions; only 8% of kids from vanadium-supplemented goats died during this time. Vanadium-deficient goats had only 55% the life-span of control goats. Also, skeletal deformations were seen in the forelegs, and forefoot tarsal joints were thickened.

Uthus and Nielsen (47) reported that, when compared to controls fed 1 μg vanadium/ g of diet, vanadium deprivation (2 ng vanadium/g diet) increased thyroid weight and thyroid weight/body weight ratio and tended to decrease growth of rats. Vanadium deprivation also depressed red blood cell glucose 6-phosphate dehydrogenase and cecal total carbonic anhydrase (48). Uthus and Nielsen (47) also found that, as dietary iodine increased from 0.05 to 0.33 to 25 μg/g, thyroid peroxidase activity decreased, and the decrease was more marked in the vanadium-supplemented (38.1 to 12.3 to 3.5 mGU/mg protein) than the vanadium-deprived (18.7 to 10.2 to 6.8 mGU/mg protein) rats. Also, as dietary iodine increased, plasma glucose increased in the vanadium-deprived rats, but decreased in the vanadium-supplemented rats. Although supplemented controls in recent vanadium deprivation studies were fed amounts of vanadium that may have had pharmacologic effects, some true deficiency signs were probably produced. It is unlikely the diets lacked any nutrient that caused such marked deficiency signs, especially the skeletal deformations, which were prevented by pharmacologic action of the small vanadium supplements used.

VI. BIOCHEMICAL FUNCTION OF VANADIUM

A defined biochemical function for vanadium in higher animals, and thus humans, has not been described. Recently, however, functional roles for vanadium have been defined for some algae, lichens, fungi, and bacteria. These roles may provide clues as to the nature of the biological function of vanadium in humans; thus, they will be briefly described here.

A. Haloperoxidases

Haloperoxidases catalyze the oxidation of halide ions by hydrogen peroxide, thus facilitating the formation of a carbon–halogen bond. In 1984, vanadium was found to be essential to enzymatic activity of a bromoperoxidase from the brown algae *Ascophyllum nodosum* (9). Since then vanadium-dependent bromoperoxidases have been found in a number of marine brown algae, marine red algae, and terrestrial lichens (49). Vanadium-dependent iodoperoxidases have also been detected in brown seaweeds (49), and a chloroperoxidase has been identified in the fungus *Curvularia inaequalis* (50). The molecular and structural characteristics of the haloperoxidases apparently differ with the source of the enzyme; structural and kinetic characteristics of some vanadium bromoperoxidases are shown in Table 2. The mechanism of action of vanadium in the haloperoxidases has not been firmly established. However, findings to date do not favor a mechanism in which V^{5+} is reduced to V^{4+} or V^{3+} and reoxidized to V^{5+} by H_2O_2. Rather, in the bromoperoxidases, H_2O_2 reacts with vanadium as V^{5+} to form a dioxygen species which reacts with bromide to yield an oxidized bromine species (51), the intermediate that forms the carbon-halogen bond. A suggested mechanism for dioxygen formation and substrate bromination is shown in Figure 2.

B. Nitrogenase

Conversion of atmospheric nitrogen to ammonia by nitrogen-fixing microorganisms is catalyzed by the enzyme nitrogenase. Vanadium-dependent nitrogenases have recently been characterized for *A. vinelandii* (nitrogenase Avl) and *A. chroococcum* (nitrogenase Acl) (52); some properties of these enzymes are shown in Table 3. The reduction of dinitrogen by nitrogenase involves the sequential MgATP-dependent transfer of electrons from an iron–protein to a vanadium–iron–cofactor center at the substrate-binding site in nitrogenase (52).

TABLE 2 Some Structural and Kinetic Characteristics of Vanadium Bromoperoxidases

Source	Molecular mass subunits (kDa)	pH optimum	k_m for H_2O_2 (μM)	k_m for Br^- (mM)
X. parietina	65	5.5	870	0.03
C. rubrum	58	7.4	17	2
C. pilulifera	64	6.0	92	11
L. saccharina	66, 64	6.5	27	1
A. nodosum I	67	6.0	27	14.8
A. nodosum II	70	7.2	27	6.7

Source: From Ref. 49.

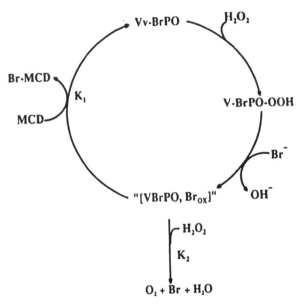

FIGURE 2 Mechanistic scheme for dioxygen formation and monochlorodimedone (2-chloro-5,5-dimethyl-1,3-dimedone, MCD) bromination through the action of a haloperoxidase. In this scheme, vanadium bromoperoxidase (V–BrPO), with vanadium in the 5+ valence state, catalyzes the oxidation of bromide by hydrogen peroxide; this results in an intermediate depicted (but not definitively identified) as "[VBrPO, BR$_{ox}$]," which brominates MCD. (From Ref. 51.)

C. Amavadine

Vanadium is found in high concentrations in a few species of the mushroom genus *Amanita*. The isolation and structure determination of a vanadium-containing compound found in mushrooms and named amavadine has been reviewed (20). The proposed structure of amavadine is shown in Figure 3. The physiologic function of amavadine is unknown. Wever and Kustin (20) suggested that amavadine acts as a cofactor with a protective

TABLE 3 Some Physicochemical Properties of the VFe Proteins in Nitrogenases of *A. vinelandii* (nitrogenase AvI^v) and *A. chroococcum* (nitrogenase AcI^v)

	AvI^v	AcI^v
Native M$_r$	200,000	210,000
Subunit structure	$\alpha_2\beta_2(\gamma_2)$	$\alpha_2\beta_2(\gamma_2)$
Subunit M$_r$	$2 \times 52,000$	$2 \times 50,000$
	$2 \times 55,000$	$2 \times 55,000$
		$2 \times 14,000$
Metal and S^{2-} content (g-atom/mol)		
Vanadium	0.7 ± 0.3	2 ± 0.3
Iron	9 ± 2	19 ± 2
S^{2-}	ND	20 ± 2

Source: From Ref. 52.

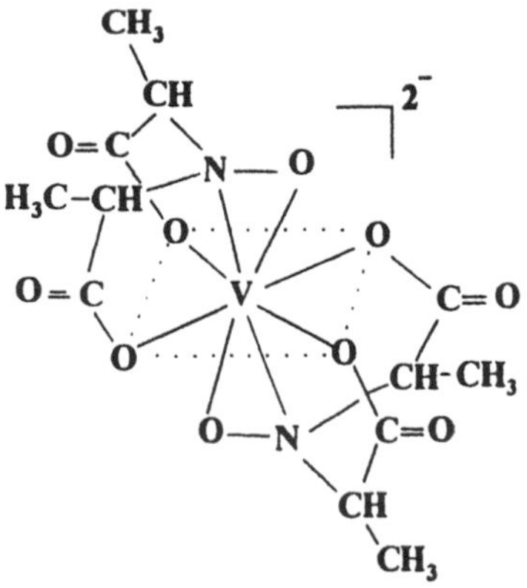

FIGURE 3 The structure of amavadine as proposed by Bayer et al. (53). Although vanadium exists in the 4+ valence state, amavadine does not contain the VO group. Amavadine represents one of the most stable vanadium (4+) complexes known.

oxidase or peroxidase function. However, the electrochemistry of amavadine is such that it may function in electron-transfer reactions through a V^{5+}/V^{4+} redox couple (54).

D. Vanadobin

Some ascidians accumulate vanadium to amounts that exceed that present in sea water by 4 million times. The function of this high concentration of vanadium in ascidian blood cells (vanadocytes) remains unexplained. Suggested functions for vanadocytes include production of the cellulose of the tunic, reversibly trapping oxygen under conditions of low oxygen tension, and acting as an antimicrobial agent (55). A substance has been isolated from ascidian blood cells that can maintain the vanadium ion in the vanadyl form and has a specific affinity for the vanadium ion; this substance has been named vanadobin (55). The physiologic role and structure of vanadobin remain undetermined.

VII. ASSESSMENTS OF VANADIUM STATUS

Because no function for vanadium in higher animals has been defined, a biochemical indicator of vanadium status does not exist. Byrne and Kučera (25) found human serum vanadium concentrations ranged from 0.014 to 0.222 (mean 0.071) ng/mL in nonexposed adults near Ghent, Belgium, and human whole-blood vanadium concentrations ranged from 0.024 to 0.226 (mean 0.056) ng/mL in nonexposed children and adults near Prague, Czechoslovakia. The range of concentrations in potentially exposed children near Prague was similar (0.018–0.239 ng/mL), but the mean value was higher (0.099 ng/mL). Perhaps vanadium concentrations in blood or serum significantly above or below those given for nonexposed individuals indicate an abnormal vanadium status.

VIII. PHARMACOLOGY AND TOXICOLOGY OF VANADIUM

Numerous biochemical and physiologic functions for vanadium have been suggested based on its in-vitro and pharmacologic actions; these have been discussed in several reviews

(15,16,37,56) and are too extensive to discuss in detail here. In-vitro studies with cells and pharmacologic studies with animals have shown that vanadium has insulin-mimetic properties, numerous stimulatory effects on cell proliferation and differentiation, effects on cell phosphorylation/dephosphorylation, inhibitory effects on the motility of sperm, cilia, and chromosomes, effects on glucose and ion transport across the plasma membrane, interfering effects on intracellular ionized calcium movement, and effects on oxidation–reduction processes. In-vitro cell-free systems have shown that vanadium inhibits numerous ATPases, phosphatases, and phosphoryl transfer enzymes (56). The pharmacologic action of vanadium receiving the most attention recently is its ability to mimic insulin. New findings in this area occur regularly; thus, even a recent review (57) of this subject may be out of date.

Vanadium is a relatively toxic element. The threshold level for toxicity apparently is near 10 to 20 mg/day or 10 to 20 μg/g of diet; this is supported by animal findings (37) and the following human findings. Schroeder et al. (58) fed 15 patients 4.5 and 9 mg vanadium/day as diammonium oxytartratovanadate for 6 to 16 months without apparent detrimental effect. However, serum cholesterol was reduced slightly by the treatment, so the vanadium supplement was not inactive. Curran et al. (28) fed each of five subjects 13.5 mg/day in three divided doses as diammonium oxytartratovanadate for 6 weeks; no sign of intolerance or toxicity was found. On the other hand, Somerville and Davies (59) gave each of 12 patients 13.5 mg vanadium/day for 2 weeks, and then 22.5 mg vanadium/day for 5 months; five patients exhibited gastrointestinal disturbances and five patients exhibited green tongue. Dimond et al. (60) gave ammonium vanadyl tartrate orally to six subjects for 6–10 weeks in amounts ranging from 4.5 to 18 mg vanadium/day; green tongue, cramps, and diarrhea were observed at the larger doses.

From their in-depth study of vanadium toxicity, Proescher et al. (61) concluded that vanadium is a neurotoxic and a hemorrhagic-endotheliotoxic poison with nephrotoxic, hepatotoxic, and probably leukocytotoxic components. Thus, it is not surprising that a variety of toxicity signs exist and that they can vary among species and with dosage. Some of the more consistent signs include depressed growth, diarrhea, depressed food intake, and death.

IX. FUTURE RESEARCH NEEDS

The primary research need for vanadium in nutrition is the identification of an essential biochemical function in higher animals. This is necessary to disentangle pharmacologic from nutritional observations in order to assess the nutritional importance of vanadium. Determination of a defined function also would facilitate other research related to the nutritional aspects of vanadium, including the determination of status assessment indicators and safe and adequate intakes. Furthermore, until a defined function is described, it is unlikely that vanadium will be unequivocally accepted as an essential nutrient for higher animals.

If vanadium has a function in humans, it most likely is very specialized; thus, its nutritional requirement would be very small. One might predict that vanadium has nutritional characteristics similar to those of iodine. Even though the iodine requirement is small (150 μg/day), deficiencies of this element occur frequently. The daily intake of vanadium can easily be below 10 μg/day (25), a level which has been suggested as the possible requirement (11); deficiency of vanadium is possible. Furthermore, because vanadium is so pharmacologically active, a beneficial action, such as the anticariogenic effect of fluoride or the anticarcinogenic action of selenium, may be found for the element. The result would be enhanced nutritional interest in vanadium. For this reason, vanadium should not at this time be dismissed as nutritionally unimportant.

REFERENCES

1. Priestley J, Gamgee A. On the physiological action of vanadium. Phil Trans R Soc Lond [Biol] 1876; 166:495–556.
2. Jackson DE. The pharmacological action of vanadium. J Pharmacol 1912; 3:477–514.
3. Henze M. Untersuchungen über das Blut der Ascidien I. Mitt. Die Vanadiumverbindung der Blutkörperchen. Hoppe-Seylers Z Physiol Chem 1911; 72:494–501.
4. Henze M. Untersuchungen über das Blut der Ascidien. Hoppe-Seylers Z Physiol Chem 1912; 79:215–228.
5. Cantley LC Jr, Josephson L, Warner R, Yanagisawa M, Lechene C, Guidotti G. Vanadate is a potent (Na,K)-ATPase inhibitor found in ATP derived from muscle. J Biol Chem 1977; 252: 7421–7423.
6. Rifkin RJ. In vitro inhibition of Na^+-K^+ and Mg^{2+} ATPases by mono, di, and trivalent cations. Proc Soc Exp Biol Med 1965; 120:802–804.
7. Shechter Y, Karlish SJD. Insulin-like stimulation of glucose oxidation in rat adipocytes by vanadyl (IV) ions. Nature 1980; 284:556–558.
8. Heyliger CE, Tahiliani AG, McNeill JH. Effect of vanadate on elevated blood glucose and depressed cardiac performance of diabetic rats. Science 1985; 227:1474–1477.
9. Vilter H. Peroxidases from Phaephyceae: a vanadium (V)-dependent peroxidase from *Asocphyllum nodosum*. Phytochemistry 1984; 23:1387–1390.
10. Bertrand D. Survey of contemporary knowledge of biogeochemistry. 2. The biogeochemistry of vanadium. Bull Am Mus Nat His 1950; 94:403–456.
11. Nielsen FH, Uthus EO. The essentiality and metabolism of vanadium. In: Chasteen ND, ed. Vanadium in Biological Systems. Dordrecht, Netherlands: Kluwer, 1990:51–62.
12. Nielsen FH. The importance of diet composition in ultratrace element research. J Nutr 1985; 115:1239–1247.
13. Nechay BR, Nanninga LB, Nechay PSE, et al. Role of vanadium in biology. Fed Proc 1986; 45: 123–132.
14. Kustin K, Macara I. The new biochemistry of vanadium. Comments Inorg Chem 1982; 2:1–22.
15. Boyd DW, Kustin K. Vanadium: a versatile biochemical effector with an elusive biological function. Adv Inorg Biochem 1984; 6:311–365.
16. Nechay BR. Mechanisms of action of vanadium. Annu Rev Pharmacol Toxicol 1984; 24: 501–524.
17. Degani H, Gochin M, Karlish SJD, Schechter Y. Electron paramagnetic resonance studies and insulin-like effects of vanadium in rat adipocytes. Biochemistry 1981; 20:5795–5799.
18. Liochev SI, Fridovich I, Vanadate-stimulated oxidation of NAD(P)H in the presence of biological membranes and other sources of O_2^-. Arch Biochem Biophys 1990; 279:1–7.
19. Fantus IG, Kadota S, Deragon G, Foster B, Posner BI. Pervandate [peroxide(s) of vanadate] mimics insulin action in rat adipocytes via activation of the insulin receptor tyrosine kinase. Biochemistry 1989; 28:8864–8871.
20. Wever R, Kustin K. Vanadium: a biologically relevant element. Adv Inorg Chem 1990; 35: 81–115.
21. Heydorn K. Factors affecting the levels reported for vanadium in human serum. Biol Trace Elem Res 1990; 26/27:541–551.
22. Myron DR, Givand SH, Nielsen FH. Vanadium content of selected foods as determined by flameless atomic absorption spectroscopy. Agric Food Chem 1977; 25:297–300.
23. Ishida O, Kihira K. Tsukamoto Y, Marumo F. Improved determination of vanadium in biological fluids by electrothermal atomic absorption spectrometry. Clin Chem 1989; 35:127–130.
24. Byrne AR, Versieck J. Vanadium determination at the ultratrace level in biological reference

materials and serum by radiochemical neutron activation analysis. Biol Trace Elem Res 1990; 26/27:529–540.

25. Byrne AR, Kučera J. New data on levels of vanadium in man and his diet. In: Momčilović B, ed. Trace Elements in Man and Animals 7. Zagreb: IMI, 1991:25.18–25.20.

26. Byrne AR, Kosta L. Vanadium in foods and in human body fluids and tissues. Sci Tot Environ 1978; 10:17–30.

27. Myron DR, Zimmerman TJ, Shuler TR, Klevay LM, Lee DE, Nielsen FH. Intake of nickel and vanadium by humans. A survey of selected diets. Am J Clin Nutr 1978; 31:527–531.

28. Curran GL, Azarnoff DL, Bolinger RE. Effect of cholesterol synthesis inhibition in normo-cholesteremic young men. J Clin Invest 1959; 38:1251–1261.

29. Hansard SL II, Ammerman CB, Henry PR. Vanadium metabolism in sheep. II. Effect of dietary vanadium on performance, vanadium excretion and bone deposition in sheep. J Animal Sci 1982; 55:350–356.

30. Conklin AW, Skinner CS, Felten TL, Sanders CL. Clearance and distribution of intratracheally instilled [48]vanadium compounds in the rat. Toxicol Lett 1982; 11:199–203.

31. Parker RDR, Sharma RP. Accumulation and depletion of vanadium in selected tissues of rats treated with vanadyl sulfate and sodium orthovanadate. J Environ Pathol Toxicol 1978; 2: 235–245.

32. Roschin AV, Ordzhonikidze EK, Shalganova IV. Vanadium—toxicity, metabolism, carrier state. J Hyg Epidemiol Microbiol Immunol 1980; 24:377–383.

33. Bogden JD, Higashino H, Lavenhar MA, Bauman JW Jr, Kemp FW, Aviv A. Balance and tissue distribution of vanadium after short-term ingestion of vanadate. J Nutr 1982; 112:2279–2285.

34. Wiegman TB, Day HP, Patak RV. Intestinal absorption and secretion of radioactive vanadium ($^{48}VO_3^-$) in rats and effect of Al(OH)$_3$. J Toxicol Environ Health 1982; 10:233–245.

35. Patterson BW, Hansard SL II, Ammerman CB, Henry PR, Zech LA, Fisher WR. Kinetic model of whole-body vanadium metabolism: studies in sheep. Am J Physiol 1986; 251:R325–R332.

36. Chasteen ND, Lord EM, Thompson HJ. Vanadium metabolism. Vanadyl (IV) electron para-magnetic resonance spectroscopy of selected tissues in the rat. In: Xavier AV, ed. Frontiers in Bioinorganic Chemistry. Weinheim: VCH, 1986:133–141.

37. Nielsen FH. Vanadium. In: Mertz W, ed. Trace Elements in Human and Animal Nutrition. Vol. 1. San Diego, CA: Academic Press, 1987:275–300.

38. Edel J, Sabbioni E. Vanadium transport across placenta and milk of rats to the fetus and newborn. Biol Trace Elem Res 1989; 22:265–275.

39. Sabbioni E, Marafante E. Metabolic patterns of vanadium in the rat. Bioinorg Chem 1978; 9:389–407.

40. Sabbioni E, Marafante E. Relations between iron and vanadium metabolism: *in vivo* incorpora-tion of vanadium into iron proteins of the rat. J Toxicol Environ Health 1981; 8:419–429.

41. Harris WR, Friedman SB, Silberman D. Behavior of vanadate and vanadyl ion in canine blood. J Inorg Biochem 1984; 20:157–169.

42. Butler A, Carrano CJ. Coordination chemistry of vanadium in biological systems. Coord Chem Rev 1991; 109:61–105.

43. Sabbioni E, Marafante E. Progress in research on newer trace elements: the metabolism of vanadium as investigated by nuclear and radiochemical techniques. In: Howell J McC, Gaw-thorne JM, White CL, eds. Trace Element Metabolism in Man and Animals (TEMA-4). Canberra: Australian Academy of Science, 1981:629–631.

44. Hansard SL II, Ammerman CB, Fick KR, Miller SM. Performance and vanadium content of tissues in sheep as influenced by dietary vanadium. J Animal Sci 1978; 46:1091–1095.

45. Hopkins LL Jr, Tilton BE. Metabolism of trace amounts of vanadium 48 in rat organs and liver subcellular particles. Am J Physiol 1966; 211:169–172.

46. Anke M, Groppel B, Gruhn K, Langer M, Arnhold W. The essentiality of vanadium for animals. In: Anke M, Baumann W, Bräunlich H, Brückner C, Groppel B, Grün M, eds. 6th Int. Trace Element Symp. 1989. Vol. 1. Mo, V. Jena: Friedrich-Schiller-Universität, 1989:17–27.

47. Uthus EO, Nielsen FH. Effect of vanadium, iodine and their interaction on growth, blood

variables, liver trace elements and thyroid status indices in rats. Magnesium Trace Elem 1990; 9:219–226.

48. Poellot RA, Seaborn CD, Uthus EO. The effect of vanadium deprivation in thyroxine replete-thyroidectomized rats. Proc ND Acad Sci 1992; 46:75.

49. Wever R, Krenn BE. Vanadium haloperoxidases. In: Chasteen ND, ed. Vanadium in Biological Systems. Dordrecht, Netherlands: Kluwer, 1990:81–97.

50. van Schijndel JWPM, Vollenbroek EGM, Wever R. The chloroperoxidase from the fungus *Curvularia inaequalis*; a novel vanadium enzyme. Biochim Biophys Acta 1993; 1161:249–256.

51. Soedjak HS, Butler A. Mechanism of dioxygen formation catalyzed by vanadium bromoperoxidase from *Macrocystis pyrifera* and *Fucus distichus*: steady state kinetic analysis and comparison to the mechanism of V-BrPO from *Ascophyllum nodosum*. Biochim Biophys Acta 1991; 1079:1–7.

52. Eady RR. Vanadium nitrogenases. In: Chasteen ND, ed. Vanadium in Biological Systems, Drodrecht, Netherlands: Kluwer, 1990:99–127.

53. Bayer E, Koch E, Anderegg G. Amavadin, an example for selective binding of vanadium in nature: Studies of its complexation chemistry and a new structural proposal. Angew Chem Int Ed Engl 1987; 26:545–548.

54. Frausto da Silva JJR. Vanadium in biology—the case of the *Amanita* toadstools. Chem Spec Bioavail 1989; 1:139–150.

55. Michibata H, Sakurai H. Vanadium in ascidians. In: Chasteen ND, ed. Vanadium in Biological Systems. Dordrecht, Netherlands: Kluwer, 1990:153–171.

56. Willsky GR. Vanadium in the biosphere. In: Chasteen ND, ed. Vanadium in Biological Systems. Dordrecht, Netherlands: Kluwer, 1990:1–24.

57. Shechter Y, Meyerovitch J, Farfel Z, et al. Insulin mimetic effects of vanadium. In: Chasteen ND, ed. Vanadium in Biological Systems. Dordrecht, Netherlands: Kluwer, 1990:129–142.

58. Schroeder HA, Balassa JJ, Tipton IH. Abnormal trace metals in man—vanadium. J Chron Dis 1963; 16:1047–1071.

59. Somerville J, Davies B. Effect of vanadium on serum cholesterol. Am Heart J 1962; 64:54–56.

60. Dimond EG, Caravaca J, Benchimol A. Vanadium. Excretion, toxicity, lipid effect in man. Am J Clin Nutr 1963; 12:49–53.

61. Proescher F, Seil HA, Stillians AW. A contribution to the action of vanadium with particular reference to syphilis. Am J Syph 1917; 1:347–405.

23
Arsenic

Manfred Anke, M. Glei, W. Arnhold, C. Drobner, and M. Seifert
Friedrich Schiller University, Jena, Germany

I. INTRODUCTION

Arsenic, described by Albertus Magnus in about 1250, has played an important role in the cultural history of mankind. Pure metallic arsenic is not poisonous, but it oxidizes in moist air to form arsenic trioxide, a toxic compound. Because of its properties as a scentless and tasteless powder, arsenic trioxide became a murderous weapon, "king of poisons" (1). Testing of a potential essentiality of As was successful only in the 1970s. Deficiency symptoms were observed in rats, goats, mini-pigs, and chicks (2).

II. CHEMICAL PROPERTIES AND OCCURRENCE

Arsenic (atomic mass 74.92) is an anisotopic element similar to phosphorus. Elemental arsenic exists at room temperature as metallic gray and yellow arsenic. Gray arsenic is the common stable form. The valencies of arsenic compounds are $+5$, $+3$, and -3, with $+3$ being the most common valency (3).

The 16-km-thick earth crust contains about 5.5 mg As/kg. Arsenic occurs in the elemental form in fly ash and forms intermetallic compounds with antimony and copper. The sulfides realgar (As_2S_2), orpiment (As_2S_3), arsenopyrite (FeSAs), cobaltite (CoFe AsS), and pyrargyrite (Ag_3AsS_3) are most widespread (3). Arsenic oxide usually occurs as a by-product of copper, lead, and nickel smelting. Coal contains between 0.5 and 93 mg As/kg, with a mean value of 18 mg/kg; brown coal contains up to 1500 mg/kg (4).

III. CONCENTRATION IN FOOD AND FEED

The arsenic content of plants is determined by the geological origin of the soil, arsenic emissions, arsenic content of fertilizers and herbicides, and the plant species. Its concentration varies from 0.01 to about 5 ppm. Plants growing on arsenic-rich soils can accumulate extremely high arsenic levels. Bermuda grass may accumulate up to 45 mg arsenic/kg dry matter. As a rule, plant stems contain more arsenic than leaves. After fertilizing with arsenic-rich flue ash, only the first cutting of crops is usually arsenic-enriched. Without rain, 50% of the monosodium methane arsenate used as a herbicide is absorbed by Johnson grass after 6 h, and 90% after 155 h. All arsenic-containing herbicides increase the arsenic content of herbage fruits and vegetables. Vegetables from old orchard soils treated with arsenic-containing insecticides were not richer in arsenic than control plants (5).

On average, the geological origin of the site has an effect on the arsenic concentration in plants. Krause (6) was able to demonstrate this influence by means of indicator plants, including wheat, rye, acre red clover, and meadow red clover. The age of plants also has a significant effect on their arsenic content. Meadow fescue, wheat, and rye reduced their arsenic content to 25% within 30 days. Plants take up arsenic passively along with water. Mushrooms as well as soybeans, cabbage, and cress seem to be arsenic accumulators (7). Most feed- and foodstuffs contain < 3 mg As/kg dry matter. The following arsenic amounts must be reckoned with: forage plants 100–1000 µg/kg dry matter, cereals 50–400 µg/kg dry matter, vegetables 50–800 µg/kg dry matter, fruit 30–1000 µg/kg dry matter, meat 25–500 µg/kg dry matter, milk 80–800 µg/kg dry matter, eggs 40–400 µg As/kg dry matter. Marine foodstuffs are considerably richer in arsenic. As a rule, they have the following arsenic concentrations, with the main amounts occurring as arsenobetaine: fish 2–80 mg/kg dry matter, oysters 3–10 mg/kg dry matter, mussels 10–20 mg/kg dry matter, fish meal for animal production 2.6–19 mg/kg dry matter. The highest biological concentration, 1100 mg/kg, was found in seafood that lives at the bottom of the sea (8).

IV. METABOLISM

A. Intake

The arsenic intake of adults is determined primarily by the proportion of seafood in the diet. On average, adults from Japan consumed 161, 329, and 273 µg/day, and those from Norway 154 µg/day. The arsenic consumption of adults varied between 4 and 84 µg/day in all other countries in which mainly terrestrial foodstuffs are consumed. This amounted to 31–55 µg/day in the United States, 81 µg/day in the United Kingdom, and 19–83 µg/day in Germany (9). The ingestion of certain drinking water or the inhalation of industrial dust can lead to considerable arsenic exposure.

B. Absorption

The arsenic in air may be absorbed to a considerable extent, as was shown by the correlation between the arsenic content of air and arsenic excretion in workers of a copper-smelting plant (10). Skin absorption is more rapid for trivalent than for pentavalent arsenic. Absorption is faster through skin with lesions than through normal skin (11).

Compounds that enter the gastrointestinal tract are subjected to the action of bacteria and enzymes, and after absorption they must pass through the liver before reaching the general circulation. This process can alter the chemical form of arsenic compounds. This is not true for arsenobetaine, but for the inorganic portion in the food. Hens absorbed more [76]As from As_2O_3 than goats. Absorption, incorporation, and excretion are slowed by the interposition of rumen flora. Arsenic-deficient goats absorbed more arsenic than corresponding control animals (12,13).

C. Tissue Incorporation and Concentration

Absorbed arsenic is incorporated into different tissues depending on time. In hens and goats, skeletal muscles stored most of the retained [76]As (31–60%) at all time points from 45 min to 96 h after oral intake. The concentrations in skeleton (25–9%), liver (11–2%), blood (12–2%), lungs (8–0%), kidneys (8–1%), feathers (32–4%), and ovary (8–2%) followed. The arsenic content incorporated into the egg was extremely low and increased with time. The [74]As incorporation into the downy feathers of hens reached its peak 12 h after oral intake, that of the hair of goats 48 h after intake (12,13). Preferred accumulation in skin and hair was also registered in mice and golden hamsters (14). Lindgren and Dencker (15) found [76]As in the epididymis, thyroid, skin, and the lens of mice and golden hamsters 4 or 30 days after injection. Fifty-percent of [74]As was strongly bound to the rough microsomal membranes in the liver of marmorset monkeys (16). Rats accumulate less of arsenobetaine arsenic in the organs than that of cacodylic acid, for example. Both As(III) and As(V) are transported to the embryo in mice and monkeys. Arsenite was transferred more slowly to the embryo than arsenate. The teratogenicity of arsenic has been described for hamsters, rats, and mice (5).

It was shown in animal experiments with kids and adult female goats that tissues and fluids differ in their indication of arsenic status. Furthermore, arsenic incorporation depends on age. Much arsenic is incorporated into the tissues during pregnancy and lactation; arsenic transfer via milk is low. Newborn babies and animals store 2 to 10 times more arsenic in the tissues than adults (2). Liver, kidney, milk, and hair best reflected the arsenic status of adult goats fed either 350 μg or <35 μg As/kg dry matter. Cardiac muscle, colostrum, aorta, and pancreas were unsuitable as indicators of arsenic status.

In a study with healthy adult human tissues, the mean arsenic concentration of most tissues was reported to be between 40 and 90 μg/kg dry matter. The variability was extremely high. Skin (120 μg/kg dry matter), nails (360 μg/kg dry matter), and hair (659 μg/kg dry matter) were substantially richer in arsenic than other tissues. In other investigations, the arsenic content of hair varied between 8 and 600 μg/kg and that of fingernails between 280 and 1200 μg/kg. The arsenic content of human hair and nails has excited considerable interest because of its value in the diagnosis of arsenic poisoning. The median arsenic content in 1000 samples of human hair was 510 μg/kg dry matter. The median concentrations for males and females were 620 and 370 μg/kg dry matter. Values higher than about 3 ppm indicate potential poisoning.

The normal arsenic content of nails is 0.4–1.1 ppm. Arsenic exposure during the growth of the nail can be determined by means of the arsenic content of different segments of finger- and toenails. Normal values of 0.001 to 0.008 ppm arsenic were found in the enamel of human teeth and 0.06 ppm arsenic in the tooth.

Levander et al. (17) summarized the arsenic content of human organs of normal and arsenic-exposed persons. The lungs of normal versus arsenic-exposed persons contained 80–170 μg and 2300–2600 μg/kg fresh weight. Also, 90–300 and 4400–6900 μg As/kg fresh weight were found in the livers of these groups. Liver tissue concentration ranged between 2.3 and 12 μg As/kg wet weight (18). Between 0.09 and 5.5 μg/L (mean 0.96 μg/L) were found in the serum, and between 0.43 and 20 μg/kg wet weight (mean 4.4 μg/kg) in packed blood cells. The blood levels of unexposed persons were reported to be 1.9–2.0 μg/L, 6–8 μg/L, 5.1 μg/L (range 0.5–32), and 19 μg/L (range 2–40) (18).

Normal urine levels vary between 1 and 80 μg/L and are generally lower than 10 μg/L. The milk of Greek and Indian women contained 0.6–6 and 0.2–1.1 μg As/L, respectively. There were no differences between the arsenic contents of colostrum and mature milk. Normal milk of cows and goats contains 15–60 μg As/L. The feeding of nontoxic arsenic doses to cows (0.05–1.25 mg/kg body weight) for 8 weeks did not increase the arsenic content of the milk. These results suggest a blood–mammary barrier to arsenic. The most likely explanation is that an active transport mechanism is saturated at normal plasma concentrations. Aliphatic organic and inorganic arsenic use the same transport mechanism (5,19).

D. Excretion

Urinary excretion of arsenic rises with increasing arsenic intake, so the total urinary excretion provides a useful index of arsenic exposure. In humans the renal excretion rate depends on the form of the arsenic taken in. After 4 days the amount of arsenic excreted in urine was 46%, 78%, and 75% of the single oral dose (500 μg arsenic) in the case of Na-arsenite, monomethyl-arsonate, and cacodylate. Cacodylate was excreted unchanged, monomethylarsonate was slightly (13%) methylated, while roughly 75% of the arsenic excreted after the ingestion of Na-arsenite was methylated arsenic (20). After oral intake of As(III) they found 51% dimethylarsinic, 21% monomethylarsonic compounds, and 27% inorganic arsenic in urine. The excretion of inorganic [74]As in man is best represented by a three-component exponential function. Sixty-six percent of the arsenic had a half-life of 2.1 days, 30%, 9.5 days, and 4%, 38 days (21).

Fish arsenite is excreted in its original form via urine by humans. No metabolic changes occurred in the human body. At the end of the first day, 50% of the fish arsenic was already excreted renally. Up to the 8th day, 76% of arsenic left the body renally after a single arsenic dose. Only 0.3% of the fish arsenic was found in the feces (22). The direct renal excretion of arsenobetaine is not accompanied by an increase of the inorganic and methylated arsenic, respectively (23).

Arsenic excretion via gall bladder is influenced by the form of intake and the chemical structure. It is very low in the case of oral intake, but increases to <10% of the injected amount in case of intravenous application in rats (24,25). The arsenic of such organic compounds as arsanilic acid used as growth stimulants for pigs and poultry is similarly well absorbed and disappears rapidly from the tissues, mostly into the feces. When these forms of arsenic are fed in the recommended amounts, the element does not accumulate in the tissues to excessive concentrations. Five to seven days after taking an arsenic-rich ration, the arsenic concentration of muscle and adipose tissue had decreased (0.5 mg/kg of body weight and 2.0 mg/kg in liver and kidneys). Monosodium methanearsonate, a herbicide, accumulates in crawfish, but this arsenic concentration is not dangerous for humans (26).

E. Metabolic Transformations

1. Reductive Biomethylation

Gosio (27) first pointed out that a mold, *Penicillium brevicaule* (*Scopulariopsis brevicaulis*), produces the garlic odor of wallpapers with arsenic-containing paints (Scheele's green, Schweinfurt green). Challenger et al. (28) identified the volatile substance as trimethylarsine. Several strains of the fungi of soil (*Aspergillus*, *Fusarium*, *Penicillia*) can produce trimethylarsine from most different arsenic compounds. Several fungi isolated from sewage can also reduce arsenic compounds to trimethylarsine. This process takes place under aerobic conditions. It is of interest that some fungi can methylate arsonic acids with aromatic substituents to form organoarsines. Such aromatic arsonic acids are in widespread use as food additives. The bimethylation of arsenic under anoxic conditions by methanogenic bacteria is carried out in two methylative steps to dimethylarsinic acid as in the aerobic system, but then reduction to dimethylarsine occurs rather than further methylation. Dimethylarsine is a highly reactive substance. This explains the tendency for dimethylarsine to be rapidly transformed into nonvolatile materials in sewage sludge (5).

The inclusion of arsonic acids in swine diets increased the dry matter and volatile solids destruction of swine waste in anaerobic storage systems, while it increased the retention of nitrogen.

2. Biosynthesis of Structurally Complex Organoarsenic Compounds

Algae in the low-phosphate oceans absorb arsenate and are forced to detoxify it immediately in order to survive. Each of the intermediates of arsenic detoxification is toxic and cannot be allowed to accumulate. The structures of the intermediates in the pathway are shown below (29). Arsenic is changed into arsenobetaine and detoxicated in a complicated process (30–32). The selenium content of the water may influence the arsenic metabolism of marine diatoms and algae (33).

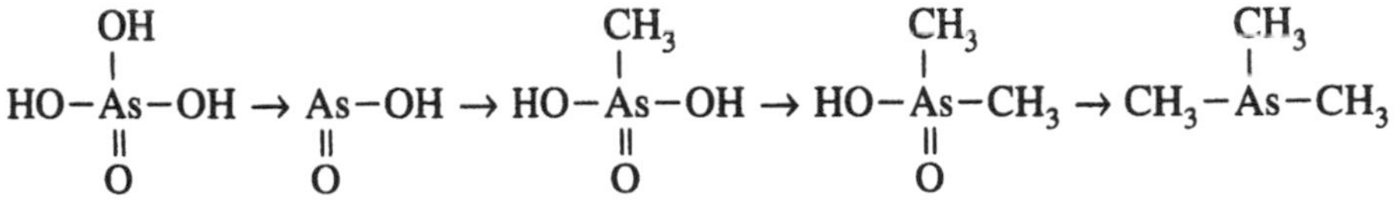

$$\underset{\underset{O}{\overset{\parallel}{}}}{\overset{\overset{OH}{\overset{|}{}}}{HO-As-OH}} \rightarrow \underset{\underset{O}{\overset{\parallel}{}}}{As-OH} \rightarrow \underset{\underset{O}{\overset{\parallel}{}}}{\overset{\overset{CH_3}{\overset{|}{}}}{HO-As-OH}} \rightarrow \underset{\underset{O}{\overset{\parallel}{}}}{\overset{\overset{CH_3}{\overset{|}{}}}{HO-As-CH_3}} \rightarrow \overset{\overset{CH_3}{\overset{|}{}}}{CH_3-As-CH_3}$$

V. ESSENTIALITY

The essentiality of arsenic has not been proven definitely. With regard to the arsenic supply of animals and humans, there must be a distinction among arsenic-deficient rations with <35 $\mu g/kg$ dry matter, normal arsenic rations of 250 to 500 $\mu g/kg$, and therapeutic doses of 3.5 to 5 mg/kg dry matter (5).

The essentiality of arsenic has been investigated in goats, mini-pigs, rats, and chickens (2,34–51). It was demonstrated that arsenic-poor diets with <35 $\mu g/kg$ dry matter slowed growth in goats, which was mainly observed during intrauterine development and after weaning. Arsenic deficiency impairs the success of the first service and the conception rate significantly. Arsenic-deficient animals absorbed significantly more fetuses than control animals, and the offspring had a considerably higher mortality rate during the second lactation. The animals died suddenly. The mitochondria of the cardiac muscle of arsenic-deficient goats showed ultrastructural changes.

The arsenic requirement of goats, mini-pigs, rats, and chicks was estimated to be <50 $\mu g/kg$ ration dry matter. The daily requirement of an adult man has been estimated to be 6 $\mu g/1000$ kcal, or 12–25 $\mu g/day$, based on experiments with animals. The arsenic requirements of animals and humans are met by the feedstuffs, foodstuffs, and water normally consumed.

VI. TOXICOLOGY

Compounds of arsenic (V)—inorganic and organic—are less toxic than those of arsenic (III); organic compounds are less toxic than inorganic ones, and insoluble compounds are less toxic than soluble ones. Arsenic (III) is the active form of arsenic, and it combines with the sulfhydryl groups of many enzymes (dihydrolipoate dehydrogenase, pyruvate dehydrogenase, monoamine oxidase, succinate oxidase, DNA polymerase). The formation of acetyl lipoate, or acetyl-CoA is inhibited.

Arsenic (V) substitutes for phosphorus, disrupting oxidative phosphorylation. The blockade of adenosine triphosphatase leads to an energy loss in the cells, with the inhibition of cell partition and transport of Na^+ and K^+ through the cell membrane. The inhibition of cellular oxidative processes results in capillary injury and tissue hypoxia.

Arsenic is also seen as a general inducer of genes involved in proliferation, recombination, amplification, and activation of viruses (18).

Arsine, with its typical garlic odor, is a strong hemolytic poison. Erythrocytes are the target. A symptom-free interval in which the toxically active compound diarsin ($H-As=As-H$) is formed following inhalation. AsH_3 induces a decrease of the erythrocyte-reduced glutathione followed by the decomposition of blood cells (52,53).

A. Acute Toxicity

The most striking systemic effects of an acute intoxication with inorganic arsenic are gastrointestinal, cardiovascular, neurologic, and hematologic symptoms.

> Gastrointestinal symptoms of acute arsenic poisoning: nausea, stomachache, sickness, diarrhea,
> Cardiovascular symptoms: depolarization of the myocardium, arrhythmia with characteristic changes of the electrocardiogram (longer OT interval, abnormal T-wave),
> Neurologic symptoms after the intake of 1 mg inorganic As/kg body weight/day are often encephalopathy with headaches, signs of disorientation, hallucinations and seizures until coma.
> Hematologic changes such as anemia and leucopenia have been described.

B. Chronic Toxicity

The chronic intoxication after oral intake corresponds with the hyperkeratotic and melanosislike skin changes after inhalation. According to epidemiologic studies, the maximum dose which does not lead to observed adverse effects is 0.001 mg As/kg/day. There are no comprehensive investigations into the effect of organic arsenic compounds on human health. Encephalopathy was diagnosed in 1.5% of 10,000 patients who were treated with typarsamid against trypanosoma; 3–4% suffered from atrophy of the optic nerve. Dermatitis and hepatitic as well as adverse hematologic effects occurred seldom (10). The intake of methylated arsenic compounds found in seafood is harmless if eating habits are normal.

VII. PERSPECTIVES AND FUTURE RESEARCH NEEDS

Evidence for the essentiality of arsenic rests primarily on the depressed growth rate and impaired reproduction observed in the goat, pig, chick, and rat. Other responses to arsenic supplementation have varied in nature and severity depending in part on the concentrations of other dietary components, including zinc, arginine, choline, and methionine (54). There is evidence that arsenic intake affects taurine and polyamine concentrations in plasma and tissues. One must consider the possibility that arsenic exerts pharmacologic effects at the concentrations fed. There is need for research directed toward an elucidation of the biochemical mechanisms by which arsenic exerts the physiologic effects observed. Dietary essentiality will be proven by demonstration that arsenic is part of an essential metabolic pathway.

REFERENCES

1. Leschke E. Klinische Lehrkurse. Münchner Med Wschr 1933; 11:54–60.
2. Anke M, Krause K, Groppel B. The effect of arsenic deficiency on growth, reproduction, life expectancy and disease symptoms in animals. In: Hemphill DD, ed. Trace Substances in Environmental Health—XXI. Columbia: University of Missouri, 1987:533–550.
3. Falbe J, Regitz M. Römpp Chemie Lexikon. 9. Aufl. Stuttgart, New York: George Thieme, 1989.
4. Peterson PJ, Girling CA, Benson LM, Zieve R. Metalloids. In: Lepp NW, ed. Effect of Heavy Metal Pollution on Plants. Vol. 1. London: Applied Science, 1981:213ff, esp. 299–322.
5. Anke M. Arsenic. In: Mertz W, ed. Trace elements in Human and Animal Nutrition. Vol. 2. 5th ed. Orlando, FL: Academic Press, 1986:347–372.
6. Krause U. The site-specific arsenic supply of ruminants in the GDR. In: Anke M, Baumann W, Bräunlich H, Brückner Chr, Groppel B, eds. 5. Spurenelementsymposium, Universität Leipzig, Universität Jena, 1986:856–863.
7. Kabata-Pendias A, Pendias H. Trace Elements in Soils and Plants. 2d ed. Boca Raton, FL: CRC Press, 1992.
8. Anke M. Arsen: Biotransformation, Stoffwechsel, Lebensnotwendigkeit, Versorgung und Bedarf. Mengen- und Spurenelemente 1985; 5:420–436.
9. Parr RM, Crawley H, Abdulla M, Iyengar GV, Kumpulainen J. Human dietary intakes of trace elements: A global literature survey mainly for the period 1970–1991. NAHRES-12. Vienna: IAEA 1992.
10. Marquardt H, Schäfer SG. Lehrbuch der Toxikologie. Mannheim, Leipzig, Wien, Zürich: B J Wissenschaftsverlag, 1994.
11. U.S. Environmental Protection Agency. An exposure and risk assessment for arsenic. Washington, DC: EPA Office for Water Regulations and Standards, 1981.
12. Anke M, Hoffman G, Grün M, Groppel B, Riedel E. Absorption, distribution and excretion of arsenic-76 in hens and ruminants. In: The Use of Isotopes to Dedect Moderate Mineral Unbalances in Farm Animals. IAEA 1982; TEC DOC 267:135–146.
13. Hoffman G, Anke M, Grün M, Groppel B, Riedel E. Absorption, distribution and excretion of [76]arsenic in hens and ruminants. In: Anke M, Schneider HJ, Brückner Chr, eds. 3. Spurenelementsymposium—Arsen, Universität Leipzig, Universität Jena, 1980:41–48.
14. Starkenstein E, Rost E, Pohl J. Toxikologie, Berlin: Urban and Schwarzenberg, 1929.
15. Lindgren A, Dencker L. Preliminary study on the long time retention of arsenite and arsenate in the epididymis, thyroid and lens in mice. In: Anke M, Schneider HJ, Brückner Chr, eds. 3. Spurenelementsymposium—Arsen, Universität Leipzig, Universität Jena, 1980:57–63.
16. Vahter M, Marafante E, Lindgren A, Dencker L. Tissue distribution and subcellular binding of arsenic in marmoset monkeys after injection of [74]As-arsenite. Arch Toxicol 1982; 51:65–77.
17. Levander OA, et al. Arsenic. Washington, DC: National Academy of Sciences, 1977.
18. Iffland R. Arsenic. In: Seiler HG, Sigel A, Sigel H, eds. Handbook on Metals in Clinical and
19. Tölgyesi G, Bokori J. Aufnahme und Ausscheidung subtoxischer Arsenmengen durch das Rind. In: Anke M, Schneider HJ, Brückner Chr, eds. 3. Spurenelementsymposium—Arsen, Universität Leipzig, Universität Jena 1980:65–68.
20. Tam GKH, Charbonneau SM, Lacroix G, Bryce F. In vitro methylation of [74]As in urine, plasma and red blood cells of human and dog. Bull Environ Contam Toxicol 1979; 22:69–71.
21. Pomroy C, Charbonneau SM, McCullough RS, Tam GKH. Human retention studies with [74]As. Toxicol Appl Pharmacol 1980; 53:550–556.

22. Tam GKH, Charbonneau SM, Bryce F, Sandi E. Excretion of a single oral dose of fish-arsenic in man. Bull Environ Contam Toxicol 1982; 28:669–673.

23. Foa V, Colombi A, Maroni M. The speciation of the chemical forms of arsenic in the biological monitoring of exposure to inorganic arsenic. Sci Total Environ 1984; 34:241–259.

24. Cikrt M, Bencko V. Fate of arsenic after parenteral administration to rats, with particular reference to excretion via bile. J Hyg Epidemiol Microbiol Immunol 1974; 18:129–136.

25. Klaassen CD. Biliary excretion of arsenic in rats, rabbits, and dogs. Toxicol Appl Pharmacol 1974; 29:447–457.

26. Abdelghani AA, Anderson AC, Hughes J, Englande AJ. Uptake, distribution and excretion of monosodium methanearsonate by Crawfish (*Procambarus* sp). In: Anke M, Schneider HJ, Brückner Chr, eds. 3. Spurenelementsymposium—Arsen, Universität Leipzig, Universität Jena 1980:147–153.

27. Gosio B. Action de quelques maissiures sur les composes fixes d'arsenic. Arch Ital Biol 1893; 18:253–265.

28. Challenger F, Higginbottom C, Ellis L. J Chem Soc 1933:95–101.

29. Benson AA, Cooney RV, Summons RE. Arsenic metabolism—a way of life in the sea. In: Anke M, Schneider HJ, Brückner Chr, eds. 3. Spurenelementsymposium—Arsen, Universität Leipzig, Universität Jena 1980:139–145.

30. Benson AA, Katayama M, Knowles FC. Arsenate metabolism in aquatic plants. Appl Organo-metallic Chem 1988; 2:349–352.

31. Cooney RV, Mumma RO, Benson AA. Arsoniumphospholipid in algae. Proc Natl Acad Sci (USA) 1978; 75:4262–4264.

32. Benson AA. Arsenic depuration via the tridacna gill membrane. Z Naturforsch 1990; 45c:793–796.

33. Katayama M, Sugawa-Katayama Y, Benson AA. Effect of selenium on arsenic metabolism in *Cylindrotheca fusiformis*. Appl Organmetallic Chem 1990; 4:213–221.

34. Krause U. Die biologische Bedeutung des Arsens. Thesis, Univesity of Leipzig, Germany, 1987.

35. Anke M, Grün M, Partschefeld M. The essentiality of arsenic for animals. In: Hemphill DD, ed. Trace Substances Environ Health X. Columbia: University of Missouri, 1976:403–409.

36. Anke M, Hennig A, Grün M, Partschefeld M, Groppel B, Lüdke H. Arsen—ein neues essen-tielles Spurenelement. Arch Tierern 1976; 26:742–743.

37. Anke M, Grün M, Partschefeld M, Groppel B, Hennig A. Essentiality and function of arsenic. In: Kirchgessner M, ed. Trace Element Metabolism in Man and Animals. Tech Universität München, Freising-Weihenstephan 1977; 3:248–252.

38. Anke M, Groppel B, Grün M, Hennig A, Meissner D. The influence of arsenic deficiency on growth, reproductiveness, life expectancy and health of goats. In: Anke M, Schneider HJ, Brückner Chr, eds. 3. Spurenelementsymposium—Arsen, Universität Leipzig, Universität Jena 1980:25–32.

39. Anke M, Schmidt A, Groppel B, Kronemann H. Further evidence for the essentiality of arsenic. In: Anke M, Baumann W, Bräunlich H, Brückner Chr, eds. 4. Spurenelementsymposium, Universität Leipzig, Universität Jena 1983:97–104.

40. Anke M, Groppel B, Kronemann H. Significance of newer essential trace elements (like Si, Ni, As, Li, V...) for the nutrition of man and animals. In: Brätter P, Schramel P, eds. Trace Elements—Analytical Chemistry in Medicine and Biology, vol. 3 1984:421–464.

41. Anke M, Schmidt A, Groppel B, Kronemann H. Importance of arsenic for fauna. In: Pais I, ed. New Results in the Research of Hardly Known Trace Elements. Budapest: University Horticul-ture Budapest, 1985:61–71.

42. Anke M, Schmidt A, Kronemann H, Krause U, Gruhn K. New data on the essentiality of arsenic. In: Mills CF, Bremner I, Chesters JK, eds. Trace Elem Man Animals 1985; 5:151–154.

43. Nielsen FH. Evidence of the essentiality of arsenic, nickel, and vanadium and their possible nutritional significance. In: Draper HH, ed. Advances in Nutritional Research. Vol. 3. New York: Plenum Press, 1980:157–172.

44. Nielsen FH. Ultratrace elements in Nutrition. Annu Rev Nutr 1984; 4:21–41.

45. Uthus EO, Nielsen FH. Arsenic deprivation and arsenic-zinc interactions in the chick. In: Anke M, Schneider HJ, Brückner Chr, eds. 3. Spurenelementsymposium—Arsen, Universität Leipzig, Universität Jena 1980:33–39.

46. Schmidt A, Anke M, Groppel B, Kronemann H. Histochemical and ultrastructural findings in As-deficiency. Mengen- und Spurenelemente 1983; 3:424–425.

47. Schmidt A, Anke M, Groppel B, Kronemann H. Effects of As-deficiency on skeletal muscle, myocardium and liver. A histochemical and ultrastructural study. Exp Pathol 1984; 25:195–197.

48. Anke M, Groppel B, Krause U. The essentiality of the toxic elements cadmium, arsenic, and nickel. In: Momcilovic B, ed. Trace Elements in Man and Animals, Zagreb 1991:11-6–11-8.

49. Anke M, Schmidt A, Krause U, Groppel B, Gruhn K, Hoffmann G. Arsenmangel beim Wiederkäuer. Mengen- und Spurenelemente 1986; 6:225–245.

50. Uthus EO, Nielsen PH. Effects in chicks of arsenic, arginine, and zinc and their interaction on body weight, plasma uric acid, plasma urea, and kidney arginase activity. Biol Trace Elem Res 1985; 7:11–20.

51. Uthus EO, Cornatzer WE, Nielsen FH. Consequences of arsenic deprivation in laboratory animals. In: Lederer WH, Fensterheim RJ, eds. New York: Van Nostrand Reinhold, 1983:173–189.

52. Forth W, Henschler D, Rummel W, Starke K. Allgemeine und spezielle Pharmakologie und Toxikologie. Mannheim, Leipzig, Wien, Zürich: B J Wissenschaftsverlag, 1992.

53. Tsalev DL, Zaprianov ZK. Atomic Absorption Spectrometry in Occupational and Environmental Health Practice. Vol. I, pp. 87, 216; Vol. II, p. 13; Boca Raton, FL: CRC Press, 1983.

54. Nielsen FH. Nutritional requirements for boron, silicon, vanadium, nickel, and arsenic: current knowledge and speculation. FASEB J 1991; 5:2661–2667.

24

Mineral–Ion Interaction as Assessed by Bioavailability and Ion Channel Function

Boyd L. O'Dell
University of Missouri, Columbia, Missouri

I. INTRODUCTION

The physiologic interaction of two or more mineral ions in the diet can have significant effects on health and welfare. While interactions involving dietary essential elements may be either detrimental or beneficial, the major concern is that an antagonistic element may induce a deficiency of its counterpart nutrient whose concentration in the diet is borderline. Assessment of such in-vivo interactions will be considered here under the concept of bioavailability. While interaction may occur at various sites, the major one that limits bioavailability occurs at the site of absorption in the intestinal mucosa. It should be noted that we know little about the mechanisms involved in the absorption of mineral elements. Besides the intestinal mucosa, interactions occur at ion channels in the plasma membranes of many cell types. An understanding of these interactions may provide a model for the interactions that occur at the absorption level. Present knowledge of interactions at ion channels is based on in-vitro experiments; consequently, such interactions may have little or no physiologic significance. Nevertheless, understanding the function of ion channels could be instructive with regard to the mechanisms involved in intestinal absorption. In-vitro mineral ion interactions are discussed under the topic, ion channels.

II. MINERAL ELEMENT INTERACTION

Clearly, there are interrelationships in the metabolism of the mineral elements consumed. One ion may be essential for the absorption and utilization of another; conversely, an ion may adversely affect the absorption and utilization of one or more other ions. The term *interaction* is used to describe such interrelationships among mineral elements and may be defined as the effect of one element on one or more other elements as revealed by physiologic or biochemical consequence. At the molecular level, such interactions must occur at specific sites on proteins, such a enzymes, receptors, or ion channels.

There are two major types of interactions, positive and negative. The former is commonly synergistic, while the latter is antagonistic. Within the two types there may be multiple or one-on-one interactions. The latter may be one-way or reciprocal. These types of interactions are illustrated in Figure 1. In this illustration, zinc interacts negatively with both copper and iron, while copper has a positive effect on the metabolism of iron. There is a reciprocal interaction between zinc and iron. The multiple nature of interactions is illustrated by the fact that excess zinc inhibits the absorption and function of copper, which in turn is essential for iron utilization. All physiologic responses to such ion interactions are concentration dependent, and in the ideal model, the antagonistic effects are overcome by higher concentrations of the inhibited ion(s).

The possible number and degree of mineral-ion interactions is extremely large and complex; for this reason, a theoretical basis for the prediction and study of interactions is much needed. An extremely helpful theory, based on the chemical and physical properties of the elements, was proposed in 1970 (1). According to this theory, ions with similar electronic configurations of their outer orbitals, i.e., with the same angular distribution of the electron orbitals, are likely to interact competitively. Most of the recognized essential trace metals are in the first transition series of the Periodic Table and the closely related IIB elements. Thus, they are found most commonly among the elements that have unfilled $3d$ orbitals. The electron orbital relationships of these elements and those of the second and third series, which have unfilled $4d$ and $5d$ orbitals, respectively, are shown in Figure 2. As an example, consider molybdenum (atomic number 42), an essential element in the second series, and its antagonist, tungsten (atomic number 74), in the third series. Both have five electrons in their d orbitals and are chemically similar, exhibiting the same valences and

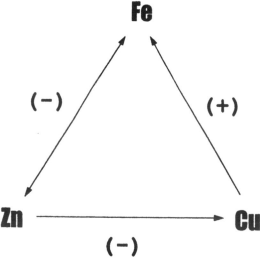

FIGURE 1 Types of ion interactions that affect bioavailability. These examples include positive, negative, reciprocal, and multiple interactions.

Transition Series	---------------------------------Elements III-VIIIB--------------------------------								IB	IIB
1st, 3d	21 Sc^1	22 Ti^2	23 V^3	24 Cr^5	25 Mn^5	26 Fe^6	27 Co^7	28 Ni^8	29 Cu^{10}	30 Zn^{10}
2nd, 4d	39 Y^1	40 Zr^2	41 Nb^4	42 Mo^5	43 Tc^5	44 Ru^7	45 Rh^8	46 Pd^{10}	47 Ag^{10}	48 Cd^{10}
3rd, 5d	57 La^1	72 Hf^2	73 Ta^3	74 W^4	75 Re^5	76 Os^6	77 Ir^7	78 Pt^9	79 Au^{10}	80 Hg^{10}

FIGURE 2 Elements of the first, second, and third transition series and the closely related IIB elements as they occur in the Periodic Table. Most of the recognized essential trace mineral elements are found in the first series, and their best-known antagonists have closely related electron orbitals. The atomic number is shown above the element symbol and the number of d electrons as a superscript. The putatively essential elements are shaded.

forming octahedral complexes with oxygen and sulfur. The elements are similar chemically and interact at the biological level, tungsten interfering with the function of molybdenum. Molybdenum forms biologically active complexes with proteins, but there is no evidence that tungsten does so. There is a strong interaction between copper and zinc bioavailability, as discussed later under copper bioavailability. This appears to be related to the relationship of the ion orbitals. Zn^{2+} has its $3d$ orbitals filled; i.e., it is a d^{10} ion. Cu^{1+} is also d^{10}, and both Cu^{1+} and Zn^{2+} form tetrahedral complexes. Cu^{2+} loses one of its d orbital electrons to become a d^9 ion, and it forms square-planar complexes. Based on this relationship, one would predict that Zn^{2+} is antagonistic to Cu^{1+} rather than Cu^{2+}.

Generally, ions of the transition elements readily form coordinate covalent bonds, complexing with ligands that are rich in the electron donor atoms O, N, and S, which are commonly found in proteins. The transition elements have specific coordination numbers, usually 4 or 6, and commonly form tetrahedral, square-planar or octahedral complexes. For example, Zn^{2+} prefers the tetrahedral, Cu^{2+} the square-planar, and Fe^{2+} the octahedral configuration. Cu^{1+} has the same configuration as Zn^{2+} and forms tetrahedral complexes. Thus, Cu^{1+} would be expected to interact with Zn^{2+} and Cd^{2+}, both of which have the same d-orbital configuration. While this paradigm has been helpful in the prediction of interactions, it is not foolproof, and research has led to unexpected results. There are numerous reviews of ion interactions as they relate to nutrition (2–5).

III. BIOAVAILABILITY AND ASSESSMENT OF INTERACTIONS

A. Definitions

Mineral interaction in animal nutrition has been studied largely by measuring the effect of dietary concentration of one ion on the physiologic or biochemical response to another. A high concentration of an antagonistic element decreases the biologic effectiveness of its target element—i.e., decreases its bioavailability. Bioavailability of an element is defined as the proportion of the element consumed that is utilized for a biochemical or physiologic function. It is made up of two major components, absorption and assimilation:

$$\% \text{ bioavailability} = \% \text{ absorption} \times \% \text{ assimilation} \times 10^{-2}$$

By assimilation is meant the incorporation of the absorbed element into a physiologically active form, e.g., a metalloenzyme, an ion channel, a structural unit, or a functional depository. Stated another way, bioavailability is the proportion of a dietary nutrient that is available for a metabolic function. There is no absolute measure of bioavailability. Bio-availability of an element in a food is expressed relative to a standard, usually a pure chemical form that is readily absorbed.

Absorption is usually the major component of bioavailability, but assimilation is significant in the case of some nutrients. The assimilation component is composed of transport, cellular uptake, and finally incorporation into a molecularly active form. While absorption of an ion can be determined with some precision, direct measurement of assimilation is difficult, if not impossible. Practically, assimilation of a nutrient is the difference between its bioavalability and its absorption, bioavailability being assessed by an overall biochemical or physiologic parameter. Differences in assimilation can be important components of bioavailability, as shown by the examples of selenium and zinc. Absorption of ^{75}Se-selenite and ^{75}Se-selenomethionine, as determined by whole-body counting, was not significantly different, 92% versus 95% (6). On the other hand, retention of ^{75}Se from selenomethionine during the first week after administration was significantly greater than that from selenite, showing a distinct difference between these sources with regard to combined absorption and assimilation. Clearly, the assimilation of dietary se-lenium depends in part on its chemical form. Zinc provides an example in which utilization is affected specifically by another dietary component, 2-picolinic acid (7). This compound increased zinc absorption in rats by nearly 60%, but it also increased urinary excretion so that there was no net effect on retention. Under this condition, measurement of zinc absorption alone would be misleading and give an inaccurate measure of bioavailability. The assessed bioavailability of an element depends in part on the parameter used in its determination and is most sensitively determined by use of the first limiting biochemical or physiologic parameter.

The bioavailability of an element is affected by intrinsic or inherent physiologic factors (see Table 1), as well as by extrinsic or dietary factors. While the intrinsic factors have a marked effect on bioavailability, the primary nutritional and interaction concerns relate to extrinsic factors. Clearly, the effects of extrinsic factors must be measured under well-defined and controlled conditions. All of the intrinsic factors, including sex, physio-logic status, and particularly nutritional status, must be considered.

B. Methods

The best methods for assessment of bioavailability are based on one or more indices of nutritional status with regard to the limiting element. This means that the person or animal is deprived of the specific nutrient before or during the assessment period. The accuracy of

TABLE 1 Bioavailability: Intrinsic Factors and Indices of Nutritional Status

Intrinsic factors	Indices of nutritional status
Age	Growth rate
Sex	Tissue element concentration
Genetics	Metal-dependent enzymes
Nutritional status	Metalloprotein concentration
Physiologic function	Chemical balance
Physiologic stress	Pathologic signs

the assay depends on the index of status used and the precision with which it can be assessed. Supplementation of the diet with graded levels of the limiting nutrient improves nutritional status, depending on its bioavailability. In the case of supplementation with an essential ion, the presence of an antagonist decreases the physiologic or biochemical response to the element and thus its bioavailability. Good indices of status are not available for all mineral elements, but commonly used indicators are listed in Table 1. The slope ratio method constitutes the most rigorous experimental design and method for treatment of data. In this design, graded levels of the standard and test sources of the nutrient are fed, and an index of nutritional status is measured. The slopes over the linear portions of the respective responses are determined, and the ratio of the slopes is considered the relative bioavailability. In this technique, illustrated in Figure 3 (left), the ratio of the suppressor, in this case phytate, to the nutrient zinc remains constant.

In contrast to this example, in which the ratio remained constant, in the typical ion-interaction experiment the diet concentration of the antagonistic ion remains constant and the ratio varies. For this reason the usual slope ratio method is not directly applicable and has not been used for quantitation of ion interactions. Figure 3 (right) depicts zinc–copper interaction, measured by hemoglobin production, in chicks fed a diet limiting in copper. The negative physiologic effect of excess zinc decreased as the dietary copper concentration increased, i.e., as the zinc:copper ratio decreased. Although they are not commonly used, ratios of the reciprocals of the slopes might be useful in the quantitation of such ion interactions.

The growth rate of immature animals fed limiting quantities of an essential element is a good measure of absorption and assimilation. Of course, it cannot be used for evaluation

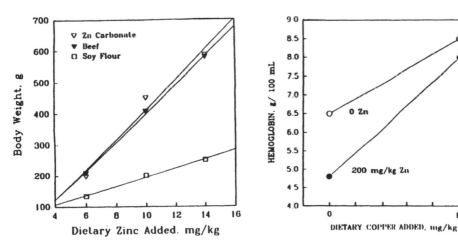

FIGURE 3 Slopes of response curves for the evaluation of bioavailability. Left: Three-week weights of chicks fed an egg white-based diet supplemented with zinc carbonate, dried beef, or soy flour as the source of zinc are plotted versus zinc added to the diet. The ratios of the slopes, beef/carbonate and soy flour/carbonate, were 0.97 and 0.31, respectively. (Data from Ref. 90, with permission.) Right: Hemoglobin concentration in blood of chicks fed a purified diet low in copper. Addition of 200 mg/kg zinc accentuated anemia, and copper supplementation, with and without zinc addition, restored hemoglobin to near normal level. The reciprocal of the ratio, 200/0 mg/kg zinc, is 0.62. (Data from Ref. 5, Table V.)

of bioavailability in mature animals, and other criteria must be applied. These include tissue concentrations of specific metalloproteins and metalloenzymes, such as hemoglobin for iron, Cu,Zn-superoxide dismutase for copper, and glutathione peroxidase for selenium. Tissue concentration of the limiting element, particularly concentrations in storage tissues, provide indices of nutritional status. Notably useful storage sites are liver for copper and iron, and bone for zinc. Besides ion concentrations in physiologic fluids and hair, chemical balance provides the only feasible technique now available for assessment of bioavailability in mature animals and humans. To be valid, this method must involve intakes of the element that are less than that required to maintain balance under the conditions imposed. Use of stable or radioactive isotopes can augment the information obtainable by this and other techniques. It is notable that the dietary requirement to maintain balance changes with depletion, i.e., with nutritional status.

C. Macro-Element Interactions

Physiologic and pharmacologic interactions between pairs of the essential macro-elements, sodium-potassium, calcium-magnesium, and phosphorus-magnesium, have been recognized for many years. However, the nutritional implications of the interactions have received little attention. Recognized interactions among the major elements are depicted by Figure 4.

1. Sodium–Potassium

In 1928, Addison (8) reported that potassium reduced blood pressure in hypertensive patients while sodium increased it. This and related studies stimulated research relating these elements to blood pressure and cardiovascular disease. High sodium chloride intake, 3–10% of diet, by rats increased systolic pressure and mortality rate, and supplementation of these diets with potassium chloride substantially reduced mortality (9). Using a genetically derived strain of salt-sensitive rats, it was observed that sodium chloride was hypertensinogenic and potassium chloride was antihypertensinogenic (10). Increasing the potassium:sodium ratio protected against hypertension. These experiments involved excessively high levels of salt but nevertheless suggest an interaction between sodium and potassium as measured by the blood pressure response.

2. Calcium–Phosphorus

The calcium:phosphorus ratio in the human skeleton is near 2:1, and a similar dietary ratio is considered ideal for many animals. Early studies with rats showed that the most favorable ratio was between 1 and 2 (11). Growth rate and bone ash decreased as the ratio decreased from 1 to 0.25, as well as when it increased toward 5. A recent study has narrowed the desirable range (12). Growth rate was depressed at a ratio of 1.6 but not at 1.3, while bone

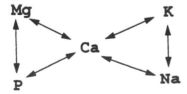

Figure 4   Interactions between and among the major mineral elements. Although depicted as reciprocal antagonisms, the elements are not necessarily equally and reciprocally antagonistic.

ash was unaffected in this range. The ratio in the typical human diet is 1:1 or less, due primarily to the normally high phosphorus level. Increasing dietary phosphorus 2.5-fold, from 800 to 2000 mg/day, did not change calcium absorption or balance in adult humans (13,14). However, with constant dietary calcium and protein, increasing phosphorus intake reduced urinary calcium excretion and increased calcium retention at high protein levels (15).

3. Calcium–Magnesium

Excessive dietary calcium decreases magnesium absorption and status in animals (16–19). The signs of magnesium deficiency, including lowered growth rate and soft tissue calcification, are aggravated by high dietary levels of calcium in several species, including the dog, rat, and guinea pig. As shown in Figure 5, the dietary magnesium concentrations required for maximal growth rate of the guinea pig is increased by excessive calcium in the diet.

4. Phosphorus–Magnesium

Consumption of excess phosphorus as well as of calcium accentuates the signs of magnesium deficiency, primarily by decreasing magnesium absorption (17–19). The effects of calcium and phosphorus are additive (Figure 5).

D. Micro-Element Interactions

Commonly recognized in-vivo interactions involving the essential micro-elements are depicted in Figure 6. The more significant nutritionally important interactions are one-way, and they are discussed below from the standpoint of the limiting nutrient.

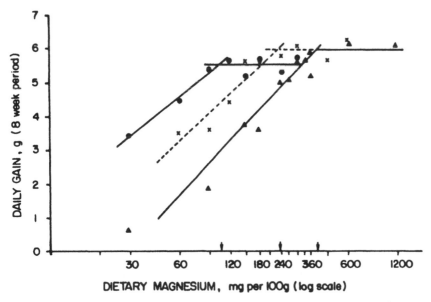

FIGURE 5 Effect of excess dietary concentration of calcium and phosphorus on magnesium bioavailability in guinea pigs. At near normal levels, 0.9% calcium and 0.8% phosphorus (●), magnesium requirement was 1.0 g/kg diet; at 3.2% calcium and 0.8% phosphorus (×), 2.4 g/kg; at 2.5% calcium and 1.7% phosphorus (▲), 4.0 g/kg. (From Ref. 91.)

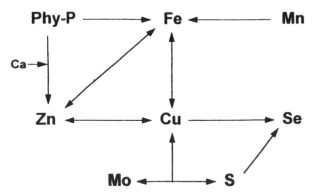

FIGURE 6 Interactions involving the essential trace elements. Phy-P designates both phytate and inorganic phosphate. The effect of phytate on zinc is accentuated by calcium.

1. Iron

The absorption and utilization of iron are affected negatively by excess of several dietary components, including zinc, manganese, and copper. Phosphate, in its inorganic as well as organic (phytate) form, also interacts with iron. Excess dietary zinc causes anemia and generally impairs iron utilization. The anemia appears to be largely the result of the effect of excess zinc on copper metabolism, inducing a secondary copper deficiency. Copper is essential for iron absorption and utilization, and thus for hemoglobin formation and the prevention of anemia (20–22). In copper deficiency there is failure of iron mobilization from some tissues, resulting in iron accumulation (20–22). Excess zinc tends to reduce tissue iron concentrations (23,24). If the only effect of excess zinc were the induction of copper deficiency, one would expect increased tissue iron concentrations. Hence, the mechanism must involve also a direct antagonistic effect of zinc on iron metabolism. High zinc (0.75% of diet) intake by rats did not affect iron absorption but decreased its incorporation into ferritin and other storage proteins (25).

Excessive intake of manganese interferes with iron metabolism. When iron intake was minimal, a small excess of manganese (45 mg/kg) caused anemia and low serum iron in lambs (26). Tissue iron concentrations were reduced by high levels of manganese (26,27). The antagonistic effect of manganese appears to reside at the iron absorption site. In iron deficiency, both manganese and iron absorption were enhanced; manganese supplementation decreased iron absorption in iron-deficient animals (28).

There is evidence that high dietary copper has a direct antagonistic effect on iron metabolism. In iron-depleted rats fed a diet limiting in iron (15 mg/kg), low levels of dietary copper, up to 5 mg/kg, improved hemoglobin repletion, but there was progressive lack of improvement from 7.5 to 20 mg/kg of copper, suggesting antagonism (29). Recent evidence in the rat supports the concept that copper is a direct antagonist of iron metabolism (30).

Inorganic phosphate depresses iron absorption and utilization (31,32). Phytate, inositol hexaphosphate, also decreases iron bioavailability (31,33), although not all investigators have confirmed this observation (34). Phytate appears to depress absorption of ferrous iron, even as the ascorbate complex, but not of hemoglobin iron (35).

2. Copper

The bioavailability of copper is affected negatively by zinc, iron, and a copper–molybdenum–sulfur complex. In practice, probably the most significant interaction among trace elements in monogastric animals is the negative effect of excess zinc on copper absorption and utilization. Early observations (24,36,37) showed that high dietary levels of zinc induce signs of copper deficiency, including anemia and decreased activity of cytochrome C oxidase. The effects were reversed or prevented by copper supplementation. Antagonistic effects of zinc on copper have also been observed with normal dietary levels of zinc when the copper level was limiting. This is illustrated in Figure 7. Besides the effect on growth rate and elastin crosslinking, slight excesses of zinc aggravate other signs of copper deficiency, including low heart and liver superoxide dismutase activities as well as low total liver copper concentration (38–40).

The interaction of zinc and copper is also manifested in plasma concentrations of the ions. In zinc-deficient animals the plasma copper concentration increases as plasma zinc decreases (39,41). It is generally assumed that this aspect of zinc–copper antagonism is mediated via metallothionein. Zinc induces this metal-binding protein in mucosal cells, and zinc–metallothionein accumulates when zinc is in excess. Metallothionein binds copper more strongly than zinc, so the latter is replaced by copper. According to this concept, copper metallothionein is excreted unabsorbed when the mucosal cells are sloughed, thereby reducing the absorption of copper (42). However, in a recent study (42a), a high dietary zinc level induced high metallothionein in the mucosa and signs of copper deficiency, but the mucosal copper concentration was not changed. Thus, zinc may affect copper absorption by another mechanism. During the absorption process in vivo, copper may be compartmentalized so as not to contact metallothionein; the ions may interact at the luminal absorption site.

Although copper deficiency in adult humans is rare, it has been induced by zinc therapy (43). Hypocupremia, microcytosis, and neutropenia occurred in a sickle cell

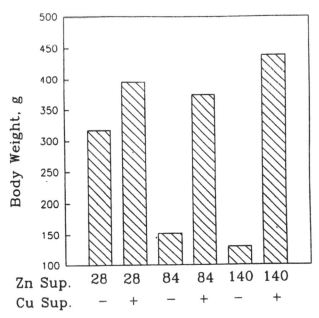

FIGURE 7 Zinc–copper interaction in chicks, as shown by the effect on growth rate. Growing chicks were fed a milk-based diet supplemented with three levels of zinc, 28, 84, and 140 mg/kg, with and without a copper supplement. The zinc supplements were within or only slightly above normal diet concentrations, and the basal diet was marginally deficient in copper. (Data from Ref. 38.)

anemia patient treated with zinc as an antisickling agent. Copper therapy corrected the signs of copper deficiency.

There is increasing evidence, particularly in ruminant animals, that excess iron interacts negatively with copper (3). High dietary iron:copper ratios also reduced the hepatic storage of copper in guinea pigs (44) and pigs (45). The mechanism of the iron–copper interaction is unknown, but it is potentiated in the rat as well as in ruminants by the presence of sulfide in the digestive tract (3).

Another interaction of considerable practical importance in the production of ruminant animals is the multiple interaction of Cu–Mo–S (3). Ingested molybdenum reacts in the rumen with endogenous sulfide to form tetrathiomolybdate or oxythiomolybdates, which in turn react with copper to form insoluble complexes. The complexes have been identified as copper thiomolybdates, $Cu(MoO_nS_{4-n})$ (35a). There is good evidence that tetrathiomolybdate decreases copper absorption (35b and references therein). These reactions are normally of little importance in monogastric animals, but if thiomolybdate is introduced directly into the blood, copper utilization is impaired.

3. Zinc

In spite of the strong negative effect of zinc on copper bioavailability, the converse effect of copper on zinc is minimal under physiologic conditions. In rat intestinal segments, a high (50:1) copper:zinc ratio significantly decreased zinc absorption compared to more physiologic ratios (46). There are few studies involving high copper:zinc ratios in intact animals, but excess dietary copper potentiated the teratogenicity of zinc deficiency in the rat (47).

The effect of excess iron on zinc bioavailability is not clear. There was increased zinc absorption in iron-depleted animals (48,49), and decreased zinc absorption when a high level of ferrous iron was administered as a single dose with zinc (50,51). However, high iron:zinc ratios did not affect zinc absorption when the zinc was supplied in a food or total meal (52). No detrimental effect of high dietary iron on zinc status was observed in infants (53) or in growing rats (54). On balance, it appears unlikely that the common dietary iron supplements adversely affect zinc absorption and utilization.

Although copper and iron interact minimally with zinc to decrease absorption and utilization, organic phosphate in the form of phytate has a major deleterious effect. Phytate (inositol hexa- and pentaphosphates) forms stable and insoluble complexes with zinc. This decreases the absorption of zinc and induces zinc deficiency when the dietary level of the element is near the requirement (55–58). The detrimental effect of phytate on zinc bioavailability is aggravated by excess dietary calcium (56–59). The effect of phytate is alleviated by chelating compounds, such as EDTA ($K_d = 3 \times 10^{-17}$), that form a reasonably high-affinity but soluble complex with zinc (59). Calcium alone does not interact significantly with zinc, but there is a strong multiple interaction of zinc, calcium, and phytate. It appears that a highly insoluble Ca–Zn–phytate complex is formed in the intestine, impairing zinc absorption. Complex formation is detrimental when dietary zinc is limiting and the phytate:zinc molar ratio is at or above approximately 15. Excess Ca accentuates the negative effect and must be factored into the equation relating phytate and zinc. Because of their high phytate content, and possibly because of other zinc-binding components, foods of plant seed origin generally exhibit low zinc bioavailability (60–63).

4. Selenium

Extremely high dietary levels, 100 times the usual concentrations, of copper or zinc induced signs of selenium deficiency in chicks (64). The resulting exudative diathesis was prevented by supplementary selenium. Dietary copper at 200 mg/kg had no effect on ^{75}Se-selenite absorption in the rat, but it lowered the ^{75}Se found in liver, heart, and lungs while increasing it in testis (65). Slight excesses of copper and zinc have no practical effect on selenium bioavailability.

Considering the chemical similarity of selenium and sulfur, one might expect metabolic antagonism. This concept is supported by the observation that Na_2SO_4 decreased the effectiveness of Na_2SeO_3 in preventing white muscle disease in lambs and calves (66,67). However, if there is antagonism between sulfur and selenium, the speciation or chemical form of selenium involved affects the degree of interaction. Addition of K_2SO_4 to an organic source of selenium did not accentuate the signs of selenium deficiency in lambs (68). The effect of speciation is also demonstrated by the fact that methionine does not alter selenite biopotency, but increases that of selenomethionine (69).

IV. ION CHANNELS AND ASSESSMENT OF INTERACTIONS

Interaction of ions occurs at, or in, ion channels, but the nutritional and physiologic significance of these interactions is unknown. Nevertheless, the mechanisms involved may shed light on interactions of physiologic significance that occur at other sites.

A. Definition and Description of Ion Channels

Ion channels are selectively permeable areas of plasma membranes. During the past 50 years the concept of ion channels has moved from a biophysical notion to the identification of the molecular components of several channels, i.e., structures of the protein subunits of the membrane complexes. Ion channels were first found in excitable tissue, and those most commonly studied in mammals occur in the central nervous system (CNS). Ion channels may be classed as ligand gated (agonist sensitive) or voltage gated (potential sensitive); specific channels that accommodate sodium, potassium, calcium, or chloride ions have been studied in depth. Table 2 lists examples of the two classes of commonly recognized ion channels. While it is beyond the scope of this chapter to discuss these channels in detail, it is of special interest that the movement of chloride across the apical membrane of secretory epithelial cells of the airways and pancreas is defective in cystic fibrosis patients. There are normally two types of chloride channels in these cells: One is activated by calcium and one by a c-AMP dependent process. Only the latter type of channel is impaired in cystic fibrosis.

In addition to ion channels, there are ion pumps that require the direct expenditure of energy in the form of ATP to transport ions across membranes and maintain cellular ion balance. These pumps are commonly phosphorylating adenosine triphosphatases (P-ATPase), such as Na,K-ATPase, which pumps Na^+ out of cells in exchange for K^+, and Ca-ATPase, which pumps Ca^{2+} out of cells in exchange for protons. There are also ion exchangers, such as the Na–Ca antiporter, that facilitate the exchange of ions without the direct expenditure of energy. Specific ions are known to inhibit ion pumps, but interactions at the level of ion pumps is beyond the scope of this chapter.

Ion transport through specific channels plays a key role in numerous aspects of cell regulation. For example, in neurons the action potential is initiated by increased Na^+ permeability and associated rapid depolarization. Under these conditions Ca^{2+} also enters the cell through voltage-sensitive calcium channels. The increased intracellular Ca^{2+}

TABLE 2   Voltage- and Ligand-Gated Ion Channels

Ion transported	Ligand	Source
Voltage-gated		
Na$^+$	—	Muscle, CNS (71)
K$^+$	—	CNS (72)
Ca^{2+}	—	Muscle, CNS (71)
Ligand-gated		
Na$^+$, K$^+$	Acetylcholine	Muscle and nerve
Na$^+$, K$^+$, Ca^{2+}	Glutamate (NMDA[a])	Neuron (73,74)
Na$^+$, K$^+$	Glutamate (kainate and AMPA[b])	Neurons (73)
K$^+$	Ca-activated	CNS, red cells (72)
Cl$^-$	GABA$_A$[c]	Neurons (CNS)
Cl$^-$	Glycine	Neurons (CNS)
Cl$^-$	c-AMP, Ca^{2+}	Epithelial cells (89)

[a]N-methyl-D-aspartate (NMDA) is an agonist for one glutamate receptor subtype.
[b]α-Amino-3-hydroxy-5-methyl-isoxazole-4-propionate (AMPA) and kainate are agonists for specific subtypes of the glutamate receptor.
[c]γ-Aminobutyric acid (GABA) is an agonist for the GABA$_A$ receptor.
Source: Adapted from Ref. 70.

concentration activates various biochemical processes. Following activation, the potassium channel allows outward movement of K$^+$ and repolarization of the cell (71). Figure 8 depicts the overall subunit structures of sodium and calcium channels. The sodium channel is composed of three polypeptide subunits, α, β$_1$, and β$_2$, and the calcium channel of five polypeptides. There is considerable similarity of amino acid sequence between calcium channel α$_1$ and sodium channel α. Each has four homologous domains, and it is postulated that there are six transmembrane segments per domain. The potassium channel is similar except that it has only one such domain (71).

B.   Specific Ion Interactions

While the discussion of in-vivo ion interactions was separated into major and minor elements, such distinction is less pertinent in the case of ion channels because they accommodate both classes of ions at catalytic concentrations. The commonly recognized ion channels are permeable primarily to ions that are nutritionally classified as major elements, including calcium, sodium, potassium, and chloride. Within the cell these ions perform regulatory roles at extremely low concentrations, levels that are highly analogous to those at which the minor elements perform catalytic or cofactor roles. In this sense the major elements serve as catalysts or second messengers. For example, the free calcium ion concentration in extracellular fluids, such as plasma, is approximately 10,000 times the intracellular concentration, 1000 μM versus 0.1 μM. The intracellular concentration of calcium may rise as much as 10-fold following cell stimulation, the surge or "puff" serving as a cell signal or second messenger. Interactions at the ion channels involve minor as well as major elements. It must be recognized that the interactions observed have been made with in-vitro systems, and there is no evidence that they are either significant or applicable in vivo. Specific examples of in-vitro interactions are discussed by ion channel.

Na⁺ channel

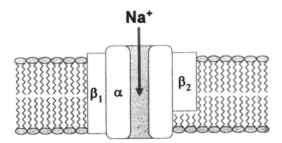

Ca²⁺ channel

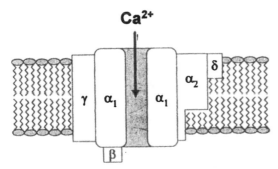

FIGURE 8 Proposed subunit structures of sodium and calcium channels. Depicted are three subunits and the pore for a sodium channel, and five subunits and the pore for a calcium channel. The amino acid sequences suggest that sodium α and calcium α_1 subunits traverse the membrane six times in each of four homologous domains (71). (Adapted from Ref. 71.)

1. Calcium Channel

Calcium enters cells by way of both voltage- and ligand-gated channels, and by a process of facilitated diffusion (75–77). Voltage-operated calcium channels are found primarily in excitable cells, such as neurons in the CNS. The movement of calcium through these channels is inhibited by several divalent cations, notably the essential elements magnesium and manganese (75). Examples of ions that inhibit both voltage-gated and ligand-gated calcium channels are listed in Table 3.

Several different ions inhibit both types of channels. Most are trace elements, some of known and some of unknown function. A notable exception is the major element magnesium, which bears a remarkably similar ionic structure to that of calcium. Zinc is conspicuous because of its inhibition of ligand-gated calcium channels at low concentrations, 3–10 μM. The inhibitory effect of magnesium on ligand-gated channels is voltage sensitive, while that of zinc, added in vitro, is independent of membrane potential (73,74).

2. Sodium Channel

Interactions of ions at or in sodium, potassium, and chloride channels are summarized in Table 4. Calcium was observed to inhibit the voltage-gated sodium channel in renal tubular

TABLE 3 Ion Interactions at Calcium Channels

Inhibitory ion	Ligand	Channel location
Voltage-gated Ca^{2+} channel		
Mg^{2+}	—	Neurons (75)
Mn^{2+}	—	Neurons (75), cerebellum (77)
Cd^{2+}	—	Neurons (75), cerebellum (77)
Ni^{2+}	—	Neurons (75)
Co^{2+}	—	Neurons (75), cerebellum (77)
Ligand-gated Ca^{2+} channel		
Zn^{2+}, Cd^{2+}	Vasopressin	Hepatocytes (78)
Ni^{2+}, Co^{2+}	Vasopressin	Hepatocytes (78)
Mg^{2+}	NMDA[a]	Neurons: spinal cord (79), hippocampal (80)
Zn^{2+}	NMDA[a]	Neurons: cortical (81,82), hippocampal (83)

[a]Magnesium inhibition of the NMDA channel is voltage dependent, while that of zinc is independent of membrane potential.

cells (84). The sodium permeability of the apical (luminal) membrane was reduced when the intracellular free calcium concentration was increased. Both magnesium and zinc decrease the movement of calcium, and probably of sodium, through the N-methyl-D-aspartate (NMDA) subtype of the glutamate receptor channel (79–82).

3. Potassium Channels

There are several types of potassium channels, including voltage-dependent and calcium-activated potassium channels (72). Cesium ions are nonspecific blockers of most types of potassium channels. Notably, sodium inhibits the calcium-activated potassium channel in erythrocyte membranes (86).

TABLE 4 Ion Interactions at Sodium, Potassium, and Chloride Channels

Inhibitory Ion	Ligand	Location
Sodium channels		
Ca^{2+}	VG[a]	Renal epithelium1 (84)
Mg^{2+}	NMDA[b]	Neurons: spinal cord (79), hippocampal (80)
Zn^{2+}	NMDA[b]	Neurons: cortical (81,82), hippocampal (83)
Potassium channels		
Cd^{2+}	Ca^{2+}	Gastric smooth muscle (85)
Na^+, Cs^+	Ca^{2+}	Erythrocytes (86)
Chloride channels		
Zn^{2+}, Cd^{2+} Ni^{2+}, Mn^{2+}	GABA	Neurons: spinal cord (87)
Zn^{2+}		Neurons: hippocampal (88)

[a]A voltage-gated channel.
[b]Magnesium inhibition of the NMDA channel is voltage dependent, while that of zinc is independent of membrane potential.

4. Chloride Channel

The GABA$_A$ receptor transports chloride ions and serves as an inhibitor of neuronal activity. This chloride channel is inhibited by zinc and other transition element ions (87). There is also a voltage-gated chloride channel that is inhibited by Zn^{2+} (88).

The physiologic significance of the ion interactions observed in vitro is unknown, but there is no evidence for the impairment of ion channel function by competitive ions in vivo. The significance of the observed interactions lies primarily in the insight they provide with regard to mechanisms of ion interactions at the cell level. From the standpoint of overall ion interaction, they may be instructive with regard to mechanisms of ion absorption at specific sites in the intestine.

V. CONCLUSIONS AND PERSPECTIVES

Mineral ions of similar electron structure in the outer d orbitals tend to interact by competing for sites on proteins that play catalytic, membrane transport, or other functional role at the molecular level. When one of the competing, or antagonistic, ions is essential but present in the diet at a low or limiting concentration and the other is in excess, function of the organism may be impaired and deficiency signs produced. Present knowledge suggests that nutritionally the most significant ion interactions occur at intestinal absorption sites. Clearly, there are interactions beyond mucosal absorption, but there is minimal evidence for interactions at the level of catalytic sites. On the other hand, there is strong in-vitro evidence that ion interactions occur at plasma membrane ion channels.

Little is known about the mechanism involved in mineral ion absorption, a basic concept that deserves research attention. There is a dearth of information about the structure and function of intestinal mucosa absorption sites. This is in marked contrast to the extensive knowledge of ion channels and their mechanisms of function. The well-defined ion channels should be explored as models of absorption sites. Another area of increasing interest and one that offers promise of providing insight into the mechanisms of membrane transport and the interactions at that level is genetics. For example, it has been shown recently (92) that a yeast gene encodes a protein required for copper transport and that deletion of the gene impairs ferrous ion uptake. Considering the more practical aspects of mineral interaction, it is obvious that there are few quantitative data relative to magnitude of the many mineral interactions that have been identified in vivo.

REFERENCES

1. Hill CH, Matrone G. Chemical parameters in the study of in vivo and in vitro interactions of transition elements. Fed Proc 1970; 29:1474–1481.
2. Kirchgessner M, Schwarz FJ, Schnegg A. Interactions of essential metals in human physiology. In: Prasad AS, ed. Clinical, Biochemical and Nutritional Aspects of Trace Elements. Vol I. New York: Alan R. Liss, 1982:477–512.
3. Mills CF. Dietary interactions involving the trace elements. Ann Rev Nutr 1985; 5:173–193.
4. O'Dell BL. Bioavailability of and interactions among trace elements. In: Chandra RK, ed. Trace Elements in Nutrition of Children. Nestle Nutrition. New York: Vevey/Raven Press, 1985:41–62.
5. Hill CH. Mineral interrelationships. In: Prasad AS, ed. Trace Elements in Human Health and Disease. Vol. II. New York: Academic Press, 1976:281–300.
6. Thomson CD, Stewart DH. Metabolic studies of ^{75}Se-selenomethionine and ^{75}Se-selenite in the rat. Br J Nutr 1973; 30:139–147.

7. Seal CJ, Heaton FW. Chemical factors affecting intestinal absorption of zinc in vitro and in vivo. Br J Nutr 1983; 50:317–324.

8. Addison WLT. The use of sodium chloride, potassium chloride and potassium bromide in cases of arterial hypertension which are amenable to potassium chloride. Can Med Assoc J 1928; 18:281–285.

9. Meneely GR, Ball COT. Experimental epidemiology of chronic sodium chloride toxicity and the protective effect of potassium chloride. Am J Med 1958; 25:713–725.

10. Dahl LK, Leitl G, Heine M. Influence of dietary potassium and sodium/potassium molar ratios on the development of salt hypertension. J Exp Med 1972; 136:318–330.

11. Bethke RM, Kick CH, Wilder W. The effect of calcium-phosphorus relationship on growth, calcification, and blood composition of the rat. J Biol Chem 1938; 98:389–403.

12. Ketaren PP, Batterham ES, Dettman EB, Farrell DJ. Phosphorus studies in pigs. 2. Assessing phosphorus availability for pigs and rats. Br J Nutr 1993; 70:269–288.

13. Spencer H, Menczel J, Lewin I, Samachson J. Effect of high phosphorus intake on calcium and phosphorus metabolism in man. J Nutr 1965; 86:125–132.

14. Spencer H, Kramer L, Osis D, Norris C. Effect of phosphorus on the absorption of calcium and on the calcium balance in man. J Nutr 1978; 108:447–457.

15. Hegsted M, Shuette SA, Zemel MB, Linkswiler HM. Urinary calcium and calcium balance in young men as affected by level of protein and phosphorus intake. J Nutr 1981; 111:553–562.

16. Tufts EV, Greenberg DM. The biochemistry of magnesium deficiency. II. The minimum requirement magnesium requirement for growth, gestation and lactation and the effect of the dietary calcium thereon. J Biol Chem 1937; 122:715–726.

17. O'Dell BL, Morris ER, Regan WO. Magnesium requirement of guinea pigs and rats. Effect of calcium and phosphorus and symptoms of magnesium deficiency. J Nutr 1960; 70:103–111.

18. Bunce GE, Chiemchaisri Y, Phillips PH. The mineral requirements of the dog. IV. Effect of certain dietary and physiologic factors upon magnesium deficiency syndrome. J Nutr 1962; 76:23–29.

19. Toothill J. The effect of certain dietary factors on the apparent absorption of magnesium by the rat. Br J Nutr 1963; 17:125–134.

20. Lee CR, Nacht S, Lukens JN, Cartwright GE. Iron metabolism in copper-deficient swine. J Clin Invest 1968; 47:2058–2069.

21. Marston HR, Allen SH, Swaby SL. Iron metabolism in copper-deficient rats. Br J Nutr 1971; 25:15–30.

22. Evans JL, Abraham PA. Anemia, iron storage and ceruloplasmin in copper nutrition in the growing rat. J Nutr 1973; 103:196–201.

23. Cox DH, Harris DL. Effect of excess dietary zinc on iron and copper in the rat. J Nutr 1960; 70:514–520.

24. Magee AC, Matrone G. Studies on the growth, copper metabolism and iron metabolism of rats fed high levels of zinc. J Nutr 1960; 72:233–242.

25. Cox DH, Harris DL. Reduction of liver xanthine oxidase activity and iron storage proteins in rats fed excess zinc. J Nutr 1962; 78:415–418.

26. Hartman RH, Matrone G, Wise GH. Effect of high dietary manganese on hemoglobin formation. J Nutr 1955; 57:429–439.

27. Matrone G, Hartman RH, Clawson AJ. Studies of manganese-iron antagonism in the nutrition of rabbits and baby pigs. J Nutr 1959; 67:309–317.

28. Thompson ABR, Olatunbosun P, Valberg LS. Interrelation of intestinal transport system for manganese and iron. J Lab Clin Med 1971; 78:642–655.

29. Fritz JC, Pla GW, Harrison BN, Clark GA, Smith EA. Measurement of the bioavailability of iron, using the rat hemoglobin repletion test. J Assoc Offic Anal Chem 1977; 61:709–714.

30. Gordon DT. Interactions among iron, zinc and copper. Proceedings of Minisymposia, American Institute of Nutrition. Nutrition 1987; 1987:27–31.

31. Hegsted DM, Finch CA, Kinney TD. The influence of diet on iron absorption. The interrelationship of iron and phosphorus. J Exp Med 1949; 90:147–156.

32. Peters T, Apt L, Ross JF. Effect of phosphates upon iron absorption studies in normal human subjects and in an experimental model using dialysis. Gastroenterology 1971; 61:315–322.

33. Apte SV, Venkatachalam PS. Iron absorption in human volunteers using high phytate cereal diet. Indian J Med Res 1962; 50:516–520.

34. Cowan JW, Esfahani M, Salji JP, Azzam SA. Effect of phytate on iron absorption in the rat. J Nutr 1966; 90:423–427.

35. Turnbull A, Cleton F, Finch CA. Iron absorption. II. The absorption of hemoglobin iron. J Clin Invest 1962; 41:1897–1907.

35a. Dick AT, Dewey DW, Gawthorne JM. Thiomolybdates and the copper-molybdenum interaction in ruminant nutrition. J Agr Sci (Cambridge) 1975; 85:567–568.

35b. Mason J, Lamand CA, Kelleher CA. The fate of ^{99}Mo-labeled sodium tetrathiomolybdate after duodenal administration in sheep: the effect on ceruloplasmin diamine oxidase activity and plasma copper. Br J Nutr 1980; 43:515–523.

36. Smith SE, Larson EJ. Zinc toxicity in rats. Antagonistic effect of copper on liver. J Biol Chem 1946; 163:29–38.

37. VanReen R. Effects of excessive dietary zinc in the rat and the interrelationship with copper. Arch Biochem Biophys 1953; 46:337–344.

38. O'Dell BL. Dietary interactions of copper and zinc. In: Hemphill DD, ed. Trace Substances in Environmental Health. Vol 1. Columbia, MO: University of Missouri, 1967:134–140.

39. Murthy L, Klevay LM, Petering HG. Interrelationships of zinc and copper nutriture in the rat. J Nutr 1974; 104:1458–1465.

40. L'Abbe MR, Fischer PWF. The effects of high dietary zinc and copper deficiency on the activity of copper-requiring metalloenzymes in the growing rat. J Nutr 1984; 114:813–822.

41. O'Dell BL, Reeves PG, Morgan RF. Interrelationships of tissue copper and zinc concentrations in rats nutritionally deficient in one or the other of these elements. In: Hemphill DD, ed. Trace Substances in Environmental Health. Vol X. Columbia, MO: University of Missouri, 1976: 411–421.

42. Hall AC, Young BW, Bremner I. Intestinal metallothionein and the mutual antagonism between copper and zinc in the rat. J Inorg Biochem 1979; 11:57–66.

42a. Reeves PG, Rossow KL, Bobilya DJ. Zinc-induced metallothionein and copper metabolism in intestinal mucosa, liver and kidney of rats. Nutr Res 1993; 13:1419–1431.

43. Prasad AS, Brewer GJ, Shoomaker EB, Rabbani P. Hypocupremia induced by zinc therapy in adults. JAMA 1978; 240:2166–2168.

44. Smith CH, Bidlack WR. Interrelationships of dietary ascorbic acid and iron on the tissue distribution of ascorbic acid, iron and copper in female guinea pigs. J Nutr 1988; 110:1398–1408.

45. Hedges JD, Kornegay ET. Interrelationships of dietary copper and iron as measured by blood parameters, tissue stores and feedlot performance of swine. J Animal Sci 1973; 37:1147–1154.

46. Van Campen DR. Copper interference with the intestinal absorption of zinc-65 by the rat. J Nutr 1969; 97:104–108.

47. Reinstein NH, Lonnerdal B, Keen CL, Hurley LS. Zinc-copper interactions in the pregnant rat: fetal outcome and maternal and fetal zinc, copper and iron. J Nutr 1984; 114:1266–1279.

48. Pollack S, George JN, Reba RC, Kaufman RM, Crosby WA. The absorption of non-ferrous metals in iron deficiency. J Clin Invest 1965; 44:1470–1473.

49. Flanagan PR, Harst J, Valberg LS. Comparative effects of iron deficiency induced by bleeding and a low-iron diet on the intestinal absorptive interactions of iron, cobalt, manganese, zinc, lead and cadmium. J Nutr 1980; 110:1754–1763.

50. Solomons NW, Jacob RA. Studies on the bioavailability of zinc in humans: effects of heme and nonheme iron on the absorption of zinc. Am J Clin Nutr 1981; 34:475–482.

51. Meadows NW, Grainger SL, Ruse W, Keeling PWN, Thompson RPH. Oral iron and the bioavailability of zinc. Br Med J 1983; 287:1013–1014.

52. Sandstrom B, Davidson L, Cederblad A, Lonnerdal B. Oral iron, dietary ligands and zinc absorption. J Nutr 1985; 115:411–414.

53. Yip R, Reeves JD, Lonnerdal B, Keen CL, Dallman PR. Does iron supplementation compromise zinc nutrition in healthy infants? Am J Clin Nutr 1985; 42:683–687.

54. Storey ML, Greger JL. Iron, zinc and copper interactions: chronic versus acute responses of rats. J Nutr 1987; 117:1434–1442.

55. O'Dell BL, Savage JE. Effect of phytic acid on zinc availability. Proc Soc Exp Biol Med 1960; 103:304–306.

56. Likuski HJA, Forbes RM. Mineral utilization in the rat. IV. Effect of calcium and phytic acid on the utilization of dietary zinc. J Nutr 1965; 85:230–234.

57. Oberleas D, Muhrer ME, O'Dell BL. Effects of phytic acid on zinc availability and parakeratosis in swine. J Animal Sci 1962; 21:57–61.

58. Turnlund JR, King JC, Keyes WR, Gorig B, Michel MC. A stable isotope study of zinc absorption in young men: effects of phytate and α-cellulose. Am J Clin Nutr 1984; 40:1071–1077.

59. Oberleas D, Muhrer ME, O'Dell BL. Dietary metal complexing agents and zinc availability in the rat. J Nutr 1966; 90:56–62.

60. O'Dell BL, Burpo CE, Savage JE. Evaluation of zinc availability in foodstuffs of plant and animal origin. J Nutr 1972; 102:653–660.

61. Momcilovic B, Belonje B, Giroux A, Shah BG. Bioavailability of zinc in milk and soy protein-based infant formulas. J Nutr 1976; 106:913–917.

62. Forbes RM, Weingartner KE, Parker HM, Bell RR, Erdman JW. Bioavailability to rats of zinc, magnesium and calcium in casein-, egg- and soy protein-containing diets. J Nutr 1979; 109:1652–1660.

63. Hunt JR, Johnson PE, Swan PB. Dietary conditions influencing relative zinc availability from foods to the rat and correlations with in vitro measurements. J Nutr 1987; 117:1913–1923.

64. Jensen LS. Precipitation of a selenium deficiency by high dietary levels of copper and zinc. Proc Soc Exp Biol Med 1975; 149:113–116.

65. Rahim AGA, Arthur JR, Mills CF. Effects of dietary copper, cadmium, iron, molybdenum and manganese on selenium utilization by the rat. J Nutr 1986; 116:403–411.

66. Muth OH, Schubert JR, Oldfield JE. White muscle disease (myopathy) in lambs and calves. VII. Etiology and prophylaxis. Am J Vet Res 1961; 22:466–469.

67. Hentz HF, Hogue DE. Effect of selenium, sulfur and sulfur amino acids on nutritional muscular dystrophy in the lamb. J Nutr 1964; 82:495–497.

68. Whanger PD, Muth OH, Oldfield JE, Weswig PH. Influence of sulfur on incidence of white muscle disease in lambs. J Nutr 1969; 97:553–562.

69. Sunde RA, Gutzke GE, Hoekstra WG. Effect of dietary methionine on the biopotency of selenite and selenomethionine in the rat. J Nutr 1981; 111:76–86.

70. Barnard EA, Darlison MG, Marshall J, Satelle DB. Structural characteristics of cation and anion channels directly operated by agonists. In: Keeling D, Benham C, eds. Ion Transport. New York: Academic Press, 1989:159–181.

71. Catterall WA. Structure and function of voltage-sensitive ion channels. Science 1988; 242:50–61.

72. Rudy B. Diversity and ubiquity of K channels. Neuroscience 1988; 25:729–749.

73. Cotman CW, Bridges RJ, Taube JS, Clark AS, Geddes JW, Monaghan DT. The role of the NMDA receptor in central nervous system plasticity and pathology. J NIH Res 1988; 1:65–74.

74. Reynolds IJ. Modulation of NMDA receptor responsiveness by neurotransmitters, drugs and chemical modification. Life Sci 1990; 47:1785–1792.

75. Reuter H. Calcium channel modulation by neurotransmitters, enzymes and drugs. Nature 1983; 301:569–574.

76. Hosey MM, Lazdunski M. Calcium channels: molecular pharmacology, structure and regulation. J Membrane Biol 1988; 104:81–105.

77. Carboni E, Wojcik WJ. Dihydropyridine binding sites regulate calcium influx through specific voltage-sensitive calcium channels in cerebellar granule cells. J Neurochem 1988; 50:1279–1286.

78. Hughes BP, Barritt GJ. Inhibition of the liver cell receptor-activated Ca^{2+} inflow system by metal inhibitors of voltage-operated Ca^{2+} channels but not by other inhibitors of Ca^{2+} inflow. Biochim Biophys Acta 1989; 1013:197–205.
79. Mayer ML, Westbrook GL, Guthrie PB. Voltage-dependent block by Mg^{2+} of NMDA responses in spinal cord neurons. Nature 1984; 309:261–263.
80. Ascher P, Nowak L. Electrophysiological studies of NMDA receptors. Trends Neurosci 1987; 10:284–288.
81. Peters S, Koh J, Choi DW. Zinc selectively blocks the action of N-methyl-D-aspartate on cortical neurons. Science 1987; 236:589–593.
82. Christine CW, Choi DW. Effect of zinc on NMDA receptor-mediated channel currents in cortical neurons. J Neurosci 1990; 10:108–116.
83. Westbrook GL, Mayer ML. Micromolar concentrations of Zn^{2+} antagonize NMDA and GABA responses of hippocampal neurons. Nature 1987; 328:640–643.
84. Frindt G, Windhager EE. Regulatory role of calcium in sodium transport. In: Bolis CL, Helmreich EJM, Passow H, eds. Information and Energy Transduction in Biological Membranes. New York: Alan R. Liss, 1984:403–406.
85. Mitra R, Morad M. Ca^{2+} and Ca^{2+}-activated K^+ currents in mammalian gastric smooth muscle cells. Science 1985; 229:269–272.
86. Schwarz W, Passow H. Ca^{2+}-activated K^+ channels in erythrocytes and excitable cells. Annu Rev Physiol 1983; 45:359–374.
87. Celentano JJ, Gyenes M, Gibbs TT, Farb DH. Negative modulation of the γ-aminobutyric acid response by extracellular zinc. Mol Pharmacol 1991; 40:766–773.
88. Franciolini F, Nonner W. Anion and cation permeability of a chloride channel in rat hippocampal neurons. J Gen Physiol 1987; 90:453–478.
89. Frizzell RA. Cystic fibrosis: a disease of ion channels? TINS 1987; 10:190–193.
90. Hempe JM, Zinc bioavailability in the chick. Ph.D. dissertation, University of Missouri, Columbia, MO, 1987.
91. O'Dell BL, Morris ER. Relationship of excess calcium and phosphorus to magnesium requirement and toxicity in guinea pigs. J Nutr 1963; 81:175–181.
92. Dancis A, Yuan DS, Haile D, et al. Molecular characterization of a copper transport protein in *S. cerevisiae*: an unexpected role for copper in iron transport. Cell 1994; 76:393–402.

25

Radiotracers for Nutritionally Essential Mineral Elements

Kurt R. Zinn

University of Alabama at Birmingham, Birmingham, Alabama

I. INTRODUCTION*

Many radioactive isotopes, also referred to as radioisotopes or radionuclides, are readily available from commercial sources or research centers. However, certain radionuclides with research potential are not readily available. In the latter case, experimentalists require additional knowledge in order to make special requests or to determine if certain production routes are applicable for their research purposes. This chapter focuses on the radioisotopes that are unique and particularly applicable to mineral nutrition research. Other radio-nuclides widely utilized in the life sciences are included in tables.

While this chapter focuses on radioactive isotopes, it is recognized that enriched stable isotopes of natural low abundance are alternative tracers for certain elements. They have the advantage of avoiding the use of radioactivity, but are more expensive due to the initial cost of the enriched isotope, as well as the difficulties in ultimately measuring the enriched isotope. Typically, measurement of stable isotope concentration requires either neutron activation or mass spectrometry techniques. Enriched stable isotopes are not feasible tracers for all minerals, since not all elements have isotopes of low abundance. Also, the large mass of enriched stable isotope often required for accurate measurement may prevent their use as a tracer. This is not a limitation for radioactive isotopes. Safety for human studies is the main advantage of the use of enriched stable isotopes.

---

*A list of abbreviations is provided in Table 1 and a glossary of terms in Table 2.

TABLE 1 Abbreviations

Term	Abbreviation	Term	Abbreviation
Activity (radioactivity)	A	Isometric transition	IT
Alpha decay	α decay	Kiloelectron-volt	KeV (1E3 eV)
Alpha particle	α	Megabecquerel	MBq (1E6 Bq)
Becquerel	Bq	Microcurie	μCi (1E-6 Ci)
Beta minus decay	β^- decay	Microgram	μg (1E-6 g)
Beta plus decay	β^+ decay	Millicurie	mCi (1E-3 Ci)
Curie	Ci	Milligram	mg (1E-3 g)
Day(s)	d	Minute(s)	m
Disintegrations per second	dps	Neutron	n
Decay constant, radioactive	λ	Neutron cross section	σ
Electron capture	EC	Neutron flux	Φ
Electron volt	eV	Positron decay	β^+ decay
exp-(x)	$e^{-(x)}$	Proton	p
Fast	F	Resonance	r
Gamma ray	γ	Resonance integral	RI
Gram	g	Second(s)	s
Half-life	$t_{1/2}$	Thermal	T
Hour(s)	h	Time, irradiation	t_i
Internal conversion	IC	Time, decay	t_d

TABLE 2 Glossary of Terms

Term (abbreviation)	Definition
Becquerel (Bq)	Unit of radioactivity as defined by the International System of units. One becquerel is equal to one disintegration per second.
Beta minus decay (β^- decay)	Mode of radioactive decay in which an electron is ejected from the nucleus, and a neutron is converted to a proton.
Curie (Ci)	Traditional unit of radioactivity. One curie is equal to 3.7×10^{10} becquerels or disintegrations per second.
Electron capture (EC)	Mode of radioactive decay in which a proton captures an orbital electon and becomes a neutron.
Internal conversion (IC)	A mechanism to release excess energy from the atomic nucleus. This process competes with gamma-ray emission.
Isomeric transition (IT)	Mode of radioactive decay for metastable (m) states where only gamma rays are emitted.
Neutron cross section (σ)	Probability that a nuclear reaction will occur. Unit is the barn (b); 1 barn $= 1 \times 10^{-24}$ cm^2.
Neutron flux (Φ)	A measurement of neutrons available for nuclear reactions, expressed as neutrons cm^{-2} s^{-1}.
No-carrier-added	Term used to describe high-specifiy-activity radioisotopes produced by transmutation reactions. Carrier refers to nonradioactive element.
Positron decay (β^+ decay)	Mode of radioactive decay in which a positively charged electron is emitted from the nucleus, and a proton is converted to a neutron.

II. APPLICATIONS

Radionuclides have three general, and sometimes overlapping applications in life sciences research: (a) tracers of metabolic processes, (b) analytical reagents, and (c) diagnostic and therapeutic agents in nuclear medicine. These three general applications of radionuclides in life sciences have evolved for several reasons. First, radionuclides have extensive applications because they are relatively inexpensive compared to nonradioactive tracers and other analytical technology. Second, radionuclides are easily detected and quantitated by several methods, including autoradiography (film or automated instrumentation), liquid scintillation counting, gamma cameras, gamma-ray counting with Na-I detectors, or gamma-ray spectroscopy with intrinsic germanium detectors. Third, the use of radionuclides eliminates the analytical blank in most experiments. Several books detail the application of radioisotopes in life science research (1–4).

A. Tracers of Metabolic Processes

Radionuclides have found widespread application as tracers in the study of metabolic processes. In general, it is assumed that the radionuclide itself is truly a tracer for the element studied. For the most part this is true; radioactive atoms for a particular element are biologically and chemically indistinguishable from the naturally occurring isotopes of the element. Isotope effects, due to difference in mass, will not be discussed in this chapter because of the minimal effects observed among the mineral elements. Examples of radiotracers used in biological research are ^{45}Ca and ^{47}Ca, whose use in calcium research ranges from absorption and bone metabolism to the role in signal transduction. Similarly, ^{32}P, as phosphate, is a tool for studying phosphorus metabolism, protein phosphorylation in metabolic regulation, and nucleotide metabolism. Specific examples are discussed in Section V.

B. Analytical Reagents

Radionuclides also find extensive applications in life science research as analytical reagents. Examples in molecular biology research include ^{32}P- and ^{35}S-labeled compounds as analytical tools for sequencing genes or measuring mRNA levels. Another extensive application is the use of radiotracers in competitive binding assays. Related radioimmunoassays, involving radioiodinated compounds (with ^{125}I or ^{131}I) or tritiated (^{3}H-labeled) compounds, are commonplace.

C. Nuclear Medicine

Nuclear medicine is a specialty that employs radioisotopes for diagnosis and therapy of certain diseases. Nuclear medicine is included in this discussion because it represents a potential source of radionuclides, analytical instrumentation, and research collaboration for other life science researchers. Examples of radioisotopes that are commonly used in nuclear medicine include the iodine radionuclides ^{131}I and ^{123}I, and ^{99}Mo, which is used to prepare ^{99}Mo/^{99m}Tc generators. ^{131}I is commonly used to diagnose and treat thyroid disease, e.g., in the treatment of thyroid cancer. Radionuclides that have potential therapeutic applications in nuclear medicine have been reviewed (5,6). With the emergence of positron emission tomography (PET) as a clinical tool for in vivo imaging, additional radionuclides and capabilities have become available for nutrition researchers. These include ^{18}F-labeled 2-deoxyglucose, using for imaging the increased metabolism in cancer cells, ^{11}C compounds, and mineral element radionuclides such as the ^{62}Zn/^{62}Cu generator and high-specific-activity ^{64}Cu. At the end of 1994, there were approximately 60 PET centers open or in construction in the United States, many of which have cyclotrons on site for radionuclide production.

III. PRODUCTION OF RADIONUCLIDES

A. Fission

Fission of ^{235}U yields a complex mixture of radionuclides from which certain radionuclides are purified for commercial applications. For example, ^{99}Mo, a radionuclide used for ^{99m}Tc generators, is produced by the fission method. ^{99}Mo is particularly well suited for nuclear medicine applications because it decays to another shorter-lived or daughter radionuclide, ^{99m}Tc (half-life 6 h), which is eluted from the generator for the radiopharmaceutical preparation and subsequent use in patient imaging. Another useful radioisotope available from fission is ^{131}I.

B. Neutron Reactions

Radionuclides are most commonly produced by bombardment of target elements with neutrons. Neutrons for this purpose are derived mainly from fission of ^{235}U in nuclear reactors (nonpower reactors) that are specifically designed for research or radionuclide production.

Neutron bombardment reactions are of two general types: one involving neutron capture and the other, neutron transmutation reactions. These reactions are also referred to as thermal-neutron and fast-neutron reactions, respectively. In neutron capture reactions (also called n,γ reactions), the target nucleus captures a neutron and immediately ejects one or more gamma rays. The resulting radionuclide is one neutron heavier, but still of the same atomic number. An example of a thermal neutron reaction is the neutron capture reaction of ^{23}Na, namely, ^{23}Na + ^{1}n → ^{24}Na + γ. The number of capture gamma rays emitted is of no significance to the product, hence there is no attempt to keep track of them in the nuclear reaction notation for most applications. Consequently, the reaction is abbreviated as ^{23}Na$(n,\gamma)^{24}$Na. Neutron-capture reactions involving elemental targets occur with thermal and resonance neutrons. Resonance neutrons, also referred to as epithermal neutrons, are of intermediate energy, having greater energy than thermal neutrons but less energy than fast neutrons. Typically, neutron-capture reactions produce radionuclides of low specific activity, depending on the exact conditions. Enriched isotopes allow increased selectivity in the production of certain (n,γ) radionuclides due to the increase in the number of target atoms for the desired reaction.

Transmutation reactions, the second type of neutron reaction, are those in which the neutron interacts with the target nucleus, and a particle is ejected. The two reactions of primary importance are the (n,p) and (n,α) reactions, in which a proton and an alpha particle, respectively, are ejected from the nucleus. The significance of this kind of nuclear reaction is that the radionuclide produced is of a different atomic number (element) than the target, and therefore a high specific activity of the new radioactive element can be attained. Examples of radionuclides produced in this manner are ^{32}P by irradiation of elemental sulfur, via ^{32}S$(n,p)^{32}$P; and ^{35}S by irradiation of chloride (e.g., KCl), via ^{35}Cl$(n,p)^{35}$S.

1. Neutron Reaction, Example Calculation

A particular element may undergo multiple neutron reactions. Table 3 is a worksheet that calculates the radioactivities induced from neutron irradiation of zinc. The worksheet is separated into columns, denoted by letters, and rows, denoted by numbers. For this

TABLE 3ᴬ Example Worksheet for Calculation of Activities Induced by Neutron Irradiation of Zinc

A	B	C	D	E	F	G	H	I	J	K	L	M

Row 2–17:

Element =	Zinc			
Atomic weight =	65.39			
Target weight =	1.00E+02	mg		
Irradiation time =	1.50E+02	h		
Decay time =	2.40E+01	h		
Thermal flux =	2.30E+14	neutrons cm⁻² s⁻¹		
Resonance flux =	1.11E+13	neutrons cm⁻² s⁻¹		
Fast flux =	8.70E+13	neutrons cm⁻² s⁻¹		

Isotopes	Abundances
Zn-64	0.486
Zn-66	0.279
Zn-67	0.041
Zn-68	0.188
Zn-70	0.006
	1.000 = Total abundance

Worksheet Column (Row 18 onward)

Target isotope (A)	Reaction (B)	Product isotope (C)	Half-life (D, E)	Decay constant (s⁻¹) (F)	Thermal (T) or fast (F) cross section (barn) (G)	Resonance integral (barn) (H)	Production rate (s⁻¹) (I)	Sample production rate (atoms/s) (J)	End of irradiation activity (μCi) (K)	Decay-corrected activity (μCi) (L)	Decay modes and main gamma rays (keV) (M)
Slow reactor neutron reactions:											
Zn-64	(n,γ)	Zn-65	243.9 d	3.29E-08	(T)7.26E-01	1.42E+00	1.83E-10	8.18E+10	3.89E+04	3.88E+04	E.C., B^+; 1115
Zn-68	(n,γ)	Zn-69m	13.76 h	1.40E-05	(T)6.99E-02	2.23E-01	1.86E-11	3.21E+09	8.68E+04	2.59E+04	I.T.; 439
Zn-70	(n,γ)	Zn-71m	3.94 h	4.89E-05	(T)8.70E-03	4.00E-02	2.45E-12	1.35E+07	3.65E+02	5.36E+00	B^-; 386, 487, 512
Fast reactor neutron reactions:											
Zn-64	(n,p)	Cu-64	12.70 h	1.52E-05	(F)3.10E-02		2.70E-12	1.21E+09	3.26E+04	8.80E+03	B^-; 511, 1346
Zn-67	(n,p)	Cu-67	61.90 h	3.11E-06	(F)1.07E-03		9.31E-14	3.52E+06	7.73E+01	5.91E+01	B^-; 185

ᵃTable format courtesy of Dr. Michael Glascock, University of Missouri Research Reactor.

example, a * indicates multiplication, and / indicates division. Rows 2–17 of Table 3 includes parameters that can be changed for different conditions. This particular example uses 1.00E+2 mg, that is, 1.00×10^2 mg or 100 mg, as the target mass of zinc to be irradiated (see column C, row 6; hereafter C6). The naturally occurring isotopic abundances are listed, but isotopically enriched targets could be used. Other parameters that could be varied are the irradiation time (C8), decay time (C9), and neutron fluxes (C12, C13, C14). The neutron fluxes listed in this example are flux profiles for the University of Missouri Research Reactor (MURR) flux trap, the highest available flux at MURR. Rows 25–36 of Table 3 list the major neutron reactions (B) with stable zinc isotopes (A), the product radioisotopes (C), and their half-lives (D, E). Information necessary for calculating induced activity include the decay constant for the product radioisotope (F), the thermal or fast neutron cross section for the reaction (G), and the resonance neutron integral (H), if applicable. Cross-section information is available from literature reports (7,8).

Formulas are necessary for calculation of rows 25–36 for columns F, I, J, K, and L. Example calculations are provided below. The decay constant, F26, is calculated as (0.693/(D26*24*3600)) = 3.29E−8. The production rate, I26, is calculated by the following formula for thermal neutron reactions: ((G26*C12)+(H26*C13))*1E−24 = 1.83E−10. The term 1E−24, which is 1×10^{-24}, is included because 1 barn is equal to 1E−24 cm². For a fast-neutron reaction, such as I34, the following formula is used: (G35*C14)*1E−24. The sample production rate in atoms per second, J26, is calculated by the following formula: I26*((C6/C5)*6.022E+20*H5). The sample production rate is essentially the production rate multiplied by the number of atoms available for reaction. The other neutron reactions must use the appropriate isotopic abundance for the target nucleus instead of H5. The end of irradiation activity, K26, is calculated by the following formula: (J26*(1 − exp−(F26*C8*3600))/37000. The 3600 value is required to convert the irradiation time (C8) from hours to seconds, while the 37000 value is necessary to convert dps to microcuries. Finally, the decay corrupted activity, L26, is calculated as follows: K26*(exp−(F26*C9*3600)). The 3600 value is required again to convert the decay time (C9) from hours to seconds.

A final point should be mentioned with respect to radionuclides produced by neutron bombardment. Any known or unknown impurities in the irradiated target element can potentially produce significant quantities of radionuclides besides those of interest. These radioimpurities are minimized by use of high-purity targets.

C. Charged-Particle Reactions

Radionuclides are also produced by charged-particle reactions at major accelerator centers or compact cyclotrons. Charged-particle nuclear reactions are usually transmutation reactions, and the product radionuclide has a different atomic number than the target isotope. Therefore, high specific activities can be attained by reactions that include spallation (p,n), (p,α), (d,p), (d,n), and (d,α). Spallation reactions are extremely high-energy reactions whereby the target nucleus is transmuted to a product nucleus that is 10–20 mass units lower. Accelerator-produced radioisotopes and production methods have been reviewed (9,10). The technology involved in PET radioisotopes, and cyclotrons for their production, has been reviewed recently (11,12).

Charged particles produced in accelerators, by their very nature, are fundamentally different from neutrons that carry no charge. Nuclear reactions that involve charged particles require them to have sufficient threshold energy to interact with the target nucleus.

Since charged particles may not have sufficient energy for full penetration of the target, all target atoms may not experience the same charged-particle flux or intensity. Additionally, as charged particles lose their energy in the target, the probability (or cross section) for a particular nuclear reaction changes. Charged-particle reactions are discussed in detail by Ehmann and Vance (4).

IV. RADIOACTIVITY

A. Modes of Radioactive Decay

1. Beta Minus (β^-) Decay

Radioactive isotopes are not stable because they contain an imbalance between neutrons and protons in the nucleus. They decay to attain greater stability, ultimately to stable isotopes. As a general rule, reactor-produced radioisotopes have an excess of neutrons and decay by loss of electrons from the nucleus, i.e., β^- decay. During the process of β^- decay, a neutron is converted to a proton, and the atomic number of the decayed nucleus is increased by one unit, changing to the element with the next higher atomic number element. β^- particles emitted from the nucleus have a range in energy, the maximum being characteristic of a given radioisotope. Radioisotopes that decay primarily by β^- emission, with no gamma-ray emission, are listed in Table 4.

2. Positron (β^+) Decay

Radioisotopes arising from charged-particle reactions are usually neutron deficient and generally decay by positron emission, abbreviated β^+ decay. In β^+ decay a proton is changed into a neutron and a positron is emitted; the atomic number is decreased by one unit. With both kinds of beta decay, the mass number (total protons plus neutrons) remains unchanged.

TABLE 4 Radionuclides That Decay Without Gamma-Ray Emissions

Nuclide	Half-life	β-Maximum endpoint energy (MeV) or other decay[a]	Method of production[b]
^{3}H	12.26 y	0.0186	R
^{14}C	5730 y	0.156	R
^{32}P	14.28 d	1.710	R
^{33}P	24.4 d	0.248	R
^{32}Si	100 y	0.221	A
^{35}S	87.9 d	0.167	R
^{36}Cl	3.08×10^5 y	β^- 98.1%: 0.714 EC 1.9%	R
^{41}Ca	1.04×10^5 y	EC	R
^{45}Ca	165 d	0.252	R
^{49}V	337 d	EC	A
^{55}Fe	2.7 y	EC	R, A
^{63}Ni	92 y	0.067	R

[a]Nuclides listed in this table decay by β^- emission unless otherwise noted.
[b]Nuclear reactor (R) and accelerator (A).

3.   Electron Capture (EC)

A third kind of radioactive decay is electron capture, a process by which an inner-orbital electron combines with a nuclear proton to form a neutron. The result is the conversion of a proton into a neutron, and a decrease of one in atomic number.

4.   Alpha (α) Decay

The final method of radioactive decay that results in particle emission from the nucleus is alpha decay. This type of decay occurs only for elements of high atomic weight, and it results in a decrease of two units in atomic number and four in mass number.

5.   Gamma-Ray Emission

Radionuclides may undergo radioactive decay by one or more of the routes listed above. Once a radioactive isotope has undergone decay by the above routes, there may still be excess energy in the nucleus. This excess energy is removed by gamma-ray emission, and such emissions often accompany the radioactive decay modes listed above. Several radio-isotopes of interest that emit gamma rays are listed in Tables 5–7 along with gamma-ray abundances or branching ratios. The abundance or branching ratio refers to the proportion of radioactive decay that results in gamma-ray emission. Gamma-ray emissions alone may represent a mode of radioactive decay for a radioactive species, which is referred to as isomeric transition (IT). Radionuclides that decay by IT have no particle emissions from the nucleus, and are referred to as metastable (m) states. An example is ^{99m}Tc, the most widely used radioisotope in nuclear medicine, which decays 99+% by IT. More than one mode of decay may occur for radioisotopes in metastable states. It is important to recognize that gamma rays always arise from an excited nucleus. Also, the excited nucleus can remove excess energy by a process other than gamma-ray emission. This is called internal conversion and involves the transfer of energy from the nucleus to an inner-orbital electron, which is then ejected from the atom. These electrons, termed conversion electrons, are mono-energetic, in contrast to the electrons emitted during β^- or β^+ decay, which have a range of energies.

B.   Rate of Radioactive Decay

The rate of radioactive decay can be represented by the equation $-dN/dt = \lambda N$. In this equation the rate ($-dN/dt$) is equal to the decay constant (λ) multiplied by the number of radioactive nuclei (N). The decay constant (λ) is equal to (ln 2/half-life). The integrated form of the above equation is $N = N_{t=0}(e^{-\lambda t})$, which can take another form, $A_t = A_{t=0}(e^{-\lambda t})$, in which A represents radioactivity. The latter form is the equation used to correct for radioactive decay. For example, the radioactivity, A_t, at some time, t, is equal to the initial activity, $A_{t=0}$, multiplied by the factor $e^{-\lambda t}$, where t equals the time of decay.

C.   Specific Activity

Specific activity is the amount of radioactivity per unit of mass, the latter commonly expressed as milligrams or millimoles of the element (or compound). Radioactivity is typically reported as curies (Ci) or becquerels (Bq), e.g., mCi/mg or mCi/mmol. Biological applications usually require radioisotopes of high specific activity, and, more particularly, samples with a high proportion of radioactive atoms. It is not obvious whether a given specific activity reflects the proportion of radioactive atoms directly, since radioactivity,

TABLE 5 Radionuclides That Decay with Gamma-Ray Emissions: Half-Lives Less than 10 Days

Nuclide	Decay model[a]	Half-life	Key gamma-rays, keV (% abundance)[b]	Method of production[c]
^{11}C	β^+	20.38 m	511	A
^{13}N	β^+	9.96 m	511	A
^{15}O	β^+	122 s	511	A
^{18}F	β^+	109.8 m	511	A
^{24}Na	β^-	14.96 h	*1368.6 (100)	R
^{31}Si	β^-	2.62 h	1266.2 (0.07)	R
^{34m}Cl	β^+ 53%, IT 47%	31.99 m	*511	A
^{38}Cl	β^-	37.2 m	*1642.7 (31)	R, A
^{38}K	β^+	7.6 m	511	A
^{42}K	β^-	12.36 h	1524.6 (18.8)	R
^{48}Cr	EC	21.6 h	*112.5 (95)	A
^{52}Mn	EC 72%, β^+ 28%	5.59 d	511	A
^{56}Mn	β^-	2.58 h	*1810.7 (27.19)	R
^{64}Cu	EC 41%, β^+ 19% β^- 40%	12.7 h	511 1345.8 (0.48)	R
^{67}Cu	β^-	61.92 h	*184.6 (48.7)	R, A
^{55}Co	β^+ 77%, EC 23%	17.5 h	*511	A
^{56}Ni	EC	6.1 d	*158.4 (98.8)	A
^{65}Ni	β^-	2.52 h	*1481.8 (23.5)	R
^{69m}Zn	IT 99+%	14.0 h	438.6 (94.8)	R
	(^{69}Zn decays by β^- with half-life of 56 m)			
^{72}As	β^+ 77%, EC 23%	26.0 h	*511	A
^{73}Se	β^+ 65%, EC 35%	7.1 h	511	A
^{76}As	β^-	26.3 h	*559.1 (44.6)	R
^{82}Br	β^-	35.3 h	*554.4 (70.7)	R
^{123}I	EC	13.2 h	*159.1 (83)	A
^{124}I	β^+ 25%, EC 75%	4.15 d	*602.7 (61)	A
^{131}I	β^-	8.04 d	*364.5 (81.2)	R

[a]Abbreviations for radioactive decay: β^-, beta minus; β^+, beta plus, positron; EC, electron capture; IT, isomeric transition.
[b]Nuclides with multiple gamma-ray emissions are indicated by *.
[c]Nuclear reactor (R) and accelerator (A).

and hence the specific activity of a given isotope, is dependent on the half-life of the isotope as well as the proportion of radioactive atoms in the sample. Therefore, it is often more useful to convert specific activity to the fraction of atoms that are radioactive. Such a calculation is provided below using ^{75}Se as the example.

1. Specific Activity Calculation

In a sample of radioactive selenium (1000 Ci/g) containing ^{75}Se as the only radioactive isotope, what proportion of the atoms are ^{75}Se? To address this question one must know how many atoms are in 1 mCi of ^{75}Se. A mCi is defined as 3.7E+7 (3.7×10^7) disintegrations per second. The half-life of ^{75}Se is converted to seconds (Eq. 1) and the decay constant is calculated (Eq. 2). The number of nuclei is calculated by use of Eq. 3.

TABLE 6 Radionuclides That Decay with Gamma-Ray Emissions: Half-Lives Greater than 10 Days

Nuclide	Decay model[a]	Half-life	Key gamma-rays, keV (% abundance)[b]	Method of production[c]
^{22}Na	β^+ 90.5%, EC 9.5%	2.60 y	511 (179.8)	A
			1274.5 (99.9)	
^{26}Al	β^+ 82%, EC 18%	7.3E+5 y	1808.7 (99.7)	A
^{48}V	β^+ 49.6%, EC 50.4%	16 d	883.5 (100)	A
			1312.1 (97.5)	
^{51}Cr	EC	27.7 d	320.1 (10.1)	R
^{54}Mn	EC	312 d	834.8 (99.98)	R
^{59}Fe	β^-	44.5 d	*1099.3 (56.5)	R
^{56}Co	EC 81%, β^+ 19%	77.7 d	*1238.3 (68.42)	A
^{57}Co	EC	271.8 d	*122.1 (85.9)	A
^{58}Co	EC 85%	70.8 d	810.7 (99.45)	R
^{60}Co	β^-	5.271 y	1173.2 (99.9)	R
			1332.5 (99.9)	
^{65}Zn	EC 98.5%, β^+ 1.467	243.9 d	1115.5 (50.7)	R, A
^{74}As	EC 37%, β^+ 31%, β^- 32%	17.7 d	*595.8 (59.4)	R
^{75}Se	EC	118.5 d	*136 (59)	R
			264.7 (59.2)	
^{109}Cd	EC	462.6 d	88.03 (3.61)	R
^{113}Sn	EC	115.1 d	*391.7 (64)	R
^{115m}Cd	β^-	44.6 d	*933.85 (2.0)	R
^{125}I	EC	60.1 d	*35.5 (6.7)	R
			27.5 (73)	

[a]Abbreviations for radioactive decay: β^-, beta minus; β^+, beta plus, positron; EC, electron capture; IT, isomeric transition.
[b]Nuclides with multiple gamma-ray emissions are indicated by *.
[c]Nuclear reactor (R) and accelerator (A).

The half-life ($t_{1/2}$) of ^{75}Se in seconds (s) is:

$$t_{1/2} = 120 \text{ d} \cdot \frac{24 \text{ h}}{\text{d}} \cdot \frac{60 \text{ m}}{\text{h}} \cdot \frac{60 \text{ s}}{\text{m}} = 1.0368\text{E}+7 \text{ s} \tag{1}$$

The decay constant, λ, for ^{75}Se is calculated as:

$$\lambda = \frac{\ln 2}{t_{1/2}} = \frac{0.693}{1.0368\text{E}+7 \text{ s}} = 6.684\text{E}-8 \text{ s}^{-1} \tag{2}$$

The number of atoms, N, in 1 mCi of ^{75}Se is determined:

$$N = \frac{(-dN/dt)}{\lambda} = \frac{3.7\text{E}+7 \text{ dps}}{6.684\text{E}-8 \text{ s}^{-1}} = 5.536\text{E}+14 \text{ atoms} \tag{3}$$

The fraction of selenium atoms present as ^{75}Se is determined from the ratio of the number of ^{75}Se atoms to the total number of Se atoms, according to Eq. 4. For the purposes of this example it is assumed that the selenium target is 100% enriched ^{74}Se.

$$\frac{5.536\text{E}+14 \text{ atoms } ^{75}\text{Se}}{8.138\text{E}+15 \text{ atoms Se total}} = 0.068, \text{ or} \cdot 100 = 6.80\% \tag{4}$$

TABLE 7 Radionuclides That Decay to Radioactive Daughters

Parent nuclide	Parent half-life (gamma rays,[a] abundance)	Daughter nuclide	Daughter half-life/ main decay[b]	Method of production[c]
^{28}Mg	20.9 h (*400 keV, 35.9%)	^{28}Al	2.24 m/β^-	R, A
^{38}S	2.8 h	^{38}Cl	37.2 m/β^-	A
^{47}Ca	4.5 d (1297 keV, 74.9%)	^{47}Sc	3.42 d/β^-	R
^{52}Fe	8.3 h	^{52m}Mn	21.1 m/β^+ EC 98.3%, IT 1.7%	A
^{62}Zn	9.13 h (144.7 keV, 83%)	^{62}Cu	9.7 m/β^+ 97.8%	A
^{66}Ni	2.3 d	^{66}Cu	5.1 m/β^-	A
^{72}Se	8.4 d (46.0 keV, 58.8%)	^{72}As	26 h/β^+ 77%, EC 23.8%	A
^{77}Br	57 h (*239 keV, 23.1%)	^{77m}Se	17.6 s/IT	A
^{99}Mo	2.75 days	^{99m}Tc	6.0 h/IT	R

[a]Nuclides with multiple gamma rays are indicated by *.
[b]Abbreviations for radioactive decay: β^-, beta minus; β^+, beta plus, positron; EC, electron capture; IT, isomeric transition.
[c]Nuclear reactor (R) and accelerator (A).

The numerator is the number of atoms in 1 mCi of ^{75}Se and the denominator is the total number of Se atoms in 1 μg of the original sample (^{74}Se) that now contains 1 mCi/μg. Conversion of ^{74}Se to ^{75}Se does not change the number of atoms in the sample. Thus a radioactive ^{75}Se sample with the specific activity of 100 Ci/g Se has 6.8%, or 6.8 out of every 100 selenium atoms, present as ^{75}Se at that particular time. To put this value in perspective, the highest specific activity of ^{32}P available for molecular biology research contains about 30% of radioactive phosphorus atoms. In general, radioisotopes of high specific activity are produced directly by fission, neutron transmutation reactions, and charged-particle reactions. Also, radioisotopes that decay to radioactive daughters provide a source of high-specific-activity isotopes, since all of the daughter atoms in the sample are radioactive.

The mass of 1 mCi of ^{75}Se is determined by Eq. (5):

$$\text{mass} = \frac{N \text{ atoms}}{\text{Avogadro's number}} \cdot \text{atomic weight}$$

$$= \frac{5.536E+14 \text{ atoms}}{6.022E+23 \text{ atoms/mol}} \cdot \frac{75 \text{ g}}{\text{mol}} = 6.8E-8 \text{ g} \tag{5}$$

D. Safety

Only trained individuals wearing appropriate radiation monitors should work with radioisotopes. Training may consist of formal courses or supervised "hands-on" instruction. Most institutions require training, or documentation thereof, as part of the approval process for use of radioisotopes. Institutions are licensed for possession and use of radioisotopes by state or federal agencies. As part of the control process, a radiation safety officer is normally assigned. Typically a local committee administers the license, approving experiments and individual authorizations.

An important consideration in the use of radioisotopes is the principle of ALARA, or *As Low As Reasonably Achievable*. Such procedures minimize both radiation exposure and expense. According to ALARA, all reasonable efforts are made to keep radiation exposure as far below the allowed limits as practical. Three factors that are important in ALARA are time, distance, and shielding. The time in handling the radioisotope should be minimized, and where possible, the distance between the radioisotope and the individual should be maximized. Appropriate shielding should be utilized to reduce exposure. Additionally, care must be taken to prevent the accidental ingestion of radioisotopes, or the contamination of personnel or facilities. The probability of these errors can be reduced by using radioisotopes only in restricted, surveyed areas, by individuals wearing proper attire (laboratory coats, gloves, safety glasses or goggles), and using techniques that prevent the spread of radio-active contamination.

E. Measurement

Various personnel monitors are utilized to measure radiation exposure. These monitors include film badges, pocket ionization chambers, and TLD (thermoluminescent dosimetry) ring badges. These monitors must be worn properly in order to be effective. Another mechanism for determining exposure to radioisotopes of iodine, for example, is to monitor externally the region of the thyroid gland which accumulates iodine specifically. Questions about personnel dosimetry should be directed to the radiation safety office at the institution where the radioactivity will be used.

Radioisotopes are most often measured in laboratory settings with Geiger-Müller detectors, primarily because these instruments are relatively inexpensive. These detectors are gas filled, with detection of radioisotopes based on gas ionization. Both β^- and gamma radiations are detected. However, care should be taken to make certain the detector's end window (or wall) is capable of transmitting the β^- particle of interest.

Accurate measurement of radioactivity is most often accomplished by use of auto-radiography, liquid scintillation counting, or gamma counting. Radioisotopes that decay without gamma-ray emissions are measured by autoradiography or liquid scintillation counting; examples are ^{32}P, ^{35}S, ^{14}C, and ^{3}H (see Table 4). Radioisotopes that decay by way of gamma-ray emissions can be measured with either liquid scintillation or gamma counting. The gamma counter employs a solid Na-I scintillation detector, and has some capability to distinguish gamma rays of different energy. For in vivo applications, such as nuclear medicine studies, a gamma camera is utilized. The gamma camera also utilizes a large Na-I detector. Several books provide more detailed discussions about liquid scintillation counting and gamma counting (1–4).

The most sophisticated technique for measuring gamma-emitting radioisotopes is high-resolution gamma-ray spectroscopy. An intrinsic germanium detector is commonly utilized, which has approximately 10-fold better energy resolution than a Na-I detector. Gamma rays that differ in energy by just a few keV can be completely resolved with this technique. A major advantage is that multiple gamma-emitting radioisotopes can be measured simultaneously. An example of a gamma-ray spectrum is shown in Figure 1. The sample contained ^{47}Ca, ^{59}Fe, ^{65}Zn, and ^{67}Cu. Each spike on the plot represents a distinct gamma-ray energy. A scanning instrument that incorporates high-resolution gamma-ray detection has been reported (13).

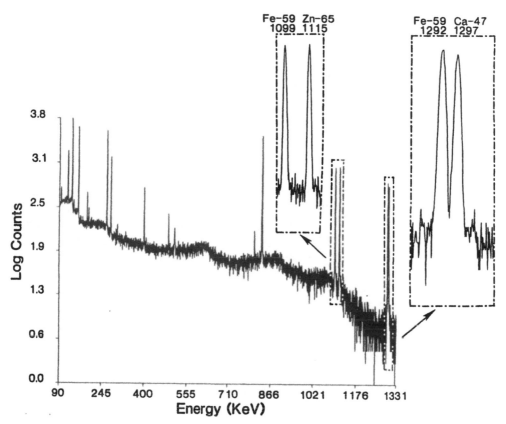

FIGURE 1 Gamma-ray spectrum of a sample containing four radioisotopes: ^{47}Ca, ^{59}Fe, ^{65}Zn, and ^{67}Cu.

V. RADIONUCLIDES APPLICABLE TO NUTRITION RESEARCH

Many radionuclides are available as tracers for the study of mineral element metabolism. Some of the commonly used radioisotopes are listed in Tables 4–7. Radiotracers for selected elements will be discussed in greater detail in the following sections.

A. Radiotracers for Macro-Elements

1. Sodium and Potassium

The best, short-lived, gamma-emitting radiotracers for sodium and potassium are ^{24}Na and ^{42}K, with half-lives of 15 and 12.5 h, respectively. These two radiotracers are readily produced at low specific activity via neutron-capture reactions. Nitrate or carbonate salts of the respective element are suitable targets. Processing involves only dissolution in water. For higher specific activity, an alternative method to produce no-carrier-added ^{24}Na is via an (n,p) reaction on magnesium, or via an (n,α) reaction on aluminum.

When a longer half-life is required, an alterntive tracer of sodium is ^{22}Na (half-life 2.6 years), which is also a gamma emitter. A recently reported alternative radiotracer for potassium is ^{38}K (half-life 7.6 min). It can be produced at compact cyclotrons (14).

2. Calcium and Magnesium

The most viable radiotracer for magnesium is ^{28}Mg (half-life 20.9 h), which can be produced at reactors or accelerators (15,16). This gamma-emitting radionuclide is listed in Table 7, since its decay product is also radioactive. The most viable choice for a gamma-emitting radiotracer for calcium is ^{47}Ca (17), also listed in Table 7. An enriched target of ^{46}Ca is required for the reactor production of ^{47}Ca. It is important to realize that enriched ^{46}Ca also contains a small amount of ^{44}Ca, which produces ^{45}Ca upon neutron irradiation. While the concentration of ^{45}Ca might be minimal at the end of neutron irradiation, the relative percentage of the radioactivity present as ^{45}Ca increases with decay time, since its half-life is much longer than that of ^{47}Ca. Other long-lived radioimpurities may also become more important with decay time. As Zinn determined (unpublished data), a commercial ^{47}Ca sample contained ^{85}Sr (half-life 64.8 days). As a rule of thumb, irradiation of 1 μg of 35%-enriched ^{46}Ca in the highest neutron flux at the Missouri University Research Reactor for 1 week produces approximately 15 μCi of ^{47}Ca, indicating that the ^{47}Ca has low specific activity. If gamma rays are not required for experimental measurements, or when a longer-lived calcium radiotracer is needed, ^{45}Ca is the more appropriate choice of isotope. ^{45}Ca has a half-life of 145 days, is more readily available commercially, and is available with a higher specific activity.

3. Chloride

The only long-lived radiotracer for chloride is ^{36}Cl (Table 4), which decays without gamma-ray emission. A gamma-emitting radiotracer for chloride is ^{38}Cl (half-life 37.2 min), which can be easily produced in research reactors. ^{38}Cl is also the decay product of ^{38}S, listed in Table 7, and would be available from a generator as a no-carrier-added radioisotope. Another alternative radioisotope of chloride is ^{34m}Cl (half-life 34 min), which has been produced for PET applications (18). For certain applications a bromide radiotracer may be substituted for a chloride radiotracer (19). There are several viable bromide radiotracers, including ^{82}Br (19), ^{75}Br, ^{76}Br, and ^{77}Br (20–22).

B. Radiotracers for Trace Elements

1. Iron

The two most commonly used radiotracers for iron are ^{55}Fe and ^{59}Fe (Table 6). Both of these radioisotopes can be produced by neutron-capture reactions. With this mode of production the specific activities are generally low, but they can be greatly increased by using enriched targets of ^{54}Fe and ^{58}Fe, respectively. ^{59}Fe of high specific activity can also be produced by a fast-neutron reaction on ^{59}Co. An alternative radiotracer for iron developed for PET applications is ^{52}Fe, which has a half-life of 8.3 h (Table 7). Production of ^{52}Fe is via transmutation reactions, and therefore very high specific activity can be achieved (23,24).

The results of an in vivo experiment involving ^{59}Fe as radiotracer are shown graphically in Figure 2. Isotope retention was based on measurement of the 1099-KeV gamma-ray emission of ^{59}Fe, using an intrinsic germanium detector. The ^{59}Fe retention was highest in the rats consuming the lowest dietary iron (25 μg/g) and lowest in those consuming 250 μg/g.

2. Copper

Radioactive tracers for copper include ^{62}Cu, ^{64}Cu, and ^{67}Cu. ^{62}Cu (half-life 9.7 min) is the decay product of radioactive ^{62}Zn (Table 7), and therefore is available from a generator

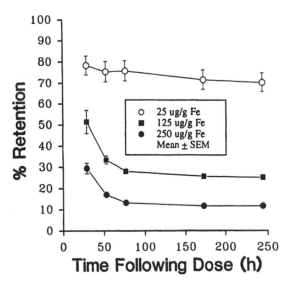

FIGURE 2 Retention of an orally administered dose of ^{59}Fe by rats previously fed three different dietary concentrations of iron. Male weanling (21-day) Sprague-Dawley rats were fed diets differing only in iron concentration, namely, 25, 125, or 250 μg/g. After 10 days, the rats were gavaged with 0.2 MBq of ^{59}Fe and whole-body measurements were made for 10 days.

(25). The principal application of ^{62}Cu thus far has been for PET imaging. ^{64}Cu (Table 5) of low specific activity is easily produced at reactors by the action of thermal neutron reaction on ^{63}Cu, ^{63}Cu (n,γ) ^{64}Cu. High-specific-activity ^{64}Cu can also be produced by fast-neutron reaction, ^{64}Zn(n,p) ^{64}Cu, using natural zinc (26), or by charged-particle reactions (27). Zinn et al. (26) have developed a new method for producing and purifying ^{64}Cu, and have attained a ^{64}Cu specific activity of 1.8×10^6 Ci/g at the end of neutron irradiation. This specific activity is equivalent to 46% radioactive copper atoms. Reactor-produced ^{64}Cu has been utilized successfully for PET imaging (28). ^{67}Cu is the longest-lived radiotracer for copper (half-life 62 h), and it has the additional advantage that it decays with highly abundant gamma rays. ^{67}Cu can be produced in nuclear reactors by the reaction ^{67}Zn(n,p) ^{67}Cu, and also in accelerators (29,30).

3. Zinc

The best choice of radioisotope for zinc depends on the half-life and specific activity required for the experiment. ^{62}Zn is an accelerator-produced radioisotope (half-life 9.3 h) that emits 144.7-keV gamma-rays (83% abundant). Whole-body scanning in animals with ^{62}Zn has been reported (31). A zinc radiotracer with a slightly longer half-life (14 h) is ^{69m}Zn, which also emits gamma rays (438 keV, 94.8%). ^{69m}Zn is reactor produced, and its production is significantly increased by use of an enriched ^{68}Zn target. Alternatively, no-carrier-added ^{69m}Zn can be produced by a fast-neutron activation of enriched ^{69}Ga. Production by this route offers the advantage that the ^{69m}Zn is free of undesired zinc radio-impurities. The longest-half-life radiotracer of zinc is ^{65}Zn, which can be produced in reactors or accelerators. Reactor production of ^{65}Zn typically results in a low-specific-activity radioisotope. On the other hand, ^{65}Zn produced in accelerators is usually high specific activity. Often ^{65}Zn is a byproduct of the production of other radioisotopes in accelerators. For example, production of ^{62}Zn produces significant activities of no-carrier-added ^{65}Zn.

4.   Selenium

The most widely used radiotracer of selenium is ^{75}Se (half-life 120 days). This radionuclide is produced at MURR by long-term neutron irradiation of enriched ^{74}Se. Alternative radiotracers for selenium are ^{72}Se and ^{73}Se. ^{72}Se is an accelerator-produced radionuclide and is available from Los Alamos National Laboratory. Production of ^{73}Se, including ^{73}Se-labeled selenomethionine, has been described (32,33). One short-lived radiotracer of selenium is ^{77m}Se, which is available as the decay product of ^{77}Br (see Table 7).

^{75}Se is useful for the study of mammalian selenoproteins. An example of how ^{75}Se can be used to identify selenoproteins in tissue homogenates is illustrated in Figure 3. The data were collected using a Na-I detector (gamma counter) after slicing the two SDS-PAGE lanes into 2-mm pieces. The smallest proteins migrate the greatest distance from the top of the gel, and appear on the right side of the plots. The rats were previously injected

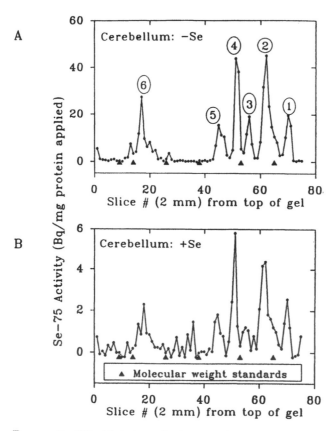

FIGURE 3 ^{75}Se-labeled proteins in rat cerebellum. A. Rats fed a selenium-deficient diet ($-$Se, 0.01 μg Se/g). B. Rats fed a similar selenium-adequate diet ($+$Se, 0.2 μg Se/g). Each plot represents one cerebellum homogenate and shows labeled proteins separated by SDS-PAGE according to size. The positions of molecular-weight standards from left to right (97.4, 66.2, 45.0, 31.0, 21.5, and 14.4 kDa) are indicated by solid triangles.

(intraperitoneal) with 14.5 MBq of ^{75}Se-selenious acid. ^{75}Se was associated with six SDS-PAGE peaks. Four of the protein peaks had apparent molecular weights of 18, 21, 24, and 61 kDa; the values determined for the remaining two ranged between 12.9 and 13.8 kDa and between 14.6 and 15.8 kDa.

5. Manganese

The most widely used radiotracer for manganese is ^{54}Mn, which has a half-life of 312 days. This radionuclide is produced in reactors by the fast-neutron reaction, ^{54}Fe$(n,p)^{54}$Mn. Alternative, shorter-lived radiotracers for manganese are ^{56}Mn, ^{52m}Mn (23,24), and ^{52}Mn (34). ^{52}Mn and ^{54}Mn have been used in a dual-label experiment in humans to determine absorption of manganese (34).

6. Other Radionuclides

An economical radiotracer for molybdenum is ^{99}Mo from spent nuclear medicine generators (35). A radiotracer of fluorine, ^{18}F, is produced in cyclotrons, but can also be produced in nuclear reactors (22,36). A radiotracer for vanadium is ^{48}V (37). The lead radionuclide, ^{212}Pb, is available from a generator system (38,39).

7. Accelerator Mass Spectrometry

A recently evolving, highly sensitive analytical method called accelerator mass spectrometry (AMS) now allows the ultralow measurement of certain long-lived radionuclides that are useful as tracers in biological research (40). Radionuclides that have been measured by AMS include ^{14}C, ^{26}Al, ^{36}Cl, and ^{41}Ca (41,42). One radionuclide with potential for AMS measurement is ^{79}Se.

VI. SOURCES OF INFORMATION

Commercially available radionuclides are listed (43–44), and a complete listing of U.S. research reactors has been published (45). The latter reference (45) provides information on the available neutron flux for the listed facilities. Many of these facilities irradiate targets for research or commercial applications, and have scientific staff available to answer questions. Additional computerized sources of information provided by the U.S. government are FIE and FEDIX (46). The MVRR is the highst neutron flux reactor at a U.S. university, and produces many research isotopes (47).

Five government laboratories currently supply radioisotopes through a coordinating office (48). A catalog is available. The U.S. government laboratories include the following: Argonne National Laboratory (49), Brookhaven National Laboratory (50), Idaho National Engineering Laboratory (51), Los Alamos National Laboratory (52), Oak Ridge National Laboratory (53), and Westinghouse Hanford Company (54).

Other accelerator centers are included in a Department of Energy publication (55). A complete listing of PET centers is maintained by the Institute for Clinical PET (56).

Applications of isotopes in the life sciences were recently reviewed by the Institute of Medicine (57).

REFERENCES

1. Wang CH, Willis DL, Loveland WD. Radiotracer methodology in the Biological, Environmental, and Physical Sciences. Englewood Cliffs, NJ: Prentice-Hall, 1975.

2. Friedlander G, Kennedy JW, Macias ES, Miller JM. Nuclear and Radiochemistry. 3d ed. New York: John Wiley, 1981.

3. Slater RJ, ed. Radioisotopes in Biology, a Practical Approach. New York: Oxford University Press, 1990.

4. Ehmann WD, Vance DE. Radiochemistry and Nuclear Methods of Analysis. New York: Wiley, 1991.

5. Mausner LF, Straub RF, Srivastava SC. Production and use of prospective radionuclides for radioimmunotherapy. In: Srivastava SC, ed. Radiolabeled Monoclonal Antibodies for Imaging and Therapy. New York: Plenum Press, 1988:149–163.

6. Volkert WA, Goeckeler WF, Ehrhardt GJ, Ketring AR. Therapeutic radionuclides: production and decay property considerations. J Nucl Med 1991; 32:174–185.

7. Glascock MD. Tables for neutron activation analysis. Columbia, MO: University of Missouri, 1991. [Internet = http://www.missouri.edu/~murrwww/naa_over.html]

8. International Atomic Energy Agency. Handbook on Nuclear Activation Cross-Sections: Neutron, Photon, and Charged Particle Nuclear Reaction Cross-Section Data. Technical Report Series No. 156. Vienna: International Atomic Energy Agency, 1974. [Internet = http://www.nndc.bnl.gov/] and [http://www.dne.bnl.gov/CoN/index.html]

9. Ruth TJ, Pate BD, Robertson R, Porter JK. Radionuclide production for the biosciences. Int J Radiat Appl Instrum Part B, Nucl Med Biol 1989; 16(4):323–336.

10. Mausner LF, Mirzadeh S, Schnakenberg H, Srivastava SC. The design and operation of the upgraded BLIP facility for radionuclide research and production. Int J Radiat Appl Instrum Part A, Appl Radiat Isot 1990; 41:367–374.

11. Saha GB, MacIntyre WJ, Go RT. Cyclotrons and positron emission tomography, radiopharmaceuticals for clinical imaging. Sem Nuclear Med 1992; 22:150–161.

12. Kairemo KJA. Positron emission tomography of monoclonal antibodies. Acta Oncologica 1993; 32:825–830.

13. Zinn KR, Morris JS, Fairfax CA, Berliner RR, Liu HB, Brugger RM. The development of a rectilinear scanner utilizing high resolution gamma-ray detection. J Radioanalyt Nuclear Chm Articles 1992; 157:15–25.

14. Tarkanyi F, Kovacs Z, Qaim SM, Stocklin G. Production of ^{38}K via the ^{38}Ar (p,n)-process at small cyclotron. Int J Radiat Appl Instrum Part A, Appl Radiat Isot 1992; 43:503–507.

15. Kolar ZI, Van Der Velden JA, Vollinga RC, Zandbergen P, de Goeij JJM. Separation of ^{28}Mg from reactor-neutron irradiated Li-Mg alloy and redetermination of it half-life. Radiochim Acta 1991; 54:167–170.

16. Van Der Velden JA, Kolar ZI, Flik G, Polak P, De Goeij JJM, Wendelaar Bonga SE. Magnesium transport between carp and water studied with ^{28}Mg^{2+} as radiotracer. Int J Radiat Appl Instrum Part A, Appl Radiat Isot 1991; 42(4):347–352.

17. McElroy ST, Link JE, Dowdy RP, Zinn KR, Ellersieck MR. Influence of age and magnesium on calcium metabolism. J Nutr 1991; 121:492–497.

18. Lagunas-Solar MC, Carvacho OF, Cima RR. Cyclotron production of PET radionuclides: ^{34m}Cl (33.99 min; β+53%; IT 47%) with protons on natural isotopic chlorine-containing targets. Int J Radiat Appl Instrum Part A, Appl Radiat Isot 1992; 43(11):1375–1381.

19. Cash D, Serfözö P, Zinn KR. Use of ^{82}Br$^-$ radiotracer to study transmembrane halide flux: The effect of a tranquilizing drug, chlordiazepoxide, on channel opening of a GABA$_A$ receptor. J Membrane Biol 1995; 145:257–266.

20. Grant PM, Whipple RE, Barnes JW, Bentley GE, Wanek PM, O'Brien HA. The production and recovery of ^{77}Br at Los Alamos for nuclear medicine studies. J Inorg Nuclear Chem 1981; 43:2217–2222.

21. Hutter JL, Ruth TJ, Martin PW. Production of ^{77}Br for TDPAC studies. Int J Radiat Appl Instrum Part A, Appl Radiat Isot 1992; 43(11):1393–1398.

22. Qaim SM. Recent developments in the production of ^{18}F, ^{75,75,77}Br, and ^{123}I. Int J Radiat Appl Instrum Part A, Appl Radiat Isot 1986; 37(8):803–810.

23. Ku TH, Richards P, Stand LG, Prach T. Preparation of ^{52}Fe and its use in a ^{52}Fe/^{52m}Mn generator. Radiology 1979; 132:475–477.

24. Steyn GF, Mills SJ, Nortier FM, Simpson BRS, Meyer BR. Production of ^{52}Fe via proton-induced reactions on manganese and nickel. Int J Radiat Appl Instrum Part A, Appl Radiat Isot 1990; 41(3):315–325.

25. Zweit J, Goodall R, Cox M, et al. Development of a high performance zinc-62/copper-62 radionuclide generator for positron emission tomography. Eur J Nuclear Med 1992; 19: 418–425.

26. Zinn KR, Chaudhuri TR, Cheng TP, Meyer WA, Morris JS. Production of no-carrier-added ^{64}Cu from zinc metal irradiated under boron shielding. Cancer 1994; 73:774–778.

27. Sweit J, Smith AM, Downey S, Sharma HL. Excitation functions for deuteron induced reactions in natural nickel: production of no-carrier-added ^{64}Cu from enriched ^{64}Ni targets for positron emission tomography. Int J Radiat Appl Instrum Part A, Appl Radiat Isot 1991; 42(2):193–197.

28. Anderson CJ, Connett JM, Schwarz SW, et al. Copper-64 labeled antibodies for PET imaging. J Nuclear Med 1992; 33:1685–1691.

29. Mirzadeh S, Mausner LF, Srivastava SC. Production of no-carrier-added ^{67}Cu. Int J Appl Instrum Part A, Appl Radiat Isot 1986; 37(1):29–36.

30. Dasgupta AK, Mausner LF, Srivastava SC. A new separation procedure for ^{67}Cu from proton irradiated Zn. Int J Radiat Appl Instrum Part A, Appl Radiat Isot 1991; 42(4):371–376.

31. Bauer R, Brummerstedt E, Jensen M, Mejborn H, Smith M. Reduced rate of uptake of zinc ions in a calf affected with the lethal syndrome A46 relative to clinically normal calves using whole body radio-isotope scanning of ^{62}Zn. APMIS 1992; 100:347–352.

32. Blessing G, Lavi N, Qaim SM. Production of ^{73}Se via the ^{70}Ge(α,n)-process using high current target materials. Int J Radiat Appl Instrum Part A, Appl Radiat Isot 1992; 43(3):455–461.

33. Plenevaux A, Guillaume M, Brihaye C, Lamaire C, Cantineau R. Chemical processing for production of no-carrier-added selenium-73 from germanium and arsenic targets and synthesis of L-2-amino-4-([^{73}Se]methylseleno) butyric acid (L-[^{73}Se]selenomethionine). Int J Radiat Appl Instrum Part A, Appl Radiat Isot 1990; 41(9):829–838.

34. Davidsson L, Cederblad A, Hagebo E, Lönnerdal B, Sandström B. Intrinsic and extrinsic labeling for studies of manganese absorption in humans. J Nutr 1988; 118:1517–1521.

35. El-Kolaly MT, Mausner LF, Srivastava SC. Spent ^{99}Mo/^{99m}Tc generator as an economical source of ^{99}Mo. Int J Radiat Appl Instrum Part B, Nuclear Med Biol 1990; 17(2):229–232.

36. Ramirez FDM, Bulbulian S, Collins CH, Collins DE. A simplified procedure for fluorine-18 production using a nuclear reactor. Int J Radiat Appl Instrum Part A, Appl Radiat Isot 1992; 43(11):1403–1406.

37. Edel J, Sabbioni E. Vanadium transport across placenta and milk of rats to the fetus and newborn. Biol Trace Element Res 1989; 22:265–275.

38. Atcher RW, Friedman AM, Hines JJ. An improved generator for the production of ^{212}Pb, and ^{212}Bi from ^{224}Ra. Int J Radiat Appl Instrum Part A, Appl Radiat Isot 1988; 39(4):283–286.

39. Hassfjell SP, Hoff P. A generator for production of ^{212}Pb and ^{212}Bi. Int J Radiat Appl Instrum Part A, Appl Radiat Isot 1994; 45(10):1021–1025.

40. Vogel JS, Turteltaub KW. Accelerator mass spectrometry in biomedical research. Nuclear Instrum Meth B: Proc. 6th Int. AMS Conf., Australia. In press. [Internet = http://www-ep.es.llnl.gov/www-ep/cams.html]

41. Johnson RR, Berkovits D, Boaretto E, et al. Calcium resorption from bone in human studied by ^{41}Ca tracing. Nuclear Instrum Meth B: Proc. 6th Int. AMS Conf., Australia. In press.

42. Elmore D. Calcium-41 as a long-term biological tracer for bone resorption. Nuclear Instrum Meth Phys Res 1990; B52:531–535.

43. Chem Sources, 1996 Edition. Fernandina Beach, FL: Chemical Sources International.

44. Guide to scientific products, instruments, and services. Science 259 suppl., 1993.

45. American Nuclear Society. Research, Training, Test and Production Reactor Directory. 3d ed. La Grange Park, IL: American Nuclear Society, 1988. [Internet = http://web.fie.com/htdoc/fed/

doe/any/edu/menu/any/doemnrt/htm] A list of research reactors, with internet links, is located at [http://thiapc1.phsics.utoledo.edu/deg/reactors.html]

46. FEDIX. Federal Information Exchange, Inc. 555 Quince Orchard Road, Suite 200, Gaithersburg, MD. Phone 301-975-0103; FAX 301-975-0109. [Internet (FIE) = http://web.fie.com/index.htm]; [Internet (FEDIX) = http://web.fie.com/htdoc/fed/all/any/any/menu/any/index/htm]

47. MURR, University of Missouri, Research Reactor Facility, Columbia, MO, 65211. Phone (573) 882-4211. [Internet = http://www.missouri.edu/~murrwww/].

48. U.S. Department of Energy, Office of Isotope Production and Distribution, Room A430 GTN, Washington, DC 20585. Phone 301-903-5161. [Internet = http://www.mwanal.lanl.gov/CST/CST-11/DOE_description.html]

49. Argonne National Laboratory, Chemistry Division, Bldg. 211, 9700 South Cass Avenue, Argonne, IL 60439-4835. Phone 630-252-3571 (For Pb-212 only).

50. Brookhaven National Laboratory, Isotope Distribution Office, Medical Department, Bldg 490, Upton, NY 11973. Phone 516-344-4461.

51. Idaho National Engineering Laboratory, EG&G-Idaho, Incorporated, Radioisotopes and Irradiation Services, P.O. Box 1625, Idaho Falls, ID 83415-7133. Phone 208-533-4326.

52. Los Alamos National Laboratory, Chemical Science and Technology Division, CST-DO, MS J514, Los Alamos, NM 87545. Phone 505-665-1486. [Internet = http://mwanal.lanl.gov/CST/CST-11/isotopes.html]

53. Oak Ridge National Laboratory, Isotope Distribution Office, P.O. Box 2009, Oak Ridge, TN 37831-8044. Phone 423-574-6984.

54. Pacific Northwest National Laboratory (PNNL), Isotope Program Office, Battelle Blvd., Richland, WA 99352. Phone 509-376-1939.

55. U.S. Department of Energy. Nuclear Physics Accelerator Facilities of the World. Washington, DC: U.S. Dept. of Energy, Office of Energy Research, 1991, Call No. DOCS-MF E 1.19:0532 T.

56. Institute for Clinical PET. 11781 Lee Jackson Memorial Highway, Suite 360, Fairfax, VA 22033. Phone (703) 691–2255.

57. Adelstein SJ, Manning FJ, eds. Isotopes for Medicine and the Life Sciences. Washington DC: Committee on Biomedical Isotopes, Division of Health Science Policy, Institute of Medicine, National Academy Press, 1994.

Index